Thoracic Anesthesia

Second Edition

6

Thoracic Anesthesia
Second Edition

Edited by

Joel A. Kaplan, M.D.

Horace W. Goldsmith Professor and Chairman
Department of Anesthesiology
Mount Sinai School of Medicine
New York, New York

Churchill Livingstone
New York, Edinburgh, London, Melbourne, Tokyo

Library of Congress Cataloging-in-Publication Data
Thoracic anesthesia / edited by Joel A. Kaplan. — 2nd ed.
       p. cm.
    Includes bibliographical references and index.
    ISBN 0-443-08712-1
    1. Chest—Surgery. 2. Anesthesiology. I. Kaplan, Joel A.
    [DNLM: 1. Anesthesia. 2. Thoracic Surgery. 3. Thorax—drug
effects.   WF 980 T4855]
    RD536.T453   1991
    617.9'6754—dc20
    DNLM/DLC
    for Library of Congress   91-15791
                                                                     CIP

© **Churchill Livingstone Inc. 1991, 1983**

Distributed in the United Kingdom by Churchill Livingstone, Robert Stevenson House, 1–3 Baxter's Place, Leith Walk, Edinburgh EH1 3AF, and by associated companies, branches, and representatives throughout the world.

Accurate indications, adverse reactions, and dosage schedules for drugs are provided in this book, but it is possible that they may change. The reader is urged to review the package information data of the manufacturers of the medications mentioned.

The Publishers have made every effort to trace the copyright holders for borrowed material. If they have inadvertently overlooked any, they will be pleased to make the necessary arrangements at the first opportunity.

Acquisitions Editor: *Toni M. Tracy*
Copy Editor: *David Terry*
Production Designer: *Jill Little*
Production Supervisor: *Sharon Tuder*

Printed in the United States of America

First published in 1991   7 6 5 4 3 2 1

To Louis Ganz,
beloved husband, father, father-in-law,
and grandfather.
He will be remembered for his inquisitive mind
and dedication to finding the ultimate solution
to even the most complex of problems.

Contributors

Aliasghar Aghdami, M.D.
Professor and Clinical Director, Department of Anesthesiology, Virginia Commonwealth University Medical College of Virginia School of Medicine, Richmond, Virginia

Jeffrey Askanazi, M.D.
Director of Research, Division of Critical Care Medicine, Department of Anesthesiology, Albert Einstein College of Medicine of Yeshiva University; Director, Nutrition Support Service, Division of Critical Care, Montefiore Medical Center, Bronx, New York

Steven J. Barker, Ph.D., M.D.
Associate Professor and Acting Chair, Department of Anesthesiology, University of California, Irvine, College of Medicine, Irvine, California

Jonathan L. Benumof, M.D.
Professor, Department of Anesthesiology, University of California, San Diego, School of Medicine, La Jolla, California

James W. Bland, Jr., M.D.
Professor, Department of Anesthesiology, and Associate Professor, Department of Pediatrics, Emory University School of Medicine; Chief, Department of Anesthesiology, Henrietta Egleston Hospital for Children, Atlanta, Georgia

Philip G. Boysen, M.D.
Professor, Departments of Anesthesiology and Medicine, University of Florida College of Medicine; Assistant Chief, Anesthesia Services, and Chief, Respiratory Care Services, Veteran Affairs Medical Center, Gainesville, Florida

Jay B. Brodsky, M.D.
Professor, Department of Anesthesia, Stanford University School of Medicine, Stanford, California

Keith K. Brosius, M.D.
Assistant Professor, Departments of Anesthesiology and Pediatrics, Emory University School of Medicine; Staff Anesthesiologist and Intensivist, Departments of Anesthesiology and Pediatrics, Henrietta Egleston Hospital for Children, Atlanta, Georgia

Sorin J. Brull, M.D.
Assistant Professor, Department of Anesthesiology, Yale University School of Medicine; Attending Anesthesiologist, Department of Anesthesia, Yale-New Haven Hospital, New Haven, Connecticut

Christopher W. Bryan-Brown, M.D.
Professor, Department of Anesthesiology; Vice Chairman of Clinical Affairs, Anesthesiology/Critical Care Medicine, Department of Anesthesiology, Albert Einstein College of Medicine of Yeshiva University, Bronx, New York

Wilfred A.P. Demajo, M.D.
Assistant Professor, Department of Anaesthesia, University of Toronto Faculty of Medicine; Associate Director, Surgical Intensive Care Unit, General Division, The Toronto Hospital, Toronto, Ontario, Canada

John B. Downs, M.D.
Professor and Chairman, Department of Anesthesiology, University of South Florida College of Medicine, Tampa, Florida

W. Thomas Edwards, Ph.D., M.D.
Associate Professor, Department of Anesthesiology, University of Washington School of Medicine; Director, Pain Relief Services, Harborview Medical Center, Seattle, Washington

Jan Ehrenwerth, M.D.
Professor, Department of Anesthesiology, Yale University School of Medicine; Attending Anesthesiologist, Department of Anesthesia, Yale-New Haven Hospital, New Haven, Connecticut

James B. Eisenkraft, M.D.
Professor, Department of Anesthesiology, Mount Sinai School of Medicine, New York, New York

Brendan T. Finucane, M.D., F.R.C.P.C.
Professor and Chairman, Department of Anaesthesia, University of Alberta Faculty of Medicine; Anaesthetist-in-Chief, Department of Anaesthesia, University of Alberta Hospitals, Edmonton, Alberta, Canada

Thomas J. Gal, M.D.
Professor, Department of Anesthesiology, University of Virginia School of Medicine, Charlottesville, Virginia

T. James Gallagher, M.D.
Professor, Departments of Anesthesiology and Surgery, University of Florida College of Medicine; Chief, Division of Critical Care Medicine, Department of Anesthesiology, Shands Teaching Hospital and Clinics, Gainesville, Florida

Alexander W. Gotta, M.D.
Clinical Professor, Department of Anesthesiology, and Vice Chairman for Academic Affairs, State University of New York Health Science Center at Brooklyn College of Medicine, Brooklyn, New York

Anita V. Guffin, M.M.S.
Assistant Professor, Department of Anesthesiology, Mount Sinai School of Medicine, New York, New York

James R. Hall, M.D.
Associate Professor, Department of Anesthesiology, Emory University School of Medicine, Atlanta, Georgia

Roger A. Johns, M.D.
Assistant Professor, Department of Anesthesiology, University of Virginia School of Medicine, Charlottesville, Virginia

Joel A. Kaplan, M.D.
Horace W. Goldsmith Professor and Chairman, Department of Anesthesiology, Mount Sinai School of Medicine, New York, New York

Richard L. Keenan, M.D.
Professor and Chairman, Department of Anesthesiology, Virginia Commonwealth University Medical College of Virginia School of Medicine, Richmond, Virginia

Thomas J. Mancuso, M.D.
Assistant Professor, Departments of Anesthesiology and Pediatrics, Emory University School of Medicine; Staff Anesthesiologist and Intensivist, Departments of Anesthesiology and Pediatrics, Henrietta Eagleston Hospital for Children, Atlanta, Georgia

H. Michael Marsh, M.M.M.B.
Professor and Chairman, Department of Anesthesiology, University of Michigan Medical School, Ann Arbor, Michigan

Christine H. Murphy, M.D.
Staff Radiologist, Department of Radiology, St. Joseph's Hospital, Atlanta, Georgia

Michael R. Murphy, M.D.
Associate Professor, Department of Anesthesiology, Emory University School of Medicine, Atlanta, Georgia

Steven M. Neustein, M.D.
Assistant Professor, Department of Anesthesiology, Mount Sinai School of Medicine, New York, New York

Alan L. Plummer, M.D.
Associate Professor, Division of Pulmonary Diseases and Critical Care, Department of Medicine, Emory University School of Medicine, Atlanta, Georgia

Linda J. Riemersma, Pharm.D.
Adjunct Associate Professor, Department of Anesthesiology, Emory University School of Medicine; Critical Care Specialist, Department of Pharmaceutical Services, Emory University Hospital, Atlanta, Georgia

Robert S. Shapiro, M.D.
Assistant Professor, Department of Radiology, Mount Sinai School of Medicine, New York, New York

Lawrence C. Siegel, M.D.
Assistant Professor, Department of Anesthesia, Stanford University School of Medicine, Stanford, California

Bjørn Skeie, M.D.
Visiting Research Fellow, Department of Anesthesiology, Albert Einstein College of Medicine of Yeshiva University, Bronx, New York

Robert A. Smith, M.S.
Assistant Professor, Department of Anesthesiology, University of South Florida College of Medicine, Tampa, Florida

Theodore C. Smith, M.D.
Professor, Department of Anesthesiology, Loyola University of Chicago Stritch School of Medicine, Maywood, Illinois; Chief, Department of Anesthesiology, E.A. Hines, Jr., Veterans Affairs Hospital, Hines, Illinois

Eldar Søreide, M.D.
Visiting Research Fellow, Department of Anesthesiology, Albert Einstein College of Medicine of Yeshiva University, Bronx, New York

Donald S. Stevens, M.D.
Assistant Professor, Department of Anesthesiology, University of Massachusetts Medical School; Associate Director, Acute Pain Management Service, University of Massachusetts Medical Center, Worcester, Massachusetts

Stephen R. Tosone, M.D.
Associate Professor, Department of Anesthesiology, Emory University School of Medicine; Chief, Department of Anesthesiology, Grady Memorial Hospital, Atlanta, Georgia

W. Ross Tracey, Ph.D.
Postdoctoral Fellow, Department of Pharmacology, University of Virginia School of Medicine, Charlottesville, Virginia

Kevin K. Tremper, Ph.D., M.D.
Professor and Chair, Department of Anesthesiology, University of Michigan Medical School, Ann Arbor, Michigan

Roger S. Wilson, M.D.
Associate Professor, Department of Anaesthesia, Harvard Medical School; Medical Director, Respiratory/Surgical Intensive Care Unit; Anesthetist, Department of Anesthesia, Massachusetts General Hospital, Boston, Massachusetts

Preface to the Second Edition

The second edition of *Thoracic Anesthesia* was written for the purpose of further improving anesthetic management for patients undergoing noncardiac thoracic surgery. Since the publication of the first edition of *Thoracic Anesthesia* in 1983, the field has continued to grow at a very rapid pace. In order to maintain its place as the standard reference textbook in the subspecialty, this edition has been completely revised, expanded, and updated. The material in this book was written by the acknowledged experts in each specific area of thoracic anethesia. It is the most authoritative and up-to-date collection of material in the field. Each chapter aims to provide the scientific foundation in the area as well as the clinical basis for practice. All of the chapters have been coordinated in an effort to avoid unnecessary duplication and conflicting opinions. Whenever possible, material has been integrated from the fields of anesthesiology, pulmonary medicine, thoracic surgery, critical care medicine, and pharmacology to present a complete clinical picture. Thus, this book should continue to serve as the definitive text in the field for anesthesia residents, thoracic anesthesia fellows and attendings, thoracic surgeons, intensivists, and others interested in the management of patients for noncardiac thoracic surgery.

The content of the book ranges from the preoperative assessment of the thoracic surgical patient, to the anesthetic, monitoring, and intraoperative support needed, plus the postoperative care of the patient in the intensive care unit. The book is organized into four parts, consisting of twenty-six chapters and hundreds of illustrations. The four major areas covered are (1) preoperative assessment and management; (2) respiratory physiology and pharmacology; (3) specific anesthetic considerations; and (4) postoperative management. Throughout, the emphasis is on the understanding of respiratory physiology and how disease states in an open-chest patient with one-lung ventilation may alter this physiology. The latest techniques and equipment are discussed in the areas of intraoperative monitoring, endobronchial intubation, tracheostomy, and mechanical ventilation. All aspects of patient care are presented in the belief that preoperative and postoperative management of the patient are as important as intraoperative management.

The first edition of *Thoracic Anesthesia* began with forewords written by Professor Mushin from England and Dr. Lichtmann and colleagues from the George Washington University School of Medicine. Dr. Mushin pointed out that "thoracic anesthesia is still a rapidly developing science" and that "it is almost impossible for anyone not a specialist in this field to keep abreast of new developments." Thus, "there is a continued need to set down the accumulated experience of those who work in this field so that their great skill and knowledge can be disseminated both to their colleagues and to the rising generation of anesthesiologists." This edition of *Thoracic Anesthesia* is a continuation of the effort to keep anesthesiologists informed of the latest developments in the field.

Dr. Lichtmann and colleagues discussed the events immediately following the assassination attempt of President Reagan in 1981, leading to his emergency thoracic surgical procedure. They discussed the development of thoracic anesthesia techniques and their application in this highly successful operative procedure. It is well recognized that they made a significant contribution to saving the President's life. In fact, the development of the subspecialty of thoracic anesthesia has been responsible for reducing mortality and improving care for all patients undergoing noncardiac thoracic surgery, and has been one of the major forces behind the surgeon's ability to handle bigger challenges with better results.

I gratefully acknowledge the contributions made by the authors of the individual chapters. They are the experts who have made the field of thoracic anesthesia come alive at the major medical centers and are the teachers of our young colleagues practicing anesthesiology around the world. This book would not have been possible without their hard work and expertise.

My sincere appreciation also goes to my secretaries, Joanie Esbri-Cullen and Margorie Fraticelli, whose long hours helped make this text a reality. In addition, thanks are in order for the secretaries of the contributing authors who sent us the original manuscripts from their institutions. I would also like to thank Toni Tracy, President of Churchill Livingstone Inc., for her support with this project, and David Terry for his hard work in putting together all the pieces of the book.

Finally, my thanks go to Norma for again acting as Editor-in-Chief!

Joel A. Kaplan, M.D.

Preface to the First Edition

This book was written to improve anesthesia care for all patients undergoing thoracic surgery. The text reflects the experience of the Division of Cardiothoracic Anesthesia at the Emory University School of Medicine, as well as that of experts from the University of California-San Diego, Harvard University, Loyola University, Mount Sinai School of Medicine, and the University of Florida. The book presents methods, materials, philosophies, attitudes, and fundamentals whose use will provide safe, individualized anesthetic care.

The scope of this book ranges from the historical background to the modern practice of thoracic anesthesia and surgery, including new modes of postopertive ventilation and oxygenation. The book focuses on the patient undergoing a thoracotomy, beginning with the preoperative evaluation and preparation for surgery and continuing through to the intraoperative management and postoperative respiratory care. It is organized into five parts, consisting of twenty-one chapters and hundreds of illustrations and x-rays. The five major areas covered are (1) thoracic anesthesia and surgery; (2) assessment of the patient; (3) cardiopulmonary physiology; (4) specific anesthetic considerations; and (5) postoperative intensive care. Throughout, the emphasis is on understanding respiratory physiology and how disease states and an open chest with one-lung ventilation may alter this physiology. The latest techniques and equipment are discussed in the areas of intraoperative monitoring, endobronchial intubation, pulmonary lavage, tracheostomy, pacemakers, and mechanical ventilators. All apsects of patient care are presented in the belief that preoperative and postoperative management of the patient are as important as intraoperative management.

The material in this book is an overview of the highly specialized field of thoracic anesthesia. Many medical disciplines including surgery, radiology, pediatrics, and internal medicine have contributed to the development of this text and the new subspecialty in thoracic anesthesia. Therefore, this work may serve as a source book for use by anesthesia residents and fellows, anesthesiologists interested in the field of thoracic anesthesia, intensivists, thoracic surgeons, pulmonary medicine specialists, and other physicians dealing with thoracic surgical patients.

I gratefully acknowledge the help of my fellow anesthesiologists at Emory for the expertly written chapters they have contributed to this book. In addition, I would like to thank my colleagues in surgery and medicine for their outstanding contributions, and most of all, I wish to express my deep appreciation to the expert anesthesiologists from other institutions whose contributions give this text balance.

My sincere appreciation goes, in addition, to my executive secretary Patricia Bailey, to Judy Hawkins and Cindy Lewis, and to the rest of our secretarial staff who spent many long hours preparing this manuscript for publication.

And, finally, my thanks to my wife, Norma, who again managed to edit a manuscript between tennis sets!

Joel A. Kaplan, M.D.

Contents

PREOPERATIVE ASSESSMENT AND MANAGEMENT

1. Evaluation of Pulmonary Function Tests and
   Arterial Blood Gases / 1
   Philip G. Boysen, M.D.

2. Radiology of the Chest / 19
   *Robert S. Shapiro, M.D., Christine H. Murphy, M.D., and
   Michael R. Murphy, M.D.*

3. Preparation of the Patient with Chronic
   Pulmonary Disease / 83
   H. Michael Marsh, M.M.M.B., and Anita V. Guffin, M.M.S.

4. Acquired Immunodeficiency Syndrome and
   Hepatitis: Risks to Patient and Physician / 95
   Alexander W. Gotta, M.D.

RESPIRATORY PHYSIOLOGY AND PHARMACOLOGY

5. Metabolic and Hormonal Functions of the Lung / 115
   Roger A. Johns, M.D., and W. Ross Tracey, Ph.D.

6. Systemic Oxygen Transport / 143
   Christopher W. Bryan-Brown, M.D.

7. Respiratory Physiology During Anesthesia / 165
   Thomas J. Gal, M.D.

8. Physiology of the Lateral Decubitus Position,
   the Open Chest, and One-Lung Ventilation / 193
   Jonathan L. Benumof, M.D.

9. Bronchodilators and Bronchoactive Drugs / 223
   Alan L. Plummer, M.D., and Linda J. Riemersma, Pharm.D.

10. Pharmacologic Preparation of the Patient
    for Thoracic Surgery / 255
    Theodore C. Smith, M.D.

SPECIFIC ANESTHETIC CONSIDERATIONS

11. Monitoring of Oxygenation and Ventilation / 285
    Kevin K. Tremper, Ph.D., M.D., and Steven J. Barker, Ph.D., M.D.

12. Anesthesia for Thoracic Diagnostic Procedures / 321
    Jan Ehrenwerth, M.D., and Sorin J. Brull, M.D.

13. Choice of Anesthetic Agents for Intrathoracic
    Surgery / 347
    Lawrence C. Siegel, M.D., and Jay B. Brodsky, M.D.

14. Endobronchial Intubation / 371
    Roger S. Wilson, M.D.

15. Anesthesia for Esophageal and Mediastinal
    Surgery / 389
    James B. Eisenkraft, M.D., and Steven M. Neustein, M.D.

16. Anesthetic Management of Therapeutic Procedures of the
    Lungs and Airway / 419
    James B. Eisenkraft, M.D., and Steven M. Neustein, M.D.

17. Tracheostomy and Tracheal Reconstruction / 441
    Roger S. Wilson, M.D.

18. Thoracic Trauma / 463
    Brendan T. Finucane, M.D.

19. Anesthesia for Pediatric and Neonatal
    Thoracic Surgery / 485
    *James W. Bland, Jr., M.D., Thomas J. Mancuso, M.D.,
    Keith K. Brosius, M.D., and Stephen R. Tosone, M.D.*

20. Pulmonary Transplantation / 555
    Wilfred A.P. Demajo, M.D.

POSTOPERATIVE MANAGEMENT

21. Management of Pain after Thoracic Surgery / 563
    Donald S. Stevens, M.D., and W. Thomas Edwards, Ph.D., M.D.

22. Routine Postoperative Respiratory Care / 593
    John B. Downs, M.D., and Robert A. Smith, M.S.

23. Etiology and Treatment of Respiratory Failure / 619
    T. James Gallagher, M.D.

24. Techniques of Ventilation and Oxygenation / 649
    James R. Hall, M.D.

25. Nutritional Care of the Thoracic Surgical Patient / 681
    Eldar Søreide, M.D., Bjørn Skeie, M.D., and Jeffrey Askanazi, M.D.

26. Complications of Thoracic Surgery / 709
    Aliasghar Aghdami, M.D., and Richard L. Keenan, M.D.

INDEX / 725

1
EVALUATION OF PULMONARY FUNCTION TESTS AND ARTERIAL BLOOD GASES

Philip G. Boysen, M.D.

The anesthesiologist is often asked to evaluate the thoracotomy patient after the necessary data have been collected. The most common reason for performing a thoracotomy, other than for cardiac surgical procedures, is for the evaluation or resection of a mass in the lung. Lung cancer is a particularly dangerous neoplastic disease since symptoms develop after a prolonged period of time, during which the lesion has had the opportunity to increase in size and metastasize. Screening techniques on the whole have been inadequate. A yearly chest x-ray is now deemed useless as a form of screening for lung cancer. Periodic cytopathologic examinations in high-risk patients have been useful in some series, but the specimens require specialized handling and a high level of expertise is necessary to make an early diagnosis. Furthermore, the occurrence of lung cancer has been closely linked to cigarette smoking and, thus, coexistent disease is common. Specifically, chronic obstructive pulmonary disease (COPD) may be well advanced before the realization that an intrapulmonary mass is present and growing.[1,2] Therefore, the anesthetic risk is closely linked to the severity of underlying lung disease (see Chapter 3).

COPD and concurrent coronary artery disease, as well as other systemic diseases, pose additional problems in the evaluation and treatment of lung cancer. This is particularly true because surgical resection for cure of lung cancer remains the best hope for survival of any individual patient. Since excision of the tumor may also involve the loss of functional lung tissue, the compromised patient is at risk for an increased occurrence of both morbidity and mortality. Thus, the evaluation of the lung generally proceeds along physiologic lines and specific data are accumulated to predict both postoperative pulmonary function and the occurrence of complications.

Carcinoma of the lung is characterized by four different histopathologic cell types: (1) epidermoid, or bronchogenic, carcinoma; (2) adenocarcinoma; (3) alveolar cell carcinoma; and (4) undifferentiated carcinoma. The last cell type is further distinguished by cellular morphology into large cell and small cell (also known as oat cell) cancer varieties. Oat cell carcinoma is perhaps the one pulmonary malignancy that may not be amenable to surgical extirpation, because of the propensity for this particular cancer to metastasize before the clinical diagnosis of carcinoma of the lung is made. Blind bilateral iliac crest biopsies reveal bony metastases in up to 50 percent of newly diagnosed patients. For this reason, the tendency is to refer these patients for antineoplastic therapy rather than to submit them to surgery.

DIAGNOSIS AND EVALUATION OF RESECTABILITY

When first asked to evaluate these patients, the anesthesiologist may find that attempts at histopathologic diagnosis have already been made, usually by flexible fiberoptic bronchoscopy with biopsy. Needle biopsy of the mass is also possible if the lesion is contiguous with the pleural space and the chest wall. If no histopathologic diagnosis has been made, the anesthesiologist may be asked to assist in further procedural studies to attempt to make a tissue diagnosis. Since there is a tendency for these cancers to invade contiguous areas, especially the mediastinum, and to metastasize to distant organs, a sequential approach is usually advised. Even if previously performed, a bronchoscopy is often repeated and may include a rigid bronchoscopic examination as well as flexible fiberoptic bronchoscopy. If this is negative, the next step will vary depending on whether the lesion is on the right or left side. On the right side, mediastinoscopy is particularly efficacious because of the takeoff angle of the right main stem bronchus and its position in the mediastinum. Visibility in this area is generally very good and biopsy is possible because of the anatomic access. A left-sided lesion is generally approached by a limited thoracotomy (mediastinotomy) rather than by a mediastinoscopy. This provides better access, a better view of the underlying area, and the ability to obtain tissue for diagnosis. If both bronchoscopy and mediastinoscopy or a limited thoracotomy (Chamberlain procedure) are negative by pathologic examination, the surgeon will proceed to thoracotomy. The anesthesiologist is challenged to give adequate anesthesia for this stepwise sequence of procedures, realizing that the accumulated data may negate the ability to proceed with full thoracotomy and resection. While these steps, in combination with preoperative evaluation of imaging studies, may define the ability to resect a carcinoma, the physiologic evaluation helps define whether the patient will tolerate a resection of lung tissue and whether the patient will suffer from increased morbidity and/or mortality.

EVALUATION OF LUNG FUNCTION

Spirometry

Spirometry is clearly the benchmark study for the evaluation of pulmonary function.[3-5] This form of testing is quite simple and reproducible. The patient is instructed to inhale to total lung capacity (TLC). Following this, he forcibly exhales as much of the gas in his lungs as can be accomplished in one breath. Thus, lung volume moves from TLC to residual volume (RV) and this change is designated as the vital capacity. The forced maneuver accentuates the possibility of uncovering obstruction of the airways. The forced vital capacity (FVC) is determined by using a system that plots exhaled lung volume versus time (Fig. 1-1). This is usually displayed and recorded as the spirometric tracing and is used to generate specific parameters that relate to lung function. Typically, the patient is asked to perform this maneuver three times to establish the reproducibility of the effort and assess maximal lung function. At this maximal effort, the patient approaches a limiting envelope that cannot be exceeded because of the nature of the airway physiology. Recently, efforts have been made to standardize testing techniques,[6-8] and equipment has been reviewed to assure reproducibility.[9-11]

Once adequate baseline function has been established, particularly if there is a history of broncho-

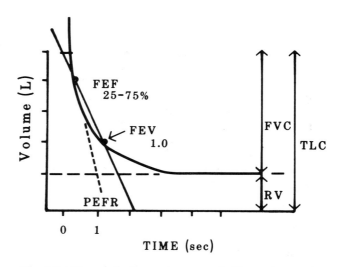

Fig. 1-1. The expiratory spirogram plotting volume versus time and the derived data (including the forced expiratory flow [FEF] from 25 to 75 percent) of the forced vital capacity (FVC), the forced expiratory volume at 1 second (FEV_1), and the peak expiratory flow rate (PEFR).

spasm or cigarette smoking, a nebulized bronchodilator is administered.[12,13] After allowing a sufficient interval for this drug to take effect, three subsequent spirometric examinations are again completed. Demonstration of an acute bronchodilator response implies improved outcome with preoperative therapy, and identifies patients who may become bronchospastic in the perioperative period. Conversely, bronchoprovocation has become an important epidemiologic tool, but, as yet, has no defined place in assessing the surgical patient.

Airway collapse is sometimes confirmed by comparing a slow vital capacity (SVC) to the FVC. In normal patients, the SVC and FVC are identical. With COPD, the FVC maneuver accentuates airway collapse.[14] Dynamic airway compression is particularly problematic for the emphysematous patient, since destruction of lung tissue results in loss of elastic recoil pressure (Fig. 1-2). When pleural pressure becomes mainly positive during forced exhalation, the airways not supported by cartilaginous tissue are collapsed. For patients with asthma and chronic bronchitis, lumenal changes associated with bronchial musculature and airway secretions obstruct air flow during exhalation.

If performance of this simple spirometric test is satisfactory, numeric data can be generated from these curves. First, the FVC during the best spirometric attempt is measured. The force expiratory volume at 1 second (FEV_1) relates volume to time, and is, therefore, a measurement of air flow obstruction. Even more valuable is the ratio between the FEV_1 and the FVC. This FEV_1 to FVC ratio is the hallmark of COPD when it is diminished.[15,16] An analysis of midflow is also performed. The maximum mid-expiratory flow rate is a measurement of air flow through the mid-50 percent of the exhaled vital capacity.

To make an assessment, most of these data are reported as absolute values and are compared with demographic data that were generated by studying normal populations.[17,18] It is important to realize that earlier data were generated without the exclusion of cigarette smokers.[19,20] Likewise, a small female may appear to be more severely compromised based on these data than may actually be the case.[21,22] Other than these exceptions, the data are very useful in comparing the patient's lung function to what might be expected for the patient's sex, height, and weight among the normal population.

Another test useful in evaluating patients preoperatively is the maximum voluntary ventilation (MVV).[23-25] As opposed to spirometry, which evaluates only one breath, the patient is asked to inhale and exhale repeatedly for a specified period of time. The maximal amount of gas that can be moved in and out

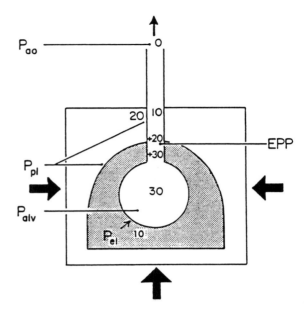

Fig. 1-2. The forces acting in the chest during a forced expiratory effort are depicted. The heavy arrows indicate compression of the thorax by contraction of the expiratory muscles. P_{pl} is the pleural pressure, in this case 20 cmH_2O. P_{el} is elastic recoil pressure of the lung, in this case 10 cmH_2O. P_{alv} is pressure in the alveolus, $P_{alv} = P_{pl}$ (20) + P_{el} (10) = 30 cmH_2O. Note that the pressure in the airways drops from the alveolar pressure (30 cmH_2O) to the mouth or P_{ao} (or atmospheric pressure). EPP indicates the equal pressure point (ie, the point in the airway at which the intramural and extramural pressures are equal), in this case 20 cmH_2O. Further downstream from the equal pressure point, toward the airway opening, there is a transmural pressure tending to narrow or close the airway. (From Cherniack et al,[85] with permission.)

of the lungs on a prolonged basis (10 to 15 seconds) is reported as the MVV. This is a nonspecific test that evaluates a variety of factors important to lung function. Obviously, the patient who has obstruction to air flow will have difficulty maintaining adequate gas flow during repeated inspiratory and expiratory attempts. Similarly, patients who are nutritionally depleted or suffer from wasting of the respiratory muscles will have difficulty approximating normal values. Although criticism has been leveled at the MVV because of its nonspecificity, it has been repeatedly shown to have a predictive value in preoperative thoracotomy patients. It has been suggested that it is necessary to perform this test to uncover some of the respiratory variables that may influence outcome.

Additional data can be generated by recording flow

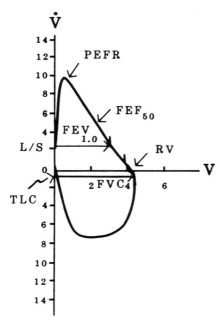

Fig. 1-3. Normal flow-volume loop showing peak expiratory flow rate (PEFR), forced expiratory volume at one second (FEV₁), and forced vital capacity (FVC). FEF, forced expiratory flow.

versus volume during a forced exhalation rather than volume versus time.[26] This exhaled maneuver is usually combined with an inspiratory attempt at achieving vital capacity, which generates a flow-volume loop that begins and ends at TLC (Fig. 1-3). The equipment necessary to perform this test is more sophisticated and more expensive, but the data generated are similar to the spirometric data with the added advantage of being able to more adequately evaluate the upper airway. Time marks during the exhaled maneuver allow not only the measurement of the FVC, but also the measurement of the FEV_1 and the peak expiratory flow rate. Maximum midflows are more adequately examined and the forced expiratory flow between 25 and 75 percent of the exhaled vital capacity is both numerically and graphically demonstrated.

Obstruction of the upper airways tends to appear as characteristic patterns depending on whether the obstruction is variable or fixed.[27] In the case of an extrathoracic obstruction (eg, obstruction because of a laryngeal tumor or mass), the impediment to air flow is usually seen during inspiration. The clinical correlate of this is the patient with extrathoracic airway obstruction who also has stridor. If the airway obstruction is fixed, there will be a fixed flow that cannot be exceeded, depending on the size of the orifice. Conversely, in the case of an intrathoracic obstruction of the airway, such as an intratracheal mass, the majority of the limitation to air flow occurs during exhalation. This is because the intrathoracic lesion is sur-

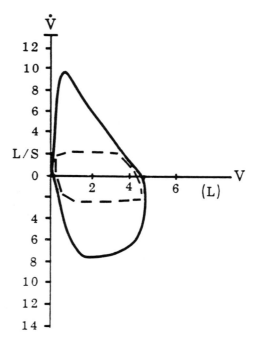

Fig. 1-4. Changes in the flow-volume loop with upper airway obstruction. The dashed line (exhalation) shows intrathoracic obstruction and the dashed line (inhalation) shows extrathoracic obstruction. Fixed obstruction throughout the respiratory cycle results in a "square" loop. The peak inspiratory and expiratory flow are fixed at approximately 34 L/s.

rounded by negative intrapleural pressure that becomes more negative during spontaneous inspiration (Fig. 1-4). This has the effect of enlarging the orifice during inspiration and constricting the orifice during forced exhalation when pleural pressure becomes positive. In the case of an extrathoracic obstruction, the drop in pleural pressure associated with inspiration causes a negative intraluminal pressure and accentuates the closure or collapse of the upper airway. In the case of the fixed obstruction (ie, during both inspiration and expiration), the flow-volume loop assumes a characteristic square shape, indicating that air flow is impeded throughout the respiratory cycle.

Lung Volumes

The second set of useful tests are used for the determination of lung volumes. These tests are used only in a supportive capacity and can be determined by any of three different techniques: body plethysmography, nitrogen washout, or helium dilution. The two gas dilution techniques are most commonly used and are based on the measurement of insoluble gases, such as helium, or the measurement of exhaled nitrogen, which is normally 80 percent of the resident gas in the lung.[28,29] These tests can be done either on a single inspired breath or with multiple breath techniques,[30] the latter being the most common.

To determine lung volumes using helium, the patient is connected to a closed circuit system in which helium is used as the reference gas (Fig. 1-5). The subject breathes quietly from a spirometer that contains approximately 10 percent helium in air and is connected to a carbon dioxide absorber. Over several minutes, equilibrium is reached such that the concentration of helium is the same in both the patient's lung and the gas reservoir. During the course of quiet breathing, sufficient oxygen is introduced into the system to keep expiratory lung volume constant. To calculate the lung volume, the volume of gas in the spirometer used in the test, the deadspace of the mechanical system, the beginning helium concentration, and the concentration of helium at equilibrium must be known. Knowing these data, functional residual capacity (FRC) can be calculated. The second dilutional technique is referred to as *nitrogen washout* (Fig. 1-6). The patient breathes 100 percent oxygen and washes the nitrogen out of the lungs during quiet respiration. All exhaled gases are collected, and total volume and concentration of nitrogen are measured.

To accurately determine FRC, it is important that

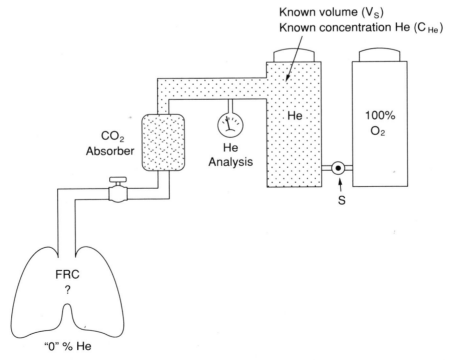

Fig. 1-5. Diagram of closed-circuit helium dilution technique for measuring lung volume. The helium in the spirometer at the beginning of the test (known volume and concentration) is "diluted" in proportion to the unknown volume in the lung (FRC). (From Tisi,[86] with permission.)

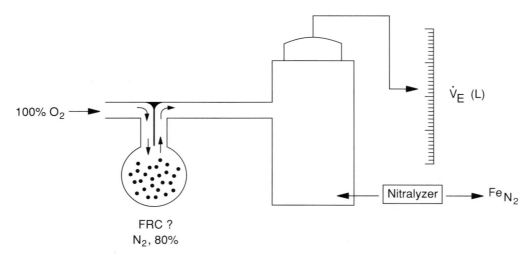

Fig. 1-6. Diagram of open-circuit N_2 washout method for measuring lung volume. All the N_2 in the subject's lung at the beginning of the test (known concentration, unknown volume) is "washed out" of the lungs by 100 percent O_2 and collected in a spirometer. (From Tisi,[86] with permission.)

the patient be connected into either the open or closed circuit at a specific point during tidal breathing. This can be accomplished by observational techniques during which the operator assesses end-expiration before beginning the study, or by using a solenoid system that electronically connects the patient into the circuit at the end of a tidal breath. Once the FRC has been calculated, the remaining compartmentalization of lung volumes can be accomplished by an analysis of spirometric tracings during several specific maneuvers. In addition to asking the patient to exhale from TLC to residual volume, the tidal volume is assessed during normal breathing and graphically displayed. The vital capacity is composed of the inspiratory capacity, the tidal volume, and the expiratory reserve volume. The inspiratory capacity includes the tidal volume and the inspiratory reserve volume, and the TLC is the sum of the inspiratory capacity and the FRC.

Determination of lung volumes using body plethysmography is a direct application of Boyle's law, which states that the volume of gas in a closed space varies inversely with the pressure to which it is subjected.[31,32] In this case, the volume of gas in the lungs is determined with the body in an airtight chamber. The patient sits in the plethysmograph, breathing through a mouthpiece that has a sensitive shutter system. The box is vented so that warmed air can escape during the time the patient is performing a test. Once a baseline is established, the measurement of lung volume can be accomplished. As the patient breathes quietly through the mouthpiece, gas in the lungs is at atmospheric pressure when there is no air flow (ie, at end-inspiration and then at end-expiration). A shutter closes at the end of a normal expiration, and traps the

gas in the chest at that specific lung volume. When this occurs, the patient is asked to make inspiratory and expiratory efforts against the occluded airway, and the intrathoracic gas volume is alternately compressed and decompressed. These pressure changes are related to the pressure changes at the mouth, which should now be equal to alveolar pressure, and changes in the thoracic gas volume, as reflected by changes of pressure within the box. The slope of the pressure volume line ($\Delta P/\Delta V$) is used to calculate the intrathoracic gas volume (Fig. 1-7). Simultaneous measurement of airflow at the mouth allows calculation of airways resistance.

Diffusing Capacity

The third form of assessment that is usually included in a battery of pulmonary function tests is the assessment of diffusing capacity.[33] This test is also widely available and has been related to postoperative function and used in predicting postoperative morbidity and mortality. There are a variety of techniques that have been suggested to perform this test. In essence, it is an attempt to estimate the status of the lung in terms of its diffusion characteristics and, of course, the physiologic gases (oxygen and carbon dioxide) are of the most interest. However, for purposes of accomplishing the study, a nonphysiologic gas (ie, carbon monoxide, D_{CO}) is used because of its affinity for hemoglobin. It is assumed that the principles of calculation for diffusing capacity are the same no matter which gas is being used. Whatever technique is used, there must be some estimate of the gas that is diffusing across the alveolar capillary membrane and the pressure differential, which is driving

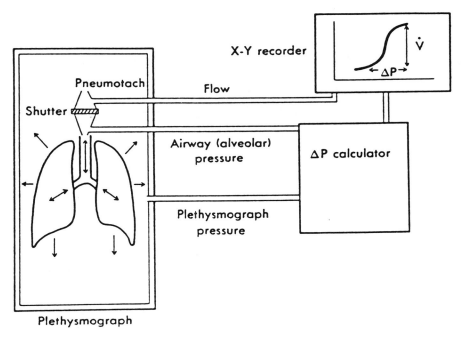

Fig. 1-7. Diagrammatic representation of the measurement of airway resistance by the body plethysmograph method: Airway resistance = atmospheric pressure − alveolar pressure/flow. Flow ($\dot{V}$) is measured directly by means of the pneumotach. The pressure differential between the chamber and the alveoli is measured as follows: plethysmograph pressure is monitored by means of a sensitive manometer in the chamber; alveolar pressure is measured as airway pressure during intervals when no gas flow is occurring. A shutter occludes the airway momentarily, usually at end-expiration, and a manometer monitors the falling pressure. The pressure differential is calculated and delivered to an appropriate display device (X-Y recorder, oscilloscope). (From Ruppel,[87] with permission.)

this gas flow, in order to calculate the diffusing capacity. It is, therefore, necessary to measure partial pressures of the tracer gas in both the alveolus and the pulmonary capillaries. As mentioned, carbon monoxide is particularly useful for making this measurement due to its high affinity for hemoglobin. As carbon monoxide diffuses into the pulmonary capillary bed, it is rapidly taken up by hemoglobin so that the partial pressure of carbon monoxide in the pulmonary capillary space is essentially zero. An exhaled sample is used to measure the mean alveolar carbon monoxide tension and, thus, provides the driving pressure by estimating the gradient for carbon monoxide. Both steady state and single-breath techniques make specific assumptions in order to estimate the diffusing capacity.[34–36]

Interpretation of Pulmonary Function Tests

Although an analysis of these data is meant to demonstrate physiologic abnormalities, there are certain diagnostic conclusions that can be reached in the face of confirming evidence found on history and physical

examinations.[37,38] Abnormal spirometric data can basically be divided into two different varieties: obstructive ventilatory defects and restrictive ventilatory defects (Fig. 1-8). The restrictive physiology is characteristically demonstrated with a reduction in the FVC. Physiologic restriction can be extrinsic or intrinsic to the lung and can be due to a variety of causes. In either event, if there is no obstruction to air flow, the FEV_1/FVC ratio should be normal in the face of a significant reduction in the FVC. Corroborative evidence pointing to extrinsic or intrinsic defects can be obtained by examining changes in lung volumes and the diffusing capacity. An intrinsic defect is usually correlated with a concentric reduction in lung volumes, such that all lung volumes are decreased by approximately the same percentage (Fig. 1-9). An extrinsic ventilatory defect, on the other hand, characteristically shows preservations of the smaller lung volumes, such as the residual volume (and the FVC), with major limitations in the TLC. Examples of extrinsic ventilatory defects include obesity, diaphragmatic paralysis, abnormalities of the spine or chest wall (eg, kyphoscoliosis), an accumulation of pleural or ascitic fluid, and other similar abnormalities. An

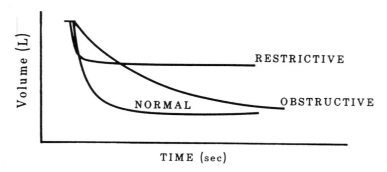

Fig. 1-8. Spirometric tracings, representing exhaled volume versus time, can be categorized as restrictive or obstructive abnormalities.

example of an intrinsic restrictive ventilatory defect is diffuse interstitial fibrosis, in which there is not only a loss in all lung volumes, but a clear impediment to diffusing capacity and gas exchange. Conversely, an extrinsic restrictive ventilatory defect should show normal diffusing capacities when corrected for inspired gas volume.

The hallmark of expiratory air flow obstruction is analysis of the FEV_1/FVC ratio which, even in elderly patients, should exceed 70 percent. Both the FEV_1 and the FEV_1/FVC ratio are reduced whether air flow obstruction is due to asthma, chronic bronchitis, or emphysema. Supporting evidence of a specific type of air flow obstruction is obtained by analyzing the lung

volumes and diffusing capacity. The patient with emphysema is markedly hyperinflated, traps gas, and has a characteristic x-ray film showing hyperlucent lung fields and flat diaphragms due to the gas trapping. In its purest form, emphysema does not respond to bronchodilators and, on clinical examination, there is minimal bronchospasm. In addition, the diffusing capacity is usually low, not because of abnormal gas exchange, but because of the ongoing destructive process in the emphysematous lung. In this case, there is a loss of effective surface area for gas transfer that diminishes the diffusing capacity for reasons other than infiltrative abnormalities at the alveolar capillary membrane. The patient with chronic bronchitis

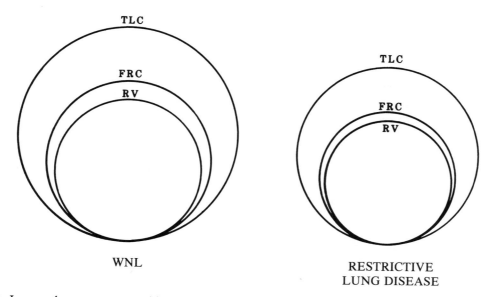

Fig. 1-9. Lung volumes represented by circles under normal circumstances with concentric reduction in all lung volumes characteristic of an intrinsic restrictive defect. WNL, within normal limits; TLC, total lung capacity; FRC, functional reserve capacity; RV, residual volume.

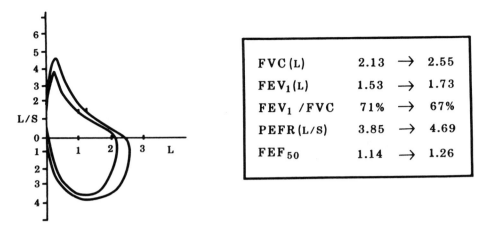

FVC (L)	2.13	$\rightarrow$	2.55
FEV$_1$ (L)	1.53	$\rightarrow$	1.73
FEV$_1$ /FVC	71%	$\rightarrow$	67%
PEFR (L/S)	3.85	$\rightarrow$	4.69
FEF$_{50}$	1.14	$\rightarrow$	1.26

Fig. 1-10. Comparison of flow-volume loops before and after the administration of a nebulized bronchodilator. Note the marked increase in both the FEV$_1$ and FVC, with little change in the FEV$_1$/FVC ratio. Both the peak flow (PEFR) and midflows (FEF$_{50}$) also show dramatic increases.

has a greater tendency to wheeze, and there is often a 10 percent or greater response to bronchodilators when spirometry is repeated. There can also be marked gas trapping during the course of the disease, but this is not as evident as in the emphysematous patient. This patient has more of a tendency to be hypoxic, often retains carbon dioxide, and has a stormy clinical course characterized by copious sputum production and frequent episodes of infection and respiratory failure. It is essential that this type of patient be adequately assessed prior to surgery and that adequate bronchodilator and antibiotic therapy be instituted to improve the chance of maximizing remaining lung function postoperatively to avoid life-threatening infection or bronchospasm. The asthmatic patient also has a tendency toward bronchospasm, but it is episodic. Younger asthmatics, in particular, often have symptom-free interludes and, during these periods, all measurements of pulmonary function testing are usually normal.

During acute episodes, obstruction to air flow is demonstrated as a reduction in the FEV$_1$ and the FEV$_1$/FVC ratio, and there may be other abnormalities consistent with hyperinflation and gas trapping (Fig. 1-10). With adequate therapy, these abnormalities can usually be reversed, and the improvement in pulmonary function parameters parallels the improvement in clinical findings. Individuals with asthma often have a tendency to wheeze because of some type of triggering episode, and bronchoprovocation has been used as a diagnostic technique.[39,40] Examples would be the bronchospastic response to cold air, exercise, or the inhalation of a variety of bronchospastic-provoking antigens or allergens. In addition, these patients are particularly prone to severe bronchospasm during anesthetic induction because of ma-

nipulation of the upper airway and intubation of the trachea. In this case, bronchospasm tends to be mediated by an intense vagal parasympathetic response that can be blocked, to some extent, by the administration of atropine or an atropine analog, such as ipratropium bromide. Thus, an attempt should be made preoperatively to provide a wheeze-free interval for these patients by the use of beta$_2$-adrenergic drugs and, often, by the addition of inhaled atropine or atropine analogs. These drugs should aid in facilitating anesthetic induction so that manipulation of the airway can be accomplished without severe consequences (see Chapter 9).

EVALUATION FOR THORACOTOMY

Basic Pulmonary Function Testing

In addition to physiologic assessment and analysis of diagnostic pattern, routine pulmonary function testing has been used to establish increased risk in patients who undergo thoracotomy. Routine pulmonary function testing with both lungs intact was first suggested as a predictive mechanism by Gaensler et al, who reported a series of 644 patients undergoing thoracoplasty mainly for tuberculosis therapy.[41] The first to demonstrate the importance of the MVV (then called *maximal breathing capacity*), these investigators reported that values less than 50 percent of predicted were associated with a higher degree of morbidity and mortality. Since many of these patients had restrictive physiology, it is not surprising that Gaensler et al also noted that an FVC less than 30 percent of the predicted value was associated with a 40 percent mortality. Both of these parameters have been confirmed by subsequent testing. Mittman reported a retrospective analysis of 199 patients who underwent thoracotomy and analyzed the data from the 28 patients who died.[42] He confirmed that an MVV less than 50 percent of the predicted value was associated with high mortality. He also showed that electrocardiograph evidence of premature ventricular contractions or recent myocardial infarction was associated with a poor prognosis. As for pulmonary function testing, Mittman showed that an abnormal nitrogen washout test or evidence of hyperinflation manifested by an increase in the RV/TLC ratio identified those patients with a poor prognosis. The criteria he proposed were sensitive but nonspecific, and application of these restrictive criteria would have denied surgery to a number of people who successfully underwent thoracotomy and lung resection in his own series. Boushy et al did a retrospective analysis of 142 patients and emphasized the relationship between COPD, the impact of pulmonary function abnormalities, and lung resection.[43] These investigators reported that an FEV$_1$ less than 2 L in patients over 60 years of age resulted in a 40 percent incidence of postoperative respiratory failure. An additional analysis of 743 patients by Lockwood defined high risk as being an FVC less than 1.85 L, a residual volume greater than 3.3 L, an FEV$_1$ less than 1.2 L, or an RV/TLC ratio greater than 47 percent.[44] Additionally, he found that if the FEV$_1$/FVC ratio was less than 35 percent and the MVV was less than 28 L/min, there was a high incidence of both morbidity and mortality. It is clear from the analysis of these data that there is no specific test that can be used to predict morbidity and mortality. It is probable that the most sensitive tests are the FEV$_1$, or the FEV$_1$ as a percentage of FVC (FEV$_1$/FVC ratio), and the MVV. These data are useful because it appears from the accumulated literature that patients capable of passing all of the pulmonary function criteria listed in Table 1-1 should be able to withstand resection of normal and malignant tissue, even if a pneumonectomy is necessary, and should be able to survive with the postoperative lung function that remains.[44] This last point deserves further emphasis because, despite improved imaging techniques, the extent of surgery necessary to remove the tumor is often not known

prior to the actual examination of the open chest. For this reason, all patients should be evaluated as though a pneumonectomy might eventually be necessary, realizing that every attempt will be made to resect only the cancerous lesion and a minimal amount of remaining lung tissue from that operative side.

The listed criteria should be assessed in terms of both morbidity and mortality. If mortality is basically a result of acute cor pulmonale because of inadequate remaining functional lung tissue, then the ability to assess the amount each lung contributes to overall lung function is important to the patient's outcome. This appears to be the case, and the FEV$_1$ and MVV appear to be the measurements best able to predict postoperative lung function and survival. In terms of morbidity, however, the MVV and D$_{CO}$ have recently been confirmed as good prognostic indicators. Severe hyperinflation, identified by an increased RV/TLC ratio, and restrictive physiology with reduced FVC also relate to postoperative morbidity. Due to pain and disruption of thoracic anatomy, a superimposed, although transient, restrictive defect is common and may overwhelm the ability of the compromised patient to maintain oxygenation and ventilation after surgery.[45]

Evaluation of Split Lung Function

It is not generally appreciated that the double-lumen tube (DLT) was originally designed to isolate the left and right lungs in order to measure exhaled gas volume from each side.[46] In later years, different designs followed the original double-lumen Carlen's tube. Recently, the DLT has become an essential feature of one-lung anesthesia, synchronous independent lung ventilation, and control of massive hemoptysis (see Chapter 14).

Early investigators advocated the use of this tube to measure split lung function. The tube was placed in an awake patient under topical analgesia and minimal sedation. Exhaled gas from the isolated lungs flowed into separate spirometers, hence the term *bronchospirometry*.[47] Thus, the fraction or percentage of the FVC that came from each lung could be evaluated, and a post-pneumonectomy vital capacity could be predicted. Because of the limitations to air flow due to the size of each individual lumen, an FEV$_1$ cannot be assessed, but once the fraction that each individual lung contributes to overall function is ascertained, simple multiplication provides predictive data for all measured ventilatory parameters.

Placement of a DLT in an awake, even cooperative, patient is difficult and requires considerable skill; therefore, a less invasive ventilatory test has been suggested. The lateral position test takes advantage of the

TABLE 1-1. Pulmonary Function Criteria Indicating Increased Risk

FVC < 50% of predicted
FEV$_1$ < 50% of predicted or < 2.0 L
MVV < 50% of predicted or < 50 L/min
D$_{CO}$ < 50% predicted
RV/TLC > 50%

fact that blood flow and ventilation shift to the dependent lung in a spontaneously breathing patient in the lateral decubitus position.

During quiet breathing, a baseline slope is constructed for the supine, right lateral, and left lateral decubitus positions.[48,49] The shift in each baseline during lateral positioning, compared with the supine position, is used to assess the contribution of each lung to overall pulmonary function. Success with this technique has been mixed, and mediastinal involvement with the tumor prevents normal anatomic and physiologic changes necessary to complete the calculations.[50,51]

In similar fashion, isolation of blood flow to each lung was attempted to assess split lung function. A special catheter was designed with an inflatable balloon large enough to occlude all blood flow to one lung.[52–54] Under fluoroscopic guidance, the catheter was advanced into the pulmonary artery of the diseased lung and temporary unilateral balloon occlusion (TUPAO) isolated the uninvolved lung. Since resection of functional lung tissue in an already compromised patient may result in postoperative acute cor pulmonale and hypoxemic respiratory failure, such an evaluation has a sound physiologic basis. Furthermore, the addition of low levels of exercise allows prognostic evaluation of exercise function postresection. If the mean pulmonary artery pressure, at rest or with exercise, exceeds 30 mmHg, or if the arterial oxygen tension falls below 45 mmHg, survival following pneumonectomy is unlikely.

Since pulmonary artery catheterization is also invasive and requires considerable skill, less invasive methods are desirable. For this reason, the techniques of radiospirometry and perfusion scanning became popular.[55,56] For radiospirometry, a radioactive isotope is injected that is rapidly cleared by the lungs. A split function crystal and gamma camera is centered over the mediastinum so that background counts and right versus left radioactive counts can be manipulated to determine the percentage of function from each lung. Using only perfusion scanning, a more stable and less expensive isotope can be used, either microionized albumin labeled with iodine 131 or technetium 99, and similar predictive information can be obtained. Whichever technique for assessing fractional or split lung function is used, the calculation to predict postoperative function is similar. For example, to calculate the predicted postoperative FEV_1, the equation is as follows:

$$\text{Predicted Postoperative } FEV_1 = \text{Preoperative } FEV_1 \times \text{Percent Function Uninvolved Lung}$$

The predicted postoperative FEV_1 compatible with long-term survival is 1,000 mL,[46] possibly as low as 800 mL.[56] To refine predictive techniques, it has been suggested that the preoperative predicted FEV_1 also be taken into account in addition to the absolute preoperative FEV_1 limitation of 2.0 L and postoperative limitation of 800 mL. Using this concept, it has been suggested that the predicted preoperative FEV should exceed 40 percent of the predicted preoperative FEV estimated on age, sex, and body weight. This extends the likelihood of successful resection to individuals of both sexes with smaller body mass and stature.[57,58]

Allowances can also be made for surgical intervention that may not require a pneumonectomy.[59] If lobectomy seems a likely possibility, the added function attributed to lung tissue remaining on the operative side can also be estimated.[60] The simplest technique relies on the number of bronchopulmonary segments usually found in each lung. If, for example, the right upper lobe will be resected and there are three segments in that lobe compared with 10 segments in that lung (ie, 7 of 10 bronchopulmonary segments will remain), the following formula may be used:

$$\text{Predicted Postoperative } FEV_1 = \text{Function [Nonoperative Lung]} + \text{Remaining Function [Operative Lung]} = \text{Preoperative } FEV_1 \times \text{Percent Perfusion [Nonoperative Lung]} + \text{Preoperative } FEV_1 \times 7/10 \times \text{Percent Perfusion [Operative Lung]}$$

Immediate postoperative lung function may more closely approximate predicted postpneumonectomy function due to trauma and edema in remaining lung tissue on the operative side. Resolution takes place so that by 3 months postoperatively, lung function closely approximates predicted data.[60,61]

EXERCISE TESTING

With the availability of noninvasive respiratory gas monitoring and pulse oximetry, there is a renewed interest in exercise testing as a means of predicting postoperative morbidity and mortality. As noted above, the major emphasis in prethoracotomy function testing has focused on (1) ventilatory measurements combined with the addition of split function assessment, and (2) the prediction of postoperative pulmonary hypertension and cor pulmonale. Exercise testing has had similar goals. The concept of using exercise as a testing modality is attractive because of the integration of ventilation, gas exchange, cardiac output, and peripheral muscle utilization of oxygen. Also, exercise results in increased flow into the pulmonary vascular bed, much like the diversion of cardiac output into remaining lung vasculature after resection.[62,63] Although recent data are promising, the most efficacious means of exercise testing and the development of a specific protocol have yet to be confirmed.

Olsen has recently reviewed available data, and suggested classifying protocols as constant or incremental and the end point as maximal or submaximal (Fig. 1-11).[64] Testing can be categorized as (1) simple tests of exercise tolerance, (2) protocols designed to predict postoperative pulmonary hypertension, and (3) the measurement of oxygen consumption ($\dot{V}O_2$) to predict morbidity and mortality.

Early investigators used all types of testing systems, either in an inclusive battery of pulmonary function tests or as a sole means of evaluation. In 1955, Gaensler et al reported results of a series of 460 patients who were exercised to a submaximal steady state, including 5.7 percent with abnormal pulmonary function.[41] They found no correlation between postoperative disability and a 180 ft/min walk. Olsen has estimated that this level would correlate to a $\dot{V}O_2$ of 800 mL/min (12 mL/kg/min) and a work rate of 25 W (150 kp·m/min for a man weighing 70 kg), assuming a walk at 2 mph at zero grade.[64] This minimal work level is usually the beginning effort in a graded exercise protocol.

A series of 213 patients, all of whom underwent pneumonectomy, was reported by Van Nostrand et al.[65] A large number of these patients had abnormal pulmonary function (31.4 percent), and predictive postoperative data were used to exclude candidates for resection. In addition, they devised a stair climb of two flights requiring a work rate of 320 kp·m/min, or 52 W, for a 70-kg man. This is also equivalent to an estimated $\dot{V}O_2$ of 1.1 L/min or 16 mL/kg/min. From the group of exercised patients, these investigators reported no improvements in discerning high-risk patients versus other studies despite a 13 percent mortality and a 40 percent rate of deaths attributable to cardiorespiratory insufficiency.

A group of 75 pneumonectomy patients subjected to graded exercise testing was reported by Reichel.[66] Postoperative mortality was 24 percent, and another 17 percent suffered major complications. Airflow obstruction for the entire study group was mild to moderate. Incremental exercise included six stages with an increase in duration, speed, and grade, culminating in a 3 mph pace at a 10 percent grade. This corresponds to 600 kp·m/min (25 mL/kg/min), still considered a low level of fitness. Of the four patients unable to complete stage 1 (2 mph on a level slope for 4 minutes), two died and another had major complications.

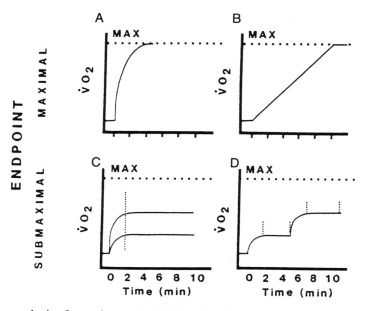

WORKRATE

CONSTANT   INCREMENTAL

Fig. 1-11. (A–D) An analysis of exercise protocols, based on the end point (maximal or submaximal) and the work rate (constant or incremental), for the total exercise period.

The 11 patients who exercised to completion of the protocol experienced no morbidity or mortality.

An additional study, by Berggren et al in 1984, evaluated patients with spirometry and cycle ergometry.[67] The exercise protocol began with 50 W for 6 minutes, and increased by 10 W increments to a maximal heart rate of 170 beats/min. They reported a 15.9 percent perioperative mortality rate, and a 32 percent 5-year survival rate. In the group undergoing lobectomy, the postoperative mortality was 7.7 percent in those who could perform work at 83 W for 6 minutes. This equates to an estimated $\dot{V}O_2$ of 1.4 L/min or 20 mL/kg/min. Mortality was also related to poor baseline pulmonary function.

Bagg exercised 30 patients by subjecting them to a 12-minute walk.[68] He measured the distance patients could walk on a level indoor surface and recorded subjective symptoms (ie, dyspnea). Such testing failed to discriminate preoperatively between the 7 patients who suffered postoperative morbidity and the 15 who did not. Thus, the use of exercise tolerance tests, if low levels of exercise are used, is problematic because of conflicting results. Furthermore, it is not clear that these studies are useful if baseline pulmonary function testing is normal.

A second line of investigation has sought to use exercise as a means of predicting which patients might have pulmonary hypertension after lung resection. An increase in pulmonary vascular resistance (PVR) would result in cor pulmonale, which has been demonstrated to be a major cause of morbidity and mortality in clinical studies and animal experiments.[69] At least four studies have also combined exercise with TUPAO, a technique already discussed as a determi-

nant of split lung function.[52,53,68,69] Uggla used steady state, submaximal work loads in his study such that a $\dot{V}O_2$ of 810 mL/min or 12 mL/kg/min was sustained during TUPAO. He concluded that these additional data better defined risk in a group of patients with moderate to severe pulmonary function deficits.[53]

More recently, Fee et al used pulmonary artery balloon flotation catheters to collect hemodynamic data during exercise.[70] In this study, 45 patients were separated into two groups based on the severity of spirometric data and arterial blood gas analysis. Two work loads were imposed, 2 mph at 4 percent grade and 4 mph at 4 percent grade, with an intervening 45 minute rest period. Corresponding work rates for these two levels are 164 kp · m/min (27 W) and 328 kp · m/min (54 W), respectively. Estimates for $\dot{V}O_2$ are 830 mL/min (12 mL/kg/min) and 1.1 L/min (16 mL/kg/min). Review of postoperative outcome led the investigators to the conclusion that if PVR was greater than 190 dynes · sec · cm^{-5} during exercise, morbidity and mortality would be increased. In fact, seven of 25 survivors exceeded this PVR limit. However, of five such patients who failed to survive surgery, two had only an open biopsy. Therefore, these studies confirm the fact that postoperative pulmonary hypertension is of grave concern.[71–73] The current frequency of postoperative morbidity and mortality due to these hemodynamic changes is currently unknown.

The actual measurement of $\dot{V}O_2$ offers a direct method of categorizing work levels and performance, and technical advances have made these data easily obtainable. A summary of recently available data is presented in Table 1-2. In the 19 patients studied by Eugene et al, preoperative spirometry failed to pre-

TABLE 1-2. Summary of Exercise Testing Data for Thoracotomy Patients

	Eugene et al[74]	Coleman et al[75]	Smith et al[76]	Bechard and Wetstein[77]	Miyoshi et al[78]	Olsen et al[79]	Boysen et al[80]
Number of Patients	19	59	22	50	33	29	17
Spirometry baseline	32	—	23	38	—	97	100
Type of exercise[a]	B	A & B	B	B	D	C	B
Surgery Pneumonectomy	6	10	4	10	—	8	3
Lobectomy	12	—	12	28	—	13	14
Morbidity (%)	16	3.5	9	4	12	24	47
Mortality (%)	—	40	50	12	45	25	0
Complications predicted	Yes	No	Yes	Yes	Yes	Yes	No

[a] For an analysis of exercise protocols *A* to *D*, see Figure 1-11.

dict deaths.[74] All three patients who died demonstrated a $\dot{V}O_2$max less than 1.0 L/min, whereas the 15 survivors exceeded this level. Nonfatal morbidity was not reported.

Coleman et al subjected surgical candidates to low levels of stair-climbing exercises and to an incremental protocol to $\dot{V}O_2$max.[75] The $\dot{V}O_2$max did not differ significantly between the two groups separated by the incidence of postoperative complications. Both the FEV_1 and the FVC were significantly lower in the group with postoperative complications. Conflicting data were reported by Smith et al, who showed that preoperative pulmonary function testing, combined with quantitative lung scanning, did not predict postoperative complications.[76] If the $\dot{V}O_2$max was less than 15 mL/kg/min, 6 of 6 patients suffered complications; when $\dot{V}O_2$max exceeded, 20 mL/kg/min, only 1 of 10 patients suffered a nonfatal complication. Similarly, Bechard and Wetstein determined $\dot{V}O_2$max during cycle ergometry in a group of 50 consecutive patients with compromised pulmonary function.[77] Complications occurred in 12 percent. There were 2 fatalities and 5 patients who suffered survivable complications with $\dot{V}O_2$max less than 10 mL/kg/min. Since none of these complications was predicted by preoperative spirometry, they suggest that exercise testing should be routinely performed to ascertain if patients fall below this critical level. Using a similar protocol, Miyoshi et al could not preoperatively separate survivors from nonsurvivors by baseline pulmonary function of $\dot{V}O_2$max, although the difference in the FEV_1/FVC ratio was statistically significant between the groups.[78] Of the 8 patients with complications, generation of high levels of blood lactate at submaximal exercise levels separated the 4 survivors from the 4 nonsurvivors. Their data suggest that in-hospital mortality can be predicted by the "$\dot{V}O_2$/BSA at la-20," which indicates anaerobic metabolism even at low levels of exercise.

Two recent studies have concentrated on exercise testing in high-risk patients as defined by abnormal spirometry. Olsen et al were successful in identifying postoperative complications using constant work loads and submaximal effort (type C).[79] Boysen et al could not generate the same results using incremental, maximal effort (type D) and calculating the $\dot{V}O_2$max.[80] The latter study enrolled 72 patients, but only 17 (24 percent) were able to complete a treadmill protocol designed to achieve $\dot{V}O_2$max. Because of the severity of pulmonary dysfunction, it may be necessary to alter protocols to achieve submaximal steady state or to employ tests that use a bicycle ergometer.

In addition to allowing an integrative assessment of cardiopulmonary function, exercise testing allows for separation of cardiac versus pulmonary limitation (Table 1-3).[81] Such testing, however, has been dependent on the ability to exercise incrementally to maximum performance. Measurement of $\dot{V}O_2$max is then assessed as a function of MVV and the heart rate at peak performance.[82] Further differentiation is provided by defining the anaerobic threshold (AT) during exercise, although the prognostic significance of this information for thoracotomy patients is unknown.[83] The AT is the level of exercise oxygen consumption above which aerobic energy production is supplemented by anaerobic mechanisms, and is associated with rising arterial lactate. It has been suggested that the AT can be noninvasively approximated.

In general, a reasonable protocol would begin with measurement of resting pulmonary function to include (1) spirometry before and after a trial of inhaled bronchodilators, (2) lung volumes, (3) diffusing capacity, and (4) arterial blood gas analysis. The MVV is measured as part of spirometric testing. Exercise testing is designed to include breath-by-breath measurement of respiratory gas exchange and airflow, pulse oximetry, and, in some circumstances, an indwelling arterial (radial artery) catheter. Once instrumented

TABLE 1-3.   Differentiation of Cardiac Versus Pulmonary Impairment by Exercise Testing

Measured Parameter	Cardiac	Pulmonary
$\dot{V}O_2$max	Decreased	Decreased
$\dot{V}_E$max/MVV	50%	80–90%
$\dot{V}O_2$max/heart rate (O_2 pulse)	Decreased	May decrease
$\dot{V}O_2$max/AT	Decreased	Indeterminate
PaO_2/SaO_2	Maintained	Decreases
$PaCO_2$	Maintained or decreased	Often decreases
V_D/V_T	Normal = decreased	Often increases

exercise begins at low levels, it is increased incrementally with the intention to determine $\dot{V}O_2$max and the AT. If the exercising subject can achieve the AT and $\dot{V}O_2$max without a fall in arterial oxygen saturation (SaO_2), respiratory impairment is not a factor in functional limitation. A fall in the SaO_2 during exercise indicates vascular or parenchymal lung disease (or a right-to-left intracardiac shunt). Indeed, Markos et al showed a highly significant relationship between arterial oxygen desaturation ($SaO_2 < 2$ percent) from the established baseline at rest and the incidence of postthoracotomy morbidity.[84]

If the $\dot{V}O_2$max and the AT are not attained because of dyspnea, impaired ventilation is a major factor. Further differentiation is possible by analyzing the degree of exercise intolerance in light of baseline pulmonary function data. Cardiac patients use less than 50 percent of their ventilatory capacity during exercise. However, the patients, limited because of pulmonary compromise, use greater than 50 percent of their FVC and MVV as they reach maximal exercise tolerance. There is, however, an increase in heart rate at low work levels or oxygen consumption (ie, the heart rate/$\dot{V}O_2$ ratio is increased). This relationship is often expressed as the inverse ratio ($\dot{V}O_2$/heart rate) and is called the *oxygen pulse*. In some cases, these patients also show a rise in the end-tidal and arterial carbon dioxide tension since alveolar ventilation may not be adequately matched to carbon dioxide production. The normal response to exercise is a fall in the PCO_2 and a fall in dead space-to-tidal volume ratio (V_D/V_T).

ARTERIAL BLOOD GAS ANALYSIS

Although a complete consideration is beyond the scope of this discussion, blood gas analysis is pertinent to thoracic anesthesia. Preoperative resting arterial blood gas analysis is useful to (1) give an indication of the severity of gas exchange abnormalities in the patient with chronic lung disease, (2) indicate which patients may be at particular risk for hypoxia during one-lung anesthesia, and (3) provide guidelines for postoperative management. It should be obvious from the previous discussion that resting blood gas analysis does not provide information as to the physiologic consequences of stress. Many patients with normal or near-normal arterial oxygen tension and arterial oxygen saturation will desaturate even with low levels of exercise.

The patient with chronic lung disease may be compromised because of low arterial oxygen tension and elevated carbon dioxide tension. For the surgical patient, the latter situation is of grave concern, because

hypercarbia indicates respiratory failure with both lungs intact. Surgical intervention is, therefore, usually unwarranted. Carbon dioxide retention usually occurs when the FEV_1 deteriorates to 800 to 1,000 mL. In the face of this degree of abnormal lung mechanics and carbon dioxide retention, it is unlikely that a patient will survive thoracotomy even if only small amounts of lung tissue are resected.

Arterial oxygen desaturation is also related to altered lung mechanics and to alterations in pulmonary blood flow. In fact, an inverse relationship is well established. In the presence of arterial oxygen desaturation, there is an immediate rise in PVR. A simple method of evaluating gas exchange and oxygenation is based on Dalton's law of partial pressure. This law states that the pressure exerted by each component gas in ambient air is additive and the sum equals the barometric pressure. This concept applies to alveolar gas and, thus, an approximation of the oxygen tension of alveolar gas is possible. The following equation is used to characterize inspired gas:

$$P_IO_2 = (P_B - 47 \text{ mmHg}) \, F_IO_2$$

where P_IO_2 = partial pressure of oxygen in inspired air, P_B = barometric pressure, F_IO_2 = fraction of inspired air that is oxygen.

The vapor pressure of water (47 mmHg) is subtracted from the barometric pressure because, by convention, alveolar gas is characterized as a "dry gas." With an intact upper airway, gas is saturated with water vapor as it enters the tracheobronchial tree. In the intubated patient with a mechanical bypass of the upper airway, this assumption is incorrect. Having calculated the P_IO_2, the next step is to estimate the oxygen tension of alveolar gas, as follows:

$$P_AO_2 = P_IO_2 - PaCO_2/0.8$$
$$\text{At sea level, } P_AO_2 = (P_B - 47)F_IO_2 - PaCO_2/0.8, \text{ or}$$
$$= 150 - 40/0.8$$
$$= 100 \text{ mmHg}$$

Comparing the calculated P_AO_2 to the measured PaO_2 provides the alveolar-to-arterial gradient for oxygen tension, commonly referred to as the $(A-a)DO_2$. Changes in cardiac output and F_IO_2 can widen this gradient, but it otherwise will reflect the degree of intrapulmonary shunt. For example, given a patient suspected of alveolar hypoventilation due to drug overdose, the following arterial blood gas analysis is obtained: $PaO_2 = 45$ mmHg, $PaCO_2 = 80$ mmHg, and pH = 7.17.

The low pH corroborates the clinical suspicion that this is an acute process. Using the alveolar air equation is useful when answering the question concerning the appropriateness of the PaO_2, given the degree of hypoventilation.

$$P_IO_2 = (P_B - 47) \, F_IO_2$$
(assume sea level, breathing room air)
$$P_IO_2 = (760 - 47) \, 21 = 150$$
then $P_AO_2 = P_IO_2 - PaCO_2/0.8$
$$P_AO_2 = 150 - 80/0.8$$
$$P_AO_2 = 50$$

Since the $PaO_2 = 45$ mmHg, the $(A-a)DO_2 = 5$ mmHg. Thus, there is no abnormality in gas exchange; rather, the hypoxemia is due to alveolar hypoventilation. Consider also the following example of a COPD patient in respiratory distress who is wheezing, cyanotic, and tachycardic: $PaO_2 = 30$ mmHg, $PaCO_2 = 65$ mmHg, and pH = 7.30.

The near-normal pH indicates some degree of renal compensation for the respiratory abnormality. The PaO_2 of 30 mmHg is consistent with clinical findings, but not with the degree of alveolar hypoventilation. Again, assume the patient is at sea level breathing room air:

$$P_AO_2 = P_IO_2 - PaCO_2/0.8$$
$$P_AO_2 = 150 \ - 65/0.8$$
$$P_AO_2 = 70 \text{ mmHg}$$

Comparison of the P_AO_2 and the measured PaO_2 indicates a difference of 40 mmHg. Therefore, the hypoxemia is due to a combination of alveolar hypoventilation and ventilation-perfusion abnormalities, both characteristic of the COPD patient in respiratory failure. The COPD patient in a steady state (but not in respiratory failure) will still manifest evidence of shunt due to ventilation-perfusion abnormalities.

The patient with borderline levels of arterial oxygen saturation is particularly prone to hypoxemia during one-lung anesthesia. With collapse of one lung there are alterations in ventilation-perfusion relationships, further complicated by reactive changes in perfusion. Fortunately, in some cases, an elevation in cardiac output protects against serious complications. Careful monitoring is necessary to assure that adequate oxygenation is maintained by applying positive end-expiratory pressure to the functioning or dependent lung or continuous positive airway pressure to the operative lung. Deciding which maneuver or combination of maneuvers to use in negating ventilation-perfusion abnormalities is often a question of monitoring the results of empiric therapy (see Chapter 8). In the immediate postoperative period, the lobectomy patient may have atelectasis, edema, or both in the remaining lung or on the operative side. Supplemental oxygen, lung inflation, and adequate pain relief may be necessary to avoid hypoxemia.

REFERENCES

1. Kohman LJ, Meyer JA, Ikins PM, et al: Random versus predictable risks of mortality after thoracotomy for lung cancer. J Thorac Cardiovasc Surg 91:551–554, 1986.
2. Ginsberg RJ, Hill LD, Eagan RT, et al: Modern 30-day operative mortality for surgical resections in lung cancer. J Thorac Cardiovasc Surg 86:654–658, 1983
3. Hutchinson J: On the capacity of the lung and on the respiratory functions with the view of establishing a precise and easy method of detecting disease by the spirometer. Trans Med Chir Soc Lond 29:137–252, 1946
4. Anthonisen NR, Wright FC, Hodgkin JE: Prognosis in chronic obstructive pulmonary disease. Am Rev Respir Dis 133:14–20, 1986
5. Wells H, Stead WW, Rossing TD, et al: Accuracy of air improved spirometer for recording fast breathing. J Appl Physiol 14:451–454, 1959
6. Gardner RM: ATS statement—snowbird workshop on standardization of spirometry. Am Rev Respir Dis 119:831–838, 1979
7. Crapo RO, Morris AH, Gardner RM: Reference spirometric values using techniques and equipment that meets ATS recommendations. Am Rev Respir Dis 123:659–664, 1981
8. Hankinson JL, Gardner RM: Standard waveforms for spirometric testing. Am Rev Respir Dis 126:362–364, 1982
9. Gardner RM, Clausen JL, Catton DJ, et al: Computer guidelines for pulmonary laboratories. Am Rev Respir Dis 134:628–629, 1986
10. Gardner RM, Clausen JL, Epler G, et al: Pulmonary function laboratory personnel qualifications. Am Rev Respir Dis 134:623–624, 1986
11. Gardner RM, Clausen JL, Crapo RO, et al: Quality assurance in pulmonary function laboratories Am Rev Respir Dis 134:626–627, 1986
12. Berger R, Smith D: Acute postbronchodilator changes in pulmonary function parameters in patients with chronic airway obstruction. Chest 93:541–546, 1988
13. Light RW, Conrad SA, George RB: The one best test for evaluating effects of bronchodilator therapy. Chest 72:512–516, 1977
14. Cherniack RM, Cherniack L, Naimark A: Respiration in Health and Disease. 2nd Ed. WB Saunders, Philadelphia, 1972
15. Clausen JL, Farins LP (eds): Pulmonary Function Testing—Guidelines and Controversies. Academic Press, San Diego, 1982
16. Cotes JE: Lung Function: Assessment and Application in Medicine. 4th Ed. Blackwell Scientific Publications, Oxford, 1979
17. Becklake MR: Concepts of normality applied to the measurement of lung function. Am J Med 80:1158–1163, 1986
18. Ferris BG, Jr: Epidemiology standardization project. Am Rev Respir Dis 37:185–191, 1978
19. Morris JF, Koskie A, Johnson LC: Spirometric standards for healthy non-smoking adults. Am Rev Respir Dis 103:57–67, 1971

20. Tashkin DP, Clark VA, Coulson AN, et al: Comparison of lung function in young nonsmokers and smokers before and after the initiation of the smoking habit. Am Rev Respir Dis 128:12–16, 1984

21. Aitkin ML, Schoene RB, Franklin J, et al: Pulmonary function at the extremes of stature. Am Rev Respir Dis 131:161–168, 1985

22. Lapp NL, Amandus HE, Hall R, et al: Lung volumes and flow rates in black and white subjects. Thorax 29:185–188, 1974

23. Needham CD, Rogan MC, McDonald I: Normal standards for lung volumes, intrapulmonary gas mixing and maximal breathing capacity. Thorax 9:313–325, 1954.

24. McKenzie DK, Gandevia SC: Strength and endurance of inspiratory, expiratory and limb muscles in asthma. Am Rev Respir Dis 134:999–1006, 1986

25. Roussos C: Function and fatigue of respiratory muscles. Chest 88:124–132, 1985

26. Knudson RJ, Lebowitz MD, Hobberg CJ, et al: Changes in the normal maximal expiratory flow-volume curve with growth and aging. Am Rev Respir Dis 127:725–734, 1983

27. Miller RD, Hyatt RE: Evaluation of obstructing lesions of the trachea and larynx by flow-volume loops. Am Rev Respir Dis 108:475–481, 1973

28. Boren NG, Kory RC, Syner JC: The Veterans Administration–Army cooperative study of pulmonary function: the lung volumes and its subdivisions in normal man. Am J Med 41:96–114, 1966

29. Crapo RO, Morris AH, Clayton PD, et al: Lung volumes in healthy non-smoking adults. Bull Eur Physiopathol Respir 18:419–425, 1982

30. Brugman TM, Morris JF, Temple WP: Comparison of lung volume measurements by single-breath helium and multiple-breath nitrogen equilibration methods in normal subjects and COPD patients. Respiration 49:52–60, 1986

31. DuBois AB, Botelho SY, Bedell GN, et al: A rapid plethysmographic method for measuring thoracic gas volume: a comparison with a nitrogen washout method for measuring functional residual capacity in normal subjects. J Clin Invest 35:222–326, 1956

32. Short S, Milic-Emili J, Martin JG: Reassessment of body plethysmographic techniques for measurement of thoracic gas volumes in asthmatics. Am Rev Respir Dis 126:515–520, 1982

33. Comroe JH, Jr: Pulmonary diffusing capacity for carbon monoxide (DL_{CO}). Am Rev Respir Dis 111:225–230, 1975

34. Burrows B, Kasik JE, Niden AN, et al: Clinical usefulness of the single-breath diffusing capacity test. Am Rev Respir Dis 84:789–792, 1961

35. Knudsen RJ, Kalterborn WT, Knudson DE, et al: The single-breath carbon monoxide diffusing capacity: reference equations derived from a healthy non-smoking population and the effects of hematocrit. Am Rev Respir Dis 135:805–811, 1987

36. Crapo RO, Morris AH: Standardized single-breath normal values for carbon monoxide diffusing capacity. Am Rev Respir Dis 123:185–189, 1981

37. Rosenberg E, Ernso P, Leech J, et al: Specific diffusing capacity (DLNA) as a measure of the lung diffusing characteristics: predictor formulas for young adults. Lung 164:207–214, 1986

38. Ayers LN, Ginsberg MC, Fein J, et al: Diffusing capacity, specific diffusing capacity and interpretation of diffusion defects. West J Med 123:255–260, 1975

39. Alberts WM, Goldman AC: Clinical use of methacholine bronchial challenge testing. South Med J 80:827–831, 1987

40. Myers JR, Carrow WM, Braman SS: Clinical applications of methacholine inhalational challenge. JAMA 246:225–280, 1981

41. Gaensler EA, Cusell DW, Lindgren I, et al: The role of pulmonary insufficiency in mortality and invalidism following surgery for pulmonary tuberculosis. J Thorac Cardiovasc Surg 29:163–187, 1955

42. Mittman C: Assessment of operative risk in thoracic surgery. Am Rev Respir Dis 84:197–207, 1961

43. Boushy SF, Billig DM, North LB, et al: Clinical course related to preoperative and postoperative pulmonary function in patients with bronchogenic carcinoma. Chest 59:383–391, 1971

44. Lockwood P: Lung function test results and the risk of postthoracotomy complications. Respiration 30:529–542, 1973

45. Wahi R, McMurtrey MJ, Decaro LF, et al: Determinants of perioperative morbidity and mortality after pneumonectomy. Ann Thorac Surg 48:33–37, 1989

46. Carlens E, Hanson HE, Nordenstrom B: Temporary unilateral occlusion of the pulmonary artery. J Thorac Surg 22:527–536, 1951

47. Neuhaus H, Cherniak NS: A bronchospirometric method of estimating the effect of pneumonectomy on the maximum breathing capacity. J Thorac Cardiovasc Surg 55:144–148, 1968

48. Marion JM, Alderson PO, Lefrak SS, et al: Unilateral lung function: comparison of the lateral position test with radionuclide ventilation-perfusion studies. Chest 69:5–9, 1976

49. Walkup RH, Vossel LF, Griffin JP, et al: Prediction of postoperative pulmonary function with the lateral position test: a prospective study. Chest 47:24–27, 1960

50. Schoonover GA, Olsen GN, Habibian MR, et al: Lateral position test and quantitative lung scan in the preoperative evaluation for lung resection. Chest 86:854–859, 1984

51. Jay SJ, Stonehill RB, Kiblani SO, et al: Variability of the lateral position test in normal subjects. Am Rev Respir Dis 121:165–167, 1980

52. Laros CD, Swierenga J: Temporary unilateral pulmonary artery occlusion in the preoperative evaluation of patients with bronchial carcinoma. Med Thorac 24:269–283, 1967

53. Uggla LG: Indication for and results of thoracic surgery with regard to respiratory and circulatory function tests. Acta Chir Scand 111:197–212, 1956

54. Olsen GN, Block AJ, Swenson EW, et al: Pulmonary function evaluation of the lung resection candidate: a prospective study. Am Rev Respir Dis 111:379, 1975

55. Kristersson S, Lindell S, Swanberg L: Prediction of pul-

monary function loss due to pneumonectomy using ^{133}Xe-radiospirometry. Chest 62:694–698, 1972

56. Olsen GN, Block AJ, Tobias JA: Prediction of postpneumonectomy pulmonary function using quantitative macroaggregate lung scanning. Chest 66:13–16, 1974

57. Boysen PG, Block AJ, Olsen GN, et al: Prospective evaluation for penumonectomy using the Tc[99] quantitative perfusion lung scan. Chest 72:422–425, 1977

58. Gass GD, Olsen GN: Preoperative pulmonary function testing to predict postoperative morbidity and mortality. Chest 89:127–135, 1986

59. Wernly JA, DeMeester TR, Kirchner PT, et al: Clinical value of quantitative ventilation-perfusion lung scans in the surgical management of bronchogenic carcinoma. J Thorac Cardiovasc Surg 80:535–543, 1980

60. Ali ML, Mountain CF, Ewer MS, et al: Predicting loss of pulmonary function after pulmonary resection for bronchogenic carcinoma. Chest 77:337–342, 1980

61. Boysen PG: Pulmonary resection and postoperative pulmonary function. Chest 77:718–719, 1980

62. Harrison RW, Adams WE, Long ET, et al: The clinical significance of cor pulmonale in the prediction of cardiopulmonary reserve following extensive pulmonary resection. J Thorac Surg 36:352–368, 1958

63. DeGraff AC, Taylor HF, Ord JW, et al: Exercise limitation following extensive pulmonary resection. J Clin Invest 44:1514–1522, 1965

64. Olsen GN: The evolving role of exercise testing prior to lung resection. Chest 95:218–225, 1989

65. Van Nostrand D, Kjelsberg MD, Humphrey EW: Preresectional evaluation of risk from pneumonectomy. Surg Gynecol Obstet 127:306–312, 1968

66. Reichel J: Assessment of operative risk of pneumonectomy. Chest 62:570–576, 1972

67. Berggren H, Ekroth R, Malmberg R, et al: Hospital mortality and long-term survival in relation to preoperative function in elderly patients with bronchogenic carcinoma. Ann Thorac Surg 38:633–636, 1984

68. Bagg LR: The 12-min walking distance: its use in the preoperative assessment of patients with bronchial carcinoma before lung resection. Respiration 46:342–345, 1984

69. Soderholm B: The hemodynamics of the lesser circulation in pulmonary tuberculosis: the effect of exercise, temporary unilateral pulmonary artery occlusion, and operation. Scand J Clin Lab Invest, Suppl. 26:1–98, 1957

70. Fee JH, Holmes EC, Gerwirtz HS, et al: Role of pulmonary resistance measurement in preoperative evaluation of candidates for lung resection. J Thorac Cardiovasc Surg 75:519–524, 1975

71. Taube K, Konietzko N: Prediction of postoperative cardiopulmonary function in patients undergoing pneumonectomy. J Thorac Cardiovasc Surg 28:348–351, 1980

72. Loddenkemper R, Gabler A, Gobel D: Criteria of functional operability in patients with bronchial carcinoma: preoperative assessment of risk and prediction of postoperative function. J Thorac Cardiovasc Surg 31:334–337, 1983

73. Brundler H, Chen S, Perruchoud AP: Right heart catheterization in the preoperative evaluation of patients with lung cancer. Respiration 48:261–268, 1985

74. Eugene J, Brown SE, Light RW, et al: Maximum oxygen consumption: a physiologic guide to pulmonary resection. Surg Forum 33:260–262, 1982

75. Coleman NC, Schraufnagel DE, Rivington RN, et al: Exercise testing in evaluation of patients for lung resection. Am Rev Respir Dis 125:604–606, 1982

76. Smith TP, Kinasewitz GT, Tucker WY, et al: Exercise capacity as a predictor of post-thoracotomy morbidity. Am Rev Respir Dis 129:730–734, 1984

77. Bechard D, Wetstein L: Assessment of exercise oxygen consumption as a preoperative criterion for lung resection. Ann Thorac Surg 44:344–349, 1987

78. Miyoshi S, Nakahara K, Ohno K, et al: Exercise tolerance test in lung cancer patients: the relationship between exercise capacity and post-thoracotomy hospital mortality. Ann Thorac Surg 44:487–490, 1987

79. Olsen CN, Weiman DS, Bolton JWR, et al: Submaximal invasive exercise testing and quantitative lung scanning in the evaluation for tolerance of lung resection. Chest (in press)

80. Boysen PG, Clark CA, Block AJ: Graded exercise testing and postthoracotomy complications. J Cardiothorac Anesth 4:68–72, 1990

81. Loke J: Distinguishing cardiac versus pulmonary limitation in exercise performance. Chest 83:441–442, 1983

82. Jones NL, Jones T, Edwards RHT: Exercise tolerance in chronic airway obstruction. Am Rev Respir Dis 103:447–491, 1971

83. Wasserman K, Whipp BJ, Koyal SN, et al: Anaerobic threshold and respiratory gas exchange during exercise. J Appl Physiol 35:236–243, 1973

84. Markos J, Mullin BP, Hillman DR, et al: Preoperative assessment as a predictor of mortality and morbidity after lung resection. Am Rev Respir Dis 139:902–910, 1989

85. Cherniak RM: Pulmonary Function Testing. p. 44. WB Saunders, Philadelphia, 1977

86. Tisi GM: Pulmonary Physiology in Clinical Medicine. 2nd Ed. p. 65. Williams & Wilkins, Baltimore, 1983

87. Ruppel G: Manual of Pulmonary Function Testing. p. 34. CV Mosby, St. Louis, 1975

2

RADIOLOGY OF THE CHEST

Robert S. Shapiro, M.D.
Christine H. Murphy, M.D.
Michael R. Murphy, M.D.

PRINCIPLES OF RADIOLOGIC INTERPRETATION

Chest radiography is a routine and essential part of the preoperative evaluation and the postoperative management of the patient undergoing thoracic surgery. Many decisions made and courses of action taken during and after surgery are the result of chest film interpretation. Even for the relatively inexperienced interpreter, a well-exposed, properly positioned posteroanterior (PA) and lateral examination on a cooperative patient can provide a wealth of information and a rather secure feeling that significant pathology may be recognized. Similarly, obtaining and interpreting the history, physical examination, and laboratory data on a cooperative patient can be relatively easy. The greatest challenges arise when faced with obtaining and interpreting data on acutely ill patients. Unfortunately, all too often the only radiograph obtainable on a thoracic surgery patient (especially in the acute postoperative period) is the bedside portable. Such a radiograph is often confusing and less than optimal due to the altered consciousness of the patient, the physical alterations from surgical intervention, and the limitations of portable technique. However, it is heartening that an acquaintance with the basics of radiographic physics (why you see what you see) and a familiarity with normal "shadows" as

they are altered by surgery and film technique, coupled with a disciplined, systematic approach to each film, will render significant and useful information from even the most confusing and less-than-optimal study.

The x-ray is a form of electromagnetic energy, similar in many respects to visible light, radiating from its source in all directions and being absorbed in varying degrees by objects it encounters. The shorter wave length of an x-ray is the medically useful property that allows it to penetrate body tissues that are opaque to light. Radiographic film allows visualization of degrees of penetration as different shades of gray. The white-gray-black value or *radiographic density* of an object is a function of its thickness, as well as its composition (physical density plus atomic number). There is a finite limit on standard radiographs to the perception of changing shades of gray. Therefore, objects of similar composition and thickness appear the same shade of gray. The margins or *interface* between different tissues, likewise, can only be seen if they differ significantly in radiographic density. Most of the body tissues consist predominantly of water and are considered "water density." Only air, fat, and bone or calcium differ significantly in composition from the rest of the body tissues, allowing radiographic appreciation of their interfaces.[1] When two tissues of the same radiographic density abut each other, their interface is lost and they are said to "sil-

19

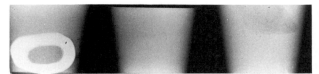

Fig. 2-1. Three cups of water, each containing a piece of body tissue, were radiographed. The cup on the left holds a piece of bone, the one in the center contains a piece of muscle, and the one on the right has a piece of fat floating in the water. The bone and fat are visible because they differ from water significantly in composition (radiographic density). The muscle-water interface is not visible because, for radiographic purposes, muscle is primarily water density. Also, notice the sharp water-air interface that is visible because of significant differences in radiographic density between air and water. (From Squire and Ettinger,[78] with permission.)

houette'' each other.[2] Figures 2-1 and 2-2 illustrate the concepts of radiographic density and interface. With the advent of computed tomography (CT), much more subtle changes in x-ray beam attenuation can be displayed on an expanded gray scale, and many more tissue interfaces become apparent. The chest film is a static, two-dimensional image of a three-dimensional being in constant flux. The image, therefore, is a *summation* of the penetration of objects superimposed in a single plane at a single instant.

Just applying the concepts of *radiographic density*, *interface*, and *summation* will explain many shadows on a radiograph. For example, consider the paired bronchus and vessel near the hilum in Figure 2-3. In Figure 2-3A, the small vessel (water density) appears denser than the much larger descending pulmonary artery (also water density). This is because it is seen on-end and, therefore, appears much thicker (effect of summation) in the frontal plane. Could this vessel be a metastatic nodule? It would be highly unlikely because metastases grow roughly as a sphere, and a soft-tissue sphere of approximately 4 mm in diameter would not be that dense. However, a calcified sphere or granuloma could be (effect of composition). The bronchus on-end, being of air density, is normally seen only near the hilum, where it is large enough to have a wall of such thickness that it can be resolved. Small air-filled bronchi are not normally seen because they are adjacent to air-filled alveoli and their *interface* is silhouetted. What happens to the interface or margins of these structures in various disease states? Figure 2-3B shows the same patient in congestive heart failure with early interstitial edema. The vessel is now larger than its paired bronchus, partially due to vascular engorgement. Also, as fluid (water density) escapes from the capillaries into the interstitium, it

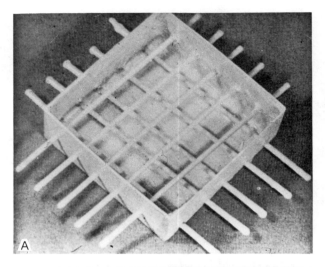

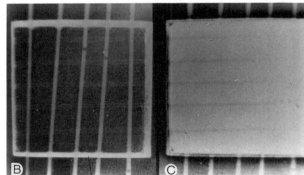

Fig 2-2. (A) A box constructed with straws piercing each side in a perpendicular fashion. Straws running in one direction were filled with water, while those at right angles remained filled with air. **(B)** Radiograph of the box in Fig. A. The air-filled straws are relatively invisible against the air background except for the fine lines produced by their paper walls. **(C)** Radiograph of the same box after it has been filled with water. Notice that the air-filled straws are visible, but the water-filled straws, being of the same radiographic density as the box, are now silhouetted and, therefore, invisible. (From Squire and Ettinger,[78] with permission.)

appears as thickening of the wall of the vessel and the bronchus (perivascular and peribronchial cuffing). The wall or interface also becomes less distinct (perihilar haze). As the failure progresses, edema fluid fills the alveoli and obscures the vessel interface (silhouette sign) (Fig. 2-3C). Note that air not only in the major bronchus but also in smaller bronchi becomes even more apparent (the ''air bronchogram'') as the alveoli become filled with fluid.

Total lung congestion, as in Figure 2-4, permits

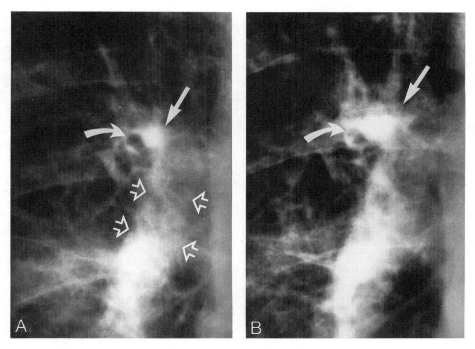

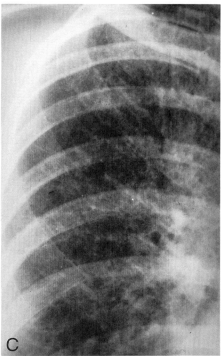

Fig. 2-3. **(A)** A coned-down view of the right hilum demonstrating the relative radiographic density of a small vessel on-end (*closed arrow*), the larger descending pulmonary artery (*open arrows*), and a bronchus on-end (*curved arrow*) as they are affected by summation. **(B)** A coned-down view of the same right hilum after development of interstitial edema. The vessel on-end (*straight arrow*) is now larger due to vascular engorgement and perivascular edema. The wall of the bronchus (*curved arrow*) is also thickened by interstitial edema. **(C)** Development of alveolar edema obscures or silhouettes the blood vessels while making air in multiple small bronchi visible as small black circles and lines within the infiltrate.

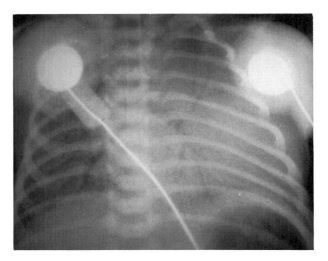

Fig. 2-4. Totally congested and therefore opacified lungs in a newborn, demonstrating extensive branching air bronchograms. Note the similarity to the air-filled straws in Figure 2-2C.

branching bronchi to be visualized as clearly as branching blood vessels are seen in a normally aerated lung. Could the lung in Figure 2-4 be totally atelectatic from proximal bronchial obstruction? No, because then the bronchi would also be airless and, therefore, invisible like the blood vessels.

From understanding radiographic density, summation, and interface, the next step to understanding why you see what you see is to recognize the effects of technique, such as penetration and projection, in altering the appearance of familiar anatomy, making it appear unfamiliar or abnormal. If a film is properly exposed, relative densities can be relied on; however, if it is underexposed, objects that are usually translucent become opaque. Conversely, overexposed radiographs will make some objects relatively invisible. Figure 2-5 shows a properly exposed PA and lateral study in a healthy adult. Note that the spine can be seen through the mediastinum to the degree that disk spaces can be faintly identified. By seeing pulmonary vessels, surrounded by air, through the heart and the domes of the diaphragm, it can usually be assumed that there are probably no alveolar consolidations in the lower lobes, even without the aid of the lateral film.

A property of light rays that also applies to x-rays is magnification. As a hand placed between a light source and a paper is moved farther away from the paper, the shadow of the hand is magnified. Similarly, structures in the chest that are farthest from the film are the most magnified. A PA chest film refers to the photon beam traversing the patient from the posterior chest wall to the anterior chest wall to reach the film.

This projection is preferred because the heart, a relatively anterior structure, is closest to the film. It is, therefore, least magnified and its size is more truly represented. Along the same line, most lateral views are taken with the left side adjacent to the film to prevent cardiac magnification. Unfortunately, portable films usually must be taken anteroposteriorly (AP), and the heart appears enlarged relative to the chest wall.

Not only does the direction of the beam in the frontal plane change the appearance of the mediastinum, but degrees of rotation (obliquity) or lordosis of the patient will distort the image. Rotational distortion can be assessed by evaluation of the relationship of an anterior structure, the clavicles, to a posterior structure, the posterior spinous process of the vertebrae. On a nonrotated view, the spinous process should be seen midway between the medial ends of the clavicles. Note their position in Figure 2-5 and then in Figure 2-6. Lordosis, a common problem in semierect portable views, occurs when the patient's chest is angled in relation to the beam, as in Figure 2-7. Note that both rotation and lordosis can cause apparent mediastinal widening.

On the lateral view (Fig. 2-5B), it can be seen that even with good inspiration, a substantial portion of the lower lobes projects below the domes of the diaphragm on a frontal view. Lordosis, rotation, and AP projection can even further increase the amount of lung tissue hidden by the diaphragm. In an underexposed film, where the lung cannot be seen through the diaphragm and heart, a significant portion of the lower lobes cannot be readily assessed for infiltrate, atelectasis, or other pathology without a lateral view.

In the ideal chest film, a patient takes a deep breath for the exposure and the domes of the diaphragm project at the 10th or 11th posterior ribs in an adult (Fig. 2-5A), or the 8th to 9th posterior ribs in a small child. However, the ability to take and hold a deep breath is, as would be expected, often inversely related to the debility of the patient. Hypoinflation can markedly change the appearance of the chest; the mediastinum widens, the heart and hila enlarge, the lungs become more opaque, and the diaphragm hides more of the lungs (Fig. 2-8). If the ribs are not counted, hypoinflation can easily be confused with congestive heart failure, pneumonia, mediastinal hematoma, and many other conditions.

The tendency when viewing a film is to let the eye drift about erratically and be drawn to areas of obvious pathology. This should not be fought, but once the mass lesion in the lung has been seen, the entire film should be scanned in a set manner to avoid missing the metastasis in a rib. The easiest method is to look *at* specific structures, comparing sides for symmetry,

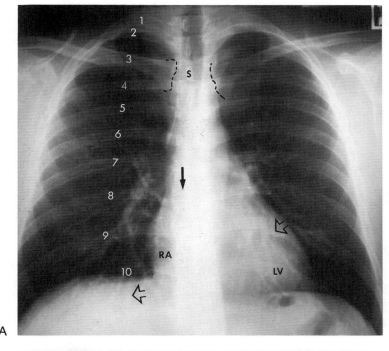

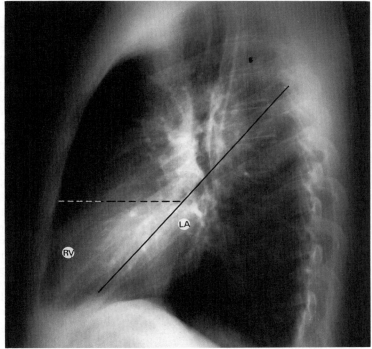

Fig. 2-5. (A) Properly exposed and positioned PA and lateral chest films of a healthy man. The disk spaces (*closed arrow*) can be seen through the mediastinum on the PA view. The blood vessels surrounded by air (*open arrows*) are seen through the heart and diaphragm. The posterior spinous process of T_3 (*S*) is midway between the medial ends of the clavicles (*dotted lines*), indicating that there is no significant obliquity or rotation. The posterior ribs are numbered with the diaphragm at the 10th, indicating a good inspiration. The cardiac chambers that are border-forming on each view are labeled. **(B)** Lateral view shows the approximate locations of the minor fissure (*dotted line*) and major fissures (*solid line*). *RA*, right atrium; *RV*, right ventricle; *LA*, left atrium; *LV*, left ventricle.

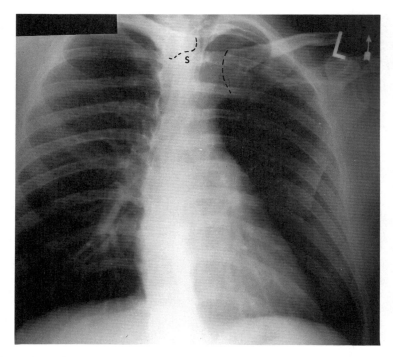

Fig. 2-6. An oblique view of the same person shown in Figure 2-5. The chest is rotated to the left, distorting the apparent size and shape of the heart and other mediastinal structures. Compare the position of the medial ends of the clavicles (*dotted lines*) to the vertebral spinous process (*S*) here and in Figure 2-5.

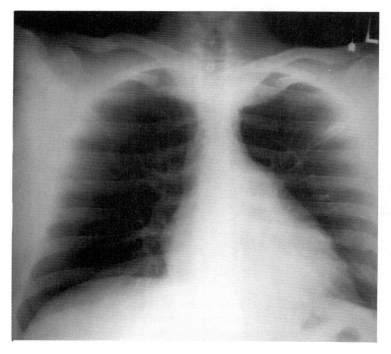

Fig. 2-7. A lordotic view of the person in Figure 2-5. Note the position and appearance of the clavicles in both views. Lordosis distorts and magnifies the cardiac shadow and also places a greater portion of the lung bases behind the domes of the diaphragm.

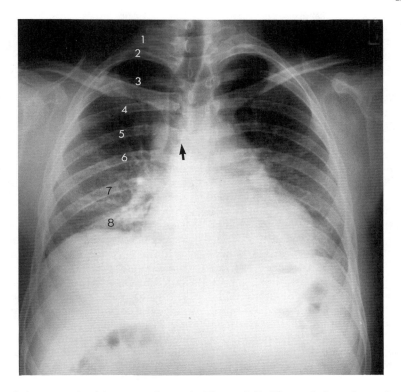

Fig. 2-8. A film of the same healthy man shown in Figure 2-5. The technique is unchanged except for moderate hypoinflation and an AP projection on the current study. The posterior right ribs are labeled, revealing the diaphragm to now be at the level of the 8th rib. The hypoaerated lungs and widened mediastinum can mimic disease such as congestive heart failure or pneumonia. Note the position of the carina (*arrow*) on a portable examination.

and then look *through* them at others.[3] For example, the bony thorax and soft tissues may be scanned first, comparing sides, then looked through to assess lung parenchyma, the hila, and peripheral pulmonary vasculature. Finally, the mediastinum and cardiac configuration may be examined. After the heart has been observed for size, shape should be noted and then looked through for valvular calcifications. A system should be developed and used every time, so that, after the film has been studied, it is certain that such things as tracheal deviation, the position of the stomach bubble, and mediastinal air have been seen. In the postoperative study, the position of tubes and lines must be added to the list of items to scan. Remembering that the x-ray beam goes from the gown on the anterior chest wall to the gown posteriorly, and through any extraneous surgical dressings or tubing, may prevent coming to the wrong conclusion. Particularly on a portable examination, these artifacts may simulate pathology. In the later section on extraalveolar air, a skin fold is shown mimicking a pneumothorax (see Fig. 2-31A). Many shadows that at

first glance appear to be pathologic can be explained by tracing their margins back to overlapping normal anatomy.

Figure 2-5 illustrates the normally appearing cardiac chambers that are border-forming in each view. Also, in Figure 2-5B, the positions of the major and minor fissures are indicated. The superior extent of the lower lobe is at the level of the hila or above. Therefore, an infiltrate in the superior segment of the lower lobe, a common place for aspiration, will appear as a perihilar infiltrate in the frontal plane. It is important to become familiar with the position of the other lobes in both planes. Knowing that an infiltrate silhouettes a certain portion of the mediastinum or diaphragm allows correct identification of the lobe. For example, consolidation or atelectasis of the right middle lobe will obscure the right heart border.

Abnormalities found on chest films taken in the intraoperative or postoperative period cannot always be assumed to be reflective of an acute process. Before delving into a discussion of acute pathology, the value of prior films must be explored. It has been said jokingly in radiologic circles that when faced with an unexplained finding on a film, the thing to do to avoid displaying ignorance is to ask for "another view." It is no joke, however, that the most informative, timesaving, and cost-beneficial "other view" is the old film. It will often save the patient needless further workup.

When evaluating preoperative films in anticipation of surgery, or when comparing them to postoperative studies, two major assessments should be made. First, does the film reveal chronic pathology that may complicate anesthesia or postoperative recovery? This would, of course, include many types of chronic pulmonary or cardiac disease. Of particular importance in thoracic surgery patients would be recognition of any complications of the disease for which the patient is having surgery. For example, abnormalities of the esophagus such as carcinoma, stricture, or hiatal hernia, and severe motility disorders such as achalasia are usually not apparent on plain chest films—unless the esophagus becomes so obstructed and dilated that it is seen as a fluid-filled mass in the mediastinum. However, a frequent complication of these conditions is recurrent aspiration. While aspiration is often clinically apparent, it may be silent or undiagnosed. If serial preoperative films are reviewed, a pictorial history of recurrent basilar infiltrates may lead to a suspicion of chronic aspiration. The patient's lungs would likely be chronically inflamed and infected, altering the ability to clear secretions and increasing

the chances of postoperative complications such as pneumonia and atelectasis. If lung damage is severe enough, large main pulmonary arteries reflecting pulmonary arterial hypertension and even cor pulmonale may be seen.

The second major value of a preoperative film is that pathology can be assessed that would be confusing or misleading when viewed postoperatively on a portable examination. For example, chest wall deformities such as scoliosis or pectus excavatum, by narrowing the PA diameter of the chest, change the appearance of the lung and mediastinum. Note in Figure 2-9A the accentuation of right lower lung markings and apparent cardiac enlargement, in the PA projection, in this otherwise healthy individual with severe pectus excavatum. Without a lateral view, such as on a portable examination, pneumonia or heart disease might be erroneously diagnosed. More severe thoracic cage deformities would not only present a confusing picture on a portable radiograph, but might also pose considerable problems in positioning the patient for anesthesia and surgery. Along the same line, arthritic changes such as severe cervical or thoracic spondylosis, or ankylosing spondylitis, while not necessarily confusing on portable examinations, should also be looked for preoperatively to avoid difficulty with or complications from intubation. Two other examples of diseases that tend to "muddy the water" when viewing portable examinations are chronic ob-

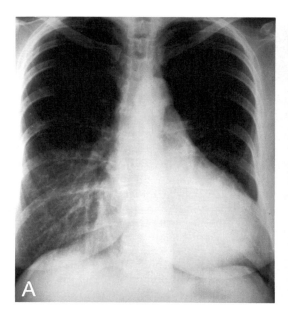 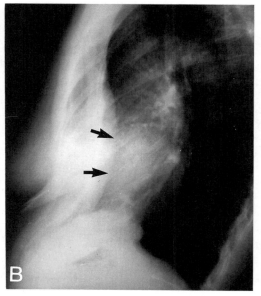

Fig. 2-9. (A) PA and **(B)** lateral views of a healthy woman with a severe pectus excavatum simulating cardiomegaly and right lung pathology. The posterior extent of the sternum is indicated by arrows.

structive pulmonary disease (COPD) and mitral valvular disease. Recognition of the pulmonary parenchymal and vascular changes seen preoperatively in these conditions may help avoid misinterpretation of postoperative studies, especially when evaluating the films for signs of congestive heart failure. This is illustrated in greater detail in the section *Pulmonary Edema* later in this chapter.

The following sections review many of the acute changes in the chest film in the intraoperative and postoperative period relating to surgical alteration or complicating disorders.

INFILTRATES

The term *infiltrate* is used loosely to include all acute pulmonary parenchymal densities that may be encountered on postoperative radiographs. Unfortunately, most infiltrates seen on a single radiograph are by themselves very nonspecific. With alveolar infiltrates, the radiographic density is the same whether the alveoli are filled with edema, blood, pus, or any other water density substance. Likewise, interstitial infiltrates from edema can be indistinguishable from other types of interstitial disease, such as fibrosis or even lymphangitic spread of carcinoma. These limitations strengthen the argument for the importance of comparison with prior films.

When assessing an infiltrate, the clue to its nature may lie in recognition and correlation of other radiographic findings and clinical data. This will become more apparent in the following discussion of specific infiltrates.

Atelectasis

Atelectasis is by far the most common infiltrate found on postoperative radiographs, especially in the first 48 hours.[4] Multiple factors such as pain, decreased consciousness, and intubation decrease the ability to cough, clear secretions, or expand the chest. Chronic hypoinflation may produce well-defined, thin, dense lines parallel or oblique to the diaphragm. These are easily recognized as linear or "plate-like" atelectasis (Fig. 2-10). Acute hypoinflation more typically appears as patchy infiltrates that can be indistinguishable from edema or pneumonia. Occasionally, air bronchograms may be apparent as the peripheral alveoli collapse around patent bronchi. With acute hypoinflation, as in Figure 2-8, counting ribs and identifying crowded vessels should lead to a suspicion of volume loss rather than an inflammatory process or pulmonary edema. However, coexisting pneumonia or edema can be difficult to exclude in the presence of marked hypoinflation. Rapid changes in configuration or location, or disappearance after physical therapy, are also indications that atelectasis rather than pneumonia is present.[5]

Lobar collapse implies a proximal obstruction and produces an airless lobe so that neither blood vessels nor air bronchograms are seen. Lobar atelectasis occurs frequently after thoracic or abdominal surgery and typically involves the lower lobes, especially the left lower lobe.[6] In a supine patient, a large heart may directly compress the left lower lobe bronchus, creating atelectasis. In open heart surgery, topical cooling of the heart is frequently used and has been shown to affect the left phrenic nerve, producing temporary paralysis of the left leaf of the diaphragm.[7] In these

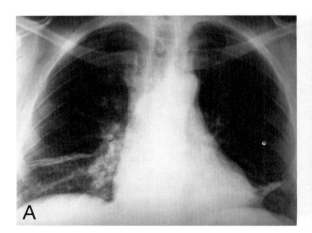
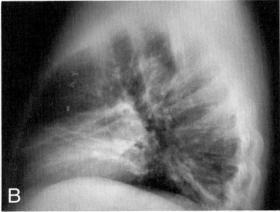

Fig. 2-10. (A) PA and **(B)** lateral views that demonstrate dense bands of linear or "plate-like" atelectasis produced by chronic hypoinflation.

cases, poor diaphragmatic excursion combined with increased or thickened secretions may predispose to mucus plugs, creating lobar atelectasis. The mucus plugs may be in the mainstem bronchi or in more peripheral branches. In the latter case, air bronchograms of the first and second bronchial divisions may be observed ending abruptly, as in Figure 2-11. In this case of left lower lobe atelectasis, note the benefit of a well-penetrated study in identifying the collapsed lobe. A hallmark of lower lobe atelectasis or consolidation is a change in density of portions of the cardiac shadow. If the film is not sufficiently penetrated so that this differential can be appreciated, then this important finding will be missed. In lobar atelectasis, the silhouette sign plays an important role. As can be seen in Figure 2-11, the medial aspect of the diaphragm is not apparent, since it is silhouetted by the collapsed lobe. In Figure 2-12, various degrees of upper lobe collapse are illustrated. Note the silhouette effect produced by adjacent atelectasis simulating mediastinal widening. Figure 2-12 also illustrates other signs of lobar atelectasis reflecting the effects of volume loss. These include elevation of the ipsilateral

diaphragm and shift of the mediastinum to the involved side. The hilum will also shift toward the atelectatic lobe. However, this is often difficult to detect on a portable examination. Following wedge resection or lobectomy, the remaining lung on the ipsilateral side may not fully re-expand or may collapse secondary to a mucus plug or inadequate function of chest tubes. This is illustrated in Figure 2-13.

Total lung atelectasis, a less frequent problem postoperatively than lobar atelectasis, also implies a mechanical obstruction to a major bronchus. In addition to formation of mucus plugs, foreign bodies such as poorly placed endotracheal tubes or aspirated teeth should be suspected with these large areas of collapse (Fig. 2-14). An adequately penetrated film is necessary for identification of the tip of the endotracheal tube and any radiopaque foreign body. Proper and improper placement of endotracheal tubes will be further discussed in a subsequent section.

Films taken immediately after extubation or removal of mechanical ventilation will often show increased density of the lungs and an apparent increase in the cardiac size due to hypoinflation. This may be

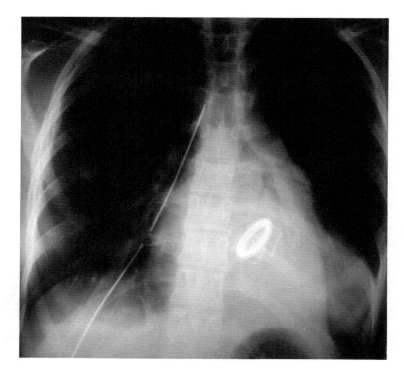

Fig. 2-11. This portable examination obtained following mitral valve surgery reveals atelectasis of the left lower lobe. The mechanism of bronchial obstruction is probably a combination of mucus plugging and direct compression by the enlarged heart. Note the abrupt cut-off of proximal air bronchograms, the changing density in the heart shadow, and the loss of definition of the medial aspect of the left hemidiaphragm as it is silhouetted by the airless lobe.

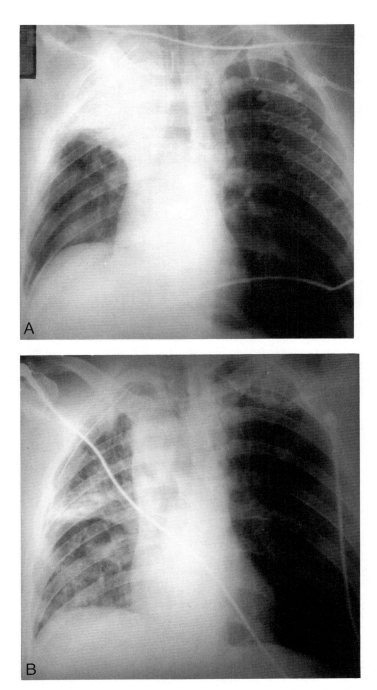

Fig. 2-12. **(A)** A postoperative portable examination on this patient reveals total atelectasis of the right upper lobe. The volume loss is compensated by elevation of the ipsilateral hemidiaphragm and mediastinal shift toward the atelectasis. **(B)** Following vigorous respiratory therapy, the right upper lobe atelectasis in panel A has partially resolved. The portion of dense atelectasis remaining medially simulated mediastinal widening.

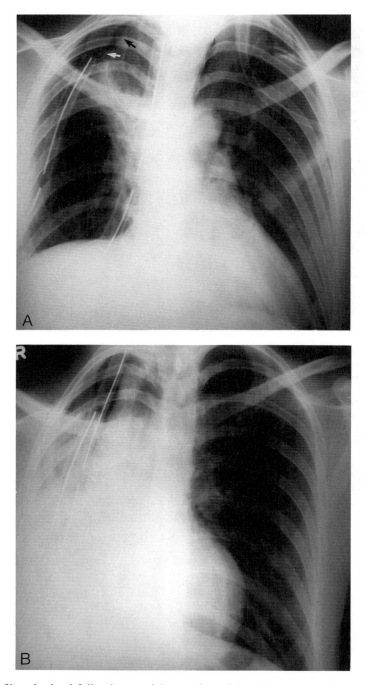

Fig. 2-13. (A) This film obtained following partial resection of the right upper lobe reveals a small residual pneumothorax (*arrows*). The infiltrate surrounding the sutures is probably a combination of atelectasis and localized hemorrhage. The remaining lung is relatively clear. **(B)** Several hours later, a film obtained because of changing auscultatory findings reveals interval collapse of the remaining right lung with compensatory hyperexpansion of the left lung. The mediastinum also has shifted significantly to the right. This is a true shift, although it is somewhat accentuated by the great change in obliquity from one film to the other. Note the position of the clavicles.

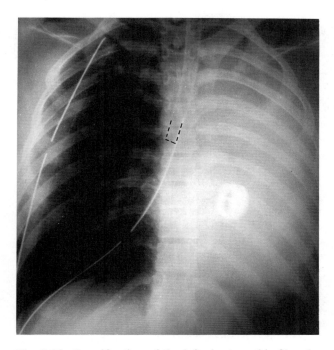

Fig. 2-14. Opacification of the left chest on this film obtained immediately after surgery is due to total atelectasis of the left lung from bronchial obstruction secondary to right main-stem bronchus intubation. There is overexpansion of the right lung and mediastinal shift to the left. The tip of the endotracheal tube (retouched) projects to the right, with leftward bowing of the tube.

misinterpreted radiographically as congestive heart failure while the patient is improving clinically (Fig. 2-15). Conversely, infiltrates due to atelectasis may rapidly disappear after the patient is placed on ventilatory assistance. Comparing the overall degree of inspiration (counting ribs) in films obtained during and after assisted ventilation may help avoid erroneous diagnoses and mistreatment.[6]

Pneumonia

The two most frequent causes of community-acquired pneumonia are *Mycoplasma pneumoniae* and *Streptococcus pneumoniae*. Hospital-acquired pneumonias are due to anaerobes or gram-negative bacteria, especially *Pseudomonas aeruginosa* in patients on respirators.[8,9] Patients with the acquired immunodeficiency syndrome are most commonly infected with *Pneumocystis carinii*.[9] Radiographic patterns of pneumonia are often divided into three major categories, reflecting the mode of spread of the infiltrate.[10] Viral and mycoplasma pneumonias (not usually a problem in postoperative patients) tend to produce primarily bilateral interstitial infiltrates. *P carinii* pneumonia initially produces bilateral interstitial infiltrates, which can progress to air-space consolidation. Lobar pneumonias, classically represented by *S pneumoniae* (formerly *Diplococcus pneumoniae*) and *Klebsiella pneumoniae*, spread contiguously in all directions within a lobe and initially present as a round or

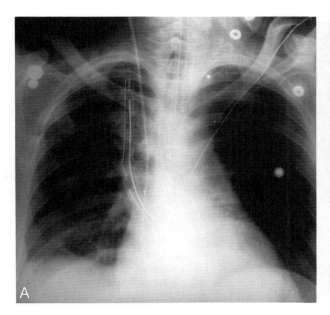
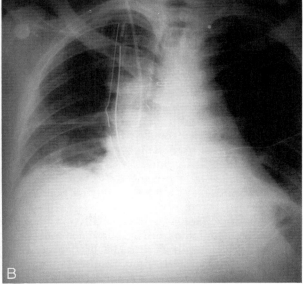

Fig. 2-15. (A) A film obtained shortly after cardiac surgery reveals relatively clear lungs and a small effusion. **(B)** This film taken after extubation reveals moderate hypoinflation and an accentuated pleural effusion, while the patient was making an uneventful recovery.

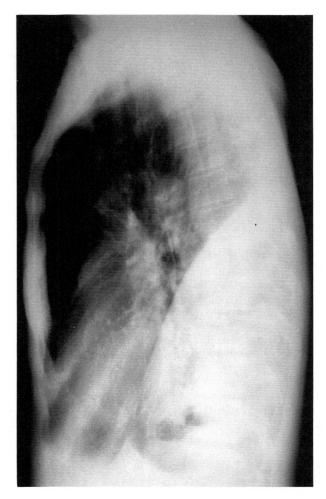

Fig. 2-16. This lateral view of a patient with *Klebsiella* pneumonia demonstrates total consolidation of the left lower lobe characteristic of lobar pneumonia.

masslike infiltrate progressing to consolidation of the entire lobe (Fig. 2-16). *S pneumoniae*, while commonly seen in the emergency room, is not often a problem postoperatively. *K pneumoniae* is more frequently hospital-acquired than other lobar pneumonias. A characteristic feature of advanced *Klebsiella* infection is volume expansion of a lobe, producing bulging or convex fissures.

Most other pneumonias, and especially most hospital-acquired pneumonias, are of the bronchopneumonia pattern. They begin as a tracheobronchitis with radiographic changes of interstitial inflammation (peribronchial and perivascular fluid accumulation) that may be indistinguishable from interstitial pneumonitis or pulmonary interstitial edema. The infection spreads along the bronchial tree, producing

patchy and even nodular-appearing infiltrates as alveolar involvement progresses in an acinar distribution (Fig. 2-17). There is eventual coalescence into larger areas of consolidation, but they are rarely as homogenous as lobar pneumonias. Bronchopneumonia is often bilateral and may first appear as perihilar infiltrates. While peripheral air bronchograms are the hallmark of alveolar consolidation, differentiating it from atelectasis, they often are not as apparent in early bronchopneumonia as in lobar pneumonia.

Many hospital-acquired infections are also suppurative and will produce necrotic areas of abscess formation. Radiographically, these may appear as scattered lucencies within the infiltrate (microabscesses) or as large abscess cavities with fluid levels. However, air-fluid levels that simulate abscess cavities can occur in bullae in patients with COPD (Fig. 2-18). Fluid within bullae can accompany an infectious process or be seen in these patients when they are in congestive heart failure. Septic emboli, as from urinary tract infections or intravenous catheter sites, present as peripherally located nodules that then coalesce into infiltrates indistinguishable from primary pneumonic infections. These septic emboli may also cavitate.

P aeruginosa is the most serious pulmonary infection occurring in patients on assisted ventilation. While it is frequently found in tracheal aspirates, not all patients are clinically affected by its presence. However, when pneumonitis occurs, the mortality rate is as high as 70 percent in some series.[6,8,11,12] *P aeruginosa* infection is seen radiographically as a bronchopneumonia as well as septic emboli. Its early presentation can be as in Figure 2-17. Later, with areas of alveolar coalescence, it is indistinguishable from any other diffuse air space infiltrate.

Pulmonary Edema

Pulmonary edema, the efflux of fluid from the pulmonary capillaries to the interstitium and alveoli, occurs whenever there is an imbalance between the normal hydrostatic and oncotic pressures in the lung or whenever there is an alteration in capillary permeability. Minor variations in hydrostatic or oncotic pressure, or changes in capillary permeability, are corrected by the pulmonary lymphatics, which can remove up to 200 mL/min of interstitial fluid accumulation in a normal lung. However, when the lymphatics are insufficient or overwhelmed, pulmonary edema will ensue. With slight increases in interstitial fluid, and often before most radiographic changes occur, patients may experience dyspnea due to the decreased compliance of the lungs. In patients receiving assisted ventilation, this decreased compliance may become apparent prior to changes in gas exchange or

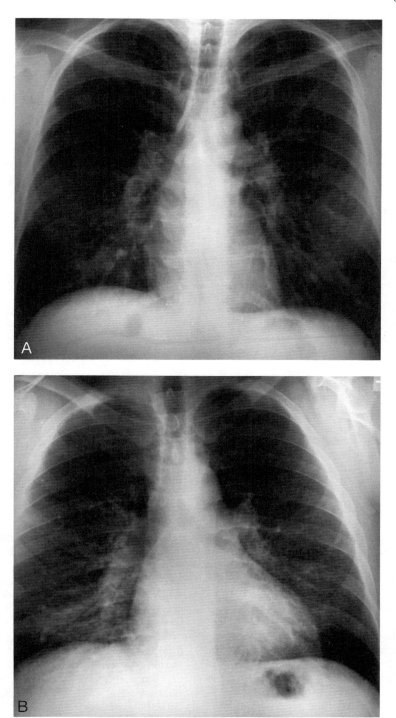

Fig. 2-17. Two early cases of bronchopneumonia. **(A)** The scattered bilateral small pulmonary nodules represent the early appearance of bronchopneumonia in this patient. There was subsequent coalescence into large areas of consolidation. **(B)** This predominantly perihilar and lower lobe interstitial infiltrate progressed to areas of alveolar consolidation.

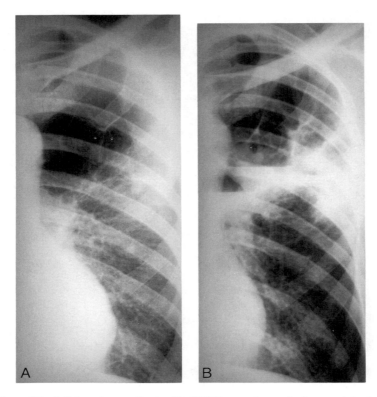

Fig. 2-18. **(A)** A view of the left lung in a patient with COPD reveals marked upper lobe bullous emphysema. **(B)** An acute infection produces fluid within these bullae as well as a surrounding infiltrate. These fluid-filled bullae could be confused with abscess cavities.

changes on the film. When interstitial fluid tension increases, some alveoli are filled while others collapse, so the radiographic alveolar opacity is a combination of edema and microatelectasis. Initiation of ventilatory assistance may prevent or reverse this microatelectasis and produce a radiographic picture of improvement before it exists clinically.[13] Of the major mechanisms of pulmonary edema (Table 2-1), the one that can be differentiated from the others radiographically is increased capillary hydrostatic pressure. Pulmonary venous hypertension (PVH) produces increased capillary hydrostatic pressure. In most instances, this is secondary to left heart failure or obstruction. However, in patients receiving parenteral fluids, hypertransfusion or fluid overload can also lead to PVH and then to edema, mimicking "cardiac" pulmonary edema.[14] Visualization of engorged pulmonary vasculature is the primary radiographic method of separating cardiac edema and overload from other causes of edema and other nonedema infiltrates.[15]

What, therefore, are the radiographic findings of PVH? In the normal erect individual, blood flow to the lungs, being influenced by gravity, is greatest in the lung bases; therefore, the diameter of lower lobe vessels is normally greater than that of upper lobe vessels. When there is an impediment to the drainage of pulmonary blood back into the heart (as in mitral valvular disease or left ventricular dysfunction) or an overall increase in fluid in the body (as in iatrogenic fluid overload), the pressure in the pulmonary veins increases. This is observed radiographically as enlargement of the pulmonary blood vessels. Although all the pulmonary veins enlarge, this is best appreciated in the upper lobes because these vessels are not obscured by the cardiac silhouette. Also, because the capillary hydrostatic pressure is already greatest in the bases and the earliest edema occurs there, the resulting basilar lung "stiffness" and poor gas exchange cause the pulmonary arterial blood flow to be redistributed to the upper lobes. This redistribution causes the upper lobe vasculature to appear even more prominent. To assess developing pulmonary venous hypertension and pulmonary arterial blood flow redistribu-

TABLE 2-1. Mechanisms of Pulmonary Edema

I. Increased capillary hydrostatic pressure
    Left ventricular failure
    Mitral valve obstruction
    Pulmonary venous obstruction
    Hypertransfusion

II. Increased capillary permeability
    Toxic inhalants
    Circulating toxins
    Immunologic reactions
    Drug idiosyncrasy
    Infections
    Radiation injury
    Uremia
    Adult respiratory distress syndrome
    Disseminated intravascular coagulation

III. Lymphatic insufficiency
    Chronic lung damage or disease
IV. Decreased plasma osmotic pressure
    Debilitated states producing hypoalbuminemia

V. Unknown or speculative
    High altitude
    Neurogenic
    Narcotic overdose
    Cardioversion
    Pulmonary embolism

(Adapted from Shapiro and Hublitz,[77] with permission.)

tion, the upper lobe vessels must be carefully evaluated for changes in size from one film to another.[16]

Since detecting pulmonary venous hypertension is of great diagnostic importance in radiographically categorizing causes of pulmonary edema, it follows that patients suspected of having edema should be radiographed in an upright position whenever possible. This is often more easily said than done. Nevertheless, every effort should be made to support the patient for an upright view if the film findings are to hold any weight in clinical decisions concerning the etiology of pulmonary edema.[15]

Differentiation of heart failure from fluid overload is usually not possible radiographically. There should be clinical suspicion of the possibility of hypertransfusion any time developing pulmonary vascular engorgement, with or without edema, is found in a postoperative patient, especially if there is no known history of heart disease.[14]

Up to this point in the discussion, changes in heart size have been ignored in assessing pulmonary edema. Although cardiac enlargement is a classic finding in cardiac failure, it may be absent in acute dysfunction such as myocardial infarction or dysrhythmia. Conversely, it may be present without failure. Also, be-

cause of the lack of reliability in evaluating subtle changes in heart size on portable radiographs taken in various degrees of hypoinflation, lordosis, and rotation, this sign is often not helpful.[5]

Failure is often not isolated to the left heart; clinically, it is the signs of right heart failure such as jugular and hepatic engorgement and pedal edema that are most obvious. In the chest film, evidence for right heart failure includes increasing size of systemic veins, specifically the superior vena cava and azygos.[17] With iatrogenic fluid overload, the systemic as well as the pulmonary vasculature will also be engorged; therefore, this is not a differential point between overload and failure.

The typical progression from well-defined pulmonary vessels, to enlargement of these vessels, to early edema producing haziness and poor definition of vessel-air interface, and then to alveolar filling has, in part, been illustrated in Figure 2-3. The classic radiographic appearance of cardiac failure is exemplified in Figure 2-19. At the same time that the interstitial fluid is producing perivascular and peribronchial cuffing, fine dense lines may also be seen running horizontally in the periphery of the lung base (Kerley B lines), representing fluid in the intralobular septae.[18] These can be very dramatic in upright views (Fig. 2-20), but are reportedly rarely identified on portable examination and, therefore, are of less value in assess-

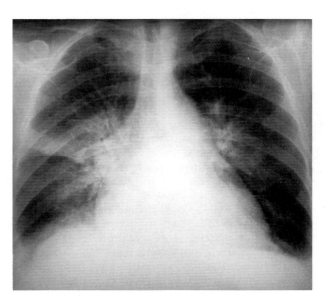

Fig. 2-19. Advanced congestive heart failure is exemplified here by cardiomegaly, prominent upper lobe vessels, bilateral small pleural effusions, and pulmonary edema, typically greatest in the perihilar and basilar areas.

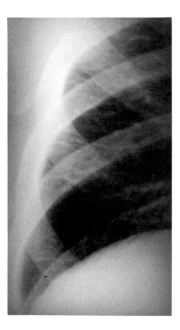

Fig. 2-20. A coned-down view of the lung periphery in a patient with interstitial edema. Thin but dense horizontal lines (Kerley B) are very apparent in this upright view, but are uncommonly appreciated on portable examinations.

ing the postoperative patient.[19,20] Development of pleural fluid is commonly associated with pulmonary edema, but in a postoperative thoracic surgery patient, in whom effusions are very common, this sign is not reliable.

As previously alluded to in the discussion of the value of prior films, COPD can produce confusing patterns of pulmonary edema. COPD produces areas of destruction of normal lung parenchyma with loss of vascularity to these areas. Radiographically, paucity, stretching, and attenuation of vessels are seen in the area of greatest emphysema, with increased density of the remaining lung due to crowding and fibrosis. Typically, severe COPD produces an elongated mediastinum with a small cardiac silhouette due to downward displacement of the diaphragm. The central pulmonary arteries may be enlarged due to pulmonary arterial hypertension from the chronic lung disease. Congestive heart failure developing in this setting often presents a very atypical pattern. Assessment of cardiac enlargement by common criteria (transverse diameter of the heart > 50 percent of the transverse diameter of the chest) will not be accurate in these patients due to hyperinflation. Findings of pulmonary vascular engorgement may be altered or

absent due to the chronically altered blood flow. The typical localization of pulmonary edema in the perihilar and lower lung zones in patients with otherwise normal pulmonary parenchyma cannot be expected in patients with chronic lung disease. In general, pulmonary edema can only occur in otherwise relatively normal lung tissue. It will not occur in bullae or fibrosis or where there is absent pulmonary vasculature. Therefore, edema in chronic lung patients will be patchy and asymmetric, and can even be unilateral.[21,22] Figure 2-21 demonstrates an unusual distribution of pulmonary edema to the upper lobes due to the patient's lower lobe emphysema. As fluid fills the interstitium in these patients, it may appear as a nodular or even miliary prominence of the already chronically increased interstitial densities. A high index of suspicion and close observation of changing interstitial patterns is needed to diagnose congestive heart failure in a patient with COPD. Minor changes in compliance due to interstitial edema in these already compromised lungs may be sufficient to produce acute respiratory failure. It is not uncommon to see a patient with severe COPD develop acute respiratory failure and have the chest examination show little, if any, change. It has also been postulated that with the

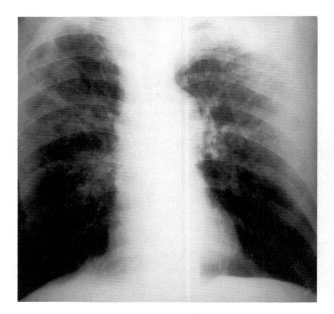

Fig. 2-21. This patient has COPD with lower lobe emphysema. Superimposed congestive heart failure has an atypical appearance due to the underlying lung disease. Here, the cardiac enlargement usually associated with failure is not apparent, and the pulmonary edema is predominantly upper lobe rather than basilar.

alteration in lymphatic drainage created in COPD, there is decreased ability to compensate for minor variations in interstitial fluid. This places the patient with COPD at a greater risk for developing edema with mild degrees of overtransfusion.[21]

Atypical patterns of pulmonary edema are also seen in other types of chronic pulmonary vascular or parenchymal derangement, such as Swyer-James syndrome, or congenital and acquired heart disease with altered flow patterns.[21,22] Mitral valvular disease is the classic example. Assessing the portable film in patients with mitral valve disease poses two threats to misdiagnosis. First, the chronic changes of cardiomegaly, pulmonary vasculature redistribution, and interstitial edema and fibrosis will mimic acute failure if previous "baseline" films are not reviewed. Second, as in other patients with parenchymal disease, if acute edema does occur, it may be atypical in location and distribution. With the blood flow in chronic mitral disease markedly shifted to the upper lung zones due to fibrosis and scarring of lower lobes from chronic edema, it logically follows that any blood flow-directed condition, whether it be edema, emboli from venous thrombosis, or septic emboli, would selectively involve the upper lung areas.

Other causes of segmentally decreased pulmonary blood flow, such as pulmonary emboli, will present as an area devoid of infiltrate in patients with diffuse edema. In fact, this finding of a lucent area in otherwise congested lungs in a patient with no known prior chronic lung disease is a good indication that the patient may have experienced a pulmonary embolus.[22]

In all the other causes of pulmonary edema in which the mechanism is other than increased capillary hydrostatic pressure (Table 2-1), radiographic signs of pulmonary venous hypertension and cardiomegaly are absent unless the patient has coexisting heart disease. The appearance of the infiltrate, however, is indistinguishable from edema associated with pulmonary venous hypertension. Also, as previously mentioned, evolving interstitial-to-alveolar edema can look quite similar to evolving bronchopneumonia or aspiration in some instances. Therefore, the clue to the etiology lies not in the infiltrate per se, but in the temporal sequence of its appearance, its distribution, and its associated clinical setting.

A decrease in plasma oncotic pressure (item IV, Table 2-1) is an uncommon cause of edema. However, if patients are nutritionally debilitated by their disease, such as those with long-standing or progressive esophageal disorders, and they receive large volumes of noncolloidal fluids during surgery, decreased oncotic pressure may be a possible cause of developing pulmonary edema.[13]

Aspiration

Infiltrates from aspiration vary according to the chemical makeup of the aspirant. Aspiration of low pH fluids, typically stomach contents, classically produces hypoxia and respiratory distress (Mendelson's syndrome) within 1 to 2 hours.[23,24] Radiographs taken within 30 minutes may show little or no change, but, within 2 to 4 hours, there is rapid appearance of diffuse alveolar infiltrates. These may involve all lobes, particularly the right middle lobe and superior segments of the lower lobes. The infiltrate is actually a localized pulmonary edema due to shift of fluid into the lungs secondary to chemical damage to alveoli and capillaries.[25] The pattern can be indistinguishable from other forms of pulmonary edema. The initial infiltrate from aspiration of gastric contents will also begin to clear rapidly, often within 24 to 36 hours. Increasing or recurrent infiltrates strongly suggest the presence of a secondary infection. Persistent areas of atelectasis may also suggest the presence of retained food particles.[5] Figure 2-22 shows a typical progression.

Adult Respiratory Distress Syndrome

In recent years, a fairly characteristic constellation of clinical, radiographic, and pathologic findings has been increasingly described in patients developing respiratory insufficiency following severe trauma, major surgery, or other critical illness. Because the condition has been frequently associated with certain diseases (Table 2-2), they have been considered predisposing or causative. Various terms reflecting this association have been proposed (Table 2-3).[26-28] However, the term *adult respiratory distress syndrome* (ARDS) has gained the most universal acceptance, probably because its inherent vagueness encompasses these others. This would seem appropriate in that the significance of the syndrome is that, despite the multitude of associated diseases, the rather uniform pulmonary pathophysiologic response suggests that there must be a common mechanism or that the ability of the lung to react is severely limited. ARDS is included under pulmonary edema secondary to increased capillary permeability by some investigators who feel that damage to pulmonary microvasculature represents the key event.[29]

Following the initial insult (eg, trauma, hemorrhage, surgery, shock, sepsis) there is a latent period of variable duration, typically 12 to 24 hours, after which clinical symptoms of tachypnea, dyspnea, cyanosis, and decreased PaO_2 develop. During the next several hours of rather catastrophic clinical deteriora-

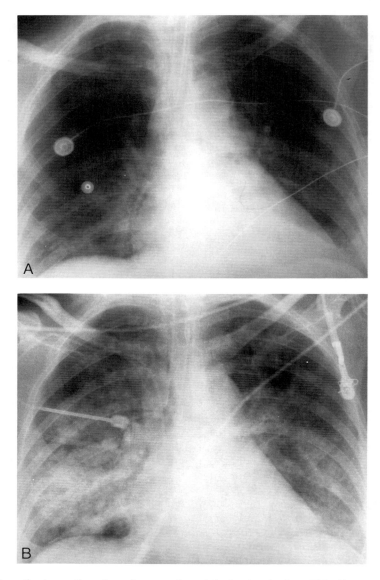

Fig. 2-22. (A) This patient was thought to have aspirated during intubation. This film, obtained immediately afterward, reveals only minimal infrahilar infiltrates, although clinically there was severe respiratory embarrassment. **(B)** A film 4 hours later shows interval development of extensive alveolar consolidation as pulmonary edema develops in response to the pulmonary damage. Unless secondary infection develops or the damage is severe enough to lead to ARDS, the edema usually begins clearing within 24 to 48 hours with appropriate supportive therapy.

tion, the chest film typically shows no appreciable change.[29] If the chest film was clear initially, it should remain so. Immediate or concomitant development of infiltrates should suggest conditions other than ARDS, such as aspiration, edema, or hemorrhage. If these conditions are pre-existing, they may of course be radiographically apparent, but the lack of change in light of increasing respiratory embarrassment is the hallmark of superimposed ARDS. One other condition, pulmonary embolization, may produce confusion at this stage, since it also presents with acute respiratory distress and a normal or stable chest film.

TABLE 2-2. Diseases Associated with or Known to Precipitate Adult Respiratory Distress Syndrome

Trauma
Shock (hypovolemic or endotoxic)
Overhydration
Extracorporeal perfusion (cardiopulmonary bypass)
Embolism
    Fat
    Amnionic fluid
Aspiration
    Chemicals
    Low pH fluids
Viral pneumonia
Radiation pneumonitis
Burns and smoke inhalation
Carcinomatosis
Bowel infarction
Clostridial sepsis
Gram-negative sepsis
Pancreatitis
Drug abuse
Eclampsia
Oxygen toxicity
Disseminated intravascular coagulation
Transfusion of mismatched blood
Heat stroke
High-altitude pulmonary edema

(Data from Refs. 26, 27, and 28.)

TABLE 2-3. Synonyms for the Term *Adult Respiratory Distress Syndrome*

Adult hyaline membrane disease
Adult respiratory insufficiency syndrome
Bronchopulmonary dysplasia
Congestive atelectasis
Da Nang lung
Fat embolism
Hemorrhage lung syndrome
Oxygen toxicity
Postperfusion lung syndrome
Posttransfusion lung
Posttraumatic atelectasis
Posttraumatic pulmonary insufficiency
Progressive pulmonary consolidation
Progressive respiratory distress
Pulmonary edema
Pulmonary hyaline membrane disease
Pulmonary microembolism
Respirator lung
Shock lung
Solid lung syndrome
Stiff lung syndrome
Traumatic wet lung
Transplant lung
Wet lung
White lung syndrome

(Data from Refs. 27, 28, and 29.)

Early signs of pulmonary embolization are discussed in a later section, and these, if present, may help in differentiation. Later stages of pulmonary embolization with infarction will produce focal rather than diffuse infiltrates not usually confused with ARDS.[28] Small pleural effusions common to pulmonary embolization are absent in ARDS, but in thoracic surgery patients, in whom pleural effusion is often present postoperatively, a slight increase may go unnoticed.

As clinical symptoms of increasing respiratory insufficiency (often requiring ventilatory assistance) progress, radiographic changes become apparent. The first film changes consist of patchy, ill-defined, bilateral pulmonary infiltrates. These will rapidly increase and coalesce, producing a pattern indistinguishable from other types of generalized alveolar pulmonary edema with diffuse air bronchograms.

Following the development of diffuse infiltration, the radiographic picture changes little over the next few days to weeks. After 7 to 10 days, changes in the chest film usually indicate complications.[29] Due to the decreased compliance of the lungs, complications from ventilatory assistance, especially positive end-expiratory pressure (PEEP), are common, and the films should be closely studied for signs of interstitial air or pneumomediastinum. Sudden deterioration may mean a tension pneumothorax. Also, the congested lungs are highly susceptible to infection, especially from gram-negative organisms such as *Pseudomonas*. Areas of increasing consolidation, a mottled appearance suggesting microabscesses, or increasing effusion (empyema) should lead to a suspicion of superimposed pneumonia.[30]

If the patient survives and the alveolar infiltrates regress, there may be complete clearing or development of an interstitial pattern of pulmonary scarring and fibrosis. Table 2-4 summarizes the typical sequence of clinical, radiographic, and pathologic findings in ARDS. In Figure 2-23, a typical radiographic progression is illustrated.

Pulmonary Hemorrhage

The infiltrate from intrapulmonary hemorrhage is typically a dense alveolar consolidation rapidly appearing and fairly rapidly clearing. Focal hemorrhage from contusion due to surgery or trauma can usually be suspected by its location (Fig. 2-24). Occasionally, patients receiving anticoagulant therapy or those with coagulation disorders will develop pulmonary parenchymal hemorrhages without pulmonary contusion. These typically are rapidly progressing fluffy alveolar infiltrates. They are usually bilateral and sym-

TABLE 2-4. Typical Sequence of Findings in Adult Respiratory Distress Syndrome

Clinical	Radiologic	Pathologic
Primary insult and latent period (approximately 24 h)	Normal or unchanging	Microemboli, periarteriolar hemorrhage
Onset of tachypnea, dyspnea, decreased PaO_2, decreased $PaCO_2$ (next 6–12 h)	Normal or unchanging	Early interstitial edema, foci of intra-alveolar edema and hemorrhage
Progression of clinical symptoms requiring assisted ventilation (occurs usually 36–48 h after initial insult)	Perihilar haze or vague bilateral infiltrates progressing rapidly to diffuse alveolar opacification	Progression of diffuse alveolar edema and hemorrhage
Persistent arterial oxygen desaturation, respiratory and metabolic acidosis, loss of lung compliance, usually requiring PEEP therapy (36–72 h after initial insult)	Diffuse bilateral alveolar opacification with obvious air bronchograms, but lack of pleural effusion	Solid, "beefy" or "liverlike" lungs with thickened alveolar septa, alveolar hemorrhage and edema, and formation of hyaline membranes
Progressive respiratory failure requiring greater positive-pressure ventilation (may last for several days or even weeks)	Persistent diffuse alveolar opacification with little change	Prominent hyaline membranes
Development of fever and increased tracheobronchial secretions	Developing focal areas of denser consolidation or areas of mottled lucency, developing effusion	Superimposed inflammatory changes with microabscesses and necrosis, empyema
Sudden deterioration in blood gases or development of soft-tissue crepitation	Interstitial air, pneumomediastinum, subcutaneous emphysema, tension pneumothorax	Extra-alveolar air from ruptured peripheral alveoli
If patient recovers, there may be symptoms of chronic pulmonary disease	Normal or varying degrees of interstitial infiltrate	Varying degrees of pulmonary fibrosis

(Data from Refs. 26, 27, 28, and 29.)

metric and can be confused with pulmonary edema. Clinical findings such as a drop of hematocrit and occasional gross hemoptysis will be more helpful in identifying the etiology of the infiltrate than will its appearance. In a patient with clinical evidence of disseminated intravascular coagulation (DIC), the acute development of bilateral alveolar infiltrates should suggest the possibility of pulmonary hemorrhage[31] (Fig. 2-25).

Small areas of hemorrhage usually resolve completely over a few days. Massive or repetitive pulmonary hemorrhage will produce interstitial fibrosis. Delay in clearing may mean superimposed ARDS, particularly in patients with DIC.[32]

Pulmonary Embolus

The typical radiographic appearance immediately following pulmonary embolus is the absence of change in the chest film.[33] This lack of change in light of a sudden deterioration in blood gases and an increase in respiratory effort is characteristic and should acutely suggest pulmonary embolization. As previously mentioned, in the appropriate clinical setting, early ARDS is also a possibility at this stage.

Although the chest film may be unchanged, the radiologic study that does show immediate changes of pulmonary embolization is the radionuclide lung scan. Segmental perfusion defects with a normal chest film and normal ventilation studies are considered almost pathognomonic of pulmonary embolization.[34] With pre-existing pulmonary disease, such as severe COPD, the scan is less specific and angiography may be necessary for diagnosis. Plain film changes that may occur and are suggestive or supportive of the clinical diagnosis of pulmonary embolization include mild diaphragmatic elevation, small areas of atelectasis, and a small effusion. Unfortunately, these subtle findings are usually lost among the similar coexisting postoperative changes.[35] With massive or recurrent embolization, changes in the vasculature have been described, including enlargement of the main pulmonary artery, vessel cutoff or lack of normal tapering, and "anemia" or decrease in caliber and number of peripheral vessels in a segment of the lung.[33]

If the embolus significantly reduces blood flow in the pulmonary circulation of a lung segment, such that systemic bronchial collaterals cannot maintain oxygenation to that segment, then it dies or infarcts. An infarcted segment of lung will develop an infiltrate

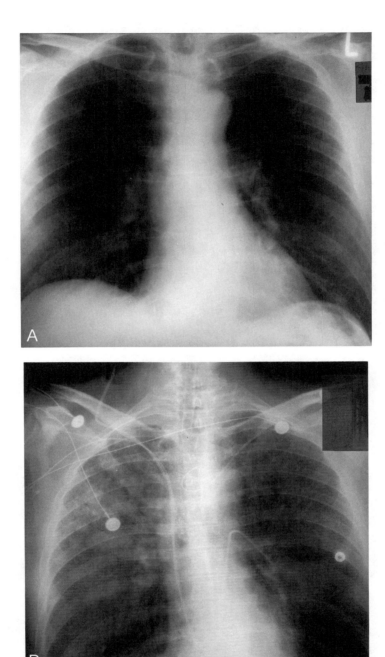

Fig. 2-23. (A) A patient with severe sepsis began experiencing increasing respiratory difficulty. The initial chest film was clear. **(B)** Forty-eight hours later, patchy bilateral infiltrates began to appear and respiratory failure was sufficient to necessitate intubation. Also note the Swan-Ganz (S-G) catheter tip in a slightly too peripheral location in the left lung. A left brachial venous catheter is coiled back on itself overlying the mediastinum. (*Figure continues.*)

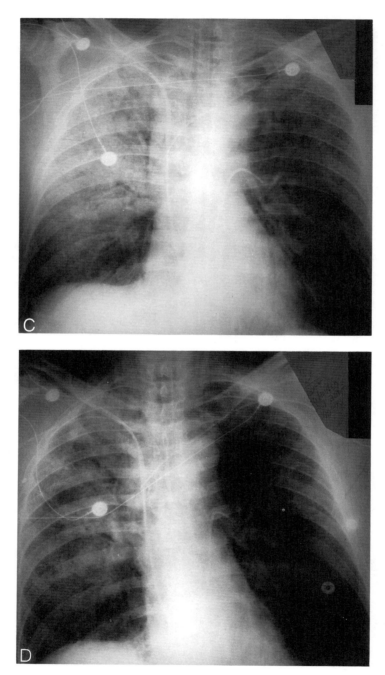

Fig. 2-23 *(Continued)*. **(C)** The following day, some of the infiltrates further coalesced with obvious air-bronchograms. Note the now correct positions of the S-G catheter and the central venous line. **(D)** The next day, with institution of PEEP, the infiltrates appeared somewhat improved, but note the development of vertical lines of subcutaneous air in the neck. This air suggests barotrauma; such a patient should be closely followed radiographically and clinically for signs of mediastinal air or pneumothorax. (*Figure continues.*)

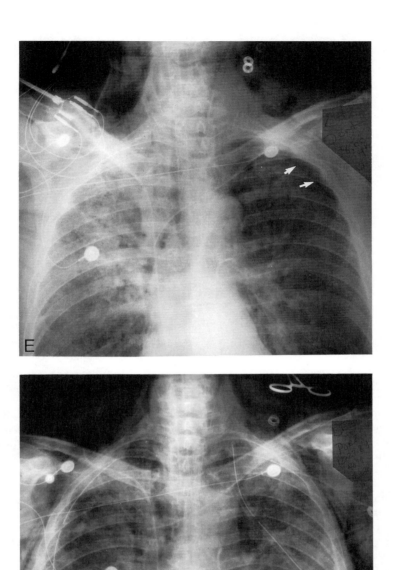

Fig. 2-23 (*Continued*). **(E)** The following evening, the subcutaneous air was more apparent bilaterally. A left pneumothorax had by then developed (*arrows*), and a right pneumothorax soon followed. **(F)** Bilateral chest tubes were placed because of pneumothoraces. The extra-alveolar air was then quite extensive. The diffuse infiltrates stabilized and remained until the patient's death several days later. Death was attributed to severe sepsis complicated by ARDS.

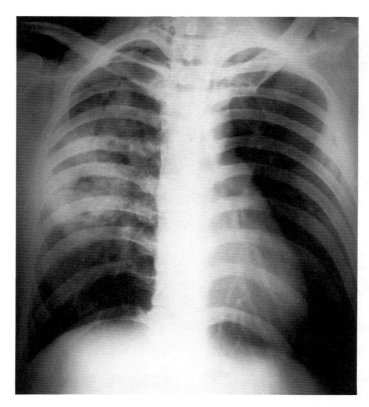

Fig. 2-24. This patient was involved in a motor vehicle accident and received blunt trauma to the right chest. This film was obtained immediately on admission. The rounded area of consolidation represents localized pulmonary contusion with hemorrhage. Also note the subcutaneous air, suggesting rupture of the lung or trachea. A pneumothorax subsequently became apparent.

due to edema and hemorrhage. The classic description of an infiltrate from pulmonary infarction is a conical or triangular alveolar consolidation with its base adjacent to a pleural surface and its apex pointing toward the hilum. Unfortunately, this classic appearance is rare.[33] More commonly, the infiltrate is nonhomogenous or patchy and of an irregular configuration. It will be pleural based; however, this does not always mean the lateral pleural surface seen in tangent on a frontal projection. It may abut the anterior or posterior pleura, a major fissure, or even an interlobar septation, and will appear to be centrally rather than peripherally located. Radiographic resolution of a pulmonary infarction is a slow process, unlike other types of edema and hemorrhage. As it resolves, it may retract into a visible parenchymal scar.[33] Pulmonary infarction can occasionally be the result of direct occlusion of pulmonary vessels by peripherally placed pulmonary arterial catheters, illustrated in the section *Monitoring and Life Support Devices* (see Fig. 2-54).

The incidence of venous thrombosis and subsequent pulmonary embolization in patients immobilized during surgery, and relatively immobilized in an extended recovery period, has been reported to be as high as 14 percent in one series.[13] It has been frequently stressed that a high index of suspicion must be maintained based on clinical findings, in light of the absence and nonspecificity of radiographic findings, in order to properly identify and treat pulmonary embolization. Reasonable suspicion should promptly lead to further radiologic studies such as radionuclide lung scanning or angiography. Figure 2-26 illustrates a typical sequence of films in a patient with pulmonary embolization and infarction.

Summary

When assessing the appearance of the lungs in the intraoperative or postoperative period, a mental checklist may lead to a proper diagnosis or at least narrow the differential.

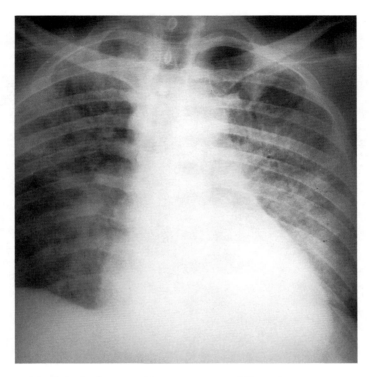

Fig. 2-25. This patient with clinical evidence of DIC developed diffuse alveolar pulmonary hemorrhage. The infiltrate itself is indistinguishable from pulmonary edema or infection.

1. What is the clinical picture and what is its temporal relationship to the developing infiltrate?

   Infiltrates developing rapidly after clinical deterioration or a hypoxic event are typical in aspiration of gastric contents. Edema from fluid overload or acute cardiac decompensation often is radiographically apparent within a few hours of the onset of changing clinical symptoms, whereas abrupt clinical deterioration, respiratory distress, or hypoxia with a relatively normal radiograph would suggest ARDS or pulmonary embolization. These infiltrates often lag behind the clinical onset of symptomatology for 24 to 48 hours or more.

   In contrast, a stable or improving patient who has just been extubated or removed from assisted ventilation may develop infiltrates. These are more likely areas of atelectasis. Changing areas of subsegmental or microatelectasis from hypoinflation usually do not present significant clinical symptomatology. Large areas of atelectasis, lobar or whole lung, will be symptomatic; however, their radiographic appearance is usually specific enough not to be confused with other conditions, such as pneumonia, ARDS, or emboli. However, it must be remembered that atelectasis may complicate or co-exist with these other conditions.

2. When assessing the temporal sequence of appearance, what has been the rate of change on serial films?

   Edema, once apparent, will develop rapidly within a few hours. It may also clear fairly rapidly (24 to 48 hours) following appropriate therapy, such as digitalization and/or diuretics. Pneumonias show less rapid change and will often radiographically lag behind clinical resolution. ARDS, once it is radiographically apparent, may evolve quickly; however, it then stabilizes with little change over a long period of time (days to weeks).

3. What is the predominant location or distribution of the infiltrate and how does this relate to underlying lung disease, the preoperative chest film, or the patient's position?

   Both aspiration and edema are gravity-dependent, and, in the supine patient, will often present in the perihilar and lower lung zones. Localized infiltrates are more typical of pneumonia, contusion, and embolus. Diffuse patterns are more characteristic of edema, massive aspiration, or ARDS. Occasionally, some pneumonias may present a diffuse pattern. In patients with underlying COPD, a normally diffuse process, such as edema from con-

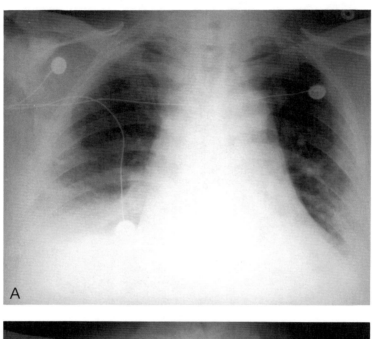

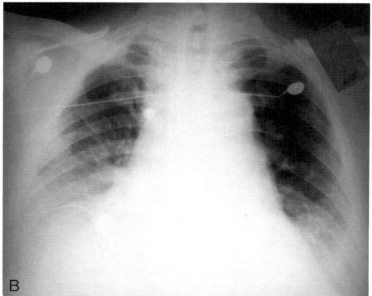

Fig. 2-26. **(A)** This semierect portable examination on a patient post-open heart surgery was obtained after extubation. The study was underexposed, but demonstrated mild hypoinflation, bilateral effusions, and postsurgical mediastinal widening. Clinically, the patient was doing well. **(B)** The patient suddenly developed respiratory distress and hypoxia. This film was obtained immediately, and again reveals bilateral effusions and hypoinflation but essentially little change. (*Figure continues.*)

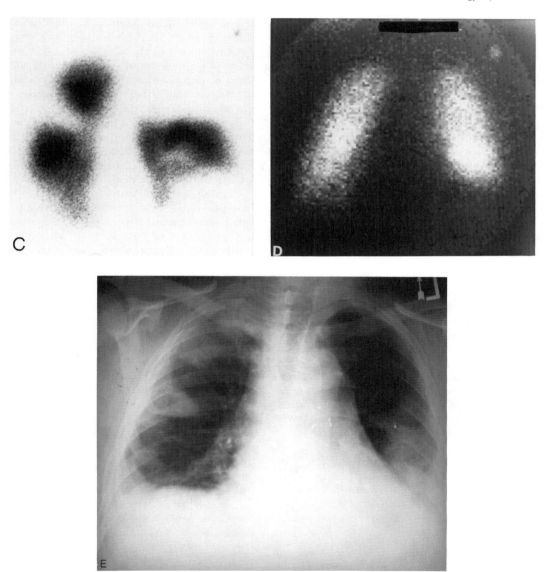

Fig. 2-26 (*Continued*). **(C)** PA view from a perfusion lung scan on the same patient showing large segmental perfusion defects in both lungs. **(D)** A normal ventilation scan obtained at the same time as the film in Fig. C. **(E)** Three days after the patient began anticoagulant therapy for pulmonary embolization, the chest film demonstrated segmental areas of infarction. These slowly resolved over the next 2 weeks.

gestive heart failure, may appear as a patchy or segmentalized infiltrate.

4. In addition to the pulmonary parenchymal changes, what changes have occurred in other structures, such as the pulmonary vasculature, heart, or pleura, that would aid in the differential diagnosis?

Accurate assessment of changing pulmonary vas-culature, and occasionally of changes in heart size, is the key to differentiating types of pulmonary edema or differentiating edema from other diffuse processes. If cardiac failure or acute fluid overload are to be differentiated from other types of edema, every effort must be made to obtain an erect film. Although small effusions are difficult to assess on the portable film, they are usually present with recent thoracic surgery. Increasing effusion may indicate infection with empyema or, possibly, superimposed pulmonary embolization. Effusion is noticeably absent in uncomplicated ARDS.

5. In assessing a newly apparent infiltrate, has there been recent manipulation of the patient or his support equipment?

   This will be elaborated on in subsequent sections; however, placement or removal of tubing and catheters may produce various complicating pulmonary or pleural densities. Also, in assessing changing infiltrates, interval administration of physical therapy may produce significant clearing of atelectasis or change in its distribution.

6. To assess an infiltrate, it must first be localized. Under ideal conditions, an erect film with good inspiration and proper exposure would be expected. Unfortunately, this is not always possible. While obliquity is not desirable for assessing the mediastinum, it can be useful in assessing infiltrates. If an upright film in deep inspiration cannot be obtained, the patient can purposely be positioned obliquely to assess lower lobes that may be hidden behind the domes of the diaphragm or the cardiac silhouette. Lordosis is also not often desirable since it can hide the lower lobes; however, it can be useful in bringing out a right middle lobe infiltrate or an apical density, if one is suspected on a routine portable. When erect PA and lateral films cannot be obtained, decubitus views can often be managed. A decubitus view, while primarily used in conjunction with assessing pleural effusion, can also assess the underlying lung, often obscured by fluid. The side up on a decubitus study can expand more fully on inspiration and can be better assessed as the fluid falls toward the mediastinum.

EXTRA-ALVEOLAR AIR

Extra-alveolar air is a very common complication of various surgical manipulations, trauma, and ventilatory assistance. Its presence can be inconsequential, as in small amounts of subcutaneous emphysema, or life-threatening, as in a tension pneumothorax. The various types of extra-alveolar air include pneumothorax, pneumomediastinum, pneumopericardium, pneumoperitoneum and retroperitoneum, pulmonary subpleural and interstitial air, and subcutaneous air.

In the adult, there is potential free communication between the mediastinum and the soft tissues of the neck and chest wall, and intra- or retroperitoneal spaces. Also, collections of subpleural or interstitial air from rupture of alveoli can track along vascular sheaths to the mediastinum. Mediastinal air can also rupture into the pleural space, producing a pneumothorax. In the absence of direct traumatic or surgical penetration of the pericardium in the adult, there is no communication between it and other portions of the mediastinum. In the newborn there is often no plane of communication from the mediastinum to the neck; therefore, a tension pneumomediastinum can occur in this age group, when it is not seen in adults. Also in newborns, pneumomediastinum can lead to pneumopericardium without implying penetrating injury to the pericardium.

Because of the communication among these various potential spaces, radiographic evidence of air in one space should raise suspicion for subsequent appearance of air in others. For instance, in barotrauma with rupture of a subpleural alveolar air space, air can dissect along the pulmonary interstitium to the mediastinum (pneumomediastinum), around the lung (pneumothorax), into the soft tissue of the neck and chest wall (subcutaneous air), and even below the diaphragm (pneumoperitoneum or pneumoretroperitoneum). Even small amounts of extra-alveolar air can be radiographically apparent due to the differences in radiographic density between air and soft tissue. As extra-alveolar air dissects tissue planes, it produces interfaces between adjacent soft tissue structures that were not previously discernible.

Extra-alveolar air in nonsurgical or nontraumatized patients is most often due to spontaneous rupture of bullae or blebs, rupture of alveoli in acute asthmatic attacks, or pleural-based cavitating processes such as necrotizing pneumonia, metastasis, or pulmonary infarct rupturing into the pleural space.[5] The incidence of tension pneumothorax in these instances is low. In traumatic or iatrogenic causes of extra-alveolar air, however, the incidence of respiratory embarrassment due to tension pneumothorax is high.[36] Iatrogenic causes of extra-alveolar air are primarily direct surgical manipulation (including pleural tap, catheter or line placement, closed chest massage) or as a result of mechanical ventilation. The increasing use of high levels of PEEP may produce a pneumothorax by direct rupture of the visceral pleura; however, more commonly, the increased pressure produces rupture of pleural-based alveoli (barotrauma) with the subsequent dissection of extra-alveolar air as described above.[36–38]

Interstitial Air

Interstitial air, the earliest evidence of alveolar rupture due to barotrauma, is reported with some frequency in newborns on PEEP for hyaline membrane disease (Fig. 2-27), but it is often not appreciable in

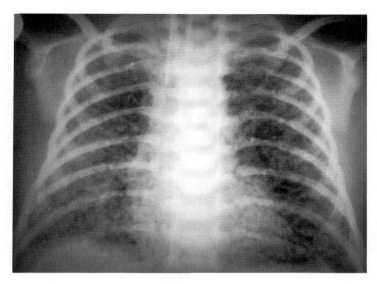

Fig. 2-27. A newborn infant on PEEP for hyaline membrane disease developed extensive interstitial air, producing the "bubbly" pattern seen here.

adults.[37,39] Interstitial or subpleural collection of air within normal lung tissue is relatively inapparent; however, most instances of interstitial air from barotrauma occur in diffusely consolidated lungs, and the air will be seen as a bubbly pattern within the infiltrate. It can easily be confused with air bronchograms or bullous lesions with surrounding infiltrate. However, if collections of subpleural air or peripheral interstitial air are apparent, they should be taken as an indicator of impending pneumomediastinum with a possibility of subsequent tension pneumothorax.[36,37]

Subcutaneous Air

Subcutaneous air can be due to local disruption of tissues such as penetrating injury, surgery, tracheostomy, or chest tube insertion. Small amounts of air are inconsequential, but increasing subcutaneous air around a tube or tracheostomy site many indicate poor position of the tube or bronchopleural fistula. Subcutaneous air can dissect through the neck and produce a pneumomediastinum, or it may be the result of air dissection from a pneumomediastinum. It may be radiographically apparent before the pneumomediastinum is appreciated, especially on portable radiographs. Presence of subcutaneous air in the neck or chest without associated penetrating injury or tube placement should raise suspicions of barotrauma, and serial films should be closely scrutinized for the possible development of pneumomediastinum and pneumothorax. In patients with blunt trauma, the appearance of subcutaneous air should also signal the

possibility of coexistent pneumothorax (Fig. 2-24). Extensive subcutaneous air can greatly confuse or obscure changes in the underlying lung parenchyma (Fig. 2-23F).[5]

Pneumomediastinum

Pneumomediastinum may result from dissection of subcutaneous, interstitial, or pleural air. Tracheal or esophageal rupture can also produce pneumomediastinum and, if undetected, result in a life-threatening mediastinitis.

Small amounts of mediastinal air are best appreciated on a lateral projection. If this view can be obtained, it should be closely scrutinized following trauma or suspected esophageal or tracheal rupture. Figure 2-28 illustrates areas where mediastinal air is most apparent on the lateral view, outlining the hila and great vessels and in the anterior mediastinum.

In postoperative portable examinations, mediastinal air is usually seen as a lucent line around the heart, delineating the adjacent pleural reflection or outlining the aortic arch (Fig. 2-29). As previously mentioned, unless there is direct penetration of the pericardium, air collections around the cardiac silhouette in the adult are most likely due to pneumomediastinum and not pneumopericardium. Occasionally, a radiolucent halo around the mediastinum is appreciated in patients with diffuse pulmonary consolidation. This may be attributed to the MACH effect (a line perceived by the eye that is not truly present) or, as some investigators believe, to the pumping

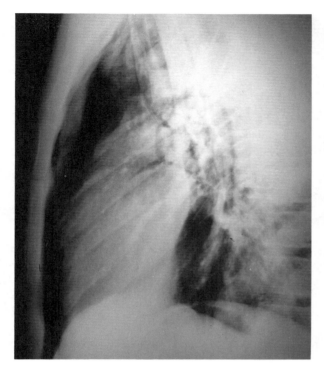

Fig. 2-28. A lateral view of a patient with extensive mediastinal air from spontaneous rupture of a bleb during an asthmatic attack. Note the thin black lines surrounding mediastinal structures and in the retrosternal area.

action of the cardiac silhouette preventing consolidation in the adjacent lung (kinetic halo).[40,41] This radiolucent halo, which is typically faint and indistinct, should not be confused with mediastinal air, which is usually a sharp, well-defined black line.[5] An example of the radiolucent mediastinal halo is seen in Figure 2-22B.

Pneumothorax

In a healthy lung, two forces maintain expansion: the pressure in a patent bronchial tree is atmospheric, while the intrapleural pressure is slightly less. The healthy lung, without associated pleural disease, will retract symmetrically with a pneumothorax, tending to preserve its normal configuration. This is illustrated in Figure 2-30A, which shows a spontaneous pneumothorax in a young adult due to rupture of an apical bleb. The intrathoracic, extrapulmonary air surrounds the partially collapsed lung on all sides, although on this upright view it is only seen along the superior and lateral margins. A word of caution to those who attempt to estimate a percentage of collapse: although the lung is only separated from the

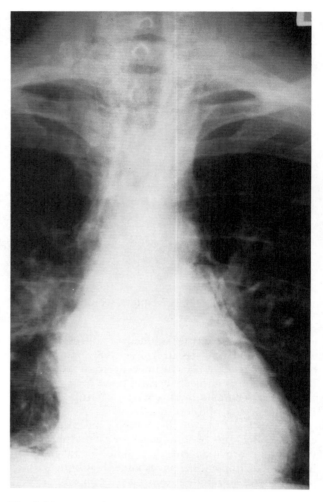

Fig. 2-29. Extensive mediastinal and some subcutaneous air in a patient with esophageal rupture. The sharp black lines of air separate mediastinal tissue planes and outline the heart and aorta.

lateral chest wall by a few centimeters, the total volume loss, considering the three-dimensional lung, is much greater than is usually reported in percentages.

When at all possible, an upright chest film, taken in forced expiration, should be used to diagnose a pneumothorax, as in Figure 2-30B. Here, the absence of pulmonary markings beyond the pleural margin is easily appreciated. The difficulty in diagnosing a pneumothorax comes when the underlying lung is not normal, an upright film is difficult to obtain, or there are overlapping artifacts such as tubing or abnormal soft tissues. In patients with emphysema and bleb formation, or in patients who are hyperinflated by a ventilator, peripheral pulmonary markings may appear

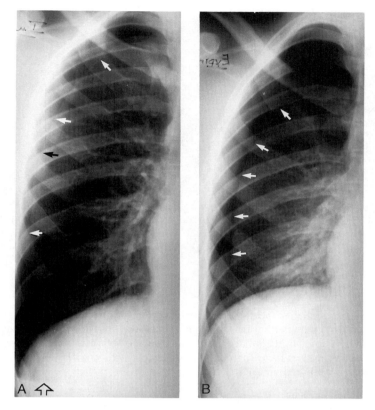

Fig. 2-30. (A) A spontaneous pneumothorax in an otherwise healthy individual. The partially collapsed lung retains its normal shape. The pleural margin (*closed arrows*) is seen as a thin white line. An air fluid level in the pleural space is indicated (*open arrow*). **(B)** A film taken during forced expiration accentuates the pneumothorax in Fig. A.

absent and may be mistaken for a pneumothorax. In this situation, it is important to carefully search for a pleural margin along the suspected pneumothorax. Artifacts such as overlying catheters and skin folds are very common on portable examinations. They may easily simulate a pleural margin and must be examined closely in this instance for pulmonary markings extending beyond their edge (Fig. 2-31). A pneumothorax may be loculated if the underlying lung or pleura does not allow the lung to collapse symmetrically. A pneumothorax can occasionally loculate along the mediastinum and simulate a large pneumomediastinum, or it can loculate subpulmonically and mimic a pneumoperitoneum.[42] A pneumothorax with associated lobar atelectasis may preferentially loculate over the atelectatic lobe instead of around the periphery of the whole lung.[43] In a supine patient, air will rise to the anterior surface and be relatively inapparent in the AP projection. Occasionally, the only sign of a pneumothorax on a supine view may be the development of a deep radiolucent

lateral costophrenic sulcus.[44] If a pneumothorax is suspected and an upright view is difficult to obtain, a lateral decubitus view with the suspected side up may demonstrate the pneumothorax. If the patient cannot be moved, a cross-table lateral view may demonstrate air collecting in the retrosternal area. This is particularly helpful in children, in whom there is normally no significant retrosternal air collection; however, in an adult, a large emphysematous retrosternal air space from COPD may present confusion.[5] Pleural fluid often accompanies a pneumothorax, and the finding of an air-fluid level extending to the pleural surface may signal a pneumothorax that is otherwise inapparent (Fig. 2-30A).

Tension pneumothorax is an infrequent complication of a pneumothorax in spontaneously breathing individuals unless there is significant trauma; however, it is a very common problem in patients receiving assisted ventilation because the air leak site is kept open as more and more air is forced through it. As air pressure increases in the pleural space, overex-

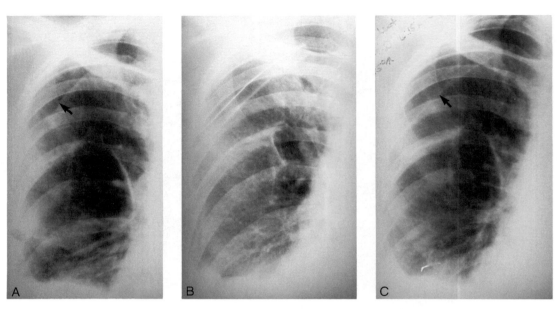

Fig. 2-31. (A) A curvilinear white line (*arrow*) at the periphery of the lung in this patient is produced by a skin fold. This was mistaken for a pneumothorax. **(B)** A chest tube was inserted as treatment for the suspected pneumothorax. **(C)** After removal of the tube, a white line produced by pleural reaction adjacent to the chest tube (*arrow*) became apparent. Artifacts such as skin folds, chest tube tracts, and overlying bandages or catheters may simulate a pleural margin.

pansion of the hemithorax with compression of adjacent structures will create serious respiratory embarrassment. Radiographic evidence of developing tension reflects this overexpansion and compression. If the lung is not significantly consolidated or "stiff," it will totally collapse into a small paramediastinal mass as tension develops. The ribs on the ipsilateral side will spread apart and the diaphragm will be depressed (Fig. 2-32). If the mediastinum is not chronically immobilized, it will shift to the opposite side and the contralateral lung and its bronchus will be compressed. Of these findings, a depression of the ipsilateral diaphragm may be the most easily assessed and reliable finding in postsurgical patients because the ipsilateral lung or pleura is often abnormal, preventing complete collapse, and the mediastinum is fixed by surgical reaction or fibrosis, preventing appreciable shift. In fact, if the diaphragm does not appear to elevate on a film done in expiration, tension should be suspected even before the diaphragm is obviously depressed. When assessing the mediastinum for shift, it must be remembered how easily patient rotation can mimic or obscure mediastinal movement (Fig. 2-6).[5] Occasionally, a tension pneumothorax may be loculated, usually in an inferior subpulmonic or paracardiac location, and the only radiographic evidence of tension may be a slight flattening of the cardiac border or a contour change in the ipsilateral diaphragm.[45]

Occasionally, with re-expansion of a pneumothorax or rapid removal of large pleural effusions, the re-expanded lung will develop unilateral alveolar pulmonary edema. Rapid resolution of this "re-expansion pulmonary edema" differentiates it from an inflammatory process.[46]

MEDIASTINUM

Not only is *apparent* mediastinal widening from magnification, hypoinflation, and rotation to be expected when comparing a portable film to a preoperative PA projection, but *actual* mediastinal widening occurs when surgical manipulation involving the heart or mediastinum creates minor degrees of hemorrhage and tissue edema. However, significant widening usually indicates gross hemorrhage and should be immediately correlated with clinical evidence of a decreasing hematocrit or increasing difficulty in ventilation or cardiovascular instability. Postoperative mediastinal hemorrhage is most common in conditions in which there are abnormally dilated vessels within the mediastinum, as is seen in pediatric cardiac surgery for correction of coarctation and in some

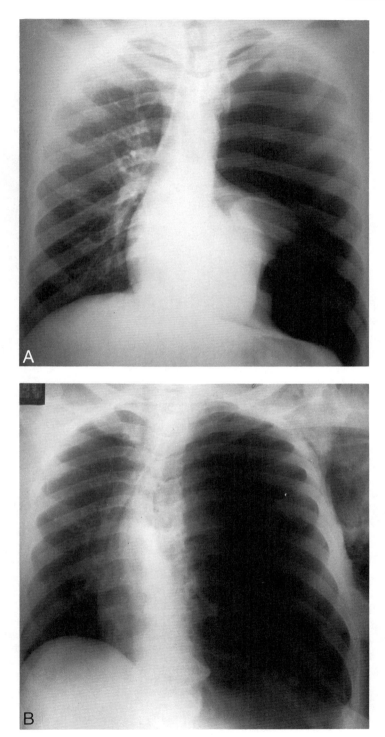

Fig. 2-32. (A & B) Two patients with tension pneumothorax. Note the total collapse of the lung with spreading of the ribs, depression of the diaphragm, and mediastinal shift. In Fig. B, the changes are most marked and there is associated subcutaneous air.

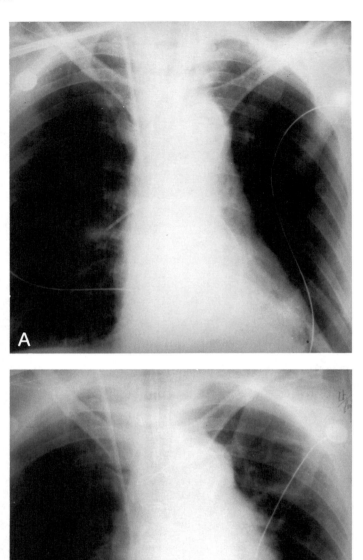

Fig. 2-33. **(A)** This film obtained shortly after open heart surgery reveals a normal-appearing mediastinum for an AP portable projection. Note the proper position of the Swan-Ganz catheter. **(B)** A film the following day, also a portable AP projection without significant change in magnification or rotation, shows significant enlargement of the mediastinum secondary to hemorrhage.

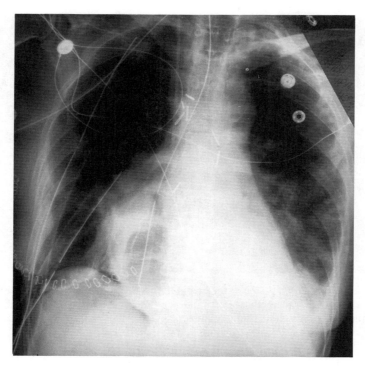

Fig. 2-34. This portable examination following distal esophageal resection for carcinoma reveals a nasogastric tube coursing to the right in a widened mediastinum. It identifies the location of the intrathoracic stomach. The mottled density of the mediastinum is due to gas within the stomach and should not be mistaken for other postoperative pathology.

shunts.[47] Occasionally, misplaced catheters can infuse fluid into the mediastinum, creating enlargement, but they more often drain into the pleural space, creating rapidly progressive pleural effusions. Figure 2-33 demonstrates postoperative mediastinal hemorrhage.

If surgery involves esophageal resection with gastric pull-through or colonic interposition, the mediastinum will, of course, be enlarged. The intrathoracic stomach or colon may present as a solid mass or be filled with multiple air spaces which, on an upright film, will present as multiple air-fluid levels. These typically project to the right side and, on a lateral view, the colon interposition is usually in the retrosternal area, while the gastric pull-through is in the midmediastinum. Note in Figure 2-34 the nasogastric tube outlining the course of the interposition on this postoperative film.

Computed tomography (CT) and magnetic resonance imaging (MRI) have revolutionized the evaluation of the mediastinum. With conventional radiography, mediastinal processes are detected when they produce a contour abnormality of the lung-mediastinal interface. By virtue of its cross-sectional imaging plane and superior contrast resolution, CT can

often provide much more information.[48] In the preoperative evaluation, CT can reveal the exact nature and location of a mass producing mediastinal widening (Fig. 2-35). When sudden mediastinal widening occurs, both CT and MRI are highly accurate in diagnosing aortic aneurysms (Fig. 2-36) and aortic dissection (Fig. 2-37).[49,50]

PLEURAL FLUID

Small amounts of pleural fluid accumulation are common following most types of thoracic surgery; unless an embolus or empyema is suspected, usually no workup is required. Rapid or significant accumulation of fluid should, however, lead to suspicion of postoperative complications such as hemorrhage. If a thoracentesis confirms hemorrhage and the hematocrit after the initial tap appears to stabilize, a further modest increase in fluid may not necessarily mean further bleeding. Blood is a pleural irritant and will induce an effusion following intrapleural hemorrhage.[51] Occasionally, misplaced catheters, especially subclavian catheters, may infuse large quantities of

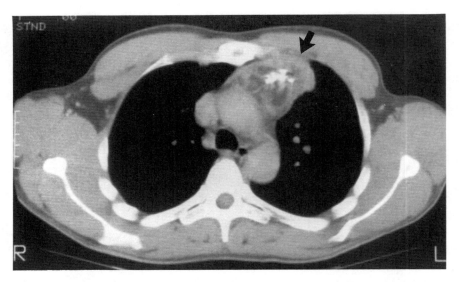

Fig. 2-35. CT scan of a patient with a widened mediastinum on chest x-ray. The scan reveals a mass located in the anterior compartment of the mediastinum (*arrow*). The presence of calcium, fat, and soft tissue densities within the mass correctly indicated a mediastinal teratoma.

fluid into the pleural space over a short period of time (Fig. 2-38).

Pleural effusions associated with heart failure or pulmonary embolus are usually small and, on a portable projection, may be missed. Also, their additive effect on already existent small postoperative effusions is usually not detectable.

On an upright study, the earliest evidence of effusion is blunting of the posterior sulcus on the lateral view and, as the effusion increases slightly, blunting of the lateral angles on a PA projection. The typical appearance is a meniscus (Fig. 2-19 and see Fig. 2-43A). On well-penetrated portable erect or semi-erect studies, small effusions can also be seen blunting the lateral angles or opacifying the lung base due to layering in the posterior sulcus.

In relatively supine views, the typical meniscus is lost and fluid layering along the posterior gutters produces a density to the lower hemithorax that fades out imperceptibly on its upper margin and produces in-

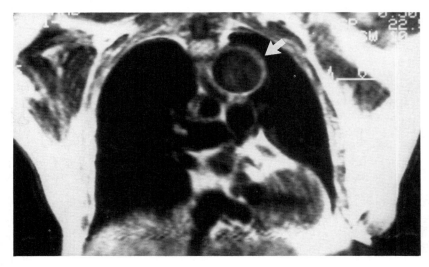

Fig. 2-36. MRI scan oriented in the coronal plane reveals the presence of an aneurysm of the aortic arch (*arrow*).

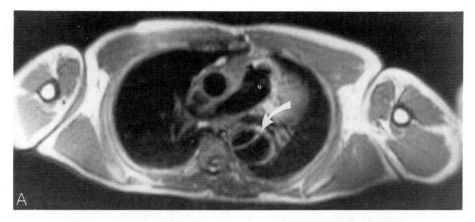

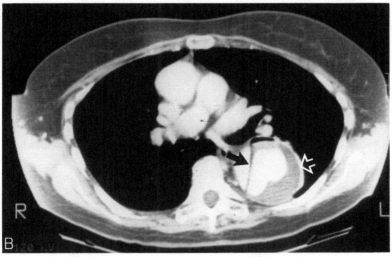

Fig. 2-37. (A) MRI scan oriented in the transaxial plane reveals the presence of a flap within the aorta (*arrow*). This is diagnostic of an aortic dissection. **(B)** CT scan in a different patient reveals the presence of a flap (*black arrow*) within the aorta. Thrombus (*open arrow*) is also noted within the aorta.

distinctness of the hemidiaphragms along its lower margin (Fig. 2-39 and see Fig. 2-42A). Decubitus views, when feasible, will confirm these effusions. Obtaining both decubitus views is helpful in that the dependent side shows layering of fluid laterally while the nondependent side shows layering of fluid against the mediastinum, allowing for better visualization of any underlying lung pathology.

On an upright view, more than approximately a centimeter of space between the top of the stomach bubble and the hemidiaphragm on the left is considered abnormal. Widening may indicate a subphrenic process, but more commonly represents a subpulmonic collection of pleural fluid. The distance between the projected diaphragm and stomach bubble on a supine view is variable and does not carry the

same significance. Subpulmonic fluid on the right may be more difficult to assess and quantitate as illustrated in Figure 2-40.

Total opacification of a hemithorax can be caused by a number of conditions, including massive effusion. Decubitus views are not helpful in evaluating fluid in a total "whiteout." Typically, massive fluid accumulations cause volume expansion of the hemithorax and mediastinal shift to the contralateral side (Fig. 2-38B), while total atelectasis produces mediastinal shift to the ipsilateral side (Fig. 2-14). Unfortunately, many times when faced with total or near total opacification of one side of the chest in the acute postoperative period, there is probably a mixture of fluid, atelectasis, and even consolidation present at the same time. Consequently, even after a diligent

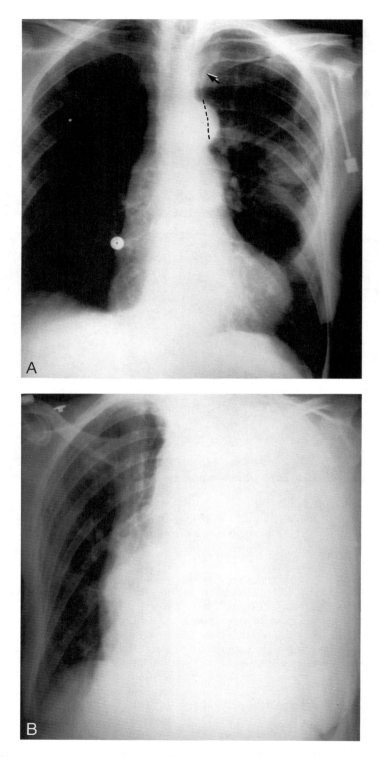

Fig. 2-38. (A) An improperly placed subclavian catheter (retouched) produced hemorrhage and infused large quantities of fluid into the left pleural space **(B)**, producing mediastinal shift and severe respiratory embarrassment.

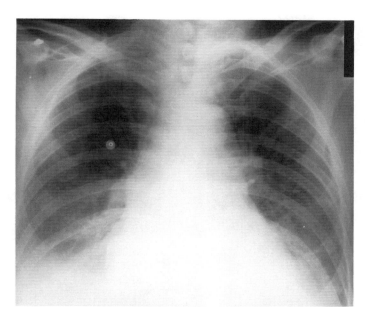

Fig. 2-39. Bilateral, moderate-sized pleural effusions in this semierect portable study are seen to blur the diaphragms and fade out imperceptibly along their superior margins.

search for blood vessels, air bronchograms, and mediastinal shift, they may still be absent. The very absence of mediastinal shift (assuming the mediastinum is not immobilized by fibrosis or surgery), however, should lead to a suspicion of more than one underlying process.

Fluid accumulations may be loculated due to preexisting pulmonary scarring or to recent surgical alteration. Peripheral loculations will appear as pleural-based soft tissue masses when seen in tangent. These same collections seen en face may also appear masslike. Fluid in the minor fissure will thicken the fissure and, if copious enough, will also present as a well-defined mass (pseudotumor) on frontal views (Fig. 2-41). Fluid layering in a major fissure on the frontal projection will be seen as a vague increased density just as fluid layering in the posterior sulcus, but its upper margin will be demarcated as a curvilinear line overlying the fifth to sixth posterior ribs. Occasionally, fluid in the major fissure will also loculate as a pseudotumor (Fig. 2-41). Fluid accumulating along the medial aspects of the lung will widen the paraspinal stripe.

It must be remembered that the presence of air within the pleural space will change the typical pleural meniscus to a sharp, straight line or air-fluid level on upright views (Fig. 2-30). Air-fluid levels in the pleural space in a single plane may be confused with air-fluid levels in lung abscesses or bullae, and a lateral view is usually recommended for differentiation.

However, when this is not possible, a distinction can usually be made in that the pleural fluid line is typically longer than an abscess cavity fluid level and extends to the lateral pleural surface.[52,53] Once again, decubitus views in place of an erect lateral may distinguish pleural from parenchymal disease.

When simple maneuvers such as decubitus views are unsuccessful in evaluating pleural densities, CT has been shown to be of value. CT can accurately diagnose and localize loculated pleural fluid collections (Fig. 2-42)[54]; it is also extremely valuable in differentiating an empyema from a lung abscess.[55] This distinction is crucial as an empyema requires chest tube drainage while a lung abscess can be treated with antibiotics. Both of these disease entities can produce cavities on conventional x-ray examinations. CT can accurately differentiate between an empyema, which is confined to the pleural space, and a lung abscess, which is an intraparenchymal process (Fig. 2-43).[55]

PERICARDIAL EFFUSION

Progressive enlargement of the cardiac silhouette in a globular configuration is the hallmark of pericardial effusion (Fig. 2-44). However, in portable examinations, assessment of changes in cardiac size and contour are limited by technique. Likewise, in the face of rapidly developing effusions or pericardial disease, restrictive pericarditis and tamponade can occur with

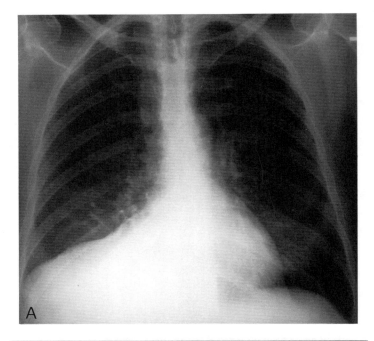

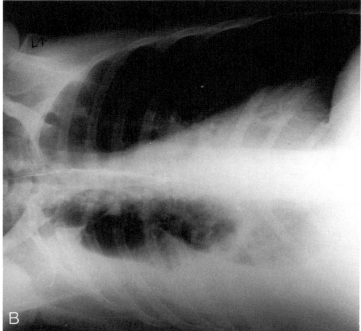

Fig. 2-40. (A) A large subpulmonic effusion on the right can mimic a high diaphragm, especially without a lateral film. **(B)** A decubitus view of the same patient reveals how large a collection of fluid can be loculated in the subpulmonic space. Also note how well the lung is expanded on the nondependent side. When assessing a lung base obscured by fluid or hypoinflation, a portable decubitus view will often show it to greatest advantage in a bedridden patient.

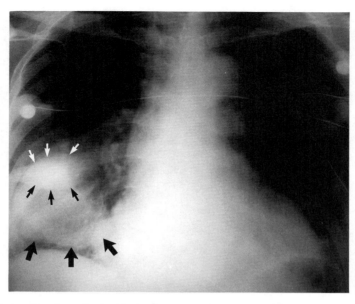

Fig. 2-41. The well-defined masses, both elliptical (*small arrows*) and round (*larger arrows*), in the right lung represent pseudotumors of loculated fluid in the minor and major fissures, respectively. These can be confirmed with a lateral view; however, the appearance of such sharply outlined homogenous masses in a patient with chronic or recent effusion should lead to suspicion of pleural fluid pseudotumor on the frontal view only.

very little change on the plain film.[56] Evidence of both systemic and pulmonary vascular engorgement from constrictive pericardiopathy should, of course, be assessed on the plain film; however, if there is clinical suspicion of pericardial disease, a much more sensitive technique is echocardiography. This procedure is noninvasive and can often be performed rapidly and easily at the bedside.

SPECIFIC POSTOPERATIVE CHANGES FROM THORACOTOMY FOR LOBECTOMY AND PNEUMONECTOMY

There are specific sequential radiographic findings that can be expected following lung resection, relating to compensatory changes in the diaphragm, pleura, mediastinum, and remaining lung. Local resection or enucleation of a small parenchymal nodule will result in hemorrhage in and around the site, occasionally simulating a remaining or recurring mass.[57] This "pseudotumor" slowly regresses over several days to a few weeks (Fig. 2-45). Similarly, any surgical manipulation of hilar structures produces perihilar infiltrate

or mass from localized edema and hemorrhage. This fuzzy and slightly full hilum should not be confused with early signs of pulmonary edema or aspiration pneumonia.

Resection of a large pulmonary segment, lobe, or entire lung will, of course, produce significant volume loss; however, this is not always apparent in the immediate postoperative studies, due to the pressure of the remaining air in the pleural space. As air is reabsorbed or aspirated through chest tubes, pleural fluid forming in response to surgery replaces the air, so volume loss again initially is not often dramatic. The resultant air-fluid level within the pleural space is best appreciated on upright views and may be a single large fluid level or multiple loculated air-fluid levels. As fluid is reabsorbed or aspirated through chest tubes, volume loss becomes apparent. Slowly, the mediastinum shifts to the ipsilateral side, the hemidiaphragm elevates, and the remaining ipsilateral lung re-expands. Eventually, the ipsilateral and contralateral remaining lung develops compensatory hyperexpansion or emphysema to fill the void. The remaining ipsilateral lobes following lobectomy may at first show diffuse opacification due to edema and residual microatelectasis.

If there is a sudden increase in the amount of intra-

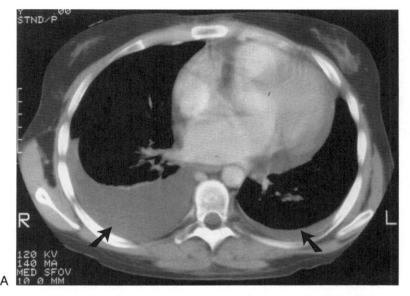

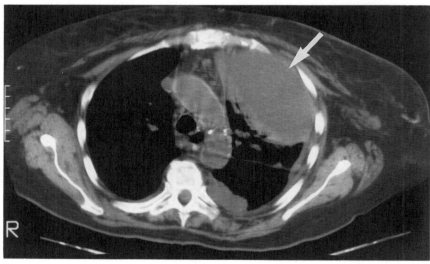

Fig. 2-42. (A) CT scan reveals bilateral, simple (nonloculated) pleural effusions forming menisci in the gravity-dependent portions of the thorax (*arrows*). **(B)** A loculated pleural effusion is present in the anterior portion of the thorax (*arrow*).

pleural air with mediastinal shift to the contralateral side, an air leak from the bronchial stump or broncho-pleural fistula should be suspected. Minor variations in the air-fluid level from film to film, however, should not cause alarm, as they are usually due to variations in patient position and variations in the daily rate of pleural absorption or chest tube aspiration of fluid versus air in the postoperative period.[57] Figure 2-46A and B represent postoperative changes acutely with

later development of a bronchopleural fistula (Fig. 2-46C and D).

Elevation of a hemidiaphragm following pneumo-nectomy or lower lobectomy may reflect diaphrag-matic or phrenic nerve damage or simply acute vol-ume loss in the thorax. On the left, acute gastric air distention may then result. Assessment of the degree of gastric dilatation on serial chest films is important so that a nasogastric tube may be appropriately

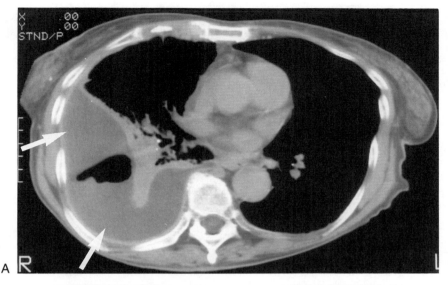

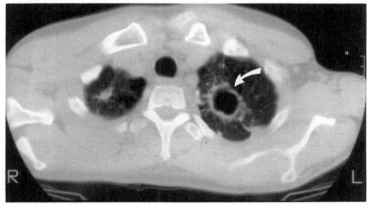

Fig. 2-43. (A) CT scan reveals fluid and air within the pleural space (*arrows*), indicative of an empyema. **(B)** CT scan reveals a cavity located within the lung parenchyma (*arrow*), indicative of a lung abscess.

placed to avoid the possible complication of gastric ischemia or rupture due to massive dilatation.

MONITORING AND LIFE SUPPORT DEVICES

In the intraoperative period, the determination of proper placement of monitoring and life support devices is usually achieved through clinical assessment of their location by physical examination or appropriate monitor readings. Only occasionally will confusing or suspicious findings suggesting malplacement or its complications lead to a call for a radiograph in the operating room. It would be inappropriately time-consuming to have radiographic confirmation of the position of every tube placed during anesthesia and surgery.

In the postoperative intensive care setting, however, radiographic monitoring of catheters and tubes becomes more appropriate, as patients and their equipment are constantly being moved and manipulated. Therefore, in a "systematic approach" to each radiograph in the postoperative period, there should be a mental "subsection" for catheters and tubes, and their possible complications.

The following sections deal with the common types of monitoring and life support equipment, their radiographic appearance, proper and improper placement, and possible complications.

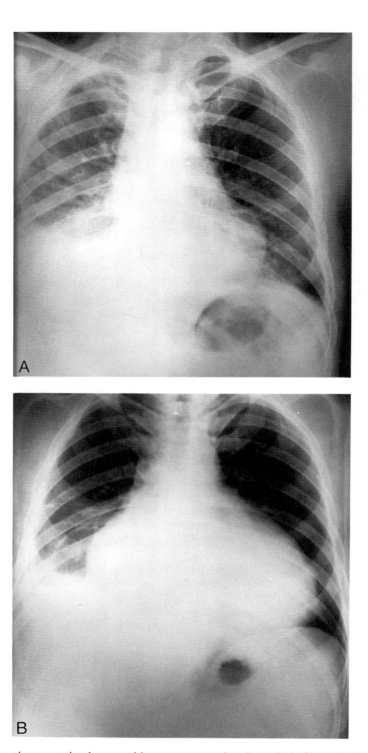

Fig. 2-44. (A) This patient sustained severe blunt trauma to the chest. This film, obtained acutely, demonstrates a large right effusion surrounding the lateral and apical margins of the lung as well as layering in the posterior gutter. With the subcutaneous and mediastinal air seen here, the patient should be suspected of having a pneumothorax, as was proven on subsequent films. Note the normal cardiac size immediately after trauma. **(B)** A few days later, serial films demonstrated progressive enlargement of the cardiac silhouette, as shown here. This rapid change, as well as the typical ''globular'' configuration, is characteristic of pericardial fluid, in this case, hemorrhage.

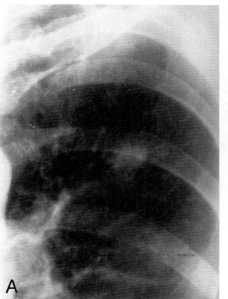
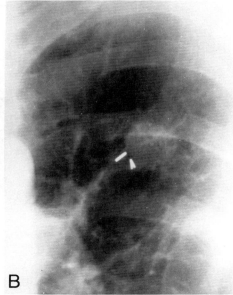

Fig. 2-45. (A) This pulmonary nodule was suspected preoperatively to represent a primary pulmonary malignancy. However, following enucleation, frozen section pathology revealed benign chronic inflammation, and further excision was not needed. **(B)** Postoperatively, the pseudotumor of hemorrhage mimics a remaining nodule. This cleared slowly over several days.

Endotracheal Tubes

Studies of the effect of flexion and extension of the neck on the position of the endotracheal tube tip indicate that it can move as much as 4 to 5 cm with vigorous head movement.[58] Therefore, the ideal position of the tip would be midway between the carina and the vocal cords, with the head in the neutral position to allow for maximal flexibility. In an adult, this is typically 5 to 7 cm above the carina. For localization purposes, there is a radiopaque stripe along the entire length, or at least at the distal tip, of most currently manufactured endotracheal tubes. (Refer to Figs. 2-15, 2-22, and 2-23 for proper placement.)

Finding the carina in a well-penetrated mediastinum is relatively easily done by following the mainstem bronchi to their junction (Fig. 2-8). An approximation of carinal position can be obtained by counting vertebrae or posterior ribs. On portable radiographs, in 95 percent of patients, the carina projects over T_5, T_6, or T_7.[59] The vocal cords overlie approximately C_5 or C_6. When assessing tube position, evaluation of the position of the patient's head in flexion or extension is also necessary, since a tip that appears in "good" position 2 or 3 cm from the carina with the head extended could slip into the right main-

stem bronchus on flexion. On many portable chest films, a portion of the mandible can be seen. In a neutral position, it overlies the lower cervical spine; with flexion, it moves over the upper thoracic spine; and, with extension, it moves above C_4 or off of the film.[59]

If the distal portion or tip of the tube should appear to bow or bend toward the right mainstem bronchus, this may also indicate a low position in patients where the carina cannot be easily visualized (Fig. 2-14). Bowing may also create an increase in the lateral wall pressure, leading to wall erosion. Erosion into the innominate artery will produce massive hemorrhage and exsanguination is a real possibility with long-term intubation or with tracheostomy.[60]

Ideally, the diameter of the tube should be one-half to two-thirds the width of the trachea. Wider tubes increase the incidence of laryngeal injury and smaller tubes have an increased airway resistance.[61] Overinflation of the balloon cuff, which may be seen radiographically as a widening or bulging of the tracheal air column near the tube tip, will likewise lead to erosion or later tracheal stenosis due to mucosal ischemia (Fig. 2-47 and see Fig. 2-52).

Overinsertion of an endotracheal tube usually results in right mainstem bronchus intubation, since the angle of takeoff of the right bronchus is more in

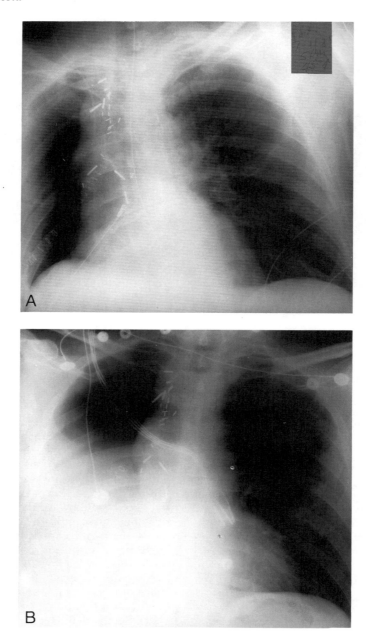

Fig. 2-46. Selected films from a series of examinations on a patient's status after recent pneumonectomy demonstrate the variations in quantity and appearance of fluid and air within the hemithorax. **(A)** This film obtained immediately after the right pneumonectomy reveals mild mediastinal shift toward the right, and primarily air without fluid in the right chest. **(B)** Two days later, fluid is seen accumulating in the right chest. The lack of an air-fluid level reflects the supine position of the patient. (*Figure continues.*)

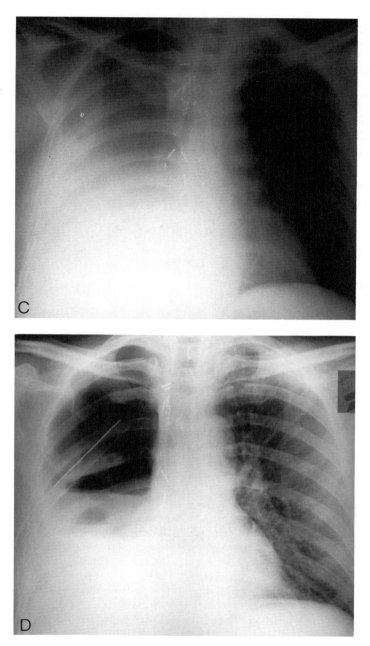

Fig. 2-46 (*Continued*). **(C)** A day later, further fluid has accumulated in the right hemithorax and the mediastinum is relatively midline. An upright film at this time would show a large air-fluid level in the apex of the hemithorax. Slowly, as air and fluid are completely reabsorbed from the pleural space over the next few weeks, there will be total opacity from fibrosis and a marked mediastinal shift into the right chest. **(D)** However, in this patient, now 1 week postoperative, a significant increase in air suggested a bronchopleural fistula and a chest tube was placed.

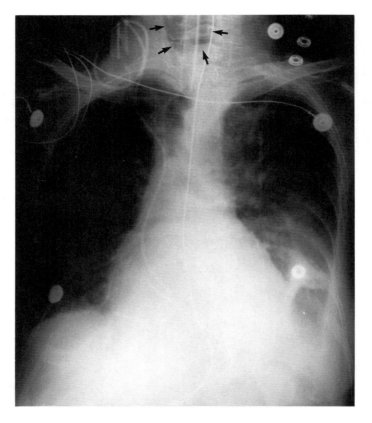

Fig. 2-47. There is malplacement of several monitoring and life support devices in this study. The endotracheal tube is somewhat high (tip at T₂), with marked overinflation of the cuff (*arrows*) in the neck. Also note the redundant Swan-Ganz catheter in the right atrium, and the redundant nasogastric tube in a previously known esophageal diverticulum.

continuity with the trachea, while the left is at a more acute angle. The radiographic findings depend on the degree of overinsertion, the duration of the misplacement, and the concentration of the inspired oxygen. Typically, varying degrees of left lung atelectasis are seen (Fig. 2-14). If the tube is low enough, the right upper lobe bronchus will also be occluded, producing right upper lobe as well as entire left lung collapse. There will be compensatory overinflation of the right middle and the right lower lobes. Following repositioning of an overinserted endotracheal tube, atelectatic segments should slowly re-expand. There may, however, be some continued opacity to the reexpanding lobe or lung for several hours to a few days. A complication of long-term lobar or total lung atelectasis or collapse would, of course, be superimposed infection. In right mainstem or bronchus intermedius intubation, because the entire tidal volume is directed at only two or three lobes, the chances of barotrauma with resulting tension pneumothorax are significantly increased, and the film should be carefully searched for signs of extra-alveolar air.[62]

A tube that is not placed deeply enough will predispose to accidental extubation. Also, if the cuff is inflated at the level of the cords (Fig. 2-47) there may be subsequent complications of ulceration and scarring. If the tube is high enough, it may be entirely excluded on the chest film and, to the unsuspecting radiologist, this will be dismissed simply as interval intentional extubation. Therefore, those who know the supposed clinical status of life-supportive devices have a special obligation to check their placement on every film reviewed.

Complications associated with intubation include aspiration or ingestion of dislodged teeth. If aspirated, they may produce atelectasis or even a ball-valve-type emphysema. Overpenetrated films are helpful in identifying their location for later removal. Unintentional esophageal intubation may produce sufficient gastric distention that decompression with a nasogastric tube is usually advisable to prevent possible spontaneous rupture and to improve diaphragmatic movement.[63] If traumatic tracheal or esophageal intubation is suspected, close observation for developing

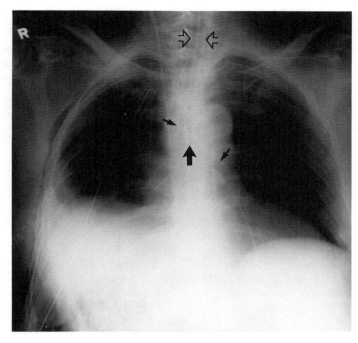

Fig. 2-48. The Robertshaw double-lumen tube is properly positioned in this patient, after partial right lung resection. Note the double-lumen tube seen through the upper trachea (*open arrows*), and the position of the carina (*large arrow*). The inferior tip of each lumen is defined by a radiopaque marker (*small arrows*). Both lungs are being adequately ventilated.

subcutaneous or mediastinal air is imperative. Undiagnosed esophageal rupture may lead to severe and often fatal mediastinitis.

Double-Lumen Endotracheal Tubes

Double-lumen endotracheal tubes greatly facilitate anesthesia when it is necessary to achieve independent control of the ventilation of each lung. Several tube designs exist. Figure 2-48 illustrates proper placement of a Robertshaw tube. The double-lumen is radiographically visible through the tracheal air column. Radiopaque markers define the terminal extent of each lumen. When correctly placed, the tip of the tracheal portion lies 1 to 2 cm above the carina, and the tip of the bronchial portion is inserted sufficiently far into the "appropriate" main bronchus for the endotracheal cuff to seal that bronchus without projecting unduly across the carinal region or occluding the orifice of the upper lobe bronchus on that side.[64]

Complications of malplacement are primarily related to inadvertent bronchial blockage (atelectasis of a lobe) or focal overexpansion (emphysema of a lobe). When evaluating placement of a double-lumen tube on an intraoperative portable film, it is important to compare the relative radiolucency of the upper to the

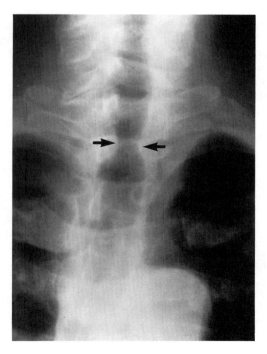

Fig. 2-49. This coned-down view of the tracheal air shadow reveals a stenosis (*arrows*) at the site of a previous tracheostomy stoma.

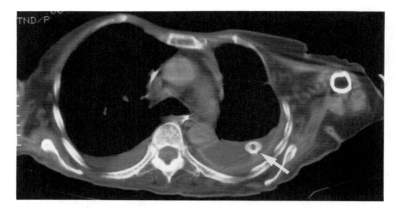

Fig. 2-50. CT scan reveals a chest tube (*arrow*) correctly positioned within a pleural fluid collection.

lower lobes. If a discrepancy exists, this may indicate poor placement. Inadvertent overventilation of a lung segment can lead to barotrauma with complications of extra-alveolar air, as discussed previously.

Tracheostomy

Tracheostomy tubes are usually opaque enough to allow fairly easy localization. The tip should ideally be one-half to two-thirds the distance between the stoma and the carina, usually around T_3 or T_4. Again, the tube width should be approximately two-thirds the tracheal diameter and the cuff should not bulge the lateral tracheal walls.[65] If a lateral view is obtainable, the tip should be pointing inferiorly and not posteriorly touching the posterior tracheal wall, which can lead to erosion and subsequent tracheo-esophageal fistula, or anteriorly leading to tracheo-innominate artery fistula.[59,66] Small amounts of subcutaneous air are common immediately following insertion. If the stoma is tightly sutured or packed, this air may, with positive-pressure ventilation, dissect into the mediastinum. Severe air leakage may indicate an improperly placed tube in the paratracheal soft tissues. Pneumothorax after tracheostomy can result from direct puncture of the lung apex at the time of insertion, from stomal air leak with pneumomediastinum or from respirator-induced pulmonary barotrauma. Mediastinal widening after tracheostomy is usually secondary to hemorrhage and should be followed closely until it stabilizes. Late complications of intubation or tracheostomy are secondary tracheal stenosis or tracheal malacia (Fig. 2-49), usually at the cuff or stomal site.[67]

Nasogastric Tubes

Large-caliber nasogastric tubes typically have a radiopaque marker running the length of the tubing. Small-caliber feeding tubes without markers may be almost invisible through the mediastinum. Newer models have a dense, 5 cm marker only at their distal tip.

Proper placement is usually clinically apparent; however, when gastric contents cannot be aspirated, tip localization can best be assessed on an overpenetrated chest or thoracoabdominal view. The gastric air bubble should be analyzed on each chest film, particularly after intubation or left lung resection, so that marked or progressive gastric dilatation can be promptly treated with nasogastric tube placement to avoid gastric ischemia and rupture.

Pleural Drainage Tubes

Most chest tubes have a radiopaque stripe along their length. The side hole is marked by a discontinuity in the stripe; this should be within the chest wall for proper drainage. Subcutaneous air is common immediately after placement, but increasing air may indicate poor position of the side hole. In the supine or semierect patient, intrapleural air collects anteriorly and superiorly, while fluid layers in the posterior gutters. Therefore, the optimal position for drainage is posterior and inferior for a hydrothorax and anterior and superior for a pneumothorax. For true localization of these tubes, a lateral film is needed, especially if it is suspected that the tubing may be tracking along the anterior or posterior chest wall outside the pleural space. If the patient is bedridden, a cross-table lateral film can be obtained when an erect lateral is not possible.

Unsuccessful pleural drainage by a chest tube may indicate improper tube placement or loculation of fluid. CT is extremely useful in determining if a chest tube is correctly located within a pleural fluid collection (Fig. 2-50).[54]

Minor pleural or parenchymal contusion along tube tracts is common. Occasionally, curvilinear pleural

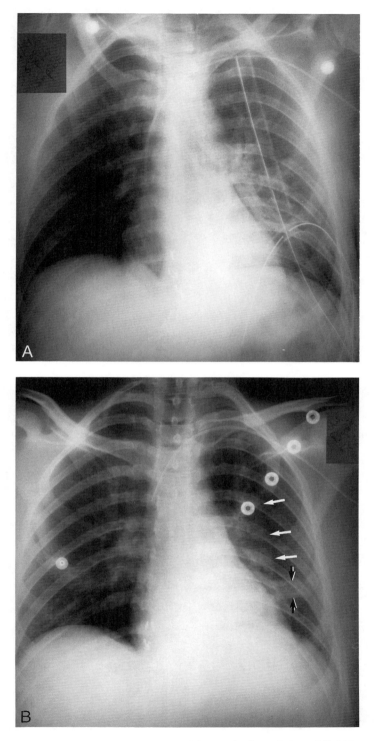

Fig. 2-51. **(A)** Two left chest tubes are properly placed for aspiration of air and fluid in a supine patient. **(B)** After the chest tubes were removed, pleural reaction along the tube tracts produced bands of density (*arrows*) that could be confused for a pleural margin in a pneumothorax or an infiltrate. Note also the proper CVP placement in this patient.

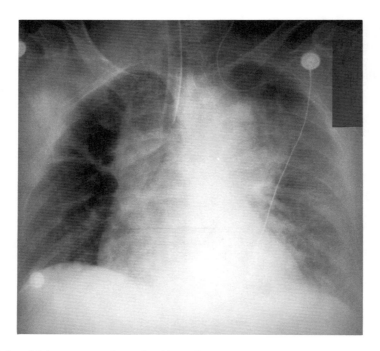

Fig. 2-52. The left brachial venous catheter in this patient was advanced into the neck veins instead of the superior vena cava, producing inaccurate CVP readings. Also note the oval radiolucency surrounding the distal end of the endotracheal tube. This represents a slightly overinflated cuff bulging the lateral tracheal walls.

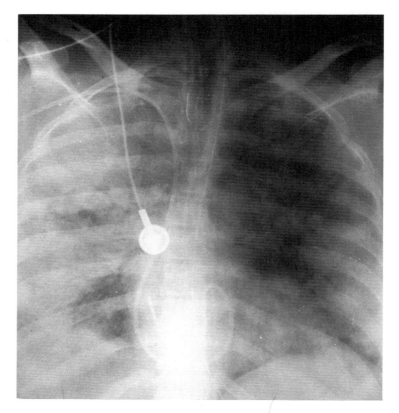

Fig. 2-53. The Swan-Ganz catheter is coiled in the right heart, increasing the chances of myocardial irritation and dysrhythmias.

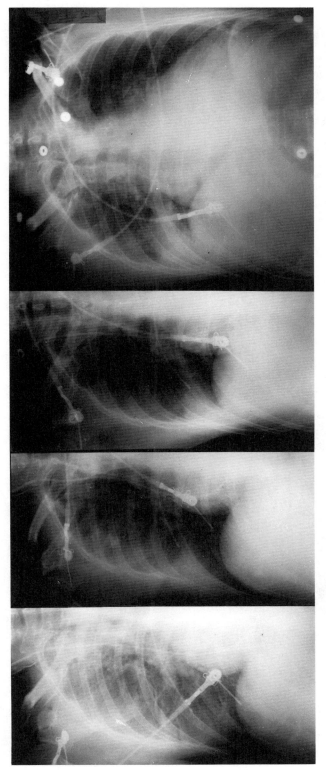

Fig. 2-54. A series of films over a 2-day period demonstrates a peripherally placed Swan-Ganz catheter within the right lung. The developing wedge-shaped, pleural-based infiltrate represents pulmonary infarction secondary to direct arterial occlusion by the catheter tip. (From Kaplan,[79] with permission.)

73

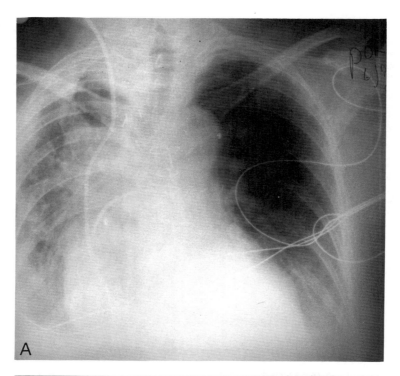

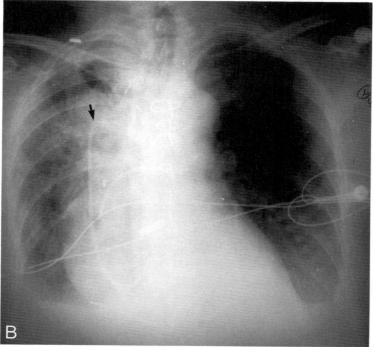

Fig. 2-55. (A) The Swan-Ganz catheter in this patient became tethered in the heart and could not be pulled free for removal. **(B)** It was, therefore, transected at the skin and allowed to retract inside the patient. The arrow marks the free proximal end in the superior vena cava. It did not migrate because of its firm attachment. Except in unusual circumstances such as this, catheter fragments loose in the veins or heart are, of course, to be strictly avoided as they will embolize to the lungs. Retrieval of loose fragments can often be accomplished by experienced angiographers using catheters, thereby avoiding further surgery.

tube tracts may simulate a pneumothorax after tube removal (Fig. 2-31C). Identifying pulmonary markings peripheral to the tube tract will avoid this confusion. If these cannot be identified, a film in forced expiration may be necessary to differentiate pneumothorax from pleural reaction. A wide tube tract may fill with fluid and appear as a band of density (Fig. 2-51). Enlarging tracts may indicate secondary infection or empyema.[65]

Central Venous Pressure Catheters

To accurately reflect central venous or right heart pressures, a catheter should ideally be positioned in the superior vena cava or right atrium so that it is proximal to any peripheral valves. Insertion of a central venous pressure (CVP) catheter directly into the internal jugular vein should accurately reflect central pressures, since there are no valves between the internal jugular vein and right heart. Although some estimation of location can be suggested by the length of tubing advanced from a certain cutaneous insertion site, kinking and misdirection are frequent enough that radiographic evaluation may be advisable whenever these catheters are placed. This is particularly advisable whenever there are unsatisfactory readings, a lack of good blood return, or suspected complications. However, fluctuations of the fluid column and ability to freely aspirate blood are not always reliable signs of proper placement, as has been frequently reported. In fact, in one prospective study, it was shown that approximately one-third of CVP catheters were incorrectly placed at the time of original insertion.[68]

The major complication from aberrant placement is mismanagement of the patient's fluids on the basis of erroneous CVP readings. This happens commonly when the tip advances into other peripheral veins, rather than into the central venous system. Typical aberrant locations include (1) a brachial or subclavian catheter going to the contralateral side or into the jugular veins (Fig. 2-52), (2) a jugular catheter going into the ipsilateral or contralateral subclavian, or (3) overinsertion into the inferior vena cava and even the hepatic veins. Besides problems with erroneous measurements, overinsertion may lead to right heart catheterization. Intracardiac positioning can lead to myocardial irritation, producing dysrhythmias and even perforation. Central venous pressure catheters have been reported extending into peripheral pulmonary artery branches. Infusion of significant amounts of fluid through these catheters can result in unilateral pulmonary edema.[69]

The percutaneous subclavian approach, because of its close proximity to the lung apex, has the added potential complication of iatrogenic pneumothorax. If this is suspected, an immediate chest film, preferably erect and in expiration, is recommended; it is imperative before attempting puncture on the opposite side because of the possibility of creating bilateral pneumothoraces. Also, a not infrequent complication of the subclavian approach is infusion of fluid into the pleural space or mediastinum (Fig. 2-38). This will mimic intrathoracic hemorrhage. When faced with a rapidly increasing effusion or mediastinal widening in a patient with a central venous catheter, particularly a subclavian catheter, malposition can be easily confirmed by injecting water-soluble contrast material through the catheter during chest film exposure.[70] This will avoid further unnecessary angiographic or surgical procedures.

Pulmonary Arterial Catheters

Pulmonary arterial catheters are radiographically distinguishable from other venous catheters by a radiopaque stripe down the center. Ideally, the catheter should traverse the right atrium and right ventri-

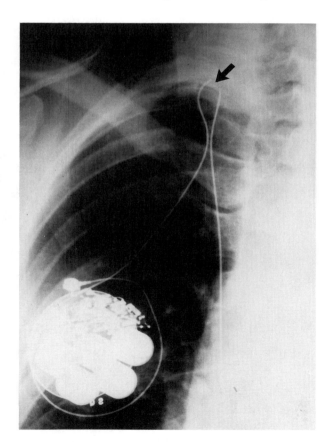

Fig. 2-56. Sharp angulation of the pacemaker lead predisposes to breakage, usually adjacent to a site of firm attachment as shown here. (From Mansour,[80] with permission.)

cle without redundancy or slack. The tip should lie in the right or left main pulmonary artery or their major descending branches, except when wedge pressure readings are being obtained (Fig. 2-33). Misdirection during insertion is less frequent than with other venous catheters, due to the flow-directed balloon. Redundancy within cardiac chambers will increase the incidence of myocardial irritation and dysrhythmias (Fig. 2-53). Also, with slack, the catheter tends to drift ''downstream'' and wedge unnecessarily.

The most significant complication is pulmonary infarction as a result of clot formation on the catheter with pulmonary embolization, or with occlusion of a pulmonary artery by the catheter itself.[71] This will happen when the tip remains in a peripheral vessel for an extended length of time or if the balloon, seen as a 1 cm radiolucency at the tip of the catheter, remains inadvertently inflated. If the catheter tip is seen projecting more than a few centimeters lateral to the cardiac silhouette when wedge pressure readings are not being taken, it is too peripheral and arterial occlusion may more likely occur. Although a tip projecting in or near the hilum would seem, at first glance, to be in a vessel large enough to make infarction unlikely, the catheter may be radiographically ''foreshortened'' in the AP projection with the tip actually in a small arterial branch. Development of an infiltrate around a peripherally located tip is indicative of an infarction (Fig. 2-54), although infarction has been reported at autopsy without previously recognized infiltrate.

Other complications, such as pulmonary artery perforation with hemorrhage or intracardiac knotting, have been reported.[72] Rarely, the pulmonary arterial catheter may become tethered in the heart, preventing easy removal (Fig. 2-55).

Transvenous Pacemakers

Proper placement of a transvenous pacemaker is best accomplished under fluoroscopic guidance. If this is not feasible, follow-up films are recommended to assure proper placement. While clinical assessment of proper pacing usually assures a good location of the electrode in the right ventricular apex, radiographs can best evaluate the course of the lead. Sharp angulation of the lead should be avoided, as this predisposes to breakage (Fig. 2-56).[73] Breakage is most common at a flexion point adjacent to a location where the lead is firmly stabilized.[74] A break may be obvious on x-ray examination, but failure to demonstrate a break radiographically does not exclude its presence, as the insulating sheath may hold the broken ends together.[73] As with central venous and pulmonary arterial catheters, excess slack increases myocardial irritation and predisposes to migration (Fig. 2-57).

If clinical evidence suggests that the electrode is in an aberrant location, both frontal and lateral films may be needed to localize it. On AP or PA projection, the tip may appear to be in the right ventricular apex, while on a lateral view it is seen in the posterior por-

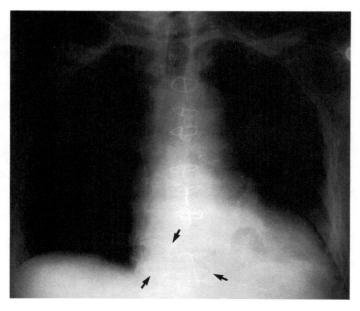

Fig. 2-57. This transvenous pacer lead is coiled in the right heart (*arrows*). Slack such as this predisposes to myocardial irritation and migration.

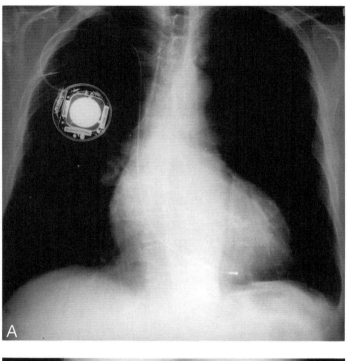

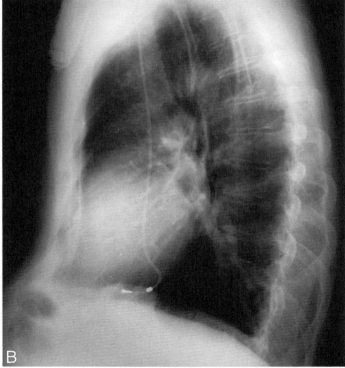

Fig. 2-58. (A) Radiographically, this pacer electrode appears to be in the right ventricular apex on this PA projection. Clinically, the electrode was not pacing adequately. **(B)** A lateral view of the same patient reveals the posterior location of the electrode within the cardiac silhouette. It is, therefore, not within the right ventricle but probably within the coronary venous system.

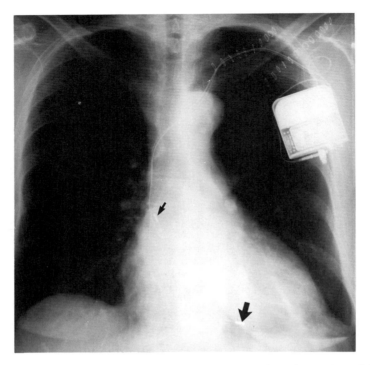

Fig. 2-59. An AV sequential pacemaker has been properly placed in this patient. The atrial electrode location is indicated (*small arrow*), and the ventricular electrode is seen in the right ventricular apex (*large arrow*).

tion of the heart, as in Figure 2-58. This posterior location usually implies placement within the coronary venous system.[73]

When ventricular pacing alone is not producing sufficient cardiac output, atrioventricular sequential pacing may be appropriate. Figure 2-59 illustrates proper placement of both atrial and ventricular leads.

Besides lead breakage and aberrant electrode placement within the heart and vessels, radiographic evidence of complications includes perforation of vessels or the myocardium. Figure 2-60 illustrates fluoroscopic confirmation of myocardial perforation, and Figure 2-61 demonstrates vessel perforation with subsequent intrathoracic but extracardiac electrode placement. With perforation or suspected injury to vessels, the radiograph should be assessed for mediastinal enlargement from hemorrhage. Superior vena caval syndrome has been reported following pacer insertion.[75] Finally, when managing patients with preexisting pacemakers, radiographs can identify the generator model and type of electrode.[76]

SUMMARY

The successful approach to chest radiology lies (1) in understanding why you see what you see in terms of radiographic density, (2) in understanding the limitations imposed on visualizing and assessing pathology due to altered techniques (the bedside portable) and the ways to circumvent these limitations in using serial films to develop a temporal sequence of a disease, and (3) in systematically scanning each part of the chest, and each tube and catheter on every film.

Finally, cooperation and communication among the various clinicians (anesthesiologist, surgeon, intensivist) and the radiologist is important. Expert interpretation without history is certainly by definition objective, but isolation of radiographic findings from other data is not in the best interest of the patient. Conversely, review of a film in light of clinical bias may produce "tunnel vision," resulting in mismanagement or overtreatment. A seemingly insignificant objective finding may take on real value within a certain clinical setting, just as a worrisome density in prejudiced eyes may dissolve into normal overlapping structures when viewed with objectivity.

The optimal approach to a film is, therefore, to view it once with objectivity and once with clinical correlation. Individually, of course, this takes discipline and strict adherence to a systematic approach. Two pairs of eyes and two points of view are often more enlightening than one. Although it is usually not routinely possible to have a team approach or joint reading of all films, when faced with a difficult or confusing clin-

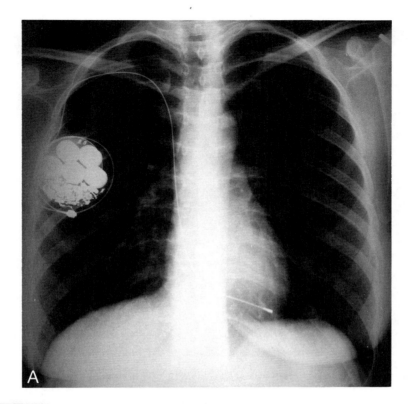

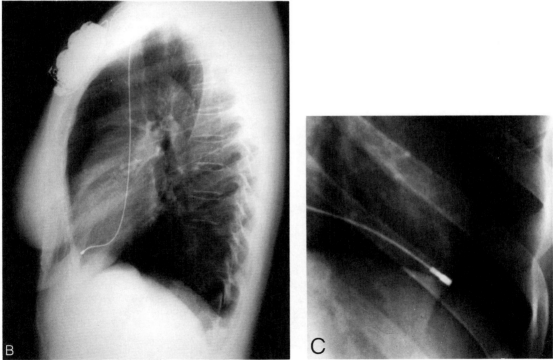

Fig. 2-60. The right ventricular electrode in this patient was felt to be too laterally positioned on the PA view **(A)** and possibly too anteriorly positioned on the lateral view **(B)**. **(C)** Fluoroscopy with spot films made in various obliquities confirmed the suspicion of myocardial perforation. Note the tip of the electrode at the surface of the cardiac silhouette.

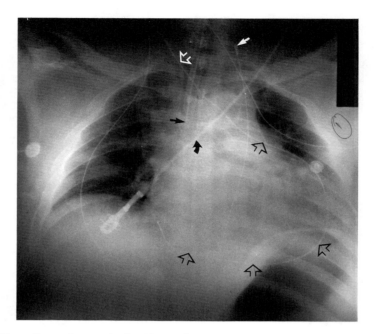

Fig. 2-61. This portable radiograph was obtained immediately after attempted placement of multiple monitoring and life support devices in a seriously ill patient who had just suffered a massive myocardial infarction. The endotracheal tube tip (*small black arrow*) is low, just above the carina (*curved black arrow*). The transvenous pacemaker lead (*open arrows*) apparently perforated a vessel in the superior mediastinum and is seen coursing in an unusual configuration around the cardiac silhouette. A lateral view (not shown) confirmed the intrathoracic but extracardiac location of the lead. The aortic counterpulsation balloon catheter is also improperly positioned. Its tip (*white arrow*) is quite superior to the normal location, the proximal descending aorta, and may be in either the carotid or vertebral artery. Also note the moderate gastric dilation, postresuscitation, in this patient.

ical or radiologic picture, direct consultation can be immensely profitable.

REFERENCES

1. Squire LF: Introduction and basic concepts. pp. 1–13. In Squire LF (ed): Fundamentals of Roentgenology. Harvard University Press, Cambridge, 1971
2. Felson B: Localization of intrathoracic lesions. pp. 22–70. In Felson B (ed): Chest Roentgenology. WB Saunders, Philadelphia, 1973
3. Squire LF: How to study a chest film. pp. 30–45. In Squire LF (ed): Fundamentals of Roentgenology. Harvard University Press, Cambridge, 1971
4. Hamilton WK: Atelectasis, pneumothorax, and aspiration as postoperative complications. Anesthesiology 22:708–722, 1961
5. Goodman LR: Cardiopulmonary disorders. pp. 93–147. In Goodman LR, Putman CE (eds): Intensive Care Radiology: Imaging of the Critically Ill. CV Mosby, St. Louis, 1978
6. McCauley RGK: Radiology in respiratory intensive care unit. Int Anesthesiol Clin 14:1–29, 1976
7. Benjamin JJ, Cascade PN, Rubenfire M, et al: Left lower lobe atelectasis and consolidation following cardiac surgery: the effect of topical cooling on the phrenic nerve. Radiology 142:11–14, 1982
8. Stevens RM, Teres D, Skillman JJ, Feingold DS: Pneumonia in an intensive care unit. Arch Intern Med 134:106–111, 1974
9. Hirschman JV, Murray JF: Pneumonia and lung abscess. pp. 1075–1081. In Braunwald E, Isselbacher KJ, Petersdorf RG (eds): Harrison's Principles of Internal Medicine. McGraw-Hill, New York, 1987
10. Fraser RG, Paré JAP: Diagnosis of Diseases of the Chest: An Integrated Study Based on the Abnormal Roentgenogram. pp. 590–605. WB Saunders, Philadelphia, 1970
11. Renner RR, Coccaro AP, Heitzman ER, et al: Pseudomonas pneumonia: a prototype of hospital based infection. Radiology 105:555–562, 1972
12. Joffe N: Roentgenologic aspects of primary pseudomonas aeruginosa pneumonia in mechanically ventilated patients. AJR 107:305–312, 1969
13. De Weese JA, Stewart S III: Pulmonary complications of nonpulmonary intrathoracic surgery. pp. 215–234. In Cordell AR, Ellison RG (eds): Complications of Intrathoracic Surgery. Little Brown, Boston, 1979

14. Westcott JL, Rudick MG: Cardiopulmonary effects of intravenous fluid overload: radiologic manifestations. Radiology 129:577–585, 1978

15. Chait A, Cohen HE, Meltzer LE, et al: The bedside chest radiograph in the evaluation of incipient heart failure. Radiology 105:563–566, 1972

16. Logue RB, Rogers JV, Gay BB, Jr: Subtle roentgenographic signs of left heart failure. Am Heart J 65:464–473, 1963

17. Preger L, Hooper TI, Steinbach HL, et al: Width of azygos vein related to central venous pressure. Radiology 93:521–523, 1969

18. Grainger RG: Interstitial edema and its radiological diagnosis: a sign of pulmonary venous and capillary hypertension. Br J Radiol 31:201–217, 1958

19. Harrison MO, Conte PJ, Heitzman ER: Radiological detection of clinically occult cardiac failure following myocardial infarction. Br J Radiol 44:265–272, 1971

20. McHugh TJ, Forrester JS, Adler L, et al: Pulmonary vascular congestion in acute myocardial infarction: hemodynamic and radiologic correlations. Ann Intern Med 76:29–33, 1972

21. Huglitz UF, Shapiro JH: Atypical pulmonary patterns of congestive failure in chronic lung disease. Radiology 93:995–1006, 1969

22. Calenoff L, Kruglik GD, Woodruff A: Unilateral pulmonary edema. Radiology 126:19–24, 1978

23. Mendelson CL: Aspiration of stomach contents into the lungs during obstetric anesthesia. Am J Obstet Gynecol 52:191–205, 1946

24. Gynum LJ, Pierce AK: Pulmonary aspiration of gastric contents. Am Rev Respir Dis 114:1129–1136, 1976

25. Wilkins RA, DeLacey GJ, Flor R, et al: Radiology in Mendelson's syndrome. Clin Radiol 27:81–85, 1976

26. Tomashefski JF, Mahajan V: Managing respiratory distress syndrome in adults. Postgrad Med 59:77–82, 1976

27. Blaisdell RW, Schlobohm RM: The respiratory distress syndrome: a review. Surgery 74:251–262, 1973

28. Putman CE, Ravin CE: Adult respiratory distress syndrome. pp. 148–162. In Goodman LR, Putman CE (eds): Intensive Care Radiology: Imaging of the Critically Ill. CV Mosby, St. Louis, 1978

29. Joffe N: The adult respiratory distress syndrome. AJR 122:719–732, 1974

30. Petty TL, Asbaugh DG: The adult respiratory distress syndrome: clinical features, factors influencing prognosis and principles of management. Chest 60:233–239, 1971

31. Putman CE, Minagi H, Blaisdel FW: The roentgen appearance of disseminated intravascular coagulation (DIC). Radiology 109:13–18, 1973

32. Robboy SJ, Minna JD, Colman RW, et al: Pulmonary hemorrhage syndrome as a manifestation of disseminated intravascular coagulation: analysis of ten cases. Chest 63:718–721, 1973

33. Fraser RG, Paré JAP: Embolic and thrombotic diseases of the lungs. pp. 804–831. In Fraser RG, Paré JAP (eds): Diagnosis of Diseases of the Chest: An Integrated Study Based on the Abnormal Roentgenogram. WB Saunders, Philadelphia, 1970

34. Neumann RD, Sostman HD, Gottschalk A: Current status of ventilation-perfusion imaging. Semin Nucl Med 10:198–217, 1980

35. Figley MM, Gerdes AJ, Ricketts HJ: Radiographic aspects of pulmonary embolism. Semin Roentgenol 2:389–405, 1967

36. Rohlfing BM, Webb WR, Schlobohm RM: Ventilator-related extra-alveolar air in adults. Radiology 121:25–31, 1976

37. Westcott JL, Cole SR: Interstitial pulmonary emphysema in children and adults: roentgenographic features. Radiology 111:367–378, 1974

38. Zimmerman JE, Goodman LR, Shahvari MBG: Effect of mechanical ventilation and positive end-expiratory pressure (PEEP) on the chest radiograph. AJR 133:811–816, 1979

39. Leeming BWA: Radiological aspects of the pulmonary complications resulting from intermittent positive-pressure ventilation (IPPV). Australas Radiol 12:361–374, 1968

40. Swischuk LE: Two lesser known but useful signs of neonatal pneumothorax. AJR 127:623–627, 1976

41. Steckel RJ: The radiolucent kinetic borderline in acute pulmonary edema and pneumonia. Clin Radiol 25:391–395, 1974

42. Kurlander GJ, Helmenn CH: Subpulmonary pneumothorax. AJR 96:1019–1021, 1966

43. Lams PM, Jolles H: The effect of lobar collapse on the distribution of free intrapleural air. Radiology 142:309–312, 1982

44. Gordon R: The deep sulcus sign. Radiology 136:25–27, 1980

45. Gobien RP, Reines HD, Schabel SI: Localized tension pneumothorax: unrecognized form of barotrauma in adult respiratory distress syndrome. Radiology 142:15–19, 1982

46. Humphreys RL, Berne AS: Rapid re-expansion of pneumothorax: a cause of unilateral pulmonary edema. Radiology 96:509–512, 1970

47. Hipona FA, Paredes S, Lerona PT: Roentgenologic analysis of common postoperative problems in congenital heart disease. Radiol Clin North Am 9:229–251, 1971

48. Baron RL, Levitt RG, Sagel SS, Stanley RJ: Computed tomography in the evaluation of mediastinal widening. Radiology 138:107–113, 1981

49. Egan TJ, Neiman HL, Herman RJ, et al: Computed tomography in the diagnosis of aortic aneurysm dissection or traumatic injury. Radiology 136:141–146, 1980

50. Geisinger MA, Risius B, O'Donnell JA, et al: Thoracic aortic dissections: magnetic resonance imaging. Radiology 155:407–412, 1985

51. Melamed M, Hipona FA, Reynes CJ, et al: The Adult Postoperative Chest. p. 307. Charles C. Thomas, Springfield, 1977

52. Friedman PJ, Hellekant ACG: Diagnosis of air-fluid levels in the thorax: radiologic recognition of bronchopleural fistula. Am Rev Respir Dis 113:159–160, 1976

53. Schachter EN, Kreisman H, Putman CE: Diagnostic problems in suppurative lung disease. Arch Intern Med 136:167–171, 1976

54. Sagel SS, Glazer HS: Lung, pleura, and chest wall. pp. 295–386. In Lee JKT, Sagel SS, Stanley R (eds): Computed Body Tomography with MRI Correlation. Raven Press, New York, 1989

55. Baber CEJ, Hedlund LW, Oddson TA, et al: Differentiating empyemas and peripheral pulmonary abscesses. The value of computed tomography. Radiology 135:755–758, 1980

56. Ellis K, Malm JR, Bowman FO, et al: Roentgenographic findings after pericardial surgery. Radiol Clin North Am 9:327–341, 1971

57. Melamed M, Hipona FA, Reynes CJ, et al: Air-fluid in the pleural space. pp. 33–208. In Melamed M, Hipona FA, Reynes CJ, et al (eds): The Adult Postoperative Chest. Charles C. Thomas, Springfield, 1977

58. Conrardy PA, Goodman LR, Laing F, et al: Alterations of endotracheal tube position—flexion and extension of the neck. Crit Care Med 4:8–12, 1976

59. Goodman LR, Conrardy PA, Laing F, et al: Radiographic evaluation of endotracheal tube position. AJR 127:433–434, 1976

60. Lane EE, Temes GD, Anderson WH: Tracheal-innominate artery fistula due to tracheostomy. Chest 68:678–683, 1975

61. Pontoppidan H, Geffin B, Lowenstein E: Acute respiratory failure in the adult. N Engl J Med 287:690–698, 1972

62. Zwillich CW, Pierson DJ, Creagh CE, et al: Complications of assisted ventilation. Am J Med 57:161–170, 1974

63. Sellery GR: Airway problems in the intensive care unit. Int Anesthesiol Clin 10:173–213, 1972

64. Black AMS, Harrison GA: Difficulties with positioning Robertshaw double-lumen tubes. Anaesth Intensive Care 3:299–311, 1975

65. Goodman LR: Pulmonary support and monitoring apparatus. pp. 29–63. In Goodman LR, Putman CE (eds): Intensive Care Radiology: Imaging of the Critically Ill. CV Mosby, St. Louis, 1978

66. Harley HRS: Ulcerative tracheo-oesophageal fistula during treatment by tracheostomy and intermittent positive-pressure ventilation. Thorax 27:338–352, 1972

67. Mulder DS, Rubush JL: Complications of tracheostomy: relationship to long-term ventilatory assistance. J Trauma 9:389–401, 1969

68. Langston CS: The aberrant central venous catheter and its complications. Radiology 100:55–59, 1971

69. Royal HD, Shields JB, Donati RM: Misplacement of central venous pressure catheters and unilateral pulmonary edema. Arch Intern Med 135:1502–1505, 1975

70. Ravin CE, Putman CE, McLoud TC: Hazards of the ICU. AJR 126:423–431, 1976

71. Roote GA, Schabel SI, Hodges M: Pulmonary complications of the flow-directed balloon-tipped catheter. N Engl J Med 290:927–931, 1974

72. Kaplan JA: pp. 85–93. In Kaplan JA (ed): Cardiac Anesthesia. Grune & Stratton, Orlando, FL, 1979

73. Hall WM, Rosenbaum HD: The radiology of cardiac pacemakers. Radiol Clin North Am 9:343–353, 1971

74. Rosenbaum HD: Roentgen demonstration of broken cardiac pacemaker wires. Radiology 84:933–936, 1965

75. Chamorro H, Rao G, Wholey MH: Superior vena cava syndrome: a complication of transvenous pacemaker implantation. Radiology 126:377–378, 1978

76. Chun PKC: Characteristics of commonly utilized permanent endocardial and epicardial pacemaker electrode systems: method of radiologic identification. Am Heart J 102:404–414, 1981

77. Shapiro JH, Hublitz UF: CRC Critical Review. Clin Radiol Nucl Med 5:389, 1974

78. Squire LF, Ettinger A: Basic Diagnostic Radiology Self-instructional Seminars. Programmed Seminars, New York, 1973

79. Kaplan JA: Hemodynamic monitoring. p. 94. In Kaplan JA (ed): Cardiac Anesthesia. Grune & Stratton, Orlando, FL, 1979

80. Mansour K: Complications of cardiac pacemakers. Am Surg 43:132, 1977

3

PREPARATION OF THE PATIENT WITH CHRONIC PULMONARY DISEASE

H. Michael Marsh, M.M.M.B.
Anita V. Guffin, M.M.S.

Survival analysis of surgical patients suggests that the major factors determining risk are age and the extent of surgical disease and dissection, balanced against physiologic reserves in the cardiopulmonary, renal, and metabolic systems, as well as the immune competence of the individual patient. Data from Knaus et al[1,2] support this conclusion, and Goldman demonstrated that associated chronic disease or emergency surgery further increases risk.[3] The risk of morbidity and mortality is also increased in thoracic surgery when the surgical lesion or the planned surgical procedure limits functional reserves or leads to the development of a secondary pneumonia or abscess.

In a study of 110,000 consecutive elective operations, chronic pulmonary disease (CPD) was second only to cardiovascular disease (CVD) in incidence, and the two were frequently associated.[4] This is not surprising, since smoking is a common etiologic factor, and smoking-related CPD is the most common of the diseases grouped under the category of chronic airway obstruction. In the series of Fowkes et al,[4] CVD was present in 22 percent, CPD in 20 percent, renal disease in 3 percent, and diabetes in 1 percent of the patients. The mortality for the population of normal patients without chronic disease in the series was 0.5 percent, while the mortality rates for patients with chronic disease were 15 percent with CVD associated with congestive heart failure (CHF), 11 percent with renal failure, 5 percent with chronic bronchitis, and 5 percent with diabetes. Alhough the presence of CVD with concurrent CHF resulted in the greatest increase in mortality, the presence of chronic bronchitis promoted an increased risk in a higher percentage of the overall population.

The incidence of postoperative pulmonary complications varies from 3 to 70 percent.[5] Studies have shown that optimal preoperative preparation can reduce this morbidity. Gracey et al reported the effects of a standardized preoperative pulmonary regimen on preoperative pulmonary function tests.[6] The regimen resulted in an improvement in lung function and the incidence of pulmonary complications was signifi-

TABLE 3-1. Pulmonary Complications in Prepared (Group A) vs. Unprepared Patients (Group B)

Operative Site	N	No. Patients with Pulmonary Complications	Severity of Complications			
			1+ Least	2+	3+	4+ Worst
Group A						
Thorax	17	4	3	1	0	0
Abdomen	5	1	1	0	0	0
Other	1	0	0	0	0	0
Total	23	5	4	1	0	0
Group B						
Thorax	17	13	1	3	5	4
Abdomen	3	1	0	0	1	0
Other	5	1	0	1	0	0
Total	25	15	1	4	6	4

(From Stein et al,[7] with permission.)

cantly decreased. Patients requiring respiratory support could be predicted based on the degree of preoperative pulmonary disease and a minimal response to the preoperative preparatory regimen.

In a group of patients with abnormal lung function, Stein et al found that 60 percent of the patients who did not receive preoperative preparation developed postoperative complications as compared to 22 percent of well-prepared patients.[7] Data from Tarhan et al in a series of 357 men with chronic obstructive pulmonary disease (COPD) demonstrated a 19 percent decrease in pulmonary complications with preoperative preparation, although no difference in overall mortality was found.[8] Multiple studies from the same institution support this finding, and the incidence of complications was greatest in patients undergoing upper abdominal and thoracic surgery (Table 3-1).[5–8]

The plan of the medical team dealing with the patient with CPD coming for thoracic surgery should be to reduce the risk as much as possible in the time available, and to place the patient into a program that, in conjunction with adequate postoperative pain relief, will maximize the speed of recovery and enhance postoperative function and exercise capacity. Thus, the pulmonary preparation for surgery encompasses the entire perioperative period, culminating in the continuance of pulmonary rehabilitation for as long as is beneficial.

There are 10 elements of the preoperative preparatory regimen which, following surgery and adequate recovery, should become the rehabilitative program. They are (1) patient and family education regarding the type of CPD present; (2) management of the reactive airway; (3) prevention of oxygen desaturation during sleep or activity; (4) respiratory muscle retraining for both strength and endurance; (5) exercise reconditioning; (6) treatment of cor pulmonale; (7) treatment of infection; (8) adequate pulmonary hygiene with the drainage and clearance of secretions; (9) adequate pain management; and (10) psychosocial management to modify behavior and increase the motivation to improve health.

The purpose of this chapter is to characterize the diseases classified as CPD, and to review their common physiologic consequences, along with those of the surgical lesion itself, and the planned thoracic surgical procedure. A program of evaluation and treatment of the thoracic surgical patient is also discussed.

CHRONIC PULMONARY DISEASE

Chronic pulmonary disease can be defined either as lung disease that causes persistent or progressive pulmonary dysfunction sufficient to limit exercise capacity and cause pulmonary hypertension, or as a disorder associated with chronic pulmonary or thoracic infection. Chronic pulmonary disease causes pathophysiologic changes decreasing the ability of the patient to withstand the stresses of anesthesia and surgery.

The diseases to be considered can be broadly grouped into four categories: (1) restrictive pulmonary diseases (eg, interstitial lung disease, diseases of the chest wall and mediastinum); (2) diseases associated with chronic airflow obstruction (eg, asthma, chronic bronchitis, emphysema, and bronchiectasis); (3) pulmonary vascular diseases excluding cor pulmonale associated with 1 or 2 (eg, primary pulmonary hypertension, pulmonary embolus); and (4) sleep-associated dysfunction excluding that seen with 1, 2, or 3 (obstructive and central sleep apnea). The etiology, natural history, pathophysiology, and management of these diseases are well described.[9,10]

PATHOPHYSIOLOGIC FEATURES OF CHRONIC PULMONARY DISEASE

Restrictive Disease

Restrictive pulmonary disease is usually due to processes that reduce the natural elasticity of the lung. The various etiologies can be divided into intrinsic or extrinsic restrictive disease, and the intrinsic form may be acute or chronic.[10]

Acute intrinsic restrictive pulmonary disease is most frequently manifestated as pulmonary edema (including neurogenic, high altitude, and opioid-induced forms). This is caused by injury to the pulmonary capillary endothelium or increases in pulmonary vascular pressures that result in the leakage of intravascular fluid into the lung. Aspiration pneumonitis and adult respiratory distress syndrome are other examples of acute intrinsic restrictive disease.[10]

Pulmonary fibrosis is the major characteristic of chronic intrinsic restrictive pulmonary disease. Progression can lead to loss of portions of the pulmonary vascular bed and the development of pulmonary hypertension with cor pulmonale. Spontaneous pneumothorax is commonly seen in the advanced stages of these diseases. Alveolar proteinosis, sarcoidosis, eosinophilia, and hypersensitivity pneumonitis fall into this category.

With extrinsic restrictive disease, the lungs are usually normal and the restriction is due to abnormalities of the pleura, thoracic cavity, or abdominal contents. The lungs are compressed, reducing lung volumes and increasing the work of breathing. This is primarily due to the abnormal, mechanical function of the chest and the increased airway resistance. Abnormalities in the chest wall may also compress the pulmonary vasculature, increasing pulmonary vascular resistance (PVR), and eventually leading to right ventricular dysfunction. Patients with extrinsic disease frequently have pulmonary infections due to the inability to produce a normal cough. These problems are seen in the presence of kyphoscoliosis, disorders of the pleura, pectus excavatum, and with abnormalities of the diaphragm such as those seen with pregnancy or obesity.[11] The restriction causes an increase in oxygen demand due to the excess work required to breath.

All types of restrictive pulmonary disease are characterized by a decrease in lung compliance. Respiratory flow rates are normal, but reductions in vital capacity and total lung volume are diagnostic of restrictive disease. Functional residual capacity is reduced toward closing volume resulting in chronic hypoxemia, and chronic hypocarbia is the end-product of the hyperventilation resulting from restrictive disease due to the characteristic breathing pattern of these patients.

Obstructive Disease

Contrary to the normal airflow seen in restrictive disease, an increased resistance to gas flow throughout the airway is seen with COPD. Patients with COPD demonstrate an increase in the size of the thoracic cavity and will likely exhibit wheezing upon exhalation.

A reactive airway and an element of reversible airway obstruction are common features of COPD. Bronchoconstriction as a result of smooth muscle contraction is the major rapidly reversible component, although vasoconstriction and reduction of edema and inflammation in the airway wall may also contribute to the relief of the obstruction, as may removal or thinning of secretions.

Changes in the transpulmonary pressure necessary to induce gas flow into and out of the lung alveoli are required to oppose both the elastic properties of the respiratory system and the flow-resistive properties of the airway.[12] Pulmonary resistance may be altered because of changes in either the airway resistance, tissue resistance, or both. Airflow obstruction can be increased by smooth muscle constriction of both large and small airways, by mucosal inflammation and edema, and/or by mucosal hypertrophy and excess mucous production with increased viscosity impeding clearance. Tissue resistance can be increased as a result of smooth muscle contraction,[13] and possibly by changes in the surfactant layer of the lung or the lung vasculature. Disease states most commonly associated with increases in pulmonary resistance are acute bronchitis, asthma, chronic bronchitis, emphysema, pulmonary vascular congestion, and pulmonary embolus.

Opposing those forces in the airway wall that tend to promote airway closure are forces tending to maintain outward traction on the wall. Lung volume is the major determinant of outward traction,[14] and the increased functional residual capacity maintained during exacerbations of asthma can be regarded as a protective response, generated in an attempt to increase outward radial traction on the airway wall.

Persistent airway obstruction leads to COPD and occurs particularly in emphysematous states. The mechanisms involved are fibrosis in the wall secondary to chronic inflammation, and loss of the elastic recoil of lung tissue as a result of lung destruction with progression of the emphysema. This type of obstruction is irreversible by bronchodilation, but varies greatly in the degree of airflow obstruction during inspiration and expiration. Increased lung volume is assumed both as a result of the loss of elastic recoil of the lung inward, and as a result of gas trapping. The latter occurs because of the increase in time constants of emptying lung units resulting from the changes in airway resistance. The result is a marked increase in the work of breathing because of the impedance of the system and the associated inefficiency of gas exchange. With the respiratory muscles at a mechanical disadvantage because of the secondary changes in chest wall shape, respiratory muscle fatigue may occur.

Patients who have serious COPD exist in a state of chronic hypoxia and CO_2 retention. Any aggravation of their compromised ventilation can result in acute hypoventilation and cardiorespiratory decompensation. Long-standing COPD causes destruction of lung parenchyma and hyperinflation of areas of the lung making disruption of the lung more likely in response to sudden changes in pressure across the lung.[15]

Pulmonary Vascular Diseases

Primary pulmonary hypertension is described as a chronic elevation of pulmonary artery pressure without identifiable cause.[16] Pathologically, the disease is described as an increased PVR resulting in an elevation in pulmonary artery pressure (PAP) to levels greater than 35 mmHg.[17] This chronic elevation in PAP leads to hypertrophy of the muscular walls of the pulmonary vasculature, resulting in hypoxemia, elevated right ventricular pressures, and eventually to right ventricular failure. The syndrome is usually observed in young women, although it may occur in either sex at any age. Primary pulmonary hypertension is often associated with Reynaud's phenomenon and various collagen vascular diseases. Diagnosis is based on the exclusion of secondary causes for the elevation in PAP, and the course of the disease is rapid, usually resulting in death within a two-year period.[18] There is a possible genetic relationship as the syndrome has been described in several members of a family over several generations.[19]

Pulmonary embolus is a more common type of pulmonary vascular disease, particularly in a hospital setting. The embolus usually arises from the venous beds of the lower extremities and may be due to venous stasis, injury to or irregularities in the vascular wall, or abnormalities in coagulation. The occurrence of an embolus results in reflex pulmonary artery vasoconstriction and an increase in dead space due to the decreased flow of blood to a portion of the lung. Hypoxia results, and, in the case of acute pulmonary embolus, hemodynamic decompensation is also seen. The causes of hypoxia in the presence of large pulmonary emboli are shown in Table 3-2.[20] Diagnosis of pulmonary embolus is difficult, as infiltrates or effu-

TABLE 3-2.   Causes of Hypoxia with Large Pulmonary Emboli

1. High pulmonary artery pressure can raise right-sided cardiac pressure and allow right-to-left shunting through a patent foramen ovale.

2. Pulmonary edema in the perfused lung due to the elevated pulmonary artery pressure.

3. The high pulmonary artery pressure can overcome hypoxic pulmonary vasoconstriction.

4. Factors released from the clot act on pulmonary blood vessels to enhance edema formation.

(Adapted from Pavlin,[20] with permission.)

sions on radiographs or positive pulmonary perfusion scans are nonspecific. More than 70 percent of pulmonary angiograms performed for diagnosis of a major pulmonary embolus demonstrate no abnormality even though classic symptoms may be present.[21]

Sleep Apnea

During normal sleep, respiratory patterns may vary, with periodic brief periods of apnea. Respiratory drive is inhibited and the normal ventilatory response to hypercapnia and hypoxia is attenuated. However, exacerbation of the periods of apnea accompanied by hypoxia and hypercapnia may lead to chronic cardiopulmonary disease.[22] Sleep apnea is defined as a failure of the automatic control of respiration that results in alveolar hypoventilation and may result in acidosis and pulmonary vasoconstriction resulting in pulmonary arterial hypertension.[23] It may be due to a loss of central nervous system drive, mechanical obstruction of the upper airway, or a combination of these factors.[24] Prolonged repetition of hypoxic and hypercapnic episodes with ensuing pulmonary hypertension may lead to right heart failure and dysrhythmias.[25] Hypercarbia or desaturation of hemoglobin associated with sleep-related disturbances can be important factors in the development of cor pulmonale, and they can exacerbate systemic hypertension and left ventricular dysfunction. These disturbances are usually seen in advanced cases of CPD and may lead to sudden death.[26]

CARDIAC DYSFUNCTION ASSOCIATED WITH CHRONIC PULMONARY DISEASE

Cor Pulmonale

Cor pulmonale, or pulmonary heart disease caused by inadequate pulmonary function, is a common feature of CPD. It is secondary to pulmonary hypertension associated with destruction of the pulmonary vascular bed, prolonged periods of oxygen desaturation, and respiratory acidosis resulting from CO_2 retention. Clinically, cor pulmonale is usually defined as right ventricular hypertrophy and dilatation, with cardiac failure secondary to pulmonary arterial hypertension due to a decrease in the cross-sectional area of the pulmonary bed. Pulmonary hypertension is defined as an elevation of the PAP above the accepted upper limit of normal, generally defined as 35/15 mmHg with a mean PAP of 20 mmHg.[27] Table 3-3 outlines the three pathologic conditions that can alter the normally low resistance pulmonary circulation into a high resistance circuit.

The onset of cor pulmonale and its manifestations is dependent on the rapidity of progression of the increase in PVR. Left ventricular dysfunction is not uncommon in CPD, but is usually associated with concurrent coronary artery disease (CAD). However, severe and chronic hypoxemia may lead to left ventricular dysfunction when cor pulmonale is advanced.

Ten to 30 percent of patients hospitalized with CHF have cor pulmonale, while 40 to 50 percent of patients dying with chronic bronchitis have evidence of associated right heart dysfunction of pulmonary origin. Cor pulmonale can be classified as acute or chronic. The acute situation arises secondary to massive pulmonary emboli decreasing the pulmonary cross-sectional area by 60 to 70 percent. This is associated with cyanosis and acute respiratory distress. There is also a rapid increase in right ventricular systolic pressure to 60 to 70 mmHg, which slowly returns toward normal with peripheral displacement of the emboli, lysis of the emboli, or increased collateral blood flow.

TABLE 3-3. Conditions Producing Pulmonary Artery Hypertension (PAH)

I. PAH produced by elevations of capillary and pulmonary venous pressure
   A. Mitral stenosis, mitral regurgitation, left atrial myxoma
   B. Hypertension, left ventricular failure
   C. Aortic stenosis or insufficiency
II. PAH produced by increases in pulmonary artery blood flow
   A. Congenital lesions: patent ductus arteriosus, atrial septal defect, ventricular septal defect, total anomalous venous return with right atrial or superior vena cava drainage, single ventricle, transposition of great vessels
   B. Acquired lesions: post-myocardial infarction ventricular septal defect
III. PAH produced by loss of arterial cross-sectional area
   A. Chronic hypoxia[a]
      1. Emphysema, chronic bronchitis, cystic fibrosis
      2. High altitude—mild PAH is a normal response—Monge's disease—chronic mountain sickness
      3. Chest and airway problems
         a. Pickwickian syndrome
         b. Kyophoscoliosis
         c. Chronic hypoxia secondary to enlarged adenoids
   B. Pulmonary fibrosis—produces fibrous occlusion and obliteration of small pulmonary arterioles with dilation of large pulmonary arteries
      1. Massive pulmonary fibrosis—silicosis and other pneumoconioses
      2. Interstitial fibrosis (fibrosing alveolitis—abnormalities of alveoli and bronchi that extend to incorporate the pulmonary arterioles in the fibrotic process
         a. Collagen disease
            1) Scleroderma
            2) Dermatomyositis
         b. Metals
            1) Berylliosis
            2) Cadmium
            3) Asbestosis
      c. Primary pulmonary disease
         1) Hamman-Rich
         2) Sarcoidosis
      d. Iatrogenic
         1) Radiation
         2) Busulfan therapy
      e. Miscellaneous
         1) Letterer-Siwe
         2) Hand-Schüller-Christian
   C. Pulmonary emboli
      1. Recurrent
         a. Thromboemboli
         b. Parasitic
            1) Bilharzia
            2) Schistosomiasis
         c. Fat and tumor emboli
         d. Sickle cell
      2. Solitary emboli
         a. Massive thromboembolism
         b. Amniotic fluid
         c. Air
   D. "Primary" pulmonary hypertension—idiopathic
      1. Primary pulmonary arterial hypertension
      2. Primary pulmonary venous hypertension
   E. Dietary causes
      1. *Crotalaria labrunoides* seeds
      2. Amniorex fumarate—European appetite suppressant
      3. Oral contraceptives
   F. Hepatic cirrhosis—possibly secondary to development of plexiform and angiomatoid lesions in the lung
   G. Filariasis—adult worms in pulmonary circulation[a]
   H. Foreign body granulomas

[a] Conditions producing cor pulmonale.
(From Reich et al,[27] with permission.)

Chronic cor pulmonale is associated with right ventricular hypertrophy and a change in shape of the right ventricle. Left ventricular dysfunction may be associated with right ventricular hypertrophy, but is not necessarily related to changes in the loading conditions of the left ventricle.[28] Chronic cor pulmonale is usually the result of long-standing pulmonary arterial hypertension,[29] and is most commonly seen in the patient with chronic bronchitis. The pulmonary vasculature may also be significantly impaired by the presence of recurrent emboli. Pulmonary vasoconstriction in the presence of the ensuing hypoxia contributes to an increase in PAP,[25] and the development of acidosis, which potentiates hypoxic pulmonary vasoconstriction.[30] The creation of an unusually high resistance in the right-sided circulation results in an increase in right ventricular work and consequent right ventricular enlargement. It is necessary for as much as 75 percent of the pulmonary circulation to be involved in order for vascular obliteration to be identified as the etiology of the pulmonary hypertension.[31,32]

Dysrhythmias

Perioperative dysrhythmias are a major complication in the patient with CPD undergoing thoracic surgical procedures. Significant dysrhythmias include supraventricular tachycardias, ventricular tachycardia or fibrillation, and conduction disturbances. Dysrhythmias are most likely to develop in patients with advanced cardiac disease, but other factors, such as the degree of surgical trauma, the effect of anesthetic and cardioactive drugs, and metabolic disorders affecting blood gases and body chemistry, also contribute to their occurrence.

Hypercarbia, hypocarbia, and hypoxia have all been shown to precipitate the development of dysrhythmias. Edwards et al showed that hyperventilation to a $PaCO_2$ of 30 or 20 mmHg (pH 7.51 and 7.61) lowered the normal serum potassium level (4.03 mEq/L) to 3.64 and 3.12 mEq/L, respectively.[33] If the potassium starts at lower levels, it is possible to decrease serum potassium into the 2.0 mEq/L range by hyperventilation, thus precipitating severe cardiac dysrhythmias. In thoracic surgery, the surgical trauma, including retraction of the heart, hemorrhage, edema, and hypoxia, may also contribute to postoperative cardiac dysrhythmias. Cardiac drugs used to treat dysrhythmias, such as digitalis, may themselves produce conduction disturbances or dysrhythmias. The release of catecholamines associated with both hypoxemia and hypocarbia is another major factor in the creation of pulmonary hypertension, and predisposes the patient to cardiac dysrhythmias, particularly when accompanied by dilation of the right atrium.

Pulmonary Edema

Hypoxemia and hypercarbia induce the retention of salt and water leading to a chronic hypervolemic state and increased cardiac output. An increase in lung water in cor pulmonale is usually considered a consequence of independent left ventricular disease or of increased capillary permeability. Pulmonary edema may be amenable to therapy and since ischemic heart disease may contribute to overall mortality in thoracic surgery, optimal preoperative therapy should include the control of heart failure using vasodilators, digitalis, and diuretics.[34] Digitalis is still used for the treatment of cor pulmonale and dysrhythmias, but great debate remains concerning its effectiveness and potential dangers,[35] since its beneficial effects in this situation are not as clearly defined as when the drug is used to treat left ventricular failure. Patients with pulmonary disease exhibit a high incidence of dysrhythmias compatible with digitalis intoxication, especially during episodes of acute respiratory failure. These episodes are usually not associated with serum digitalis levels normally seen with toxicity, suggesting that there may be an increased sensitivity to the drug during these episodes.

INCREASED RISK OF NOSOCOMIAL INFECTIONS

The risk of nosocomial infections following thoracic surgery is greatly increased in the patient with CPD due to disturbances of the pulmonary host defense mechanisms or to the immune responses to infection. Local defense mechanisms include (1) efficient nasofiltration during gas inhalation; (2) airway reflexes that protect against large particulate inhalation, as well as against aspiration; (3) the alveolar macrophage system for immunologic defense; and (4) the mucociliary blanket, which acts as a transport system to remove pathogens and particulate matter outward toward the glottis to be cleared by swallowing or coughing. Immune competence may be affected either by the CPD itself or by the use of steroids in its treatment.[36]

Hospital acquired pneumonia is common in patients with CPD undergoing surgery. Mortality with nosocomial pneumonia is approximately 20 to 25 percent. Colonization of the tracheobronchial tree can be decreased by the use of selective bowel decontamination,[37,38] and broad spectrum antibiotics are often used to treat chronic respiratory infections prior to surgery. These antibiotics may also be given to patients with a change in character of sputum, fever, or leucocytosis.[39,40] In a series of 221 patients undergoing thoracotomy, Cooper found that the use of preoperative prophylactic antibiotics decreased both pulmonary and pneumonectomy space infections.[41] Mortality was 17 percent in the group receiving no preoperative antibiotics and only 9 percent in the group receiving prophylaxis.

Respiratory infections also play a role in the development of asthma.[36] Viral infections cause acute asthma when they involve the upper respiratory tract in adults and in children under 5 years of age. Typically, these susceptible children show respiratory syncytial viral infections, have a family history of atopy, are males, have preexisting airway hyperactivity, and exhibit malaise, rhinorrhea, and excess mucous production. The association of sinusitis, nasal polyps, and acute asthma in a nonatopic adult is also well-described. Recent data suggest possible mechanisms underlying these associations.[42] These patients can be cured of their asthma when the sinusitis is treated with antibiotics.

PATHOPHYSIOLOGIC CHANGES ASSOCIATED WITH THORACIC SURGERY

The Surgical Lesion

Excision or biopsy of tumors of the lung or lesions involving the mediastinum, esophagus, pleura, diaphragm, or thoracic wall are the usual thoracic surgical procedures for which patients are being prepared. It is important that the anesthesiologist understand the implications of the surgical lesion for both the safe conduct of the initial operation and the management of postoperative recovery.[43] Patients do not always benefit from lung resection, but the surgery may be necessary for other reasons, such as control of hemoptysis. Significantly diminished pulmonary function or severe CAD should be considered relative contraindications to resection. Careful attention should be given to the surgical lesion itself as it may cause localized airway obstruction with the risk of development of a secondary infection or abscess. Plans to isolate the affected lung using double-lumen tubes or bronchial blockers should be considered (see Chapter 14).

If a lesion is cancerous, there are several extrapulmonary syndromes that may be seen and need to be addressed in the preoperative period.[44] These include increases in metabolic and hormonal manifestations, such as excess secretion of adrenocorticotropic hormone, gonadotropin, human growth hormone, gastrointestinal hormones, calcium-related hormones, or hypoglycemic factors. Carcinoid syndrome may also be seen. Neuromyopathic syndromes are associated with lung cancer in as many as 16 percent of cases and can cause peripheral neuropathy, subacute cerebellar degeneration, central sleep apnea, and encephalomyelitis. Dermatomyositis and subacute necrotizing myelopathy have also been described, and connective tissue, vascular, hematologic, and cutaneous manifestations are seen.

Adrenal hyperactivity in association with lung cancer was first described in 1928 by Brown,[45] and again in 1948 by Albright and Reifenstein.[46] Ectopic protein production is a characteristic feature of many cancerous lesions, and the adrenal hyperactivity in lung cancer is due to production of a pro-ACTH (adrenocorticotropic hormone). Although 1 to 3 percent of patients become cushingoid, a much higher percentage show muscle weakness, polyuria, and hypokalemic alkalosis. Seventy-two percent of patients with bronchogenic tumors have pro-ACTH in their blood.

In 1938, Winkler and Krenshaw described the association of lung cancer with hyponatremia and excess urine sodium.[47] Further reports from Schwartz et al support this observation.[48] An increase in ADH is seen in 60 percent of patients with small cell cancer, 40 percent with large cell cancers, 46 percent with adenocarcinoma, and 36 percent with squamous cell cancer.

Surgical Procedure

Pulmonary dysfunction during and following thoracotomy and upper abdominal surgery occurs even in otherwise normal patients. This is the result of the effects of surgery on the chest wall, the lung itself, or both. Chest wall dysfunction leads to a reduction in functional residual capacity, vital capacity, cough frequency, and tidal volume, and to an increase in respiratory rate with little change in minute volume. Respiratory rate and minute volume are decreased by the use of narcotics for pain relief, possibly leading to acute hypercarbia. In addition, resection of the lung, or loss of lung volume from secondary air space disease lead to decreases in total lung capacity and vital capacity. Gas exchange efficiency may be significantly impaired by each of these changes. Incision-associated pain and splinting, secondary respiratory muscle dysfunction, and diaphragm and abdominal muscle weakness or discoordination may lead to secretion retention with exacerbation of respiratory failure. All of these issues must be addressed in the preoperative period in order to provide adequate perioperative care.

PREPARING THE PATIENT FOR SURGERY

The risk of perioperative morbidity or mortality in the patient with CPD is primarily dependent on the severity and the effect of the disease on the physiologic reserves of cardiopulmonary function, with consideration given to age, concurrent disease, and the planned surgery. The respiratory complications associated with surgery include atelectasis, respiratory insufficiency, exacerbation of asthma, pneumothorax, effusion, pulmonary edema, or embolus. These complications occur in 5 to 7 percent of all surgical patients. Their incidence is doubled in active cigarette smokers and is roughly tripled with the use of upper abdominal or thoracic incisions for the surgical approach. Seventy percent of patients with moderate to severe COPD have complications associated with surgery, and while the mortality is relatively low, the extended hospital stay is very costly. Optimal preparation of the patient for surgery must involve the internist, surgeon, and anesthesiologist working together to maximize the patient's chances for an uneventful perioperative course.

Preoperative Evaluation

Ideally, the preoperative visit should take place 3 to 5 days before the planned surgery. Major aspects to be considered during the preoperative visit include the usual components of a general preoperative evaluation (history, physical examination, and specific symptom review), assessment of the clinical features of CPD amenable to preoperative correction (Table 3-4),[49] identification of the surgical lesion and planned surgical procedure to estimate risk, and the formulation of a planned approach to preoperative pulmo-

nary and general preparation for anesthesia and surgery and for recovery and rehabilitation.

In evaluating the severity of disease, the following issues should be addressed.

Airway Obstruction

Airway reactivity and persistent airflow limitation may be present alone or together. The presence of atopy or allergy, smoking history, secretions, cough, history of pneumonia or bronchitis, and use of bronchodilators should all be noted. Cultures of bronchial secretions may be helpful, but viral infections are often responsible for increasing airway reactivity. Flow-volume studies and bronchial provocation tests may be necessary to detect minimal dysfunction (see Chapter 1). Shortness of breath on exertion, wheezing, rhonchi, and a chronic cough with sputum production are classic features of emphysema (pink puffer or blue bloater varieties), and should definitely lead to flow-volume studies and estimation of lung volumes. The response to bronchodilators, and imaging studies to examine for bronchiectasis and bullous lung changes may be helpful.

Chronic Respiratory Insufficiency

Where history indicates a decreased performance status below 80 on the Karnofsky scale (Table 3-5),[50] arterial blood gas samples on room air or with oxygen supplementation should be obtained. Increased $_A$-aDO_2, decreased PaO_2/F_IO_2 ratio below 300, elevated

---

TABLE 3-4. Preoperative Respiratory Care Regimen

1. Stop smoking
2. Dilate the airways
   a. Beta$_2$-agonists
   b. Theophylline
   c. Steroids
   d. Cromolyn sodium
3. Loosen the secretions
   a. Airway hydration (humidifier/nebulizer)
   b. Systemic hydration
   c. ? Mucolytic and expectorant drugs
   d. Antibiotics
4. Remove the secretions
   a. Postural drainage
   b. Coughing
   c. Chest physiotherapy (percussion and vibration)
5. Increased education, motivation, and facilitation of postoperative care
   a. Psychologic preparation
   b. Incentive spirometry
   c. Exposure to secretion removal maneuvers
   d. Exercise
   e. Weight loss/gain
   f. Stabilize other medical problems

(From Benumof,[49] with permission.)

TABLE 3-5. The Karnofsky Scale of Performance

Able to carry out normal activity of daily living	100	Normal, no symptoms
	90	SOBOE
	80	SOB at rest
Unable to work; some home help	70	Self care
	60	Help needed
	50	Medical care
Needs institutional help	40	Disabled
	30	Hospitalized
	20	Active support
	10	Moribund
	0	Dead

Abbreviations: SOBOE, short of breath on exercising; SOB, shortness of breath.
(From Karnofsky et al,[50] with permission.)

$PaCO_2$ values with incomplete compensation for respiratory acidosis, and elevated hemoglobin values (greater than 17 gm percent) or carboxyhemoglobin values (greater than 2 or 3 percent) should alert the clinician to the potential for respiratory failure in the postoperative period. Respiratory muscle strength and endurance should be estimated with the use of pulmonary function tests (see Chapter 1).

Cardiac Dysfunction Associated with CPD

The presence and severity of cor pulmonale should be assessed in each patient. Those with severe emphysema may improve with the use of nocturnal or 24-hour oxygen supplementation to prevent desaturation and the associated episodic increases in mean pulmonary artery pressure. The presence of concurrent cardiac disease should be determined and the use of electrocardiography and echocardiography are helpful in the preoperative assessment.

Patients undergoing thoracic surgery are at increased risk for cardiac events, such as ischemia, infarction, and CHF, when compared with patients undergoing general abdominal surgery. This is due to the proximity of the heart to the operative field with direct traction often applied to the pericardium, to the general risk factors associated with this patient group, and to the commonly seen pulmonary-related heart disease. Further cardiac evaluation prior to thoracic surgery can be done with the use of tests such as dipyridamole-thallium imaging, holter monitoring, and exercise testing. Since patients with CPD are usually symptom-limited, submaximal exercise studies may provide false negative results.

Increased Risk of Nosocomial Infection

With regard to this risk factor, there are several tests that may help guide the clinician with perioperative management. Sputum and nasal or pharyngeal cultures, comparative chest x-rays to examine for new or changing infiltrates, tests to rule out chronic viral infections including human immunodeficiency virus, and examination of the fluid in the presence of a pleural effusion may be justified. The nutritional status of the patient should also be considered as malnutrition increases the risk of infection. In a group of 64 preoperative hospitalized patients on a surgical service, previously unrecognized malnutrition manifested by at least one abnormality in albumin levels, weight history, skin-fold measurements, transferrin levels, creatinine index, or delayed sensitivity reactions was found to be present in 97 percent.[51] Postoperative morbidity and mortality were related to the degree of preoperative malnutrition (see Chapter 25). Previous

splenectomy may also compromise the patient as it may decrease complement production. Prophylactic treatment with antibiotics in view of the use of nasogastric tubes, tracheostomy tubes, etc. should be considered.

The Surgical Lesion

Assessment of the surgical lesion should be provided by the surgeon and include the staging of lung cancer when bronchial carcinoma is present. Chest x-rays and CT scans should be available particularly with lesions of the hilar region. Fluoroscopy of the diaphragms also may be indicated in these cases. Bronchoscopy can be used to confirm the diagnosis in 60 to 70 percent of patients, and the information gained may be valuable in planning treatment. Preoperative drainage of retained secretions or lung abscesses may be helpful in preventing aspiration during surgery. Mediastinoscopy may be indicated when there is suspicion of extensive mediastinal involvement prior to resective surgery, in small cell carcinoma where peritracheal nodal involvement makes resection of the lung difficult, and in elderly patients where the surgical risk is increased by nodal involvement (see Chapter 12).

The Surgical Procedure

Thoracic surgical procedures often drastically reduce respiratory functional reserves. Careful preoperative assessment of the surgical lesion and of the potential effects of any needed lung resection is extremely important. Exacerbation of reactive airway disease is associated with certain drug combinations and with instrumentation of the airway. Bronchodilatory regimens may lead to secondary cardiac events. Other possible occurrences include corticosteroid insufficiency, rupture of lung abscesses, emptying of secretions from bronchiectatic airways, or bleeding of vascular lesions into the airway. Iatrogenic pulmonary edema is also a common event associated with pneumonectomy, when diastolic dysfunction of the left ventricle is ignored. Hypoxia from right-to-left shunting at the atrial level may also be precipitated by pneumonectomy (see Chapter 26).

Therapeutic Regimen

The initial 10-step outline for pulmonary preparation should carry over into a program for the postoperative pulmonary rehabilitation.

1. *Patient counseling.* The underlying CPD state should be known to the patient and the implications of drug therapy and the surgical procedure

should be explained. The anesthesiologist should educate the patient with regard to the anesthetic procedure, explaining the risks and benefits as well as postoperative mechanisms for pain relief. The possibility of postoperative intensive care should also be discussed.

2. *Management of the reactive airway.* Where acute curable upper respiratory infection is present, delaying elective surgery 7 to 10 days is ideal if not essential. Prophylactic antibiotic coverage to treat or prevent secondary bacterial infection is important. Smoking is best stopped 6 to 8 weeks before surgery if maximum gains in improved pulmonary function are to be achieved. However, reductions in carboxyhemoglobin levels do occur within 24 or 48 hours, and these are worthwhile. Mild chronic bronchitis with hemophilus influenza infection, and excess mucous production in the asthmatic bronchitic subgroup, may be improved by 3 to 5 days of broad spectrum antibiotic use and then a 5 day period of active pulmonary hygiene. Where bronchospasm is reversible, the use of combined medications to maintain the patient airway throughout anesthesia and the postoperative period is useful (see Chapter 9). The necessity for steroid coverage, or drug plasma levels, such as theophylline, to avoid toxicity should be noted.

3. *Management of chronic respiratory insufficiency.* Exercise desaturation or sleep-related desaturation may indicate the need for oxygen therapy on a part time or 24-hour basis. Hospital observation for 3 to 5 days is best to allow the stabilization of therapy, although surgical resection of the lung is probably contraindicated in the great majority of these patients. Where there is a tendency to nocturnal CO_2 retention or failure to respond to oxygen alone, nasal continuous positive airway pressure or nasal intermittent positive pressure ventilation may be helpful in preparing the patient for surgery.

4. *Respiratory muscle retraining for strength and endurance* and

5. *Exercise reconditioning.* These programs (points 4 and 5) should include attention to the nutritional state (see Chapter 25). Four to 6 weeks are needed to maximize benefits, but modalities are available for preparation on a short-term basis.

6. *Treatment of cor pulmonale and detection of other associated cardiac conditions.* This step is essential, and the usual drug regimens for CHF should be continued. Therapy with bronchodilators, antibiotics, physical therapy, and the administration of sodium bicarbonate may be useful. Reduction of pulmonary hypertension can be aided in this manner or by the administration of oxygen, since the primary cause of the hypertension is hypoxemia. When cor pulmonale does appear, direct cardiac therapy with vasodilators, diuretics, digitalis, and other inotropes may be necessary, and the determination of digoxin levels is suggested. The use of invasive monitoring to guide therapy preoperatively is wise in some patients. Identification of a potential patent foramen ovale, seen in 27 percent of individuals, may be useful when pneumonectomy is planned or where increased PVR is anticipated postoperatively.

7. *Adequate treatment of actual pulmonary infection.* Prophylactic antibiotic use for preventing nosocomial infections should be well understood by the anesthesiologist and deserves discussion with the surgical team involved. Specific infections must be treated with the appropriate antibiotics.

8. *Adequate pulmonary hygiene.* Chest physical therapy/deep breathing, postural drainage with or without percussion, and mechanical devices for suction or intermittent positive pressure inflation may be indicated.

9. *Adequate pain management postoperatively.* Such management is essential for good pulmonary hygiene (see Chapter 21). This may be needed on a long-term basis when the surgical cure of painful syndromes is not achieved.

10. *Psychosocial management.* This should include education for smoking cessation, control or cessation of ethanol use, maintaining optimal body weight and habitus through food intake and exercise, and examination of the living conditions of the patient that may contribute to the disease. Depression is a component of CPD that is often ignored and can contribute to a poor outcome from surgery and anesthesia. This, combined with anxiety, may increase the risk of the surgical encounter.

The responsibility of the preoperative preparation and the intra- and postoperative management of the thoracic surgical patient with CPD must be shared by the surgeon, anesthesiologist, and pulmonary medicine specialist. With careful planning and coordination of efforts, the risk of anesthesia and surgery can be significantly reduced.

REFERENCES

1. Knaus WA, Zimmermann JE, Wagner DP et al: APACHE—acute physiology and chronic health evaluation: a physically based classification system. Crit C Med 9:591–597, 1981

2. Knaus WA, Draper EA, Wagner DP et al: An evaluation of outcome from intensive care in major medical centers. Ann Int Med 104:410–418, 1986

3. Goldman L: Multifactorial index of cardiac risk in noncardiac surgery: ten year status report. J Cardiothorac Anesth 3:237–244, 1987
4. Fowkes FGR, Lunn JN, Farrell SC, et al: Epidemiology in anesthesia III: mortality risk in patients with coexisting physical disease. Brit J Anaesth 54:819–824, 1982
5. Bonner JT: Preoperative preparation. pp. 171–196. In Kaplan JA (ed): Thoracic Anesthesia. Churchill Livingstone, New York, 1983
6. Gracey DR, Divertie MB, Didier BP: Preoperative pulmonary preparation of patients with chronic obstructive pulmonary disease. Chest 76:123–129, 1979
7. Stein M, Koota GM, Simon M, et al: Preoperative pulmonary evaluation and therapy for surgery patients. JAMA 211:787–790, 1970
8. Tarhan S, Moffitt EA, Sessler A, et al: Risk of anesthesia and surgery in patients with chronic bronchitis and chronic obstructive pulmonary disease. Surgery 74:720–726, 1973
9. Baum GL, Wolinsky E (eds): Textbook of Pulmonary Diseases. 4th Ed. Little, Brown, Boston 1989
10. Stoelting RK, Dierdorf SF, McCammon RL (eds): Anesthesia and Coexisting Disease. 2nd Ed. Chs. 9, 13–17. Churchill-Livingstone, New York, 1988
11. Burwell CS: Extreme obesity associated with alveolar hypoventilation: a pickwickian syndrome. Am J Med 21:811–818, 1956
12. Taylor AE, Rehder K, Hyatt RE, et al: Clinical Respiratory Physiology. WB Saunders, Philadelphia, 1989
13. Colebatch HJH, Mitchell CA: Constriction of isolated living liquid-filled dog and cat lungs with histamine. J Appl Phys 30:691–702, 1971
14. Gunst SJ, Warner DO, Wilson TA, et al: Parenchymal interdependence and airway response to methacholine in excised dog lobes. J Appl Phys 65:2490–2497, 1988
15. Rothman HH: Acute exacerbation in chronic obstructive pulmonary disease. pp. 721–737. In Dantzker DR (ed): Cardiopulmonary Critical Care. Grune & Stratton, Orlando, FL, 1986
16. Rich S, Brudage BH: Primary pulmonary hypertension: current update. JAMA 251:2252–2254, 1984
17. Wagenvoort CA, Wagenvoort N: Primary pulmonary hypertension: a pathologic study of the lung vessels in 156 clinically diagnosed cases. Circulation 42:1163–1184, 1970
18. Legler DC: Uncommon diseases and cardiac anesthesia. pp. 785–831. In Kaplan JA (ed): Cardiac Anesthesia. WB Saunders, Philadelphia, 1987
19. Lloyd JE, Primm RK, Newman JH: Familial primary pulmonary hypertension: clinical patterns. Am Rev Respir Dis 129:194–197, 1984
20. Pavlin EG: Respiratory diseases. pp. 305–332. In Katz J, Benumof JL, Kadis LB (eds): Anesthesia and Uncommon Diseases. WB Saunders, Philadelphia, 1990
21. Greenfield LJ, Langham MR: Surgical approaches to thromboembolism. Br J Surg 71:958–970, 1984
22. Strohl KP, Saunders NA, Sullivan CE: Sleep apnea syndrome. pp. 355–402. In Saunders NA, Sullivan CE (eds): Sleep and Breathing. Marcel Dekker, New York, 1984
23. Dorland's Illustrated Medical Dictionary. 27th Ed. WB Saunders, New York, 1985
24. Bradley TD, Phillipson EA: Pathogenesis and pathophysiology of the obstructive sleep apnea syndrome. Med Clin North Am 69:1169–1185, 1985
25. Fishman, AP: Chronic cor pulmonale. Am Rev Respir Dis 114:775–794, 1976
26. Belman MJ: Pulmonary rehabilitation. pp. 1107–1121. In Baum GL, Wolinsky E (eds): Textbook of Pulmonary Diseases. Little, Brown, Boston, 1989
27. Reich DL, Brooks JL, Kaplan JA: Uncommon cardiac diseases. pp. 333–377. In Katz J, Benumof JL, Kadis LB (eds): Anesthesia and Uncommon Diseases. WB Saunders, Philadelphia, 1990
28. Baum SL, Schwartz A, Llamas R, et al: Left ventricular function in chronic obstructive lung disease. N Engl J Med 285:361–365, 1971
29. Ross JC, Newman JH: Chronic cor pulmonale. pp. 1120–1129. In Hurst JW (ed): The Heart. McGraw-Hill, New York, 1986
30. Ferrer MT: Disturbance in the circulation in patients with cor pulmonale. Bull N Y Acad Med 9:942–957, 1965
31. Dunnil MS: An assessment of the anatomical factor in cor pulmonale in emphysema. J Clin Path 14:246–258, 1961
32. Hicken P, Brewer D, Heath D: The relationship between the weight of the right ventricle of the heart and the internal surface area and number of alveoli in the human lung in emphysema. J Pathol Bacteriol 92:529–546, 1966
33. Edwards R, Winnie AL, Ramamurthy S: Acute hypocapnic hypokalemia: an iatrogenic anesthetic complication. Anesth Analg 56:786–792, 1977
34. Goldman L, Caldera DC, Nussbaum SR, et al: Multifactorial index of cardiac risk in noncardiac surgical procedures. N Engl J Med 297:845–850, 1977
35. Green LH, Smith TW: The use of digitals in patients with pulmonary disease. Ann Int Med 87:459–465, 1977
36. Hornick DB: Pulmonary host defense: defects that lead to chronic inflammation of the airway. Clin Chest Med 9:669–678, 1988
37. Salata RA, Ellner JJ: Bacterial colonization of the tracheobronchial tree. Clin Chest Med 9:623–634, 1988
38. Stoutenbeck CHP, Van Saene HKF, Miranda DR, et al: The effect of selective decontamination of the digestive tract on colonization and infection rate in multiple trauma patients. Intensive Care Med 10:185–192, 1988
39. Finlayson D: Pharmacology for the anesthesiologist, 16th annual postgraduate course: therapeutic problems in respiratory and intensive care of critically ill patients. Atlanta, 1980
40. Chodosh S, Enstein K: Comparison of ampicillin vs. tetracycline for exacerbations of chronic bronchitis. Am Rev Resp Dis 98:134, 1968
41. Cooper DKL: The incidence of postoperative infection and the role of antibiotic prophylaxis in pulmonary surgery: a review of 221 consecutive patients undergoing thoracotomy. Brit J Dis Chest 75:154–160, 1981
42. Frick WE, Busse WW: Respiratory infections: their role in airway responsiveness and pathogenesis of asthma. Clin Chest Med 9:539–550, 1988
43. Bruderman I: Bronchogenic carcinoma. pp. 1197–1237. In Baum GL, Wolinsky E (eds): Textbook of Pulmonary Diseases. Little, Brown, Boston, 1989

44. Niewehner CB, Morgan WKC: Extrapulmonary syndromes associated with tumors of the lung. pp. 1265–1287. In Baum GL, Wolinsky E (eds): Textbook of Pulmonary Diseases. Little, Brown, Boston, 1989

45. Brown WH: A case of pluriglandular syndrome: "diabetes of bearded women." Lancet 2:1022–1023, 1928

46. Albright F, Reifenstein EC (eds): The Parathyroid Glands & Metabolic Bone Disease: Selected Studies. Williams & Wilkins, Baltimore, 1948

47. Winkler AW, Crankshaw OF: Chloride depletion in conditions other than Addison's disease. J Clin Invest 17:1–6, 1938

48. Schwartz WB, Tassel D, Bartter FC: Further observations of hyponatremia and renal sodium loss probably resulting from inappropriate secretion of antidiuretic hormone. N Eng J Med 262:743–748, 1960

49. Benumof JL: Anesthesia for Thoracic Surgery. pp. 156–165. WB Saunders, Philadelphia, 1987

50. Karnofsky D, Abelmann WH, Crauer LF, et al: The use of nitrogen mustards in the palliative treatment of carcinoma with particular reference to bronchogenic carcinoma. Cancer 1:634–656, 1948

51. Mullen JL, Gertner MH, Buzy GP, et al: Implications of malnutrition in the surgical patient. Arch Surg 114: 121–125, 1979

4

ACQUIRED IMMUNODEFICIENCY SYNDROME AND HEPATITIS: RISKS TO PATIENT AND PHYSICIAN

Alexander W. Gotta, M.D.

ACQUIRED IMMUNODEFICIENCY SYNDROME

In 1968, a sexually active 15-year-old boy was admitted to the St. Louis City Hospital with extensive *Chlamydia* infection. On physical examination, a small lesion, later proven to be Kaposi's sarcoma, was noted on his thigh. Shortly thereafter, he died; at postmortem, he was found to have an unsuspected, extensive parenchymatous invasive sarcoma, an aggressive tumor, with a degree of malignancy unknown to the physicians caring for him. His disease and death remained a mystery until 1988, when preserved tissue and serum specimens were analyzed and demon-

strated a virus related to, or identical with, the human immunodeficiency virus type 1 (HIV-1). This is the first known case of the acquired immunodeficiency syndrome (AIDS).[1]

Although the disease obviously existed unrecognized, it was not until 1981 that physicians on both coasts of America reported a previously undefined syndrome among homosexuals and intravenous drug users. A report from California documented four previously healthy homosexual men who developed *Pneumocystis carinii* pneumonia, extensive mucosal candidiasis, and multiple viral infections.[2] Cytomegalovirus (CMV) was recovered from all four patients. One of the four had Kaposi's sarcoma. The investigators suggested that the syndrome was caused by CMV infection, but they were unable to state why homosexuals were suddenly susceptible. In New York, 11 cases of community-acquired *P. carinii* pneumonia were diagnosed.[3] The disease had occurred between 1979 and 1981 in young men who were drug abusers, homosexuals, or both. The patients presented with pneumonia and lymphopenia; one had Kaposi's sarcoma and eight were already dead at the time of the report. The investigators suggested that unknown factors made drug abusers and homosexuals vulnerable to *Pneumocystis* infection.

The initial reports opened the gates to a host of case presentations and investigations, leading to the recognition of a common factor tying together the victims of this syndrome—a marked alteration in the immune system of the afflicted and vulnerability to a wide range of opportunistic infections and tumors.

The appearance of this strange and hitherto unknown form of disease created apprehension, anxiety, and outright fear as it became evident that clearly defined population groups were at high risk and that certain forms of behavior were associated with the infection. Most alarming was the exponential growth of the disease, from the first few reported cases to the thousands that quickly followed. As the number of reported cases grew, so did the number of deaths. It became obvious that this was a universally fatal disease.

AIDS is caused by a retrovirus, initially termed the *human T-cell lymphotropic virus type III* (HTLV-III).[4] The lymphadenopathy virus (LAV) was soon recognized as being identical to HTLV-III,[5] and the causative agent was known for a while by the awkward title of HTLV-III/LAV. This cumbersome nomenclature has been simplified, and the former HTLV III/LAV is now known simply as the human immunodeficiency virus, or HIV. There are at least two distinct forms of HIV, called HIV-1 and HIV-2.[6–9] Each is capable of causing AIDS, but HIV-1 has been identified as causing most cases of the disease in Africa, Europe, and the Americas. This situation is complicated by the fact that HIV has the capacity in vivo to mutate to HIV subsets, and that the virulence, and its ability to cause disease progression, is a direct result of the development of virulent mutants.[10] Whether other AIDS-producing HIVs may be discovered is unknown. Because of the lag in incubation period associated with the progression of HIV infection to outright AIDS, and the relatively recent discovery of HIV-2, it is not yet apparent whether HIV-2 is as virulent as HIV-1, and whether the AIDS produced by HIV-2 is similar to that produced by HIV-1. The reasons for development of more pathogenic mutants of HIV-1 in vivo are also not understood and, thus, certain prediction of those who will proceed from HIV-1 infection to AIDS is currently not possible. Both HIV-1 and HIV-2

have been identified in the United States, both are known to have caused cases of AIDS, and both are contaminants of the American blood supply.

ORIGIN AND EPIDEMIOLOGY

HIV has probably existed in central Africa for many years, infecting inhabitants of isolated villages and establishing an equilibrium relationship with its human host. Its identity as a unique disease form and its deadly potential were obscured by the many infectious diseases present in Africa and by the failure of the disease to spread beyond the boundaries of remote habitations. However, the incursions of civilization, with road-building, contact with a variety of people of varying immunologic status, association with prostitutes, and sexual promiscuity, probably stirred the latent virus into activity, accounting for its remarkable spread throughout tropical Africa and the development of the African AIDS epidemic. While the first case of AIDS in Africa (identified retrospectively) was described in Zaire in 1976, there is evidence of the existence of the disease for years prior, since antibodies to the virus have been detected in blood drawn for other studies in central Africa in 1959.[11] Seroprevalence rates in sub-Saharan Africa now range from near zero in some areas to as high as 18 percent in others. Many of these individuals are already ill, and many have died. However, most of those infected are asymptomatic and unaware. It is estimated that 8 percent of the sub-Saharan African population will be infected with HIV by 1993, a total of 50 million people. By 1991, 1 million deaths are anticipated, with another 10 million between 1992 and 1996.[11]

The exact magnitude of HIV infection and AIDS is unknown because of the lack of reliability of public health and data-gathering services in many parts of the world. While the World Health Organization (WHO) reported 100,410 cases of AIDS in 138 countries as of July 1, 1988, the true number is undoubtedly greater by a multiple of three or even four.[12] The WHO expects an additional 1 million cases within the next 5 years. National economies will be strained as they are called on to care for the many ill; doubtless, many thousands will die unattended and unobserved. Even in economically mature and sophisticated countries, it is doubtful that the increasing demands for care for AIDS patients can be adequately met. The hospital system in New York City has been burdened almost to the breaking point by many factors, with the overwhelming cost of care for AIDS patients being a very important factor.[13]

Through August 1989, a total of 105,990 cases of AIDS had been reported in the United States and its territories. Of these, 62,464 had already died, a total case fatality rate of 58.9 percent. Of the total cases, 104,210 were adults or adolescents, of whom 58.2 percent had died, and 1,780 were less than 13 years old, of whom 54.6 percent had died. There is a distinct geographic prevalence in this country (Table 4-1). Of all reported cases, 19.8 percent have occurred in New York City, 6.4 percent in San Francisco, 7.0 percent in Los Angeles, and 2.9 percent in Houston. San Francisco, however, has the highest incidence rate, at 104.5 per 100,000 population; San Juan, Puerto Rico, is second, at 76.3, and New York City is third, at 60.9. AIDS has been reported in every state.[14]

In the five states with the highest rates of HIV infection, among men 20 to 29 years of age, the rate of infection with HIV is 3.4 percent; among men 30 to 39 years of age, it is 11.1 percent. The Commissioner of Health of New York State estimates that nearly 2 percent of women (one of 60) in New York City are infected with HIV, as are 60 percent of all intravenous drug users and 70 percent of male homosexuals and bisexuals. In Massachusetts, among parturients, the rate is one per 476 individuals (2.1 per 1,000), ranging as high as eight per 1,000 in inner city hospitals.[15] In a large center-city hospital in New York City, the rate among parturients is 20 per 1,000.[16] One thousand HIV-infected infants will be born in New York State this year.

These impressive and rapidly growing numbers make it apparent that the practicing anesthesiologist will deal with HIV-infected patients. Many will be completely unaware of their infection as they present themselves for routine surgical procedures. Others will be anesthetized for thoracic diagnostic procedures. A third group will be those with the frank disease undergoing life-lengthening procedures, or those obtaining supportive care in intensive care units. Infection is not often apparent, the disease is communicable, the immune-suppressed patient is at risk for the development of opportunistic infection, and precau-

tions for protection of both patient and health care worker are necessary.

THE DISEASE

The human organism has developed a variety of techniques to recognize and cope with foreign invaders, be they viral, bacterial, or protozoan. The cell-mediated immune system may be considered a system of checks and balances, with T4 (helper) cells of the lymphocyte series acting as guardians against such invaders. When the host is invaded, T4 cells have the capacity to recognize violations of host integrity and to use humoral transmitters to mobilize the immune system. The immune response is eventually discontinued by T8 (suppressor) cells, thus discontinuing the host defense reaction. HIV invades and inactivates T4 cells while having no effect on T8 cells, thus reducing the T4/T8 ratio, turning off the immune system, and leaving the host vulnerable to a wide variety of opportunistic infections by organisms ordinarily controlled by the intact and properly functioning immune system. Killer cells, which protect the host from tumors by scavenging and eliminating tumor cells, are also inactivated. Thus, the host is laid open to both opportunistic infections and tumors.[17]

As a retrovirus, HIV encodes its genetic information in RNA and uses reverse transcriptase, a unique viral enzyme characteristic of retroviruses, to copy its genome into DNA, which is then integrated into the host-cell genome as a provirus.[18] The infected lymphocytes are then induced to develop and express an adhesive substance on their cell membranes. Uninfected cells will adhere to infected cells and in turn become infected, causing the development of a syncytial, growing mass of infected lymphocytes.[19]

While tests for the virus antigen are available and, if uniformly reliable, could serve to indicate current infection,[20] it is much more common to search for anti-HIV antibodies as an indicator of infection. The enzyme-linked immunosorbent assay (ELISA) is most commonly used because of its low cost, simplicity, and capacity to be performed on a large scale. Positive ELISA tests may be confirmed by Western blot assays or radioimmunoprecipitation assays (RIPAs).

Antibody tests have several deficiencies limiting their value. After infection with HIV, the ELISA usually remains negative for 8 to 12 weeks, while the more sensitive RIPA will become positive in 2 to 3 weeks. However, viremia will develop in as little as 8 days.[21] Thus, there is a built-in "window in time" during which the contaminated individual will be antigen-positive—a virus shedder, capable of infecting others—and yet still negative and, therefore, undetectable by the commonly used tests. One study has

TABLE 4-1. AIDS: Current Incidence Per 100,000 Population

State	Incidence
New York	34.5
New Jersey	27.8
Florida	25.1
California	20.8
Georgia	16.6
District of Columbia	89.5
City	
San Francisco	104.5
San Juan, Puerto Rico	76.3
Jersy City	62.9
New York	60.9

(From Centers for Disease Control.[14])

demonstrated that seronegativity for antibodies may persist for as long as 14 months after infection, thus opening widely the window in time and increasing the danger of infection by infected, but unrecognized, individuals.[22]

Screening the entire American population for HIV positivity may seem an easy and effective technique for minimizing contact with infected individuals and limiting spread of the disease. The appeal of such simplistic methods is diluted by recognition of the often prolonged window in time of HIV-antigen positivity, antibody negativity, and the intrinsic defects of any screening device. While the tests are both sensitive and accurate, the rate of false positivity can be unacceptably high. If the tests are used to screen populations with a high rate of true prevalence, then the false-positive rate is low. This situation would exist if the homosexual population of San Francisco, for example, or the intravenous drug-abusing population of New York City were tested. If, however, a population is tested in which the true rate of positivity is low, the rate of false positivity may exceed 50 to 60 percent.[23] The Armed Services have developed extremely reliable testing and retesting mechanisms, reducing false positives to one per 135,187.[24] Yet, the cost of the technique (estimated at $40,000 per true positive) makes its widespread use impractical.[25] Antibodies to HIV-2 are often not detected by ELISA screening for HIV-1. If HIV-2-induced AIDS becomes more prevalent, dual screening will need to be introduced.

Risk Groups

The high risk groups for the development of AIDS are (1) male homosexuals, (2) intravenous drug abusers, (3) hemophiliacs, (4) those who have sexual contact with the previously mentioned groups, and (5) blood recipients (Table 4-2).

It may be difficult to recognize a common theme in these disparate groups. However, an important characteristic of HIV is its marked intracellular incorporation into T4 lymphocytes or related cells of the nervous system, bowel, or skin with little free virus in the plasma or other body fluids. The relatively low fluid concentration of the virus renders the disease poorly communicable, since a certain critical mass of virus apparently must be exchanged from one infected individual to another noninfected individual in order for adequate viral propagation to occur. Thus, either one bolus dose must be transferred, as with the infusion of a contaminated unit of blood or blood product, or repeated exposure to smaller amounts must occur, as in the promiscuous homosexual. While a variety of bodily fluids have been found to harbor the virus, evidence indicates that interchange of blood or blood and seminal fluid is necessary for virus transmission. Heterosexual vaginal intercourse between men and women free of venereal disease appears not to be a common means of HIV transmission.[26] Traumatic sexual contact, however, as occurs with anal intercourse, is an important means of transmission and probably explains why AIDS is so prevalent among homosexuals.[27–30] Transmission is facilitated by sexual techniques that may enhance sexual gratification but that are sufficiently traumatic to allow direct exchange of blood or intimate contact between contaminated blood and bowel epithelium. Orogenital sex has also been implicated in HIV transmission.[31] Heterosexual transmission is common in Africa, but probably reflects the high incidence of venereal diseases and ulcerative genital lesions on that continent.[32]

Alterations in the sexual practices of homosexuals have decreased the incidence of new HIV seropositivity in that population. However, since most homosexuals in large cities in the United States are already infected (70 percent estimated in New York City), the

TABLE 4-2.   AIDS Risk Groups

Group	No. of cases	Percentage of Total
Adults		
Male homo/bisexual	63,397	61
Intravenous drug user	21,370	21
Male homo/bisexual and intravenous drug user	7,379	7
Hemophilia/coagulation disorder	996	1
Heterosexual contact	4,807	5
Blood or tissue recipient	2,566	2
Undetermined	3,595	3
Total	104,210	100
Pediatric		
Hemophilia/coagulation disorder	102	6
Mother at risk	1,422	80
Blood or tissue recipient	200	11
Undetermined	56	3
Total	1,780	100

incidence of AIDS among homosexuals will continue to increase.

With the alteration in homosexual practices and the adoption of "safe sex" techniques, the homo/bisexual population is becoming less significant in HIV transmission, while intravenous drug abusers have become increasingly important as victims of AIDS.[33] In the United States, 18 percent of all cases of AIDS have occurred in intravenous drug abusers. However, in New York City, the majority of new cases now occur in this group, and it is estimated that 60 percent of drug abusers in the city are HIV-positive. The communal use of contaminated needles and syringes by drug abusers, together with an almost complete absence of sterilization procedures, guarantee that infected individuals will spread the virus to many (if not all) members of their group. Intravenous drug abusers have made no changes in their habits that would protect them from cross-contamination of HIV. Unfortunately, the drug abuser group plays a major role in heterosexual transmission of the disease to their female sexual partners and hence to their infected offspring.

One percent of AIDS in adults has occurred in hemophiliacs or patients with other clotting disorders, most of whom were infected prior to the development of effective blood screening techniques. In children, 5.8 percent of AIDS cases have occurred in those with hemophilia or other clotting deficiencies. It is expected that the incidence of new cases in these groups will decrease in time because of the more efficient elimination of contaminated blood from the donor pool.

Transfusion of contaminated blood or blood components has accounted for 2,566 cases of AIDS in adults (2 percent of all adult cases) and 200 cases in children (11 percent of all pediatric cases).[14] Most recipients of HIV-infected blood become seropositive. AIDS develops in approximately half of these recipients within 7 years.[34] Blood is now screened for HIV antibody, and positive units are not admitted to the donor pool. However, the fallibility of the ELISA will allow a few contaminated units to slip through, while the window in time of virus positivity and antibody negativity (as long as 14 months) introduces further risks. It has been estimated that 26 per 1,000,000 U of blood transfused in this country are virus-positive and antibody-negative and, thus, a great danger to recipients.[35] This estimate has been revised favorably, to one per 153,000 U transfused. However, a patient who receives the average transfusion (5.4 U) is at odds of contamination of one per 28,000.[36] The risk has been decreasing more than 30 percent per year. It is estimated that donor-recruitment practices, plus careful education and screening, eliminate 49 of every 50 donors likely to be HIV-positive and that testing is 92 to 97 percent effective, for a combined effectiveness of 99.9 percent.[36] The risk of undetected infectious units can probably be further reduced by transfusing fewer units, obtaining units from fewer donors, and depending most on a pool of true HIV-negative donors. Women should be recruited as new donors, since their incidence is significantly less than that of men. In those countries in which routine blood donor screening procedures are not performed, or not available, transfused blood represents a great hazard. The danger is amplified if the incidence of HIV positivity is also increased (as it often is). The risk of blood transfusion in many parts of the world is undefined, yet doubtless very formidable.

Methods of Transmission

HIV has been isolated from (1) seminal fluid, (2) blood, (3) tears, (4) saliva, and (5) synovial fluid.[37,38] It is reasonable to expect that HIV might be found in any human secretion or excretion, and all should be handled (when necessary) with great care. However, there has been no documented transmission of the virus by any fluid other than blood or seminal fluid. In the one well-described case in which viral transmission took place via a human bite, there was blood in the mouth of the biter, and it was almost certainly the blood, not the saliva, that served as the vehicle of transmission.[39]

AIDS is spread primarily by sexual contact, homosexual in western Europe and the United States[37] and heterosexual in Africa.[8,12,32] In the United States, the national seroprevalence rate in men is 0.29 per 1,000, while in women it is 0.02 per 1,000, for a 14.5 : 1 male to female ratio. This contrasts markedly with the 1 : 1 ratio in Africa. This difference in the sexual distribution of the disease may reflect, at least in part, the sex distribution of drug abusers, but is also, in great part, reflective of sexual habits.

The sometimes-predicted surge in heterosexual spread of AIDS in the United States has not occurred,[26] although the incidence of such transmission has increased. In the United States, heterosexual transmission almost invariably involves at least one partner with another causative factor, usually intravenous drug abuse.[40] Comingling of blood with blood or seminal fluid is an important factor in HIV transfer, and traumatic sexual practices are much more likely to be associated with the viral spread.

Venereal disease is another important cofactor, and the higher incidence of these diseases in Africa may explain the heterosexual nature of the disease on that continent. Venereal disease may alter genital mucosa, increase permeability of surface cells to the virus, and, thus, facilitate viral entry and infection. Ulcerated lesions of the genitals are closely linked to HIV transmission. Local customs with respect to male circumcision may also be important, since there is controversial evidence that absence of circumcision leads to higher rates of HIV infection, as the area under the prepuce may serve as a safe harbor for the virus.[32]

AIDS is also spread by blood or blood products, whole blood, packed red blood cells, fresh frozen plasma, cryoprecipitate, and other concentrates of clotting factors.[41–43] Transfusion of contaminated blood or blood products will introduce bolus doses of virus. Smaller but infective inocula might be introduced by needle prick[44] or the communal use of syringes used by HIV-positive subjects.[33]

The virus has been identified in saliva and tears, but there is no evidence of transmission via these vectors, nor has there been any report of virus transmission via joint fluid.

While extraordinary precautions have been recommended to prevent transmission of HIV by fomites or contact with oral, tracheal, and ocular secretions, these precautions are doubtless overdone and not indicative of any major risks in dealing with these substances.

Clinical Syndromes

Acute infection with HIV may be asymptomatic, with no obvious sign of the significant alteration in the patient's state of health, or may be associated with such nonspecific signs and symptoms as transient chills, fever, rash, and malaise, which soon disappear, leaving victims unaware of their potentially fatal illness.

An indeterminate period of quiescence usually follows contamination, during which time the virus invades and alters lymphocytes, skin, central nervous system, peripheral nerves, and bowel. Bowel mucosa may be infected by direct introduction of the virus during anal sex, or may merely share in the extensive infection of all receptive and suitable cells. It is postulated that the marked diarrhea characteristic of AIDS may be a direct result of HIV infection of bowel mucosa.[45]

The infection is extensive, with many organ systems involved and many different opportunistic infections and tumors present; thus, diagnosis may at first be quite difficult.[46] The difficulty is enhanced by the fact that detectable antibody production may lag significantly behind infection and, thus, reliable laboratory confirmation may not be readily available. The reasons for the change from asymptomatic quiescence to an often fulminant disease are poorly understood, but may be related to the development of unusually pathogenic mutants of the infective virus.[10] Because of the long period of latency, it is impossible to predict with absolute certainty the number of infected but asymptomatic patients who will eventually develop AIDS. Evidence to date indicates that HIV positivity will always lead to AIDS,[47] albeit after a variable and perhaps prolonged period of time, and that AIDS is universally fatal.

The AIDS-related complex (ARC) may be the first evidence of HIV infection. Diagnostic criteria have been developed to distinguish ARC from AIDS, the main distinction being the absence of life-threatening opportunistic infection or major tumor. This appears not to be a distinction at all, and it seems most reasonable to think of HIV positivity, ARC, and AIDS as contiguous points on a curve of death. Certain signs and symptoms in HIV antibody-positive individuals serve as harbingers of AIDS. These include (1) oral candidiasis, (2) intermittent or continuous fever for more than 1 month, (3) repeated night sweats, (4) debilitating fatigue, (5) persistent diarrhea, (6) loss of body weight of 10 percent or more, and (7) development of another venereal disease (eg, syphilis or gonorrhea). Another marker of impending AIDS development is the failure in the HIV-positive individual of T cells to produce gamma interferon when stimulated by antigen.[48] The importance of the T cell failure rests in the important role these cells play as activators of the immune system. Failure of activation leaves the body vulnerable to unrepulsed invasion by bacteria, viruses, or protozoans, and sets the stage for the characteristic opportunistic infections of AIDs.

Opportunistic Infections

The most important opportunistic infection in AIDS in the United States is *P. carinii* pneumonia. *P. carinii* is a protozoan and a common resident of the lungs of healthy and asymptomatic individuals, where it is held in check by a properly functioning intact immune system. Depression of the immune system, as might occur with HIV infection or antitumor chemotherapy, allows overgrowth of the organism and the development of a characteristic pneumonitis. In pneumocystic pneumonia, the lungs are grossly heavy, dense, and rubbery. The alveoli are clogged with a thick, gummy exudate, limiting gas exchange and causing the dyspnea typical of the infection. Silver stain and high-power microscopy reveal a protozoan curled up in its cocoonlike cyst, accounting for its name.

Tuberculosis is a major opportunistic infection in AIDS in Africa, and is assuming a more important role in AIDS in the United States. The decline in the annual incidence of tuberculosis in the United States has now stopped, and the disease is resurgent. Although all the factors for this resurgence are not readily apparent, it appears that the increase in HIV infection is of great importance. In a young person with tuberculosis, AIDS must always be suspected. The tuberculosis of the AIDS patient may be particularly virulent, and pose a risk to health care workers who care for the patient.[49] Whether other infections are particularly virulent in the AIDS patient and more readily communicable than in the non-HIV-contaminated individual is as yet unclear. Infection with *Mycobacterium avium-intracellulare*, an uncommon variant of tuberculosis, is also found commonly in AIDS patients.

CMV is the most common opportunistic infection in AIDS, and may be isolated from more than 90 percent of patients with the disease. Indeed, initially, CMV was thought to be the cause of AIDS. CMV is troublesome because of the hepatitis or retinitis associated with infection. CMV pneumonitis is uncommon, but carries a high mortality rate. Other important opportunistic infections include cryptococcosis, toxoplasmosis, candidiasis, cryptosporidiosis, and herpes simplex.

Not all pulmonary dysfunction is due to opportunistic infection. Bronchiolitis obliterans organizing pneumonia has been described in AIDS.[50] More common, however, is nonspecific interstitial pneumonitis, which may account for as many as 32 percent of instances of pneumonitis in AIDS patients.[51-53] Lymphocytic interstitial pneumonitis is characterized by interstitial accumulation of mature lymphocytes, plasma cells, and reticuloendothelial cells, and may be an unremitting process unresponsive to immunosuppressive therapy. It has also been suggested that interstitial pneumonitis usually resolves or stabilizes without specific therapy, although subsequent episodes may occur. Thus, the differential diagnosis of pneumonitis in the AIDS patient is complex, and may be quite difficult.

Kaposi's Sarcoma

Kaposi's sarcoma is an angiosarcoma that, at one time, was considered a relatively benign, slow-growing ulcer of the lower extremity of elderly Italian or other Mediterranean males. The clinical picture is different in Africa, where Kaposi's sarcoma has always been more aggressive and virulent. The Kaposi's sarcoma of AIDS resembles the African model. It is aggressive, central rather than peripheral, often found on the head and neck, including the mouth, and involves lymph nodes and parenchymatous organs. In the first known case of AIDS in the United States, a small lesion on the thigh belied the presence of massive parenchymatous infiltration with a Kaposi's tumor.

The tumor attacks young men and is found in one-third of AIDS patients, but rarely is the direct cause of death. It is suggested that HIV infection alone is not the sole cause of Kaposi's sarcoma in AIDS patients, but that unrecognized cofactors, such as another sexually transmitted agent or abuse of nitrite inhalants, must also be present.[54]

Other neoplasms commonly seen in patients with AIDS include both Hodgkin's[55] and non-Hodgkin's lymphomas. In a study in New York City, it was shown that since the beginning of the AIDS epidemic there have been large increases in non-Hodgkin's lymphomas among the population at highest risk for HIV infection (ie, men aged 25 to 54 years who have never married or who live in neighborhoods with high AIDS mortality). In this group, between 1980 and 1984, age-adjusted incidences of non-Hodgkin's lymphoma increased from 12.3 per 100,000 to 31.8 per 100,000 individuals. In addition, the proportion of cancer that was non-Hodgkin's lymphoma increased from 6.4 to 20.2 percent.[56]

Weight Loss, Diarrhea

Weight loss is caused by the profuse diarrhea characteristic of AIDS, and is aggravated by malaise, apathy, and anorexia. Diarrhea may be due to HIV infection of the bowel mucosa,[45] but is also due to overgrowth of normal bowel flora. Weight loss is worsened by difficulty in eating and is associated with extensive pharyngeal and esophageal edema due to oral and esophageal *Candida* infection.

Adenopathy

Adenopathy is diffuse and extensive due to reactive hyperplasia. Adenopathy may be present wherever lymphoid tissue is found, including tonsils and adenoids.[57,58] Theoretically, extensive tonsillar and adenoidal hypertrophy could represent an impediment to endotracheal intubation.

Neurologic Syndromes

It is now evident that HIV is neurotropic and invades cells of the central and peripheral nervous systems, causing a protean variety of nervous system signs and symptoms.[59-62] The virus has been isolated from cerebrospinal fluid, brain, spinal cord, and peripheral nerve of patients with AIDS-related neurologic complications. The neurologic syndromes in AIDS include (1) subacute encephalitis, (2) vacuolar degeneration of the spinal cord, (3) chronic meningitis, and (4) peripheral neuropathy.

At postmortem examination, evidence of subacute encephalitis has been found in up to 90 percent of AIDS patients.[63,64] Dementia is an important manifestation of AIDS encephalitis. It should be recognized that dementia in a young person with no ready explanation for its cause should be considered AIDS until proven otherwise. Alterations in ocular motor function may serve as an early prediction of AIDS dementia complex.[64]

Vacuolar degeneration of the spinal cord occurs in 20 percent of patients and is characterized by paraparesis, ataxia, and incontinence, presenting a clinical picture of weakness, unsteady gait, and loss of bowel and bladder control. Fever and nuchal rigidity are characteristic of chronic meningitis.

Peripheral neuropathies are common and may be due to direct viral invasion of the nerves.[65] HIV replication has been demonstrated in infiltrating mononuclear cells in patients with AIDS and necrotizing vasculitis of the nervous system. This finding of HIV replication in cells surrounding the vasa nervorum suggests that HIV may be directly involved in the pathogenesis of peripheral nerve vasculitis in patients with AIDS.[66] Thus, neuropathy is probably due to both direct viral nervous infection and nervous dysfunction secondary to vasculitis. Peripheral nerve dysfunction is probably caused by axonal degeneration, although demyelination may also play a role.

Neuropathies vary considerably in their clinical presentation. Anesthesiologists may be called on to deal with severe and intractable pain that is poorly responsive to analgesics and other pain control mechanisms. In a study of 40 patients with well-established AIDS, 35 percent (13 of 37 patients without exclusionary factors) had clinical and electrophysiologic evidence of a distal symmetric polyneuropathy.[65] In this study, symptoms and signs of neuropathy were mild, and consisted mainly of the diminished ankle reflexes and loss of appreciation of vibratory sensation. Painful dysesthesias were uncommon. Amplitude reduction of sural nerve action potentials distinguished patients with clinical neuropathy from those without. There was no evidence of clinical progression of the syndrome over a 6-month period. Neuropathy occurred only in patients with prolonged disease (ie, greater than 5 months), and was marked in those with severe weight loss and dementia.

Facial paralysis may be the initial manifestation of AIDS.[67] The unexplained occurrence of this unusual phenomenon, especially in an otherwise asymptomatic young person, should always cause the physician to consider HIV infection.

Psychosis

Schizophrenia[68] or other psychoses may occur in the AIDS patient, either because of a psychotic predisposition that antedates the viral infections or because the psychiatric disorder occurred as a result of HIV infection. AIDS should be suspected in every patient presenting with psychosis of unknown origin and a history of homosexual practice or intravenous drug abuse. In one study of HIV-infected homosexual men contrasted with an uninfected group and with heterosexuals, it was discovered that ambulatory homosexual men had a higher life-time prevalence of major psychiatric disorders and that a majority of the homosexual men developed a diagnosable psychiatric syndrome preceding the HIV-related illness or seropositivity.[69] The homosexual population differed significantly from the heterosexuals in the incidence of psychiatric disorder, and it appears that the psychiatric abnormalities are associated with homosexuality and high risk for AIDS, rather than AIDS itself.

Dementia

Dementia is clinically recognizable in 30 to 50 percent of patients with AIDS. Postmortem examinations of the brains of those who have died of AIDS have demonstrated histologic evidence compatible with dementia in as many as 90 percent of patients.[63,64]

Cardiac Dysrhythmias and Myocardial Dysfunction

In one study of 58 patients who died of AIDS, 26 (45 percent) had histopathologic myocarditis on postmortem examination: 15 of these 26 patients had clinical cardiac abnormalities, 6 had congestive heart failure, 4 had ventricular tachycardia, 10 had electrocardiographic (ECG) abnormalities, and 4 had pericardial abnormalities. Of the 32 patients without myocarditis, 6 (19 percent) had pericardial or ECG abnormalities or both, but none had congestive heart failure or ventricular tachycardia. Overall, clinical cardiac abnormalities were found in 21 patients (36 percent).[70] Serious cardiac abnormalities are common in patients with AIDS, and are associated with myocarditis.

Renal Failure

A variety of nephropathies may occur with HIV infection. In one major study of hospitalized patients with AIDS, 78 of 750 patients (10.4 percent) needed evaluation for renal disorders; 55 of these 78 patients (70 percent) had massive proteinuria, azotemia, or both (AIDS-associated nephropathy), and irreversible uremia developed in 43 patients. The prognosis is very poor. Maintenance hemodialysis is not effective in prolonging life, either in patients with AIDS-associated nephropathy and uremia or in patients with end-stage renal failure in whom AIDS developed during the course of maintenance dialysis. AIDS-associated nephropathy is characterized by proteinuria (>3.5 g/d of urinary protein). The histologic lesion is focal and segmental glomerulosclerosis.[71]

In children, the incidence of nephropathy is the same as in adults. Four morphologic variants have been described in children: (1) focal glomerular sclerosis, (2) mesangial hyperplasia, (3) minimal change disease, and (4) segmental necrotizing glomerulonephritis. The prognosis is as poor in children as in adults.[72]

Arthralgia

Reiter's syndrome, reactive arthritis, polymyositis, and sicca syndrome can herald the onset of clinically evident HIV infection or can occur in patients with well-developed AIDS. These arthralgias may mimic systemic lupus erythematosus.[73,74]

AIDS in Children

Children are often and increasingly innocent victims of HIV infection.[75] As of September 1989, a total of 1,780 children under the age of 13 years had developed AIDS. Of these, 971 had died, for a current case fatality rate of 54.6 percent. While the infusion of blood or blood products, either to treat hemorrhage or replace deficient clotting factors, played a role in transmitting the virus to children, this accounts for only 17 percent of all pediatric AIDS cases. Eighty percent of all pediatric AIDS cases occur in children born to mothers who have AIDS or HIV infection or who belong to a high-risk group (eg, prostitutes, intravenous drug abusers, or the sexual partners of drug abusers).

Since the incidence of in utero transmission of AIDS antibodies from mother to child is 100 percent, every baby born of an antibody-positive mother will also test positive for the presence of the antibody. In the European collaborative study of 271 children born to HIV-infected mothers in 8 European countries, the estimated vertical transmission rate of the disease from mother to child was 24 percent.[76] In the Italian portion of the multicenter study, HIV infection occurred in 32.6 percent of children born to seropositive mothers.[77] In a New York City study,[78] of those children who eventually developed AIDS, 20 percent developed the disease in the first year of life and the remainder developed it at a nearly constant rate of 8 percent per year, reaching the median at 4.8 years. One in every 62 children born in New York City has antibodies to HIV at the time of birth.

Therapy

Prevention

Since the virus is most commonly transmitted by traumatic sexual intercourse, allowing the intermingling of seminal fluid and blood or blood with blood, decreasing these practices will limit the spread of HIV. The homosexual community apparently has changed its habits, at least temporarily, with consequent reduction of HIV transmission. This group will, however, continue to be important in new AIDS cases, since so many are already infected.

Intravenous drug abusers have not changed their habits to any appreciable extent. This population, already predominant as new cases in New York City, will probably increase in importance throughout the rest of the country.

The blood supply is relatively, but not absolutely, safe. Contaminated blood and blood products still enter the transfusion pool and cannot be completely excluded using current screening devices.[79] Screening donated blood for anti-HIV antibodies and hepatitis B antigen has markedly reduced the incidence of transfusion-induced AIDS, but these cases still occur. The most effective mechanism is self-screening (ie, asking prospective donors to exclude themselves from donating blood if they belong to a high-risk group).[80] Fortunately, the incidence of seropositivity among American blood donors is declining, and is now 1.8 per 10,000.[81]

The use of autologous blood is the safest and most effective technique to protect prospective blood recipients during anesthesia and surgery since, with the use of their own blood, patients cannot be infected with anything other than what they already have.[82] In most patients, 3 or 4 U of autologous blood can be drawn preoperatively and infused as needed during an operative procedure. The use of autotransfusion devices will also minimize the use of homologous blood and the risks associated with its use. There is no evidence that blood from designated donors is safer than blood from a random pool of donors. Those who receive blood from such designated donors (eg, friends or relatives) are no safer than recipients of nonselected blood from a blood bank. While designated donor programs have their superficial appeal, their lack of efficacy, coupled with the difficult logistics of dealing with designated donors and their blood, make such programs impractical.

Prudent use of blood and blood products is mandated. The indiscriminate use of large amounts of fresh frozen plasma to cure mild coagulopathies demands careful consideration and elaboration of new transfusion policies.[83]

The development of an effective vaccine presents many problems. Among the retroviruses, the lentiviruses (such as HIV) have the ability to resist host neutralization by varying their virus envelopes, thus constantly presenting new sets of antigens to the host defense mechanisms.[84] This chameleonic capacity of the virus makes vaccine development very difficult. Since HIV induces an ineffective antibody response to its presence, it is problematic whether a vaccine will develop an effective antibody response. The problem is worsened by the fact that there is no animal model for AIDS. The chimpanzee can be infected with HIV, but survives the infection without developing AIDS. Monkeys can be infected with a similar virus, simian immunodeficiency virus, and do develop an AIDS-like disease, including encephalitis.[85] However, the only definitive animal model for HIV vaccine studies is the human being. Despite these formidable problems, vaccines are being prepared, either as purified inactive envelope glycoproteins of HIV, short synthetic peptides derived from a portion of the HIV envelope, recombinant DNA techniques, or vaccinia virus recombinants. Human trials are being conducted, but an effective vaccine is not predicted for the near future.

Treatment of Opportunistic Infection

The patients with AIDS is subject to a wide variety of opportunistic infections. While many of the varied bacterial, protozoan, viral, and fungal infections characteristic of the disease are responsive to therapy, the depressed immune system leaves the host vulnerable to repeat infection. Acyclovir, vidarabine, and ganciclovir have been recommended for herpes zoster, herpes simplex, and CMV infection.[86] Tuberculosis has been successfully treated with various combinations of isoniazid, rifampin, and ethambutol, with streptomycin as an alternative. Clotrimazole, amphotericin, and amikacin have been useful in treating candidal infections.

Unfortunately, resistance to antiviral drugs has developed. Ganciclovir-resistant CMV has been reported in immune-suppressed patients.[87] One patient was infected with a resistant virus, another was infected with a susceptible virus that became resistant, and a third was infected first by a susceptible strain and later by a genetically distinct resistant one. Herpes simplex resistant to acyclovir has been identified, and has produced devastating herpes infection in several patients.[88] It has been suggested that foscarnet may be useful in resistant viral infections because its mode of action is different from that of acyclovir or ganciclovir.[89]

Pneumonitis due to the protozoan *P. carinii* is the most important life-threatening opportunistic infection in AIDS patients in North America. Co-trimoxazole and pentamidine are equally effective, but each drug has significant toxicity. There is a high incidence of hypersensitivity reactions to co-trimoxazole, and both drugs cause neutropenia. Pentamidine has been associated with hepatic and renal dysfunction. Pentamidine must be administered by intramuscular or intravenous injection, while co-trimoxazole has the advantage of oral administration. In an attempt to localize pentamidine to the site of infection and, thus, limit serious systemic effects, it has been suggested that the drug might be aerosolized for inhalant use.[90] A preliminary report suggested significant benefit from this technique.

The Centers for Disease Control (CDC) has suggested guidelines for prophylaxis against *P. carinii* pneumonia (PCP) for those infected with HIV.[91] It is recommended that unless a contraindication exists, physicians should initiate prophylaxis against *P. carinii* pneumonia for any HIV-infected adult patient who has already had an episode of the illness, even if the patient has been receiving zidovudine (AZT). Unless contraindicated, prophylaxis should also be initiated for HIV-infected patients who have never had an episode of *P. carinii* pneumonia if their CD4+ (T4) cell count is less than 200/mm³ or if their CD4+ cells are less than 20 percent of total lymphocytes. Patients with CD4+ cell counts of less than 100/mm³ or CD4+ cells less than 10 percent and patients with oral thrush or persistent fever (temperature over 100°F) are at particularly high risk for *P. carinii* pneumonia. Suggested regimens include (1) oral trimethoprim-sulfamethoxazole (160 mg of trimethoprim and 800 mg of sulfamethoxazole) given twice daily with 5 mg of leucovorin once daily, and (2) aerosol pentamidine given as 300 mg every 4 weeks via the Respigard II jet nebulizer. The dose should be diluted in 6 mL of sterile water and delivered at 6 L/min from a 50 psi compressed air source until the reservoir is dry. Because other doses and aerosol delivery systems have not yet been adequately studied and analyzed, no recommendation regarding such systems can be made.

Since neither aerosol pentamidine nor oral trimethoprim-sulfamethoxazole prophylaxis is known to be safe in association with pregnancy, it is inadvisable to give either agent to HIV-infected pregnant women. Alternative regimens that are of unproven efficacy and safety for humans, but that might be considered for prophylaxis, include dapsone plus trimethoprim, or dapsone plus pyrimethamine, and pyrimethamine-sulfadoxine. Although *P. carinii* pneumonia is common in children with AIDS, there are insufficient data to develop guidelines for pediatric use.

If the debilitating diarrhea of AIDS is due to susceptible strains of *Salmonella* or *Shigella*, ampicillin or co-trimoxazole might be effective. However, there is evidence that some of the diarrhea of AIDS is due directly to HIV infection of bowel epithelium; thus, antibiotic therapy will be of no avail.

Treatment of HIV Infection

It is difficult to develop an effective therapeutic regimen directed specifically against HIV infection because of the propensity of the organism to sequester itself in cells spread diffusely throughout the body, cells that may be invaded by the pathogen yet resistant to the entry of therapeutic drugs. Additionally, drugs effective against HIV often have significant toxicities limiting their applicability.

Therapy has been directed at reverse transcriptase, the enzyme essential for HIV replication. The reverse transcriptase inhibitor, (azidothymidine, zidovudine, AZT), 3'-azido-3'deoxythymidine also enhances immune function.[92] The AZT cooperative group has reported that the drug decreased mortality and the frequency of opportunistic infections in patients with AIDS or ARC during a period of up to 6 months. Opportunistic infections occur less frequently with AZT, and the mortality rate was decreased. It is not known whether HIV will develop resistance to AZT, the one drug known to be effective.

Patients with AIDS-associated neuropathy have also benefited from AZT treatment.[93,94] Particular benefit was observed in children with symptomatic HIV infection, many of whom suffered from AIDS encephalopathy.[95] Since dementia is an important manifestation of AIDS encephalopathy, therapeutic efficacy can be conveniently measured by an increase in the intelligence quotient (IQ) in these children.

Unfortunately, while life may be prolonged with AZT treatment, and the quality of life improved, there is no evidence that AZT will affect the universal mortality of those with the disease. Anemia and neutropenia occur as results of AZT treatment, and can be quite troublesome. In one study of AZT therapy in AIDS and ARC, the major toxicity of the drug was anemia, with hemoglobin levels below 7.5 g/dL in 24 percent of the AZT patients and 4 percent of placebo recipients. Twenty-one percent of AZT recipients and 4 percent of placebo recipients required multiple transfusions. Neutropenia occurred in 16 percent of AZT patients and 2 percent of placebo recipients.[96]

Dideoxycytidine has also been found effective in treating HIV infection.[97] The drug is tolerated (at least short-term) by patients with AIDS or ARC, and drug levels above the in vitro virustatic concentration can be attained. After oral administration, dideoxycytidine is well absorbed and crosses the blood-brain barrier. Its toxic effects are dissimilar from AZT, and an alternating regimen of dideoxycytidine and AZT has been tolerated for up to 28 weeks.

Ampligen is a mismatched double-stranded RNA that, in patients with AIDS or ARC, appears to have the ability to restore immunologic function and to control HIV replication.[98] In vitro, ampligen reduces the amount of AZT necessary to inhibit HIV replication, and seems to have a synergistic virustatic effect.

Recombinant interferon has also proved to be valuable in AIDS, and has been found effective in containing Kaposi's sarcoma. In one study, 12 of 26 patients with Kaposi's sarcoma achieved a major response.[99]

The infusion of 55 to 500 mL of plasma from donors with high anti-HIV antibody titers into patients with advanced AIDS has produced short-term benefits. HIV antigen is cleared immediately, and the recipients' serum acquires the HIV antibody profile of the donor. Patients improved symptomatically, and the effect lasted up to 11 weeks.[100]

AIDS in the Hospital Setting

Hazards to Health Care Workers

In 1983, the first report was published of a health care worker who developed AIDS from contact with her patients and who subsequently died of the disease.[101] A female surgeon from Denmark, who was in none of the known risk groups, developed profuse wasting and diarrhea while working with the native population in Zaire. She returned to Copenhagen and died there. Postmortem examination revealed the stigmata of AIDS.

The CDC reports that as of September 19, 1988, 169 health care workers, with no evidence of high-risk behavior, had developed AIDS, ostensibly via contact necessitated by their professional activities. At the time of the report, 44 of the 169 had undergone extensive investigation, and no cause other than occupation could be ascribed to their disease.[102]

Of the 44 health care workers studied, there were 9 (20 percent) nursing assistants; 8 (18 percent) physicians, including 4 surgeons; 8 (18 percent) housekeeping/maintenance; 6 (14 percent) nurses; 4 (9 percent) clinical laboratory technicians; 2 (5 percent) respiratory therapists; 1 (2 percent) dentist; 1 (2 percent) paramedic; 1 (2 percent) embalmer; and 4 (9 percent) no patient contact.

It is evident that the nature of the work exposes the

health care provider to a real risk of contamination with HIV and the development of AIDS. How great is the risk? In a report published in 1985, among 85 health care workers and employees with exposure to specimens from AIDS patients, none developed AIDS or was positive for HIV antibodies. The study group included 31 needle-stick incidents involving 30 individuals.[103] Several reports of occupational HIV transmission then appeared, reporting a rate of nosocomial HIV transmission of less than 0.1 percent, with the rate after needle-stick exposure estimated to range from 0.1 to 0.5 percent. However, in 1988, the CDC reported that the risk, while small, is greater than initial reports had indicated.[104] In their survey of 963 health care workers exposed to blood from HIV-positive patients, 4 were found to be positive for HIV antibody, for a seroprevalence rate of 0.42 percent, with the upper limit of 95 percent confidence interval at 0.95 percent. However, all 4 seroconverted after needle exposure (ie, four of 860 exposed) for a seroprevalence rate of 0.47 percent and an upper limit of 95 percent confidence at 1.06 percent. Thus, a needle stick from an HIV-positive patient involves a risk of seroconversion of 1 in 100 to 1 in 200.

Approximately 1.5 million Americans are HIV positive, with the number increasing exponentially. Most HIV-positive individuals are not aware of their status, and do not appear ill; nor do they have any characteristics identifying their infectious state. Thus, the CDC recommends that all patients be considered as potential hazards to health care workers and that the following universal precautions be used in all patients[105]:

1. Barrier precautions should be used when contact with blood or body fluid of any patient is anticipated.
2. Gloves should be worn when handling body fluids, mucous membranes, or broken skin. There are no reported differences in barrier effectiveness between intact latex and intact vinyl used to manufacture gloves. Thus, the type of gloves selected should be appropriate to the task being performed.
3. Mask and eyewear should be worn when droplets are formed.
4. Handwashing is very important and should be done frequently, especially after patient contact.
5. Needles should be handled with great care and never recapped.
6. Mouth-to-mouth resuscitation should be minimized and adequate ventilatory equipment should always be available.
7. Health care workers with dermatitis should not be involved in direct patient care.

8. Pregnancy involves no special risks, but the pregnant health care worker should exercise all precautions.

These recommendations have been amplified by the American Society of Anesthesiologists Committee on Occupational Health on Operating Room Personnel. The Committee stresses strategies to prevent accidental needle sticks, emphasizing that needles should not be recapped, bent, broken, removed from syringes, or manipulated by hand. Puncture-proof containers must be available (and used) for disposable needles, syringes, and sharp instruments. The Committee further recommends surface cleaning with commercial disinfectants, but makes no specific recommendations.

Anesthesiologists deal constantly with bodily fluids such as blood, as they start intravenous infusions, draw arterial blood specimens, and transfuse blood or blood products or saliva, as they effect endotracheal intubation. Gloves should be worn at all times. Protective eyewear is also important, and should be used during bronchoscopy or endotracheal intubation. While eyeglasses offer a significant degree of protection, goggles (either disposable or permanent) offer the greatest protection, and may be fitted over glasses.

The procedures outlined above are applicable not only to the operating room but also to any area of patient care where health care workers may come in contact with bodily secretions or excretions. Such contact is often made in the recovery room or intensive care unit, where blood is drawn, intravenous infusions started, central monitoring introduced, and tracheas intubated and suctioned. The health care worker is most vulnerable in the hospital emergency room, or when called on to resuscitate patients in the hospital but outside of the operating room. Suitable protective equipment must be incorporated into every cardiac arrest "call-box."

The "universal precautions" may be criticized as "overkill." Most patients are not infected with HIV, and it is clear that puncture with a needle contaminated with HIV-infected blood is the major source of danger to health care workers. It should be emphasized that only blood or seminal fluid is known definitely to be a vector for the AIDS virus, and there are no established cases of HIV transmission by other bodily fluids. Nonetheless, since AIDS is universally fatal, and since health care workers have developed the disease, presumably through patient contact, prudence demands that all reasonable precautions must be taken to avoid contamination. These precautions should be used with all patients, since the majority of HIV-infected patients are not readily identifiable.

While the "universal precautions" are important for protection against infection with HIV, they are even more important for protection against hepatitis, especially hepatitis B. This disease is much more communicable than AIDS, and health care workers are very prone to infection from their patients. The development of the disease, while without the general fatality of AIDS, nonetheless is unpleasant, disruptive, and occasionally fatal.

Hazards to Patients

The risks to health care workers of acquiring AIDS from their patients have received great attention and caused great alarm. What have received little attention are the risks posed by health care workers to their immune-suppressed patients. Many physicians carry *P. carinii* within their lungs, but do not become ill because their intact immune systems hold the protozoan in check. Herpes simplex may be painful or unsightly, but immune-intact individuals bear its discomfort for only a brief period of time. Herpes may be devastating, and even lethal, in the immune-suppressed. The deadly potential of herpes is made more acute by the recently discovered resistance of the virus to previously effective drug therapy. While precautions are necessary to protect medical personnel from the patients with AIDS, the same precautions help safeguard the patient from medical personnel.

Anesthetic Management

Practicing anesthesiologists will, knowingly or unknowingly, voluntarily or involuntarily, deal with HIV-infected patients for thoracic surgery, and their contact with such patients will increase in time, as the rate of infection grows. The infected individual may be asymptomatic, with no stigmata of the disease, and require nothing other than routine anesthetic care; or may be seriously ill, and require maximum attention and anesthetic skill. Because of the wide variety of clinical manifestations, it is impossible to generalize or to advocate one anesthetic agent or technique as ideal or, conversely, to condemn any anesthetic agent or technique as completely inappropriate.

HIV-infected patients will undergo any of the operative procedures commonly used in those without the affliction, since infected patients are subject to the same disabilities as those not infected. Among the intravenous drug abuser group, trauma is very common and operative repairs for the consequences of trauma are frequent. Diagnostic procedures to confirm or deny the impression of AIDS are not as common as they were when the disease was so poorly understood and recognition was difficult. However, bronchoscopies and node biopsies are not uncommon.

Preoperative assessment of the patient with AIDS demands evaluation of the presence and nature of opportunistic infections and the appropriate therapy to control infection. The pneumonias are especially important because of their ability to interfere with ventilation. *Pneumocystis* pneumonia can make ventilation especially difficult because of the thick, tenacious, gummy secretions that fill the alveoli. The inhalation of pentamidine appears effective both in preventing *Pneumocystis* infection and in treating the established pneumonitis. Since renal dysfunction is quite common in patients with AIDS, preoperative evaluation of renal function via determination of creatinine, blood urea nitrogen, and electrolytes should be determined. It should be noted, however, that renal dysfunction of AIDS is progressive and has as yet no known therapy.

Since as many as 45 percent of patients with AIDS have cardiac infection and 36 percent have serious dysfunction, including cardiac dysrhythmias and congestive heart failure, a chest x-ray and ECG should be routine. Determination of cardiac output and ejection fraction may be indicated. The high incidence of virus-induced cardiac disease should broaden the criteria for the use of invasive monitors, especially the pulmonary artery catheter. However, invasive monitoring may be hazardous because of sympathetic dysfunction and severe hypotension.[106]

Patients with AIDS challenge physicians to exercise compassion, care, and understanding in meeting their responsibility to be of service to the terminally ill. Many of these patients are drug abusers, often addicted to a wide range of drugs, with different potentials for withdrawal. The narcotic addict is usually also an alcoholic.[107] Adequate history is mandatory to determine the polypharmacy of addiction and the nature of withdrawal should this clinical syndrome occur. In addition to dementia, the AIDS patient, facing the prospect of almost certain death in the near future, may become depressed, withdrawn, and uncommunicative, making adequate assessment very difficult, if not impossible.

Patients may be quite dehydrated because of the profound diarrhea characteristic of the disease. They are frequently malnourished because of the frequent extensive *Candida* infection of the mouth and esophagus. Adequate fluid repletion and correction of electrolyte imbalance are necessary prior to extensive anesthesia for thoracic surgery, and may require total parenteral nutrition to correct the state of malnourishment.

Management of the airway may be troublesome because of hypertrophy of tonsils and adenoids. Kaposi's sarcoma, which often is a central and aggressive tumor in the patient with AIDS, may occur in the upper airway and make intubation difficult. Oral candidiasis is a common opportunistic infection in afflicted patients, and can cause significant edema and erythema, sufficient to alter the anatomy to the extent that endotracheal intubation using conventional techniques may be difficult or impossible. In a patient with extensive oral *Candida* infection, awake visualization of the airway should be performed and ease of intubation assessed with the patient breathing spontaneously. If the anatomy is distorted by the infection, respiratory depressants and muscle relaxants should not be used until the airway is secured, either by awake intubation or tracheostomy. Guided intubation with fiberoptic laryngoscopy or bronchoscopy may be impossible because of severe anatomic deformity, erythema, and edema.

Adequate ventilation of the patient with *Pneumocystis* pneumonia may be difficult because of the thick intra-alveolar exudate limiting gas exchange. Pulse oximetry and capnography will be of particular benefit in monitoring the adequacy of ventilation.

Since HIV is blood borne and may be transmitted via the infusion of blood or blood products, it is imperative that anesthesiologists understand the risk of transfusion and develop criteria for the use of these products. Coagulopathies occur in the AIDS patient, usually platelet dysfunction and thrombocytopenia. This decrease in platelet number and activity may be due to viral suppression of bone marrow or may be due to therapy (eg, AZT). Should there be any question of platelet inadequacy, a bleeding time should be performed and platelet infusion considered to correct a prolonged bleeding time.

The choice of anesthetic agent and technique must be individualized to the patient's state of health and the surgical requirements. Inhalation anesthetics, with their negative inotropic properties, should be used with caution in the patient with a myocardium compromised by viral infection. Intravenous narcotics, with no effect on inotropy, may be the drugs of choice. Consideration should also be given to the advisability of using halogenated drugs in patients with active hepatitis B or with CMV hepatitis. Spinal or epidural anesthesia may be contraindicated because of a viral infection of the central and peripheral nervous systems and the possibility of further dissemination of the infection. This has not been demonstrated and may be of more medicolegal than medical importance. However, AIDS is progressive, and neuropathies are common. Regional anesthesia should be used if it is clearly the technique of choice and the patient has been adequately advised of the risks of the procedure and the probable increase in neurologic signs and symptoms.

HEPATITIS

Hepatitis is a group of diseases of varying degrees of severity, infectivity, and with differing prognoses depending on the viral etiologic agent. It is convenient to divide hepatitis into hepatitis A, hepatitis B, and hepatitis non-A, non-B (NANBH) (now called hepatitis C).

Hepatitis A is a parenteral viral infection spread by the fecal-oral route, usually with contaminated water as the vector. The disease occurs in epidemics or as a constant infective process, infecting close to 100 percent of the population living in a contaminated area.

Hepatitis B virus (HBV) is found in human fluids, including blood, seminal fluid, and saliva, and is transmitted from host to recipient by any of these substances. Formerly, hepatitis B was the most common infectious liver disease associated with blood transfusion. Screening donor blood for the viral particle surface antigen (HBsAg) has markedly reduced the incidence of transfusion-associated hepatitis B without any great reduction in the incidence of posttransfusion hepatitis.[108]

Posttransfusion hepatitis is now almost invariably due to NANBH. This hepatitis occurs in at least two forms; one is parenteral, fecal-oral, and occurs in epidemics,[109] the other is blood borne and spread by blood transfusion.[110]

In the United States, hepatitis B is the most common form of hepatitis, occurring in 48 percent of those afflicted; NANBH is found in 42 percent; and hepatitis A is found in 10 percent.[111]

While posttransfusion hepatitis B has been significantly reduced in the United States, the disease itself still represents a significant health hazard, especially to health care workers. While the risk of becoming HIV antibody-positive after a prick with a contaminated needle is only 1 in 100 to 1 in 200, it is estimated that 6 to 30 percent of persons who receive a needle prick exposure from an HBsAg-positive individual will become infected.[102] This probably reflects the much higher blood concentration of infective virus in the patient with hepatitis B as contrasted to the patient with AIDS. In contrast to AIDS, human saliva has been shown to be infective, and hepatitis B can be spread by human bite.[112]

In 1987, it was estimated by the CDC that 300,000 new cases of hepatitis B develop each year, with approximately 75,000 (25 percent) of infected persons developing acute hepatitis.[102] Of these infected individuals, 18,000 to 30,000 (6 to 10 percent) will become HBV carriers, at risk of developing chronic liver disease (chronic active hepatitis, cirrhosis, and primary liver cancer), and will be infectious to others.

Approximately 12,000 health care workers become infected with HBV each year, with 500 to 600 of them being hospitalized and 700 to 1,200 developing a chronic carrier state. Of these infected health care workers, approximately 250 will die proximately or remotely as a result of the infection; 12 to 15 will die from fulminant hepatitis, 170 to 200 from cirrhosis, and 40 to 50 from liver cancer. Ten to thirty percent of health care workers demonstrate serologic evidence of past or present HBV infection, with the percentage increasing directly with the number of years of practice.

An effective vaccine to prevent hepatitis B has been available since 1982, stimulating active immunity against HBV infection and providing more than 90 percent protection against hepatitis B for 7 or more years following vaccination. After infection with HBV, the vaccine is 70 to 88 percent effective when given within 1 week of exposure. When combined with hepatitis B immune globulin, prevention after exposure exceeds 90 percent. In 1987, the Department of Health and Human Services and the Department of Labor stated that hepatitis B vaccine should be provided to all health care workers regularly exposed to blood and other body fluids potentially contaminated with HBV, at no charge to the worker.[113]

Non-A, non-B hepatitis is now the prevalent form of posttransfusion hepatitis, accounting for 90 percent or more of all cases. The incubation period of both hepatitis B and NANBH overlap, that of B being 35 to 77 days and that of NANBH being 18 to 89 days.[110] Non-A, non-B hepatitis is frequently asymptomatic, or with only vague and ill-defined signs and symptoms. Fatigue, anorexia, malaise, nausea, vomiting, abdominal pain, and hepatomegaly occur to varying degrees of severity, while jaundice is present in only 39 percent.

Screening blood for NANBH previously relied upon a surrogate, alanine amino transferase (ALT), formerly known as SGPT. Unfortunately, the test is quite imprecise. While patients with NANBH may have elevated ALT levels, there are wide fluctuations in the level, and blood can still be virus-positive and infective, even when ALT levels are normal.[114,115] Nonetheless, screening for ALT-elevated blood (ie, greater than 45 IU; normal, 8 to 20 IU) can eliminate as much as 40 percent of infective blood. There is also a direct relationship between the value of ALT-elevated units

of blood administered and the development of hepatitis, with a 91 percent incidence of infection when 2 or more U of ALT-elevated blood are transfused.[116]

A test for antibody to hepatitis C or NANBH has recently been put into clinical practice. It is estimated that the routine application of this assay in donor screening will detect approximately 85 percent of those capable of transmitting NANBH and, thus, represents a significant advance over ALT testing.[117–120]

While NANBH is usually milder clinically than hepatitis B, the development of chronic hepatitis and cirrhosis is more common, and the disease represents a significant risk for severe morbidity and mortality.[121,122]

There is no effective therapy for either hepatitis B or NANBH, and prevention is still the most practical and important mechanism for preventing spread of these diseases and their fearsome consequences.[123] Recombinant interferon alfa has had some success in treating NANBH. However, therapy is not universally successful, and the relapse rate after discontinuing treatment approaches 50 percent.[124,125] The universal precautions outlined above, together with prudent policies of blood collection and use, are most effective in limiting these diseases. Autologous blood programs are highly recommended, as are intraoperative cell harvesting, reinfusion mechanisms, and the development of a pool of tried and negative blood donors.

Duty To Care

Hepatitis represents a much greater risk to health care workers than does AIDS. Nonetheless, a mystique has developed about HIV infection, creating a fear bordering on hysteria. Suitable precautions will limit, but never eliminate, the risk of these diseases. The ethical physician recognizes the duty to render care to those who need his help. The duty of care is neither debatable nor negotiable for the ethical health care worker.[126]

REFERENCES

1. Garry RF, Witte MH, Gottlieb A, et al: Documentation of an AIDS virus infection in the United States in 1968. JAMA 260:2085–2087, 1988
2. Gottlieb MS, Schroff M, Schanker HM, et al: *Pneumocystis carinii* pneumonia and mucosal candidiasis in previously healthy homosexual men. N Engl J Med 305:1425–1431, 1981
3. Masur H, Michelis MA, Greene JB, et al: An outbreak of community-acquired *Pneumocystis carinii* pneumonia. N Engl J Med 305:1431–1438, 1981

4. Broder S, Gallo RC: A pathogenic retrovirus (HTLV-III) linked to AIDS. N Engl J Med 311:1292–1297, 1984

5. Laurence J, Brun-Vezinet F, Schutzer S, et al: Lymphadenopathy-associated viral antibody in AIDS. N Engl J Med 311:1269–1273, 1984

6. Evans LA, Moreau J, Odenhouri K, et al: Simultaneous isolation of HIV-I and HIV-II from an AIDS patient. Lancet 2:1389–1391, 1988

7. Brun-Vezinet F, Rey MA, Katlama C, et al: Lymphadenopathy-associated virus type 2 in AIDS and AIDS-related complex. Lancet 1:128–132, 1987

8. Clavel F, Mansinho K, Chamaret S, et al: Human immunodeficiency virus type 2 infection associated with AIDS in West Africa. N Engl J Med 316:1180–1185, 1987

9. Albert J, Bottiger B, Biberfeld G, Fenyo EM: Replicative and cytopathic characteristics of HIV-2 and severity of infection. Lancet 1:852–853, 1989

10. Cheng-Mayer C, Seto D, Tateno M, Levy JA: Biologic features of HIV-1 that correlate with virulence in the host. Science 240:80–82, 1988

11. Ronald AR, Ndinya-Achola JO, Plummer FA, et al: A review of HIV I in Africa. Bull NY Acad Med 64:480–490, 1988

12. Mann JM, Chin J: AIDS: a global perspective. N Engl J Med 319:302–303, 1988

13. New York Times, January 7, 1989, p. 31

14. Centers for Disease Control: HIV/AIDS surveillance. AIDS cases reported through August 1989. 1–16, September, 1989

15. Hoft R, Berardi VP, Weiblen BJ, et al: Seroprevalence of human immunodeficiency virus among childbearing women. N Engl J Med 318: 525–530, 1988

16. Landesman S, Minkoff H, Holman S, et al: Serosurvey of human immunodeficiency virus infection in parturients. JAMA 258:2701–2703, 1987

17. Seligmann M, Chess L, Fahey JL, et al: AIDS—an immunologic reevaluation. N Engl J Med 311:1286–1292, 1984

18. Steis R, Broder R: AIDS: a general overview. p. 322. In DeVito VT, Hellman S, Rosenberg SA (eds): AIDS, Etiology, Diagnosis, Treatment and Prevention. Lippincott, Philadelphia, 1985

19. Sande MA: AIDS: an introduction. Bull NY Acad Med 64:462–463, 1988

20. Stute R: HIV antigen detection in routine blood donor screening. Lancet 1:566, 1987

21. Gaines H, von Sydow M, Sonnerborg A, et al: Antibody response in primary human immunodeficiency virus infection. Lancet 1:1249–1253, 1987

22. Ranki A, Valle S, Krohn M, et al: Long latency precedes overt seroconversion in sexually transmitted human-immunodeficiency-virus infection. Lancet 2:589–593, 1987

23. Meyer KB, Pauker SG: Screening for HIV: can we afford the false positive rate? N Engl J Med 371:238–241, 1987

24. Burke DS, Brundage JR, Redfield RR, et al: Measurement of the false positive rate in a screening program for human immunodeficiency virus infections. N Engl J Med 319:961–964, 1988

25. Weiss R, Thier SO: HIV testing is the answer—what's the question? N Engl J Med 319:1010–1012, 1988

26. Handsfield HH: Transmission of human immunodeficiency virus (HIV). N Engl J Med 318:1202, 1988

27. Lorian V: AIDS, anal sex, and heterosexuals. Lancet 1:1111, 1988

28. Kingsley LA, Detels R, Kaslow R, et al: Risk factors for seroconversion to human immunodeficiency virus among male homosexuals. Lancet 1:345–349, 1987

29. Goedert JJ, Sarngadharan MG, Biggar RJ, et al: Determinants of retrovirus (HTLV-III) antibody and immunodeficiency conditions in homosexual men. Lancet 2:711–716, 1984

30. Coates RA, Calzavara LM, Read SE, et al: Risk factors for HIV infection in male sexual contacts of men with AIDS or an AIDS-related condition. Am J Epidemiol 128:729–739, 1988

31. Goldberg DJ, Green St, Kennedy GH, et al: HIV and orogenital transmission. Lancet 2:1363, 1988

32. Simonsen JN, Cameron DW, Gakinya MN, et al: Human immunodeficiency virus infection among men with sexually transmitted diseases. N Engl J Med 319:274–278, 1988

33. Ron A, Rogers DE: AIDS in New York City: the role of intravenous drug users. Bull NY Acad Med 65:787–800, 1989

34. Ward JW, Bush TJ, Perkins HA, et al: The natural history of transfusion-associated infection with human immunodeficiency virus factors influencing the rate of progression to disease. N Engl J Med 321:947–952, 1989

35. Ward JW, Homberg SD, Allen JR, et al: Transmission of human immunodeficiency virus (HIV) by blood transfusions screened as negative for HIV antibody. N Engl J Med 318:473–478, 1988

36. Cumming PD, Wallace EL, Schorr JB, Dodd RY: Exposure of patients to human immunodeficiency virus through the transfusion of blood components that test antibody-negative. N Engl J Med 321:941–946, 1989

37. Friedland GH, Klein RS: Transmission of the human immunodeficiency virus. N Engl J Med 317:1125–1135, 1987

38. Seifert MH: Transmission of human immunodeficiency virus (HIV). N Engl J Med 318:1203, 1988

39. Anonymous: Transmission of HIV by human bite. Lancet 2:522, 1987

40. Allen JR: Heterosexual transmission of human immunodeficiency virus (HIV) in the United States. Bull NY Acad Med 64:464–479, 1988

41. Curran JW, Lawrence DN, Jaffee H, et al: Acquired immunodeficiency syndrome (AIDS) associated with transfusion. N Engl J Med 310:69–75, 1984

42. Delpre G, Ilfeld D, Pitlik S, et al: AIDS after coronary bypass surgery. Lancet 1:103, 1984

43. Deresinski SC, Cooney DP, Auerbach DM, et al: AIDS transmission via transfusion therapy. Lancet 1:102, 1984

44. Anonymous: Needlestick transmission of HTLV-III from a patient infected in Africa. Lancet 2:1376–1377, 1984

45. Nelson JA, Wiley CA, Reynolds-Kohler C, et al: Human

immunodeficiency virus detected in bowel epithelium from patients with gastrointestinal symptoms. Lancet 1:259–262, 1988

46. Valle SL, Saxinger C, Ranki A, et al: Diversity of clinical spectrum of HTLV-III infection. Lancet 1:301–304, 1985

47. Rees M: Describing the AIDS epidemic. Lancet 2:98–99, 1987

48. Murray HW, Hillman JK, Rubin BY, et al: Patients at risk for AIDS-related opportunistic infections. N Engl J Med 313:1504–1510, 1985

49. Varteresian-Karanfil L, Josephson A, Fikrig S, et al: Pulmonary infection and cavity formation caused by *Mycobacterium tuberculosis* in a child with AIDS. N Engl J Med 319:1018–1019, 1988

50. Allen JN, Wewers MD: HIV-associated bronchiolitis obliterans organizing pneumonia. Chest 96:197–198, 1989

51. Suffredini AF, Ognibene FP, Lack EE, et al: Nonspecific interstitial pneumonitis: a common cause of pulmonary disease in the acquired immunodeficiency syndrome. Ann Intern Med 107:7–13, 1987

52. Grieco MH, Chinoy-Acharya P: Lymphocytic interstitial pneumonia associated with the acquired immune deficiency syndrome. Am Rev Respir Dis 131:952–955, 1985

53. Solal-Celigny P, Coudere LJ, Herman D, et al: Lymphoid interstitial pneumonitis in acquired immunodeficiency syndrome-related complex. Am Rev Respir Dis 131:956–960, 1985

54. Haverkos HW, Amal Z, Drotman DP, Morgan M: Kaposi's sarcoma in homosexual men with AIDS, by race. Lancet 2:1075, 1988

55. Lopez-Herce JA, Cid J, Sanudo EF, et al: AIDS and Hodgkins disease. Lancet 2:1104–1105, 1986

56. Kristal AR, Nasca PC, Burnett WS, Mikl J: Changes in the epidemiology of non-Hodgkin's lymphoma associated with epidemic human immunodeficiency virus (HIV) infection. Am J Epidemiol 128:711–718, 1988

57. France AJ, Kean DM, Douglas RHB, et al: Adenoidal hypertrophy in HIV-infected patients. Lancet 2:1076, 1988

58. Barzan L, Carbone A, Saracchini S, et al: Nasopharyngeal lymphatic tissue hypertrophy in HIV infected patients. Lancet 1:42–43, 1989

59. Resnick L, Di Marzo-Veronese F, Schupbach J, et al: Intra-blood-brain-barrier synthesis of HTLV-III specific IgG in patients with neurologic symptoms associated with AIDS or AIDS-related complex. N Engl J Med 313:1498–1504, 1985

60. Ho DD, Rota TR, Schooley RT, et al: Isolation of HTLV-III from cerebrospinal fluid and neural tissues of patients with neurologic syndromes related to the acquired immunodeficiency syndrome. N Engl J Med 313:1493–1497, 1985

61. de la Monte SM, Moore T, Hedley-White ET: Vacuolar encephalopathy of AIDS. N Engl J Med 315:1549–1550, 1986

62. Black PH: HTLV-II, AIDS, and the brain. N Engl J Med 313:1538–1540, 1985

63. Lantos PL, Tighe JR, Bateman NT: Post-mortem neuropathological studies in AIDS. Lancet 2:1075–1076, 1988

64. Currie J, Benson E, Ramsden B, et al: Eye movement abnormalities as a predicator of the acquired immunodeficiency syndrome dementia complex. Arch Neurol 45:949–953, 1988

65. So YT, Holtzman DM, Abrams DI, Olney RK: Peripheral neuropathy associated with acquired immunodeficiency syndrome. Arch Neurol 45:945–948, 1988

66. Gherardi R, Lebargy F, Gaulard P, et al: Necrotizing vasculitis and HIV replication in peripheral nerves. N Engl J Med 321:685–686, 1989

67. Belec L, Georges AJ, Vuillecard E, et al: Peripheral facial paralysis indicating HIV infection. Lancet 2:1421–1422, 1988

68. Thomas CS: HIV and schizophrenia. Lancet 2:101, 1987

69. Atkinson JH, Grant I, Kennedy CJ, et al: Prevalence of psychiatric disorders among men infected with human immunodeficiency virus. Arch Gen Psychiatry 45:859–864, 1988

70. Reilly JM, Cunnion RE, Anderson, DW, et al: Frequency of myocarditis, left ventricular dysfunction and ventricular tachycardia in the acquired immune deficiency syndrome. Am J Cardiol 62:789–793, 1988

71. Rao TKS, Friedman EA, Nicastri AD: The types of renal disease in the acquired immunodeficiency syndrome. N Engl J Med 316:1062–1068, 1987

72. Strauss J, Abitbol C, Zilleruelo G, et al: Renal disease in children with the acquired immunodeficiency syndrome. N Engl J Med 321:625–630, 1989

73. Kaye BR: Rheumatologic manifestations of infection with human immunodeficiency virus (HIV). Ann Intern Med 111:158–167, 1989

74. Itescu S, Branato LJ, Winchester R: A sicca syndrome in HIV infection: association with HLA-DR5 and CD8 lymphocytosis. Lancet 2:466–468, 1989

75. Scott GB, Buck BE, Leterman JG, et al: Acquired immunodeficiency syndrome in infants. N Engl J Med 310:76–81, 1984

76. Peckham CS, Senturia AE, Ades ML, et al: Mother-to-child transmission of HIV infection. Lancet 2:1039–1043, 1988

77. Tovo PA, de Martino M, Caramsi G, et al: Epidemiology, clinical features and prognostic factors of paediatric HIV infection. Lancet 2:1043–1046, 1988

78. Auger I, Thomas P, De Gruttola V, et al: Incubation periods for paediatric AIDS patients. Nature 336:575–577, 1988

79. Bove JR: Transfusion-associated hepatitis and AIDS. N Engl J Med 317:242–245, 1987

80. Menitove JE: The decreasing risk of transfusion-associated AIDS. N Engl J Med 321:966–968, 1989

81. Ness PM, Douglas DK, Harper M: Declining prevalence of HIV-positive seropositive blood donors. N Engl J Med 321:615, 1989

82. Committee on Public Health, New York Academy of Medicine: Statement on sources of blood for transfusion. Bull N Y Acad Med 64:595–600, 1988

83. NIH Consensus Conference: Fresh frozen plasma. JAMA 253:551–553, 1985

84. Sarma PS, Cremer KJ, Gruber J: Acquired immunodeficiency syndrome: progress and prospects for vaccine development. J Natl Cancer Inst 80:1193–1197, 1988

85. Letvin NL, Daniel MD, Sehgal PK, et al: Induction of AIDS-like disease in macaque monkeys with T-cell tropic retrovirus STLV-III. Science 230:71–73, 1985

86. Young LS: Treatable aspects of infection due to human immunodeficiency virus. Lancet 2:1503–1506, 1987

87. Erice A, Chou S, Biron KK, et al: Progressive disease due to ganciclovir-resistant cytomegalovirus in immunocompromised patients. N Engl J Med 320:289–293, 1989

88. Erlich KS, Mills J, Chatis P, et al: Acyclovir-resistant herpes simplex virus infections in patients with the acquired immunodeficiency syndrome. N Engl J Med 320:293–296, 1989

89. Chatis PA, Miller CH, Schrager LE, Crumpacker CS: Successful treatment with foscarnet of an acyclovir-resistant mucocutaneous infection with herpes simplex virus in a patient with acquired immunodeficiency syndrome. N Engl J Med 320:297–300, 1989

90. Montgomery AB, Debs RJ, Luce JM, et al: Aerosolized pentamidine as sole therapy for *Pneumocystis carinii* pneumonia in patients with acquired immunodeficiency syndrome. Lancet 2:480–483, 1987

91. Centers for Disease Control: Guidelines for prophylaxis against *Pneumocystis carinii* pneumonia for persons infected with human immunodeficiency virus. JAMA 262:335–340, 1989

92. Fischl MA, Richman DD, Grieco H, et al: The efficacy of azidothymidine (AZT) in the treatment of patients with AIDS and AIDS-related complex. N Engl J Med 317:185–191, 1987

93. Yarchoan R, Berg G, Brouwers P, et al: Response of human-immunodeficiency-virus associated neurological disease to 3′-azido-3′-deoxythymidine. Lancet 1:123–125, 1987

94. Schmitt FA, Bigley JW, Mckinnon R, et al: Neuropsychological outcome of zidovudine (AZT) treatment of patients with AIDS and AIDS-related complex. N Engl J Med 319:1573–1578, 1988

95. Pizzo PA, Eddy J, Falloon J, et al: Effect of continuous infusion of zidovudine (AZT) in children with symptomatic HIV infection. N Engl J Med 319:889–896, 1988

96. Richman DD, Fischl MA, Grieco MH, et al: The toxicity of azidothymidine (AZT) in the treatment of patients with AIDS and AIDS-related complex. N Engl J Med 317:192–197, 1987

97. Yarchoan R, Perno CF, Thomas RV, et al: Phase I studies of 2′-3′-dideoxycytidine in severe human immunodeficiency virus infection as a single agent and alternating with zidovudine (AZT). Lancet 1:76–80, 1988

98. Mitchell WM, Montefiori DC, Robinson WE, et al: Mismatched double stranded RNA (ampligen) reduces concentration of zidovudine (azidothymidine) required for in-vitro inhibition of human immunodeficiency virus. Lancet 1:890–892, 1987

99. de Wit R, Schattenkerk JME, Boucher CAB, et al: Clinical and virological effects of high-dose recombinant interferon-alpha in disseminated AIDS-related Kaposi's sarcoma. Lancet 2:1214–1217, 1988

100. Jackson GG, Perkins JT, Rubenis M, et al: Passive immunoneutralization of human immunodeficiency virus in patients with advanced AIDS. Lancet 2:647–652, 1988

101. Bygbjerg IC: AIDS in a Danish surgeon (Zaire, 1976). Lancet 1:925, 1983

102. Centers for Disease Control: Guidelines for prevention of transmission of human immunodeficiency virus and hepatitis B to health care and public-safety workers. MMWR 38:5–6, 1989

103. Hirsch MS, Wormser GP, Schooley RT, et al: Risk of nosocomial infection with human T-cell lymphotropic virus III (HTLV III). N Engl J Med 312:1–4, 1985

104. Marcus R: Surveillance of health care workers exposed to blood from patients infected with human immunodeficiency virus. N Engl J Med 319:1118–1123, 1988

105. MMWR 37:377–382, 387–388, 1988

106. Craddock C, Pasvol G, Bull R, et al Cardiorespiratory arrest and autonomic neuropathy in AIDS. Lancet 2:16–18, 1987

107. Stimmel B, Vernace S, Tobias H: Hepatic dysfunction in heroin addicts: the role of alcohol. JAMA 222:811–812, 1972

108. Seeff LB, Wright EC, Zimmerman HJ, McCollum RW: VA cooperative study of post-transfusion hepatitis, 1969–1974. Incidence and characteristics of hepatitis and responsible risk factors. Am J Med Sci 270:355–362, 1975

109. Khuroo MS: Study of an epidemic of non-A, non-B hepatitis. Am J Med 68:818–824, 1980

110. Hoofnagle JH, Gerety RJ, Tabor E, et al: Transmission of non-A, non-B hepatitis. Ann Intern Med 87:14–20, 1977

111. Alter MJ, Gerety RJ, Smallwood LA, et al: Sporadic non-A, non-B hepatitis: frequency and epidemiology in an urban U.S. population. J Infect Dis 145:886–893, 1982

112. Cancio-Bello T, de Medina M, Shorey J, et al: An institutional outbreak of hepatitis B related to a human biting carrier. J Infect Dis 146:652–656, 1982

113. U.S. Department of Labor, U.S. Department of Health and Human Services Joint Advisory Notice: Protection against occupational exposure to hepatitis B virus (HBV) and human immunodeficiency virus (HIV). Federal Register 52:41818–41824, 1987

114. Tabor E, Seeff LB, Gerety RJ: Chronic non-A, non-B hepatitis carrier state. N Engl J Med 303:140–143, 1980

115. Realdi G, Alberti A, Rugge M, et al: Long-term followup of acute and chronic non-A, non-B post-transfusion hepatitis: evidence of progression to liver cirrhosis. Gut 23:270–275, 1982

116. Aach RD, Szmuness W, Mosley JW, et al: Serum alanine aminotransferase of donors in relation to the risk of non-A, non-B hepatitis in recipients. N Engl J Med 304:989–994, 1981

117. Stevens CE, Talyor PE, Pindyck J, et al: Epidemiology of hepatitis C. JAMA 263:49–53, 1990

118. Alter HJ, Purcell RH, Shih JW, et al: Detection of antibody to hepatitis C virus in prospectively followed transfusion recipients with acute and chronic non-A, non-B hepatitis. N Engl J Med 321:1494–1500, 1989

119. Van Der Poel CL, Reesink HW, Schaasberg W, et al: Infectivity of blood seropositive for hepatitis C virus antibodies. Lancet 1:558–560, 1990

120. Menitove JE, Richards WA, Destree M: Early US experience with anti-HCV kit in blood donors. Lancet 1:750, 1990

121. Koretz RL, Suffin SC, Gitnick GL: Post-transfusion chronic liver disease. Gastroenterology 71:797–803, 1976

122. Knodell RG, Conrad E, Ishak KG: Development of chronic liver disease after acute non-A, non-B post-transfusion hepatitis. Gastroenterology 72:902–909, 1977

123. Sherlock S, Thomas HC: Treatment of chronic hepatitis due to hepatitis B virus. Lancet 2:1343–1346, 1985

124. Davis GL, Balart LA, Schiff ER, et al: Treatment of chronic hepatitis C with recombinant interferon alfa: a multi-center randomized, controlled trial. N Engl J Med 321:1501–1506, 1989

125. DiBisceglie AM, Martini P, Kassianides C, et al: Recombinant interferon alfa therapy for chronic hepatitis C: a randomized, double-blind, placebo-controlled trial. N Engl J Med 321:1506–1510, 1989

126. Bayer R: AIDS and the duty to treat: risk, responsibility, and health care workers. Bull N Y Acad Med 64:498–505, 1988

5

METABOLIC AND HORMONAL FUNCTIONS OF THE LUNG

Roger A. Johns, M.D.
W. Ross Tracey, Ph.D.

Once viewed as an organ involved solely in gas exchange, the lung is now regarded as an active metabolic organ that plays an important role in maintaining cardiovascular homeostasis. The anatomic location of the lungs serves to make this possible, as it ensures that the lungs receive the entire cardiac output. Therefore, the lungs are in an optimal position to actively modulate the chemical composition of the blood. This may be achieved via the removal, metabolism, or activation of a wide variety of substances present in the circulation (eg, norepinephrine, 5-hydroxytryptamine [5-HT], angiotensin II, bradykinin). In addition, vasoactive (eg, endothelium-derived relaxing factor [EDRF], eicosanoids) and immunoregulatory substances (eg, eicosanoids, adenine nucleotides) are released into the vasculature where they elicit localized or systemic effects. Table 5-1 lists some of the compounds that are either acted on by or released from the lungs.

METABOLIC AND SECRETORY COMPONENTS OF THE LUNG

The lung contains at least 40 different cell types, of which only a small proportion are primarily involved with the metabolic and hormonal characteristics of this organ. These include the vascular endothelium, Clara cells, K cells, type II pneumocytes, and mast cells.

Vascular Endothelium

The vascular endothelium comprises approximately 30 percent of the cellular composition of the human lung parenchyma (Table 5-2).[1] These cells are responsible for a major portion of the metabolic activity of the lungs and also fulfill important secretory functions. The pulmonary endothelial cells are joined by tight intercellular junctions and form a continuous

TABLE 5-1. Handling of Biologically Active Compounds by the Lung

Compounds selectively cleared and/or metabolized
  Norepinephrine
  5-HT (serotonin)
  Adenosine triphosphate
  Adenosine diphosphate
  Adenosine monophosphate
  Adenosine
  Bradykinin
  Angiotensin I (converted to angiotensin II)
  Atrial natriuretic peptides
  Prostaglandins E_1, E_2, and $F_{2\alpha}$
  Morphine
  Steroids

Compounds unaffected by the lung
  Epinephrine
  Dopamine
  Isoproterenol
  Angiotensin II
  Substance P
  Oxytocin
  Vasopressin
  Eledoisin
  Bombesin
  Vasoactive intestinal peptide
  Gastrin
  Prostaglandin A_1, A_2, I_2 (prostacyclin)
  Thromboxane A_2

Compounds released from the lung
  Adenosine
  Prostaglandin I_2, E, and F
  Endothelium-derived relaxing factor
  Leukotriene A_4, B_4, C_4, D_4, and E_4
  Histamine
  5-HT
  Heparin
  Plasminogen activator

lining of the pulmonary vasculature.[2,3] This monolayer of cells acts as part of a physical barrier (the alveolar-capillary membrane) between the blood and the outside environment[2] and also functions in the transport of water, solutes, and respiratory gases. The pulmonary endothelium is unique mainly because of its extensive surface area, the fact that it is exposed to the entire cardiac output, and its anatomic location in the circulatory system.

TABLE 5-2. Cellular Composition of Alveolar Region of Human Lung

Cell Type	Cells ($n \times 10^6$)	Percentage of Total Lung Cells
Interstitial cells	84	36
Endothelial cells	68	30
Alveolar type II cells	37	16
Macrophages	23	9
Alveolar type I cells	19	8

(From Crapo et al,[1] with permission.)

The metabolic function of the pulmonary endothelium depends on the interplay among blood flow, transit time, perfusion, and surface area. The human pulmonary capillary bed is the largest capillary bed in the body, estimated to have a total surface area at rest of 50 to 70 m^2, which, at 75 percent total lung capacity, may expand to 90 m^2.[4] In addition, the surface of the pulmonary endothelial cells is covered by many projections (Fig. 5-1) and invaginations (caveolae) (Fig. 5-2) that serve to further increase the total surface area. The total perfused endothelial surface area (and therefore the total surface area available for metabolism) is under active control. Physiologic and pathophysiologic changes in pulmonary arterial pressure can lead to recruitment of portions of the pulmonary vasculature that are normally poorly perfused. Endothelial uptake and surface metabolism of blood-borne substances are influenced by transit time; therefore, changes in blood flow (which affect transit time) directly influence metabolism.

In particular, the pulmonary endothelium removes compounds such as norepinephrine and 5-HT from the blood,[5] synthesizes and releases vasoactive agents such as prostacyclin (PGI_2)[6–8] and EDRF,[6,9,10] and metabolizes other compounds such as the adenine nucleotides.[5] The pulmonary endothelium also converts inactive peptides to metabolites with vasoactive properties (angiotensin I to angiotensin II)[11,12]; conversely, vasoactive peptides such as bradykinin are inactivated.[11,12] In addition to these activities, the endothelium is involved in the metabolism of xenobiotics (ie, chemicals foreign to the body) via several metabolic enzyme systems, which include the cytochrome P-450 mono-oxygenases.[13,14] The pulmonary cytochrome P-450 mono-oxygenase system may also be important in producing endogenous vasoactive compounds.[15]

Clara Cells

Clara cells are nonciliated, columnar cells that line the terminal bronchioles and that may project into the airway lumen. These are secretory cells that have a high level of metabolic activity, as demonstrated by cytochemical and ultrastructural studies.[16] The secretory functions of the Clara cell are poorly understood, and they have been variously suggested to secrete pulmonary surfactant, components of the bronchiolar periciliary fluid, cholesterol, and carbohydrates.[17]

There is substantial evidence to suggest that these cells represent a primary site of cytochrome P-450-dependent metabolism in the lung. Cytochrome P-450 isozymes have been localized in Clara cells,[18,19] and these cells have been demonstrated to exhibit cytochrome P-450-like metabolic activity.[20] The cytochrome P-450 mono-oxygenase system provides a ma-

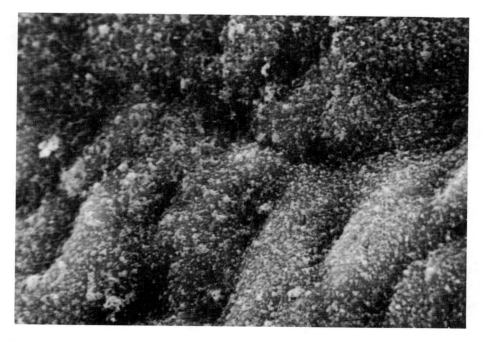

Fig. 5-1. Scanning electron photomicrograph demonstrating surface projections of pulmonary endothelial cells ($\times$ 2,500). (From Tracey et al,[68] with permission.)

jor route for the oxidative metabolism of xenobiotics. This pathway, although primarily involved in detoxification, may also lead to the formation of metabolites that are more toxic than the parent compound. Therefore, the Clara cell, while an important pulmonary site for the inactivation of xenobiotics, may also be the initial site of parenchymal injury induced by the metabolic activation of certain agents of environmental (eg, paraquat, carbon tetrachloride) or clinical (eg, bleomycin) origin. In addition, the ability of Clara cells to metabolize exogenous substances may indicate that these cells are an important site for the metabolic activation of certain carcinogens.

K Cells

K cells are specialized basal epithelial cells of the lung that are derived from an endocrine cell line referred to as APUD (amine precursor, uptake, and decarboxylation). These cells are found alone or in groups, referred to as *neuroepithelial bodies*, that are localized most frequently in subsegmental bronchi, primarily at or near bifurcation points; they are rarely found in terminal bronchioles.[17] In humans and other species, K cells are most prevalent in the fetal lung and are only infrequently found in the adult lung.[17]

K cells are believed to contain the peptides bombesin,[21] leu-enkephalin,[22] somatostatin,[23] and calci-

tonin,[24] as well as 5-HT and catecholamines.[25,26] However, it is unclear whether K cells serve primarily as a paracrine (ie, exerting local effects) or an endocrine (ie, exerting systemic effects) function. Since these cells are occasionally located in close association with sensory nerve endings, substances released from these cells might also affect neuronal function.

The K cells are suspected to be involved in several pulmonary disorders. For example, the K cell is the site of origin of small cell lung carcinomas and of carcinoid tumors of the lung,[17,26] both of which may produce abnormal quantities of the chemical mediators produced by the K cell. Exposure to hypoxia has been reported to elicit K cell degranulation,[27–29] and various other environmental stimuli, such as nitrogen dioxide[30] and asbestos,[31] are able to induce K cell proliferation.

Type II Pneumocytes

The type II pneumocyte is the well-known primary producer of pulmonary surfactant. However, as with the K cell, the metabolic and hormonal roles of this cell type are poorly understood. Nevertheless, due to the presence of a cytochrome P-450 mono-oxygenase system,[19,20] type II pneumocytes may be responsible for the metabolism of xenobiotics. In addition, other investigators have postulated a role for the type II pneumocyte in defending the lung against oxidant injury.[32,33]

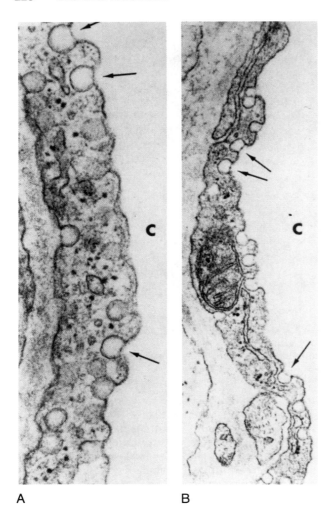

A   B

Fig. 5-2. (A & B) Transmission electron photomicrographs demonstrating caveolae in pulmonary capillary endothelial cells. The luminal stoma of the caveola is spanned by a delicate membrane composed of a single lamella (*arrows*) in contrast to the bilamellar cell and caveolae membranes. *C*, capillary lumen. Fig. A, × 68,000; Fig. B, × 44,000. (From Ryan and Ryan,[279] with permission.)

Mast Cells

Mast cells are found in the airway lumen, beneath the capsule of mucous glands, in the connective tissue surrounding small airways and blood vessels, and beneath the pleura.[34] These cells contain an immense repertoire of bioactive compounds (Table 5-3) that, when released in sufficient quantity, may cause bronchospasm as well as vasoconstriction or vasodilation.[34–36] Although mast cells are not normally involved in the regulation of bronchiolar or vascular tone, they assume an important role in pulmonary

TABLE 5-3. Mast Cell-Derived Mediators

Preformed and rapidly released mediators
  Histamine
  Eosinophil chemotactic factor
  Neutrophil chemotactic factor
  Kininogenase
  Arylsulfatase A
  Exoglycosidases
  5-HT

Mediators generated de novo
  Superoxide radical
  Leukotrienes C, D, and E
  Prostaglandins
  Thromboxanes
  Hydroxyeicosatetraenoic acids
  Hydroperoxyeicosatetraenoic acids
  Prostaglandin-generating factor
  Platelet-activating factor
  Adenosine

Granule-associated mediators
  Heparin
  Tryptase
  Chymotrypsin
  Arylsulfatase B

(Data from Friedman and Kaliner[34] and Marom and Casale.[46])

diseases or syndromes of immune or atopic etiology (eg, asthma, anaphylaxis).

TYPES OF METABOLIC PROCESSES WITHIN THE LUNG

Several different processes are responsible for the metabolic functions of the lung. These include metabolism of humoral substances at the cell surface, specific uptake mechanisms for humoral substances (which may be followed by intracellular metabolism), and synthesis and release of vasoactive compounds. These processes may apply to some or all of the metabolically active pulmonary cell types, but they are most important in the pulmonary endothelium, which is in intimate contact with the blood passing through the pulmonary circulation. A brief overview of these processes is given here; a more specific discussion relating to the metabolism of various compounds can be found later in this chapter.

Metabolism of Humoral Substances at the Cell Surface

Associated with the luminal plasma membrane of the pulmonary endothelial cells are several enzymes responsible for the metabolism of the adenine nucleotides, bradykinin, and angiotensin I. The enzymes that handle the adenine nucleotides, adenosine triphosphatase (ATPase) and 5'-nucleotidase, appear to

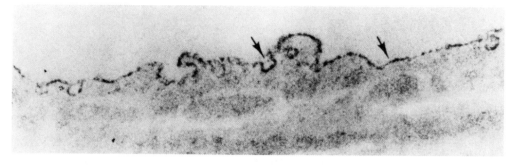

Fig. 5-3. Immunocytochemical localization of angiotensin-converting enzyme in pulmonary endothelial cells. The reaction product is localized on the luminal surface of the endothelial cells (*arrows*) (× 81,000). (From Ryan and Ryan,[12] with permission.)

reside solely in the endothelial caveolae.[37,38] On the other hand, angiotensin-converting enzyme (ACE), the enzyme responsible for the conversion of angiotensin I to angiotensin II and the inactivation of bradykinin, appears to be less restricted in its distribution, having been localized both in the caveolae and on the endothelial projections (Fig. 5-3).[39] A well-known class of drugs used in the treatment of hypertension, the ACE inhibitors (eg, captopril, enalapril, lisinopril) prevents the conversion of angiotensin I to angiotensin II (and the inactivation of bradykinin) by ACE.

Specific Uptake Mechanisms for Humoral Substances That Undergo Subsequent Intracellular Metabolism

Norepinephrine (but not epinephrine or isoproterenol) and 5-HT are the compounds primarily handled via this pathway. The uptake of both compounds by the endothelium relies on a carrier-mediated and sodium-dependent transport process that is saturable and temperature dependent.[40] However, the sites of 5-HT and norepinephrine uptake are distinct, as neither amine inhibits the uptake of the other.[41] Uptake of norepinephrine occurs mainly in the pre- and postcapillary vessels and the pulmonary veins,[42] while 5-HT uptake is primarily confined to the arterioles and capillaries.[43,44] The uptake process is blocked by cocaine, chlorpromazine, tricyclic antidepressants (eg, imipramine, desipramine, amitriptyline), certain steroids (eg, estradiol and corticosterone), anoxia, hyperoxia, and hypothermia.[11,40] Anesthetic gases (nitrous oxide, halothane) can partially reduce norepinephrine uptake, and exposure to environmental agents such as paraquat and monocrotaline results in decreased 5-HT extraction.[40] In fact, in various experimental models, 5-HT and/or norepinephrine extraction is used as a sensitive index of endothelial functional integrity.[45]

Once within the endothelial cell, norepinephrine

and 5-HT are deaminated by monoamine oxidase (MAO); norepinephrine is further metabolized by catechol-o-methyltransferase (COMT).[11] The characteristics of the uptake process itself are similar to those for the accumulation of 5-HT and norepinephrine by nerve endings and synaptosomes (uptake 1, neuronal), but also shares characteristics with uptake 2 (extraneuronal), that is, the subsequent intracellular metabolism by MAO and COMT.[40]

Synthesis and Release of Compounds

The lung may be defined as an endocrine organ by virtue of the fact that humoral agents are released from or produced within the lung which may then act on distant parts of the body, particularly, the cardiovascular system. Examples of these compounds are PGI_2 and angiotensin II. The lung is also an important shock organ in humans, as indicated by the vast array of potent vasoactive compounds released from the lung during anaphylaxis, which include 5-HT, histamine, thromboxane, leukotrienes, platelet-activating factor, and kinins. The lung also regulates its own circulation through the release of locally acting substances such as EDRF, adenosine, and, possibly, endothelium-derived contracting factor(s) (EDCF). The recently described constrictor peptide, endothelin,[46] may also prove to be an important product of the pulmonary endothelium; however, a physiologic role for this substance has yet to be demonstrated.

PROCESSING AND ACTION OF SPECIFIC FACTORS

Eicosanoids

The term *eicosanoids* refers to a group of compounds derived from the metabolism of arachidonic acid (eicosatetraenoic acid), a component of mem-

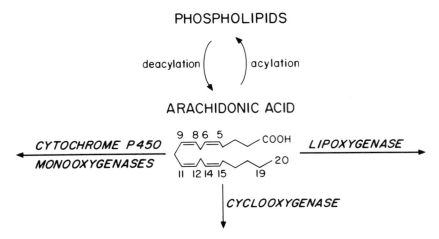

Fig. 5-4. Metabolic pathways for the metabolism of arachidonic acid to eicosanoids. (From Johns and Peach,[15] with permission.)

brane lipids. These compounds are continuously produced at a low rate, since membrane lipids are constantly being turned over under normal basal metabolic conditions. Arachidonic acid is present in its esterified form in the cell membrane, and is released following the activation of a phospholipase A_2, or the sequential action of phospholipase C and diacylglycerol lipase. After release from its glycerol backbone, arachidonic acid can be metabolized via three major pathways, the cyclo-oxygenase pathway, the lipoxygenase pathway, or the cytochrome P-450 mono-oxygenase pathway (Fig. 5-4). Metabolites arising from these pathways are biologically active, and elicit responses that include dilation or constricton of pulmonary vessels and bronchi, and regulation of pulmonary immune responses. Several of the cell types found within the lungs contain the full complement of enzymes required for the synthesis of these metabolites, as well as those enzymes necessary for their subsequent inactivation. Thus, the lung is capable of finely regulating the levels of various eicosanoids in the cardiovascular system, and may even use these compounds as a means of regulating its own perfusion. The lung has played a historic role in the understanding of the synthesis, metabolism, and actions of the eicosanoids, perhaps due to its propensity for the production of these compounds in response to a wide variety of stimuli.

Cyclo-Oxygenase Pathway

The metabolism of arachidonic acid via cyclo-oxygenase results in the formation of the cyclic endoperoxides, PGG_2 and PGH_2 (Fig. 5-5). The endoperoxides are highly unstable and are further metabolized

to the relatively more stable prostaglandins, such as PGD_2, PGE_2, and $PGF_{2\alpha}$, as well as thromboxane A_2 (TXA_2) and prostacyclin (PGI_2). This group of eicosanoids has potent, varied, and often opposing actions in both the pulmonary vasculature and airways, including eliciting vasoconstriction (TXA_2, $PGF_{2\alpha}$, PGE_2, PGD_2) or vasodilation (PGI_2, PGE_1), promoting TXA_2 or inhibiting (PGI_2) platelet aggregation, or causing bronchoconstriction ($PGF_{2\alpha}$, PGD_2, TXA_2) or bronchodilation (PGE_2).[47–50]

Probably the most important pulmonary cell type responsible for the synthesis and release of cyclo-oxygenase products is the endothelium. All of the major prostaglandins have been demonstrated in endothelial cell culture preparations using chromatographic and/or prostaglandin bioassays; however, the endothelium primarily produces PGI_2.[15] PGI_2 is continuously released from the lung, and it is known that PGI_2 production can be up-regulated via increases in blood flow and shear stress,[51,52] leading to subsequent pulmonary vasodilation. Increasing the rate of respiration can also increase the release of both PGI_2 and TXA_2, PGI_2 release being preferentially increased over that of TXA_2.[53] This increase in PGI_2 release in fact may be due to respiration-induced alterations in pulmonary hemodynamics, ie, local blood flows and shear stresses. Under varying experimental conditions, human lungs have been demonstrated to produce PGI_2, PGD_2, PGE_1, PGE_2, and $PGF_{2\alpha}$.[54,55]

Cyclo-oxygenase metabolites are handled by the lung via a combination of an active, carrier-mediated transport process and intracellular metabolism.[55,56] Ferreira and Vane were the first to study the metabolism of prostaglandins in the pulmonary circulation in vivo.[57] These investigators found that more than 90

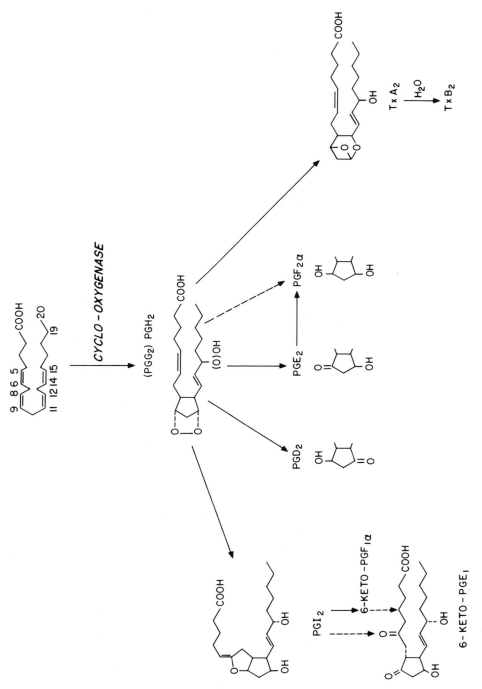

Fig. 5-5. The cyclo-oxygenase pathway for arachidonate metabolism. (From Johns and Peach,[15] with permission.)

percent of PGE_1, PGE_2, or $PGF_{2\alpha}$ was removed on one passage through the lung. On the other hand, PGA_1 and PGA_2,[58] as well as PGI_2,[59] survive passage through the pulmonary circulation essentially unchanged. The survival of PGA_1 and pulmonary extraction of PGE_1 have been confirmed in the human lung.[60] Although it is unclear whether the lung is able to extract TXA_2 from the pulmonary circulation, this compound is highly unstable and believed to be hydrolytically inactivated to TXB_2 while still in the circulation.[54] Nevertheless, TXB_2 is subject to pulmonary extraction, albeit via a mechanism that may be distinct from that responsible for the uptake of prostaglandins, since PGE_1, PGE_2, and $PGF_{2\alpha}$ do not prevent its uptake.[61] It is clear that within the closely related group of cyclo-oxygenase products, only certain members are subject to the selective uptake mechanisms of the lung. Following their removal from the pulmonary circulation, the prostaglandins are metabolized and inactivated intracellularly; however, the pulmonary cell types responsible for this inactivation have yet to be elucidated.

Lipoxygenase Pathway

Like the products of the cyclo-oxygenase pathway, the lipoxygenase metabolites are derived from the metabolism of arachidonic acid; in this case, via the enzyme 5-lipoxygenase (Fig. 5-6). The action of 5-lipoxygenase leads to the production of 5-hydroperoxyeicosatetraenoic acid (5-HPETE), which is then acted on by a dehydrase to yield the unstable intermediate, leukotriene (LT) A_4. LTA_4 may then be converted to LTB_4 or, via a second pathway, to the sulfidopeptide leukotrienes, LTC_4, LTD_4, and LTE_4 (historically known as slow-reacting substance of anaphylaxis).

The leukotrienes are important regulators of immune function within the lung, as well as potent activators of airway and vascular smooth muscle. LTB_4 is both chemotactic and chemokinetic for leukocytes, particularly neutrophils, and is also able to elicit neutrophil degranulation.[49,56,62] In addition, LTB_4 may also cause vasoconstriction and bronchoconstriction.[63–65] LTC_4 and LTD_4 are able to induce profound changes in the pulmonary vasculature, including an increase in vascular permeability.[62] These compounds are potent constrictors of both the pulmonary arteries[66,67] and veins,[67,68] although they appear to preferentially constrict the pulmonary veins.[69] The leukotrienes have been suggested to play a role in various pulmonary syndromes, such as the adult respiratory distress syndrome,[70,71] hypoxic pulmonary vasoconstriction (HPV),[72] and persistent pulmonary hypertension of the neonate.[73] Bronchoconstriction is also a characteristic action of the sulfidopeptide leuko-

trienes,[74,75] indicating that these compounds may be important mediators in asthma. While the actions of LTC_4 and LTD_4 are mediated by TXA_2 in some animal models,[56,62] this is not the case in the human lung.

In keeping with the hypothesis that the leukotrienes may play a role in HPV, hypoxia has been reported to stimulate leukotriene release from the lung,[76] although others have reported that decreased oxygen tensions inhibit leukotriene release.[68,77,78] Leukotriene release from lung parenchyma has also been demonstrated following antigen challenge.[77–79]

The cellular source of the leukotrienes has not been definitively localized. Mast cells, which are present in large numbers in the lung parenchyma, are likely a major source of these compounds, as are eosinophils, neutrophils, and macrophages.[62] Pulmonary arteries[80,81] and veins[68] from various species have also been demonstrated to release leukotrienes, but it is unclear whether this release reflects production from the smooth muscle, adventitial layer, or contaminating mast cells (which are likely to be present in the media). It is unlikely that the endothelium is the source of leukotrienes, since the endothelium appears to lack LTA_4 synthetase and requires the transfer of LTA_4 from another source (eg, neutrophils) prior to being able to synthesize these mediators.[82–84] Bronchial tissue has also been reported to release leukotrienes,[79] although, as with vascular tissue, they may actually be derived from contaminating mast cells.

The leukotrienes do not appear to be subject to an active uptake mechanism comparable to that which removes prostaglandins from the pulmonary circulation. The pulmonary metabolism of leukotrienes is a complex and poorly understood process. Human lung tissue primarily converts LTC_4 to LTD_4,[85] whereas pulmonary neutrophils are a likely site of inactivation of LTB_4 and LTC_4.[86,87] A more complete discussion of the metabolism of the leukotrienes can be found in Garcia et al,[62] Hammarstrom et al,[88] Drazen and Austen,[89] and Bray.[90]

Cytochrome P-450 Mono-Oxygenase Pathway

Cytochrome P-450-dependent metabolism of arachidonic acid can proceed via one of three major pathways to form several different types of hydroxy-or dihydroxyeicosatetraenoic acids or unstable epoxyeicosatetraenoic acids (Fig. 5-7), many of which are capable of modulating smooth muscle tone. The ability of the lung to synthesize and release these compounds has received little attention; therefore, a clear understanding of these capabilities awaits further investigation. The role of pulmonary cytochrome P-450 in the metabolism of xenobiotics is discussed below in the section *Metabolism of Xenobiotics*.

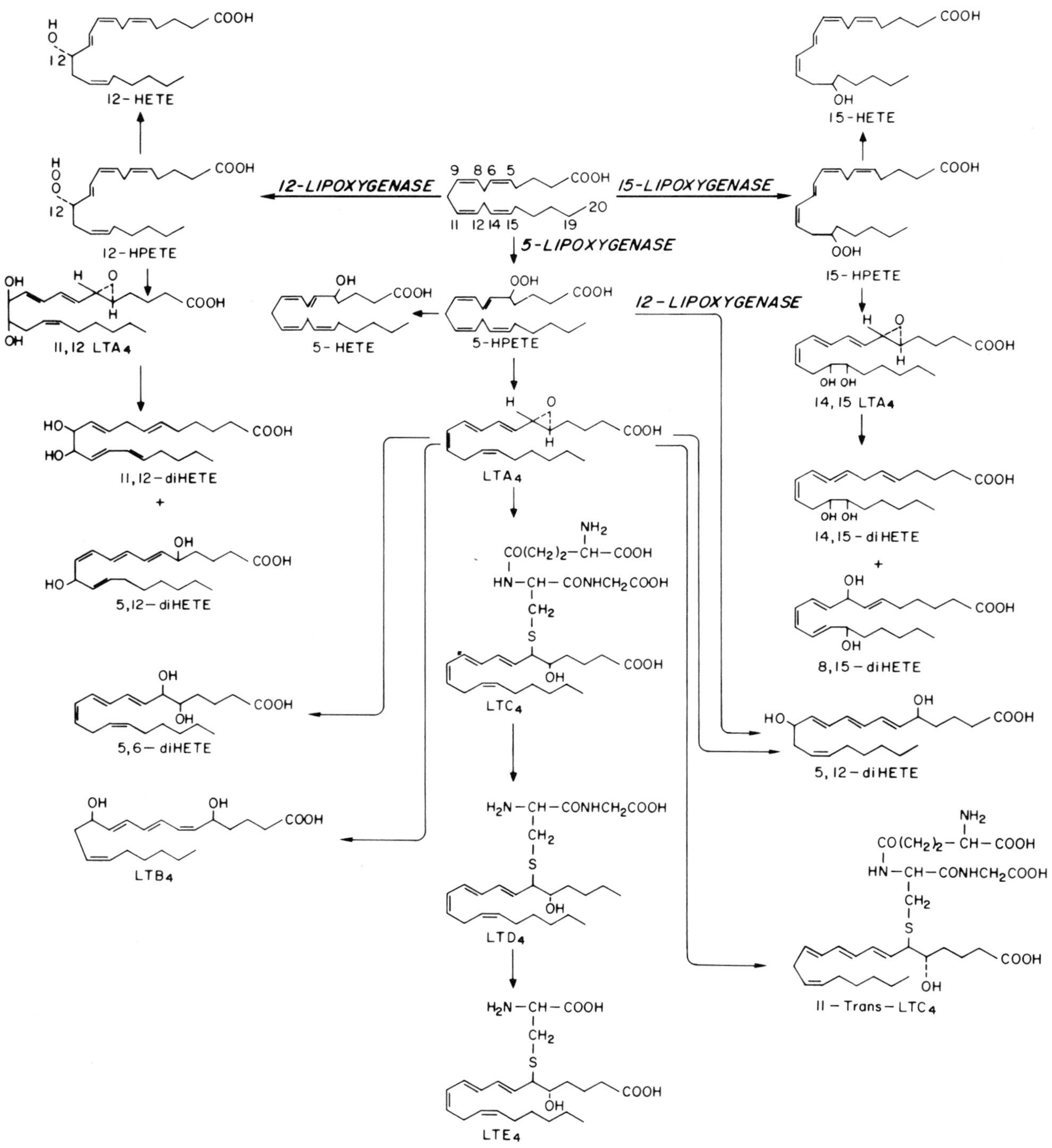

Fig. 5-6. The lipoxygenase pathway for arachidonate metabolism. (From Johns and Peach,[15] with permission)

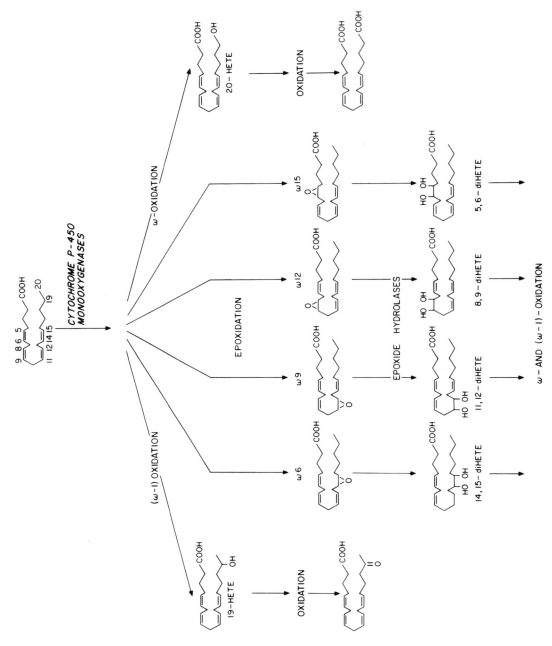

Fig. 5-7. The cytochrome P-450 pathway for arachidonate metabolism. (From Johns and Peach,[15] with permission.)

The Lipoxin Pathway

The lipoxins (LxA_4 and LxB_4) are a fourth class of arachidonic acid metabolites formed by the sequential actions of a 15-lipoxygenase and a 5-lipoxygenase.[91] The lipoxins were originally isolated from human leukocytes that were incubated with 15-HPETE,[91,92] and subsequently were shown to be produced by alveolar macrophages under similar conditions.[93] The vascular endothelium contains both 15- and 5-lipoxygenase activities,[94,95] raising the possibility that the pulmonary endothelium may either produce lipoxins or provide the necessary substrate (15-HPETE) for lipoxin production by circulating leukocytes. These compounds are mentioned here because they have potent vasodilatory and bronchoconstrictive properties.[96,97] However, a physiologic (or pathophysiologic) role for these compounds has yet to be conclusively demonstrated. In addition, assuming that these compounds are present physiologically, it is also unknown whether the lung has the capacity to inactivate or remove them from the circulation. Further research is obviously required in this area, but it is conceivable that the lipoxins represent an additional humoral mediator produced by the lung.

Platelet-Activating Factor

Platelet-activating factor (PAF) is a family of structurally related acetylated phospholipids that has biologic activities similar to those associated with acute allergic and inflammatory reactions and has a wide range of pathophysiologic effects on the lung. PAF is not an eicosanoid, but is included here because it is also released from membrane phospholipids by phospholipase A_2. It causes pulmonary hypertension, increased airway resistance, decreased dynamic compliance, airway hyperreactivity, edema, and pulmonary inflammatory cell accumulation in both experimental animals and humans.[98] PAF has been proposed as an important mediator in chronic obstructive airway disease and asthma.[97–100]

Peptides

A wide variety of bioactive peptides have been found to be present in the lung (Table 5-4). These substances are not unique to the pulmonary circulation but are also present in several other organ systems, particularly the nervous system and gastrointestinal tract. It is not surprising that the lung contains several peptides also found in the upper gastrointestinal tract, as the lung is derived from the embryonic foregut.[101] Those peptides of more defined physiologic or clinical importance are discussed below.

TABLE 5-4.   Bioactive Peptides in the Lung

Angiotensin II
Bradykinin
Substance P
Vasoactive intestinal peptide
Neuropeptide Y
Atrial natriuretic peptides
Bombesin-like peptide
Cholecystokinin
Enkephalins
Eosinophil-chemotactic peptides
Neurotensin
Spasmogenic lung peptide
Eledoisin
Adrenocorticotropic hormone
Somatostatin

Adrenocorticotropic Hormone

Adrenocorticotropic hormone (ACTH) has been found in normal lung[102] and in increased amounts in bronchial tumors and in lung from chronic smokers.[103–105] Intrapulmonary ACTH may play an important role in lung maturation. Hypophysectomized fetal sheep have a decreased surfactant production and delayed pulmonary maturation, even following administration of exogenous cortisol. The administration of exogenous ACTH, however, increases surfactant biosynthesis and enhances pulmonary compliance, implying an effect independent of corticosteroids.[106] ACTH has also been shown to inhibit ACE and may play a role in regulating angiotensin metabolism in the lung.[107]

Angiotensin

Angiotensin I is converted to its active form, angiotensin II, during passage through the pulmonary circulation[108] (Fig. 5-8). This conversion is due to ACE, a carboxypeptidase located within the caveolae intracellulares and on the projections of the endothelial cells lining the pulmonary vasculature (Fig. 5-3).[109] While ACE is present in endothelium and other tissues throughout the body, the fact that the pulmonary circulation receives the entire cardiac output makes the lung a primary regulator of the angiotensin system. Angiotensin II is a highly potent vasoconstrictor whose production is increased in hypoxic lung.[110,111] Inhibition of ACE reduces pulmonary artery pressure and vascular resistance.[112] Angiotensin II also stimulates the production of prostacyclin, a cyclo-oxygenase metabolite of arachidonic acid with potent vasodilating and platelet antiaggregation effects.[113] While 20 percent of angiotensin I will be converted to angiotensin II in a single pass through the pulmonary circulation,[108] angiotensin II is not metabolized within the lung, but is allowed to pass freely to the systemic circulation.

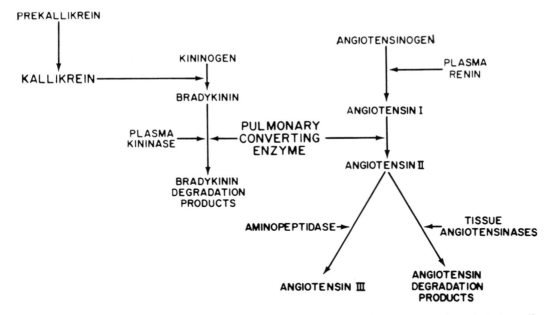

Fig. 5-8. Synthesis and metabolism of angiotensin II and bradykinin. (From Block and Stalcup,[45] with permission.)

Bradykinin

Bradykinin is produced in the lungs, as in the rest of the body, through metabolism of plasma and tissue kininogens. Bradykinin is also inactivated in the lung by the same dipeptidylcarboxypeptidase, ACE (Fig. 5-8), which is responsible for the conversion of angiotensin I to angiotensin II.[114] Bradykinin is a potent vasodilator of the pulmonary circulation, mediated in part by EDRF (see below). If the endothelium is damaged or destroyed, bradykinin manifests itself as a potent vasoconstrictor.[115] In addition, bradykinin stimulates the metabolism of arachidonic acid in pulmonary endothelial cells, causing the release of a variety of vasoactive eicosanoids.[9,116,117] Bradykinin constricts bronchial smooth muscle and increases pulmonary microvascular permeability.[118]

Atrial Natriuretic Peptide

Atrial natriuretic peptide (ANP) is a recently discovered hormone produced by atrial myocytes that links the heart, kidneys, adrenals, blood vessels, and brain in a complex hormonal system related to volume and pressure homeostasis.[119] ANP is a potent vasodilator that decreases aldosterone secretion from the adrenal gland and increases renal natriuresis. Its natriuretic and diuretic effects are further potentiated by the release of arginine vasopressin from the pituitary. Active metabolism of ANP by the lungs may help to regulate its multiple actions.[120]

ANP may play an important role in modulating the pulmonary circulation in normal and disease states, since the lung is the first organ through which ANP passes after it is released from the heart. ANP is a vasodilator of the intact pulmonary vascular bed[121] and of isolated pulmonary arteries.[122] Hypoxia stimulates the release of ANP from the heart,[123] and ANP has also been shown to decrease the hypoxic pulmonary vasoconstrictor response.[124] Several studies have demonstrated an increase in ANP release in chronic pulmonary hypertension,[125,126] suggesting that ANP could modulate the elevated pulmonary vascular tone in these patients.

Vasoactive Intestinal Peptide

The biologic activity of vasoactive intestinal peptide (VIP) was discovered in the lung prior to its isolation and chemical identification from the intestine.[127,128] Nerve fibers and nerve terminals containing VIP are present in several structures of the lung, including bronchial and pulmonary blood vessels, bronchial smooth muscle, and bronchial submucosal glands. Many of these nerve fibers originate from microganglia within the lung, providing a source of intrinsic innervation of pulmonary structures.[129,130] VIP has also been found in mast cells of the lung.[131] It is a potent pulmonary vasodilator[132,133] as well as a relaxant of airway smooth muscle.[133,134] Decreased biologic activity of VIP may be a contributing factor to the pathogenesis of cystic fibrosis and bronchial asthma.[129,130,135–137]

Summary of Physiologic Actions of Peptides in the Lung

Several of the peptides occurring in the lungs have vasoactive and bronchoconstrictive properties. Angiotensin II, spasmogenic lung peptide, substance P, and bombesin are pulmonary vasoconstrictors,[129,130,138–140] while VIP and ANP are potent pulmonary vasodilators.[132] Bombesin, substance P, cholecystokinin, and spasmogenic lung peptide all induce bronchoconstriction.[129,139] Activated complement C5a is capable of increasing pulmonary microvascular permeability and may be important in mediating pulmonary edema in a variety of disease states.[101,141] Substance P and VIP also stimulate bronchial secretion,[105] while bombesin and ACTH have been strongly implicated in the regulation of normal growth and development of the fetal lung.[105] Kinins may be generated by lung tissues during IgE-mediated allergic responses. Eosinophil- and granulocyte-stimulating chemotactic peptides and kinins are mediators of anaphylaxis and acute inflammation.[105,142]

In conclusion, a multitude of bioactive peptides have been localized in the lung. These compounds are both constrictors and dilators of vascular and bronchial smooth muscle and are capable of influencing pulmonary vascular permeability and inflammatory responses within the lung. The exact role of these agents in normal pulmonary homeostasis continues to be studied.

Other Nonpeptide Substances

Catecholamines

As discussed earlier, the pulmonary endothelium is responsible for the uptake and inactivation of norepinephrine. More than 30 percent of this catecholamine is removed from the venous blood in a single passage through the lungs.[26] The carrier-mediated uptake is saturable, sodium dependent, and temperature dependent.[12,40,143,144] The specificity of this uptake process is demonstrated by the inability of the lung to remove epinephrine or dopamine from the circulation; isoproterenol is also not affected by this uptake mechanism.[11,26,40,43] Once within the endothelial cell, norepinephrine is metabolized via MAO and COMT to inactive metabolites (Fig. 5-9).[11,36,40] Several different

drugs can significantly reduce the pulmonary removal and/or metabolism of norepinephrine. These drugs include estradiol and corticosterone, imipramine, cocaine, halothane, and nitrous oxide.[11,40,145] In addition to the obvious autonomic neuronal sources of norepinephrine within the lung, catecholamines are also produced within the tracheobronchial tree by the K cells.[26]

5-Hydroxytryptamine

Like norepinephrine, 5-HT is cleared from the pulmonary circulation via endothelium-dependent mechanisms.[5,12,40,144] These mechanisms reflect a primary process of uptake rather than enzymatic degradation (Fig. 5-10), and are virtually identical to those responsible for norepinephrine extraction. However, there are some significant differences; for instance, unlike norepinephrine, 5-HT is essentially completely removed from the circulation (ie, as much as 98 percent) during one passage through the lung.[11,26,143] In addition, although the mechanisms of norepinephrine and 5-HT uptake are comparable, the sites of uptake appear to be different, as suggested by the inability of each amine to inhibit the uptake of the other.[144,145] 5-HT uptake is inhibited by cocaine, chlorpromazine, and tricyclic antidepressants (imipramine, amitriptyline).[11,40] Both K cells and mast cells represent pulmonary sources of 5-HT.[26,34,36]

Histamine

Histamine differs from norepinephrine and 5-HT in that histamine is not removed from the pulmonary circulation to any appreciable degree.[40,143] The lack of pulmonary metabolism of histamine apparently reflects the absence of an uptake mechanism, as pulmonary homogenates are quite capable of inactivating histamine.[11,40,143] Given that pulmonary mast cells contain significant stores of this agent, the absence of a pulmonary uptake mechanism for histamine may have important pathophysiologic consequences arising from the resulting vulnerability of the airways and pulmonary vessels to endogenously released histamine.

Adenine Nucleotides

Adenine nucleotides (adenosine triphosphate [ATP], adenosine diphosphate [ADP], adenosine monophosphate [AMP]) are substantially (40 to 90 percent) removed from the pulmonary circulation during one passage through the lung.[5,11,26,146] Cellular uptake is not required as these compounds are metabolized at

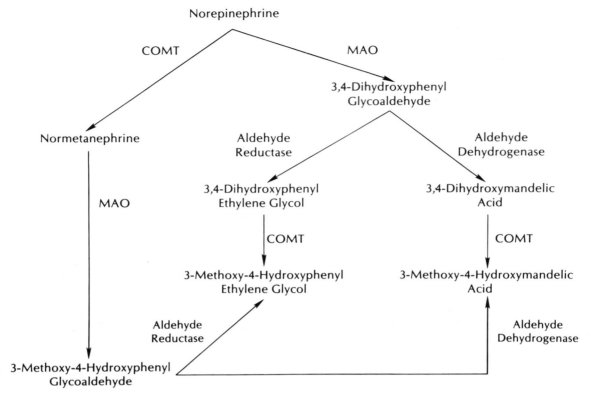

Fig. 5-9. Metabolism of norepinephrine. MAO, monoamine oxidase; COMT, catechol-o-methyl transferase.

the pulmonary endothelial surface by 5'-nucleotidase and ATPase[5,146] localized in the endothelial caveolae.[37,38] Adenosine, which is produced during the degradation of the adenine nucleotides, is taken up by the endothelial cells via a saturable process that is inhibited by dipyridamole.[147] Once within the endo-

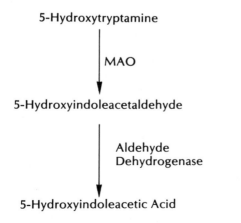

Fig. 5-10. Metabolism of serotonin (5-HT). MAO, monoamine oxidase.

thelial cell, adenosine may subsequently be used in the formation of intracellular nucleotides, primarily ATP.[146] This metabolic pathway also represents the conversion of endothelium-dependent vasodilators (ATP, ADP) to endothelium-independent vasodilators (AMP, adenosine) and is therefore capable of regulating the extracellular concentration of these agents as well as the associated biologic responses. Not only does the endothelium efficiently remove adenosine and adenine nucleotides from the circulation, it may release adenosine after exposure to hypoxia[148] (and various other stimuli),[146] which could explain the increase in pulmonary adenosine levels observed during acute alveolar hypoxia.[149]

Acetylcholine

Acetylcholine is a potent, endothelium-dependent pulmonary vasodilator, and is mentioned here due to the fact that clinical administration of this compound or its analogs may have potential benefits in conditions in which pulmonary hypertension is a problem. However, the physiologic pulmonary actions of this compound are restricted to sites of neuronal release, as it is rapidly degraded by synaptic acetylcholinesterase, and any acetylcholine that might enter the vasculature is equally rapidly degraded by blood-borne cholinesterases.[143] A more comprehensive review of the pharmacologic effects of acetylcholine on the pulmonary circulation can be found in a review by Peach et al.[150]

Endothelium-Derived Relaxing and Contracting Factors

In the past several years, the vascular endothelium, including that of the lung, has been found to produce several potent vasodilating and vasoconstricting substances. Most prominent among these is EDRF, which was discovered by Furchgott and Zawadzki in 1980 when they observed that the relaxation of strips of rabbit aorta by acetylcholine was dependent on the presence of the endothelium.[151] Subsequently, a wide variety of agents have been found to require a func-

tionally intact endothelium to produce vascular relaxation. These include several potent vasodilators present in the pulmonary circulation, such as bradykinin, histamine, substance P, vasoactive intestinal peptide, ATP, ADP, thrombin, calcitonin gene-related peptide, arachidonic acid, and trypsin. In addition, several contractile agents, including norepinephrine, 5-HT, and vasopressin, act on the endothelium to release EDRF, which modulates their direct contractile actions on the vascular smooth muscle.[15,150,152–156]

EDRF is a labile, extremely potent vasodilator with a biologic half-life estimated at between 6 and 70 seconds.[157–159] It is released from the endothelium under basal conditions as well as in response to the agonists mentioned above, thereby mediating their vasodilating actions. EDRF is produced from L-arginine by a calcium, calmodulin, and NADPH-dependent enzyme, EDRF synthase. Once produced, EDRF is transferred from the endothelium to the vascular smooth

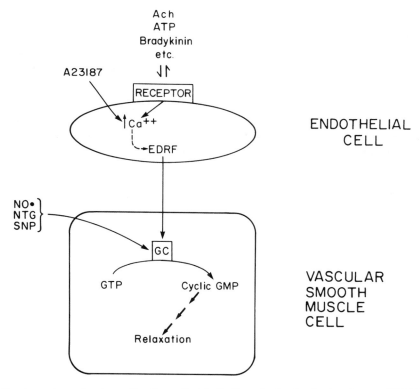

Fig. 5-11. Synthesis and mechanism of action of endothelium-derived relaxing factor (EDRF). Agents that release EDRF directly (eg, the calcium ionophore, A23187) or through endothelial cell receptors (eg, acetylcholine [ACH], adenosine triphosphate [ATP], bradykinin) elicit an increase in intracellular calcium that correlates with EDRF release. EDRF is transferred to the vascular smooth muscle where it activates soluble guanylate cyclase (GC), causing an increase in cyclic guanosine monophosphate (GMP) that subsequently leads to vascular relaxation. Nitric oxide (NO), nitroglycerin (NTG), and sodium nitroprusside (SNP) also cause relaxation through elevation of cyclic GMP, but do not require the endothelium.

muscle, where it activates soluble guanylate cyclase (Fig. 5-11). This activation leads to an increase in smooth muscle cyclic guanosine monophosphate concentration, which subsequently elicits vascular relaxation.[9,164–167] The production of EDRF is inhibited by both high and low oxygen tensions, which may be particularly important in the pulmonary circulation.[151,168,169] The specific chemical identity of EDRF still is a subject of intense investigation. Recently, a great deal of evidence has suggested that EDRF is nitric oxide or a similar nitroso compound,[170–180] although this is still an area of some controversy.[181–187] In addition, experimental evidence suggests that there may be more than one EDRF, and several investigators have postulated the existence of an endothelium-derived hyperpolarizing factor (EDHF).[188–190]

EDRF is similar to prostacyclin in that it is a potent inhibitor of platelet aggregation,[179,191] as well as an endothelium-derived vasodilator. In addition to this antiaggregatory effect, EDRF has also been shown to inhibit platelet adhesion.[192,193]

The role of EDRF and the endothelium in pulmonary vascular physiology and pathophysiology has recently been reviewed.[150] Basal release of EDRF may be important in the maintenance of the low vascular resistance of the normal pulmonary circulation. Flow-dependent dilation in several vascular beds has been shown to be the result of EDRF release from the endothelium in response to shear stress.[194–196] Thus, the pulmonary endothelium may also be important to the ability of the pulmonary circulation to accommodate increases in flow with only moderate increases in pulmonary artery pressure.

Studies in isolated pulmonary vessels[168] and in intact perfused lungs[197] have suggested that hypoxic inhibition of EDRF production may be one factor contributing to the hypoxic pulmonary vasoconstrictor response. The endothelium has also been shown to reduce hypoxia-induced vasoconstriction of the pulmonary venule.[198]

The endothelium is damaged or functionally impaired in a wide variety of pulmonary disease states. Such damage can significantly alter the wide-ranging metabolic functions of the pulmonary endothelium discussed in this chapter. Endothelial damage and impaired EDRF production or activity have been proposed as contributing factors in both acute and chronic pulmonary hypertension. Esterly et al reported anatomic changes in the endothelium secondary to pulmonary hypertension.[199] They observed an early hyperplastic reaction of endothelial cells at 2 weeks following increased pulmonary artery pressure and flow, followed by endothelial cell injury and degeneration over the subsequent 2 months. Ultrastructural changes also have been reported in the pulmonary artery endothelium of lung biopsy specimens from patients with pulmonary hypertension due to congenital heart defects.[200]

Endothelial damage also plays a significant role in the manifestations of pulmonary hyperoxia and oxygen toxicity.[150] Following hyperoxic exposure, there is clear anatomic evidence of endothelial cell injury,[201] altered endothelial cell metabolism,[202] and impaired relaxation to endothelium-dependent vasodilators.[203] Endothelial cell injury is also a factor in the pulmonary hypertension due to endotoxemia.[150]

In addition to their ability to mediate vascular smooth muscle relaxation, endothelial cells release factors that cause vascular smooth muscle contraction.[204] While less is known about EDCFs than EDRFs, it appears that there are at least three different types of EDCFs.[204] These include metabolites of arachidonic acid, an unidentified unstable factor released from anoxic or hypoxic endothelial cells, and a recently characterized polypeptide known as endothelin.[204] Endothelin is a 21-amino acid peptide released from the endothelium, which is an extremely potent constrictor of vascular smooth muscle.[46] This peptide has been a subject of intense investigation since its recent isolation from pulmonary endothelium and the identification of the gene responsible for its production. The true physiologic importance of endothelin remains to be established; however, it may be involved in long-term regulation of blood vessel tone.

Another important metabolic function of the endothelium is its ability to modulate cell growth within the vessel wall.[205–207] In its basal state, the endothelium produces heparin-like factors that inhibit smooth muscle proliferation.[208] When the endothelial cell is replicating or injured, it produces a variety of growth factors (eg, platelet-derived growth factor and epidermal growth factor)[205,209] and stops producing antiproliferative factors. This production of growth factors and inhibition of antiproliferative factors may play a role in the hypertrophy and hyperplasia of the vasculature in conditions such as chronic hyperoxia, hypoxia, and lung injury.[150]

METABOLISM OF XENOBIOTICS

The lungs are in an optimal position to be involved in the metabolism of both blood-borne and environmental xenobiotics. Venous drainage from the entire body perfuses the alveolar-capillary unit. The thin and apposed epithelial-endothelial cellular structure of the alveolar-capillary unit provides an enormous surface area to the air on one side and to the blood on the other.

A wide variety of drugs and chemicals are actively taken up and/or metabolized by the lungs. Some of these compounds, which are chemically similar to en-

**TABLE 5-5. Metabolic Enzyme
Pathways Present in Lung**

Cytochrome P-450 mixed function oxygenase
Amine oxidase
Glutathione-S-epoxide transferase
Glutathione-S-aryl transferase
Epoxide hydrolase
Glucuronyl transferase
Nitro reductase
Sulfotransferase
N-methyltransferase

(Modified from Philpot et al,[263] with permission.)

**TABLE 5-6. Xenobiotics
Metabolized by the Lung**

Drug	Reference
Amphetamine	264,265
Metaraminol	266, 267, 268
Isoproterenol	269
Chlorphentermine	270
Chlorpromazine	265
Diphenhydramine	265
Imipramine	271
Mescaline	272
Methadone	273
Fentanyl	230
Meperidine	230
Propranolol	229
Bupivacaine	224
Lidocaine	225

dogenous hormones and substances metabolized by the lungs, share endothelial cell-localized enzymes, receptors, binding sites, and transport mechanisms. Most agents, however, are taken up into epithelial and endothelial cells by simple diffusion. Numerous metabolic enzyme systems have been detected within the lung (Table 5-5) and provide the means for metabolism of these substances.

The most studied, and perhaps most important, route of metabolism is via the family of cytochrome P-450 mono-oxygenase enzymes. The lung is known to be a rich source of at least three different isozymes of cytochrome P-450.[210–212] Consequently, the lung is actively involved with xenobiotic metabolism. As was mentioned earlier, several pulmonary cell types are rich sources of cytochrome P-450 enzymes or cytochrome P-450-like activity, namely, the Clara cell,[18,19] the type II pneumocyte,[19,20] and the endothelium.[13,14] In addition, the medial layer of the pulmonary vasculature may also contain a functional cytochrome P-450 system, assuming that the data obtained from systemic vessels can be extrapolated to the pulmonary vasculature.[213,214] Therefore, the lung has the capacity to metabolize xenobiotics presented to it from either the atmospheric environment (via the Clara cell and the type II pneumocyte) or the blood (via the endothelium). Although both cytochrome P-450 and NADPH cytochrome P-450 reductase are present in Clara cells and type II pneumocytes, NADPH cytochrome P-450 reductase has not been localized to endothelial cells.[13] Thus, it is possible that this enzyme system may be nonfunctional in the endothelium. In contrast, however, cytochrome P-450-dependent mono-oxygenase activity has been reported in isolated endothelial cells.[215,216]

Isozymes of cytochrome P-450 may be involved in protective mechanisms within the lung and, conversely, may also play a role in the development of pulmonary toxicity arising from the metabolism of xenobiotics. For example, Mansour and colleagues recently demonstrated that induction of certain pulmonary cytochrome P-450 isozymes led to a reduction in the pathophysiologic changes induced by exposure to

hyperoxia.[217,218] On the other hand, although the cytochrome P-450 system generally produces metabolites that are less toxic than the parent compounds, the pulmonary damage induced by agents such as paraquat, nitrofurantoin, mitomycin C, benzo(a)pyrene, and 4-ipomeanol reflects the cytochrome P-450-dependent production of toxic metabolites.[5,219] It has also been postulated that cytochrome P-450 metabolites may be involved in the regulation of pulmonary vascular tone during HPV,[220,221] although the results of a recent study do not support this hypothesis.[68] A great deal of further investigation is required to clarify the understanding of the potential physiologic and pathophysiologic roles of the cytochrome P-450 mono-oxygenase system of the lung.

Many of the drugs known to be metabolized by the lung are of interest to anesthesiologists (Table 5-6). These include sympathomimetics, antihistamines, morphine-like analgesics, tricyclic antidepressants, and local anesthetics. The metabolism of some of these drugs leads to the production of metabolites associated with lung injury (Table 5-7).

There is evidence that a few of these agents (amphetamine, metaraminol, isoproterenol) are taken up by specific carrier-mediated uptake mechanisms; however, for most drugs, uptake is nonspecific. To be effectively removed, these compounds have certain

**TABLE 5-7. Metabolized Xenobiotics
Associated With Lung Injury**

Drug	Reference
Bleomycin	274, 275
Nitrofurantoin	276
Mitomycin C	277
Paraquat	278
Carbon tetrachloride	26

common physicochemical properties. Most are basic amines with a pK_a greater than 8, and all are lipophilic. These drugs also often possess a charged cationic group at physiologic pH.[5] The cationic component of these amines is attracted to the multiple anionic domains on the endothelial cell membrane; thereafter, the lipophilic component facilitates entry into the cell.[222,223]

Bupivacaine and lidocaine are two lipophilic basic amines that undergo extensive pulmonary uptake on passage through the pulmonary circulation. Rothstein et al[224] observed an 81 percent extraction of bupivacaine on a single pass through the rabbit pulmonary circulation in vivo. Similar results have been observed with lidocaine.[225–227] Propranolol is another hydrophobic amine with local anesthetic properties that is taken up by the lung in a manner similar to lidocaine and bupivacaine.[5] The uptake of all of these agents is decreased by a reduction in temperature.[228] The uptake of propranolol appears to be saturable, as first-pass uptake is markedly decreased in patients regularly taking this drug.[229]

Several narcotic agents used in anesthesia are also lipophilic basic amines. Roerig et al[230] studied the first-pass uptake of fentanyl, meperidine, and morphine in patients prior to elective surgery. They found rapid uptake of fentanyl and meperidine, but no significant uptake of morphine. These differential effects can be explained by the physicochemical differences between these basic amines. Fentanyl and meperidine are orders of magnitude more lipid soluble than morphine. Morphine is also a less basic amine (pK_a = 7.9) compared with fentanyl (pK_a = 8.4) and meperidine (pK_a = 8.5). This extensive uptake of fentanyl and meperidine clearly has a major effect on the peak concentrations of these drugs seen by other organ systems.

Certain anesthetic agents have also been shown to inhibit lung metabolism. Halothane and nitrous oxide decrease 5-HT and norepinephrine uptake by pulmonary endothelial cells in a competitive and rapidly reversible manner.[231–234] Halothane and pentobarbital inhibit the synthesis of lung proteins,[235,236] and ketamine has been shown to competitively and reversibly inhibit lung 5-HT metabolism.[237]

PHYSIOLOGIC AND PATHOPHYSIOLOGIC IMPLICATIONS

Hypoxic Pulmonary Vasoconstriction

The mechanism of HPV remains unknown. Investigations have focused on either the direct effects of hypoxia on pulmonary vascular smooth muscle or the indirect effects of hypoxia mediated through a wide array of neurohumoral agents.[238] Hypoxia may cause pulmonary vasoconstriction through either the production of a vasoconstrictor or the inhibition of a tonically released vasodilator. Many of the agents discussed in this chapter, including histamine, bradykinin, 5-HT, angiotensin II, and prostaglandins, have been studied extensively as potential mediators of HPV.[72,238] While many of these substances can modulate pulmonary vascular tone and may contribute to the HPV response, none is essential. Several investigators have suggested that the sulfidopeptide leukotrienes may mediate the HPV response[239–242]; however, more recent investigations have disputed this hypothesis.[68,77,243–250] The potent endothelium-derived vasoconstrictor, endothelin, is unlikely to be involved in HPV due to its slow response time and prolonged duration of action.

The pulmonary endothelium may, however, have a significant role to play in HPV. Experimental evidence suggests that hypoxia inhibits the production and/or release of EDRF from the endothelium, thereby leading to pulmonary vasoconstriction.[168,197] Loss of basal EDRF production in pathologic situations where the endothelium is damaged may also lead to augmented HPV.[198]

Acute Lung Injury

Many of the mediators discussed in this chapter are under intense investigation to determine their role in the mechanisms of acute lung injury and the adult respiratory distress syndrome. The complex metabolic activities of the lung are significantly altered in acute lung injury. This can result in increases in the amounts of prostaglandins, thromboxanes, leukotrienes, platelet-activating factor, activated complement, thrombin, and oxygen free radicals.[251] The quantities of other factors derived from the endothelium, including EDRF and endothelin, may be markedly reduced or enhanced. The extensive literature linking many of these substances to the pulmonary and systemic responses of acute lung injury has been reviewed.[139]

The primary changes following acute lung injury are vascular in nature, including endothelial cell damage and pulmonary hypertension. This is associated with airway constriction and alveolar duct closure, intravascular coagulation, complement activation, and aggregation of granulocytes and platelets.[139,251,252] This acute phase of injury is followed by a reparative phase in which alveolar type II cells replicate to replace damaged alveolar type I cells, with subsequent inflammatory cell infiltration and fibrosis.[251,253] The pulmonary vasculature exhibits structural changes with loss of precapillary units and hypertrophy of vascular smooth muscle.[251,254,255]

Arachidonate metabolites may contribute to these events through direct actions, causing vascular and bronchial constriction or dilation, endothelial cell damage, and increases in microvascular permeability. In addition, eicosanoids may have indirect effects through the stimulation of complement, leukocytes, and platelets.[256] Leukotrienes may contribute to acute lung injury through their actions of chemotaxis, increased permeability, and pulmonary vasoconstriction.[257] As discussed above, platelet-activating factor has been implicated as a mediator in several experimental models of acute lung injury. Its exogenous administration has been shown to cause alveolar capillary damage, high-permeability pulmonary edema, pulmonary vasoconstriction, and bronchoconstriction.[258]

Conversely, some metabolic products of the lung may help to modulate or prevent lung injury.[251] Vasoactive intestinal peptide is an endogenous bronchodilator and vasodilator that may counteract the effects of leukotrienes and other bronchoconstrictors during lung injury. Prostacyclin, in addition to being a strong relaxant of vascular smooth muscle and an inhibitor of thromboxane generation, also inhibits polymorphonuclear leukocyte aggregation, lysosomal enzyme release, and platelet aggregation. In several experimental studies of acute lung injury, prostacyclin has been shown to prevent the development of pulmonary vascular permeability and pulmonary hypertension, and to exert a stabilizing activity on polymorphonuclear leukocytes.[259] The production of leukotrienes and their subsequent effects of vasoconstriction and increased pulmonary vascular permeability are also inhibited.[259]

Pulmonary Embolism

Several aspects of pulmonary metabolism contribute to the response of the lung to thromboembolism. The activation of fibrinolysis and an increase in prostacyclin formation help to decrease the effects of emboli and maintain normal ventilation-perfusion balance. Other factors, such as neutrophil chemotaxins, adherence-inducing agents, and oxygen-derived free radicals, may be detrimental. The production of the superoxide radical from activated leukocytes, for example, may directly inactivate EDRF and damage the endothelium, thereby contributing to pulmonary hypertension. The balance between the varied metabolic effects during pulmonary embolism contributes to the degree to which pulmonary vascular resistance will increase, as well as the development of lung vascular injury and tissue edema.[260]

Pulmonary Metabolic Processes as Clinical Indicators of Lung Function

Recently, the understanding of pulmonary metabolism has been applied to an evaluation of pulmonary endothelial function in vivo. Indicator dilution techniques have been used to assess 5-HT, prostaglandin E_1, or norepinephrine uptake in normal individuals and in patients with pulmonary disease. Observed decreases in uptake or clearance of these substances by the lungs have proven to be early indicators of pulmonary endothelial cell dysfunction, an initial derangement of many types of lung injury. These techniques are undergoing refinement and may soon be of significant diagnostic and prognostic value.[261,262]

CONCLUSIONS

Beyond its respiratory functions, the lung has important and wide-ranging metabolic and hormonal activity. It is the site of production, activation, and metabolism of multiple agents, including eicosanoids, peptides, and amines, as well as recently discovered endothelium-derived dilating and constricting factors (EDRF, EDCF, EDHF, endothelin). These autacoids and hormones have multiple functions both within and outside the lung. Included among them are potent vascular and bronchial dilators and constrictors, immunoregulators, modulators of vascular growth and hypertrophy, activators and inhibitors of platelet aggregation, and mediators of permeability. The lungs are also capable of affecting the disposition of a number of exogenous compounds and drugs by extracting and/or metabolizing these substances during their passage through the pulmonary vasculature. These agents contribute to the normal pulmonary vascular tone and the ability of the pulmonary vasculature to accommodate changes in flow in response to physiologic and pathophysiologic stimuli.

REFERENCES

1. Crapo JD, Barry BE, Gehr P, et al: Cell number and cell characteristics of the normal human lung. Am Rev Respir Dis 125:332–337, 1982
2. Simionescu M: Cell organization of the alveolar-capillary unit: structural-functional correlations. pp. 13–36. Said SI (ed): The Pulmonary Circulation and Acute Lung Injury. Mount Kisco, NY Futura Publishing, 1985
3. Smith U, Ryan JW: Electron microscopy of endothelial and epithelial components of the lungs: correlations of structure and function. Fed Proc 32:1957–1966, 1973
4. Weibel ER, Gomez DM: The architecture of the human lung. Science 137:577–585, 1962

5. Ryan US, Grantham CJ: Metabolism of endogenous and xenobiotic substances by pulmonary vascular endothelial cells. Pharmacol Ther 42:235–250, 1989

6. Johns RA, Izzo NJ, Milner PJ, et al: Use of cultured cells to study the relationship between arachidonic acid and endothelium-derived relaxing factor. Am J Med Sci 31:287–292, 1988

7. van Grondelle A, Worthen GS, Ellis D, et al: Altering hydrodynamic variables influences PGI_2 production by isolated lungs and endothelial cells. J Appl Physiol 57:388–395, 1984

8. Gryglewski RJ, Korbut R, Dietkiewicz A: Generation of prostacyclin by lungs in vivo and its release into the arterial circulation. Nature 273:765–767, 1978

9. Johns RA, Peach MJ: Parabromophenacyl bromide inhibits endothelium-dependent arterial relaxation and cyclic GMP accumulation by effects produced exclusively in the smooth muscle. J Pharmacol Exp Ther 244:859–865, 1988

10. Ignarro LJ, Buga GM, Chaudhuri G: EDRF generation and release from perfused bovine pulmonary artery and vein. Eur J Pharmacol 149:79–88, 1988

11. Said SI: Metabolic functions of the pulmonary circulation. Circ Res 50:325–333, 1982

12. Ryan JW, Ryan US: Pulmonary endothelial cells. Fed Proc 36:2683–2691, 1977

13. Serabjit-Singh CJ, Nishio SJ, Philpot RM, Plopper CG: The distribution of cytochrome P-450 monooxygenase in cells of the rabbit lung: an ultrastructural immunocytochemical characterization. Mol Pharmol 33:279–289, 1988

14. Dees JH, Masters BSS, Muller-Eberhard U, Johnson EF: Effect of 2,3,7,8-tetrachlorodibenzo-p-dioxin and phenobarbital on the occurrence and distribution of four cytochrome P-450 isozymes in rabbit kidney, lung and liver. Cancer Res 42:1423–1432, 1982

15. Johns RA, Peach MJ: Metabolism of arachidonic acid and release of endothelium-derived relaxing factors. pp. 65–89. In Vanhoutte PM (ed): Relaxing and Contracting Factors. Humana, Clifton, NJ, 1988

16. Widdicombe JG, Pack RJ: The Clara cell. Eur J Respir Dis 63:202–220, 1982

17. Gail DB, Lenfant CJM: Cells of the lung: biology and clinical implications. Am Rev Respir Dis 127:366–387, 1983

18. Serabjit-Singh CJ, Wolf CR, Philpot RM, Plopper CG: Cytochrome P-450: localization in rabbit lung. Science 207:1469–1470, 1980

19. Devereux TR, Serabjit-Singh CJ, Slaughter SR, et al: Identification of cytochrome P-450 isozymes in nonciliated bronchiolar epithelial (Clara) and alveolar type II cells isolated from rabbit lung. Exp Lung Res 2:221–230, 1981

20. Devereux TR, Fouts JR: Xenobiotic metabolism by alveolar type II cells isolated from rabbit lung. Biochem Pharmacol 30:1231–1237, 1981

21. Wharton J, Polak JM, Bloom SR, et al: Bombesin-like immunoreactivity in the lung. Nature 273:769–770, 1978

22. Cutz E, Chan W, Track NS: Bombesin, calcitonin, and leuenkephalin immunoreactivity in endocrine cells of human lung. Experientia 37:765–767, 1981

23. Dayer AM, Rademakers A, DeMey J, Will JA: Serotonin, bombesin, and somatostatin-like immunoreactivity in neuroepithelial bodies (NEBs) of rhesus monkey fetal lung. Fed Proc 43:880, 1984

24. Becker KL, Monaghan KG, Silva OL: Immunocytochemical localization of calcitonin in Kulchitsky cells of human lung. Arch Pathol Lab Med 104:196–198, 1980

25. Hage E, Hage J, Juel G: Endocrine-like cells of the pulmonary epithelium of the human adult lung. Cell Tissue Res 178:39–48, 1977

26. Mihm FG: Non-respiratory functions of the lung. pp. 1–7. In 40th Annual Refresher Course Lectures and Clinical Update Programs. Lecture 155. American Society of Anesthesiologists, Chicago, IL, 1989

27. Bonikos DS, Bensch KG: Endocrine cells of bronchial and bronchiolar epithelium. Am J Med 63:765–771, 1977

28. Becker KL, Silva OL: Hypothesis: the bronchial Kulchitsky (K) cell as a source of humoral biologic activity. Med Hypotheses 7:943–949, 1981

29. Keith IM, Will JA: Hypoxia and the neonatal rabbit lung: neuroendocrine cell numbers, 5-HT fluorescence intensity, and the relationship to arterial thickness. Thorax 36:767–773, 1981

30. Kleinerman J, Marchevsky AM, Thornton J: Quantitative studies of APUD cells in airways of rats. Am Rev Respir Dis 124:458–462, 1981

31. Johnson NF, Wagner JC, Wills HA: Endocrine cell proliferation in the rat lung following asbestos inhalation. Lung 158:221–228, 1980

32. Forman HJ, Fisher AB: Antioxidant enzymes of rat granular pneumocytes. Lab Invest 41:1–6, 1981

33. Freeman BA, Mason RJ, Crapo JD: Induction of antioxidant enzymes in alveolar type II cells following exposure of rats to hyperoxia. Am Rev Respir Dis 123:230, 1981

34. Friedman MM, Kaliner MA: Symposium on mast cells and asthma: human mast cells and asthma. Am Rev Respir Dis 135:1157–1164, 1987

35. Wasserman SI: The lung mast cell: its physiology and potential relevance to defense of the lung. Environ Health Perspect 35:153–164, 1980

36. Marom Z, Casale TB: Mast cells and their mediators. Ann Allergy 50:367–370, 1983

37. Ryan JW, Smith U: Metabolism of adenosine 5'-monophosphate during circulation through the lungs. Trans Assoc Am Physicians 84:297–306, 1971

38. Smith U, Ryan JW: Pinocytotic vesicles of the pulmonary endothelial cells. Chest 59:125–155, 1971

39. Ryan US, Frokjaer-Jensen J: Pulmonary endothelium and processing of plasma solutes: structure and function. pp. 37–60. In Said SI, Vane J (eds): The Pulmonary Circulation and Acute Lung Injury. Futura Publishing, Mount Kisco, NY, 1985

40. Jonod AF: 5-hydroxytryptamine and other amines in

the lungs. pp. 337–349. In Fishman AP, Fisher B (eds): Handbook of Physiology. Section 3: The Respiratory System. Vol I. Circulation and Nonrespiratory Functions. American Physiological Society, Bethesda, MD, 1985

41. Alabaster VA, Bakhle YS: Removal of 5-hydroxytryptamine in the pulmonary circulation of rat isolated lungs. Br J Pharmacol 40:468–482, 1970

42. Nicholas TE, Strum JM, Angelo LS, Junod AF: Site and mechanism of uptake of ^{3}H-1-norepinephrine by isolated perfused rat lungs. Circ Res 35:670–680, 1974

43. Strum JM, Junod AF: Radioautographic demonstration of 5-hydroxytryptamine-^{3}H uptake by pulmonary endothelial cells. J Cell Biol 54:456–467, 1972

44. Fisher AB, Pietra GG: Comparison of serotonin uptake from the alveolar and capillary spaces of isolated rat lung. Am Rev Respir Dis 123:74–78, 1981

45. Block ER, Stalcup SA: Today's practice of cardiopulmonary medicine: metabolic functions of the lung: of what clinical relevance? Chest 81:215–223, 1982

46. Yanagisawa M, Kurihara H, Kimura S, et al: A novel potent vasoconstrictor peptide produced by vascular endothelial cells. Nature 332:411–415, 1988

47. Hanley SP: Prostaglandins and the lung. Lung 164:65–77, 1986

48. Kadowitz PJ, Spannhake EW, Hyman AL: Prostaglandins evoke a whole variety of responses in the lung. Environ Health Perspect 35:181–190, 1980

49. Kadowitz PJ, Lippton, HL, McNamara DB, et al: Action and metabolism of prostaglandins in the pulmonary circulation. pp. 333–356. In Oates JA (ed): Prostaglandins and the Cardiovascular System. Raven Press, New York, 1982

50. Ogletree ML: Pharmacology of prostaglandins in the pulmonary microcirculation. Ann N Y Acad Sci 384:191–206, 1982

51. Frangos JA, Eskin SG, McIntire LV, Ives CL: Flow effects on prostacyclin production by cultured human endothelial cells. Science 227:1477–1479, 1985

52. Reeves JT, van Grondelle A, Voelkel NF, et al: Prostacyclin production and lung endothelial cell shear-stress. Prog Clin Biol Res 136:125–131, 1983

53. Korbut R, Boyd J, Eling T: Respiratory movements alter the generation of prostacyclin and thromboxane A_2 in isolated rat lung: the influence of arachidonic acid pathway inhibitors on the ratio between pulmonary PGI_2 and TXA_2. Prostaglandins 21:491–503, 1981

54. Robinson C, Hardy CC, Holgate ST: Pulmonary synthesis, release, and metabolism of prostaglandins. J Allergy Clin Immunol 76:265–271, 1985

55. Eling TE, Ally AI: Pulmonary biosynthesis and metabolism of prostaglandins and related substances. Environ Health Perspect 55:159–168, 1984

56. Bakhle YS, Ferreira SH: Lung metabolism of eicosanoids: prostaglandins, prostacyclin, thromboxane, and leukotrienes. pp. 365–386. In Fishman AP, Fisher AB (eds): Handbook of Physiology. Section 3: The Respiratory System. Vol. 1. Circulation and Nonrespiratory Functions. American Physiological Society, Bethesda, MD, 1985

57. Ferreira SH, Vane JR: Prostaglandins. Their disappearance from the release into the circulation. Nature 216:868–873, 1967

58. McGiff JC, Terragno NA, Strand JC, et al: Selective passage of prostaglandins across the lung. Nature 223:742–745, 1969

59. Dusting GJ, Moncada S, Vane JR: Recirculation of prostacyclin (PGI_2) in the dog. Br J Pharmacol 64:315–320, 1978

60. Hammond GL, Cronau LH, Whitaker D, Gillis CN: Fate of prostaglandins E_1 and A_1 in the human pulmonary circulation. Surgery 81:716–722, 1977

61. Hoult JRS, Robinson C: Selective inhibition of thromboxane B_2 accumulation and metabolism in perfused guinea pig lung. Br J Pharmacol 78:85–88, 1983

62. Garcia JGN, Noonan TC, Jubiz W, Malik AB: Leukotrienes and the pulmonary microcirculation. Am Rev Respir Dis 136:161–169, 1987

63. Lawson C, Bunting S, Holzgrefe H, Fitzpatrick F: Leukotriene B_4 and 20-hyroxyleukotriene B_4 contract guinea pig trachea strips *in vitro*. J Pharmacol Exp Ther 237:888–892, 1986

64. Tracey WR, Eyre P: Effects of bradykinin and leukotrienes B_4 and D_4 on the bovine bronchial artery *in vitro*: role of the endothelium. Agents Actions 25:195–204, 1988

65. Hanna CJ, Bach MK, Pare PD, Schellenberg RR: Slow-reacting substances (leukotrienes) contract human airway and pulmonary vascular smooth muscle *in vivo*. Nature 290:343–344, 1981

66. Hand JM, Will JA, Buckner CK: Effects of leukotrienes on isolated guinea pig pulmonary arteries. Eur J Pharmacol 76:439–442, 1981

67. Ohtaka H, Tsang JY, Foster A, et al: Comparative effects of leukotrienes on porcine pulmonary circulation *in vitro* and *in vivo*. J Appl Physiol 63:582–588, 1987

68. Tracey WR, Bend JR, Hamilton JT, Paterson NAM: Role of lipoxygenase, cyclooxygenase and cytochrome P-450 metabolites in contractions of isolated guinea pig pulmonary venules induced by hypoxia and anoxia. J Pharmacol Exp Ther 250:1097–1104, 1989

69. Schellenberg RR, Foster A: Differential activity of leukotrienes upon human pulmonary vein and artery. Prostaglandins 27:475–482, 1984

70. Editorial review. Lancet 8476:301–303, 1986

71. Stephenson AH, Lonigro AJ, Hyers TM, et al: Increased concentrations of leukotrienes in bronchoalveolar lavage fluid of patients with ARDS or at risk for ARDS. Am Rev Respir Dis 138:714–719, 1988

72. Voelkel NF: Mechanisms of hypoxic pulmonary vasoconstriction. Am Rev Respir Dis 133:1186–1195, 1986

73. Stenmark KR, James SL, Voelkel NF, et al: Leukotriene C_4 and D_4 in neonates with hypoxemia and pulmonary hyertension. N Engl J Med 309:77–80, 1983

74. Dahlen S-E, Hedqvist P, Hammarstrom S, Samuelsson B: Leukotrienes are potent constrictors of human bronchi. Nature 288:484–486, 1980

75. Adelroth E, Morris MM, Hargreave FE, O'Byrne PM: Airway responsiveness to leukotrienes C_4 and D_4 and to methacholine in patients with asthma and normal controls. N Engl J Med 315:480–484, 1986

76. Morganroth ML, Stenmark KR, Zirrolli JA, et al: Leukotriene C_4 production during hypoxic pulmonary vasoconstriction in isolated rat lungs. Prostaglandins 28:867–875, 1984

77. Paterson NAM: Influence of hypoxia on histamine and leukotriene release from dispersed porcine lung cells. J Appl Physiol 61:1790–1795, 1986

78. Peters SP, Lichtenstein LM, Adkinson NF, Jr: Mediator release from human lung under conditions of reduced oxygen tension. J Pharmacol Exp Ther 238:8–13, 1986

79. Undem BJ, Pickett WC, Lichtenstein LM, Adams GK III: The effect of indomethacin on immunologic release of histamine and sulfidopeptide leukotrienes from human bronchus and lung parenchyma. Am Rev Respir Dis 136:1183–1187, 1987

80. Piper PJ, Antoniw JW, Stanton AWB: Release of leukotrienes from porcine and human blood vessels by immunological and nonimmunological stimuli. Ann NY Acad Sci 524:133–141, 1988

81. Piper PJ, Galton SA: Generation of leukotriene B_4 and leukotriene E_4 from porcine pulmonary artery. Prostaglandins 28:905–914, 1984

82. Feinmark SJ, Cannon PJ: Endothelial cell leukotriene C_4 synthesis results from intercellular transfer of leukotriene A_4 synthesized by polymorphonuclear leukocytes. J Biol Chem 261:16466–16472, 1986

83. Claesson H-E, Haeggstrom J: Human endothelial cells stimulate leukotriene synthesis and convert granulocyte released leukotriene A_4 into leukotrienes B_4, C_4, D_4 and E_4. Eur J Biochem 173:93–100, 1988

84. Ibe BO, Campbell WB: Synthesis and metabolism of leukotrienes by human endothelial cells: influence on prostacyclin release. Biochim Biophys Acta 960:309–321, 1988

85. Aharony D, Dobson PT, Krell RD: In vitro metabolism of [^{3}H]-peptide leukotrienes in human and ferret lung: a comparison with the guinea pig. Biochem Biophys Res Commun 131:892–898, 1985

86. Brom J, Konig W, Stuning M, et al: Characterization of leukotriene B_4-omega-hydroxylase activity within human polymorphonuclear granulocytes. Scand J Immunol 25:283–294, 1987

87. Lee CW, Lewis RA, Corey EJ, et al: Oxidative inactivation of leukotriene C_4 of stimulated human polymorphonuclear leukocytes. Proc Natl Acad Sci USA 79:4166–4170, 1982

88. Hammarstrom S, Orning L, Bernstrom K: Metabolism of leukotrienes. Mol Cell Biochem 69:7–16, 1985

89. Drazen JM, Austen KF: Leukotrienes and airway responses. Am Rev Respir Dis 136:895, 998, 1987

90. Bray MA: Leukotrienes in inflammation. Agents Actions 19:87–99, 1986

91. Serhan CN, Hamberg M, Samuelsson B: Lipoxins: novel series of biologically active compounds formed from arachidonic acid in human leukocytes. Proc Natl Acad Sci USA 81:5335–5339, 1984

92. Serhan CN, Hamberg M, Samuelson B: Trihydroxytetraenes: a novel series of compounds formed from arachidonic acid in human leukocytes. Biochem Biophys Res Commun 118:943–949, 1984

93. Kim SJ: Formation of lipoxins by alveolar macrophages. Biochem Biophys Res Commun 150:870–876, 1988

94. Hopkins NK, Oglesby TD, Bundy GL, Gorman RR: Biosynthesis and metabolism of 15-hydroperoxy-5,8,11,13-eicosatetraenoic acid by human umbilical vein endothelial cells. J Biol Chem 259:14048–14053, 1984

95. Revtyak GE, Johnson AR, Campbell WB: Cultured bovine coronary arterial endothelial cells synthesize HETEs and prostacyclin. Am J Physiol 254:C8–C19, 1988

96. Lefer AM, Stahl GL, Lefer DJ, et al: Lipoxins A4 and B4: comparison of eicosanoids having bronchoconstrictor and vasodilator actions but lacking platelet aggregatory activity. Proc Natl Acad Sci USA 85:8340–8344, 1988

97. Dahlen S-E, Raud J, Serhan CN, et al: Biological activities of lipoxin A include lung strip contraction and dilation of arterioles in vivo. Acta Physiol Scand 130:643–647, 1987

98. McManus LM, Deavers SI: Platelet activating factor in pulmonary pathobiology. Clin Chest Med 10:107–117, 1989

99. Barnes PJ: Platelet-activating factor and asthma. Allergy Clin Immunol 81:12, 1988

100. Page CP: The role of platelet-activating factor in asthma. J Allergy Clin Immunol 81:144, 1988

101. Said SI: Peptides, endothelium and pulmonary vascular reactivity. Chest 4:207S–209S, 1985

102. Clements JA, Funder JW, Tracey K, et al: Adrenocorticotropin, β-endorphin, and β-lipotropin in normal thyroid and lungs: possible implications for ectopic hormone secretion. Endocrinology 111:2097–2102, 1982

103. Gerwitz G, Yalow RS: Ectopic ACTH production in carcinoma of the lung. J Clin Invest 53:1022–1032, 1974

104. Yalow RS, Eastridge CE, Higgins G, et al: Plasma and tumor ACTH in carcinoma of the lung. Cancer 44:1789–1792, 1979

105. Dey RD, Said SI: Lung peptides and the pulmonary circulation. pp. 101–122. In Said SI, Vane J (eds): The Pulmonary Circulation and Acute Lung Injury. Futura Publishing, New York, 1985

106. Liggins GC, Kitterman JA, Campos GA, Clements JA: Pulmonary maturation in the hypophysectomized ovine fetus: differential responses to adrenocorticotropin and cortisol. J Dev Physiol 3:1–14, 1981

107. Verma PS, Miller RL, Taylor RE, et al: Inhibition of canine lung angiotensin converting enzyme by ACTH and structurally related peptides. Biochem Biophys Res Commun 104:1484–1488, 1982

108. Ryan JW, Stewart JM, Leary WP, Ledingham JG: Metabolism of angiotensin I in the pulmonary circulation. Biochem J 120:221–223, 1970

109. Ryan JW, Smith U: A rapid, simple method for isolating pinocytotic vesicles and plasma membrane of lung. Biochem Biophys Acta 249:177–180, 1971
110. Allison DJ, Clay T: Angiotensin II release from the hypoxic lobe of the intact dog lung. J Physiol (Lond) 260:32P–33P, 1976
111. Berkov S: Hypoxic pulmonary vasoconstriction in the rat: the necessary role of angiotensin II. Circ Res 35:256–261, 1974
112. Niarchos AP, Roberts AJ, Laragh JH: Effects of the converting enzyme inhibitor (SQ 20881) on the pulmonary circulation in man. Am J Med 67:785–791, 1979
113. Gryglewski RJ, Splawinski J, Korbut R: Endogenous mechanisms that regulate prostacyclin release. Adv Prostaglandin Thromboxane Res 7:777–787, 1980
114. Ryan U: Processing of angiotensin and other peptides by the lungs. Ch. 10. In Fishman AP, Fisher AB (eds): Handbook of Physiology, Section 3: The Respiratory System. Vol. 1. Circulation and Nonrespiratory Functions. American Physiological Society, Bethesda, MD, 1985
115. Chand N, Altura BM: Acetylcholine and bradykinin relax intrapulmonary arteries by acting on endothelial cells: role in lung vascular diseases. Science 213:1376–1379, 1981
116. Vargaftig BB, Dao Hai N: Selective inhibition by mepacrine of the release of "rabbit aorta contracting substance" evoked by the administration of bradykinin. J Pharm Pharmacol 24:159–161, 1972
117. Barst RJ, Stalcup SA, Mellins RB: Bradykinin-induced changes in circulating prostanoids in unanesthetized sheep. Fed Proc 42:302, 1983
118. Johnson AR: Effects of kinins on organ systems. pp. 357–399. In Erdos EG (ed): Handbook of Experimental Pharmacology, Vol. 25 (suppl.). Springer-Verlag, Berlin, 1979
119. Needleman P, Greenwald JE: Atriopeptin: a cardiac hormone intimately involved in fluid, electrolyte, and blood-pressure homeostasis. N Engl J Med 314:828–834, 1986
120. Turrin M, Gillis CN: Removal of atrial natriuretic peptide by perfused rabbit lungs *in situ*. Biochem Biophys Res Commun 140:868–873, 1986
121. Kadowitz PJ, Needleman P, Hyman Al: Vasodilator actions of atriopeptin II in the feline pulmonary vascular bed. Circulation 70:II–34, 1984
122. Ignarro LJ, Wood DS, Harbison RG, Kadowitz PJ: Atriopeptin II relaxes and elevates cGMP in bovine pulmonary artery but not vein. J Appl Physiol 60:1128–1133, 1986
123. Baertschi AJ, Hausmaninger C, Walsh RS, et al: Hypoxia-induced release of atrial natriuretic factor (ANF) from the isolated rat and rabbit heart. Biochem Biophys Res Commun 140:427–433, 1986
124. Tadepalli AS, Krueger AD: Effect of synthetic human atrial natriuretic peptide on hypoxic pulmonary vasoconstriction. Fed Proc 46:518, 1987
125. Adnot S, Chabrier PE, Andrivet P, et al: Atrial natriuretic peptide concentrations in pulmonary hemodynamics in patients with pulmonary artery hypertension. Am Rev Respir Dis 136:951–956, 1987
126. Burghuber OC, Hartter E, Punzengruber C, et al: Human atrial natriuretic petide secretion in precapillary pulmonary hypertension. Chest 92:31–37, 1988
127. Said SI, Mutt V: Long acting vasodilator peptide from lung tissue. Nature 224:699–700, 1969
128. Said SI, Mutt V: Polypeptide with broad biological activity: isolation from small intestine. Science 169:1217–1218, 1970
129. Said SI: Vasoactive peptides and the pulmonary circulation. Ann NY Acad Sci 384:207–212, 1982
130. Said SI: Vasoactive peptides in the lung, with special reference to vasoactive intestinal peptide. Exp Lung Res 3:343–348, 1982
131. Cutz E, Chan W, Track NS, et al: Release of vasoactive intestinal polypeptide in mast cells by histamine liberators. Nature 275:661–662, 1978
132. Hamasaki Y, Saga T, Mojarad M, Said SI: VIP counteracts leukotriene D₄-induced contractions of guinea pig trachea lung and pulmonary artery. Trans Assoc Am Physicians 96:406–611, 1983
133. Mojarad M, Said SI: Vasoactive intestinal peptide (VIP) dilates pulmonary vessels in anesthetized cats. Am Rev Respir Dis 123:239, 1981
134. Diamond L, Szarek JL, Gillespie MN, Altiere RJ: In vivo bronchodilator activity of VIP in the cat. Am Rev Respir Dis 128:827–832, 1983
135. Matsuzaki Y, Hamasaki Y, Said SI: Vasoactive intestinal peptide: a possible transmitter of non-adrenergic relaxation of guinea pig airways. Science 210:1252–1253, 1980
136. Said SI: Influence of neuropeptides on airway smooth muscle. Am Rev Respir Dis 136:552–558, 1987
137. Said SI: Vasoactive intestinal peptide: a brief review. J Endocrinol Invest 9:191–200, 1986
138. Kulik TJ, Johnson DE, Elde RP, Lock JE: Pulmonary vascular effects of bombesin and gastrin-releasing peptide in conscious newborn lambs. J Appl Physiol 55:1093–1097, 1983
139. Said SI: Peptides and lipids as mediators of acute lung injury. In Zapol WR, Falke KJ (eds): Acute Respiratory Failure. In Lenfant C (ed): Lung biology in Health and Disease Series. Marcel Dekker, New York, 1984
140. Worthen GS, Tanaka DT, Gumbay RS, et al: Substance P causes pulmonary vasoconstriction in rabbits. Am Rev Respir Dis 129:A337, 1984
141. O'Brodovich HM, Stalcup SA, Pang LM, Lipset JS: Bradykinin production and increased pulmonary endothelial permeability during acute respiratory failure in unanesthetized sheep. J Clin Invest 67:514–522, 1981
142. Desai U, Kruetzer DL, Showell H, et al: Acute inflammatory pulmonary reactions induced by chemotactic factors. Am J Pathol 96:71–83, 1979
143. Vane JR: Metabolic activities of the lung. Excerpta Medica 78:1–10, 1980
144. Hechtman HB, Shepro D: Lung metabolism and systemic organ function. Circ Shock 9:457–467, 1982

145. Gillis CN: Metabolism of vasoactive hormones by lung. Anesthesiology 39:626–632, 1973

146. Pearson JD, Gordon JL: Nucleotide metabolism by endothelium. Ann Rev Physiol 47:617–627, 1985

147. Fitzgerald GA: Dipyridamole. N Engl J Med 316:1247–1257, 1987

148. Shryock JC, Rubio R, Berne RM: Release of adenosine from pig aortic endothelial cells during hypoxia and metabolic inhibition. Am J Physiol 254:H223–H229, 1988

149. Mentzer RM JR, Rubio R, Berne RM: Release of adenosine by hypoxic canine lung tissue and its possible role in pulmonary circulation. Am J Physiol 229:1625–1631, 1975

150. Peach MJ, Johns RA, Rose CE, Jr: The potential role of interactions between endothelium and smooth muscle in pulmonary vascular physiology and pathophysiology. pp. 643–697. In Weir EK, Reeves JT (eds): Pulmonary Vascular Physiology and Pathophysiology. Marcel Dekker, New York, 1989

151. Furchgott RF, Zawadzki JV: The obligatory role of endothelial cells in the relaxation of arterial smooth muscle of acetylcholine. Nature 288:373–376, 1980

152. Furchgott RF: Role of endothelium in response of vascular smooth muscle. Circ Res 53:557–573, 1983

153. Furchgott RF: The role of the endothelium in the responses of vascular smooth muscle to drugs. Annu Rev Pharmacol Toxicol 24:175–197, 1984

154. Peach MJ, Loeb AL, Singer HA, Saye JA: Endothelium-derived relaxing factor. Hypertension 7:194–1100, 1985

155. Peach MJ, Singer HA, Loeb AL: Mechanisms of endothelium-dependent vascular smooth muscle relaxation. Biochem Pharmacol 34:1867–1874, 1985

156. Busse R, Trogisch G, Bassenge E: The role of endothelium in the control of vascular tone. Basic Res Cardiol 80:475–490, 1985

157. Angus JA, Cocks TM: Endothelium-derived relaxing factor. Pharmacol Ther 41:303–352, 1989

158. Griffith TM, Edwards DH, Lewis MJ, et al: The nature of endothelium-derived relaxing factor. Nature 308:645–647, 1984

159. Gryglewski RJ, Palmer RMJ, Moncada S: Superoxide anion is involved in the breakdown of endothelium-derived vascular relaxing factor. Nature 320:454–456, 1986

160. Busse R, Mülsch A: Calcium-dependent nitric oxide synthesis in endothelial cytosol is mediated by calmodulin. FEBS 265:133–136, 1990

161. Singer HA, Peach MJ: Calcium and endothelial-mediated vascular smooth muscle relaxation in rabbit aorta. Hypertension, suppl. II4:II-19-II-25, 1982

162. Bredt DS, Snyder SH: Isolation of nitric oxide synthetase, a calmodulin-requiring enzyme. Proc Natl Acad Sci USA 87:682–685, 1990

163. Loeb AL, Izzo NJ, Johnson RM, et al: Intracellular calcium transients associated with endothelium-derived relaxing factor release may be mediated by inositol 1,4,5, trisphosphate pp. 205–210. In Fiskum R (ed): Proceedings of the George Washington University VII International Symposium: Cell Calcium Metabolism 1987. Plenum Press, New York, 1989

164. Holzmann S: Endothelium-induced relaxation by acetylcholine associated with larger rises in cyclic GMP in coronary arterial strips. J Cyclic Nucl Res 8:409–419, 1982

165. Rapoport R, Murad F: Endothelium-dependent and nitrovasodilator-induced relaxation of vascular smooth muscle: role of cyclic GMP. J Cyclic Nucleotide Prot Phosphoryl Res 9:196–281, 1983

166. Furchgott R, Jothianandan D: Relation of cyclic GMP levels to endothelium-dependent relaxation by acetylcholine in rabbit aorta. Fed Proc 42:619, 1983

167. Ignarro LJ, Kadowitz PJ: The pharmacological and physiological role of cyclic GMP in vascular smooth muscle relaxation. Ann Rev Pharmacol Toxicol 25:171–191, 1985

168. Johns RA, Linden JM, Peach MJ: Endothelium-dependent relaxation and cyclic GMP accumulation in rabbit pulmonary artery are selectively impaired by hypoxia. Circ Res 65:1508–1515, 1989

169. De Mey JG, Vanhoutte PM: Anoxia and endothelium-dependent reactivity of the canine femoral artery. J Physiol 335:65–74, 1983

170. Palmer RM, Ferrige AG, Moncada S: Nitric oxide release accounts for the biological activity of endothelium-derived relaxing factor. Nature 327:524–526, 1987

171. Palmer RM, Rees DD, Ashton DS, Moncada S: L-arginine is the physiological precursor for the formation of nitric oxide in endothelium-dependent relaxation. Biochem Biophys Res Commun 153:1251–1256, 1988

172. Palmer RM, Ashton DS, Moncada S: Vascular endothelial cells synthesize nitric oxide from L-anginine. Nature 333:664–666, 1988

173. Ignarro LJ, Buga GM, Wood KS, et al: Endothelium-derived relaxing factor produced and released from artery and vein is nitric oxide. Proc Natl Acad Sci USA 84:9265–9269, 1987

174. Ignarro LJ, Byrns RE, Buga GM, Wood KS: Endothelium-derived relaxing factor from pulmonary artery and vein possesses pharmacologic and chemical properties identical to those in nitric oxide radical. Circ Res 61:866–879, 1987

175. Ignarro LJ, Buga GM, Byrns RE, et al: Endothelium-derived relaxing factor and nitric oxide possess identical pharmacologic properties as relaxants of bovine arterial and venous smooth muscle. J Pharmacol Exp Ther 246:218–226, 1988

176. Ignarro LJ, Byrns RE, Buga GM, et al: Pharmacological evidence that endothelium-derived relaxing factor is nitric oxide: use of pyrogallol and superoxide dismutase to study endothelium-dependent and nitric oxide-elicited vascular smooth muscle relaxation. J Pharmacol Exp Ther 244:181–189, 1988

177. Ignarro LJ, Gold ME, Buga GM, et al: Basic polyamino acids rich in arginine, lysine, or ornithine cause both enhancement of and refractoriness to formation of endothelium-derived nitric oxide in pulmonary artery and vein. Circ Res 64:315–329, 1989

178. Ignarro LJ: Endothelium-derived nitric oxide: actions and properties. FASEB J 3:31–36, 1989

179. Moncada S, Radomski MW, Palmer RM: Endothelium-derived relaxing factor. Identification as nitric oxide and role in the control of vascular tone and platelet function. Biochem Pharmacol 37:2495–2501, 1988

180. Kelm M, Feelisch M, Spahr R, et al: Quantitative and kinetic characterization of nitric oxide and EDRF released from cultured endothelial cells. Biochem Biophys Res Commun 154:236–244, 1988

181. Hoeffner U, Boulanger C, Vanhoutte PM: Proximal and distal dog coronary arteries respond differently to basal EDRF but not to NO. Am J Physiol 256:H828–H831, 1989

182. Marshall JJ, Wei EP, Kontos HA: Independent blockade of cerebral vasodilation from acetylcholine and nitric oxide. Am J Physiol 255:H847–H854, 1988

183. Tracey WR, Linden JL, Peach MJ, Johns RA: Comparison of spectrophotometric and biological assays for nitric oxide and EDRF: nonspecificity of the diazotization reaction for nitric oxide and failure to detect EDRF. J Pharmacol Exp Ther 252:922–928, 1990

184. Beny JL, Brunet PC: Neither nitric oxide nor nitroglycerin accounts for all the characteristics of endothelially mediated vasodilation of pig coronary arteries. Blood Vessels 25:308–311, 1988

185. Long CJ, Shikano K, Berkowitz BA: Anion exchange resins discriminate between nitric oxide and EDRF. Eur J Pharmacol 142:317–318, 1987

186. Myers PR, Guerra R, Jr, Harrison DG: Release of NO and EDRF from cultured bovine aortic endothelial cells. Am J Physiol 256:H1030–H1037, 1989

187. Shikano K, Ohlstein EH, Berkowitz BA: Differential selectivity of endothelium-derived relaxing factor and nitric oxide in smooth muscle. Br J Pharmacol 92:483–485, 1987

188. Taylor SG, Weston AH: Endothelium-derived hyperpolarizing factor: a new endogenous inhibitor from the vascular endothelium. Trends Pharmacol Sci 9:272–274, 1988

189. Chen G, Suzuki H, Weston AH: Acetylcholine releases endothelium-derived hyperpolarizing factor and EDRF from rat blood vessels. Br J Pharmacol 95:1165–1174, 1988

190. Feletou M, Vanhoutte PM: Endothelium-dependent hyperpolarization of canine coronary smooth muscle. Br J Pharmacol 93:515–524, 1988

191. Hawkins DJ, Meyrick BO, Murray JJ: Activation of guanylate cyclase and inhibition of platelet aggregation by endothelium-derived relaxing factor released from cultured cells. Biochim Biophys Acta 969:289–296, 1988

192. Radomski MW, Palmer RM, Moncada S: Comparative pharmacology of endothelium-derived relaxing factor, nitric oxide and prostacyclin in platelets. Br J Pharmacol 92:181–187, 1987

193. Radomski MW, Palmer RM, Moncada S: The anti-aggregating properties of vascular endothelium: interactions between prostacyclin and nitric oxide. Br J Pharmacol 92:639–646, 1987

194. Kaiser L, Hull SS, Sparks HV: Methylene blue and ETYA block flow-dependent dilation in canine femoral artery. Am J Physiol 250:H974–H981, 1986

195. Kaiser L, Sparks HV: Mediation of flow-dependent arterial dilation by endothelial cells. Circ Shock 18:109–114, 1986

196. Rubanyi GM, Romero JC, Vanhoutte PM: Flow-induced release of endothelium-derived relaxing factor. Am J Physiol 250:H1145–H1149, 1986

197. Brashers VL, Peach MJ, Rose CE, Jr: Augmentation of hypoxic pulmonary vasoconstriction in the isolated perfused rat lung by in vitro antagonists of endothelium-dependent relaxation. J Clin Invest 82:1495–1502, 1988

198. Tracey WR, Hamilton JT, Craig ID, Paterson NAM: Effect of endothelial injury on the responses of isolated guinea-pig pulmonary venules to reduced oxygen tension. Am Rev Respir Dis 140:68–74, 1989

199. Esterly JA, Glagov S, Ferguson DJ: Morphogenesis of intimal obliterative hyperplasia of small arteries in experimental pulmonary hypertension. Am J Pathol 52:325–327, 1968

200. Rabinovitch M, Bothwell T, Hayakawa BN, et al: Pulmonary artery endothelial abnormalities in patients with congenital heart defects and pulmonary hypertension. Lab Invest 55:632–653, 1986

201. Kistler GS, Caldwell PRB, Weibel ER: Development of fine structural damage to alveolar and capillary lining cells in oxygen-poisoned rat lungs. J Cell Biol 32:605–628, 1967

202. Commisky JM, Simon LM, Theodore J, et al: Bioenergetic alterations in cultivated pulmonary artery and aortic endothelial cells exposed to normoxia and hypoxia. Exp Lung Res 2:155–163, 1981

203. Coflesky JT, Evans JN: Hyperoxia alters endothelial-dependent relaxation and pharmacologic sensitivity of pulmonary arteries. Am Rev Respir Dis 133:A159, 1986

204. Rubanyi GM: Endothelium-derived vasoconstrictor factors. pp. 61–74. In Ryan US (ed): Endothelial Cells. Vol. 3. CRC Press, Boca Raton, FL, 1988

205. DiCorleto PE: Cultured endothelial cells produce multiple growth factors for connective tissue cells. Exp Cell Res 153:167–172, 1984

206. Campbell JH, Campbell GR: Endothelial cell influences on vascular smooth muscle phenotype. Ann Rev Physiol 48:295–306, 1986

207. Clowes AW, Karnovsky MJ: Suppression by heparin of smooth muscle cell proliferation in injured arteries. Nature 265:625–626, 1977

208. Castellot JJ, Rosenberg RD, Kamovsky MJ: Endothelium, heparin, and the regulation of cell growth. pp. 118–128. In Jaffe E (ed): Biology of Endothelial Cells. Martinus Nijihoff, Boston, 1984

209. DiCorleto PE, Gajdusec CM, Schwartz SM, Ross R: Biochemical properties of the endothelium-derived growth factor: comparison to other growth factors. J Cell Physiol 114:339–345, 1983

210. Domin BA, Serabjit-Singh CJ, Vanderslice RR, et al: Tissue and cellular differences in the expression of cytochrome P-450 isozymes. pp. 219–224. In Paton W,

Mitchell J, Turner P (eds): Proceedings of the IUPHAR, 9th International Congress of Pharmacology. Macmillan Press, London, 1984

211. Vanderslice RR, Domin BA, Carver GT, Philpot RM: Species-dependent expression and induction of homologues of rabbit cytochrome P-450 isozyme 5 in liver and lung. Mol Pharmacol 31:320–325, 1987

212. Bend JR, Hook GER, Easterling RE, et al: A comparative study of the hepatic and pulmonary microsomal mixed-function oxidase systems in the rabbit. J Pharmacol Exp Ther 183:206–217, 1972

213. Juchau MR, Bond JA, Benditt EP: Aryl 4-monooxygenase and cytochrome P-450 in the aorta: possible role in atherosclerosis. Proc Natl Acad Sci USA 73:3723–3725, 1976

214. Serabjit-Singh CJ, Bend JR, Philpot RM: Cytochrome P-450 monooxygenase system: localization in smooth muscle of rabbit aorta. Mol Pharmacol 28:72–79, 1985

215. Abraham NG, Pinto A, Mullane KM, et al: Presence of cytochrome P-450–dependent monooxygenase in internal cells of the hog aorta. Hypertension 7:899–904, 1985

216. Baird WM, Chemerys R, Grinspan JB, et al: Benzo (a) pyrene metabolism in bovine aortic endothelial and bovine lung fibroblast-like cell cultures. Cancer Res 40:1781–1786, 1980

217. Mansour H, Levacher M, Azoulay-Dupuis E, et al: Genetic differences in response to pulmonary cytochrome P-450 inducers and oxygen toxicity. J Appl Physiol 64:1376–1381, 1988

218. Mansour H, Brun-Pascaud M, Marquetty C, et al: Protection of rat from oxygen toxicity by inducers of cytochrome P-450 system. Am Rev Respir Dis 137:688–694, 1988

219. Serabjit-Singh CJ, Wolf CR, Philpot RM: Cytochrome P-450: localization in rabbit lung. Science 207:1469–1470, 1980

220. Sylvester JT, McGowan C: The effects of agents that bind to cytochrome P-450 on hypoxic pulmonary vasoconstriction. Circ Res 43:429–437, 1978

221. Miller MA, Hales CA: Role of cytochrome P-450 in alveolar hypoxic pulmonary vasoconstriction in dogs. J Clin Invest 64:666–673, 1979

222. Simionescu M, Simionescu N: Endothelial surface domains in pulmonary alveolar capillaries. pp. 35–62. In Ryan US (ed): Pulmonary Endothelium in Health and Disease.

223. Pietra GG, Sampson P, Lanken PN, et al: Transcapillary movement of cationized ferritin in the isolated perfused rat lung. Lab Invest 49:54–61, 1983

224. Rothstein R, Cole JS, Pitt BR: Pulmonary extraction of [³H]bupivacaine: modification by dose, propranolol and interaction with [¹⁴C]5-hydroxytryptamine. J Pharmacol Exp Ther 240:410–414, 1987

225. Post C, Andersson RGG, Ryrfeldt A, Nilsson E: Transport and binding of lidocaine by lung slices and perfused lungs of rats. Acta Pharmacol Toxicol 43:156–163, 1978

226. Jorfeldt L, Lewis DH, Lofstrom JB, Post C: Lung uptake of lidocaine in healthy volunteers. Acta Anaesth Scand 23:567–584, 1979

227. Jorfeldt L, Lewis DH, Lofstrom JB, Post C: Lung uptake of lidocaine in man as influenced by anaesthesia, mepivacaine infusion or lung insufficiency. Acta Anaesth Scand 27:5–9, 1983

228. Dollery CT, Junod AF: Concentration of (L)-propranolol in isolated perfused lungs of rat. Br J Pharmacol 57:67–71, 1976

229. Geddes DM, Nesbitt K, Traill T, Blackburn JP: First pass uptake of ¹⁴C-propranolol by the lung. Thorax 34:810–813, 1979

230. Roerig DL, Kotrly KJ, Vucins EJ, et al: First-pass uptake of fentanyl, meperidine, and morphine in the human lung. Anesthesiology 67:466–472, 1987

231. Bakhle YS, Block AJ: Effects of halothane on pulmonary inactivation of noradrenaline and prostaglandin E₂ in anesthetized dogs. Clin Sci Mol Med 50:87–90, 1976

232. Cook DR, Brandon BW: Enfluane, halothane, and isoflurane inhibit removal of 5-hydroxytryptamine from the pulmonary circulation. Anesth Analg 61:671–675, 1982

233. Naito H, Gillis CN: Effects of halothane and nitrous oxide on removal of norepinephrine from the pulmonary circulation. Anesthesiology 39:575–580, 1973

234. Watkins CA, Wartell SA, Rannels P: Effect of halothane on metabolism of 5-hydroxytryptamine by rat lungs perfused in situ. Biochem J 210:157–166, 1983

235. Rannels DER, Roake GM, Watkins CA: Additive effects of pentobarbital and halothane to inhibit synthesis of lung proteins. Anesthesiology 57:87–93, 1982

236. Rannels DE, Christopherson R, Watkins CA: Reversible inhibition of protein synthesis in lungs by halothane. Biochem J 210:379–387, 1983

237. Martin DC, Carr AM, Livingston RR, Watkins CA: Effects of ketamine and fentanyl on lung metabolism in perfused rat lungs. Am J Physiol 257:E379–E384, 1989

238. Archer SL, Weir EK, McMurtry IF: Mechanisms of acute hypoxic and hyperoxic changes in pulmonary reactivity. pp. 241–290. In Weir EK, Reeves JT (eds): Pulmonary Vascular Physiology and Pathophysiology. In Lenfant C (ed): Lung Biology in Health and Disease. Marcel Dekker, New York, 1989

239. Ahmed T, Oliver W, Jr: Does slow-reacting substance of anaphylaxis mediate hypoxic pulmonary vasoconstriction? Am Rev Respir Dis 127:566–571, 1983

240. Morganroth ML, Reeves JT, Murphy RC, Voelkel MF: Leukotriene synthesis and receptor blockers block hypoxic pulmonary vasoconstriction. J Appl Physiol 56:1340–1346, 1984

241. Goldberg RN, Suguihar C, Ahmed T, et al: Influence of an antagonist of slow reacting substance of anaphylaxis on the cardiovascular manifestations of hypoxia in piglets. Pediatr Res 19:1201–1205, 1985

242. Raj JU, Chen P: Role of eicosanoids in hypoxic vasoconstriction in isolated lamb lungs. Am J Physiol 253:H626–H633, 1987

243. Rengo F, Trimarco B, Ricciardelli B, et al: Effects of disodium cromoglycate on hypoxic pulmonary hypertension in dogs. J Pharmacol Exp Ther 211:686–689, 1979

244. Mammel MC, Edgren BE, Gordon MJ, Boros SJ: Failure of two leukotriene synthesis inhibitors to reverse hypoxic pulmonary vasoconstriction. Clin Res 34:153A, 1986

245. Leffler CW, Mitchell JA, Green RS: Cardiovascular effects of leukotrienes in neonatal piglets. Role in hypoxic pulmonary vasoconstriction? Circ Res 55:780–787, 1984

246. Schuster DP, Dennis DR: Leukotriene inhibitors do not block hypoxic pulmonary vasoconstriction in dogs. J Appl Physiol 62:1808–1813, 1987

247. Garrett RC, Foster S, Thomas HM: Lipoxygenase and cyclooxygenase blockade by BW 755C enhances pulmonary hypoxic vasoconstriction. J Appl Physiol 62:129–133, 1987

248. Ovetsky RM, Sprague RS, Stephenson AH, et al: Inhibition of leukotriene synthesis does not alter the pulmonary stress response to alveolar hypoxia. Am Rev Respir Dis 135:A127, 1987

249. McCormack DG, Paterson NAM: The contrasting influence of two lipoxygenase inhibitors on hypoxic pulmonary vasoconstriction in anesthetized pigs. Am Rev Respir Dis 139:100–105, 1989

250. Naeije R, Leeman M, Lejeune P: Effects of diethylcarbomazine and cromolyn sodium on hypoxic pulmonary vasoconstriction in dogs. Bull Eur Physiopathol Respir 22:75–80, 1986

251. Said SI: The pulmonary circulation and acute lung injury: introduction and overview. pp. 3–10. In: The Pulmonary Circulation and Acute Lung Injury. Futura Publishing, Mt. Kisko, NY, 1985

252. Tate RM, Repine JE: Neutrophils and the adult respiratory distress syndrome. Am Rev Respir Dis 128:552–559, 1983

253. Rinaldo JE, Rogers RM: Adult respiratory distress syndrome: changing concepts of lung injury and repair. N Engl J Med 206:900–909, 1982

254. Jones R, Zapol WM, Reid L: Progressive and regressive structural changes in rat pulmonary arteries during recovery from prolonged hyperoxia. Am Rev Respir Dis 125:227, 1982

255. Reid L: The pulmonary circulation: remodeling in growth and disease. Am Rev Respir Dis 119:531–546, 1979

256. Snapper JR, Brigham KL: Arachidonate products as mediators of diffuse lung injury. pp. 321–336. In Said SI (ed): The Pulmonary Circulation and Acute Lung Injury. Futura Publishing, Mt. Kisko, NY, 1985

257. Reeves JT, Stenmark KR, Voelkel MF: Possible role of leukotrienes in the pathogenesis of pulmonary hypertensive disorders. pp. 337–356. In Said SI (ed): Pulmonary Circulation and Acute Lung Injury. Futura Publishing, Mt. Kisko, NY, 1985

258. Mojarad M, Cox CP, Said SI: Platelet activating factor (PAF) and acute lung injury. pp. 375–386. In Said SI (ed): The Pulmonary Circulation and Acute Lung Injury. Futura Publishing, Mt. Kisko, NY, 1985

259. Hirose T: Prostacyclin as a modulator of acute lung injury. pp. 455–467. In Said SI (ed): The Pulmonary circulation and Acute Lung Injury. Futura Publishing, Mt. Kisko, NY, 1985

260. Malik AB, Johnson A: Role of humoral mediators in the pulmonary vascular response to pulmonary embolism. pp. 445–468. In Weir EK, Reeves JT (eds): Pulmonary Vascular Physiology and Pathophysiology. In Lung Biology in Health and Disease. Marcel Dekker, New York, 1989

261. Pitt BR, Lister G: Interpretation of metabolic function of the lung. Influence of perfusion, kinetics, and injury. Clin Chest Med 10:1–12, 1989

262. Dawson CA, Roerig DJ, Linehan JH: Evaluation of endothelial injury in the human lung. Clin Chest Med 10:13–24, 1989

263. Philpot RM, Anderson MW, Eling TE: Uptake, accumulation and metabolism of chemicals by the lung. pp. 123–171. In Bakhle YS, Vane JR (eds): Metabolic Functions of the Lung. Marcel Dekker, New York, 1977

264. Anderson MW, Orton TC, Pickett RD, Eling TE: The accumulation of amines in the isolated perfused rabbit lung. J Pharmacol Exp Ther 189:456–466, 1974

265. Bend JR, Serabjit-Singh CJ, Philpot RM: The pulmonary uptake, accumulation, and metabolism of xenobiotics. Ann Rev Pharmacol Toxicol 25:97–125, 1985

266. Davila T, Davila D: Uptake and release of ^{3}H-metaraminol by rat lung. The influence of various drugs. Arch Int Pharmacodyn 215:336–344, 1975

267. Junod AF: Uptake, metabolism and efflux of ^{14}C-5-hydroxytryptamine in isolated, perfused rat lungs. J Pharmacol Exp Ther 183:341–355, 1972

268. Alabaster VA, Bakhle YS: The removal of noradrenaline in the pulmonary circulation of rat isolated lungs. Br J Pharmacol 40:468–482, 1983

269. Briant RH, Blackwell EW, Williams FM, et al: The metabolism of sympathomimetic bronchodilator drugs by the isolated perfused dog lung. Xenobiotica 3:787–799, 1973

270. Minchin RF, Madsen BW, Ilett KF: Effect of desmethylimipramine on the kinetics of chlorophenteramine accumulation in isolated perfused rat lung. J Pharmacol Exp Ther 211:514–518, 1979

271. Junod AF: Accumulation of ^{14}C-imipramine in isolated perfused rat lungs. J Pharmacol Exp Ther 183:182–187, 1972

272. Roth RA, Roth JA, Gillis CN: Disposition of ^{14}C-mescaline by rabbit lung. J Pharmacol Exp Ther 200:394–401, 1977

273. Wilson AGE, Law FCP, Eling TE, Anderson MW: Uptake, metabolism and efflux of methadone in 'single pass' isolated rabbit lungs. J Pharmacol Exp Ther 199:360–367, 1976

274. Catane R, Schwade JG, Turrisi AT, et al: Pulmonary toxicity after radiation and bleomycin: a review. Int J Radiat Oncol Biol Phys 5:1513–1518, 1979

275. Catravas JD, Lazo JS, Gillis CN: Biochemical markers

of bleomycin toxicity: clearance of [14C]-5-hydroxytryptamine and [3H]norepinephrine by rabbit lung in vivo. J Pharmacol Exp Ther 217:524–529, 1981

276. Boyd MR, Stiko AW, Sasme HA: Metabolic activation of nitrofurantoin-possible implications for carcinogenesis. Biochem Pharmacol 28:601–606, 1979

277. Jarasch ED, Bruder G, Heid HW: Significance of xanthine oxidase in capillary endothelial cells. Acta Physiol Scand, suppl. 548:39–46, 1986

278. Smith LL: The identification of an accumulation system for diamines and polyamines into the lung and its relevance for paraquat toxicity. Arch Toxicol, suppl. 5:1–14, 1982

279. Ryan US, Ryan JW: Correlations between the fine structure of the alveolar-capillary unit and its metabolic activities. pp. 197–242. In Bakhle YS, Vane JR (eds): Metabolic Functions of the Lung. Marcel Dekker, New York, 1977

6

SYSTEMIC OXYGEN TRANSPORT

Christopher W. Bryan-Brown, M.D.

Anesthesiologists have more influence on the patient's outcome by maintaining systemic oxygen transport during and after a surgical procedure than by any other action they may take. Failure to keep the body perfused with an appropriate volume and flow of oxygenated blood has been shown to be associated with increased mortality, postoperative organ failure, poor wound healing, and sepsis,[1-6] particularly in the already compromised patient. For example, monitoring to ensure that properly oxygenated blood is circulating in the periphery by pulse oximetry has resulted in a significant reduction in preventable anesthetic mishaps since 1984.[7]

Under conditions of normal physiology, the respiratory system is geared so that ventilation, cardiac output, and the distribution of blood flow are matched to provide for tissue oxygen requirements.[8] Thus, if the metabolic rate of a region of the body increases, ventilation and cardiac output will also increase proportionately to deliver the necessary increment of oxygen, while local vasodilatation will direct the increased flow to the appropriate tissues. After a few minutes, a new equilibrium will have been reached and, because of the coupling of the various components of the delivery system, mixed venous and arterial blood gas values will return to their values prior to the increased demand. In this chapter, the processes involved in transporting oxygen from the lungs to the tissues, the inter- and intraorgan distribution of oxygen, how the train of physiologic events changes in shock and stressed states, the reactions to failure of the various components, and how the various systems might best be monitored, are described.

BACKGROUND

Barcroft, in his dissertations on oxygen insufficiency, described the components of oxygen transport.[9,10] He realized that the oxygenation of the blood was only part of the picture, and that both flow and content had to be considered. A subject could be "within a measurable distance of death" from "anoxaemia" and recover, unless "elderly or unsound." Barcroft did not describe the instrument to measure that "distance," except to state that the oxygen insufficiency had to be more than enough to produce coma. Fortunately, he did provide the classification of *hypoxia (anoxaemia)* into the categories *hypoxic (anoxic)*, *anemic (anaemic)*, and *stagnant*, which are still in use today. Adequate oxygen transport required adequate oxygenation of the arterial blood to saturate enough hemoglobin, adequate hemoglobin and adequate flow. Nunn and Freeman, nearly half a century later, again pointed out that all three components were needed for oxygen delivery, and that, for instance, an anemic patient would be further jeopardized by hypoxia.[11] The difficulty in this ostensibly simple concept is that the definition of "adequate" has only just begun to be supported by data over the past few years.

Two other types of hypoxia were recognized in the earlier years of oxygen physiology, although their significance was not readily understood in clinical medicine. In 1920, *affinity hypoxia* was described as "alteration of the dissociation curve of oxyhaemoglobin, so that this gives of its oxygen less easily than usual" in an editorial in the *Lancet*,[12] probably quoting J.S. Haldane. Again the clinical recognition did not come

143

to light for many years until 1953, when two Scottish physicians noted a defect in the gas transport function of stored red blood cells. Valtis and Kennedy, in their publication in the following year, showed how a three-unit transfusion of stored blood was sufficient to temporarily reduce the arteriovenous oxygen content difference [C(a − v̄)O$_2$] by approximately 1 mL/dL.[13] Although the postoperative patient tends to be hypermetabolic and to have a reduced C(a − v̄)O$_2$, the effect was more marked in transfused patients.

Histotoxic anoxia was recognized by Peters and Van Slyke as an oxygen deprivation caused by a cell not being able to use oxygen.[14] Cyanide poisoning was given as a typical example. Current theories tend to center around distributional phenomena (eg, maldistribution, loss of autoregulation in the microcirculation, or microembolism) to explain why cells do not pick up sufficient oxygen in shock states.[15] Recent experimental work reemphasizes that cell damage may also be a factor in septic shock.[16] The loss of adenosine from the mitochondrial nucleotide pool during hypoxia has also been suggested as another cause of insufficient oxygen utilization when more oxygen becomes available.[17] If the cell switches over to anaerobic metabolism (Pasteur effect), there is a loss of adenosine from the mitochondria to the cytosol as the transfer mechanisms break down. Acidosis further exacerbates the overall loss by encouraging the deamination of adenosine to inosine. If more oxygen returns to the cell, there is then a shortage of substrate to make adenosine triphosphate by means of oxidative phosphorylation in the mitochondria. Nucleotides are further lost as inosine is oxidized to uric acid via the xanthine oxidase pathway, releasing oxygen free radicals, which in turn may further exacerbate tissue damage.

The distribution of blood flow to the various organ systems of the body is governed by a balance of neurohumoral stimuli. The concept of *supply dependency* has shaped much of the more teleologic thinking as to the mechanism whereby oxygen is distributed to tissues most in need.[18] Supply-dependent organs are those that, under normal circumstances, use most of the oxygen available. They tend to function near the *critical point*, where further oxygen utilization will diminish the oxygen tension low enough to reduce uptake. If a greater amount of metabolic work is to be maintained, an increased delivery is required, which usually is achieved by more blood flow. Examples of supply-dependent organs would be the heart and brain. Supply-independent organs normally have blood flow and oxygen supply far greater than required for their energy needs, such as the kidneys and skin. When hypovolemia or hypoxia occurs, the reaction of the body is to direct blood flow from supply-independent organs to supply-dependent organs, thus changing the overall priority to survival rather than function.[19] However, as pointed out by Laver, survival may well be determined by the proper oxygenation of a few grams of tissue.[20]

August Krogh was the first physiologist to show that the distribution of blood flow within organs was an actively controlled process and not due to a passive vasodilation.[21] He demonstrated in a muscle preparation that vasodilation occurred in response to demand, with the opening of previously closed capillaries and an increase in diameter of those already open. From his observations, he postulated that there were three mechanisms whereby the oxygen supply to a tissue could be boosted: *increased volume of flow* in dilated vessels, *increased flow velocity*, and *recruitment* of previously unopened vessels. Thus, a larger capillary surface area could be available for the diffusion of oxygen into the tissue and more oxygen delivered to the capillaries.

Some changes have occurred in the perception of recruitment, at least in muscle. The original observations of Krogh were made with the unphysiologic perfusate of india ink. He used it to demonstrate the openness of capillaries, and it probably did not behave like blood. More recent in vivo observations suggest that, at rest, flow velocities in the microcirculation are very inhomogeneous. In response to demand, the flow velocities in the slower elements speed up, and the flow becomes homogeneous.[22] In contrast, tissues with a very low metabolic demand, such as fascia and tendon, have been observed to have intermittent flows, with periods of no flow predominating.[23] In 1971, Folkow et al suggested that the exchange surface area could be under the control of precapillary sphincters and their activity could be modulated by local metabolic means.[24] Despite much research, precapillary sphincters have been found in only a few very specific tissues and are not applicable as a general mechanism.[25]

The control of blood distribution within the microcirculation is only partially understood. It is easy to make the observation that a hypoxic tissue regulates its own vascular tone and then allocates blood flow to the cells with the greatest metabolic requirement. The mechanisms whereby these processes are effected have been much harder to elucidate. When they cease to function properly, uncontrolled blood flow decreases the efficiency of oxygen delivery and a "physiologic shunt" develops, giving rise to regional hypoxia and a higher than expected venous oxygen content. Regional tissue hypoxia could result from local obstruction or an uncontrolled local increase in resistance. Blood would tend to flow more through the remaining capillaries,[15] which become like the "thoroughfare vessels" originally described in the mesentery.[26] On the other hand, vasodilator therapy can also unbalance the flow distribution by bringing about a more homogeneous flow when there is not a homogeneity of metabolism. The effect can then be that excessive and inadequate oxygen delivery occurs side by side, particularly when flow is limited by the physical narrowing of the supplying arteries. This has become known as a *steal syndrome*.[27] Vasodilation may actually divert blood away from areas receiving a barely adequate flow into areas that do not need more. The ways that this deficit is overcome are either by an overall greater flow or by a restoration of autoregulation.

OXYGEN DELIVERY

The convection of oxygen from the lungs to the tissues is the product of blood flow and oxygen content. The conventional formula is

$$\dot{D}O_2 = \dot{Q} \times CaO_2 \tag{1}$$

where $\dot{D}O_2$ is the oxygen delivery, $\dot{Q}$ is the cardiac output, and CaO_2 is the arterial oxygen content. CaO_2 is usually calculated as the product of the hemoglobin concentration ([Hb]), which represents the major part of the carrying capacity, and the saturation (SaO_2), which quantifies how fully the hemoglobin is loaded. A usually small increment, derived from the tension (PaO_2), is added to account for dissolved oxygen.

$$\begin{align} CaO_2 = \\ ([Hb] \times 1.34 \times SaO_2/100) + (PaO_2 \times 0.00314) \tag{2} \\ \text{(combined)} \qquad\qquad \text{(dissolved)} \end{align}$$

The factor 0.00314 is the solubility of oxygen expressed as gas volume (STP) in milliliters per 100 milliliters of blood per millimeter of mercury partial pressure at 37°C (mL/dL/mmHg) The factor 1.34 is an estimate, established as a standard in the early 1900s by such researchers as Haldane, for the oxygen-combining capacity of a gram of hemoglobin ($mL_{(STP)}/g$). Values from 1.33 to 1.36 will be found in the scientific literature of the past few decades. In 1963, the precise determination of the molecular weight of hemoglobin led to the stoichiometric calculation of 1.39. This figure has always proved higher than investigators have measured. Nunn has suggested that as the measurement of [Hb] is validated on the International Cyanmethemoglobin Standard, which in turn is based on iron content, methemoglobin and other non-oxygen-combining pigments are included.[28] This inflates the measured hemoglobin concentration, so the observed combining capacity is less than 1.39. With current methods of hemoglobinometry, a value of approximately 1.31 may be closer to previous proposals.[29]

Adequate perfusion of tissues also requires a sufficient head of pressure to overcome vascular resistance, and a sufficient blood volume to ensure that all vascular beds can be filled. Because the circulation can make adjustments that keep the more obvious metabolically active tissue functioning despite an overall deficit, shortfalls are easily missed in the clinical situation. The following sections will be devoted to the components of oxygen delivery and how they can be assessed and optimized.

Oxygen Tension

The normal arterial oxygen tension (PaO_2) in the healthy nonsmoking person tends to decline with age. Marshall and Wyche analyzed 12 studies involving 1,209 air-breathing patients and derived the following regression equation:

$$PaO_2 = (102 - 0.33\,[A]) \pm 10 \text{ mmHg} \tag{3}$$

where [A] is the subject's age in years.[30] Because the range given is two SD, Nunn pointed out that this ought to be used as a reference range, as 5 percent of normal people will be outside the confidence limits.[31] It is also possible for a normal person aged 70 years to have a PaO_2 the same as one aged 20 years. Almost all normal individuals should have a PaO_2 above 70 mmHg.

The range of inspired oxygen tensions (P_1O_2) that have been experienced by human beings is shown in Table 6-1. Although acclimatized humans have successfully managed with a P_1O_2 of 43 mmHg on the summit of Mt. Everest,[32] most people are unconscious from hypoxic hypoxia by the time it is as low as 57 mmHg, even when the arterial carbon dioxide tension ($PaCO_2$) is kept from falling to levels that will diminish cerebral perfusion.[33] The highest human habitation is approximately 18,000 ft (5,500 m), where barometric pressure is half normal, although a few people have lived higher for considerable periods (J.B. West, personal communication). While these remarkable feats of endurance indicate what is possible to survive, there is marked redistribution already occurring in the circulation when the PaO_2 is as low as 50 mmHg,[19] which is approximately related to a P_1O_2 in the mid-90s. As the P_1O_2 is elevated above normal, various pulmonary deficits arise that make this a largely temporizing maneuver for increasing arterial oxygenation.[34-36] Hunt and Goodson have suggested that administering supplemental oxygen to postsurgical patients maintaining their PaO_2 levels in the 150 to 200 mmHg range for 48 hours can promote wound healing and reduce postoperative sepsis.[37] This can

TABLE 6-1. **Moist Inspired Oxygen Tensions (P_iO_2) and Important Related Physiologic Events**

mmHg		kPa[a]
43	Summit of Mt. Everest—29,028 ft (8,848 m). (West et al[32])	5.7
57	Loss of consciousness (Siesjö et al[33])	7.6
65	Cerebral blood flow ↑ 70%	8.7
70	Highest human habitation—18,000 ft (5,500 m)	9.3
72	Cerebral blood flow ↑ 35%	9.6
96	Marked redistribution of circulation (Heistad and Abboud[19]) SaO_2 approximately 85%; altitude of 12,000 ft (3,943 m)	13
149	Air at 1 atmosphere	20
178	Tracheal mucus flow ↓ 16% (Laurenzi et al[34])	24
356	Safe limit for pulmonary toxicity (Clark and Lambertsen[35]) Pulmonary "shunt" ↑ (Monaco et al[36]) Optimum for wound healing (Hunt and Goodson[37])	48
713	Vascular resistance ↑ (Lambertsen[38]) Cardiac output ↓ (Plewes and Fahri[39])	95
1,470	Oxygen convulsions; CNS O_2 toxicity (Bert[41])	195
2,000	Normal oxygen transport without Hb (Boerema et al[42])	267

Abbreviations: CNS, central nervous system; Hb, hemoglobin.
[a] 1 kPa = 7.5 mmHg.

often be done by using 50 percent oxygen by face mask.

When 100 percent oxygen is breathed, the peripheral vascular resistance increases.[38] Plewes and Fahri were able to show that while the CaO_2 increased, $\dot{D}O_2$ remained constant, since the cardiac output was found to decrease proportionally.[39] When these inspired oxygen fractions (F_iO_2) are used, PaO_2 values over 500 mmHg may be produced, which can downgrade autoregulation in the microcirculation. Using surface tissue polarographic electrodes, Carlsson et al were able to demonstrate the development of a patchy hypoxia in the human cerebral cortex.[40] Thus, small areas of almost zero oxygen tension are adjacent to areas with supranormal values, indicating maldistribution.

Central nervous system toxicity (convulsions) can occur when two atmospheres of oxygen are breathed; this is termed the *Bert effect*.[41] When the inspired oxygen tension reaches three atmospheres, hemoglobin becomes superfluous, as there is enough dissolved oxygen to meet metabolic requirements.[42] The human experience has mainly consisted of anecdotal reports on the maintenance of very severely anemic patients who refused blood transfusion on religious grounds. The use of hyperbaric oxygenation for other therapeutic purposes does not seem to have fulfilled initial promises. The best indications currently are life-threatening carbon monoxide poisoning and cerebral air embolism.[43]

The relevance of this information is that there are few clinical reasons why the PaO_2 should ever need to be above 200 mmHg. Conditions that might benefit from higher levels are cardiogenic shock,[44] severe anemia, or regional ischemia. In a patient with an intact cardiovascular system, a safe lower limit is not easily defined. When the PaO_2 falls to 70 mmHg, hemoglobin remains approximately 95 percent saturated, trivially lower than normal (Fig. 6-1). This has become a frequently stated goal in the treatment of hypoxic patients. Although this level is not supported with good data, it seems to have been arrived at by delphic decision making. At lower levels, coronary sinus blood flow increases, although a significant increase in cerebral blood flow does not usually occur until the PaO_2 goes below 50 mmHg.[33] If a patient is symptomatic with angina pectoris or cardiac dysrhythmias, supplemental oxygen is obviously indicated.

Oxygen-Hemoglobin Dissociation

The relationship of oxygen tension (PO_2) to the saturation of hemoglobin within the erythrocyte and oxygen is shown in Figures 6-1 and 6-2. This is for standard conditions: pH = 7.4 (H^+ = 40 nmol/L), PCO_2 = 40 mmHg (5.3 kPa), and temperature (T) = 37°C. As

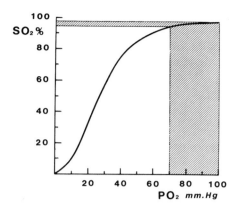

Fig. 6-1. A standard oxyhemoglobin dissociation curve. When the oxygen tension (PO_2) falls from 100 to 70 mmHg (13.3 to 9.3 kPa), the saturation (SO_2) only falls 3 percent. This is the normal physiologic range for PaO_2, and demonstrates the loading portion of the curve. (From Bryan-Brown,[160] with permission.)

shown in Figure 6-1, the fall in SO_2 when the PO_2 decreases from 100 to 70 mmHg is only 3 percent. This is the range of PaO_2 seen in most air-breathing individuals, and an indication that 70 mmHg should be enough to meet oxygen delivery needs in an intact circulation. Thus, the loading of the hemoglobin molecule with oxygen is accomplished even with a mild hypoxic hypoxia. Figure 6-2 also shows the characteristics of the "unloading" portion of the curve. Under normal circumstances, the mixed venous oxygen tension ($P\overline{v}O_2$) and saturation ($S\overline{v}O_2$) are approximately

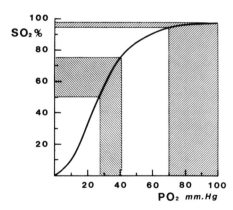

Fig. 6-2. Standard oxyhemoglobin dissociation curve, comparing the normal loading and unloading portions. When the PO_2 is 40 mmHg (5.3 kPa), the hemoglobin is one-quarter desaturated. When the PO_2 drops to 27 mmHg (3.6 kPa), a further quarter of the hemoglobin is desaturated. This is the $P\overline{v}O_2$ range over which there is a normal physiologic reserve.

40 mmHg (5.3 kPa) and 75 percent, respectively. Thus, only a quarter of the hemoglobin capacity for oxygen has been used. When half the capacity has been used ($S\overline{v}O_2 = 50$ percent), the PO_2 has only fallen to 27 mmHg (3.6 kPa), which is usually well tolerated. As the pH is lower and PCO_2 is higher in the tissues, the PO_2 will have a greater value than shown from the standard curve, as these factors will shift the curve to the right (Bohr effect).[45] This *right shift* is considered an aid to oxygen utilization in the tissues in hypoxic conditions. It will cause hemoglobin to have only a slightly lower affinity for oxygen in the *loading* part of the curve, but a much lower affinity in the *unloading* portion. Thus, a slight decrement in SaO_2 is more than made up for by the greater amount of oxygen available in the tissues before the oxygen tension reaches hypoxic levels. This compensation becomes ineffective as the PaO_2 drops below 50 mmHg (6.7 kPa), and loading and unloading begin to occur on the same gradient.

The position of the curve is usually described by the P_{50}, which is the PO_2 when the hemoglobin is 50 percent saturated with oxygen. The standard value for P_{50} is approximately 27 mmHg (3.6 kPa). The relationship of the major factors that shift the oxyhemoglobin dissociation curve are quantified in the Bellingham formula[46]:

$$P_{50} = \log(26.6 + 0.5[MCHC - 33] \\ + 0.69[2,3\text{-}DPG - 14.5] + 0.0013BE \\ + 0.48[pH - 7.4] + 0.024[T - 37]) \quad (4)$$

where MCHC is the mean corpuscular hemoglobin concentration, 2,3-DPG is 2,3-diphosphoglycerate in micromoles per gram of hemoglobin (μmol/g Hb), and BE is base excess in millimoles per liter (mmol/L). The effect of carbon dioxide tension differences from 40 mmHg (5.3 kPa) can be accounted for by BE, which is governed by the relationship of PCO_2 to pH.[47]

Perutz has proposed a molecular mechanism whereby hemoglobin changes its affinity for oxygen.[48–50] The molecule can exist in either a relaxed (R structure) or tight (T structure) form. In the relaxed form, oxygen can get at the heme moiety more easily and is more firmly bound, that is, affinity is greater. When various agents, such as hydrogen ion (H^+), 2,3-DPG, carbon dioxide, or chloride, increase in concentration, hydrogen bonds (salt bridges) develop between various sites on the alpha and beta chains, making it more difficult for oxygen to reach the binding site. This is the tight configuration (T structure). An elevation of temperature also facilitates hydrogen bonding. Oxygen itself promotes the relaxing of the molecule, so that when desaturation of oxyhemoglobin begins, the affinity decreases; therefore, smaller decrements in PO_2 are needed to remove a given amount of oxygen. This explains the steepening of the oxyhemoglobin dissociation curve in the unloading region. Carbon monoxide is a very powerful relaxing agent. When half the hemoglobin is carboxyhemoglobin (HbCO), the P_{50} of the remaining hemoglobin is approximately half normal.[51] Thus, in carbon monoxide poisoning, a patient has both an *anemic* and an *affinity hypoxia*.

When the hydrogen bonds are disrupted, protons (H^+) are released. Thus, oxyhemoglobin is a stronger acid and, therefore, a weaker buffer than deoxyhemoglobin. As oxygen is released in the tissues, protons are incorporated into the hydrogen bonds. The effects of carbon dioxide production are buffered both by this and carbaminohemoglobin formation. The pH of the venous blood is usually only a few hundredths of a pH unit below the arterial value. When [Hb] is in the normal range, if the respiratory quotient (RQ) is 0.7, the venous blood would have the same pH value as the arterial.

The main factors that alter the affinity of hemoglobin for oxygen are listed with their mechanisms in Table 6-2. Some of the compensatory mechanisms for restoring the P_{50}, when it is an appropriate physio-

logic or therapeutic response, are also shown.[52] The various ligands squeeze oxygen out of the hemoglobin molecule, while at the same time, oxygen tends to release the ligands. A lower pH will decrease glycolysis; thus, in chronic acidosis, 2,3-DPG production will decrease, returning the P_{50} to normal. Conditions giving rise to increased deoxyhemoglobin levels (eg, anemia, hypoxia, and low-output cardiac failure) will allow more 2,3-DPG to become bound to the hemoglobin molecule. The concentration of free, 2,3-DPG in the erythrocyte cytosol will fall, so production and total concentration will increase.

The clinical relevance of this information seems obvious. With chronic hypoxia, a person should be able to deliver more oxygen or oxygen at a higher tension in the tissues by right-shifting the oxyhemoglobin dissociation curve, thereby improving survival when oxygen delivery is compromised. Acute alkalosis or the use of stored blood may create an affinity hypoxia. Unfortunately, in the normal individual, the position of the oxyhemoglobin dissociation curve seems to be a minor factor influencing body function and, in the critically ill patient, despite much experimental evidence, it does not seem to affect outcome.[53,54].

TABLE 6-2.   Factors Affecting Oxyhemoglobin Dissociation[a]

Factor	P_{50}	Mechanism	Compensation
Acidosis	↑	H^+ creates hydrogen bonds (salt bridges) promoting T structure	PFK activity ↓, glycolysis ↓, 2,3-DPG production ↓
Carbon dioxide	↑	Carbamino compound formation and H^+ promoting T structure	Same
2,3-DPG	↑	Heterotopic ligand promoting T structure	Free 2,3-DPG decreases 2,3-DPG production
Chloride	↑	Increases salt bridges in Hb	
MCHC	↓	Intraerythrocyte buffering ↑, mean H^+ ↓ promotes R structure	
Temperature	↑	Increases effect of CO_2 and directly promotes T structure	[2,3-DPG] ↓
[Hb] ↓, PaO_2 ↓, cardiac failure	↑	Deoxyhemoglobin ↑, bound 2,3-DPG ↑, 2,3-DPG production ↑	
Banking blood	↓	Hydrolysis of 2,3-DPG	Store blood near neutral pH with phosphate and adenine
Mean phosphate ↓	↓	2,3-DPG production ↓	Phosphate administration
Mean glucose ↑	↓	Glycolization of hemoglobin	Control blood glucose
Carbon monoxide	↓	HbCO promotes R structure	Elevate P_IO_2

Abbreviations: PFK, phosphofructokinase; for definition of R and T structures, see text; for other abbreviations and symbols, see Appendix 6-1.
[a] Also see Bryan-Brown.[52]

Hemoglobin Concentration and Hematocrit

The conventional relationship between ([Hb]) and the hematocrit is $1:3$. Except in some anemias, this is sufficiently accurate for clinical and research purposes, and will be assumed in the discussion below.

Comroe, in a fit of physiologic abstraction, calculated that a resting air-breathing man with no hemoglobin would require a cardiac output of 83 L/min to provide enough oxygen for basal metabolic requirements, if every molecule of oxygen were used.[55] If the $P\bar{v}O_2$ were to be kept at 40 mmHg, then a cardiac output of 133 L/min would be needed. The breathing of pure oxygen would reduce the cardiac output requirement by 80 percent. This is still beyond the capacity of the best-trained athlete.

The range of values encountered in humans can be considerable. There is an often-raised question as to how much the [Hb] should be before a patient is anesthetized or to optimize $\dot{V}O_2$ and $\dot{D}O_2$ in the critically ill patient. Anemia and polycythemia have to be considered from the point of view of both gross convection (oxygen movement from lungs to tissues) and their effects on the distribution of oxygen in the microcirculation. Some of the effects are shown in Table 6-3.

The lowest acceptable preoperative [Hb] was stated a century ago by Miculicz to be 30 percent of normal (approximately 4.5 g/dL).[56] His patients were receiving chloroform, with air as the carrier gas. He had noted that when the [Hb] fell to 20 percent of normal, his patients died in respiratory failure. Since this initial well-founded observation, recommendations have been frequent, but not based on any sound statistics until the last few years.[57] A consensus developed that the minimal safe [Hb] prior to surgery was probably 9 to 10 g/dL. Carson et al seemed to confirm this in a study of operative mortality in relation to anemia.[58] Unfortunately, as many of the patients were actively bleeding and of a persuasion to refuse blood transfusion, hypovolemia seems to be another possible etiology for poor outcome in this series. Messmer has now established the criteria and safety of deliberate preoperative hemodilution to 10 g/dL as a technique for both improving blood flow and economizing on blood transfusion.[59] He had previously found that increased blood flow was needed to maintain $\dot{V}O_2$ when the [Hb] was below 9 g/dL.[60]

Surgical patients have survived a [Hb] around 2 g/dL.[61-63] Volume support, a high F_IO_2, and mild hypo-

TABLE 6-3. Hemoglobin Concentration and Hematocrit and Significant Physiologic Events

[Hb] (g/dL)		Hct (%)
2	Limit of survival (Nearman and Eckhauser[61] and Harris[62])	6
4	Lowest elective preoperative (Miculicz[56])	12
5	Collagen formation normal (Zederfeldt[64])	15
6	Wound PO_2 maintained (Hunt and Goodson[37])	18
7	Cerebral ERO_2 decreases (Borgström et al[66])	21
9	$\dot{V}O_2 \uparrow$ because cardiac work $\uparrow$ (Cain[65]) Increased flow needed to maintain $\dot{V}O_2$ (Messmer[60]) Increased postoperative mortality (Carson et al[58])	27
10	Preoperative hemodilution (Messmer[59])	30
12	Optimum in surgical shock (Wilson and Walt[67] and Czer and Shoemaker[68])	36
14	Maximum $\dot{D}O_2$ for $M\dot{V}O_2$ (Richardson and Guyton[70])	42
15	Cerebral thromboembolism increases (Pearson and Weatherly-Mein[71])	45
16	O_2 transport capacity $\downarrow$	48
19	High altitude dwellers (15,000 ft or 4,600 m)[73]	57
>20	Progressive cardiac decompensation	>60

Abbreviations: [Hb], hemoglobin concentration; Hct, hematocrit; for other abbreviations and symbols, see Appendix 6-1.

thermia seem to have been the ingredients for success.[61-63] Very low [Hb] does not seem to interfere with either collagen formation[64] or wound healing,[37] and it appears that the surgical tradition that anemia delays wound healing was based on patients with either malnutrition or hypovolemia.

In severe anemia, the efficiency of oxygen delivery decreases. This observation was made by Cain in experimental circumstances,[65] and is a finding in humans anemic to the critical point, when extraction ratios (ERO$_2$) can approach the normal range.[63] This produces what initially seems like a paradoxically high P$\bar{v}$O$_2$. Experimental evidence indicates that this becomes a measurable phenomenon when the [Hb] is below 7 g/dL,[66] and will be further discussed in the section *Hemodilution*.

The optimum value for survival in surgical patients with shock has been found in the 11 to 12 g/dL range.[67,68] An earlier study on acute respiratory failure patients had indicated that a Hct over 40 percent was associated with the highest survival,[69] but this was a retrospective review in an era when stress ulceration and gastric hemorrhage were prevalent disorders. Much survival literature is confusing because of the admixture of low Hct with hypovolemia. Whereas a loss of red blood cell mass of 70 percent can be tolerated, profound shock can result from as little as a 30 percent loss of blood volume.

The erythrocytes normally contribute approximately half the viscosity of the blood. As hematocrit rises, oxygen-carrying capacity increases, but the blood takes more energy to circulate. From their investigations, Richardson and Guyton were able to show that the optimum balance for most $\dot{D}O_2$ for least myocardial oxygen uptake (M$\dot{V}$O$_2$) occurred when the Hct was in the 40 to 45 percent range.[70] As the hematocrit rises further, the incidence of thromboembolic phenomena increases.[71] It should be noted that exercise performance may be improved with a [Hb] over 16 g/dL,[72] a point appreciated by the "blood-doping" athlete, but not sufficiently investigated to report on in other hyperdynamic conditions. Even higher Hcts are encountered in people living at higher attitudes as a compensation for hypoxic hypoxia.[73]

Sickle cell disease provides an interesting problem in oxygen delivery. The blood viscosity of a homozygotic (HbSS) patient with an Hct in the 18 to 24 percent range can be as high as that of someone with an Hct of 45 percent with normal hemoglobin (HbA).[74] The sickle erythrocytes are much stiffer than normal erythrocytes, and may not readily pass through the narrower capillaries in the microcirculation. The addition of normal red blood cells to correct the anemia may push up the viscosity. If the Hct goes over 35 percent, the viscosity may become unacceptably high

and be enough to provoke a crisis.[75-77] Patients with [Hb] less than 7.0 g/dL undergoing major surgical procedures should probably be transfused prior to surgery. If 50 percent of the red blood cells contain HbA, the rheologic characteristics of the blood may improve markedly in the deoxyhemoglobin state. If blood transfusion is considered desirable, then the [Hb] should be kept down to the 11 g/dL range, and if the plan is to have 50 percent HbA, then exchange transfusion may be contemplated.[78] Another plan for a less severe case could be to maintain the patient in a volume-expanded state, and replace surgical blood losses with blood. Because of the dangers of transmitting diseases with blood transfusion, and the paucity of data to show it makes a major difference to patient outcome, a conservative approach is probably desirable.

From a clinical standpoint there is no specific number that could be used to designate a patient's [Hb] below which elective surgery should be postponed for reasons of safety. Patients with end-stage renal disease frequently have successful surgery with a [Hb] less than 7 g/dL. Those who have lost blood during surgery and refuse transfusion have overcome the stress of an operation with similar levels. On the other hand, patients with cardiac or coronary arterial disease do not seem to withstand anemia so readily, and will be better off with a [Hb] greater than 11 g/dL.

The one caveat in assessing the preoperative need for any [Hb] concerns hypovolemia. Classically, dehydration has been well known to give a misleadingly high value, but what is less well appreciated is that in the critically ill and trauma population, even severe hypovolemia may not manifest a low [Hb].[79-81]

Blood Volume

When the blood volume decreases, reflex circulatory and neurohumoral adjustments occur that seem to maintain vital functions, albeit with less reserve. Thus, when a hypovolemic patient is anesthetized or is stressed by illness or trauma, the hypovolemia is unmasked as the patient develops cardiovascular collapse or multiple system failure. The prompt restoration of blood volume, according to a well-developed protocol, reduces mortality and morbidity in the acute surgical patient.[5,6,82-84] For the anesthesiologist, hypovolemia should be an avoidable condition, but the diagnosis is not always easily made because of the physiologic compensations.

The reaction of the body to hypovolemia tends to direct the delivery of oxygen (blood flow) to maintain supply-dependent tissues.[85-87] In this it is very similar to hypoxic hypoxia.[19] A slight but significant difference is that, in hypovolemia, the diminution of flow to supply-independent tissues is further reduced. Potentially, this can convert them to supply dependency and take the $\dot{D}O_2$ below the critical point, causing hypoxic damage. While this is happening, the conventional "vital signs" of a patient can continue to be in the normal range. In one investigation using healthy volunteers, an acute hemorrhage of more than 20 percent of the predicted blood volume produced a fall in mean blood pressure (BP) of 15 mmHg, whereas the cardiac output was reduced 41 percent.[88] In another study, Price et al showed that with a lesser hemorrhage of 15 to 20 percent of predicted blood volume, there was no significant alteration of hemodynamic variables.[89] The splanchnic blood volume was reduced by 40 percent, but with no appreciable increase in vascular resistance. In critically ill patient populations, it is very possible to have patients with 20 to 40 percent reductions from a predicted blood volume, yet have their hemodynamic pressure and flow variables within normal parameters.[79–81,90] It is not usual for patients in this state to be able to compensate for further stress, and they will often exhibit their deficit with cardiovascular collapse on the induction of anesthesia, when sympathetic tone is reduced. It is also noteworthy that in acutely ill patients with seemingly adequate cardiovascular variables, fluid loading with crystalloid and colloid solutions can augment $\dot{D}O_2$ and $\dot{V}O_2$ further,[80,91] particularly in hypovolemic patients. This probably indicates that an oxygen debt is being repaid and that current metabolic needs are being supplied.

The skin and splanchnic system make up a reservoir that can replace an approximate 20 percent loss of blood volume without any loss of intrinsic splanchnic function. The moment-to-moment control of the blood pressure and systemic blood volume is in part achieved by adjustments in sympathetic tone that result in the transfer of blood to and from the capacitance vessels in the splanchnic system and skin.[92–95] Total hepatic flow is reduced when enough blood is lost to reduce the blood pressure,[96] and liver size diminishes radiographically.[97] Laboratory investigations in a canine shock model suggest that hepatic blood flow has to be reduced to at least 40 percent of normal before there is any indication of hypoxic change.[98] Liver oxygenation is reduced by halothane[99] and, to a lesser extent, enflurane,[100] but apparently not isoflurane.[99] There are no good data as to whether this should be a consideration for choice of anesthetic agent when high-blood-loss surgery is to be performed.

The viability of the liver and intestines does not seem to be compromised by hypovolemia, unless there is vascular disease affecting the blood supply. Gut and liver function may be less effective, giving rise to a picture of stress ulceration, malabsorption, the transgression of bowel flora outside the bowel wall, and mild hepatic failure. On the other hand, the blood flow to the pancreas may be much more severely reduced in some shock states, particularly hemorrhage.[101] It has been postulated that this can further jeopardize the patient by the release of lysosomal enzymes, which in turn produce a *myocardial depressant factor* that lessens myocardial contractility. The clinical significance of this factor is still under consideration, even though it is becoming diluted as a host of other factors and mediators have appeared on the shock scene.[102]

While a decrease in skin blood flow per se is seldom a cause for concern, it may be an indicator of poor oxygen delivery or hypovolemia. Visual signs such as pallor and poor capillary refill are hard to quantitate. A higher than normal temperature gradient between the core and the skin has been shown to correlate well with the severity of the circulatory deficit, and has been used by monitoring the dorsum of the big toe with a thermistor.[103] A more sophisticated approach has been to compare the PO_2 of the arterial blood with that measured by a transcutaneous oxygen electrode.[104,105] This gradient is usually very small unless blood flow to the skin is decreased.

The kidney reacts to hypovolemia with a reduction in urine output and sodium retention. In critical illness or following a drop in blood pressure, the renin-angiotensin system is activated, both intrinsically and because of increased sympathetic tone, with a decrease in renal blood flow.[106] Antidiuretic hormone is also secreted in response to decreased blood pressure and a loss of distending pressure in the great veins and right atrium. Renal insufficiency due to poor kidney perfusion can occur with hypovolemia in the absence of hypotension. In one study, 50 percent of the patients who developed renal failure following a major hemorrhage had no recorded episode of hypotension.[107]

Valeri et al also found that the P_{50} was lower in hypovolemic patients, which was attributed to the greater desaturation of circulating hemoglobin in the tissues.[108] Their 2,3-DPG concentrations were higher than normal, which agrees with the observations made when the ratio of deoxyhemoglobin to oxyhemoglobin in the circulation rises.[46] This is further evidence of hypovolemia promoting hypoxia.

The cardiovascular assessment of hypovolemia is difficult in the pre- and postoperative periods when the patient has an intact or even overactive sympathetic nervous system. It was pointed out by Landis and Hortenstine that an elevated central venous pressure (CVP) was not an unexpected finding in hypovolemia, as the immediate adjustments to changes in blood volume were sympathetically mediated.[109] A clinical application of this information was developed by Weil et al, who suggested that since the CVP could be high in hypovolemia, a period of volume loading of the circulation should be tried.[110] If the CVP fell or did not rise, hypovolemia was the probable diagnosis. More volume loading was the indicated therapy, until the patients' systems were functioning normally or the CVP began to rise. In a series of hypovolemic patients, Baek et al found that there was no correlation between CVP or pulmonary artery occlusion (wedge) pressure and blood volume.[80] When patients with an abnormally high CVP were loaded with a standard volume of fluid, it fell in over half the patients. The patients in whom the CVP fell also had a marked increase in cardiac output, $\dot{D}O_2$, $\dot{V}O_2$, and stroke work with a decrease in vascular resistances. Blood volume measurements showed a 20 percent deficit, while the group in whom the CVP rose had a blood volume in the normal range. The "vital signs" of the two groups were similar.

From a practical standpoint, hypovolemia is so prevalent in the ill or traumatized hospital population[81,90] that it ought to be one of the first considerations when a system goes into failure. When shock resuscitation is carried out, the goals should be to meet the supply-dependent oxygen requirements of the body. Since metabolic requirements are usually higher at this time, supranormal values are found to maximize survival.[5,84,111] A reasonable aim would be to try to increase the $\dot{V}O_2$ to 120 percent of basal, initially by appropriate volume expansion and, if necessary, by inotropic agents. A cardiac output of 150 percent of resting value and a blood volume of 110 percent of predicted may be required to achieve this. Monitoring $\dot{V}O_2$ is currently the most realistic way that oxygen debts can be avoided throughout the perioperative period,[4,5,112] and it may also confirm that a patient has an adequate blood volume when other circulatory parameters are in the desired range.

Blood Pressure

Most tissues autoregulate their blood flow over a wide range of blood pressures according to their metabolic or functional needs. When the oxygen supply is not enough to meet demand, the vascular system supplying the deprived area dilates so that blood flow increases. Overriding this system, the sympathetic nervous system imposes further direction, prioritizing blood flow and oxygen delivery to organ systems with the most pressing need and mobilizing blood from capacitance vessels. Approximately 60 percent of the systemic blood volume is in small veins and venules (<2 mm diameter). Much of this can also

be mobilized. Thus, sympathetic tone can effectively make up 20 percent of the estimated blood volume (approximately 1 L in a normal man) to maintain or augment circulatory function.[113] The limiting factor is time when this alpha$_1$-adrenergic effect is being used to compensate for large deficits. There is a gradual return of blood flow to such tissues as resting muscle and the splanchnic area, and this initial protective mechanism is lost.[94,95] This could be either from the down regulation of alpha$_1$-receptors or the accumulation of vasodilators such as acidosis or adenosine. Many anesthetic techniques, agents, and adjuvants alter sympathetic tone and have a direct effect on vascular smooth muscle. They therefore have the potential for profoundly altering both the delivery of oxygen to organs and within tissues as well as causing cardiovascular collapse.

The cerebral circulation maintains a fairly constant blood flow, governed by oxygen requirements, over a wide range of blood pressure. Lassen demonstrated a plateau effect between a mean BP of 50 to 150 mmHg.[14] Above and below these bounds blood flow varies with pressure as the resistance vessels are beyond the limits of vasoconstriction or vasodilation. This traditional viewpoint has been criticized by Heistad and Kontos,[115] who felt that Lassen's work did not take into account that his protocol used drugs to raise and lower the blood pressure that can affect the cerebral vascular resistance. The result was an exaggeration of the flatness in the autoregulation (plateau) part of the flow-pressure curve. A reduction of cerebral blood flow (CBF) by about one-fifteenth for every 10 mmHg drop in mean BP in the autoregulatory phase would seem to be more likely. Maximum cerebrovascular dilation occurs when the mean BP is down to 40 mmHg.[116] Local distribution seems to be under metabolic control, with the production of vasodilation by adenosine in relatively hypoxic regions.[117]

If a patient has cerebrovascular disease, a fall in mean BP has to be regarded as a potential risk that may give rise to regional ischemia and hypoxic brain damage. Some of the original workers on CBF recognized that the autoregulatory range shifted to a higher level in essential hypertension.[118] Thus, the hypertensive patient becomes more sensitive to the dangers of hypotension. With successful management of hypertension with good blood pressure control, the autoregulatory range shifts back toward normal.[119] By extrapolation from laboratory work, this process is likely to take 2 to 3 months; thus, anyone whose hypertension is recently under treatment has to be considered at the same risk as a hypertensive patient.

The effect of inhalation anesthetics is to reduce the range of the autoregulatory phase so that CBF is more closely proportional to the blood pressure. Halothane and enflurane have a greater effect than an equipotent dose of isoflurane and, in the normal blood pressure range, there is a proportionately greater than normal flow for the cerebral metabolic rate of oxygen ($CMRO_2$).[120,121] This greater flow may be protective, as vasodilator drugs tend to make the distribution of oxygen within tissues less efficient by reducing microvascular autoregulation. The result is a decreased ERO_2. It would, therefore, be prudent in the management of head injury patients undergoing surgery for other conditions to avoid deep anesthesia with inhalation agents. Opioid anesthesia seems to leave cerebral autoregulation largely intact.[122]

The normal autoregulatory range for the coronary arterial system is a mean BP of 60 to 180 mmHg.[123] As the left ventricular perfusion is mainly during diastole, it mostly relies on the maintenance of diastolic pressure. The overriding stimulus for coronary vasodilation appears to be a greater metabolic requirement for oxygen.[124]

The renal circulation has a similar pattern of autoregulation to the brain, but with the autoregulatory phase failing when the mean BP goes below 70 mmHg.[106,123] The kidney has a strong override from the sympathetic nervous system and renin-angiotensin mechanism that may mask intrinsic requirements for more $\dot{D}O_2$.[125]

From the clinical standpoint, drugs that manipulate the blood pressure may also alter or interfere with the distribution of blood so that some tissues may be inadequately supplied with oxygen. The first action in the acutely hypotensive patient with no preceding history of longstanding cardiac disease is to increase intravascular volume with fluid loading. Increased preload and filling of the ventricles should augment cardiac output and blood pressure.[110] As a temporary maneuver, the pharmacologic contraction of the venous capacitance vessels can also boost cardiac filling. In one study, it was found that when the blood pressure was restored with dihydroergotamine and etilofrine, the former mobilized blood by limb and cutaneous venoconstriction while the latter contracted the splanchnic veins.[126] There was a reduction of blood flow through the areas involved, but the full significance of this on patient outcome is still speculative.

Cardiac Output

The patient in cardiac failure or with a low cardiac output presents with similar compensations to one suffering from hypoxia, hypovolemia, or hypotension. In a study of patients with mild ($\dot{Q} > 2.5$ L/min/m^2), moderate ($\dot{Q} = 2.5 - 2.0$ L/min/m^2), and severe ($\dot{Q} < 2.0$ L/min/m^2) disease, Leithe et al compared regional blood flows with those of normal subjects ($\dot{Q} \approx 3.5$ L/min/m^2).[127] As cardiac output decreased there was a proportional increase in systemic, hepatic, renal, and limb vascular resistance with a concomitant decrease in blood flow. The kidney produced a slight exception in severe failure with a modest, but significant increase in blood flow above that in moderate heart failure. There was a considerable range of blood pressures in this patient population. When the cardiac output was limited, flow to the measured systems was not related to blood pressure, only to the diminution of total flow.

The pharmacologic support of cardiac output has both beneficial and unwanted effects.[128] Mueller has suggested that the best plan of action when using inotropes and vasoconstrictors is to precisely define the deficit that needs correction.[129] The aim is to get the desired result without increasing workload on the heart enough to produce myocardial ischemia. If inotropy is required, a drug such as dobutamine would be indicated, as it causes a minimal tachycardia. If an increase in blood pressure is needed, it can be caused by small doses of norepinephrine or dopamine. Dopamine has the advantage of suppressing the renin-angiotensin axis; thus, it can produce inotropy while also increasing renal and splanchnic blood flow.

When increased cardiac output is attempted with the addition of vasodilators to reduce afterload, myocardial ischemia may be exacerbated with sodium nitroprusside, which is primarily an arteriolar vasodilator. The administration of nitroglycerin, which has a greater effect on the venous capacitance system, is associated with less ST segment depression on the electrocardiogram.[130] Tissue oxygenation (striated-muscle, myocardium, and subcutaneous tissue), in general, is better for a given mean BP decrease with nitroglycerin than with sodium nitroprusside.[131] The reason suggested is that venous pressure is lower, and therefore the perfusion gradient and blood flow is higher. Unfortunately, the vasodilation by nitrates and phosphodiesterase inhibitors tends to favor limb blood flow, and may even decrease blood flow to the renal and hepatic-splanchnic regions.[128] Hydralazine and nifedipine appear to decrease resistance in all regions, and would, therefore, be more likely to improve systemic oxygen delivery.

The clinical message inherent in these observations is that when cardiac output is augmented pharmacologically, the additional flow does not get equally distributed to all systems, and to some may even be less. The support of oxygen transport to the tissues in cardiac failure is, therefore, a delicate balancing act in which those caring for the patient have taken over or have a controlling influence over the distribution of available oxygen.

HYPERDYNAMIC STATES

A hyperdynamic state exists when the cardiac output appears abnormally high for the metabolic needs of the patient. This is usually seen in the recovery period from an insult such as severe stress, hemorrhage, or trauma, and during sepsis or anemia. Although the mechanisms may be variable, the overall effect is an increased oxygen delivery with an inefficient oxygen utilization ($\dot{D}O_2 \uparrow$ and $ERO_2 \downarrow$). This, therefore, gives rise to an unexpectedly high mixed venous oxygen level ($P\bar{v}O_2$, $S\bar{v}O_2$, or $C\bar{v}O_2$), which originally introduced the concept of *histotoxic anoxia*.[14] The same effect is seen as an increased supply dependency in the tissues, as more $\dot{D}O_2$ is needed to maximize $\dot{V}O_2$. It is also possible, when the cardiac output is insufficient, for the $S\bar{v}O_2$ to be normal or high because of the reduced ERO_2 in the stressed patient.[132] The use of venous oxygen monitoring needs to be coupled with oxygen uptake to ensure correct interpretation and an adequately oxygenated patient.

In summary, the hyperdynamic state consists of (1) increased energy expenditure to maintain ionic gradients, (2) glycolysis and lactic acidosis, and (3) increased cardiac output with loss of autoregulation in the microcirculation. "Steal" syndromes develop in compromised and damaged tissues.

Sepsis

The septic patient provides a striking example of disorganized peripheral oxygen transport. The observation that it took more oxygen delivery to maintain uptake became readily apparent when routine cardiac output monitoring became a standard procedure in many critical care units. This was a result of the introduction of the thermodilution cardiac output catheter. Figure 6-3 shows $\dot{D}O_2$ and $\dot{V}O_2$ data from initial resuscitation for an episode of sepsis to a moribund state with multiple systems organ failure 10 days later. As the patient's condition deteriorated, the gradient of $\dot{V}O_2$ to $\dot{D}O_2$ (availability) gradually decreased until more than twice the $\dot{D}O_2$ was needed to maintain the initial $\dot{V}O_2$. Peirce[133] even suggested, from an analysis of data from Powers et al,[134] that the human metabolism in the critically ill might convert to *oxygen conformity*, that is, that the metabolic rate would depend on the available oxygen. While supply-dependent oxygen uptake was confirmed in other studies of acute respiratory distress patients,[135,136] it was partly explained away as a quirk from the use of the indirect Fick method of calculating $\dot{V}O_2$:

$$\dot{V}O_2 = \dot{Q} \times C(a - \bar{v})\,O_2 \qquad (5)$$

Cardiac output ($\dot{Q}$) is a common factor in the calculation of both $\dot{D}O_2$ (Eq. 1) and $\dot{V}O_2$ (Eq. 5). In septic

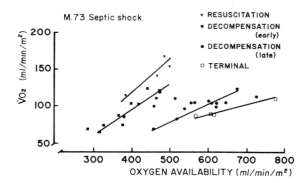

Fig. 6-3. Data from a septic patient who developed multiple systems organ failure. Over the course of 10 days, until he died, he demonstrated progressive supply dependency. Increasing $\dot{D}O_2$ (availability) was needed to maintain even an inadequate $\dot{V}O_2$. (From Bryan-Brown,[161] with permission).

ventilated patients, on a moment-to-moment basis during the respiratory cycle, the cardiac output can vary as much as 70 percent.[137] Since the arteriovenous oxygen content difference [$C(a - \bar{v})\,O_2$] remains fairly constant, if there is a large variation in $\dot{Q}$, $\dot{D}O_2$ and $\dot{V}O_2$ will rise and fall together. This explanation has been partially refuted by the observation that the $\dot{V}O_2$ is cardiac output dependent when the $\dot{V}O_2$ is measured directly.[138] Accuracy in the measurement of $\dot{V}O_2$ is very hard to achieve. Even in the critically ill it is markedly variable.[139] Direct measurement may be confounded by oxygen uptake in the lung, which can become a highly metabolic tissue in the adult respiratory distress syndrome (ARDS) accompanying pneumonia. This has been clearly demonstrated in dogs with pneumonia[140] and in humans. Smithies et al found up to 80 mL of $\dot{V}O_2$ difference between the direct airway measurement and the indirect Fick method in patients with ARDS.[141] The clinical implication is that, as directly measured $\dot{V}O_2$ is the sum of pulmonary and systemic oxygen uptake, in ARDS or pneumonia the contribution of the lung may produce uncertainty as to the real value of systemic oxygen uptake.

The hallmark of life-threatening pathologic supply dependency in sepsis and ARDS is an inability to increase the ERO_2 when $\dot{D}O_2$ decreases. This established belief was confirmed by Gutierrez and Pohill, who found that it was associated with a 70 percent mortality as opposed to 30 percent in those with a normal response.[142] Bihari et al also demonstrated the poor outcome in a group of patients who were critically ill with ARDS.[143] Those who were supply dependent died when $\dot{D}O_2$ was increased with prostacyclin. The suggestion by this group of investigators was that because the patients were not having these cellular oxygen needs met, they were going into a progressive oxygen debt. Confirmatory support for this idea comes from the observation that when the cardiac output is boosted by fluid loading, patients with elevated lactate levels decrease their serum lactate concentrations as $\dot{V}O_2$ increases.[91]

Cain has pointed out that most of the evidence points to two kinds of supply dependency.[144] The normal physiologic variety occurs when $\dot{D}O_2$ is below the critical point. $\dot{V}O_2$ is linearly related to $\dot{D}O_2$ and can be extrapolated back to approximately zero. At the critical point, further oxygen delivery leads to a progressively decreasing ERO_2. The pathologic variety is generally associated with a high resting metabolic rate, ARDS, and sepsis. The patient does not appear to be able to mobilize any microcirculatory reserve to increase extraction, and extraction remains low over a wide range of $\dot{D}O_2$.

Taylor et al have listed the factors that could cause loss of capillaries capable of being perfused in ARDS.[15] They include platelet and complement activation, thromboxane, oxygen radicals, lymphocyte damage, microembolization by leukocytes, and macroembolization by clotting and edema. Metabolic changes, which could compromise autoregulation, include adenosine, epinephrine, alpha-adrenergic stimulation, temperature, mitochondrial damage, and acidemia.

Clinically, there are few treatment measures that seem to be successful in reversing an established pathologic supply dependency. This may be because the precise mechanisms that bring it about and the reasons that the condition has such a high mortality have not yet been elucidated. The best outcome appears to be resuscitation by increasing $\dot{D}O_2$ until the $\dot{V}O_2$ is well above normal resting levels.[3,5]

Hemodilution

Hemodilution is becoming an accepted technique of intraoperative patient care in order to reduce the use of blood products while at the same time possibly improving tissue oxygenation. Before the beginning of the operation, patients are bled into bypass pumps, bags, or reservoirs, and the plasma volume is expanded with a variety of crystalloid or colloid solutions to maintain the blood volume at least at normal levels. When the patients require more oxygen-carrying capacity, their own blood is returned. The effects of isovolemic hemodilution on oxygen delivery are not as simple as might be expected.

The flow of blood through the microcirculation is governed by the Hagen-Poiseuille relationship:

$$Flow = \frac{Radius^4 \times \Delta P \times \pi}{Viscosity \times Length \times 8} \qquad (6)$$

At a Hct of 45 percent, approximately half the viscosity is due to erythrocytes. If the Hct is reduced to 20 percent, the viscosity is about halved,[145] so a decrease in Hct should greatly enhance flow. Furthermore, since blood is a non-Newtonian fluid, as flow increases, viscosity becomes relatively even lower because shearing forces reduce the ability of the various components to adhere to each other. Rouleaux formation is much less, and the greater ease with which red blood cells are deformed facilitates their passage through the capillary circulation. These factors should make hemodilution very attractive as a method of increasing blood flow, except for the reduction in oxygen content. The maximum oxygen carriage for the least cardiac work is in the 40 to 45 percent Hct range.[70] On the other hand, the maximum red blood cell flux for a given driving force is in the 27 to 33 percent Hct range, depending on the diluent used for isovolemic hemodilution. The initial response to isovolemic hemodilution is an increase in cardiac output, initially by stroke volume, due both to an increased venous return and to increased cardiac emptying secondary to the loss of peripheral resistance.[146] Blood distribution continues to be maintained to most organs in approximately the same fraction as prior to hemodilution, except that the coronary circulation appears to be increased to a greater extent. This fits in well with the observation by Cain who showed that when the Hct was reduced to below 27 percent in lightly anesthetized, paralyzed dogs, $\dot{V}O_2$ began to rise.[65] This could only be accounted for by an increase in myocardial $\dot{V}O_2$ due to the work of pumping more blood.

Another compensation to hemodilution has been demonstrated from the classic work of Fåhraeus and Lundqvist,[147,148] who showed that the Hct and the viscosity of blood in capillary tubes was reduced. Erythrocytes tend to flow in the center of a blood vessel, where velocities are higher. The resulting plasma margination is most marked in smaller tubes, where the ratio of plasma to erythrocytes is, therefore, greater. As the viscosity of blood decreases, the speed with which the erythrocyte passes through the microcirculation becomes much greater than that of plasma. The hematocrit in the microcirculation, therefore, tends to fall proportionately less than that of the peripheral blood when the red blood cell mass is reduced.

As the hematocrit is progressively decreased to 20 percent, a hyperdynamic picture begins to appear. The capillary circulation is less capable of adjusting the red blood cell distribution, which becomes more uniform. Cain found in his anemic dogs that there was a paradoxic rise in the $P\bar{v}O_2$, even to normal levels, by the time the critical point was reached.[65] There are two probable explanations for this. Using a mathematical model, Gutierrez suggested that the transit time of the erythrocyte in the microcirculation had so decreased that there would be insufficient time for equilibration with the plasma PO_2, which would take place in the larger vessels.[149] Another theory is that the loss of control of red blood cell distribution in anemia results in the production of physiologic shunts.

Hemodilution may give rise to postoperative advantages in patients with peripheral vascular disease, such as wound healing,[150] and improved morbidity from ischemic and other complications.[151] Maximum oxygen-carrying capacity for a given arterial blood pressure probably occurs at a Hct of 33 percent, but is still above normal down to 27 percent.[152,153] Messmer suggested that hemodilution should be considered for anyone undergoing elective surgery in whom a blood loss of 1 to 2 L is anticipated. The patient should not be anemic (Hb $\geq$ 12 g/dL) nor have coronary heart disease with ischemic electrocardiographic changes, uncontrolled hypertension, hepatic or renal failure, restrictive or obstructive pulmonary disease, or coagulopathies. Age per se does not seem to be a cause for exclusion. Klövekorn et al have stated that active ischemic heart disease and poor ventricular function are clear contraindications.[154]

MONITORING

The complexity and quantity of monitoring for patients to assess the adequacy of systemic oxygen transport during thoracic surgery are often determined by local custom and considerations such as the skill of the surgeon or the experience of the anesthesiologist. It is, therefore, necessary to analyze what should be useful by examining the effects of failure of the various components.

The monitoring of inspired oxygen (F_IO_2) and pulse oximetry is fairly standard for patients undergoing thoracic surgery. Although there are no precise data as to the minimum safe level of SaO_2, most manufacturers set their default levels at 90 percent. The combination of F_IO_2 and SaO_2 should enable the anesthesiologist to set an anesthetic gas mixture and recognize acute airway problems such as accidental endobronchial intubation.

Prough and Johnston,[155] in their analysis of monitoring, agree that the monitoring of $\dot{V}O_2$ is the most physiologically reasonable, as this is a goal-oriented end point. The problem is the obviously invasive nature of the method and the considerable work involved to make frequent measurements. An oxygen debt is the product of inadequate $\dot{V}O_2$ and time.[156] In the critically ill surgical patient, the considerable

work has been shown to pay off with reduced mortality and morbidity,[5] when it is worthwhile to monitor the blood gases and cardiac output at short intervals.

When the delivery system begins to fail, there is a reduction in renal, splanchnic, and cutaneous blood flow. Pulse oximetry not only can give continuous quantitative SaO_2 information, but the pulse wave itself is a qualitative index of cutaneous blood flow. In too-light anesthesia, cutaneous blood flow is also reduced by sympathetic tone, but, in the fully anesthetized patient, a loss of wave height is very likely due to hypovolemia. Cutaneous blood flow has also been monitored by temperature[103] and transcutaneous oxygen tensions.[104,105] Urine output is the easiest guide for renal blood flow. More recently, a lack of splanchnic blood flow has been inferred from "intracellular acidosis" of the gastric mucosa.[157] The intramucosal pH (pH_i) is calculated from the plasma bicarbonate (HCO_3^-) of an arterial blood sample and the steady-state "adjusted" carbon dioxide tension ($PCO_{2(SS)}$) of a saline solution tonometered in an intragastric balloon. The Henderson-Hasselbalch equation is used:

$$pH_1 = 6.1 + \log_{10}\left(\frac{[HCO_3^-]}{PCO_{2(SS)} \times 0.03}\right) \qquad (7)$$

A pH_i of less than 7.25 is an indication of reduced perfusion.

The continuous monitoring of $S\bar{v}O_2$ with a fiberoptic pulmonary artery catheter has been found to best reflect cardiac output and oxygen delivery in the anesthetized patient.[158] A fall in $S\bar{v}O_2$ is usually associated with a significant change in cardiac output. Reinhart, on the other hand, was unable to find a clinically useful correlation in the operating room or intensive care unit.[159] He did find that the $S\bar{v}O_2$ and central venous oxygen saturation ($ScvO_2$) correlated very closely except in the most hypoxic patients, which has made way for a cheaper and almost as effective monitoring catheter. $S\bar{v}O_2$ monitoring has not become highly accepted, partly because of the extra expense needed to obtain data that may not be easy to interpret.

In the majority of patients, oxygen transport is closely related to cardiac output, which seems to remain one of the best indices to monitor in the high-risk patient. No significant change in any cardiorespiratory or renal parameter can be fully interpreted without it. This is the major reason why there is such a search for a reliable noninvasive method.

Various biochemical methods have been used to monitor oxygenation, such as intramuscular or surface electrodes, subcutaneous tonometers, noninvasive near-infrared measurement of the reduction of cytochrome aa_3 in the brain, and phosphorus magnetic resonance spectrography. So far, none of these methods has been accepted for routine use in the critical surgical patient. Lactic acidemia can be caused by hypoxia, but in most institutions is too long a procedure for real-time monitoring. The measurements of arterial and mixed venous blood gases are easily performed, and even when oxygen levels are normal, the development of an acidosis may indicate poor tissue perfusion.

CONCLUSIONS

The traditional "vital signs" of pulse, blood pressure, and respiration give very little information as to the adequacy of systemic oxygen transport. The clinical determination of adequacy is made difficult, as it is often a function of the microcirculation. When autoregulation and the reflex distribution of oxygen (blood) are diminished by chemical mediators from damaged tissues, microembolic phenomena, anesthetic agents, and other drugs, increased flow is needed to maintain oxygenation. It is, therefore, easy to be unaware that an oxygen debt is developing in a critically ill patient, because the components of the delivery system (convection) seem to be intact.

The most successful method of avoiding postoperative organ failure from ischemic and hypoxic damage in the American Society of Anesthesiologists class III and IV or otherwise compromised patient would seem to be to maintain $\dot{D}O_2$ at a level that can fulfill the needs of supply-dependent tissues.[4,5] A Hct of 30 to 33 percent (except in the patient with apparent myocardial ischemia), a blood volume slightly in excess of normal ($\approx$ 110 percent), and a cardiac output to 150 percent above the resting normal value (scaled down appropriately for the anesthesia) seem to be suitable goals. The monitoring of $\dot{V}O_2$ is needed to be sure that the expected metabolic needs are likely to be met. Increasing the inspired oxygen tension to improve oxygenation seems to be of limited value once the PaO_2 is above 200 mmHg (27 kPa) except in extreme anemia. The development of acidemia should always give rise to the suspicion of poor perfusion.

REFERENCES

1. Chang N, Goodson WH III, Gotrup F, Hunt TK: Direct measurement of wound and tissue oxygen tension in postoperative patients. Ann Surg 179:470, 1983
2. Knighton DR, Halliday B, Hunt TK: Oxygen as an antibiotic: the effect of inspired oxygen on infection. Arch Surg 119:199, 1984
3. Bland RD, Shoemaker WC, Abraham E, Cobo JC: Hemodynamic and oxygen transport patterns in surviving and non-surviving postoperative patients. Crit Care Med 13:85, 1985
4. Shoemaker WC, Appel PL, Kram HB: Tissue oxygen debt as a determinant of lethal and nonlethal postoperative organ failure. Crit Care Med 16:1117, 1988
5. Shoemaker WC, Appel PL, Kram HB: Prospective trial of supranormal values of survivors as therapeutic goals in high-risk surgical patients. Chest 94:1176, 1988
6. Charlson ME, MacKenzie CR, Gold JP, et al: The preoperative and intraoperative hemodynamic predictors of postoperative myocardial infarction or ischemia in patients undergoing noncardiac surgery. Ann Surg 210:637, 1989
7. Tinker JH, Dull DL, Caplan RA, et al: Role of monitoring devices in the prevention of anesthetic mishaps: a closed claims analysis. Anesthesiology 71:541, 1989
8. Wasserman K: Coupling of external to internal respiration. Am Rev Respir Dis, Suppl. 129:21, 1984
9. Barcroft J: On anoxaemia. Lancet 2:485, 1920
10. Barcroft J: Physiological effects of insufficient oxygen supply. Nature 106:125, 1920
11. Nunn JF, Freeman J: Problems of oxygenation and oxygen transport during haemorrhage. Anaesthesia 19:206, 1964
12. Editorial: The therapeutic use of oxygen. Lancet 2:365, 1920
13. Valtis DJ, Kennedy AC: Defective gas transport function of stored red blood cells. Lancet 1:119, 1954
14. Peters JP, Van Slyke DD: Quantitative Clinical Chemistry. Williams & Wilkins, Baltimore, 1931–1932
15. Taylor AE, Hernandez L, Perry M, et al: Overview of tissue oxygen utilization. p. 13. In Bryan-Brown CW, Ayres SM (eds): New Horizons II. Oxygen Transport and Utilization. Society of Critical Care Medicine, Fullerton, CA, 1987
16. Gutierrez G, Marini C, Acero A, Holyan A: O_2 transport and high-energy phosphate utilization during *E. coli* endotoxemia. Am Rev Respir Dis 139:A445, 1989
17. Hochachka PW, Guppy M: Metabolic Arrest and the Control of Biological Time. pp. 10–35. Harvard 1987
18. Bryan-Brown CW: Blood flow to all organs: parameters for function and survival in critical illness. Crit Care Med 16:170, 1988
19. Heistad DD, Abboud FM: Circulatory adjustments to hypoxia. Circulation 61:463, 1980
20. Laver MB: The Arthurian legend. Anesthesiology 40:523, 1974
21. Krogh A: The supply of oxygen to the tissues and the regulation of the capillary circulation. J Physiol 52:457, 1919
22. Tyml K: Capillary recruitment and heterogeneity of microvascular flow in skeletal muscle before and after contraction. Microvasc Res 32:84, 1986
23. Hills BA: Intermittent flow in tendocapillary bundles. J Appl Physiol 9:277, 1979
24. Folkow B, Sonnenschein RR, Wright DL: Loci of neurogenic and metabolic effects on precapillary vessels of skeletal muscle. Acta Physiol Scand 81:459, 1971
25. Gaehtgens P: Microcirculatory control of tissue oxygentation. p. 44 In Reinhart K, Eyrich K: Clinical Aspects of O_2 Transport and Tissue Oxygenation. Springer-Verlag, Berlin, 1989

26. Lipowsky HH, Zweifach BW: Network analysis of the microcirculation of the cat mesentery. Microvasc Res 7:73, 1974

27. Becker LC: Conditions for vasodilator-induced coronary artery steal in experimental myocardial ischemia. Circulation 57:1103, 1978

28. Nunn JF: p. 260. Applied Respiratory Physiology. 3rd Ed. Butterworth, Boston, 1987

29. Gregory IC: The oxygen and carbon monoxide capacities of foetal and adult blood. J Physiol 236:625, 1974

30. Marshall BE, Wyche MQ, Jr.: Hypoxemia during and after anesthesia. Anesthesiology 37:178, 1972

31. Nunn JF: 3rd Ed. p. 270. Applied Respiratory Physiology. Butterworth, Boston, 1987

32. West JB, Hackett PH, Maret KH, et al: Pulmonary gas exchange on the summit of Mt Everest. J Appl Physiol Respir Environ Exerc Physiol 54:678, 1983

33. Siesjö BK, Jóhannsson H, Ljunggren B, et al: Brain dysfunction in cerebral hypoxia and ischemia. p. 65. In Plum F (ed): Brain Dysfunction in Metabolic Disorders. Raven Press, New York. 1974

34. Laurenzi GA, Vin S, Guarneri JJ: Adverse effect of oxygen on tracheal mucus flow. N Engl J Med 279:333, 1968

35. Clark JM, Lambertsen CJ: Pulmonary oxygen toxicity: a review. Pharmacol Rev 23:37, 1971

36. Monaco V, Burdge R, Newell J, et al: Pulmonary venous admixture in injured patients. J Trauma 12:15, 1972

37. Hunt TK, Goodson WH: Uncomplicated anemia does not influence wound healing. p. 42. In Tuma RF, White JV, Messmer K (eds): The Role of Hemodilution in Optimal Patient Care. Zuckschwerdt, München, 1989

38. Lambertsen CJ: Physiological effects of oxygen inhalation at high partial pressures. p. 12. In Lambertsen CJ (ed): Fundamentals of Hyperbaric Medicine. Publication No. 1298. National Academy of Sciences, National Research Council, Washington, DC 1966

39. Plewes JL, Fahri LE: Peripheral circulatory response to acute hyperoxia. Undersea Biomed Res 10:123, 1983

40. Carlsson C, Eintrei C, Odman S, Lund N: Effects of increases in the inspired oxygen fraction on brain surface oxygen pressure fields and regional cerebral blood flow. Acta Anaesth Scand, Suppl. 80, 29:86, 1985

41. Bert P: Barometric Pressure. p. 709. Paris, 1878. Hitchcock MA, Hitchcock FA (translators). Undersea Medical Society, Bethesda, MD, 1978

42. Boerema I, Meyne NG, Brummelkamp WK, et al: Life without blood. J Cardiovasc Surg 1:133, 1960

43. Davis JC (ed): Hyperbaric Oxygen Therapy: A Committee Report. UMS Publication No. 30 CR (HBO). Undersea Medical Society, Bethesda, MD, 1983

44. Ayres SM, Gianelli S, Meuller H: Care of the Critically Ill. 2nd ed. Appleton-Century-Crofts, New York, 1974

45. Bohr C, Hasselbalch K, Krogh A: Ueber einen in biologischer Beiziehung wichtigen Einfluss, den die Kohlensäurespannung des Blutes auf dessen Sauerstoffbindung übt. Scand Arch Physiol 16:402, 1904

46. Bellingham AJ, Detter JC, Lenfant C: Regulatory mechanisms of hemoglobin oxygen affinity in acidosis and alkalosis. J Clin Invest 50:700, 1972

47. Severinghaus JW: Blood gas calculator. J Appl Physiol 21:1108, 1966

48. Perutz MF: Stereochemistry of cooperative effects in haemoglobin. Nature 228:726, 1970

49. Perutz MF: Regulation of oxygen affinity for hemoglobin: influence of the structure of the globin on the heme. Ann Rev Biochem 48:327, 1979

50. Perutz MF: Mechanisms regulating the reactions of human hemoglobin with oxygen and carbon monoxide. In Reinhart K, Eyrich K (eds): Clinical Aspects of O_2 Transport and Tissue Oxygenation. Springer-Verlag, Berlin, 1989

51. Roughton FJW, Darling RC: The effect of carbon monoxide on the oxyhemoglobin dissociation curve. Am J Physiol 141:17, 1944

52. Bryan-Brown CW: Oxygen transport and the oxyhemoglobin dissociation curve. p. 161. In Berk JL, Sampliner JE (eds): Handbook of Critical Care. 3rd Ed. Little, Brown, Boston, 1990

53. Valeri CR, Bryan-Brown CW, Altschule MD (eds): Function of Red Blood Cells. Crit Care Med 7:357, 1979

54. Klocke RA: Oxygen transfer from the red cell to the mitochondrion. p. 239. In Bryan-Brown CW, Ayres SM (eds): New Horizons II. Oxygen Transport and Utilization. Society of Critical Care Medicine, Fullerton, CA, 1987

55. Comroe JH: p. 183. Physiology of Respiration. 2nd Ed. Year Book Medical Publishers, Chicago, 1974

56. Miculicz P: Beilage zum Centrablatt für Chirugie (1890). Cited in Da Costa JC, Kalteyer FS: The changes induced by ether as an anaesthetic. Ann Surg 34:329, 1901

57. Rawstron RE: Preoperative haemoglobin levels. Anaesth Intensive Care 4:175, 1976

58. Carson JL, Poses RM, Spence RK, Bonavita C: Severity of anaemia and operative mortality and morbidity. Lancet 1:727, 1988

59. Messmer K: Acute preoperative hemodilution: physiological basis and clinical applications. p. 54. In Tuma RF, White JV, Messmer K (eds): The Role of Hemodilution in Optic Patient Care. Zucksehwerdt, München, 1989

60. Messmer K: Compensatory mechanisms for acute dilutional anemia. Bibl Haematol 47:31, 1981

61. Nearman HS, Eckhauser ML: Postoperative management of a severly anaemic Jehovah's Witness. Crit Care Med 11:142, 1983

62. Harris TJB, Parikh, Rao YK, Oliver RPH: Exsanguination in a Jehovah's Witness. Anaesthesia 38:989, 1983

63. Litchtenstein A, Eckhart WF, Swanson KJ, et al: Unplanned introperative and postoperative hemodilution: oxygen transport and consumption during severe anemia. Anesthesiology 69:119, 1988

64. Zederfeldt B: Studies on wound healing and trauma. Acta Chir Scan Suppl 224:1, 1957

65. Cain SM: Oxygen delivery and uptake in dogs during anemia and hypoxia. J Appl Physiol 42:228, 1977

66. Borgström L, Johansson H, Siesjö BK: The influence of acute normovolemic anemia on cerebral blood flow and

oxygen consumption of anesthetized rats. Acta Physiol Scand 93:505, 1975

67. Wilson RF, Walt AF: Blood replacement. p. 136. In Walt AF, Wilson RF (eds): Management of Trauma: Pitfalls and Practices. Lea & Febiger, Philadelphia, 1975

68. Czer LSC, Shoemaker WC: Optimal hematocrit value in critically ill postoperative patients. Surg Gynecol Obstet 147:363, 1978

69. Asmundsson T, Kilburn KH: Survival of acute respiratory failure: a study of 239 episodes. Ann Intern Med 70:471, 1969

70. Richardson TQ, Guyton AC: Effects of polycythemia and anemia on cardiac output and other circulatory factors. Am J Physiol 197:1167, 1959

71. Pearson TC, Weatherly-Mein G: Vascular occlusive episodes and venous haematocrit in primary proliferative polycythaemia. Lancet 2:873, 1978

72. Woodson RD: Hemoglobin concentration and exercise capacity. Am Rev Respir Dis 129:S72, 1970

73. Hurtado A: Animals in high altitudes: resident man. Section 4, p. 843. In Dill SB (ed): Handbook of Physiology, Adaptation to Environment. American Physiological Society, Washington, DC, 1964

74. Murphy JR, Wengard M, Brereton W: Rheologic studies of HbSS blood. Clin Med 87:475, 1976

75. Anderson R, Cassell M, Mullinax GL, et al: Effect of normal cells on viscosity of sickle-cell blood. Arch Intern Med 111:286, 1963

76. Jan K, Usami S, Smith JA: Effects of transfusion on rheologic properties of blood in sickle cell anemia. Transfusion 22:17, 1982

77. Schmalzer E, Chien S, Brown AK: Transfusion therapy in sickle cell disease. Am J Pediatr Hematol Oncol 4:395, 1982

78. Murphy SB: Difficulties in sickle cell states. p. 476. In Orkin FK, Cooperman LH (eds): Complications in Anesthesiology. JB Lippincott, Philadelphia, 1983

79. Biron PE, Howard J, Altschule MD, et al: Chronic deficits in red cell mass in patients with orthopaedic injuries (stress anemia). J Bone Joint Surg 54-A:1001, 1972

80. Baek SM, Makabali G, Bryan-Brown CW, et al: Plasma expansion in surgical patients with high central venous pressure. Surgery 78:394, 1975

81. Shippy CR, Appel PL, Shoemaker WC: Reliability of clinical monitoring to assess blood volume in critically ill patients. Crit Care Med 12:107, 1984

82. Shoemaker WC, Appel P, Czer LSC, et al: Pathogenesis of respiratory failures (ARDS) after hemorrhage and trauma: I. Cardiorespiratory patterns preceding the development of ARDS. Crit Care Med 8:504, 1980

83. Hopkins JA, Shoemaker WC, Chang PC, et al: Clinical trial of an emergency resuscitation algorithm. Crit Care Med 11:86, 1983

84. Shoemaker WC, Appel PL, Kram HB: The role of oxygen transport patterns in the pathophysiology, prediction of outcome, and therapy of shock. p. 65. In Bryan-Brown CW, Ayres SM (eds): New Horizons II. Oxygen Transport and Utilization. Society of Critical Care Medicine, Fullerton, CA, 1987

85. Wiggers CJ, Werle JM: Cardiac and peripheral resistance factors as determinants of circulatory failure in hemorrhagic shock. Am J Physiol 136:421, 1942

86. Chien S: Role of the sympathetic nervous system in hemorrhage. Physiol Rev 47:214, 1967

87. Rowell LB: Human Circulation: Regulation During Physical Stress. p. 137. Oxford University Press, New York, 1986

88. Hinshaw DB, Peterson M, Huse WM, et al: Regional blood flow in hemorrhage shock. Am J Surg 102:224, 1961

89. Price HL, Deutsch S, Marshall BE, et al: Hemodynamic and metabolic effects of hemorrhage in man with particular reference to the splanchnic circulation. Circ Res 18:469, 1966

90. Elwyn DH, Bryan-Brown CW, Shoemaker WC: Nutritional aspects of body water dislocations in postoperative and depleted patients. Ann Surg 182:76, 1975

91. Haupt MT, Gilbert EM, Carlson RW: Fluid loading increases oxygen consumption in septic patients with lactic acidosis. Am Rev Respir Dis 131:912, 1985

92. Rowell LS, Betry JMR, Blackmon JR, et al: Importance of the splanchnic vascular bed in human blood pressure regulation. J Appl Physiol 32:213, 1972

93. Johnson JM, Rowell LB, Niederberg M, et al: Human splanchnic and forearm vasoconstrictor responses to reduction of right atrial and aortic pressure. Circ Res 34:515, 1974

94. Bond RF: A review of skin and muscle hemodynamics during hypotension and shock. Adv Shock Res 8:53, 1982

95. Rowell LB, Johnson JM: Role of the splanchnic circulation in reflex control of the cardiovascular system. p. 153. In Shepard AP, Granger DN (eds): Physiology of the Intestinal Circulation. Raven Press, New York, 1984

96. Bearn AG, Billing B, Edholm OG, et al: Hepatic blood flow and carbohydrate changes in man during fainting. J Physiol 115:442, 1951

97. Glaser EM, McPherson DR, Prior KM, et al: Radiological investigation of the effects of haemorrhage on the lungs, liver and spleen with special reference to the storage of blood in man. Clin Sci 13:461, 1954

98. Kessler M, Höper J, Harrison DK, et al: Tissue O_2 supply under normal and pathological conditions. Adv Exp Med Biol 169:69, 1984

99. Gelman S, Fowler KC, Smith LR: Liver circulation and function during isoflurane and halothane anesthesia. Anesthesiology 61:726, 1984

100. Andreen M, Irestedt L: Effects of enflurane on splanchnic circulation. Acta Anaesthesiol Scand Suppl. 71:48, 1979

101. Spath JA, Jr, Gorcaysk RI, Lefer AM: Pancreatic perfusion in the pathophysiology of hemorrhagic shock. Am J Physiol 226:443, 1974

102. Parillo JE: The cardiovascular response to human septic shock. p. 285. In Fuhrman BP, Shoemaker WC (eds): Critical Care: State of the Art. Vol. 10. Society of Critical Care Medicine, Fullerton, CA, 1989

103. Joly H, Weil MH: Temperature of the great toe as an indication of the severity of shock. Circulation 39:131, 1969

104. Tremper KK, Shoemaker WC: Transcutaneous oxygen monitoring of critically ill adults with and without low flow shock. Crit Care Med 9:706, 1981

105. Barker SJ, Tremper KK. Transcutaneous oxygen tension: a physiological variable for monitoring oxygenation. J Clin Monit 2:130, 1985

106. Brenner BM, Zatz R, Ichikawa I: The renal circulation. p. 93. In Brenner BM, Rector FC, Jr (eds): The Kidney. WB Saunders, Philadelphia, 1986

107. Hou SH, Bushinsky DA, Wish JB, et al: Hospital acquired renal insufficiency: a prospective study. Am J Med 74:243, 1983

108. Valeri CR, Zaroulis CG, Fontier NL: Peripheral red cells as a functional biopsy to determine tissue oxygen tension. p. 650. In Roth M, Astrup P (eds): Alfred Benzon Symposium IV. Academic Press, San Diego, 1972

109. Landis EM, Hortenstine JC: The functional significance of venous blood pressure. Physiol Rev 30:1, 1950

110. Weil MH, Shubin H, Rosoff L: Fluid repletion in circulatory shock. Central venous pressure and other practical guides. JAMA 192:668, 1965

111. Bland RD, Shoemaker WC: Probability of survival as a prognostic and severity of illness score in critically ill surgical patients. Crit Care Med 13:91, 1985

112. Shibutani K, Komatsu T, Kubal K, et al: Critical level of oxygen delivery in anesthetized man. Crit Care Med 11:640, 1983

113. Rothe CF: Physiology of the venous return. Arch Intern Med 146:977, 1986

114. Lassen NA: Cerebral blood flow and oxygen consumption in man. Physiol Rev 39:183, 1959

115. Heistad DD, Kontos HA: Cerebral circulation. p. 137. In Shepard JT, Abboud FM (eds): Handbook of Physiology. The Cardiovascular System, Peripheral Circulation and Organ Blood Flow. Section 2, Vol. 3, Part 1. American Physiological Society, Bethesda, MD, 1983

116. Kontos HA, Wei EP, Navari RM, et al: Responses of cerebral arteries and arterioles to acute hypotension and hypertension. Am J Physiol 234:H371, 1978

117. Kontos HA: Regulation of the cerebral microcirculation in hypoxia and ischemia. p. 311. In Bryan-Brown CW, Ayres SM (eds): New Horizons II. Oxygen Transport and Utilization. Society of Critical Care Medicine, Fullerton, CA, 1987

118. Kety SS, Hafkenschiel JH, Jeffers WA, et al: The blood flow, vascular resistance and oxygen consumption of the brain in essential hypertension. J Clin Invest 27:511, 1948

119. Hoffman WE, Miletich DJ, Albrecht RF: The influence of antihypertensive therapy on cerebral autoregulation in aged hypertensive rats. Stroke 13:701, 1982

120. Miletich DJ, Iankovich AD, Albrecht RF, et al: Absence of autoregulation of cerebral blood flow during halothane and enflurane anesthesia. Anesth Analg 55:100, 1976

121. Todd MM, Drummond JC: A comparison of the cerebrovascular and metabolic effects of halothane and isoflurane in the cat. Anesthesiology 60:276, 1984

122. Jobes DR, Kennell E, Bitner R, et al: Effects of morphine-nitrous oxide anesthesia on cerebral vasodilation. Anesthesiology 42:30, 1975

123. Feigl EO: Coronary physiology. Physiol Rev 63:1, 1983

124. Duvelleroy MA, Mehmel HC, Laver MB: The hemoglobin-oxygen equilibrium and coronary blood flow: an analog model. J Appl Physiol 35:480, 1973

125. Hall JE: Regulation of renal hemodynamics. p. 242. In Guyton AC, Hall JE (eds): Cardiovascular Physiology IV: International Review of Physiology. Vol. 26. University Park Press, Baltimore, 1982

126. Stanton-Hicks M, Hock A, Stumeier KD, et al: Venoconstrictor agents mobilize blood from different sources and increase intrathoracic filling during epidural anesthesia in supine humans. Anesthesiology 66:317, 1987

127. Leithe ME, Margorien RD, Hermiller JB, et al: Relationship between central hemodynamics and regional blood flow in normal subjects and in patients with congestive heart failure. Circulation 69:57, 1984

128. Leier CV: Regional blood flow responses to vasodilators and inotropes in congestive heart failure. Am J Cardiol 62:86E, 1988

129. Mueller HS: Catecholamine support of the critically ill cardiac patient: inotropic agents versus vasopressors: alpha- or beta-adrenergic agonists or both? Intensive Crit Care Digest 5:36, 1986

130. Chiariello M, Gold HK, Leinback RC, et al: Comparison between the effects of nitroprusside and nitroglycerin on ischemic injury due to acute myocardial infarction. Circulation 54:766, 1976

131. Endrich B, Franke N, Peter K, Messmer K: Induced hypotension: action of sodium nitroprusside and nitroglycerin on the microcirculation. Anesthesiology 66:605, 1987

132. Kyff JV, Vaughn S, Yang SC, et al: Continuous monitoring of mixed venous saturation in patients with acute myocardial infarction. Chest 95:607, 1989

133. Peirce EC II: Extracorporeal membrane oxygenation for acute respiratory insufficiency: current status. p. 143. In Bregman D (ed): Mechanical Support of the Failing Heart and Lungs. Appleton-Century-Crofts, New York, 1977

134. Powers SR, Mannal R, Neclerio M, et al: Physiologic consequences of positive end-expiratory pressure (PEEP) ventilation. Ann Surg 178:265, 1973

135. Danek SJ, Lynch JP, Weg JG, et al: The dependence of oxygen uptake on oxygen delivery in the adult respiratory distress syndrome. Am Rev Respir Dis 122:387, 1980

136. Monsenifar A, Goldbach P, Tashkin DP, et al: Relationship between O_2 delivery and O_2 consumption in the adult respiratory distress syndrome. Chest 84:267, 1983

137. Snyder JV, Powner DJ: Effects of mechanical ventilation on the measurement of cardiac output by thermodilution. Crit Care Med 16:1117, 1983

138. Pepe PE, Culver BH: Independently measured oxygen consumption during reduction of oxygen delivery by positive end-expiratory pressure. Am Rev Respir Dis 132:788, 1985

139. Weissman C: Measuring of oxygen uptake in the clinical setting. p. 25. In Bryan-Brown CW, Ayres SM (eds): New Horizons II. Oxygen Transplant and Utilization. Society of Critical Care Medicine, Fullerton, CA, 1987

140. Light RB: Intrapulmonary oxygen consumption in ex-

perimental pneumococcal pneumonia. J Appl Physiol 64:2490, 1988

141. Smithies MN, Royston B, Makita K, et al: Measuring oxygen consumption in the ITU. Proceedings of Annual Meeting of Intensive Care Society, 1989

142. Gutierrez G, Pohill RJ: Oxygen consumption is linearly related to O_2 supply in critically ill patients. J Crit Care 1:45, 1986

143. Bihari D, Smithies MN, Gunson A, Tinker J: The effects of vasodilation with prostacyclin on oxygen delivery and uptake in critically ill patients. N Engl J Med 317:397, 1987

144. Cain SM: Supply dependency of oxygen uptake. p. 80. In Reinhart K, Eyrich K (eds): Clinical Aspects of O_2 Transport and Tissue Oxygenation. Springer-Verlag, Berlin, 1989

145. Tuma RF: Physiological principles related to volume expansion and hemodilution. p. 11. In Tuma RF, White JV, Messmer K (eds): The Role of Hemodilution in Optimal Patient Care. Zuckschwerdt, München, 1989

146. Sunder-Plassmann L, Klöverkorn WP, Messmer K: Präoperative Hämodilution: Grundlagen, Adaptationmechanismen und Grenzen klinischer Anwendung. Anaesthesist 25:124, 1976

147. Fåhraeus R: The suspension stability of blood. Physiol Rev 9:214, 1929

148. Fåhraeus R, Lundqvist T: The viscosity of blood in narrow capillary tubes. Am J Physiol 96:562, 1931

149. Gutierrez G: The rate of oxygen release and its effect on capillary O2 tension: a mathematical analysis. Respir Physiol 63:79, 1986

150. Bailey MJ, Johnston CLW, Yates CJP, et al: Preoperative haemoglobin as predictor of outcome of diabetic amputations. Lancet 2:168, 1979

151. Shah DM, Prichard MN, Newell JC, et al: Increased cardiac output and oxygen transport after intraoperative isovolemic hemodilution: a study in patients with peripheral vascular disease. Arch Surg 115:597, 1980

152. Laks H, Pilon RN, Klöverkorn WP, et al: Acute hemodilution: its effects on hemodynamics and oxygen transport in anesthetized man. Ann Surg 180:103, 1974

153. Martin E, Hansen E, Peter K: Acute limited normovolemic hemodilution: a method for avoiding homologous blood transfusion. World J Surg 11:53, 1987

154. Klövekorn WP, Richter J, Ott E, et al: Hemodilution in coronary bypass operations. Biblioteca Haematologica 47:297, 1981

155. Prough DS, Johnston WE: Fluid resuscitation in septic shock: no solution yet. Anesth Analg 69:699, 1989

156. Crowell A, Smith EE: Oxygen deficit and irreversible hemorrhagic shock. Am J Physiol 206:313, 1964

157. Fiddain-Green RG, Baker S: Predictive value of the stomach wall pH for complications after cardiac surgery: comparison with other monitoring. Crit Care Med 15:153, 1987

158. Waller JL, Kaplan JA, Baumann DI, Carver JM: Clinical evaluation of a new fiberoptic catheter during surgery. Anesth Analg 61:676, 1982

159. Reinhart K: Monitoring O_2 transport and tissue oxygenation in the critically ill patient. p. 195. In Reinhart K, Eyrich K (eds): Clinical Aspects of O_2 Transport and Tissue Oxygenation. Springer-Verlag, Berlin, 1989

160. Bryan-Brown CW: Physiology of respiration. In Miller TA, Rowlands BJ (eds): Physiologic Basis of Modern Surgical Care. CV Mosby, St. Louis, 1988

161. Bryan-Brown CW: Gas transport and delivery. In Shoemaker WC, Thompson WL (eds): Critical Care: State of the Art. Vol. 1. Society of Critical Care Medicine, Fullerton, CA, 1980

SUGGESTED READINGS

Bryan-Brown CW, Ayres SM (eds): New Horizons II. Oxygen Transport and Utilization. Society of Critical Care Medicine, Fullerton, CA, 1987

Nunn JF: Applied Respiratory Physiology. 3rd Ed. Butterworth, Boston, 1987

Reinhart K, Eyrich K (eds): Clinical Aspects of O_2 Transport and Tissue Oxygenation. Springer-Verlag, Berlin 1989

Snyder JV, Pinsky MR (eds): Oxygen Transport in the Critically Ill. Year Book Medical Publishers, Chicago, 1987

Tuma RF, White JV, Messmer K (eds): The Role of Hemodilution in Optimal Patient Care. Zuckschwerdt, München, 1989

Appendix 6-1.
ABBREVIATIONS AND DEFINITIONS

	Definition	Unit
O₂ Metabolism		
PaO_2 ($P\bar{v}O_2$)	Arterial (mixed venous) O_2 tension	mmHg (kPa)
SaO_2	Arterial O_2 saturation	percent
$S\bar{v}O_2$	Mixed venous O_2 saturation	
$ScvO_2$	Central venous O_2 saturation	
CaO_2 ($C\bar{v}O_2$)	Arterial (mixed venous) O_2 content $= (Hb \times SaO_2/100 \times 1.34) + (PaO_2 \times 0.003)$	mL/dL
$C(a - \bar{v})O_2$	Arteriovenous O_2 content difference	mL/dL
$\dot{Q}$	Cardiac output or flow	L/min
$\dot{Q}I$	Cardiac index	L/min · m²
$\dot{D}O_2$ ($\dot{T}O_2$)	O_2 delivery (transport) $= \dot{Q} \times CaO_2$	mL/min
$\dot{V}O_2$	O_2 utilization or uptake $= \dot{Q} \times C(a - \bar{v})O_2$	mL/min
$CMRO_2$	Cerebral $\dot{V}O_2$	mL/100 g/min
$M\dot{V}O_2$	Myocardial $\dot{V}O_2$	mL/min
ERO_2	Extraction ratio or utilization coefficient $= C(a - \bar{v})O_2/CaO_2$ or $\dot{V}O_2/\dot{D}O_2$	
P_{50}	PO_2 when $SO_2 = 50\%$ (pH = 7.4, $PCO_2 = 40$ mmHg, T = 37°C)	mmHg
P_{50iv}	PO_2 when $SO_2 = 50\%$ (ambient conditions of pH, PCO_2, and T)	mmHg
RQ	Respiratory quotient $= \dot{V}O_2/\dot{V}CO_2$	
$\dot{Q}_B$	Organ blood flow	mL/min
$\dot{Q}_B/\dot{V}O_2$	Utilization ratio	
kPa	kilopascal (SI unit)	7.5 mmHg
Circulation		
CBF	Cerebral blood flow	mL/100 g/min
CVP	Central venous pressure	mmHg
PAOP	Pulmonary artery occlusion ("wedge") pressure	mmHg
$\dot{Q}$	Cardiac output	L/min

Appendix 6-2.
TERMINOLOGY

Affinity hypoxia	Hypoxia resulting from increased oxyhemoglobin affinity (P_{50} ↓).
Critical point	The minimum oxygen delivery ($\dot{D}O_2$) that will maintain oxygen uptake ($\dot{V}O_2$).
Down regulation	The loss of sensitivity of a receptor following prolonged stimulation (particularly noted in alpha$_1$-adrenergic receptors).
Extraction ratio	Ratio of oxygen used to oxygen delivered: $ERO_2 = (CaO_2 - C\bar{v}O_2)/CaO_2$ or $\dot{V}O_2/\dot{D}O_2$.
Oxygen conformity	Metabolism is regulated by the availability of oxygen.
External respiration	Activity of respiratory and cardiovascular systems exchanging O_2 and CO_2 between the air and tissues (the transport component).
Internal respiration	O_2 utilization and CO_2 production in tissues (the metabolic component).
Respiratory quotient	Ratio of oxygen uptake to carbon dioxide output. Some nomenclatures use *RQ* for wholebody and *R* for individual tissue or reaction exchange.
Supply dependency	Condition in a tissue or organism when $\dot{V}O_2$ is limited by $\dot{D}O_2$.
Utilization ratio	Blood flow per unit of oxygen used: $\dot{Q}_B/\dot{V}O_2$.

7

RESPIRATORY PHYSIOLOGY DURING ANESTHESIA

Thomas J. Gal, M.D.

Respiratory function in the anesthetized state is characterized by an impairment of pulmonary gas exchange. To identify the mechanisms by which general anesthesia and the drugs that produce it may impair gas exchange, an understanding of respiratory physiology is essential. This chapter focuses on two principal areas of respiratory function that are significantly affected during anesthesia: the mechanical behavior of the respiratory system and the chemical regulation of respiration.

RESPIRATORY MECHANICS

Any understanding of respiratory physiology must begin with a consideration of respiratory mechanics. This area of physiology deals with the respiratory system's role as an air pump. It involves analysis of the forces responsible for the physical transport of air into and out of the gas exchange portion of the system, ie, the lung. These forces act against other elements that oppose the airflow.

Respiratory Muscles: The Force Generators

Air moves in and out of the lungs as the thoracic cavity expands and decreases in size. This volume change is accomplished by the contraction of the respiratory muscles. Functionally, they are skeletal muscles whose prime task is to rhythmically displace the chest wall. There are three major muscle groups responsible for ventilation: the diaphragm, the intercostal muscles, and the accessory muscles. Although the functions of these muscles will be considered individually, it is important to remember that they actually work together in a coordinated fashion.

The diaphragm is a dome-shaped muscle that separates the thoracic cavity from the abdomen. The muscle is somewhat unique in that its fibers radiate from a central tendon to insert peripherally on the anterolateral aspects of the upper lumbar vertebrae (crural portion) and on the xiphoid and upper margins of the lower ribs (costal portion). The motor innervation originates from the phrenic nerve that is formed by the combination of cervical roots three, four, and five. Contraction of the diaphragm causes its dome to descend, thereby expanding the chest longitudinally. The attachments to costal margins also cause the lower ribs to rise and the chest to widen. This action of the diaphragm is responsible for approximately two-thirds of quiet resting ventilation. The normal excursion of the diaphragm during such quiet breathing is approximately 1.5 cm. As the dome descends to expand the thorax, abdominal contents are displaced caudally. Thus, the fall in pleural pressure and the accompanying lung expansion produce an increase in abdominal pressure and some protrusion of the abdominal wall.

The intercostal muscles are composed of two sheet-like layers that run between the ribs and receive their innervation from nerves that exit from the spinal cord at levels from the first to eleventh thoracic segments. The external intercostals and the parasternal portion of the internal intercostals produce an inspiratory action. Their contraction elevates the upper ribs to increase the anteroposterior dimensions of the chest (pump-handle motion). The lower ribs are also raised to increase the transverse diameter of the thorax (bucket-handle motion). Although these actions of the intercostals do not play a major role in normal resting ventilation, they are important in maintaining high levels of ventilation, such as are required during exercise.

The accessory muscles contribute to inspiration by elevating and stabilizing the rib cage. The principal accessory muscles are the scalenes and sternocleidomastoids. The scalenes originate from the transverse processes of the lower five cervical vertebrae and receive innervation from the same spinal segments. The muscles slope caudally to insert on the first two ribs such that contraction elevates and fixes the rib cage. While this plays only a minor role in quiet breathing, the enlargement of the upper chest is important at high levels of ventilation. The second group of accessory muscles, the sternocleidomastoids, elevates the sternum and increases the longitudinal dimensions of the thorax. They also are only active at high levels of ventilation and assume great importance in disease states associated with severe airway obstruction.

In contrast to the active phase of inspiration, expiration is passive during quiet breathing and occurs because of the elastic recoil of the respiratory system. However, when high levels of ventilation are required, or if air movement is impeded by airway obstruction, expiration must involve active muscle contraction. This is achieved in part by the internal intercostal muscles that depress the ribs, but the major participants in active expiration are the abdominal muscles.

These muscles, which constitute the ventrolateral abdominal wall, are innervated by the lower six thoracic and first lumbar nerves. They consist of the midline rectus abdominus and laterally of the internal and external oblique and transversus abdominus. These muscles act to displace the rib cage by pulling the lower ribs downward and inward. They also pull the abdominal wall inward and thus increase intra-abdominal pressure. This displaces the diaphragm cranially into the thorax with a resultant increase in pleural pressure and decrease in lung volume at end expiration. In addition to their role as powerful muscles of expiration, the abdominal muscles are also important contributors to other respiratory activities, such as forced expiration and coughing, and the non-respiratory functions of defecation and parturition.

All measurements of pulmonary function that require patient effort are influenced by respiratory muscle strength. This can be evaluated specifically by measurements of maximal static respiratory pressures. These pressures are generated in an occluded airway during a maximal forced effort and can be measured with simple aneroid gauges.[1] The inspiratory muscles are at their optimal length near residual volume. Thus, maximal inspiratory pressure (PI_{max}) is usually measured after a forced exhalation. Similarly, maximum expiratory pressure (PE_{max}) is measured at total lung capacity where expiratory muscles are stretched to their optimum length by a full inspiration (Fig. 7-1). Typical values for PI_{max} in healthy young males are approximately -125 cmH$_2$O, while PE_{max} may be as high as $+200$ cmH$_2$O.

Values for PE_{max} less than $+40$ cmH$_2$O suggest impaired coughing ability, whereas PI_{max} values of -25 cmH$_2$O or less indicate severe inability to take a deep breath. The latter value is often used as a criterion for extubation; however, observations in healthy volunteers during partial curarization suggest that this level of ventilatory ability does not ensure adequate airway integrity.[2]

Physiologic Determinants of Lung Volumes

A young adult male of average height would be likely to have a total lung capacity (TLC) of approximately 6.5 L, a residual volume (RV) of 1.5 L, and, thus, a vital capacity (VC) of approximately 5 L. Differences in lung volumes among individuals are largely a function of differences in body size, particularly height. Other determinants of TLC include the strength of the inspiratory muscles and the elastic recoil properties of lung and chest wall. The size of the RV is influenced primarily by expiratory muscle

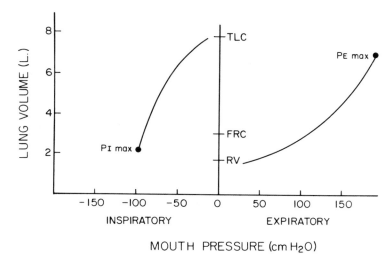

Fig. 7-1. Normal values for maximum static inspiratory (PI_{max}) and expiratory (PE_{max}) pressures measured at the mouth are plotted as a function of lung volume from residual volume (RV) to total lung capacity (TLC). FRC, functional residual capacity. (From Gal,[156] with permission.)

strength and the outward recoil of the chest wall. The limits of expiration may also be affected by dynamic airway closure, particularly with advancing age.

The volume at the end of a spontaneous exhalation during quiet breathing, functional residual capacity (FRC), corresponds to the resting volume of the respiratory system. At this volume, airway pressure is zero, a reflection of the balance between the opposing recoil characteristics of the lung and chest wall.

The respiratory system and its component lung and chest wall are elastic. That is, they tend to regain their original size and configuration following deformation when deforming forces are removed. Both lung and chest wall have positions of equilibrium. These are the volumes that they tend to assume in the absence of external forces acting on them, and the volumes to which they continuously attempt to return when displaced. The equilibrium position of the lung is at or near RV (Fig. 7-2). To sustain any volume in the lung above RV, force must be applied to the lung and the lung will recoil with an equal and opposite force. At all volumes above RV, the lung recoils inward. The equilibrium position of the chest wall is at a relatively large volume, approximately 60 percent of VC (Fig. 7-2). To sustain any volume in the chest wall below this point, the chest wall must be contracted and it will tend to recoil outward, opposite in direction from the lung. To sustain any volume above its equilibrium

point, the chest wall must be actively enlarged by inspiratory muscle contraction. Above this volume, the chest wall recoils inward, in concert with the lung.

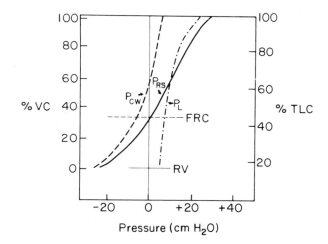

Fig. 7-2. Elastic recoil pressures showing relaxation pressure volume characteristics for the lung (P_L), chest wall (P_{CW}), and total respiratory system (P_{RS}) plotted as a function of lung volume. VC, vital capacity; TLC, total lung capacity; RV, residual volume; FRC, functional residual capacity. (From Gal,[156] with permission.)

In the intact respiratory system, the lung and chest wall are coupled and work together. Behavior of the respiratory system is determined by the individual properties of the lung and chest wall. The equilibrium position of the respiratory system will be at that volume where the tendency of the lung to recoil inward is balanced by the tendency of the chest wall to recoil outward (Fig. 7-2). To sustain any volume in the respiratory system other than this resting volume, a force must be applied to displace both lung and chest wall. The recoil pressure of the respiratory system (P_{RS}) that develops is the algebraic sum of the individual recoil pressure of the lung (P_L) and the chest wall (P_{CW}). Thus, $P_{RS} = P_L + P_{CW}$. The volume at which P_{RS} is zero is termed the *resting* or *relaxation volume* (Vr) of the respiratory system. In normal persons during quiet breathing, the volume of the lung at end expiration (FRC) approximates this Vr. Under certain circumstances, however, FRC may differ from Vr. Static factors, such as respiratory muscle tone, posture, and external forces, may reduce end-expiratory lung volume, while dynamic mechanisms may increase it.

The role of the elastic properties of the lung and chest wall and the relaxation pressure-volume characteristics of the respiratory system were delineated by having subjects relax their respiratory muscles as completely as possible while their airway was occluded at different lung volumes.[3] The pressures measured during these maneuvers reflect the elastic properties of the respiratory system to an extent to which a subject is able to truly relax the respiratory muscles of the rib cage. The extent to which respiratory muscle activity contributes to the relaxation pressures is difficult to assess. However, partial neuromuscular blockade by pancuronium produced a 15 percent decrease in FRC in six awake seated subjects.[4] The pressure-volume curve of the relaxed chest wall was shifted to the right such that its recoil or outward pull was decreased. Since lung recoil did not change, Vr or FRC was decreased. In supine subjects, partial paralysis did not affect FRC.[5] The latter observation suggests that the role of the respiratory muscles of the rib cage is less important in the supine posture.

Postural alterations on the pressure-volume relationships of the respiratory system are largely accounted for by the influence of gravity on the abdomen, which behaves mechanically like a fluid-filled container. In the erect posture, the downward pull of gravity on the abdominal contents exerts an inspiratory action on the lungs by way of the diaphragm. In contrast, the action of the rib cage is more expiratory in nature. In the supine posture, gravity also exerts a small expiratory action of the rib cage by pulling the ribs down and in, but has a marked expiratory action on the diaphragm and abdomen. The pressure-volume curve for the chest wall is thus shifted to the right, ie, it produces less opposition to the inward recoil of the lung. As a result, FRC normally decreases from approximately 50 percent of TLC in the upright position to approximately 40 percent of TLC in the supine position, and even further, to approximately 30 percent of TLC, in Trendelenburg position. Interestingly, these striking changes with posture do not appear to be manifest in patient with pulmonary emphysema. The enlarged volumes for FRC in the latter are relatively unaffected by body position.[6]

The static pressure-volume characteristics of the chest wall can be altered by externally applied forces. Restriction of the chest wall by strapping the rib cage or abdomen produces a marked decrease in FRC, primarily by limiting the tendency of the chest wall to recoil outward.[7] A somewhat similar displacement of the chest wall occurs in the seated subject submerged to the xiphoid or shoulder, much like the patient undergoing shock-wave lithotripsy. Under submerged conditions, there is a decrease in FRC that is dependent on the depth of immersion.[8] Most of the decrease in lung volume reflects the inward displacement of the abdominal contents by the higher hydrostatic pressure. The same hydrostatic pressure acting on the extremities may displace blood from the periphery to the lung and also contributes to the reduction of FRC.

Adult humans and most of the larger terrestrial mammals with relatively stiff chest walls breathe near their Vr, and FRC is approximately equal to Vr or about 50 percent of TLC. The single exception is the horse, which appears to breathe around its Vr with active inspiratory and expiratory phases such that FRC is less than Vr. This respiratory pattern is believed to minimize the high elastic work of breathing, since the latter is lowest when tidal volume is equally divided above and below Vr.[9]

During quiet breathing, ample time exists for emptying of the lungs to occur. If, however, ventilation must be increased (ie, during exercise) or emptying is delayed because of obstruction to flow, the end-expiratory lung volume may be determined by a dynamic rather than static equilibrium. In obstructive lung disease, for example, FRC is commonly increased. Although alteration in resting lung volume (Vr) may result from decreased lung elastic recoil, factors such as expiratory flow limitation may result in initiation of inspiration at an even higher dynamically determined FRC.

The human newborn provides a particularly important example of a dynamically determined end-expiratory lung volume. The chest wall of infants and neonates is highly compliant, ie, its outward recoil is exceedingly small. Although the inward recoil of the lungs is slightly less than in the adults, the lungs are relatively stiff compared with the chest wall. The static balance of elastic forces would predict an FRC at a very low lung volume (< 10 percent of TLC).[10] Since such a low lung volume seems incompatible with airway stability and adequate gas exchange, there is reason to suspect that dynamically determined FRC is substantially above the passive static Vr. Olinsky et al observed that the lung volume during apnea was lower than the usual end-expiratory level in neonates.[11] This suggests that with the usual rapid respiratory rates and relatively long time required for pulmonary emptying, the neonate might not have sufficient time to passively exhale to FRC except during apnea. Such would be the case until the chest wall developed a greater degree of outward recoil and Vr increased. Additional evidence suggests that inspiratory muscle activity and narrowing of the glottis during expiration may contribute somewhat to expiratory "braking" to terminate expiration above Vr.

Forces Involved in Breathing

Production of Airflow

Air flows in and out of the respiratory system because of differences in pressure. Flow occurs from a region of higher pressure to one of lower pressure. Basically, there are two pressure differences in the lung and another across the chest wall that tend to expand or collapse these structures. The force driving airflow is the pressure differential between the airway opening or mouth (P_m) and the pressure in the alveoli (P_{alv}). This is termed the *trans-airway pressure* (Table 7-1). The lung distends and collapses because of a pressure gradient between the alveoli (P_{alv}) and the pleural space (P_{pl}). This difference is termed *transpulmonary pressure* (P_L), ie, the pressure across the lung. The pressure across the chest wall (P_{cw}) can be reflected by the difference between the pleural pressure (P_{pl}) and the atmospheric or body surface pressure (P_{bs}).

TABLE 7-1. Transmural Pressures in the Respiratory System

Component	Symbol	Gradient
Airway	P_{aw}	$P_{alv} - P_m$
Lung	P_L	$P_{alv} - P_{pl}$
Chest wall	P_{cw}	$P_{pl} - P_{bs}$
Lungs and chest wall	Prs	$P_{alv} - P_{bs}$

Abbreviations: P_{alv}, pressure in airspaces (alveoli); P_{bs}, pressure at body surface (atmospheric); P_{pl}, intrapleural pressure (estimated as esophageal pressure); P_m, mouth pressure (airway opening).

Forces Opposing Airflow

Within the respiratory system certain elements oppose airflow and, thus, result in pressure drops. Forces opposing airflow are those resulting from the elastic, flow resistive, and inertial properties of the respiratory system. Thus, they are termed *elastance, resistance*, and *inertance*. Inertance deals with the mass of the lung, the acceleration of these tissues, and the linear acceleration of gas in the lung. It is analogous to inductance in an electrical circuit. Thus, pressure losses due to inertial forces increase progressively as respiratory frequency increases. These pressure losses are quite small and negligible during quiet breathing and in most clinical situations. However, inertance may assume some importance during very rapid breathing, such as in exercise and other physiologic testing. Elastance and its reciprocal, compliance, are reflections of the relationships of pressure to volume when there is no airflow. Hence, such measurements are referred to as static. Resistance, on the other hand, is highly dependent on the rate of change of lung volume, ie, flow. Such measurements during active breathing are referred to as dynamic.

Statics

The lung is a distensible elastic body enclosed in an elastic container, the thoracic cavity. Just as a spring is described by the force required to stretch it to a certain length, so can the respiratory system be described by the static pressure required to change its volume. This relationship between changes in volume and changes in pressure is termed *compliance* (V/P), the reciprocal of elastance. For the various components of the respiratory system, compliance is determined by relating the change in volume to a given pressure difference.

Because the pressure-volume curves for the respiratory system are curvillinear (Fig. 7-2), compliance will vary from one portion of the curve to another, depending on the range of lung volumes. Values, therefore, are usually obtained in the range of 1 L above FRC where the pressure-volume relationships are most linear.

The measurement of P_{pl} can be estimated by a special thin-walled balloon in the midesophagus. The balloon is 10 cm long and is usually filled with 0.5 mL of air.[12] A 127-cm long nasogastric tube incorporating a similar balloon is available commercially and has made the measurement more accessible to the clinician.[13] The pressure across the lung (P_L) is measured by connecting the balloon to one port of a differential pressure transducer while the other port of the transducer senses mouth pressure.

It is important to make the distinction between the terms *static* and *dynamic compliance*. When no gas flow occurs and pressure and volume are kept constant, the measurement is considered to be static compliance. Such would be the case if the patient's lung was inflated by a device, such as a super syringe, and then held. Dynamic compliance, on the other hand, relates pressure and tidal volume at the moment inspiration changes to expiration and flow ceases only momentarily. Ideally, these two compliance measurements are similar. However, if flow is impeded for some reason, as with bronchoconstriction or a kink in the endotracheal tube, dynamic compliance is influenced by resistance to flow. Therefore, it does not reflect the true static compliance and differs by an amount related to flow resistance at end inspiration. The difference between the peak dynamic pressures and a quasistatic pressure (plateau) can be readily appreciated in circuits using a ventilator equipped with an inspiratory hold or pause, by interrupting flow, or by merely clamping the expiratory tubing (Fig. 7-3). The relationship between delivered volume and plateau pressure during this pause is of-ten referred to as the *quasistatic* or *effective compliance*, while dynamic compliance relates to the relationship between delivered volume and peak dynamic pressure.

Dynamics

Airflow dynamics describes the relationships between pressure and flow in the respiratory system. Resistance, therefore, is computed from pressure differences responsible for flow (Table 7-1) and the simultaneous measurement of airflow ($R = P/\dot{V}$).

Various components of the respiratory system contribute to the total resistance to airflow. These include an elastic component in the chest wall and a nonelastic component termed *pulmonary resistance*. Approximately 40 percent of total respiratory resistance is accounted for by the chest wall. It is important to note that the "chest wall" in physiologic terms includes not only the bony thorax, but also the diaphragm and abdominal contents. Therefore, changes in muscle tone affect measurements of total respiratory system resistance.

The remaining 60 percent of total respiratory resistance is pulmonary resistance that was assumed to be essentially the same as airway resistance and, thus, a reflection of airway caliber. Recent studies in dogs, however, have shown that lung tissue contributes a significant component of pulmonary resistance during constriction[14] or bronchodilation.[15]

An important factor to consider about airway resistance (R_{aw}) is the fact that resistance to airflow is determined by the size of the airways. Airways are largest at high lung volumes and smallest at low volumes, such as residual volume. Passive changes in R_{aw} can occur with changes in lung volume in the absence of bronchodilation or constriction. Since the relationship of R_{aw} to lung volume is not linear (Fig. 7-4), the reciprocal of R_{aw}, conductance (G_{aw}), is related to lung volume in a linear fashion and is used to identify the presence of bronchoconstriction or bronchodilation. Such determinants of R_{aw} and G_{aw} are by convention made at FRC.

The gold standard for measurement of airway resistance is body plethysmography. The technique first described by DuBois et al also provides a measurement of thoracic gas volume (FRC).[16] The large body box is complex, however, and is not practical for use in anesthetized patients. Several other techniques have been utilized instead:

Forced Oscillation. Total respiratory resistance can be measured during quiet breathing by imposing rapid small sine wave oscillations at the mouth and recording the resultant sine wave flows and pressures. Such oscillations are produced by a loudspeaker or valve-

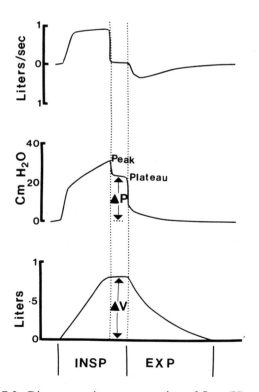

Fig. 7-3. Diagrammatic representation of flow (V), pressure (P), and tidal volume (V_T) typical of a cycle of mechanical ventilation incorporating an inspiratory pause (area enclosed between dotted lines). (From Gal,[157] with permission.)

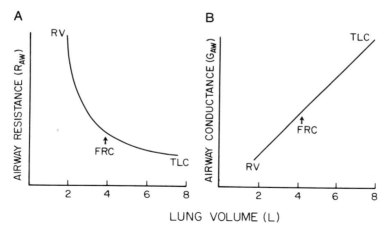

Fig. 7-4. (**A**) The hyperbolic relationship of airway resistance (R_{aw}) to lung volume is contrasted with (**B**) the linear relationship of its reciprocal airway conductance (G_{aw}). RV, residual volume; TLC, total lung capacity; FRC, functional residual capacity. (From Gal,[156] with permission.)

less pump. To measure the pressure change due to resistance, the reactance component (ie, that caused by elastance and inertance) must be eliminated. At high frequencies, the inertial properties dominate and reactance is positive. At low frequencies, reactance is influenced by the capacity of the system (elastance) and is negative. The frequency at which reactance is zero is termed the *resonant frequency* of the respiratory system (usually 3 to 8 Hz). At this frequency, elastance and inertance are 180° out of phase (ie, equal magnitude and opposite sign) and cancel out. The oscillating pressure wave is then caused by resistance alone. One of the major advantages of this technique is that it requires very little patient cooperation. However, to be a true reflection of changes in airway caliber, lung volume changes must be taken into account.

Flow-Pressure-Volume Method. Simultaneous recordings of the three variables, flow, pressure, and tidal volume, provide the basis for this analysis. The changes in pressure (ΔP) and flow ($\Delta \dot{V}$) between two points where volume is identical (V_{iso}) are used to calculate resistance. This method of analysis is termed the *isovolume technique.*

Passive Exhalation Method. The lungs fill and empty in an exponential fashion, ie, the rate of change in the variable (lung volume) is proportional to the magnitude of the variable. Such a system can be characterized by a turnover time or time constant, usually designated by the greek letter tau (τ). The latter is the time at which volume would decrease to zero if it continued to decrease at the initial rapid rate. During

one time constant, volume decreases to approximately 37 percent of its initial value of 1/e, where e = 2.71828, the base of the natural logarithm. In the respiratory system, τ is equal to the product of resistance and compliance:

$$\tau_{(s)} = R\ (cmH_2O \cdot L^{-1} \cdot s) \times C\ (L \cdot cmH_2O^{-1})$$

In this method, compliance is determined by inflation of the lung to a volume of 1.0 L and by relating this volume (1.0 L) to a pressure measured prior to exhalation. If the time interval to exhale to 370 mL (Fig. 7-5) is then measured and divided by this compli-

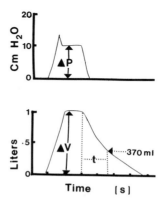

Fig. 7-5. Illustration of the passive exhalation method for estimating resistance. Compliance (C) is calculated as V/P prior to exhalation. *t*, Time constant (τ) required to exhale to 37 percent of preexpiratory volume (ie, 370 mL). Resistance (R) is calculated from the equation, R × C = *t*. (From Gal,[157] with permission.)

ance value, a calculation of total respiratory system resistance can be made.

ANESTHETIC TECHNIQUES AND THEIR EFFECT ON RESPIRATORY MECHANICS

Regional Anesthesia

Most clinicians consider regional anesthetic techniques (spinal, epidural, intercostal block) to be essentially free of clinically significant effects on respiratory mechanics. This opinion, in part, is based on the fact that there is no loss of consciousness or airway instrumentation with such techniques. It also relates to the fact that the mechanics of quiet respiration, such as tidal volume and respiratory rate, are not appreciably affected. Indeed, mid or high thoracic levels of motor block have little, if any, impact on resting ventilation, since the diaphragm is unaffected. Thus, the diaphragm is better able to descend because the abdominal wall, which is relaxed, offers less resistance. In effect, there is an increased abdominal compliance. Nevertheless, this same paralysis of abdominal muscles affects forced exhalation. For example, Egbert et al noted a 50 percent decrease in the pressure subjects could generate during a forced exhalation after a high spinal block, whereas the ability to generate a negative inspiratory pressure was virtually unimpaired.[17] As a result, inspiratory capacity was preserved while expiratory reserve volume decreased. A similar pattern was observed with the motor block associated with epidural anesthesia.[18] Likewise, a milder degree of motor blockade with intercostal block (T_6 to T_{12}) produced mild decrements in expiratory effort and flow with no effects on inspiratory function.[19]

The limitation of expiratory effort may adversely affect patients with chronic bronchitis, whose ability to generate sufficient pressure for an effective cough may be compromised. This same group of patients with chronic lung disease has demonstrated somewhat confusing changes in pulmonary ventilation after spinal anesthesia in the extreme lithotomy position.[20] Unlike normal individuals who demonstrate reductions in forced vital capacity (FVC) under the same circumstances, these patients did not experience worsening, and some showed mild improvement. This has been ascribed to an elevation of the diaphragm at end expiration that is assisted by the weight of the abdominal viscera and flexion of the thighs. Similar improvements have been noted with the "emphysema belt" and head down or leaning forward positions.[21,22] The same effect on the abdominal

viscera may adversely affect inspiratory capacity in obese patients under spinal anesthesia.[23]

General Anesthesia

General anesthesia affects the static (pressure-volume) and dynamic (pressure-flow) behavior of the respiratory system. These mechanical effects have interested clinicians and investigators because of their potential contribution to the impaired gas exchange found in anesthetized patients. Perhaps no facet of respiratory system behavior has received as much attention as the change in FRC. A decrease in FRC with induction of general anesthesia was first noted by Bergman.[24] Subsequent observations in supine anesthetized humans indicated that FRC was reduced an average of about 500 mL or 15 to 20 percent of the awake value.[25] The decreased volume is similar in magnitude to that observed when subjects go from the erect to recumbent position, as noted earlier. The magnitude of FRC reduction appears to be related to age and body habitus (ie, weight to height ratio). In fact, morbidly obese patients demonstrate a much larger decrease in FRC to approximately 50 percent of their preanesthetic values.[26]

The changes in FRC occur within 1 minute of induction of anesthesia,[27] do not appear to progress with time,[28] and are not further affected by the addition of muscle paralysis.[29] A number of factors may contribute to the FRC reduction, but the underlying mechanisms are complex and as yet not totally clear. Some of these possible causes include atelectasis, increased expiratory muscle activity, trapping of gas in distal airways, cephalad displacement of the diaphragm, decreased outward chest wall recoil, increased lung recoil, and increases in thoracic blood volume.

Atelectasis may contribute to or result from the reduction in FRC. The rapid appearance of densities on computed tomography (CT) supports this possibility.[30] The prompt development of the densities and their lack of dependence on high inspired oxygen concentrations suggest that they may be caused by compression of gas rather than resorption, as initially suggested by Dery et al.[31]

Trapping of gas behind closed distal airways does not appear to contribute to the decreased FRC because measurements of thoracic gas volume have demonstrated the FRC changes.[32] Furthermore, measurement of nitrogen washout, which measures only gas in contact with the open airways, gave similar results to those that measured total thoracic gas volume by body plethysmography.[29]

During both rapid eye movement sleep and halothane anesthesia, the tonic activity of the diaphragm decreases. Muller et al postulated that this reduced diaphragmatic tone was responsible for the FRC reduction with anesthesia.[33] The intercostal muscles appear to be even more sensitive to depression by volatile agents such as halothane.[34] This would make it attractive to hypothesize that the reduced tone of diaphragm and intercostals results in a reduced outward recoil of the chest wall. This process does not appear to progress further, since addition of neuromuscular blockade, which would be expected to diminish muscle tone further, produces no additional changes in FRC. The absence of any additional effect with paralysis also argues against any role of increased tone of the expiratory (abdominal) muscles in determining the end-expiratory lung volume.

Although the changes in FRC could reflect increased elastic recoil of the lungs, most researchers favor the hypothesis that the initial effect is a reduction of outward recoil of the chest wall. The changes in the lung are probably secondary to breathing at low lung volumes, since changes similar to those induced by anesthesia have been demonstrated with chest strapping.[35]

Another possible mechanism contributing to the reduction of FRC may involve a shift of blood from the limbs to the lung and abdomen. The blood in the lungs may have a twofold effect. First, lung congestion may decrease lung compliance and, thus, increase lung recoil. Second, the blood competes with air for intrathoracic volume. At the same time, an increase in abdominal blood volume can act to displace the diaphragm upward or the abdominal wall outward. A report by Hedenstierna et al suggested that the diaphragm was displaced cranially and that the decrease in thoracic volume at FRC was associated with a shift of blood from the thorax to the abdomen.[36] Others noted that changes in volume of the rib cage, shape and position of the diaphragm, and intrathoracic fluid (blood) and gas contributed in varying amounts to reducing FRC in different subjects.[37] In the latter study, thoracic gas volume was reduced considerably more than total thoracic volume. This suggest that there is some increase in thoracic blood volume with induction of anesthesia.

Reduction in FRC with intravenous agents differs from the more dramatic effect of inhalation anesthetics. Thiopental[27] and methohexital[38] produced changes in nonintubated subjects that were similar to those associated with normal sleep.[39] In most cases, the decrement in FRC was less than 200 mL. The relatively small magnitude of change was attributed to maintenance of rib cage activity in contrast to the marked depression seen with agents such as halothane.[34] Another intravenous agent, ketamine, also appears to have a sparing action on intercostal muscle activity and is associated with a maintenance of FRC

at awake levels in adults[40] and children.[41] In the latter group, the increased respiratory rates and prolonged passive lung emptying, as illustrated by the time constant (τ), were associated with an FRC greater than Vr.[42] The investigators speculated that the prolonged τ with ketamine anesthesia was the result of increases in respiratory system compliance (thus τ, the product of $R \times C$, is increased). With halothane, τ is shortened, presumably because respiratory system compliance decreases.

Most changes in the mechanical properties can be ascribed to the smaller size of the respiratory system under anesthesia. The increased lung elastic recoil could reduce FRC, but is most likely the result of the reduction of FRC. The data of Westbrook et al indicate that FRC and compliance are reduced proportionately.[29] This suggests that specific compliances (ie, compliance related to lung volume) in the awake and anesthetized state are rather similar.

In contrast to the pressure-volume characteristics, the pressure-flow characteristics of the respiratory system have received far less attention. Only a few studies have compared measurements of pulmonary resistance (R_L) in the awake and anesthetized states. With only one exception,[43] most researchers have noted increases in resistance following induction of anesthesia and tracheal intubation.[44–47] There are a number of problems interpreting these changes in R_L. One relates to the limitations of estimating pleural pressure from esophageal pressure, while another concerns the measurement of airway pressure at the proximal or mouth end of the tracheal tube and not the trachea beyond the distal end of the tube. In the latter case, transpulmonary pressure, the pressure drop across the lung, may be underestimated, as will be the calculated R_L. Finally, the substitution of a fixed value of tube resistance calculated in vitro must be questioned, since the latter can actually exceed the combined resistance of lungs and tube in situ.[48]

Foremost among the remaining mechanisms that might contribute to changes in pulmonary resistance with induction of general anesthesia are the physical properties of the gas mixture of volatile agent, oxygen, and nitrous oxide that differ from air and oxygen with respect to density and viscosity. Nitrous oxide is more dense than air or oxygen. Thus, resistance to turbulent flow, which is directly related to density, would increase with high concentrations of nitrous oxide in the gas mixture. In contrast, viscosity of a nitrous oxide-oxygen mixture is less than air. Thus, resistance to laminar flow might be expected to decrease. Besides being complex and impossible to predict, it is unlikely that changes in density and viscosity can account for most of the changes in R_L seen with anesthesia.

Of far greater importance is airway caliber, which,

in addition to smooth muscle tone, may be affected by accumulation of secretions, changes in lung elastic recoil, and, most importantly, lung volume. Airway caliber would be expected to be reduced by general anesthesia solely because of the reduced FRC (Fig. 7-4). Even in the absence of changes in bronchomotor tone, resistance would be expected to be passively increased by more than one-third. If the influences of tracheal intubation and airway manipulation and the opposing bronchodilating properties of inhalation anesthetics are factored in, it is no wonder that elucidation of the mechanisms controlling pulmonary resistance in the anesthetized patient has been difficult.[49]

Changes in pulmonary resistance (R_L) usually have been thought to represent changes in airway resistance (R_{aw}) and to reflect little pulmonary tissue resistance (R_{ti}). The latter depends on the pressure-volume hysteresis of lung tissue as lung volume changes. However, R_{ti} has been shown to figure prominently in decreased R_L produced by halothane in canine lungs.[14,15] These findings indicate that it is not appropriate to interpret changes in R_L as solely attributable to R_{aw}.

Muscle Relaxants

The use of muscle relaxants has transformed anesthetic practice by allowing safer levels of anesthesia to be used while providing adequate surgical conditions. Initial reports of curare with cyclopropane anesthesia extolled the drug's freedom from cardiorespiratory effects.[50] However, favorable opinion of the drug was not shared by the majority of anesthesiologists, who commonly encountered postoperative respiratory difficulty in curarized patients. It was uncertain whether respiratory problems arose purely because of peripheral muscle weakness or because of central actions of the drug—as a depressant or analgesic. This was clarified in a study by Smith et al, whose volunteers underwent curarization while awake. These investigators concluded that the drug's effects on respiration were solely attributable to muscle weakness and did not affect the central nervous system.[51] Smith et al made additional observations that suggested a possible effect on proprioception and airway mechanics.

Shortly thereafter, a number of studies appeared aimed at finding drugs that produced marked peripheral muscle paralysis (grip strength) and spared respiratory function (vital capacity). The report of Unna and Pelikan is typical of studies that attempted to find equipotent doses of relaxant drugs that decrease grip strength by 95 percent while minimally affecting vital capacity.[52] It initially appeared that depolarizing

blockers had much less ability to achieve this "respiratory sparing" action. These studies underscored the difficulty establishing equipotent doses. Recent work indicates that vital capacity was spared relative to grip strength during careful infusion of succinylcholine.[53]

Assessments of what constitutes normal ventilation in the face of neuromuscular blockade have been performed repeatedly, since restoration of adequate ventilation is of prime concern in the curarized patient. Of even more concern is the patient's ability to maintain airway integrity and cope with factors that might impede gas exchange and ventilation. A recent report has shown that the presence of adequate ventilation during recovery from neuromuscular blockade does not indicate the capability of maintaining functional integrity of the upper airway.[2] While the restoration of muscle strength is aimed at providing adequate ventilation in postoperative patients, little attention is given to assuring adequate patency of the upper airway. Pavlin et al have shown that airway protection may be inadequate when ventilation per se is deemed adequate by the time-honored criterion of a maximum inspiratory pressure of -25 cmH$_2$O.[2] The ability to swallow or maintain an unobstructed airway was associated with an inspiratory pressure of approximately twice that value. The ability to sustain a head lift for 5 seconds was uniformly associated with the ability to provide adequate airway protection. It is important to note that the performance of the head lift must be accomplished with a closed mouth, since the need to elevate the mandible is highly suspicious of the inability to maintain the airway.[54] The presence of an endotracheal tube must not obscure this observation.

Tracheal Intubation

The presence of an endotracheal (ET) tube may itself alter respiratory function in several ways. First, the ET tube imposes a mechanical burden to breathing since it acts as a fixed inspiratory and expiratory resistor that reduces upper airway caliber. This increased resistance does not appear to be of much significance during quiet breathing,[55] but begins to exert a more marked effect during maneuvers requiring greater degrees of effort.[56] Secondly, the tube bypasses the larynx and partially splints the trachea, each of which are important determinants of airflow resistance and important components of normal coughing. Finally, mechanical irritation of the larynx and trachea elicits reflexes such as coughing and constriction of airways distal to the tube. This further stimulation of the tracheobronchial tree provokes reflex mucus secretion, which tends to offset the role of the tube in promoting tracheal toilet, and may result in additional coughing and bronchoconstriction.[57]

There is little disagreement that an ET tube acts as a fixed inspiratory and expiratory resistor that may represent a burden to the spontaneously breathing patient. However, when the tube is inserted, it does not simply add to a patient's normal total airway resistance but rather substitutes for the resistance of the upper airway, ie, from the mouth to midtrachea. This portion of the respiratory tract in adults has an average volume of approximately 72 mL, whereas the internal volume of a standard 8.0 mm internal diameter tube is 12 to 15 mL.[58] However, a patient's upper airway volume may vary by as much as 50 percent with changes in head position.[58] Therefore, in some situations, the ET tube may substitute a relatively small but predictable upper airway volume and caliber for a highly unpredictable one.

Pressure-flow relationships of the respiratory system tend to be alinear, largely because of the turbulent flow patterns in the upper airway, especially at the glottis. Major changes in upper airway resistance occur throughout the respiratory cycle and are principally the result of changes in glottic cross-sectional area with movements of the vocal cords. The cross-sectional area of the glottis oscillates around a mean value of 66 mm^2 during quiet breathing, whereas pharyngeal size is almost 10 times that.[59] The cross-sectional area of the trachea is more than 150 mm^2, and may be as high as 300 mm^2.

Attempts to quantitate the actual magnitude of the airflow resistance imposed by ET tubes have largely consisted of assessing the resistance of the tube in isolation. This method, which measures the pressure drop across the tube at a constant flow rate, has been criticized because patients do not breathe with constant flow rates. Instead, flow varies in a sinusoidal fashion during inspiraton and expiration. Resistance, which is a function of flow rates, varies likewise. Furthermore, this in vitro measurement of the pressure drop during a constant flow may overestimate the actual resistance of the tube in vivo. The resistance of the tube measured in isolation in many cases actually exceeds the combined resistance of the tube in situ and the remaining respiratory system because of the abrupt change in cross-sectional area between the tube and trachea.[60]

The resistance of a tube depends somewhat on its radius of curvature in situ. In tubes that have a similar diameter and length, the pressure drop associated with a given flow will be greater in tubes with a smaller radius of curvature. Such tubes, because of their larger pressure drop, produce more resistance to breathing.[61] When inserted in a patient, the bend of a nasotracheal tube has a smaller radius of curvature than does the same tube inserted orally. Thus, an oral tracheal tube offers less resistance to breathing. The oral route also allows for insertion of a shorter tube and one of larger internal diameter. The internal diameter is probably the most important variable, since the pressure drop and its resultant resistance to breathing is related inversely to the fourth power of the radius during laminar flow and to an even greater power for turbulent flow.

The data of Sahn et al emphasizing these differences in resistance between various sizes of ET tubes have important clinical implications.[62] With flow rates such as might occur during deep breathing (1 L/s), the resistance of a 7.0-mm tube is approximately twice that of an 8.0-mm tube. On the other hand, a 9.0-mm tube produces only about one-third the airflow resistance of an 8.0-mm tube at the very same flow rates. The presence of an ET tube tends to elicit increased secretions, and its accompanying discomfort may limit the depth of inspiration. It may be speculated that both factors result in reduced lung volumes and increased lung stiffness or recoil. Observations in intubated subjects, however, fail to indicate any significant decreases in TLC or lung recoil.[56]

The resting end-expiratory position of the respiratory system, the FRC, is the volume at which the inward recoil of the lungs is opposed by an equal outward recoil of the chest wall. In infants, FRC appears to be a "dynamic" balance of forces and occurs at a higher volume than the true static FRC because of their high respiratory rates and possibly because of the high expiratory resistance associated with glottic action. The data of Berman et al suggest that the presence of an ET tube in infants significantly reduces FRC and impairs oxygenation as a result of interference with glottic action.[63]

Others have similarly hypothesized that the expiratory flow resistance imposed by normal glottic function is also an important determinant of FRC in adults. By excluding this mechanism, an ET tube could impair the ability of the glottis to decrease expiratory flow and to maintain a normal FRC. The data of Annest et al have been cited as evidence to support this possibility, since their patients exhibited an average FRC decrease of 350 mL while intubated.[64] However, in four of their nine patients, FRC during intubation was virtually identical to that after extubation. On the other hand, in a group of patients with moderate airway obstruction, FRC increased significantly by more than 30 percent following insertion of an ET tube for fiberoptic bronchoscopy.[65] The absolute magnitude of this FRC increase approached 1 L in most patients. Such an observation in bronchitic patients is in keeping with what may be expected when peripheral airway constriction occurs and airway resistance is increased. This tends to dispute the relative importance of the expiratory flow resistance from glottic narrowing in determining the normal adult FRC.

The glottic aperture increases during inspiration and decreases during expiration. The cords move toward the midline during expiration to produce a variable controlled resistance that regulates airflow. This glottic narrowing, however, primarily determines the rate at which the respiratory system returns to its resting volume (FRC), but not the actual volume.[66] Furthermore, this braking of expiratory airflow by vocal cord adduction is reduced during hyperpnea such that the audible grunting characteristic of infants would probably not be heard.[67] Only during full active expiration to residual volume does the glottic aperture narrow significantly and reach a minimal size at or near residual volume.

In keeping with this, normal healthy subjects intubated after topical anesthesia showed no significant change in FRC measurements (Fig. 7-6). This finding argues against any notion that the glottis plays as im-

portant a role in determining the FRC in adults as it may in infants. In only two subjects did the changes in FRC exceed normal variations expected with duplicate measurements. One subject showed a decrease of 17 percent, while FRC increased in another subject by 13 percent. The latter subject continued to show an increased FRC following intubation, a phenomenon that may have resulted from persistent peripheral airway constriction. In any event, while FRC or end-expiratory volume may be influenced by dynamic factors, such as overall airway resistance, it appears that in normal adults FRC is largely determined by the static balance of forces between the lung and chest wall, and is not significantly influenced by the presence of an ET tube.

Although airway constriction is most commonly inferred from spirometric indices obtained during forced expiration, the measurement of airway resistance (R_{aw}) appears to be the most sensitive and direct technique to identify airway obstruction. The upper limit of normal for R_{aw} is considered to be 2.0 cm H_2O/L/s. However, in most healthy, normal subjects it is closer to 1.0 cmH_2O/L/s (Fig. 7-7). In one study, healthy subjects exhibited increases in R_{aw} ranging

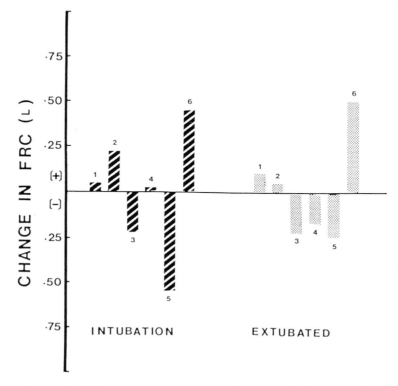

Fig. 7-6. Individual changes in FRC (compared with control) associated with tracheal intubation and extubation in six healthy subjects. (From Gal,[158] with permission.)

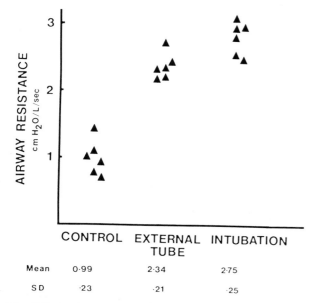

Fig. 7-7. Individual changes in airway resistance in six subjects associated with an endotracheal tube externally and in situ in the trachea. (From Gal,[158] with permission.)

from 1.2 to 1.5 cmH$_2$O/L/s (mean, 1.34 cmH$_2$O/L/s) when breathing through 8.0-mm tubes held externally.[68] With the tubes actually in place in the trachea, R_{aw} increased even more. The mean increase above control was 1.75 cmH$_2$O/L/s, resulting in an actual mean R_{aw} value of 2.75. If the increase in R_{aw} with the external tube is accepted as an estimate of tube resistance (1.35), the resistance of the airways distal to the tube can also be estimated as 2.75 − 1.35 = 1.40. In the intubated subjects, the ET tube bypasses the upper airways to the midtrachea. This segment of the airways accounts for approximately one-third of R_{aw} during mouth breathing, or approximately 0.33 cmH$_2$O/L/s in normal volunteers.[69] The R_{aw} in airways distal to the tube would be approximately 0.67 cmH$_2$O/L/s. Thus, the estimate of 1.40 cmH$_2$O/L/s in the intubated subjects suggest at least a doubling of resistance in airways distal to the tube. The most likely cause of this dramatic increase in resistance is reflex airway constriction resulting from irritation by the ET tube. Furthermore, since such responses occurred in subjects whose airways were substantially anesthetized by topical local anesthetic, it is reasonable to speculate that airway responses would be exaggerated in patients whose trachea were not anesthetized with topical anesthesia or those in whom adequate depths of general anesthesia have not been established.

CHEMICAL REGULATION OF VENTILATION

Although the analysis of the system that controls breathing can be subdivided into chemical and neural elements, clinical appraisal of the neural control system is much more difficult and hazardous. The chemical control system, which is profoundly affected by anesthesia, responds to three basic physiologic stimuli: increases in the partial pressure of CO$_2$, increases in hydrogen ion concentration (decreased blood pH), and decreases in arterial PO$_2$.

Effect of Hypercapnia

Ventilation removes metabolically produced carbon dioxide. If ventilation is reduced, arterial tension (PaCO$_2$) will rise. Similarly, if ventilation is voluntarily or reflexly increased, PaCO$_2$ will decrease. The reciprocal relationship between ventilation and CO$_2$ is described by a rectangular hyperbola. For CO$_2$ excretion (Fig. 7-8), it is apparent from the diagram that a doubling of alveolar ventilation ($\dot{V}_A$) results in halving of CO$_2$ tension, while CO$_2$ tension doubles if ventilation is halved. A normal man has an alveolar ventilation of approximately 4.4 L/min and a resting PaCO$_2$ near 40 mmHg, as shown in Fig. 7-8 as the set-point *A*.

In the same normal individual, inhalation of CO$_2$ increases ventilation, which rises in nearly linear fashion with changes in PaCO$_2$. Stimulation to breathe depends on the hydrogen ion concentration in the extracellular fluid surrounding the central nervous system (CNS) chemoreceptors near the ventral lateral surface of the medulla. The changes in hydrogen ion concentration as a result of inhalation of CO$_2$ depend somewhat on the concentration of bicarbon-

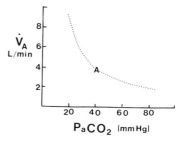

Fig. 7-8. CO$_2$ excretion hyperbola describing the reciprocal relationship between alveolar ventilation ($\dot{V}_A$) and arterial CO$_2$ tension (PaCO$_2$). The curve assumes a constant CO$_2$ production ($\dot{V}CO_2$). Note that most individuals ventilate around set-point *A*, ie, a resting $\dot{V}_A$ of 4.4 L/min and CO$_2$ of 40 mmHg.

ate in the extracellular fluid. Alterations of bicarbonate levels in blood or cerebrospinal fluid (CSF) from metabolic disturbances can, therefore, modify the ventilatory response to CO_2. The central chemoreceptors account for approximately 80 percent of the total increase in ventilation during inhalation of CO_2. The remaining 20 percent increase seems to arise from stimulation of peripheral chemoreceptors in the carotid body.

Effect of Hypoxia

The ventilatory response to decreases in inspired oxygen tension tends to be hyperbolic (Fig. 7-9), such that decreases in oxygen tension exert a greater effect on ventilation when hypoxemia is severe as opposed to mild reductions in oxygen supply. This curvilinear relationship can be conveniently converted to a straight line by plotting ventilation against the reciprocal of arterial oxygen tension ($1/PaO_2$) or, as is more common, against arterial O_2 saturation. The linear relationship with O_2 saturation suggests that ventilation may be primarily influenced by the oxygen content. Most studies, however, point to oxygen tension or partial pressure (PaO_2) rather than O_2 saturation as the stimulus to the peripheral chemoreceptors. This is underscored by the effect of inhaling carbon monoxide, which markedly affects O_2 content, but has little or no effect on ventilation, since PaO_2 is not affected.

The hypoxic ventilatory response is mediated by the peripheral chemoreceptors in the carotid body. In their absence the hypoxic ventilatory drive is lost and hypoxia may exert a depressant action on the central chemoreceptors. The carotid bodies exert only a subtle influence on resting ventilation when PaO_2 is greater than 60 mmHg. Below this, ventilation increases dramatically in hyperbolic fashion while at a PaO_2 of 200 mmHg or more the carotid body discharge diminishes to a minimal level.

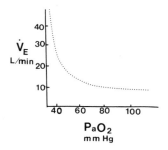

Fig. 7-9. Effects of decreasing arterial oxygen tension (PaO_2) on minute ventilation ($\dot{V}_E$). The hyperbolic plot can be linearized by plotting $\dot{V}_E$ against the reciprocal of PaO_2 or against O_2 saturation.

An important interaction occurs between the two major ventilatory stimulants of hypoxia and hypercapnia. The presence of hypoxia enhances the ventilatory response to CO_2. Similarly, an increase in CO_2 results in a greater sensitivity to hypoxia. These interactive effects require an intact central as well as peripheral chemoreceptor function.

Effect of Metabolic Acidosis

A decrease in arterial pH from metabolic acidosis with normal PaO_2 and $PaCO_2$ primarily stimulates ventilation by the effect of the acidemia on the peripheral chemoreceptors (carotid bodies). This arises from the concept that neither hydrogen nor bicarbonate ions readily cross the blood-brain barrier, and is supported by observations in dogs that carotid body denervation attenuates and delays the response.[70] Biscoe et al demonstrated in cats that a change of 0.20 pH units (7.45 to 7.25) increased carotid body neural output two to three times.[71] This doubling of ventilation is roughly equivalent to that seen when PaO_2 decreases from normal to approximately 40 or 50 mmHg.

In normal volunteers, Knill and Clement noted approximately a doubling of ventilation in normoxic normocarbic volunteers as the hydrogen ion concentration was increased approximately 13 nmol/L (about 0.12 units of pH decrease).[72] This response was attenuated by hyperoxia and enhanced by hypoxia, again attesting to the interacton of these stimuli at the peripheral chemoreceptor.

For the same degree of acidemia or pH change, the addition of CO_2 evokes a larger increment in ventilation than does the addition of fixed acid. The initial response to acute metabolic acidosis is weak, because as $PaCO_2$ decreases from carotid body stimulation, CO_2 tension in the CSF decreases and pH increases. Thus, the strong peripheral stimulation of the hydrogen ion is offset by a central alkalosis and reduced stimulus to the medullary chemoreceptors. Gradually, after several hours, bicarbonate levels decrease and permit CSF pH to decrease back toward its normal value. As a result, central chemoreceptor activity is restored to normal.

Effect of Metabolic Alkalosis

Unlike the relatively consistent compensatory mechanisms in metabolic acidosis, those associated with metabolic alkalosis are rather inconsistent and controversial. The observations indicate that metabolic alkalosis is not a well-defined limited entity, and the differences relate to the manner in which the alkalosis is produced. Respiratory compensation (ie, hypoventilation) is minimal or absent when alkalosis is associated with hypokalemia, as with diuretics. Compensation was greatest when alkalosis was induced by agents that increased buffer base in all body fluid compartments.[73]

Measurement of Ventilatory Responses

Ventilatory control mechanisms can be assessed at rest, but are usually characterized by the response to standard stimuli. These usually consist of induced changes in arterial CO_2 or O_2 tension. The output of the respiratory neurons or the ventilatory drive is usually reflected by increases in minute ventilation in normals. However, factors that increase the mechanical work of breathing may modify the ventilation that results from a given amount of respiratory stimulation in certain disease states. Thus, it is important to assess respiratory muscle strength and evaluate other aspects of respiratory mechanics by spirometry in such patients prior to interpreting ventilatory responsiveness.

Sensitivity to Carbon Dioxide

As alveolar or arterial CO_2 tension increases, the increased ventilation resulting from this acute hypercapnia is linearly related to the CO_2 stimulus. Because hypoxia affects CO_2 sensitivity, the response is usually measured with oxygen-enriched mixtures such that arterial oxygen tension is greater than 150 mmHg. Thus, the central medullary chemoreceptor activity is responsible for the increase in ventilation.

Various techniques have been used to test the chemosensitivity to carbon dioxide. The techniques, which include both steady-state and rebreathing methods, differ solely in the manner in which hypercapnia is produced.

Steady-State Technique

This method relies on measuring the ventilatory response to a steadily maintained CO_2 stimulus. Thus, ventilation and CO_2 levels are measured for 10 to 15 minutes after a gas mixture containing increased CO_2 is breathed. Usually, three such gas mixtures (3, 5, and 7 percent CO_2) are used. Each is breathed for a prolonged period to assure that $PaCO_2$ and hydrogen ion concentration have equilibrated and are similar in the environment of the medullary chemoreceptors. Such equilibration may be difficult to achieve in patients with pulmonary disease. Because of the prolonged equilibration required with the steady-state technique, a response curve generated at two levels of

CO_2 stimulation (dual isohypercapnia) has been used.[74]

Rebreathing

Because of its time-consuming nature, the steady-state method has experienced limited clinical use. Currently, the most widely used clinical technique of CO_2 response testing is the rebreathing method originally described by Read.[75] He demonstrated that the response can be determined rapidly as subjects rebreathe from a small bag or spirometer containing 7 percent CO_2 and 93 percent O_2. The rate at which alveolar and arterial CO_2 tensions rise is largely a function of the volume contained in the rebreathing bag. Usually, this is equivalent to the subject's vital capacity plus 1 L (6 to 7 L). The 7 percent CO_2 approximates mixed venous levels and expedites equilibration of CO_2 among alveolar (end-tidal), arterial, and brain compartments. This initial equilibration is further enhanced by having subjects take two or three vital capacity breaths with the CO_2 mixture prior to rebreathing. Since CO_2 is not eliminated from the system during rebreathing, arterial and alveolar CO_2 are not affected by the level or pattern of ventilation. Rather, they rise approximately 3 to 6 mmHg/min and provide an open physiologic control loop to stimulate ventilation. This open loop is advantageous because, unlike the steady-state method, changes in ventilation do not affect end-tidal or alveolar CO_2 tensions.[76] Furthermore, ventilation can be measured over a rather large range of CO_2 tensions in a brief (5 to 6 minutes) time period.

Sensitivity to Hypoxia

Steady-State Techniques

Much like the responses to CO_2, the ventilatory responses to hypoxia have been evaluated by steady-state and non-steady-state techniques. In the steady-state techniques, gas mixtures containing various concentrations of O_2 are breathed while CO_2 is added to the inspired gas as ventilation increases to hold alveolar CO_2 constant.[77] Ventilation can then be plotted as a function of oxygen tension at that particular CO_2. An alternative approach determines the influence of hypoxia on steady-state CO_2 responses. The hypercapneic inspired mixtures are breathed at high ($PO_2 = 200$ mmHg) and low ($PO_2 = 40$ mmHg) oxygen concentrations. The major difficulty with such steady-state techniques is the prolonged exposure to hypoxia that is required. Thus, their use is largely confined to the experimental laboratory area, and their clinical utility is limited at best.

Non-Steady-State Techniques

Non-steady-state tests involve rapid changes in oxygen in the inspired gas mixture. This takes advantage of the quick equilibration of peripheral chemoreceptors with inspired oxygen tension. The rapid changes in oxygen tension require a rapidly responding O_2 analyzer or an accurate responsive ear oximeter. Progressive hypoxia may be produced by rebreathing a mixture of air and CO_2. Isocapneic conditions are maintained by a soda lime CO_2 absorber.[78] Another method uses progressive addition of nitrogen to the breathing mixture in order to stimulate respiration.[79] The latter procedure is performed over a 20-minute period. To avoid any possible direct depressant effects of hypoxia on the central chemoreceptors, Edelman et al attempted to achieve a briefer exposure.[80] They used several (usually one to five) breaths of nitrogen with no attempt to control CO_2. In a matter of seconds, O_2 saturation decreased and ventilation increased. Hypoxic sensitivity is expressed as the maximal ventilation produced in response to the minimal O_2 saturation after several exposures to inspired N_2 breaths.

Sensitivity to Metabolic Acidosis

The ventilatory response to metabolic acidemia, which is a function of peripheral carotid body stimulation, has received far less attention than the responses to hypoxia and hypercapnia. Such acidosis has been produced by infusion of ammonium chloride and, more recently, by L-arginine hydrochloride.[72] The most important factor to remember with stimulation from metabolic acidosis is the significant interaction of hypoxemia and hypercapnia at the peripheral chemoreceptor. Thus, hypercapnia and hypoxia augment the response while hypocapnia and hyperoxia attenuate the stimulus to ventilation.

Ventilatory Indices of Chemosensitivity

Carbon Dioxide Response

The two basic variables of ventilatory control, ie, resting ventilation and $PaCO_2$, may be highly variable and only slightly affected when the ventilatory control system is significantly altered.[81] Nevertheless, they have been advocated as indices of ventilatory controls[82] largely because the CO_2 stimulus in most CO_2 response studies is not the same as the more relevant metabolic CO_2 stimulus.[83]

Conventional means of expressing CO_2 sensitivity use a plot of the CO_2 load or stimulus on the abscissa and ventilation on the ordinate (Fig. 7-10). The latter values are obtained from actual data points with

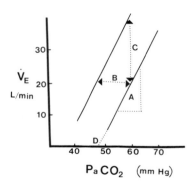

Fig. 7-10. Hypercapneic ventilatory response expressed as increase in minute ventilation ($\dot{V}_E$) as a function of increased arterial CO_2 tension ($PaCO_2$). *A*, Slope of the response; *B*, displacement of the response (ie, a change in the abscissa at a constant ordinate value); *C*, change in ordinate at a constant abscissal value; *D*, apneic threshold.

steady-state techniques, while least squares linear regression determines the plot with rebreathing data. The carbon dioxide stimulus on the abscissa has included inspired CO_2 concentration and the utilization of end-tidal tension. However, $PaCO_2$ may be the most accurate reflection of the CO_2 stimulus, particularly if pulmonary disease is present. The ordinate on the carbon dioxide ventilation plot is provided by respiratory minute volume (V_E). The hyperoxic carbon dioxide sensitivity is expressed as the increment in V_E (L/min) per increment in $PaCO_2$ (mmHg). This can be quantitated by the following equation:

$$\dot{V}_E = S\,(PaCO_2 - B)$$

where S is the slope of the relationship between $V_E/PaCO_2$ and B is the intercept on the x axis. The steeper the slope, the more vigorous the response to CO_2 (Fig. 7-10), which is a measure of the gain of the control system.

In most normal young adults, the slope of the CO_2 response ranged from 1.5 to 5.0 L/min/mmHg CO_2.[84] Much of the interindividual differences in the response related to the tidal volume response during rebreathing. In general, the lowest ventilatory responses occurred in those whose tidal volumes were smallest.[85]

Changes in CO_2 sensitivity can be indicated by slope changes in the response. However, some factors, such as pharmacologic intervention, may alter CO_2 sensitivity without changing slope. In this case, the shift of the CO_2 response can be characterized by the term *displacement* (Fig. 7-10). This is the shift across the x axis in mmHg of CO_2 at a constant ordinate (V_E) value, usually 20 or 30 L/min. Another expression for the shift of the CO_2 response curve uses a change in ordinate ($\dot{V}_E$) at a constant CO_2 value. Often, 60 mmHg is used and is referred to as the "$\dot{V}_E60$." Another interesting term represents an extrapolation of the CO_2 response curve to zero ventilation on the CO_2 axis. This *apneic threshold* represents the CO_2 level at which apnea should occur from hyperventilation. This value is not easily obtainable in awake adults and may not provide any more information than the resting $PaCO_2$.

Hypoxic Response

Ideally, the hypoxic ventilatory response should be expressed as a change in ventilation relative to a change in the stimulus (decreased O_2). However, the curvilinear nature of the relationship renders it complex and not easily characterized by a single index. One early index compared the ratio of the slopes of two CO_2 response curves, one performed in the presence of hypoxia ($PaO_2 = 40$ mmHg) and the other normoxia ($PaO_2 = 150$ mmHg).[86] This ratio has little physiologic meaning and is highly dependent on the hypercapneic response.

Severinghaus et al introduced an index terminated "$\Delta V40$" that was expressed in liters per minutes.[87] This represented the increase in minute ventilation that occurred as oxygen tension was reduced from above 200 mmHg to 40 mmHg with normocapnia. At an oxygen tension of 40 mmHg, the ventilatory response is rather steep (Fig. 7-9). Thus, the potential for error exists in estimating the actual ventilation value, since small decreases in PO_2 are associated with rather large increases in ventilation. The $\Delta V40$ can also be estimated from the two CO_2 response curves, one performed with normoxia and the other at the hypoxic level ($PaO_2 = 40$ mmHg). Ventilations measured at an isocapneic point ($PaCO_2 = 40$ mmHg) can thus be compared.

The ventilatory response to hypoxia can be linearized by plotting the reciprocal of ventilation against PO_2 or, more conveniently, by relating the change in ventilation to arterial oxyhemoglobin saturation (Fig. 7-11). Thus, the hypoxic response can be quantitated as $\Delta V/\%$ desaturation. Although the latter index is the simplest means of quantitating the hypoxic response, a more complex description of the hyperbolic relationship between ventilation (V_E) and oxygen tension (PaO_2) is equally popular. Parameter A is used to characterize the shape of the curve, which is expressed mathematically by the following equation:

$$\dot{V}_E = \dot{V}_0 + \frac{A}{PaO_2 - 32}$$

where $\dot{V}_0$ is the asymptote for ventilation and 32 is the asymptote for PaO_2 at which ventilation is assumed to be infinite. The magnitude for A is related to the briskness of the response.

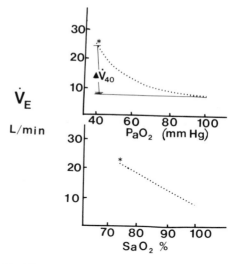

Fig. 7-11. The hyperbolic response to hypoxia can be quantitated as $\Delta V40$, the increase in ventilation ($\dot{V}_E$) at a hypoxic level ($PaO_2 = 40$ mmHg) compared with normoxia. Note the increased $\dot{V}_E$ is linearly related to arterial O_2 saturation (SaO_2 percent). At $PaO_2 = 40$, the blood is roughly 25 percent desaturated ($SaO_2 = 75$ percent). Thus, ventilation at this point and at $PaO_2 = 40$ are nearly identical (*).

In normal subjects, the ventilatory response to hypoxia appears to be more variable than the hypercapneic response. For example, while the mean value for parameter A was 186, the range of values was 69 to 410.[88] In terms of desaturation, hypoxic sensitivity ranged from 0.16 to 1.35 L/min/1% desaturation (mean, 0.6),[89] while $\Delta V40$ values ranged from 5.4 to 64.8 L/min.[90] Certain mathematic interrelationships can be constructed for these three indices. For example, since normal blood undergoes a 25 percent desaturation at a PaO_2 of 40 mmHg, the $\Delta V/1\%$ desaturation and V40 are related by a factor of 25 to 1 such that $\Delta V40/25 = \Delta V/1\%$ desaturation. Also, if $PaO_2 = 40$ mmHg is substituted into the equation containing parameter A, the following relationship results:

$$A = \Delta V40 \times 8$$

Other Indices of Respiratory Center Output

Ventilatory Drive and Timing

Traditional methods for measuring ventilatory drive have used the measurement of minute ventilation to express the effects of stimuli on respiratory system mechanics. Such measurement of the ventilatory response provides a reasonably valid reflection of respiratory drive. Further valuable analysis can be obtained by analyzing the pattern and timing of the response. Indeed, the pattern, which consists of tidal volume (V_T), can result from changes in the duration of inspiration (T_I) or by changes in mean inspiratory flow (V_T/T_I). The total duration of each respiratory cycle (T_{TOT}) is a combination of the duration of inspiration (T_I) as well as expiration (T_E). Since respiratory frequency is essentially equal to $60/T_{TOT}$, it can be altered by changes in T_I, T_E, or both. Each breathing cycle has been characterized as a result of two basic mechanisms, drive and timing.[91] The V_T/T_I reflects the activity of the driving mechanism, whereas T_I/T_{TOT}, the fraction of the total respiratory cycle occupied by inspiration, is an index of timing.

Occlusion Pressure

The negative pressure generated at the mouth during the first 100 ms of inspiration against an occluded airway has gained widespread acceptance as a clinical correlate of central respiratory drive. The occlusion pressure ($P_{0.1}$) reflects respiratory drive in normal subjects and in those with mechanical dysfunction of the respiratory system. Although the measurement has some limitations as a direct index of inspiratory neural drive, it is useful to identify whether ventilatory failure is the result of abnormal respiratory mechanics or an abnormality of respiratory control.[92]

Diaphragmatic Electromyogram

The generation of inspiratory pressure such as the $P_{0.1}$ requires intact innervation of the diaphragm. Thus, diaphragmatic electromyography appears to be a valid indicator of central chemosensitivity. However, reproducible recordings are difficult to obtain with esophageal electrodes because changes in position can often vary the magnitude of response more than ventilatory stimuli. The discomfort associated with the electrodes has also hampered their widespread use. Fortunately, changes in $P_{0.1}$ correlate favorably with this invasive technique.[93]

Control of Breathing in Normal and Disease States

Normal Variations with Age

Alterations in the ventilatory responses to hypoxia and hypercapnia have been demonstrated in many disease states. However, even in the normal population, the wide variations may be attributed to a host of factors that modify the responses. For example, advancing age is associated with a gradual decline of pulmonary function manifested by decreasing vital capacity, maximal flow rates, and arterial oxygen tension. In normal elderly patients (aged 65 to 79 years), the ventilatory responses to both hypoxia and hypercapnia were reduced to approximately half that in normal younger counterparts.[94,95] Since occlusion pressure responses were reduced to the same extent as the ventilatory responses, the differences could not be attributed to mechanical factors, but rather were the result of altered chemosensitivity.[94]

At the other extreme of age, the normal newborn sustains its higher oxygen demands per unit of mass through an increased V_E, decreased resting PCO_2, and a shift in the CO_2 response curve to the left.[96] The slope of the CO_2 response is similar to adults, but appears to be a function of gestational age. For example, slopes in term infants were five times those of preterm (29 to 32 weeks) infants.[97] In the latter group, hypoxia depressed rather than augmented the CO_2 response. The response to hypoxia in newborns is not sustained but rather is biphasic, ie, it increases initially then decreases to an intermediate level slightly above baseline.[98] The hypoxic response in adults is also biphasic, but the time course is different.[99] In infants, ventilation begins to decrease after 2 to 5 minutes of isocapneic hypoxia, whereas in adults the high level of ventilation is sustained for 20 to 25 minutes before decreasing.

Hereditary Aspects of Ventilatory Responses

Numerous observations have suggested that there is a familial influence on the determination of ventilatory drive. Low ventilatory responses to CO_2 and a diminished response to added airway resistance were characteristic of parents whose children succumbed to the sudden infant death syndrome.[100] Normal adult offspring of patients with hypercapnia caused by chronic obstructive pulmonary disease (COPD) had decreased responses to hypoxia and hypercapnia when compared with offspring of patients with similar obstruction but normocapnia.[101] For the most part, heredity appears to influence the hypoxic response more consistently than the hypercapneic response. This is evident in the case of identical twins and endurance athletes.[102] In the latter group of long-distance runners, familial factors appear to play a major role in their decreased hypoxic ventilatory response.

Acclimatization to Altitude

While the reduced hypoxic response appears to benefit the endurance athlete at sea level, at altitude, the relative hypoventilation is detrimental and more likely to be associated with acute mountain sickness.[103] Because of the low ambient O_2 tension at extreme altitude, a brisk ventilatory response is required for adequate arterial oxygenation. Schoene has demonstrated that subjects who best adjust to altitude have brisk responses to hypoxia in contrast to those of distance runners.[104] The response to hypercapnia in these same climbing subjects also tended to be significantly higher than in the runners. Subsequently, he demonstrated that exercise performance on Mt. Everest correlated with the briskness of the ventilatory response to hypoxia.[105]

Chronic Obstructive Pulmonary Disease

Hypercapnia and hypoxemia often develop in patients with COPD as their disease advances. These gas exchange abnormalities have been attributed to mechanical limitations[106] and poor matching of ventilation and perfusion,[107] as well as decreased sensitivity to hypoxia and hypercapnia as ventilatory stimuli. Patients with COPD frequently have blunted ventilatory responses. Interpretation of these responses requires indices other than minute ventilation because of the mechanical limitations imposed by disease. Other indices of respiratory center activity, such as phrenic electromyography[108] and occlusion pressure $(P_{0.1})$,[109] have been used to distinguish the patients who cannot breathe from those who will not breathe.

In patients with airway obstruction, hypercapneic ventilatory responses tend to be decreased compared with normals. In normocapneic patients, the CO_2 responses in terms of electromyographic activity[108] and occlusion pressures[109] appear to be essentially normal. The occlusion pressures $(P_{0.1})$ during quiet room air breathing and at elevated CO_2 levels are increased and suggest heightened respiratory center activity. By comparison, patients with resting hypercapnia demonstrate a reduced slope of the occlusion pressure response as well as the ventilatory response. Although their $P_{0.1}$ at rest is higher than normal individuals, the values with further increases in CO_2 are markedly depressed compared with normal individuals.[109]

Numerous observations in COPD patients have demonstrated that patients with hypercapnia tend to have a shorter duration of inspiration, smaller tidal volumes, and more rapid respiratory rates than their normocapneic counterparts.[110,111] This pattern of breathing tends to increase the dead space to tidal volume ratio. Hence, despite increases in minute ventilation, alveolar ventilation decreases, and CO_2 retention is more likely to develop. For the most part, this CO_2 retention is associated with more hypoxemia than that seen in normocapneic patients. The hypoxemia may in fact be responsible for the characteristic rapid shallow breathing pattern.[112]

In patients who are chronically hypoxemic, the normal augmentation of the hypercapneic ventilatory response by hypoxia is significantly attenuated.[113] This reduced ventilatory response correlates with the degree of airway obstruction and suggests that mechanical limitations are important. However, other investigators have shown that hypoxemic patients have reduced responses to hypoxia both in terms of ventilatory and occlusion pressure $(P_{0.1})$ responses.[114] Ventilatory responses to CO_2 are depressed in the same patients, but $P_{0.1}$ responses are not.

The decreased hypoxic response in hypoxemic patients might be likened to that which develops in high altitude dwellers or which is seen in cyanotic patients with congenital heart defects. On the other hand, it could be postulated that the decreased hypoxic response preceded the onset of lung disease and contributed to the hypoxemia.

The findings of depressed responses to hypoxia in hypoxemic patients, compared with patients without hypoxemia but with similar degrees of chronic airway obstruction, raise the question about the mechanism of CO_2 narcosis as a result of correcting hypoxemia.[114] The deleterious effects of administering oxygen-enriched mixtures to hypoxemic hypercapneic patients have been attributed to removal of the hypoxia ventilatory drive. It could, therefore, be suspected that such patients have a blunted CO_2 response but an intact hypoxic response. This is clearly not the case.[114]

The administration of an oxygen-enriched mixture ($F_IO_2 = 0.4$) to 20 patients with COPD in early stages of acute respiratory failure ($PaO_2 < 40$ mmHg; $PaCO_2 > 60$ mmHg) resulted in a 14 percent decrease in minute ventilation ($\dot{V}_E$) and a 12 percent increase in $PaCO_2$.[115] Although these average changes appear to be proportional, there was no relationship in individual patients between changes in V_E and concomitant changes in $PaCO_2$. These findings, as well as the effects of 100 percent O_2 in another group of similar patients[111] and observations in stable COPD patients,[116] suggest that hypercapnia induced by hyperoxia is not primarily related to altered respiratory drive but rather is the result of further impairment in gas exchange. The increase in alveolar O_2 tension reduces the hypoxic pulmonary vasoconstriction that normally maintains ventilation-perfusion matching. This shift of blood to poorly ventilated areas results in an increased dead space (V_D). The increase in V_D could also be partially related to the Haldane effect, which results in displacement of CO_2 from oxygenated blood and increases the arterial-alveolar CO_2 difference.

EFFECTS OF ANESTHETICS ON RESPIRATORY CONTROL

The vast majority of drugs used in the practice of anesthesiology, including the intravenous and volatile anesthetic agents, have as their principal side effect an alteration of respiratory control. This is manifested as a depressed desire to breathe that assumes great clinical relevance, since these drug effects may seriously impair ventilation in the perioperative period.

Inhalation Anesthetics

Carbon Dioxide Response

Each of the present-day halogenated inhalation agents (halothane, enflurane, and isoflurane) produces profound respiratory depression in a dose-related manner. This respiratory depression is far greater than that associated with older outmoded agents (ether, cyclopropane, or fluroxene). At concentrations that produce loss of consciousness and surgical anesthesia, tidal volume is reduced. Although respiratory rate increases, minute ventilation decreases and an elevation of CO_2 occurs in proportion to the depth of anesthesia as multiples of the minimum alveolar concentration (MAC). The extent of this hypoventilation and CO_2 retention varies with each agent. At 1.0 MAC, halothane produces a modest increase in CO_2 to approximately 45 mmHg. By comparison, the same level of isoflurane increases CO_2 to approximately 50 mmHg, while enflurane produces even more marked hypercapnia to above 60 mmHg.[117] While the effects of surgical stimulation tend to counteract this rise in CO_2, the hypercapnia tends to worsen in patients with COPD in proportion to their degree of airway obstruction.[118] In the face of an added mechanical load, these patients with COPD are unable to achieve adequate gas exchange with the rapid shallow breathing pattern associated with halothane.

The normal increase in ventilation with increasing CO_2 (ie, the slope of the response) is blunted by the inhalation anesthetics in a dose-dependent manner. Whereas sedating halothane doses (0.1 MAC) produce little or no change in the slope of the response, anesthetizing doses (> 1.0 MAC) produce significant decreases in slope. The observations of Tusiewicz et al indicate that much of this ventilatory depression is due to a reduction of rib cage recruitment that occurs at higher levels of ventilation in the awake state.[34] The latter may also help to explain the effects of surgical stimulation, which produce a decrease in resting CO_2 but no change in the slope of the CO_2 response.[119]

Information about the role of mechanical factors in the reduced CO_2 response slope in humans is sketchy. Derenne et al studied a now-obsolete agent, methoxyflurane, and noted that although the slope of the ventilatory response was decreased in the anesthetized state, the occlusion pressure response was minimally changed from the awake state.[120] They suggested that much of the ventilatory depression was due to increased lung-thorax elastance and not reduced neural drive. With enflurane, the role of mechanical factors appears to be less dramatic. Wahba concluded that both drive and timing appeared to be affected.[121] Differences in respiratory timing also appear to account for some of the difference in respiratory depression between halothane and enflurane. The latter is associated with a considerably slower breathing frequency.[122]

The absence of wakefulness with the inhalation anesthetics results in a complete dependence on the chemical regulation of ventilation. Thus, passive hyperventilation that removes the CO_2 stimulus results in apnea. Such apnea is difficult, if not impossible, to elicit in conscious subjects, but easy to achieve during anesthesia. This CO_2 level, which is 5 to 9 mmHg below the normal awake resting value, is referred to as the *apneic threshold*, a term coined by Hanks et al.[123] The apneic threshold can be estimated by linear extrapolation of the CO_2 response curve to zero ventilation (Fig. 7-10).

Hypoxic Response

Traditional views of the peripheral chemoreceptors considered them the body's last defense and resistant to drug depression. Present knowledge, however, recognizes that these structures are profoundly depressed in humans by even sedating levels of anesthesia. The initial studies in dogs by Weiskopf et al demonstrated blunting of the hypoxic response with 1.1 percent halothane.[124] Knill and Gelb noted that the response in humans was even more profound.[125] Similar effects were seen with enflurane[126] and isoflurane.[127] Noteworthy is the relatively profound depression of the response in contrast to the hypercapneic response (Table 7-2). At levels that minimally affect the CO_2 response, the hypoxic response is nearly abolished. This also appears to be true for nitrous oxide, which, at concentrations of 30 to 50 percent, has no effect on the CO_2 response, but depresses the ventilatory response to hypoxia.[128] Furthermore, it has been shown in humans[126] and dogs[125] that the normal synergistic interaction between hypoxia and hypercapnia is eliminated. Rather than acting to increase ventilation, the two stimuli act to depress ventilation in anesthetized subjects.

Like the response to hypoxia, the response to added [H+], metabolic acidemia, is mediated via peripheral chemoreceptors. Knill and Clement have shown that halothane sedation and anesthesia in humans markedly attenuate the response to acidemia and its attendant interaction with hypoxemia.[129] Thus, any patient compensation for these derangements must arise from measures instituted by the physician.

TABLE 7-2. **Ventilatory Response During Sedation and Anesthesia**

	0.1 MAC			1.1 MAC			2.0 MAC		
	H	E	I	H	E	I	H	E	I
CO_2 response slope (% awake)	100	77	130	37	37	33	—	—	17
Hypoxic response ΔV_{45} (% awake)	30	42	45	0	3	3	—	—	—

Abbreviations: MAC, minimum alveolar concentration; H, halothane; E, enflurane; I, isoflurane.
(Data from Knill et al.[125-127])

Intravenous Anesthetics

Barbiturates

Among the various CNS depressants used to achieve sedation, the barbiturates do not appear to have a significant effect on resting ventilation when used in doses that produce sedation or drowsiness. Intramuscular pentobarbital, 2 mg/kg, reduced the ventilatory response to hypoxia in 5 of 10 healthy volunteers for a period of approximately 90 minutes.[130] Sedative doses of thiopental did not significantly affect resting ventilation or the response to isocapneic hypoxia and hyperoxic hypercapnia.[131] However, hypnotic or anesthetic levels of thiopental depressed both hypoxic and hypercapneic responses to nearly the same extent (35 to 45 percent of control). In this respect, the barbiturates differ from inhalation anesthetics, since the latter agents depress hypoxic response far in excess of their effects on hypercapneic responses.

Ketamine

The dissociative anesthetic, ketamine, appears to have minimal depressant actions on respiratory control. Early observations indicated that intravenous doses of 2.2 mg/kg did not affect resting ventilation or the response to CO_2 challenge.[132] In a study of dogs anesthetized with ketamine, the hypercapneic response appeared to be increased, leading to speculation that ketamine may be a respiratory stimulant by virtue of its increased sympathetic nervous system activity.[133] However, another more precisely controlled study in dogs demonstrated that ketamine produced slight but significant depression of both hypoxic and hypercapneic responses.[134] In healthy human volunteers, 3 mg/kg of intravenous ketamine appeared to produce respiratory depression similar to that observed with premedicant doses of morphine (0.2 mg/kg).[135] In children, an intravenous bolus dose of ketamine produced nearly a 40 percent decrease in the CO_2 response slope.[136] This transient response disappeared in 30 minutes while a continuous infusion was maintained. The respiratory depression in the latter steady-state infusion period was similar to that observed in adults, namely, a rightward shift of the CO_2 response curve, but no change in slope.[135] These changes are characteristic of premedicant doses of morphine (Fig. 7-12). With higher morphine doses approaching 0.5 mg/kg, a slope change occurs and begins to resemble the other anesthetics that produce a loss of consciousness.

Lidocaine

The amide local anesthetic lidocaine has been widely used to control dysrhythmias and produce regional anesthesia, and as an adjunct in combination with other general anesthetics. Lidocaine administered as an intravenous bolus, 1.5 mg/kg, causes a transient 50 percent decrease in the slope of the CO_2 ventilatory response.[137] In the same subjects, a lidocaine infusion increased the slope. Serum lidocaine concentrations during the infusion were approximately 3 μg/mL, a level similar to that seen after epidural block and similar to concentrations associated with up to a 28 percent reduction in anesthetic requirement.[138] These same steady-state lidocaine levels also produced depression of the hypoxic ventilatory response manifested by a 20 percent reduction in parameter *A*.[139]

Impairment of Pulmonary Gas Exchange During Anesthesia

Abnormalities of pulmonary gas exchange with general anesthesia have long been recognized. Impaired oxygenation and, to some extent, CO_2 elimination appear to be a reflection of increased $\dot{V}_A/\dot{Q}$ mismatch, right to left intrapulmonary shunting, and an increase in dead space. A number of theories have been proposed to account for these changes. Foremost among them are a reduction in lung volume (FRC) and an alteration in the distribution of ventilation.

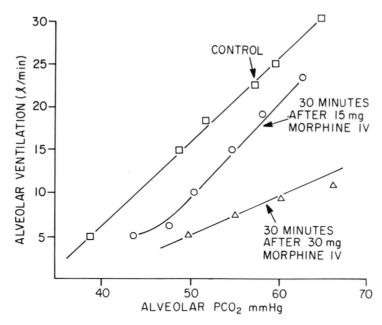

Fig. 7-12. Effects of premedicant doses of morphine (0.15 mg/kg) and larger doses on the ventilatory response to CO_2. (From Bailey and Stanley,[160] with permission.)

Reduction in Functional Residual Capacity

In supine subjects, the induction of general anesthesia reduces FRC such that end-expiratory volume decreases close to residual volume. Thus, FRC may lie below the closing capacity, ie, the volume associated with dependent airway closure or dynamic flow limitation.[140] Early observations with halothane anesthesia suggested a correlation between the degree of impaired oxygenation and the reduction in FRC and led to the hypothesis that airway closure and atelectasis were the consequences of a reduced FRC.[141]

One important aspect of the theory of airway closure lies in the assumption that closing capacity (CC) remains the same in both anesthetized and awake states. The decrease in lung compliance in the anesthetized state reflects an increased elastic recoil. Airway closure is due to a great extent to a decrease in lung elastic recoil. As a result, a decrease in CC might be expected with general anesthesia. Initial reports suggested no difference in CC between awake and anesthetized states.[142,143] Subsequent work, however, provided evidence that both FRC and CC are proportionately reduced with anesthesia.[144] These investigators used the foreign gas bolus technique, as opposed to the resident gas (N_2) technique used in the previous study, and suggested that the latter might not adequately measure CC when lung volumes are restricted. However, an additional study found no difference when the two techniques were compared.[145]

Therefore, the issue of whether awake control CC values are the same as those in anesthetized subjects is not resolved.

The degree of intrapulmonary shunting appears to correlate with the reduction in FRC[146] and with the degree of atelectasis that develops in dependent lung regions.[147] Thus, it is tempting to attribute such atelectasis simply to reduced FRC. A study in awake supine subjects with thoracoabdominal restriction argued against this simple mechanism.[148] The restriction reduced lung volume and altered pulmonary mechanics in a fashion similar to general anesthesia. FRC decreased by more than 20 percent and was matched by a reduction of CC measured by the resident gas (N_2) technique. No atelectasis was noted with CT scanning and $\dot{V}_A/\dot{Q}$ distribution and arterial blood gases were unchanged from the control state. In this respect, the awake subjects differed from the anesthetized subjects with the same decrement in FRC. The researchers concluded that the development of compression atelectasis in anesthetized patients cannot be ascribed solely to a decrease in FRC, nor can the changes in pulmonary mechanics with restriction be attributed solely to the development of atelectasis.

Intrapulmonary Gas Distribution

Ventilation is not normally uniform throughout the lung. The effects of gravity on the lung and the forces necessary to allow it to conform to the shape of the thorax result in a vertical gradient of pleural pressure.[149] The pleural pressure acting on the upper (nondependent) areas of the lung is more subatmospheric (negative) than that acting on the lower (dependent) portions. As a result, the nondependent areas are more inflated than the dependent ones (see Chapter 8, Fig. 8-4). The gradient of pleural pressure up and down the lung changes 0.4 cmH_2O/cm of lung height. Thus, in a lung 30 cm high, 7.5 cmH_2O of pressure difference exists from apex to base. In the supine position, the dorsal areas become dependent. The height of the lungs is reduced by nearly one-third; thus, the gravitational effect is somewhat diminished.

Although the nondependent areas are more distended at FRC, when the subject breathes in such that a transpulmonary pressure of 5 cmH_2O is generated, the volume change or ventilation to dependent areas is greater. This is because of the sigmoid shape of the pressure-volume curve. The larger nondependent areas have a lower regional compliance, ie, they lie on a less steep portion of the pressure-volume curve.

These regional differences in ventilation are important in matching ventilation to perfusion. The dependent or basal areas tend to be better perfused because of gravitational effects. Since the bases are also better ventilated, there is good matching of ventilation and perfusion (Fig. 7-13). Higher ventilation and blood flow are delivered to the bases. In supine, anesthetized, paralyzed humans, the ventilation or distribution of inspired gas becomes more uniform from top to bottom lung areas. Meanwhile, anesthetics produce a decrease in pulmonary artery pressure that impedes perfusion on nondependent lung regions. Increased alveolar pressures with mechanical ventilation further interfere with perfusion of nondependent areas. Thus, dependent lung areas are well perfused but rather poorly ventilated. In contrast, nondependent areas receive more ventilation but considerably less perfusion.

While lying in the lateral decubitus position, patients exhibit a greater blood flow to the dependent lung, largely because of gravitational effects. In the awake state, the normal vertical gradient of pleural pressure also allows for greater ventilation of the same dependent lung and maintenance of normal $\dot{V}_A/\dot{Q}$ distribution. This is more apparent in the large right lung, which is not subject to compression by an enlarged heart. In fact, in relatively normal persons with unilateral lung disease, respiratory gas exchange is optimal if the good lung is dependent.[150,151] Exceptions to this appear to occur in infants[152] and in patients with COPD.[153] In the latter two groups, ventilation of the dependent lung is decreased presumably because of decreased lung recoil and airway closure. Application of 10 cmH_2O of positive end-expiratory

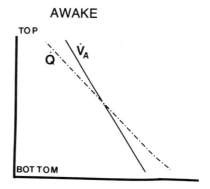

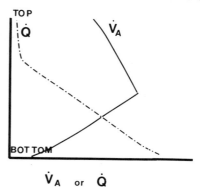

Fig. 7-13. Diagrammatic representation of the distribution of ventilation ($\dot{V}_A$) and perfusion ($\dot{Q}$) between nondependent (top) lung areas and dependent (bottom) areas. Note that $\dot{V}_A$ is distributed more uniformly from top to bottom in the anesthetized paralyzed state.

pressure restores preferential distribution of ventilation to the dependent lung.[149]

Radiographic and bronchospirometric studies show that the dependent lung receives greater ventilation and has a higher O_2 uptake in the lateral position. Although its FRC is lower than the nondependent lung, N_2 washout is also more rapid.[150] When patients are anesthetized in the lateral position during thoracic surgery, distribution of the pulmonary blood flow is similar to the awake state, ie, the dependent lung receives greater perfusion. The greater portion of ventilation, however, is switched from the dependent to the nondependent lung. In a sense, the ventilation is more uniform; this is reflected in more equal N_2 clearances for each lung.[154] This shift in distribution of ventilation results from a loss of lung volume (decreased FRC) that is unequally shared by both lungs. The dependent lung, which undergoes a greater decrease in FRC, moves to a less steep portion of the pressure-volume curve (see Chapter 8, Fig. 8-4), while the nondependent lung moves from a relatively flat portion to a steeper one. The abdominal contents as well as the mediastinum also impede dependent lung expansion. Thus, the anesthetized patient in the lateral position has a nondependent lung that is well ventilated but poorly perfused. In contrast, the well-perfused dependent lung is poorly ventilated. Opening the chest may only serve to increase the overventilation of the nondependent lung (see Chapter 8).

The increased $\dot{V}_A/\dot{Q}$ mismatching that accompanies anesthesia and paralysis appears to be largely a result of altered distribution of ventilation with a relative failure of intrapulmonary perfusion to adjust.[155] Although some of this failure of blood flow to adjust for the altered ventilation may relate to inhibition of hypoxic pulmonary vasoconstriction by the inhalation anesthetics, the altered pattern of expansion of the lung with anesthesia and paralysis may also affect the distribution of blood flow along with ventilation.

REFERENCES

1. Black LF, Hyatt RE: Maximal respiratory pressures. Normal values and relationship to age and sex. Am Rev Respir Dis 103:641–650, 1971
2. Pavlin EG, Holle RH, Schoene RB: Recovery of airway protection compared with ventilation in humans after paralysis with curare. Anesthesiology 70:381–385, 1989
3. Rahn H, Otis AB, Chadwick LE, Fenn WO: The pressure volume diagram of the thorax and lung. Am J Physiol 146:161–178, 1946
4. Detroyer A, Basteiner-Geens J: Effects of neuromuscular blockade on respiratory mechanics in conscious man. J Appl Physiol 47:1162–1168, 1979
5. Gal TJ, Arora NS: Respiratory mechanics in supine subjects during partial curarization. J Appl Physiol 52:57–63, 1982
6. Tucker DH, Sieker HO: The effect of change in body position on lung volumes and intrapulmonary gas mixing in patients with obesity, heart failure and emphysema. Am Rev Respir Dis 85:787–791, 1960
7. Scheidt M, Hyatt RE, Rehder K: Effects of rib cage or abdominal restriction on lung mechanics. J Appl Physiol 51:1115–1121, 1981
8. Agostoni E, Burtner G, Torri G, Rahn H: Respiratory mechanics during submersion and negative pressure breathing. J Appl Physiol 21:251–258, 1966
9. Koterba AM, Kosch PC, Beech J, Whitlock T: Breathing strategy of the adult horse (Equus Caballus) at rest. J Appl Physiol 64:337–346, 1988
10. Bryan AC, Wohl MEB: Respiratory mechanics in children. pp. 180–181. In Macklem PT, Mead J (eds). Handbook of Physiology. The Respiratory System. American Physiological Society, Bethesda, MD, 1986
11. Olinsky A, Bryan MH, Bryan AC: Influence of lung infla-
tion on respiratory control in neonates. J Appl Physiol 36:426–429, 1974
12. Milic-Emili J, Mead J, Turner M, et al: Improved technique for estimating pleural pressure from esophageal balloons. J Appl Physiol 19:207–211, 1964
13. Leatherman NE: An improved balloon system for monitoring intraesophageal pressure in acutely ill patients. Crit Care Med 6:189–192, 1978
14. Ludwig, MS, Dreshas O, Solway J, et al: Partitioning of pulmonary resistance during constriction in the dog: effects of volume history. J Appl Physiol 62:807–815, 1987
15. Warner DO, Vettermann J, Brusasco V, Rehder K: Pulmonary resistance during halothane anesthesia is not determined only by airway caliber. Anesthesiology 70:453–460, 1989
16. DuBois AB, Botelho SY, Comroe JH: A new method for measuring airway resistance in man using body plethysmograph values in normal subjects and in patients with respiratory disease. J Clin Invest 35:326–335, 1956
17. Egbert LD, Tamersoy K, Deas TC: Pulmonary function during spinal anesthesia: the mechanism of cough depression. Anesthesiology 22:882–885, 1961
18. Freund FG, Bonica JJ, Ward RJ, et al: Ventilatory reserve and level of motor block during high spinal and epidural anesthesia. Anesthesiology 28:834–837, 1967
19. Hecker BR, Bjurstrom R, Schoene RB: Effect of intercostal nerve blockade on respiratory mechanics and CO_2 chemosensitivity at rest and exercise. Anesthesiology 70:13–18, 1989
20. Giesecke AH, Cale JO, Jenkins MT: The prostate position, ventilation, and anesthesia. JAMA 203:389–391, 1968
21. Barach Al, Beck GJ: Ventilatory effects of head down position in pulmonary emphysema. Am J Med 16:55–60, 1954
22. Barach AL: Chronic obstructive lung disease: postural relief of dyspnea. Arch Phys Med Rehabil 55:494–504, 1974
23. Catenacci AJ, Sampathacar KR: Ventilatory studies in the obese patient during spinal anesthesia. Anesth Analg 48:48–54, 1969
24. Bergman NA: Distribution of inspired gas during anesthesia and artificial ventilation. J Appl Physiol 18:1085–1089, 1963
25. Rehder K, Marsh HM: Respiratory mechanics during anesthesia and mechanical ventilation. pp. 737–752. In Macklem PT, Mead J (eds): Handbook of Physiology. The Respiratory System. Mechanics of Breathing. American Physiological Society, Bethesda, MD, 1986
26. Damia G, Mascheroni D, Croci M, Tarenzi L: Perioperative changes in functional residual capacity in morbidly obese patients. Br J Anaesth 60:574–557, 1988
27. Bergman NA: Reduction in resting end-expiratory position of the respiratory system with induction of anesthesia and neuromuscular paralysis. Anesthesiology 57:14–17, 1982
28. Hewlett AM, Hulands GH, Nunn JF, Millwdge JS: Functional residual capacity during anesthesia. II. Spontaneous respiration. Br J Anaesth 46:486–494, 1974

29. Westbrook PR, Stubbs SE, Sessler AD, et al: Effects of anesthesia and muscle paralysis on respiratory mechanics in normal man. J Appl Physiol 34:81–86, 1973

30. Brismar B, Hedenstierna G, Lundquist H, et al: Pulmonary densities during anesthesia with muscular relaxation—a proposal of atelectasis. Anesthesiology 62:422–428, 1985

31. Dery R, Pelletier J, Jaques A, et al: Alveolar collapse induced by nitrogenation. Can Anaesth Soc J 12:531–544, 1965

32. Hedenstierna G, Lofstrom B, Lundh R: Thoracic gas volume and chest abdomen dimensions during anesthesia and muscle paralysis. Anesthesiology 55:499–506, 1981

33. Muller N, Volgyesi G, Becker L, et al: Diaphragmatic muscle tone. J Appl Physiol 47:279–284, 1979

34. Tusiewicz K, Bryan AC, Froese AB: Contributions of changing rib cage—diaphragm interactions to the ventilatory depression of halothane and anesthesia. Anesthesiology 47:327–337, 1977

35. Scheidt M, Hyatt RE, Rehder K: Effect of rib cage or abdominal restriction on lung mechanics. J Appl Physiol 51:1115–1121, 1981

36. Hedenstierna G, Strandberg A, Brismar B, et al: Functional residual capacity, thoracoabdominal dimensions, and central blood volume during general anesthesia with muscle paralysis and mechanical ventilation. Anesthesiology 62:247–254, 1985

37. Krayer S, Rehder K, Beck KC, et al: Quantification of thoracic volumes by three-dimensional imaging. J Appl Physiol 62:591–598, 1987

38. Bickler PE, Dueck R, Prutow R: Effects of barbiturate anesthesia and functional residual capacity and rib cage/diaphragm contributions to ventilation. Anesthesiology 60:147–182, 1987

39. Hudget DW, Devadatta P: Decrease in functional residual capacity during sleep in normal humans. J Appl Physiol 57:1319–1322, 1984

40. Mankikian B, Cantineau JP, Sartene R, et al: Ventilatory pattern and chest wall mechanics during ketamine anesthesia in humans. Anesthesiology 65:492–499, 1986

41. Shulman D, Bearsmore CS, Aronson HG, Godfrey S: The effect of ketamine on functional residual capacity in young children. Anesthesiology 62:551–556, 1985

42. Shuman D, Bar-yishay E, Beardsmore C, Godfrey S: Determinants of end-expiratory lung volume in young children during ketamine or halothane. Anesthesia 66:636–640, 1987

43. Gold MI, Han YH, Helrich M: Pulmonary mechanics during anesthesia. III. Influence of intermittent positive pressure ventilation and relation to blood gases. Anesth Analg 45:631–641, 1966

44. Wu N, Miller WF, Luhn NR: Studies of breathing in anesthesia. Anesthesiology 17:696–707, 1956

45. Rehder K, Mallow JE, Fibuch EE, et al: Effects of isoflurane anesthesia and muscle paralysis on respiratory mechanics in normal man. Anesthesiology 41:477–485, 1974

46. Hedenstierna G, McCarthy G: Mechanics of breathing, gas distribution, and functional residual capacity at different frequencies of respiration during spontaneous and artificial ventilation. Br J Anaesth 57:706–712, 1975

47. Dohi S, Gold MI: Pulmonary mechanics during general anesthesia. The influence of mechanical irritation on the airway. Br J Anaesth 51:205–213, 1979

48. Loring SH, Elliott EA, Drazen JM: Kinetic energy loss and convective acceleration in respiratory resistance measurements. Lung 156:33–42, 1979

49. Lehane JR, Jordan C, Jones JG: Influence of halothane and enflurane on respiratory airflow resistance and specific conductance in anesthetized man. Br J Anaesth 52:773–781, 1980

50. Griffith HR, Johnson GC: The use of curare in general anesthesia. Anesthesiology 3:418–420, 1942

51. Smith SM, Brown HO, Toman JEP, Goodman LS: The lack of cerebral effects of d-tubocurarine. Anesthesiology 8:1–13, 1947

52. Unna KR, Pelikan EW: Evaluation of curarizing drugs in man. VI. Critique of experiments on unanesthetized subjects. Ann NY Acad Sci 54:480–489, 1951

53. Williams JP, Bourke DL: Effects of succinylcholine on respiratory and non-respiratory muscle strength in humans. Anesthesiology 63:299–303, 1985

54. Kallos T: Open mouthed head lifting, a sign of incomplete reversal of neuromuscular blockade. Anesthesiology 37:650–651, 1972

55. Colgan FA, Liang JQ, Barrow RE: Noninvasive assessment by capacitance respirometry of respiratory before and after extubation. Anesth Analg 54:807–813, 1975

56. Gal TJ: Pulmonary mechanics in normal subjects following endotracheal intubation. Anesthesiology 52:27–35, 1980

57. Widdicombe JG: Mechanism of cough and its regulation. Eur J Respir Dis, Suppl. 10:11–15, 1980

58. Nunn JF, Campbell EJM, Peckett BW: Anatomical subdivision of the volume of respiratory dead space and effects of positions of the jaw. J Appl Physiol 14:174–176, 1959

59. Baier H, Wanner A, Zarzecki S, Sackner M: Relationships among glottis opening, respiratory flow, and upper airway resistance in humans. J Appl Physiol 43:603–611, 1977

60. Chang HK, Mortola JP: Fluid dynamic factors in tracheal pressure measurements. J Appl Physiol 51:218–225, 1981

61. Habib MP: Physiological implications of artificial airways. Chest 96:180–184, 1989

62. Sahn SA, Laksminarayan S, Petty TI: Weaning from mechanical ventilation. JAMA 235:2208–2212, 1976

63. Berman LS, Fox WW, Raphaely R: Optimum levels of CPAP for tracheal extubation of newborn infants. J Pediatr 89:109–112, 1976

64. Annest SJ, Gottlieb M, Paloski WH, et al: Detrimental effects of removing end-expiratory pressure prior to endotracheal extubation. Ann Surg 191:539–545, 1980

65. Matsushima Y, Jones RL, King EG, et al: Alterations in pulmonary mechanics and gas exchange during routine fiberoptic bronchoscopy. Chest 86:184–188, 1984

66. England SJ, Bartlett D: Influence of human vocal cord movements on airflow resistance during eupnea. J Appl Physiol 52:773–779, 1982

67. England SJ, Bartlett D: Changes in respiratory movements of the human vocal cords during hyperpnea. J Appl Physiol 52:780–785, 1982

68. Gal TJ, Suratt PM: Resistance to breathing in healthy subjects after endotracheal intubation under topical anesthesia. Anesth Analg 59:270–274, 1980

69. Ferris BG, Mead J, Opie LH: Partitioning of respiratory flow resistance in man. J Appl Physiol 19:653–668, 1964

70. Mitchell RA: The regulation of respiration in metabolic acidosis and alkalosis. pp. 109–131. In Brooks CMC, Kao FF, Lloyd BB (eds): Cerebrospinal Fluid and the Regulation of Ventilation. Blackwell Scientific Publications, Oxford, 1965

71. Biscoe TJ, Purves MJ, Sampson SR: The frequency of nerve impulses in single carotid body chemoreceptor afferent fibers recorded in vivo with intact circulation. J Physiol (Lond) 208:121–131, 1970

72. Knill RL, Clement JL: Ventilatory responses to acute metabolic acidemia in humans awake, sedated, and anesthetized with halothane. Anesthesiology 62:745–753, 1985

73. Goldring RM, Cannon PJ, Heineman HO, Fishman AP: Respiratory adjustment to chronic metabolic alkalosis in man. J Clin Invest 47:188–202, 1968

74. Gross JB, Zebrowski ME, Carel WD, et al: Time course of ventilatory depression after thiopental and midazolam in normal subjects and in patients with chronic obstructive pulmonary disease. Anesthesiology 58:540–544, 1983

75. Read DJC: A clinical method for assessing the ventilatory response to carbon dioxide. Australas Ann Med 16:20–32, 1967

76. Rebuck AS, Read J: Patterns of ventilatory response to carbon dioxide during recovery from severe asthma. Clin Sci 41:13–21, 1971

77. Lloyd BB, Cunningham DJC: A quantitative approach to the regulation of human respiration. pp. 331–349. In Cunningham DJC, Lloyd BB (eds): The Regulation of Human Respiration. Blackwell Scientific Publications, Oxford, 1963

78. Rebuck AS, Campbell EJM: A clinical method for assessing the ventilatory response to hypoxia. Am Rev Respir Dis 109:345–350, 1974

79. Weil JV, Byrne-Quinn E, Sodal I, et al: Hypoxic ventilatory drive in normal man. J Clin Invest 49:1061–1072, 1970

80. Edelman NH, Epstein PE, Lahiri S, Cherniack NS: The ventilatory responses to transient hypoxia and hypercapnia in man. Respir Physiol 17:302–314, 1973

81. Gross JB: Resting ventilation measurements may be misleading. Anesthesiology 61:110, 1984

82. Knill RL: Wresting or resting ventilation. Anesthesiology 59:599–600, 1983

83. Stremel RW, Huntsman DJ, Casaburi R, et al: Control of ventilation during intravenous CO_2 loading in the awake dog. J Appl Physiol 44:311–316, 1978

84. Irsigler GB: Carbon dioxide response lines in young adults: the limits of the normal response. Am Rev Respir Dis 14:529–536, 1976

85. Rebuck AS, Rigg JRA, Kangalee M, Pengelly LD: Control of tidal volume during rebreathing. J Appl Physiol 37:475–478, 1974

86. Nielson M, Smith H: Studies on the regulation of respiration in acute hypoxia. Acta Physiol Scand 24:293–313, 1952

87. Severinghaus J, Bainton CR, Carcelena R: Respiratory insensitivity to hypoxia in chronically hypoxic man. Respir Physiol 1:308–334, 1966

88. Hirschman CA, McCullough RE, Wel JV: Normal values for hypoxic and hypercapneic ventilatory drives in man. J Appl Physiol 38:1095–1098, 1975

89. Rebuck AS, Woodley WE: Ventilatory effects of hypoxia and their dependence on PCO_2. J Appl Physiol 38:16–19, 1975

90. Kronenberg RS, Hamilton FN, Gabel R, et al: Comparison of three methods for quantitating respiratory response to hypoxia. Respir Physiol 16:109–125, 1972

91. Milic-Emili J, Grunstein MM: Drive and timing components of ventilation. Chest, Suppl. 70:131–133, 1976

92. Milic-Emili J: Recent advances in clinical assessment of control of breathing. Annu Rev Resp Dis 160:1–17, 1982

93. Lopata M, Evanich MJ, Lourenco RV: Relationship between mouth occlusion pressure and electrical activity of the diaphragm: Effects of flow resistive loading. Am Rev Respir Dis 116:449–455, 1977

94. Peterson DD, Pack AI, Silage DA, Fishman AP: Effects of aging on ventilatory and occlusion pressure responses to hypoxia and hypercapnia. Am Rev Respir Dis 124:287–391, 1981

95. Kronenberg RS, Drage CW: Attenuation of the ventilatory and heart rate responses to hypoxia and hypercapnia with aging in normal men. J Clin Invest 52:1812–1819, 1973

96. Avery ME, Chernick V, Dutton RE, Permutt S: Ventilatory responses to inspired carbon dioxide in infants and adults. J Appl Physiol 18:895–903, 1963

97. Frantz ID, Adler SM, Thach BT, Taeusch HW: Maturational effects of respiratory responses to carbon dioxide in premature infants. J Appl Physiol 41:41–45, 1976

98. Rigatto H, Torreverousco R, Cates OB: Effects of O_2 on the ventilatory response to CO_2 in preterm infants. J Appl Physiol 39:896–899, 1975

99. Easton PA, Sklykerman J, Anthonisen NR: Ventilatory response to sustained hypoxia in normal adults. J Appl Physiol 61:906–911, 1986

100. Schiffman PL, Westlake RE, Santiago TV, Edelman NH: Ventilatory control of parents of victims of sudden death syndrome. N Engl Med 320:486–491, 1980

101. Mountain R, Zwillich C, Weil J: Hypoventilation in obstructive disease. The role of familial factors. N Engl J Med 298:521–525, 1978

102. Collins DD, Scoggin CH, Zwillich CW, Weil JV: Hereditary aspects of decreased hypoxic drive in endurance athletes. J Appl Physiol 44:464–468, 1978

103. Lakshminaryan S, Pierson DJ: Recurrent high altitude pulmonary edema with blunted chemosensitivity. Am Rev Respir Dis 11:869–872, 1975

104. Schoene RB: Control of ventilation in climbers to extreme altitude. J Appl Physiol 53:886–890, 1982

105. Schoene RB, Lahiri S, Hackett PH, et al: The relationship of hypoxic ventilatory response to exercise performance on Mt. Everest. J Appl Physiol 56:1478–1483, 1984

106. Brodsky JD, Macdonell JA, Cherniack RM: The respiratory response to carbon dioxide in health and in emphysema. J Clin Invest 39:724–729, 1960

107. West JB: Causes of carbon dioxide retention in lung disease. N Engl J Med 284:1232–1236, 1971

108. Lourenco RV, Miranda JM: Drive and performance of the ventilatory apparatus in chronic obstructive lung disease. N Engl J Med 279:53–59, 1968

109. Gelb AF, Klein E, Schiffman P, et al: Ventilatory response and drive in acute and chronic obstructive pulmonary disease. Am Rev Respir Dis 116:9–16, 1977

110. Surli J, Grassino A, Lorange G, Milic-Emili J: Control of breathing in patients with chronic obstructive lung disease. Clin Sci Molec Med 54:295–304, 1978

111. Aubier M, Murciano D, Milic-Emili J: Effects of administration of O_2 on ventilation and blood gases in patients with chronic obstructive lung disease during acute respiratory failure. Am Rev Respir Dis 122:747–753, 1980

112. Bradley CA, Fleetham JA, Anthonisen NR: Ventilatory control in patients with hypoxemia due to obstructive lung disease. Am Rev Respir Dis 120:21–30, 1979

113. Kepron W, Cherniack RM: The ventilatory response to hypercapnia and to hypoxemia in chronic obstructive lung disease. Am Rev Respir Dis 108:843–850, 1973

114. Bradley CA, Fleetham JA, Anthonisen NR: Ventilatory control in patients with hypoxemia due to obstructive lung disease. Am Rev Respir Dis 120:21–30, 1979

115. Aubier M, Murcinao D, Fournier M, et al: Central respiratory drive in acute respiratory failure of patients with chronic obstructive lung disease. Am Rev Respir Dis 122:191–199, 1980

116. Sassoon CSH, Hassell KT, Mahutte CK: Hyperoxic-induced hypercapnia in stable chronic obstructive pulmonary disease. AM Rev Respir Dis 135:909–911, 1987

117. Hickey RF, Severinghaus JW: Regulation of breathing: drug effects in lung biology in health and disease. pp. 1251–1312. In Horbein TF (ed): Regulation of Breathing. Marcel Dekker, New York, 1978

118. Pietak S, Weenig CS, Hickey RF, Fairley HB: Anesthetic effects on ventilation in patients with chronic obstructive pulmonary disease. Anesthesiology 42:160–166, 1975

119. Lam AM, Clement JL, Knill RL: Surgical stimulation does not enhance ventilatory chemoreflexes during enflurane anesthesia in man. Can Anaesth Soc J 27:22–28, 1980

120. Derenne JP, Couture J, Iscoe S, Whitelaw WA: Occlusion pressures in men rebreathing CO_2 under methoxyflurane anesthesia. J Appl Physiol 40:805–814, 1976

121. Wahba WM: Analysis of ventilatory depression by enflurane during clinical anesthesia. Anesth Analg 59:103–109, 1980

122. Byrick RJ, Janssen EG: Respiratory waveform and rebreathing in T-piece circuits: a comparison of enflurane and halothane waveforms. Anesthesiology 53:371–378, 1980

123. Hanks EC, Nai SH, Fink BR: The respiratory threshold during halothane anesthesia. Anesthesiology 22:393–397, 1961

124. Weiskopf RB, Raymond LW, Severinghaus JW: Effects of halothane on canine respiratory response to hypoxia with and without hypercarbia. Anesthesiology 41:350–360, 1974

125. Knill RC, Gelb AW: Ventilatory responses to hypoxia and hypercapnia during halothane sedation and anesthesia in man. Anesthesiology 49:244–251, 1978

126. Knill RL, Mannimen PH, Clement JL: Ventilation and chemoreflexes during enflurane sedation and anesthesia in man. Can Anaesth Soc J 26:353–360, 1979

127. Knill RL, Kieraszewicz HT, Dodgson BG: Chemical regulation of ventilation during isoflurane sedation and anesthesia in humans. Can Anaesth Soc J 30:607–614, 1983

128. Yacoub O, Doell D, Kryger MH, Anthonisen NR: Depression of hypoxic ventilatory response by nitrous oxide. Anesthesiology 45:385–389, 1976

129. Knill RL, Clement JL: Ventilatory responses to acute metabolic acidemia in humans awake, sedated, and anesthetized with halothane. Anesthesiology 62:745–753, 1985

130. Hirshman CA, McCullough RE, Cowen PJ, Weil J: Effect of pentabarbitone on hypoxic ventilatory drive in man. Br J Anaesth 47:963–968, 1975

131. Knill RL, Bright S, Manninen P: Hypoxic ventilatory responses during thiopentone sedation and anesthesia in man. Can Anaesth Soc J 25:366–372, 1978

132. Virtue RW, Alanis JM, Mori M, et al: An anesthetic agent; 2-orthochlorophenyl-2 methylamino cyclohexanone. HCl (CI-581). Anesthesiology 28:823–833, 1967

133. Soliman MG, Brindle GF, Kuster G: Response to hypercapnia under ketamine anesthesia. Can Anaesth Soc J 22:486–494, 1975

134. Hirshman CA, McCullough RE, Cohen DJ, Weil J: Hypoxic ventilatory drive in dogs during thiopental, ketamine, or pentobarbital anesthesia. Anesthesiology 43:628–634, 1975

135. Bourke DL, Malit LA, Smith TC: Respiratory interactions of ketamine and morphine. Anesthesiology 66:135–137, 1987

136. Hamza J, Ecoffey C, Gross JB: Ventilatory response to CO_2 following intravenous ketamine in children. Anesthesiology 70:422–425, 1989

137. Gross JB, Caldwell CB, Shaw LM, Laucks SO: The effect of lidocaine on the ventilatory response to carbon dioxide. Anesthesiology 59:521–529, 1983

138. Himes RS, DiFazio CA, Burney RG: Effects of lidocaine on the anesthetic requirements for nitrous oxide and halothane. Anesthesiology 47:437–440, 1977

139. Gross JB, Caldwell CB, Shaw LM, Apfelbaum JL: The effect of lidocaine infusion on the ventilatory response to hypoxia. Anesthesiology 61:662–665, 1984

140. Rehder K, Marsh HYM, Rodarte JR, Hyatt RE: Airway closure. Anesthesiology 47:40–52, 1977

141. Hickey RF, Visick WD, Fairley HB, Fourcade HE: Effects of halothane anesthesia on functional residual capacity and alveolar-arterial oxygen tension difference. Anesthesiology 38:20–24, 1973

142. Gilmour J, Burnham M, Craig DG: Closing capacity measurement during general anesthesia. Anesthesiology 45:477–482, 1976

143. Hedenstierna G, McCartha G, Bergstrom M: Airway closure during mechanical ventilation. Anesthesiology 44:114–123, 1976

144. Juno P, Marsh HM, Knopp TJ, Rehder K: Closing capacity in awake and anesthetized paralyzed man. J Appl Physiol 44:238–244, 1978

145. Hedenstierna G, Santesson J: Airway closure during anesthesia: a comparison between resident gas and argon bolus techniques. J Appl Physiol 47:874–881, 1979

146. Dueck R, Prutow RJ, Davies NJH, et al: The lung volume at which shunting occurs with inhalation anesthesia. Anesthesiology 69:854–861, 1988

147. Hedenstierna G, Tokics L, Strandberg A, et al: Correlation of gas exchange impairment to development of atelectasis during anaesthesia and muscle paralysis. Acta Anaesthesiol Scand 30:183–191, 1986

148. Tokics L, Hedenstierna G, Brismar B, Strandberg A: Thoracoabdominal restriction in supine men: CT and lung function measurements. J Appl Physiol 64:599–604, 1988

149. Agostoni E: Mechanics of the pleural space. Physiol Rev 52:57–128, 1972

150. Remolina C, Kahn AU, Santiago TV, Edelman NH: Positional hypoxemia in unilateral lung disease. N Engl J Med 304:523–525, 1981

151. Fishman AF: Down with the good lung. N Engl J Med 304:537–538, 1981

152. Davies H, Kitchman R, Gordon I, Helms P: Regional ventilation in infancy. Reversal of adult pattern. N Engl J Med 313:1626–1628, 1985

153. Shim C, Chun K, Williams MH, Blaufox MD: Positional effects on distribution of ventilation in chronic obstructive pulmonary disease. Ann Intern Med 105:346–350, 1986

154. Rehder K, Hatch DJ, Sesselr AD, Fowler WS: The function of each lung of anesthetized paralyzed man during mechanical ventilation. Anesthesiology 37:16–26, 1972

155. Landmark SJ, Knopp TJ, Rehder K, Sesler AD: Regional pulmonary perfusion and $\dot{V}/\dot{Q}$ in awake and anesthesized paralyzed man. J Appl Physiol 43:993–1000, 1977

156. Gal TJ: Pulmonary function testing. pp. 773–792. In Miller RD (ed): Anesthesia. 3rd Ed. Churchill Livingstone, New York, 1990

157. Gal TJ: Monitoring the function of the respiratory system. Ch. 9. In Lake CL (ed): Clinical Monitoring. WB Saunders, Philadelphia, 1989

158. Gal TJ: How does tracheal intubation alter respiratory mechanics? Probl Anesth 2:191–200, 1988

159. Benumof JL: Respiration physiology and respiratory function during anesthesia. pp. 505–549. In Miller RD (ed): Anesthesia. 3rd Ed. Churchill Livingstone, New York, 1990

160. Bailey PL, Stanley TH: Pharmacology of intravenous narcotic anesthetics. pp. 281–366. In Miller RD (ed): Anesthesia. 3rd Ed. Churchill Livingstone, New York, 1990

8

PHYSIOLOGY OF THE LATERAL DECUBITUS POSITION, THE OPEN CHEST, AND ONE-LUNG VENTILATION

Jonathan L. Benumof, M.D.

Patients undergoing thoracic surgery usually are in the lateral decubitus position under general anesthesia, have an open chest wall, and are pharmacologically paralyzed. Compared with the awake state in the upright position, all these anesthesia and surgical requirements (lateral decubitus position, general anesthesia, open pleural space, and paralysis) can cause major alterations in the distribution of perfusion ($\dot{Q}$), ventilation ($\dot{V}$), and ventilation-perfusion relationships ($\dot{V}/\dot{Q}$). The first part of this chapter discusses each of these anesthetic and surgical effects on the distribution of $\dot{Q}$, $\dot{V}$, and $\dot{V}/\dot{Q}$ during two-lung ventilation. The second part of this chapter considers the physiologic consequences of spontaneous ventilation with an open chest. Finally, a good deal of thoracic surgery must be performed with the operated lung being either nonventilated (nonmoving) and/or functionally or physically separated from the ventilated, dependent lung. This is most easily accomplished by the insertion of a double-lumen tube. Via blockade of

one airway lumen, the nondependent or surgical lung is deliberately not ventilated, and via the other airway lumen, the dependent or nonsurgical lung is ventilated (one-lung ventilation). One-lung ventilation imposes a new set of determinants on the distribution of blood flow (and, of course, ventilation), and the third part of this chapter considers the physiology of one-lung ventilation.

PHYSIOLOGY OF THE LATERAL DECUBITUS POSITION

Upright Position

Distribution of Pulmonary Perfusion

Contraction of the right ventricle imparts kinetic energy to the blood in the main pulmonary artery. Most of the kinetic energy in the main pulmonary artery is dissipated in climbing a vertical hydrostatic gradient, and the absolute pressure in the pulmonary artery (P_{pa}) decreases 1 cmH$_2$O/cm of vertical distance up the lung (Fig. 8-1). At some height above the heart, P_{pa} becomes zero (atmospheric) and, still higher in the lung, the P_{pa} becomes negative.[1] In this region, alveolar pressure (P_A) then exceeds P_{pa} and pulmonary venous pressure (P_{pv}), which is very negative at this vertical height. Since the pressure outside the vessels is greater than the pressure inside the vessels, the vessels in this region of the lung are collapsed and there is no blood flow (zone 1, $P_A > P_{pa} > P_{pv}$). Since there is no blood flow, no gas exchange is possible, and the region functions as alveolar dead space or "wasted" ventilation. Little or no zone 1 exists in the lung under normal conditions, but the amount of zone 1 lung may

be greatly increased if P_{pa} is reduced, as in oligemic shock, or if P_A is increased, as in positive-pressure ventilation.

Further down the lung, absolute P_{pa} becomes positive and blood flow will begin when P_{pa} exceeds P_A (zone 2, $P_{pa} > P_A > P_{pv}$). At this vertical level in the lung, P_A exceeds P_{pv}, and blood flow is determined by the mean $P_{pa} - P_A$ difference rather than the more conventional $P_{pa} - P_{pv}$ difference.[2] The zone 2 blood flow-alveolar pressure relationship has the same physical characteristics as a river waterfall flowing over a dam. The height of the upstream river (before reaching the dam) is equivalent to P_{pa} and the height of the dam is equivalent to P_A. The rate of water flow over the dam is only proportional to the difference between the height of the upstream river and the dam

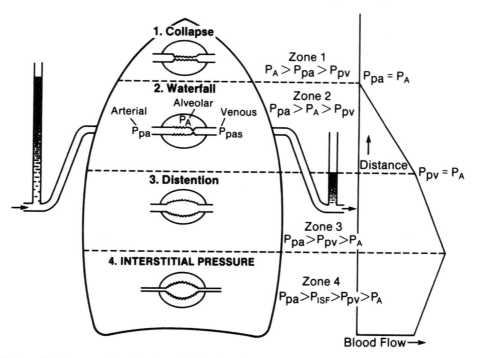

Fig. 8-1. Schematic diagram showing the distribution of blood flow in the upright lung. In zone 1, alveolar pressure (P_A) exceeds pulmonary artery pressure (P_{pa}) and no flow occurs because the intra-alveolar vessels are collapsed by the compressing alveolar pressure. In zone 2, arterial pressure exceeds alveolar pressure, but alveolar pressure exceeds venous pressure (P_{pv}). Flow in zone 2 is determined by the arterial-alveolar pressure difference ($P_{pa} - P_A$) and has been likened to an upstream river waterfall over a dam. Since P_{pa} increases down zone 2 and P_A remains constant, the perfusion pressure increases, and flow steadily increases down the zone. In zone 3, pulmonary venous pressure exceeds alveolar pressure, and flow is determined by the arterial-venous pressure difference ($P_{pa} - P_{pv}$), which is constant in this portion of the lung. However, the transmural pressure across the wall of the vessel increases down this zone so that the caliber of the vessels increases (resistance decreases); therefore, flow increases. Finally, in zone 4, pulmonary interstitial pressure becomes positive and exceeds both pulmonary venous pressure and alveolar pressure. Consequently, flow in zone 4 is determined by the arterial-interstitial pressure difference ($P_{pa} - P_{isf}$). (Adapted from West,[12] with permission.)

($P_{pa} - P_A$), and it does not matter how far below the dam the downstream riverbed (P_{pv}) is. This phenomenon has various names, including the "waterfall," "Starling resistor," "weir" (dam made by beavers), and "sluice" effect. Since mean P_{pa} increases down this region of the lung but mean P_A is relatively constant, the mean driving pressure ($P_{pa} - P_A$) increases linearly; therefore, mean blood flow increases linearly.

However, it should be noted that respiration and pulmonary blood flow are cyclic phenomena. Therefore, absolute instantaneous P_{pa}, P_{pv}, and P_A pressures are changing all the time and the relationships among P_{pa}, P_{pv}, and P_A are dynamically determined by the phase lags between the cardiac and respiratory cycles. Consequently, a given point in zone 2 may actually be in either a zone 1 or 3 condition at a given moment, depending on whether the patient is in respiratory systole or diastole or cardiac systole or diastole.

Still lower down in the lung, there is a vertical level where P_{pv} becomes positive and also exceeds P_A. In this region, blood flow is governed by the pulmonary arteriovenous pressure difference ($P_{pa} - P_{pv}$) (zone 3, $P_{pa} > P_{pv} > P_A$), for in this zone, both of these vascular pressures exceed the P_A, the capillary systems are thus permanently open and blood flow is continuous. In descending zone 3, gravity causes both absolute P_{pa} and P_{pv} to increase at the same rate so that the perfusion pressure ($P_{pa} - P_{pv}$) is unchanged. However, the pressure outside the vessels, namely, pleural pressure (P_{pl}), increases less than P_{pa} and P_{pv}, so that the transmural distending pressures ($P_{pa} - P_{pl}$ and $P_{pv} - P_{pl}$) increase down zone 3, the vessel radii increase, vascular resistance decreases, and blood flow, therefore, further increases.

Finally, whenever pulmonary vascular pressures are extremely high, as they would be in a severely volume-overloaded patient, a severely restricted and constricted pulmonary vascular bed, an extremely dependent lung (far below the vertical level of the left atrium), and in patients with pulmonary embolism and mitral stenosis, fluid may move out of the pulmonary vessels into the pulmonary interstitial compartment. The transudated pulmonary interstitial fluid may significantly alter the distribution of pulmonary blood flow.

When the flow of fluid into the interstitial space is excessive and cannot be cleared adequately by lymphatics, it will accumulate in the interstitial connective tissue compartment around the large vessels and airways, forming peribronchial and periarteriolar edema fluid cuffs. The transudated pulmonary interstitial fluid fills the pulmonary interstitial space and may eliminate the normally present negative and radially expanding interstitial tension on the extra-alve-

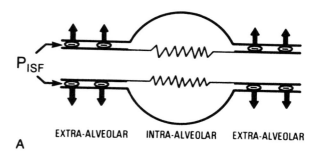

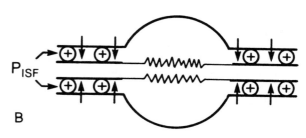

Fig. 8-2. The effect of pulmonary interstitial fluid pressure (P_{isf}) on extra-alveolar vessels. In normal lungs **(A)**, a negative P_{isf} around the extra-alveolar vessels tethers or keeps them open. When either pulmonary interstitial fluid accumulates or lung volume is extremely low, P_{isf} may become positive, exceed both pulmonary venous and alveolar pressures, and create a zone 4 **(B)** of the lung (where flow is proportional to the difference between pulmonary artery pressure and pulmonary interstitial pressure). (From Benumof,[95] with permission.)

olar pulmonary vessels (Fig. 8-2). The expansion of the pulmonary interstitial space by fluid causes pulmonary interstitial pressure (P_{isf}) to become positive and exceed P_{pv} (zone 4, $P_{pa} > P_{isf} > P_{pv} > P_A$).[3,4] In addition, the vascular resistance of extra-alveolar vessels may be increased at a very low lung volume (ie, the residual volume), where the tethering action of the pulmonary tissue on the vessels is also lost, causing P_{isf} to increase positively (see lung volume discussion below).[5,6] Consequently, zone 4 blood flow is governed by the arterio-interstitial pressure difference ($P_{pa} - P_{isf}$), which is less than the $P_{pa} - P_{pv}$ difference; therefore, zone 4 blood flow is less than zone 3 blood flow. In summary, zone 4 is a region of the lung that has transuded a large amount of fluid into the pulmonary interstitial compartment or is possibly at a very low lung volume. Both of these circumstances produce a positive interstitial pressure, causing extra-alveolar vessel compression, increased extra-alveolar vascular resistance, and decreased regional blood flow.

Following filling of the pulmonary interstitial compartment with edema fluid, fluid from the interstitial space, under an increased driving force (P_{isf}), will cross the relatively impermeable epithelial wall holes, and the alveolar space will fill. Intra-alveolar edema fluid will additionally cause alveolar collapse and atelectasis, thereby promoting further fluid accumulation.

It should now be evident that as P_{pa} and P_{pv} increase, three important changes take place in the pulmonary circulation, namely, recruitment or opening of previously unperfused vessels, distention or widening of previously perfused vessels, and transudation of fluid from very distended vessels.[7,8] Thus, as mean P_{pa} increases, zone 1 arteries may become zone 2 arteries, and as mean P_{pv} increases, zone 2 veins may become zone 3 veins. The increases in both mean P_{pa} and P_{pv} distend zone 3 vessels according to their compliance and decrease the resistance to flow through them. Zone 3 vessels may become so distended that they leak fluid and become converted to zone 4 vessels. In general, recruitment is the principal change as P_{pa} and P_{pv} increase from low to moderate levels; distention is the principal change as P_{pa} and P_{pv} increase from moderate to high levels of vascular pressure; and, finally, transudation is the principal change when P_{pa} and P_{pv} increase from high to very high levels.

Distribution of Ventilation

Gravity also causes vertical P_{pl} differences that cause, in turn, regional alveolar volume, compliance, and ventilation differences. The vertical gradient of P_{pl} can be best understood by thinking of the lung as a plastic bag filled with semifluid contents; in other words, it is a viscoelastic structure. Without the presence of a supporting chest wall, the effect of gravity on the contents of the bag would be to cause the bag to bulge outward at the bottom and inward at the top (it would assume a globular shape). With the lung inside the supporting chest wall, the lung cannot assume a globular shape. However, gravity still exerts a force on the lung to make it assume a globular shape; the force creates a relatively more negative pressure at the top of the pleural space (where the lung pulls away from the chest wall) and a relatively more positive pressure at the bottom of the lung (where the lung is compressed against the chest wall) (Fig. 8-3). The magnitude of this pressure gradient is determined by the density of the lung. Since the lung is approximately one-quarter of the density of water, the gradient of P_{pl} (in cmH_2O) will be approximately one-quarter of the height of the upright lung (30 cm). Thus, P_{pl} increases positively by 30/4 = 7.5 cmH_2O from the top to the bottom of the lung.[9]

Since P_A is the same throughout the lung, the P_{pl} gradient causes regional differences in transpul-

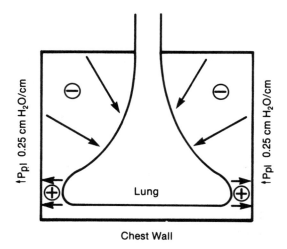

Fig. 8-3. Schematic diagram of the lung within the chest wall showing the tendency of the lung to assume a globular shape due to the lung's viscoelastic nature. The tendency of the top of the lung to collapse inward creates a relatively negative pressure at the apex of the lung, and the tendency of the bottom of the lung to spread outward creates a relatively positive pressure at the base of the lung. Thus, pleural pressure increases by 0.25 cmH_2O/cm of lung dependency. (Modified from Benumof,[123] with permission.)

monary distending pressures ($P_A - P_{pl}$). Since P_{pl} is most positive (least negative) in the dependent basilar lung regions, alveoli in these regions are more compressed, and, therefore, are considerably smaller than superior, relatively noncompressed apical alveoli (there is an approximately fourfold alveolar volume difference).[10] If the regional differences in alveolar volume are translated over to a pressure-volume curve for normal lung (Fig. 8-4), the dependent small alveoli are on the midportion and the nondependent large alveoli are on the upper portion of the S-shaped pressure-volume curve. Since the different regional slopes of the composite curve are equal to the different regional lung compliances, dependent alveoli are relatively compliant (steep slope) and nondependent alveoli are relatively noncompliant (flat slope). Thus, the majority of the tidal volume is preferentially distributed to dependent alveoli, since they expand more per unit of pressure change than nondependent alveoli.

Distribution of the Ventilation-to-Perfusion Ratio

Figure 8-5 shows that both blood flow and ventilation (both on the left vertical axis) increase linearly with distance down the normal upright lung (horizontal axis, reverse polarity).[11] Since blood flow increases from a very low value and more rapidly than ventila-

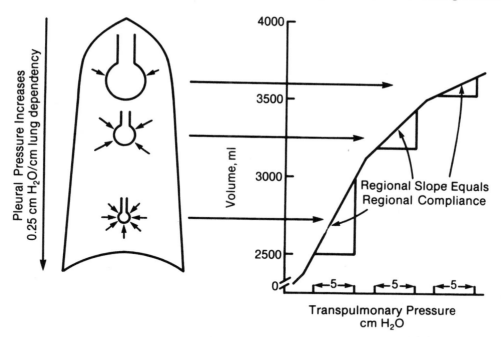

Fig. 8-4. Pleural pressure increases 0.25 cmH₂O every centimeter down the lung. The increase in pleural pressure causes a fourfold decrease in alveolar volume. The caliber of the air passages also decreases as lung volume decreases. When regional alveolar volume is translated over to a regional transpulmonary pressure-alveolar volume curve, small alveoli are on a steep (large slope) portion of the curve, and large alveoli are on a flat (small slope) portion of the curve. Since the regional slope equals regional compliance, the dependent small alveoli normally receive the largest share of the tidal volume. Over the normal tidal volume range (lung volume increases by 500 mL from 2,500 [normal FRC] to 3,000 mL), the pressure-volume relationship is linear. Lung volume values in this diagram relate to the upright position. (Modified from Benumof,[123] with permission.)

tion with distance down the lung, the ventilation-to-perfusion ($\dot{V}_A/\dot{Q}$) ratio (right vertical axis) decreases rapidly at first, then more slowly.

The $\dot{V}_A/\dot{Q}$ ratio best expresses the amount of ventilation relative to perfusion in any given lung region. Thus, alveoli at the base of the lung are somewhat overperfused in relation to their ventilation ($\dot{V}_A/\dot{Q} <$ 1). Figure 8-6 shows the calculated ventilation ($\dot{V}_A$) and blood flow ($\dot{Q}$) in liters per minute, the $\dot{V}_A/\dot{Q}$ ratio, and the alveolar PO₂ and PCO₂ in mmHg for horizontal slices from the top (7 percent of lung volume), middle (11 percent of lung volume), and bottom (13 percent of lung volume) of the lung.[12] It can be seen that the P$_A$O₂ increases by over 40 mmHg from 89 mmHg at the base to 132 mmHg at the apex, while P$_A$CO₂ decreases by 14 mmHg from 41 mmHg at the bottom to 28 mmHg at the top. Thus, in keeping with the regional $\dot{V}_A/\dot{Q}$, the bottom of the lung is relatively hypoxic and hypercarbic compared with the top of the lung.

Ventilation-to-perfusion inequalities have different effects on P$_a$CO₂ compared with P$_a$O₂. Blood passing through underventilated alveoli tends to retain its CO₂ and does not take up enough O₂; blood traversing overventilated alveoli gives off an excessive amount of CO₂, but cannot take up a proportionately increased amount of O₂ owing to the flatness of the oxyhemoglobin dissociation curve in this region. Hence, a lung with uneven ventilation-to-perfusion relationships can eliminate CO₂ from the overventilated alveoli to compensate for the underventilated alveoli. Thus, with uneven ventilation-to-perfusion relationships, P$_A$CO₂-to-P$_a$CO₂ gradients are small and P$_A$O₂-to-P$_a$O₂ gradients are usually large.

Lateral Decubitus Position: Distribution of Perfusion and Ventilation

Awake

Gravity causes a vertical gradient in the distribution of pulmonary blood flow in the lateral decubitus position for the same reason that it does in the upright position. Since the vertical hydrostatic gradient is less

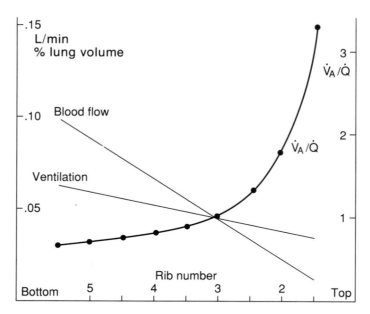

Fig. 8-5. Distribution of ventilation and blood flow (left vertical axis) and the ventilation-to-perfusion ratio (right vertical axis) in normal upright lung. Both blood flow and ventilation are expressed in liters per minute per percent alveolar volume and have been drawn as smoothed-out linear functions of vertical height. The closed circles mark the ventilation-to-perfusion ratios of horizontal lung slices (three of which are shown in Fig. 8-6). A cardiac output of 6 L/min and a total minute ventilation of 5.1 L/min were assumed. (From West,[122] with permission.)

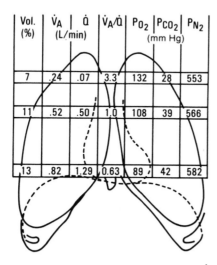

Vol. (%)	$\dot{V}_A$ (L/min)	$\dot{Q}$	$\dot{V}_A/\dot{Q}$	P_{O_2}	P_{CO_2}	P_{N_2}
				(mm Hg)		
7	.24	.07	3.3	132	28	553
11	.52	.50	1.0	108	39	566
13	.82	1.29	0.63	89	42	582

Fig. 8-6. The ventilation-to-perfusion ratio ($\dot{V}_A/\dot{Q}$) and the regional composition of alveolar gas. Values for the regional flow ($\dot{Q}$), ventilation ($\dot{V}_A$), P_{O_2}, and P_{CO_2} are derived from Figure 8-5. P_{N_2} has been obtained by what remains from the total gas pressure (which, including water vapor, equals 760 mmHg). The volume [Vol. (%)] of the three lung slices are also shown. Compared with the top of the lung, the bottom of the lung has a low $\dot{V}/\dot{Q}$ ratio and is relatively hypoxic and hypercarbic. (From West,[12] with permission.)

in the lateral decubitus position than in the upright position, there is ordinarily less zone 1 blood flow (in the nondependent lung) in the former position compared with the latter position (Fig. 8-7). Nevertheless, blood flow to the dependent lung is still significantly greater than blood flow to the nondependent lung. Thus, when the right lung is nondependent, it should receive approximately 45 percent of the total blood flow, in contrast to the 55 percent of the total blood flow it receives in the upright and supine positions.[13,14] When the left lung is nondependent, it should receive approximately 35 percent of the total blood flow, in contrast to the 45 percent of the total blood flow that it receives in the upright and supine positions.[13,14]

Since gravity also causes a vertical gradient in pleural pressure (P_{pl}) (Figs. 8-3 and 8-4) in the lateral decubitus position (as it does in the upright position, Fig. 8-8A), ventilation is relatively increased in the dependent lung compared with the nondependent lung (Fig. 8-8B). In addition, in the lateral decubitus position, the dome of the lower diaphragm is pushed higher into the chest than the dome of the upper diaphragm; therefore, the lower diaphragm is more sharply curved than the upper diaphragm. As a result, the lower diaphragm is able to contract more efficiently during spontaneous respiration. Thus, in the lateral decubitus position in the awake patient, the lower

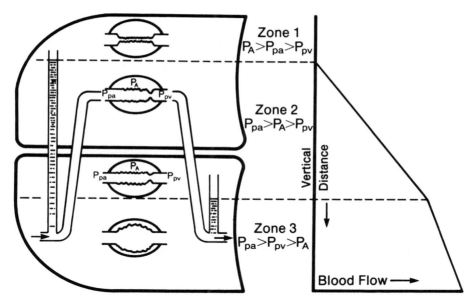

Fig. 8-7. Schematic representation of the effects of gravity on the distribution of pulmonary blood flow in the lateral decubitus position. The vertical gradient in the lateral decubitus position is less than in the upright position. Consequently, there is less zone 1 and more zone 2 and 3 blood flow in the lateral decubitus position compared with the upright position. Nevertheless, pulmonary blood flow increases with lung dependency and is greater in the dependent lung compared with the nondependent lung. P_A, alveolar pressure; P_a, pulmonary artery pressure; P_v, pulmonary venous pressure. (From Benumof,[124] with permission.)

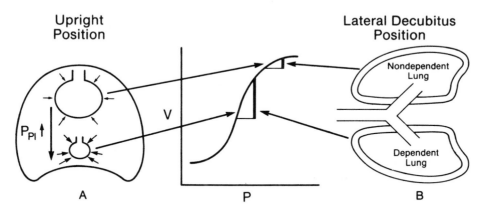

Fig. 8-8. Pleural pressure (P_{pl}) in the awake upright patient **(A)** is most positive in the dependent portion of the lung, and alveoli in this region are therefore most compressed and have the least volume. Pleural pressure is least positive (most negative) at the apex of the lung, and alveoli in this region are therefore least compressed and have the largest volume. When these regional differences in alveolar volume are translated over to a regional transpulmonary pressure-alveolar volume curve, the small dependent alveoli are on a steep (large slope) portion of the curve and the large nondependent alveoli are on a flat (small slope) portion of the curve. In this diagram, regional slope equals regional compliance. Thus, for a given and equal change in transpulmonary pressure, the dependent part of the lung receives a much larger share of the tidal volume than the nondependent part of the lung. In the lateral decubitus position **(B)**, gravity also causes pleural pressure gradients and therefore similarly affects the distribution of ventilation. The dependent lung lies on a relatively steep portion and the nondependent iung lies on a relatively flat portion of the pressure-volume curve. Thus, in the lateral decubitus position, the dependent lung receives the majority of the tidal ventilation. V, alveolar volume; P, transpulmonary pressure. (From Benumof,[124] with permission.)

lung is normally better ventilated than the upper lung, regardless of the side on which the patient is lying, although there remains a tendency toward greater ventilation of the larger right lung.[15] Since there is greater perfusion to the lower lung, the preferential ventilation to the lower lung is matched by its increased perfusion, so that the distribution of the $\dot{V}/\dot{Q}$ ratios of the two lungs is not greatly altered when the awake subject assumes the lateral decubitus position. Since perfusion increases to a greater extent than does ventilation with lung dependency, the $\dot{V}/\dot{Q}$ ratio decreases from nondependent to dependent lung (just as it does in upright and supine lungs).

Anesthetized, Closed Chest

Comparing the awake to the anesthetized patient in the lateral decubitus position, there is no difference in the distribution of pulmonary blood flow between the dependent and nondependent lungs. Thus, in the anesthetized patient, the dependent lung continues to receive relatively more perfusion than the nondependent lung. The induction of general anesthesia, however, does cause significant changes in the distribution of ventilation between the two lungs.

In the lateral decubitus position, the majority of ventilation is switched from the dependent lung in the awake subject to the nondependent lung in the anesthetized patient (Fig. 8-9).[16,17] There are several interrelated reasons for this change in the relative distribu-

tion of ventilation between the nondependent and dependent lung. First, the induction of general anesthesia usually causes a decrease in functional residual capacity (FRC), and both lungs share in the loss of lung volume. Since each lung occupies a different initial position on the pulmonary pressure-volume curve while the subject is awake, a general anesthesia-induced reduction in the FRC of each lung causes each lung to move to a lower but still different portion of the pressure-volume curve (Fig. 8-9). The dependent lung moves from an initially steep part of the curve (with the subject awake) to a lower and flatter part of the curve (after anesthesia is induced), while the nondependent lung moves from an initially flat portion of the pressure-volume curve (with the subject awake) to a lower and steeper part of the curve (after anesthesia is induced). Thus, with the induction of general anesthesia, the lower lung moves to a less favorable (flat, noncompliant) portion and the upper lung to a more favorable (steep, compliant) portion of the pressure-volume curve. Second, if the anesthetized patient in the lateral decubitus position is also paralyzed and artificially ventilated, the high curved diaphragm of the lower lung no longer confers any advantage in ventilation (as it does in the awake state), since it is no longer actively contracting.[18] Third, the mediastinum rests on the lower lung and physically impedes lower lung expansion, as well as selectively decreasing lower lung FRC. Fourth, the weight of the abdominal contents pushing cephalad against the diaphragm is

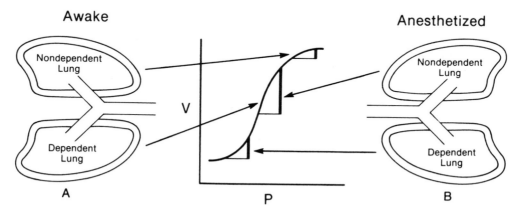

Fig. 8-9. Schematic diagram showing the distribution of ventilation in the awake patient in the lateral decubitus position **(A)** and the distribution of ventilation in the anesthetized patient in the lateral decubitus position **(B)**. The induction of anesthesia has caused a loss of lung volume in both lungs, with the nondependent lung moving from a flat, noncompliant portion to a steep, compliant portion of the pressure-volume curve and the dependent lung moving from a steep, compliant part to a flat, noncompliant part of the pressure-volume curve. Thus, the anesthetized patient in a lateral decubitus position has the majority of the tidal ventilation in the nondependent lung (where there is the least perfusion) and the minority of the tidal ventilation in the dependent lung (where there is the most perfusion). V, alveolar volume; P, transpulmonary pressure. (From Benumof,[124] with permission.)

greatest in the dependent lung, which physically impedes lower lung expansion the most and disproportionately decreases lower lung FRC. Finally, suboptimal positioning, which fails to provide room for lower lung expansion, may considerably compress the dependent lung. Opening the nondependent hemithorax further disproportionately increases ventilation to the nondependent lung.

In summary, the anesthetized patient (with or without paralysis) in the lateral decubitus position and with a closed chest has a nondependent lung that is well ventilated but poorly perfused and a dependent lung that is well perfused but poorly ventilated, resulting in an increased degree of mismatching of ventilation and perfusion. The application of positive end-expiratory pressure (PEEP) to both lungs restores the majority of ventilation to the lower lung.[14] Presumably, the lower lung returns to a steeper, more favorable part of the pressure-volume curve, and the upper lung resumes its original position on a flat, unfavorable portion of the curve.

Anesthetized, Open Chest

Compared with the condition of the anesthetized, closed-chest patient in the lateral decubitus position, opening the chest wall and pleural space alone does not ordinarily cause any significant alteration in the partitioning of pulmonary blood flow between the dependent and nondependent lungs; thus, the dependent lung continues to receive relatively more perfu-

sion than the nondependent lung. Opening the chest wall and pleural space, however, does have a significant impact on the distribution of ventilation (which must now be delivered by positive pressure). The change in the distribution of ventilation may result in a further mismatching of ventilation with perfusion (Fig. 8-10).[19]

If the upper lung is no longer restricted by a chest wall and the total effective compliance of that lung is equal to that of the lung parenchyma alone, it will be relatively free to expand and will consequently be overventilated (and remain underperfused). Conversely, the dependent lung may continue to be relatively noncompliant, poorly ventilated, and overperfused.[13] Surgical retraction and compression of the exposed upper lung can provide a partial, although nonphysiologic, solution to this problem: if expansion of the exposed lung is mechanically or externally restricted, ventilation will be diverted to the dependent, better-perfused lung.[20]

Anesthetized, Open Chest, Paralyzed

In the open-chest anesthetized patient in the lateral decubitus position, the induction of paralysis alone does not cause any significant alteration in the partitioning of pulmonary blood flow between the dependent and nondependent lungs. Thus, the dependent lung continues to receive relatively more perfusion than the nondependent lung. There are, however, strong theoretical and experimental considerations

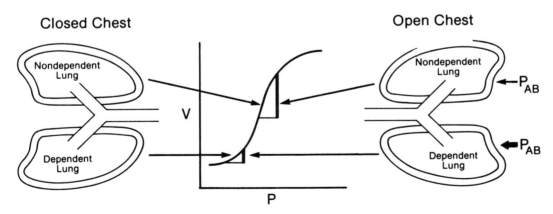

Fig. 8-10. Schematic diagram of a patient in the lateral decubitus position, comparing the closed-chest anesthetized condition with the open-chest anesthetized and paralyzed condition. Opening the chest increases nondependent-lung compliance and reinforces or maintains the larger part of the tidal ventilation going to the nondependent lung. Paralysis also reinforces or maintains the larger part of tidal ventilation going to the nondependent lung because the pressure of the abdominal contents (P_{AB}) pressing against the upper diaphragm is minimal (smaller arrow), and it is therefore easier for positive-pressure ventilation to displace this lesser resisting dome of the diaphragm. V, alveolar volume; P, transpulmonary pressure. (From Benumof,[124] with permission.)

that indicate that paralysis might cause significant changes in the distribution of ventilation between the two lungs under these conditions.

In the supine and lateral decubitus positions, the weight of the abdominal contents pressing against the diaphragm is greatest on the dependent part of the diaphragm (posterior lung and lower lung, respectively) and least on the nondependent part of the diaphragm (anterior lung and upper lung, respectively) (Fig. 8-10). In the awake, spontaneously breathing patient, the normally present active tension in the diaphragm overcomes the weight of the abdominal contents, and the diaphragm moves the most (largest excursion) in the dependent portion and least in the nondependent portion. This is a healthy circumstance because this is another factor that maintains the greatest amount of ventilation when there is the most perfusion (dependent lung) and the least amount of ventilation when there is the least perfusion (nondependent lung). During paralysis and positive-pressure breathing, the passive and flaccid diaphragm is displaced preferentially in the nondependent area, where the resistance to passive diaphragmatic movement by the abdominal contents is least; conversely, the diaphragm is displaced minimally in the dependent portion where the resistance to passive diaphragmatic movement by the abdominal contents is greatest.[21] This is an unhealthy circumstance because the greatest amount of ventilation may occur where there is the least perfusion (nondependent lung), and the least amount of ventilation may occur where there is the most perfusion (dependent lung).[21]

Summary of Physiology of Lateral Decubitus Position and the Open Chest

In summary (Fig. 8-11), the preceding section has developed the concept that the anesthetized, paralyzed patient in the lateral decubitus position with an open chest may have a considerable ventilation-perfusion mismatch, consisting of greater ventilation but less perfusion to the nondependent lung and less ventilation but more perfusion to the dependent lung. The blood flow distribution is mainly and simply determined by gravitational effects. The relatively good ventilation of the upper lung is caused, in part, by the open-chest and paralyzed conditions. The relatively poor ventilation of the dependent lung is caused, in part, by the loss of dependent-lung volume with general anesthesia and by compression of the dependent lung by the mediastinum, abdominal contents, and suboptimal positioning effects. In addition, poor mucociliary clearance and absorption atelectasis with an increased F_1O_2 may cause further dependent-lung volume loss. Consequently, two-lung ventilation under

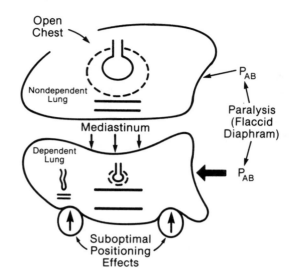

Fig. 8-11. Schematic summary of ventilation-perfusion relationships in the anesthetized patient in the lateral decubitus position who has an open chest and is paralyzed and suboptimally positioned. The nondependent lung is well ventilated (as indicated by the large dashed lines) but poorly perfused (small perfusion vessel), and the dependent lung is poorly ventilated (small dashed lines) but well perfused (large perfusion vessel). In addition, the dependent lung may also develop an atelectatic shunt compartment (indicated on the left side of the lower lung) because of the circumferential compression of this lung. (See text for detailed explanation.) P_{AB}, pressure of the abdominal contents. (From Benumof,[124] with permission.)

these circumstances may result in an increased alveolar-arterial oxygen tension difference $[P(_A - a)O_2]$ and less than optimal oxygenation.

A physiologic solution to the adverse effects of anesthesia and surgery in the lateral decubitus position on the distribution of ventilation and perfusion during two-lung ventilation would be the selective application of PEEP to the dependent lung (via a double-lumen endotracheal tube). Selective PEEP to the lower lung should increase the ventilation to this lung by moving it up to a steeper, more favorable portion of the lung pressure-volume curve. Indeed, this has been done with reasonably good success.[22] A series of 22 mechanically ventilated patients (both lungs) undergoing thoracotomy in the lateral decubitus position was divided into two groups. Group 1 patients had 10 cmH$_2$O of PEEP applied to the dependent lung while zero end-expiratory pressure (ZEEP) was applied to the nondependent lung. Group 2 (control) patients were intubated with a standard endotracheal tube, and both lungs were ventilated with ZEEP. Selective PEEP to the dependent lung in group 1 patients resulted in an adequate P_aO_2 with a lower inspired O_2 concentration during surgery and a smaller $P(_A - _a)O_2$ at the end of surgery than when both lungs were ventilated with ZEEP. Thus, even if the selective PEEP to the dependent lung increased dependent lung pulmonary vascular resistance and diverted some blood flow to the nondependent lung, the diverted blood flow could still participate in gas exchange with the ZEEP-ventilated nondependent lung.[23] However, it should be noted that this technique requires that the nondependent (and operative) lung be ventilated, which may impede the performance of surgery.

PHYSIOLOGY OF THE OPEN CHEST AND SPONTANEOUS VENTILATION

Mediastinal Shift

An examination of the physiology of the open chest during spontaneous ventilation reveals why controlled positive-pressure ventilation is the only practi-

cal way to provide adequate gas exchange during thoracotomy.[24] In the spontaneously breathing, closed-chest patient in the lateral decubitus position, gravity causes the pleural pressure in the dependent hemithorax to be less negative than in the nondependent hemithorax (Figs. 8-3, 8-4, and 8-8), but there is still negative pressure in each hemithorax on each side of the mediastinum. In addition, the weight of the mediastinum causes some compression of the lower lung, contributing to the pleural pressure gradient. With the nondependent hemithorax open, atmospheric pressure in that cavity exceeds the negative pleural pressure in the dependent hemithorax; this imbalance of pressure on the two sides of the mediastinum causes a further downward displacement of the mediastinum into the dependent thorax. During inspiration, the caudad movement of the dependent-lung diaphragm increases the negative pressure in the dependent lung and causes still further displacement of the mediastinum into the dependent hemithorax. During expiration, as the dependent-lung diaphragm moves cephalad, the pressure in the dependent hemithorax becomes relatively positive, and the mediastinum is pushed upward out of the dependent

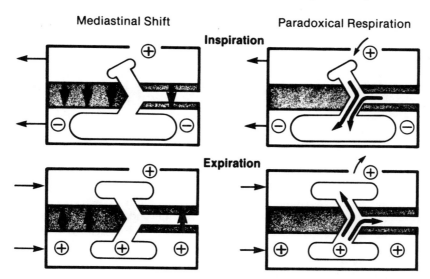

Fig. 8-12. Schematic representation of mediastinal shift and paradoxical respiration in the spontaneously ventilating patient with an open chest in the lateral decubitus position. The open chest is always exposed to atmospheric pressure ($\oplus$). During inspiration, negative pressure ($\ominus$) in the intact hemithorax causes the mediastinum to move vertically downward (mediastinal shift). In addition, during inspiration, movement of gas from the nondependent lung in the open hemithorax into the dependent lung in the closed hemithorax, and movement of air from the environment into the open hemithorax causes the lung in the open hemithorax to collapse (paradoxical respiration). During expiration, relative positive pressure ($\oplus$) in the closed hemithorax causes the mediastinum to move vertically upward (mediastinal shift). In addition, during expiration, the gas moves from the dependent lung to the nondependent lung and from the open hemithorax to the environment; consequently, the nondependent lung expands during expiration (paradoxical respiration). (From Benumof,[124] with permission.)

hemithorax (Fig. 8-12). Thus, the tidal volume in the dependent lung is decreased by an amount equal to the inspiratory displacement caused by mediastinal movement. This phenomenon is called *mediastinal shift* and is one mechanism that results in impaired ventilation in the open-chest, spontaneously breathing patient in the lateral decubitus position. The mediastinal shift can also cause circulatory changes (decreased venous return) and reflexes (sympathetic activation) that result in a clinical picture similar to shock: the patient is hypotensive, pale, and cold, with dilated pupils. Local anesthetic infiltration of the pulmonary plexus at the hilum and the vagus nerve can diminish these reflexes. More practically, controlled positive-pressure ventilation abolishes these ventilatory and circulatory changes associated with mediastinal shift.

Paradoxical Respiration

When a pleural cavity is exposed to atmospheric pressure, the lung is no longer held open by negative intrapleural pressure, and it tends to collapse because of unopposed elastic recoil.[24] Thus, the lung in an open chest is at least partially collapsed. It has long been observed during spontaneous ventilation with an open hemithorax that lung collapse is accentuated during inspiration, and, conversely, the lung expands during expiration. This reversal of lung movement with an open chest during respiration has been termed *paradoxical respiration*. The mechanism of paradoxical respiration is similar to that of mediastinal shift. During inspiration, the descent of the diaphragm on the side of the open hemithorax causes air from the environment to enter the pleural cavity on that side through the thoracotomy opening and fill the space around the exposed lung. The descent of the hemidiaphragm on the closed-chest side causes gas to enter the closed-chest lung in the normal manner. However, gas also enters the closed-chest lung (which has a relatively negative pressure) from the open-chest lung (which remains at atmospheric pressure); this results in further reduction in the size of the open-chest lung during inspiration. During expiration, the reverse occurs, with the collapsed, open-chest lung filling from the intact lung and air moving back out of the exposed hemithorax through the thoracotomy incision. The phenomenon of paradoxical respiration is illustrated in Figure 8-12. Paradoxical breathing is increased by a large thoracotomy and by increased airway resistance in the intact lung. Paradoxical respiration may be prevented either by manual collapse of the open-chest lung or, more commonly, by controlled positive-pressure ventilation.

PHYSIOLOGY OF ONE-LUNG VENTILATION

Comparison of Arterial Oxygenation and CO_2 Elimination During Two-Lung Versus One-Lung Ventilation

As discussed previously, the matching of ventilation and perfusion is impaired during two-lung ventilation in an anesthetized, paralyzed, open-chest patient in the lateral decubitus position. The reason for the mismatching of ventilation and perfusion is relatively good ventilation but poor perfusion of the nondependent lung and poor ventilation and good perfusion of the dependent lung (Fig. 8-11). The blood flow distribution was seen to be determined by gravitational effects. The relatively good ventilation of the nondependent lung was seen to be caused, in part, by the open chest and paralysis. The relatively poor ventilation of the dependent lung was seen to be caused, in part, by the loss of dependent lung volume with general anesthesia and by circumferential compression of the dependent lung by the mediastinum, abdominal contents, and suboptimal positioning effect. The compression of the dependent lung may also cause the development of a shunt compartment in the dependent lung (Fig. 8-11). Consequently, two-lung ventilation under these circumstances may result in an increased $P(A - a)O_2$ and impaired oxygenation.

If the nondependent lung is nonventilated, as during one-lung ventilation, then any blood flow to the nonventilated lung becomes shunt flow, in addition to whatever shunt flow might exist in the dependent lung (Fig. 8-13). Thus, one-lung ventilation creates an obligatory right-to-left transpulmonary shunt through the nonventilated nondependent lung, which is not present during two-lung ventilation. Consequently, it is not surprising to find that, given the same inspired oxygen concentration (F_IO_2) and hemodynamic and metabolic status, one-lung ventilation results in a much larger alveolar-to-arterial oxygen tension difference and lower P_aO_2 than does two-lung ventilation. This contention is supported by numerous studies that compared arterial oxygenation during two-lung ventilation with one-lung ventilation under a wide variety of conditions, but specifically when each of the patients served as their own control.[25–39]

One-lung ventilation has much less of an effect on P_aCO_2 in comparison with its effect on P_aO_2. Blood passing through underventilated alveoli retains more than a normal amount of CO_2 and does not take up a normal amount of O_2; blood traversing overventilated alveoli gives off more than a normal amount of CO_2 but cannot take up a proportionately increased

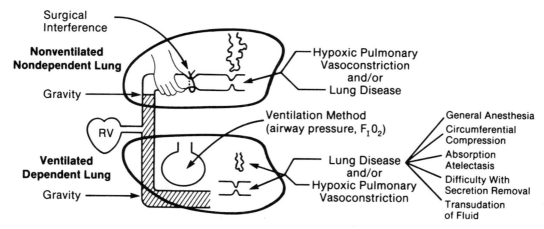

Fig. 8-13. Schematic diagram showing the major determinants of blood flow distribution during one-lung ventilation. Blood flow to the nonventilated, nondependent lung is reduced by the force of gravity, surgical interference (compression, tying off of vessels), hypoxic pulmonary vasoconstriction, and/or lung disease (vascular obliteration, thrombosis). Blood flow to the ventilated, dependent lung is increased by gravity; however, dependent-lung blood flow and vascular resistance may be altered in either direction depending on the method of ventilation (amount of airway pressure, F_IO_2, and the amount of dependent-lung disease and/ or hypoxic pulmonary vasoconstriction). Factors that may increase the amount of dependent lung disease intraoperatively are listed on the extreme right of the figure. (From Benumof,[125] with permission.)

amount of O_2 due to the flatness of the top end of the oxygen-hemoglobin dissociation curve. Thus, during one-lung ventilation, the ventilated lung can eliminate enough CO_2 to compensate for the nonventilated lung, and P_aCO_2-to-P_aCO_2 gradients are small; however, the ventilated lung cannot take up enough O_2 to compensate for the nonventilated lung, and P_AO_2-to-P_aO_2 gradients are usually large.

Blood Flow Distribution During One-Lung Ventilation

Blood Flow to the Nondependent, Nonventilated Lung

Fortunately, there are usually both passive mechanical and active vasoconstrictor mechanisms operating during one-lung ventilation that minimize the blood flow to the nondependent, nonventilated lung, thereby preventing the P_aO_2 from decreasing as much as might be expected on the basis of the distribution of blood flow during two-lung ventilation. The passive mechanical mechanisms that decrease blood flow to the nondependent lung consist of gravity, surgical interference with blood flow, and, perhaps, the amount of pre-existing disease in the nondependent lung (Fig. 8-13). Gravity causes a vertical gradient in the distribution of pulmonary blood flow in the lateral decubitus position for the same reason that it does in the

upright position (Fig. 8-7). Consequently, blood flow to the nondependent lung is less than blood flow to the dependent lung. The gravity component of blood flow reduction to the nondependent lung should be constant with respect to both time and magnitude.

Surgical compression (directly compressing lung vessels) and retraction (causing kinking and tortuosity of lung vessels) of the nondependent lung may further passively reduce nondependent lung blood flow. In addition, ligation of pulmonary vessels during pulmonary resection will greatly decrease nondependent lung blood flow. The surgical interference component of blood flow reduction to the nondependent lung should be variable with respect to both time and magnitude.

The amount of disease in the nondependent lung is also a significant determinant of the amount of blood flow to the nondependent lung. If the nondependent lung is severely diseased, then there may be a fixed reduction in blood flow to this lung preoperatively and collapse of such a diseased lung may not cause much of an increase in shunt. The notion that a diseased pulmonary vasculature might be incapable of hypoxic pulmonary vasoconstriction (HPV) is supported by the observations that administration of sodium nitroprusside and nitroglycerin (which should abolish any pre-existing HPV) to chronic obstructive pulmonary disease patients (who have a fixed reduction in the cross-sectional area of their pulmonary vascular bed) does not cause an increase in shunt,[26] whereas these drugs do increase shunt in patients with acute regional lung disease who have an otherwise normal pulmonary vascular bed.[27] If the nondependent lung is normal and has a normal amount of blood flow preoperatively, then collapse of such a normal lung may be associated with a higher nonventilated, nondependent lung blood flow and shunt. A higher one-lung ventilation shunt through the nondependent lung may be more likely to occur in patients who require thoracotomy for nonpulmonary disease.[28] However, the above theoretical relationship between the amount of nondependent lung disease and shunt during one-lung ventilation has not been systematically studied.

The most significant reduction in blood flow to the nondependent lung is caused by an active vasoconstrictor mechanism. The normal response of the pulmonary vasculature to atelectasis is an increase in pulmonary vascular resistance (in just the atelectatic lung); the increase in atelectatic lung pulmonary vascular resistance is thought to be due almost entirely to HPV.[29-31] The selective increase in atelectatic lung pulmonary vascular resistance diverts blood flow away from the atelectatic lung toward the remaining normoxic or hyperoxic ventilated lung. The diversion of blood flow minimizes the amount of shunt flow that occurs through the hypoxic lung. Figure 8-14 shows

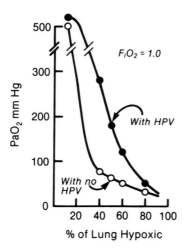

Fig. 8-14. A model of the effect of hypoxic pulmonary vasoconstriction (HPV) on P_aO_2 as a function of the percent of lung that is hypoxic. The model assumes an F_IO_2 of 1.0, a normal hemoglobin, cardiac output, and oxygen consumption. In the range of 30 to 70 percent of the lung being hypoxic, the normal expected amount of HPV can increase P_aO_2 significantly. (From Benumof,[124] with permission.)

the theoretically expected effect of HPV on arterial oxygen tension (P_aO_2) as the amount of lung that is made hypoxic increases.[32] When very little of the lung is hypoxic (near 0 percent), it does not matter, in terms of P_aO_2, whether the small amount of lung has HPV operating or not because, in either case, the shunt will be small. When most of the lung is hypoxic (near 100 percent), there is no significant normoxic region to which the hypoxic region can divert flow, and, again, it does not matter, in terms of P_aO_2, whether the hypoxic region has HPV operating or not. When the percentage of lung that is hypoxic is intermediate (between 30 and 70 percent), which is the amount of lung that is typically hypoxic during the one-lung ventilation/anesthesia condition, there is a large difference between the P_aO_2 expected with a normal amount of HPV (which is a 50 percent blood flow reduction for a single lung) compared to when there is no HPV.[32] In fact, in this range of hypoxic lung, HPV can increase P_aO_2 from hypoxemic levels to much higher and safer values. It is not surprising, then, that numerous clinical studies of one-lung ventilation have found that the shunt through the nonventilated lung is usually 20 to 30 percent of the cardiac output as opposed to the 40 to 50 percent shunt that might be expected if there was no HPV operating in the nonventilated lung.[25,28,33-39] Thus, HPV is an autoregulatory mechanism that protects the P_aO_2 by decreasing the amount of shunt flow that can occur through hypoxic lung.

Figure 8-15 outlines the major determinants of the amount of atelectatic lung HPV that might occur during anesthesia. In the following discussion, the HPV issues or considerations are numbered as they are in Figure 8-15.

1. The distribution of the alveolar hypoxia is probably not a determinant of the amount of HPV; all regions of the lung (either the basilar or dependent parts of the lungs [supine or upright] or discrete anatomic units such as a lobe or single lung) respond to alveolar hypoxia with vasoconstriction.[40]

2. As with low $\dot{V}/\dot{Q}$ ratios and nitrogen-ventilated lungs, it appears that the vast majority of blood flow reduction in acutely atelectatic lung is due to HPV, and none of the blood flow reduction is due to passive mechanical factors (such as vessel tortuosity).[29-31] This conclusion is based on the observation that re-expansion and ventilation of a collapsed lung with nitrogen (removing any mechanical factor) does not increase the blood flow to the lung, whereas ventilation with oxygen restores all of the blood flow back to precollapse values. This conclusion applies whether ventila-

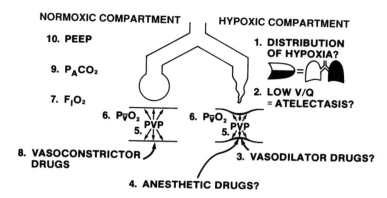

Fig. 8-15. Diagram showing many of the components of the anesthetic experience that might determine the amount of regional HPV. The clockwise numbering of considerations corresponds to the order in which these considerations are discussed in the text. $\dot{V}/\dot{Q}$, ventilation-to-perfusion ratio; PVP, pulmonary vascular pressure; $P\bar{v}O_2$, mixed venous oxygen tension; F_IO_2, inspired oxygen tension; P_ACO_2, alveolar carbon dioxide tension; PEEP, positive end-expiratory pressure. (From Benumof,[126] with permission.)

tion is spontaneous or with positive pressure, and whether the chest is open or closed.[30] In canines, a slight amount of further subacute ($>$ 30 minutes) decrease in blood flow to atelectic lung may have been due to some mechanical effect of the atelectasis on lung blood vessels.[41] However, in humans, a prolonged unilateral hypoxic challenge during anesthesia results in an immediate vasoconstrictor response with no further potentiation or diminution of the HPV response.[42]

3. Most systemic vasodilator drugs have been shown to either directly inhibit regional HPV or to have an effect in a clinical situation that is consistent with inhibition of regional HPV (ie, decreasing P_aO_2 and increasing shunt in patients with acute respiratory disease). The vasodilator drugs that have been shown to inhibit HPV or to have a clinical effect consistent with inhibition of HPV are nitroglycerin,[27,43–49] nitroprusside,[27,50–56] dobutamine,[57,58] several calcium antagonists,[59–64] and many beta$_2$-agonists (isoproterenol, ritodrine, orciprenaline, salbutamol, adenosine triphosphatase, and glucagon).[58,65–71] Aminophylline and hydralazine may not decrease HPV.[72,73]

4. The effect of anesthetic drugs on regional HPV must be considered from both experimental (animal studies) and clinical (human one-lung ventilation studies) points of view, as discussed below.
   a. *Effect of anesthetics on experimental hypoxic pulmonary vasoconstriction.* An undesirable property of general anesthesia would be inhibition of HPV in the nonventilated, nondependent lung by the anesthetic drug. All of the

inhalation and many of the injectable anesthetics have been studied with regard to their effect on HPV. These studies have been referenced in great detail by Benumof.[74] Halothane has been most extensively studied. The experimental preparations used may be divided into four basic categories: (1) in vitro; (2) in vivo-not intact (pumped perfused lungs, no systemic circulation or neural function); (3) in vivo-intact (normally perfused lungs, normal systemic circulation); and (4) humans (volunteers or patients). It appears, according to this experimental preparation breakdown, that the inhibition of HPV by halothane is a universal finding in the in vitro and in vivo-not intact preparations. However, in the more normal or physiologic in vivo-intact and human studies, halothane has caused none or only a very slight decrease in HPV response. Thus, it appears that a fundamental property of halothane is its inhibition of HPV in experimental preparations, which can be controlled for other physiologic influences (eg, pulmonary vascular pressure, cardiac output, mixed venous oxygen tension, CO$_2$ level, temperature) that can have an effect on the HPV response. In the more biologically complex in vivo-intact models, other factors seem to be involved that greatly diminish the inhibitory effect of halothane on HPV. Important methodologic differences between the in vitro and in vivo-not intact preparations and the in vivo-intact and human models that could account for the observed differences in halothane effect on HPV are presence (or absence) of perfusion pulsations, perfusion fluid composition, size of perfusion circuit, baroreceptor influences, absence of bronchial blood flow (which abolishes all central and autonomic nervous activity in the lung), chemical influences (ie, pH, PO_2), humoral influences (ie, histamine and prostaglandin release from body tissues), lymph flow influences, unaccounted-for or uncontrolled changes in physiologic variables (such as cardiac output, mixed venous oxygen tension, and pulmonary vascular pressures, which might have directionally opposite effects on HPV), and, very importantly, the use of different species.

Ether has been the next most studied drug, and it appears that the quantitative effect of ether on HPV is also dependent on the type of experimental preparation used. Thus, the in vitro and in vivo-not intact models show much more inhibition of HPV by ether than the in vivo-intact and human models. Although the number of studies involving halogenated drugs other than halothane (namely, isoflurane, enflurane, methoxyflurane, fluroxene, and trichlorethylene), has been too small to permit recognition of an experimental preparation result pattern, most of these anesthetics have demonstrated inhibition of HPV (at least in the in vitro models). Nitrous oxide seems to cause a small, somewhat consistant inhibition of HPV. All injectable anesthetics studied to date have no effect on HPV.

To summarize previous animal studies, it appears that a fundamental property of inhalational anesthetics is to decrease HPV. However, in intact animal preparations, some biologic or physiologic property seems to remove or greatly lessen the inhibitory effect of anesthetic drugs on HPV. It may be that the cause(s) of the difference in effect of anesthetic drugs on regional HPV from preparation to preparation, anesthetic to anesthetic, and species to species (see below) is closely related to the fundamental mechanism of HPV, which is still unknown.

b. *Effect of anesthetics on arterial oxygenation during clinical one-lung ventilation.* An often-made extrapolation of the much more numerous in vitro and in vivo-not intact HPV studies is that anesthetic drugs might impair arterial oxygenation during one-lung anesthesia by inhibiting HPV in the nonventilated lung. One of the previously cited studies on the effect of isoflurane on regional canine HPV was especially well controlled and showed that when all nonanesthetic drug variables that might change regional HPV are kept constant, isoflurane inhibits single-lung HPV in a dose-dependent manner.[75] Additionally, the study is valuable because the investigators offer an easily comprehensible quantitative summary of the relationship between dose of isoflurane administered and degree of inhibition of the single-lung canine HPV response. If the summary can be extrapolated or applied to the clinical one-lung ventilation situation (at least as an approximation), insights can be gained into what might be expected with regard to arterial oxygenation when such patients are anesthetized with isoflurane. To put this insight into clinical focus, it is necessary to first understand what should happen to blood flow, shunt flow, and arterial oxygenation, as a function of a normal amount of HPV, when two-lung ventilation is changed to one-lung ventilation in the lateral decubitus position. Once the stable one-lung ventilation condition has been described, it is then possible, using the data from the previously mentioned study, to see how isoflurane administration would affect the one-lung ventilation blood flow distribution, shunt flow, and the arterial oxygen tension.

  i. *Two-lung ventilation: blood flow distribution.* Gravity causes a vertical gradient in the distribution of pulmonary blood flow in the lateral decubitus position for the same reason that it does in the upright position (Fig. 8-7). From Figure 8-7 and the previous discussion, the average two-lung ventilation blood flow distribution in the lateral decubitus position would consist of 40 percent of total blood flow perfusing the nondependent lung and 60 percent of total blood flow perfusing the dependent lung (Fig. 8-16, left-hand side of figure).

  ii. *One-lung ventilation: blood flow distribution, shunt flow, and arterial oxygen tension.* When the nondependent lung is nonventilated (made atelectatic), HPV in the nondependent lung will increase nondependent lung pulmonary vascular resistance and decrease nondependent lung blood flow. In the absence of any confounding or inhibiting factors to the HPV response, a single-lung HPV response should decrease the blood flow to that lung by 50 percent.[32] Consequently, the nondependent lung should be able to reduce its blood flow

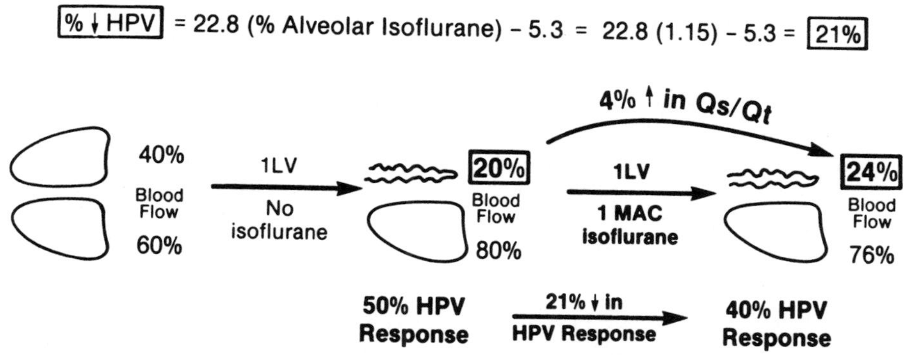

$$\boxed{\% \downarrow \text{HPV}} = 22.8 \, (\% \text{ Alveolar Isoflurane}) - 5.3 = 22.8 \, (1.15) - 5.3 = \boxed{21\%}$$

Fig. 8-16. Schematic diagram showing the effect of 1 MAC isoflurane anesthesia on shunt during one-lung ventilation (1 LV) of normal lungs. The two-lung ventilation nondependent/dependent lung blood flow ratio is 40/60 percent (left-hand side). When two-lung ventilation is converted to one-lung ventilation (as indicated by atelectasis of the nondependent lung), the HPV response decreases the blood flow to the nondependent lung by 50 percent, so that the nondependent/dependent lung blood flow ratio is now 20/80 percent (middle). According to the data of Domino et al, administration of 1 MAC isoflurane anesthesia should cause a 21 percent decrease in the HPV response, which would decrease the 50 percent blood flow reduction to a 40 percent blood flow reduction in the HPV response.[75] Consequently, the nondependent/dependent lung blood flow ratio would now become 24/76 percent, representing a 4 percent increase in the total shunt across the lungs (right-hand side). (From Benumof,[127] with permission.)

from 40 to 20 percent of total blood flow, and the nondependent-to-dependent lung blood flow ratio during one-lung ventilation should be 20 to 80 percent (Fig. 8-16, middle).

All the blood flow to the nonventilated nondependent lung is shunt flow; therefore, one-lung ventilation creates an obligatory right-to-left transpulmonary shunt flow that was not present during two-lung ventilation. If no shunt existed during two-lung ventilation conditions (ignoring the normal 1 to 3 percent shunt flow due to the bronchial, pleural, and thebesian circulations), it would be expected that the ideal total shunt flow during one-lung ventilation (that is, with intact HPV) would be a minimal 20 percent of total blood flow. With a normal hemodynamic and metabolic state, the arterial oxygen tension should be approximately 280 mmHg.[76] Other, much more complicated, models have been constructed to describe what to expect in terms of shunt during one-lung ventilation when varying degrees of shunt exist during two-lung ventilation.[77]

iii. *Effect of isoflurane on the one-lung ventilation blood flow distribution, shunt flow, and arterial oxygen tension.* Domino et al found that the percent inhibition of regional HPV response was equal to 22.8 (percent alveo-lar isoflurane) minus 5.3 (Fig. 8-16, top equation).[75] The top equation and right-hand side of Figure 8-16 show that one minimum alveolar concentration (MAC) isoflurane anesthesia would inhibit the nondependent lung HPV response by approximately 21 percent, which would decrease the nondependent lung HPV response from a 50 to 40 percent nondependent lung blood flow reduction; this, in turn, would increase nondependent lung blood flow from 20 to 24 percent of total blood flow, causing shunt to increase by 4 percent of the cardiac output and P_aO_2 to decrease a moderate amount to 205 mmHg ($F_IO_2 = 1.0$). A decrease in P_aO_2 and an increase in shunt of this magnitude is small and may not be detectable given the usual accuracy of clinical methodology. In fact, in clinical one-lung ventilation studies involving intravenously anesthetized patients with this level of shunting, administration of 1 MAC isoflurane (and halothane) anesthesia during stable one-lung ventilation conditions caused no detectable decrease in P_aO_2.[33,78] In one of these clinical studies, stable one-lung ventilation conditions in the lateral decubitus position were established in patients who were anesthetized with only intravenous drugs.[33] While stable one-lung ventilation was maintained, inhalational anesthetics were administered (halothane and isoflurane end-tidal concentrations were > 1 MAC for at least 15 minutes) and then discontinued (halothane and isoflurane end-tidal concentrations decreased to near zero). In the other study, steady-state one-lung ventilation conditions in the lateral decubitus position were established in patients who were anesthetized with only inhalational drugs (halothane and isoflurane end-tidal concentrations were > 1 MAC for more than 40 minutes).[78] While one-lung ventilation was continued, inhalational anesthesia was then discontinued, and intravenous anesthesia administered (halothane and isoflurane end-tidal concentrations decreased to near zero). There was no significant difference in P_aO_2 during inhalation anesthesia with either halothane or isoflurane compared with intravenous anesthesia during one-lung ventilation in either of the two experimental sequences. In addition, there were no significant changes in physiologic variables, such as cardiac output, pulmonary vascular pressure, and mixed venous oxygen tension, that might secondarily alter nondependent lung HPV. Thus, irrespective of whether inhalational anesthesia is administered before or after intravenous anesthesia during one-lung ventilation, inhalation anesthesia does not further impair arterial oxygenation. These findings are consistent with the interpretation that 1 MAC halothane and isoflurane in patients with a moderate level of shunting does not inhibit HPV enough to cause a significant decrease in P_aO_2 during one-lung ventilation in the lateral decubitus position. Almost identical results have been obtained during one-lung ventilation of volunteers with nitrogen (while the other lung was ventilated with 100 percent oxygen) who were alternately anesthetized with isoflurane and intravenous drugs[79] and enflurane and intravenous drugs.[80]

5. The HPV response is maximal when pulmonary vascular pressure is normal and is decreased by either high or low pulmonary vascular pressure. The mechanism for high pulmonary vascular pressure inhibition of HPV is simple: the pulmonary circulation is poorly endowed with smooth muscle and cannot constrict against an increased vascular pressure.[81–83] The mechanism for low pulmonary vascular pressure inhibition of HPV is

more complex. In order for this to occur, the hypoxic compartment must be atelectatic. Under these circumstances, when pulmonary vascular pressure decreases, it is possible for part of the ventilated lung (but not the atelectatic lung) to be in a zone 1 condition (alveolar pressure increases relative to pulmonary artery pressure) and experience a disproportionate increase in pulmonary vascular resistance, which would divert blood flow back over to the atelectatic lung, thereby inhibiting atelectatic lung HPV.[84]

6. The HPV response is also maximal when the mixed venous oxygen tension ($P\bar{v}O_2$) is normal and is decreased by either high or low $P\bar{v}O_2$. The mechanism for high $P\bar{v}O_2$ inhibition of HPV is presumably due to reverse diffusion of oxygen, causing the oxygen tension of either the vessels, interstitial or alveolar spaces, or all of these to be increased above the HPV threshold.[85] That is, if enough oxygen can get to some receptor in the small arteriole-capillary-alveolar area, then the vessels will not vasoconstrict. The mechanism for low $P\bar{v}O_2$ inhibition of HPV is a result of the low $P\bar{v}O_2$ decreasing alveolar oxygen tension in the normoxic compartment down to a level sufficient to induce HPV in the supposedly "normoxic" lung.[86,87] The HPV in the "normoxic" lung competes against and offsets the HPV in the originally hypoxic lung and results in no blood flow diversion away from the more obviously hypoxic lung.

7. Selectively decreasing the F_IO_2 in the normoxic compartment (from 1.0 to 0.5–0.3) will cause an increase in normoxic lung vascular tone, thereby decreasing blood flow diversion from hypoxic to normoxic lung.[83,87]

8. Vasoconstrictor drugs (dopamine, epinephrine, phenylephrine) seem to constrict normoxic lung vessels preferentially, thereby disproportionately increasing normoxic lung vascular resistance.[58,62,68,81] The increase in normoxic lung vascular resistance will decrease normoxic lung blood flow and increase atelectatic lung blood flow. The HPV-inhibiting effect of vasoconstrictor drugs is similar to decreasing normoxic lung F_IO_2.

9. Hypocapnia has been thought to inhibit directly regional HPV and hypercapnia to enhance directly regional HPV.[82,88] In addition, during one-lung ventilation conditions, hypocapnia can only be produced by hyperventilation of the one lung. The hyperventilation requires an increased ventilated lung airway pressure, which may cause increased ventilated lung pulmonary vascular resistance, which in turn may divert blood flow back into the hypoxic lung. Hypercapnia during one-lung ventilation seems to act as a vasoconstrictor

drug by selectively increasing ventilated lung pulmonary vascular resistance (which would divert blood flow back to the nonventilated lung). In addition, hypercapnia is ordinarily caused by hypoventilation of the ventilated lung, which greatly increases the risk of developing low $\dot{V}/\dot{Q}$ and atelectatic regions in the dependent lung. However, it should be noted as a theoretical possibility that if hypoventilation of the dependent lung is associated with decreased ventilated lung airway pressure, ventilated lung pulmonary vascular resistance may be decreased, which in turn would promote or enhance HPV in the nonventilated lung.

10. The effects of changes in airway pressure due to PEEP and tidal volume changes will be discussed in detail in the section on the methods used to ventilate the dependent lung. In brief, selective application of PEEP to just normoxic ventilated lung will selectively increase pulmonary vascular resistance in the ventilated lung and shunt blood flow back into the hypoxic nonventilated lung (ie, decrease nonventilated lung HPV).[89,90] On the other hand, high-frequency ventilation of the gas-exchanging lung is associated with a low airway pressure and an enhancement of HPV in the collapsed lung.[91]

Finally, there is some evidence that certain types of infections (which may cause atelectasis), particularly granulomatous and pneumococcal infections, may inhibit HPV.[92,93]

Blood Flow to the Dependent, Ventilated Lung

The dependent lung usually has an increased amount of blood flow due to both passive gravitational effects and active nondependent lung vasoconstrictor effects (Fig. 8-13, lower panel). However, the dependent lung may also have a hypoxic compartment (areas of low $\dot{V}/\dot{Q}$ ratio and atelectasis) that was present preoperatively or that developed intraoperatively. The dependent lung hypoxic compartment may develop intraoperatively for several reasons. First, in the lateral decubitus position, the ventilated dependent lung usually has a reduced lung volume owing to the combined factors of induction of general anesthesia and circumferential (and perhaps severe) compression by the mediastinum from above, by the abdominal contents pressing against the diaphragm from the caudad side, and by suboptimal positioning effects (rolls, packs, chest supports) pushing in from the dependent side and axilla (Fig. 8-13).[14,18,21,94] Second, absorption atelectasis can also occur in regions of the dependent lung that have low $\dot{V}/\dot{Q}$ ratios when they are exposed to a high inspired oxygen concentration.[95,96] Third,

difficulty in secretion removal may cause the development of poorly ventilated and atelectatic areas in the dependent lung. Finally, maintaining the lateral decubitus position for prolonged periods of time may cause fluid to transude into the dependent lung (which may be vertically below the left atrium) and cause further decreased lung volume and increased airway closure in the dependent lung.[97]

The development of a low $\dot{V}/\dot{Q}$ ratio and/or atelectatic areas in the dependent lung will increase vascular resistance in the dependent lung[94,98] (due to dependent lung HPV[40]), thereby decreasing dependent lung blood flow and increasing nondependent lung blood flow.[99] Stated differently, the pulmonary vascular resistance in the ventilated compartment of the lung determines the ability of the ventilated, and supposedly normoxic, lung to accept redistributed blood flow from the hypoxic lung. Clinical conditions that are independent of specific dependent lung disease, but which may still increase dependent lung vascular resistance in a dose-dependent manner, are a decreasing inspired oxygen tension in the dependent lung (from 1.0 to 0.5–0.3)[83,87,99] and a decreasing temperature (from 40° to 30°C).[100]

Miscellaneous Causes of Hypoxemia During One-Lung Ventilation

Still other factors may contribute to hypoxemia during one-lung ventilation. Hypoxemia due to mechanical failure of the O_2 supply system or the anesthesia machine is a recognized hazard of any kind of anesthesia. Gross hypoventilation of the dependent lung can be a major cause of hypoxemia. Malfunction of the dependent lung airway lumen (blockage by secretions) and malposition of the double-lumen endotracheal tube are, from experience, the most common causes of an increased $P(A-a)O_2$ and hypoxemia. Resorption of residual oxygen from the clamped nonventilated lung is time-dependent and accounts for a gradual increase in shunt and decrease in P_aO_2 after one-lung ventilation is initiated.[98] With all other anesthetic and surgical factors constant, anything that decreases the $P\bar{v}O_2$ (decreased cardiac output, increased oxygen consumption [excessive sympathetic nervous system stimulation, hyperthermia, shivering]) will cause an increased $P(A-a)O_2$.[101,102]

Management of One-Lung Ventilation

Conventional Management

The proper initial conventional management of one-lung ventilation is logically based on the preceding determinants of blood flow distribution during one-lung ventilation. In view of the fact that one-lung ventilation incurs a definite risk of causing systemic hypoxemia, it is extremely important that dependent-lung ventilation, as it affects these determinants, be optimally managed. This section considers the usual management of one-lung ventilation in terms of the most appropriate F_IO_2, tidal volume, and respiratory rate that should be used.

Inspired Oxygen Concentration

Although the theoretical possibilities of absorption atelectasis and oxygen toxicity exist, the benefits of ventilating the dependent lung with 100 percent oxygen far exceed the risks. A high F_IO_2 in the single ventilated lung may critically increase the P_aO_2 from arrhythmogenic and life-threatening levels to safer levels. In addition, a high F_IO_2 in the dependent lung will cause vasodilation, thereby increasing the dependent-lung capability of accepting blood flow redistribution due to nondependent-lung HPV.[83] Direct chemical 100 percent oxygen toxicity will not occur during the time frame of the operative period,[103] and absorption atelectasis in the dependent lung[96] is unlikely to occur in view of the remaining one-lung ventilation management characteristics (moderately large tidal volumes with intermittent positive-pressure, low-level PEEP).

Tidal Volume

The dependent lung should be ventilated with a tidal volume of approximately 10 mL/kg. Use of a tidal volume much less than 10 mL/kg might promote dependent-lung atelectasis. Use of a tidal volume much greater than 10 mL/kg might excessively increase dependent-lung airway pressure and vascular resistance,[98] thereby increasing nondependent-lung blood flow (decreasing nondependent-lung HPV).[89,104,105] If a tidal volume of 10 mL/kg causes excessive airway pressure, it should be lowered (after mechanical causes, ie, tube malfunction, have been ruled out) and the respiratory rate increased.

A dependent-lung tidal volume of 10 mL/kg represents a volume that is in the middle of a range of tidal volumes (8 to 15 mL/kg) that have been found in one study not to greatly affect arterial oxygenation during one-lung ventilation.[36] In that study, changes in P_aO_2 with alterations in the tidal volume (during stable one-lung ventilation conditions) in individual patients were variable and unpredictable in both degree and direction (although the mean value for the group did not change). Thus, it appears that changing the tidal volume from 15 to 8 mL/kg during one-lung ventilation has an unpredictable, but usually not great, impact on arterial oxygenation.[36] No dependent-lung

PEEP should be used initially because of concern of unnecessarily increasing dependent-lung vascular resistance (see the section *Selective Dependent-Lung PEEP*).

Respiratory Rate

The respiratory rate should be set so that the P_aCO_2 remains at 40 mmHg. Since a dependent-lung tidal volume of 10 mL/kg represents a 20 percent decrease from the usual two-lung tidal volume of 12 mL/kg, the respiratory rate usually needs to be increased by 20 percent in order to maintain carbon dioxide homeostasis. The trade-off between decreased tidal volume and increased respiratory rate usually results in a constant minute ventilation; although ventilation and perfusion are considerably mismatched during one-lung ventilation, and unchanged minute ventilation during one-lung ventilation (compared to two-lung ventilation) can continue to eliminate a normal amount of carbon dioxide due to the high diffusability of carbon dioxide.[98,106–108] Hypocapnia should be avoided because use of the airway pressure in the dependent lung necessary to produce systemic hypocapnia may excessively increase dependent-lung vascular resistance. Furthermore, hypocapnia may directly inhibit HPV in the nondependent lung.[82,88]

In summary, on the commencement of one-lung ventilation, 100 percent oxygen, a tidal volume of 10 mL/kg, and a 20 percent increase in respiratory rate are used as initial ventilation settings. Ventilation and arterial oxygenation are monitored by use of frequent arterial blood gases, end-tidal carbon dioxide concentration, and pulse oximetry or transcutaneous gas tensions. If there is a problem with either ventilation or arterial oxygenation, one or more of the differential lung management techniques described below is used.

Differential Lung Management

Selective Dependent-Lung PEEP

Since the ventilated dependent lung often has a decreased lung volume during one-lung ventilation (Figs. 8-11, 8-13, and 8-17A), it is not surprising that several attempts have been made to improve oxygenation by selectively treating the ventilated lung with PEEP.[14–22,38,89,104,105] An accepted risk of selective dependent-lung PEEP is that the PEEP-induced increase in lung volume can cause compression of the small dependent-lung intra-alveolar vessels and increase dependent-lung pulmonary vascular resistance; this will divert blood flow away from the ventilated lung to the nonventilated lung (Fig. 8-17B), increasing the

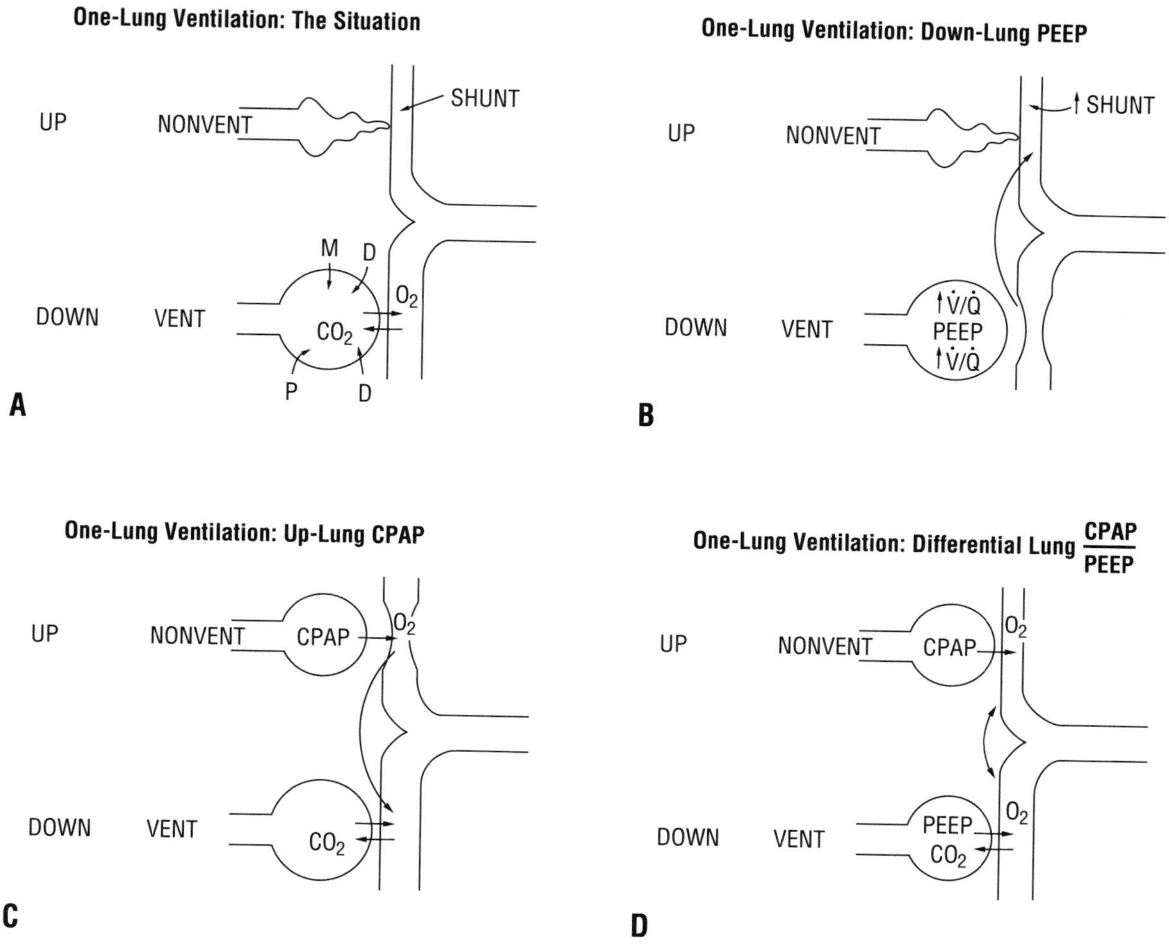

Fig. 8-17. A four-part schematic diagram showing the effects of various differential lung management approaches. **(A)** The one-lung ventilation situation. The dependent lung (DOWN) is ventilated (VENT), but is compressed by the weight of the mediastinum (M) from above, the pressure of the abdominal contents against the diaphragm (D), and by positioning effects of rolls, packs, and shoulder supports (P). The nondependent lung (UP) is nonventilated (NONVENT) and blood flow through this lung is shunt flow. **(B)** The dependent lung has been selectively treated with PEEP, which improves ventilation-to-perfusion ($\dot{V}/\dot{Q}$) relationships in the dependent lung, but also increases dependent-lung vascular resistance; this diverts blood to, and thereby increases shunt flow through, the nonventilated lung. **(C)** Selective application of continuous positive airway pressure (CPAP) to the nondependent lung permits oxygen uptake from this lung; even if the CPAP causes an increase in vascular resistance and diverts blood flow to the dependent lung, the diverted blood flow can still participate in gas exchange in the ventilated dependent lung. Consequently, selective nondependent-lung CPAP can greatly increase P_aO_2. **(D)** With differential lung CPAP (nondependent lung)/PEEP (dependent lung), it does not matter where the blood flow goes, since both lungs can participate in O_2 uptake. With this latter one-lung ventilation pattern, P_aO_2 can be restored to levels near those achieved by two-lung ventilation. (From Benumof,[126] with permission.)

shunt and decreasing the P_aO_2. The fact that increases in both PEEP and tidal volume in the dependent ventilated lung have an additive effect in decreasing P_aO_2 during one-lung ventilation greatly supports the one-ventilated lung volume versus vascular resistance hypothesis.[89,104] Therefore, the effect of dependent-lung PEEP on arterial oxygenation is a trade-off between the positive effect of increasing dependent-lung functional residual capacity (FRC) and $\dot{V}/\dot{Q}$ ratio and the negative effect of increasing dependent-lung vascular resistance and shunting blood flow to the nonventilated lung. Not surprisingly, the various one-lung ventilation-PEEP studies have included patients who have had an increase,[38,104,109] no change,[104,109–111] or a decrease[38,104,109,112] in oxygenation. It may be expected that in patients with a very diseased dependent lung (low lung volume and $\dot{V}/\dot{Q}$ ratio), the positive effect of selective dependent-lung PEEP (increased lung volume and increased $\dot{V}/\dot{Q}$ ratio) might outweigh the negative effects of selective dependent-lung PEEP (shunting of blood flow to the nonventilated, nondependent lung), whereas in patients with a normal dependent lung, the negative effects of dependent-lung PEEP would outweigh the benefits. Indeed, in one study in which 10 cmH$_2$O PEEP was selectively applied to the dependent lung, P$_a$O$_2$ increased in those patients with an initial P$_a$O$_2$ of less than 80 mmHg (F$_I$O$_2$ = 0.5), whereas P$_a$O$_2$ decreased or remained constant in patients with an initial P$_a$O$_2$ higher than 80 mmHg (F$_I$O$_2$ = 0.5).[109] Presumably, in the patients with P$_a$O$_2$ lower than 80 mmHg (F$_I$O$_2$ = 0.5), the dependent lung had a low FRC (had low $\dot{V}/\dot{Q}$ ratio and atelectatic regions) and, therefore, the positive effect of increased dependent-lung volume predominated over the negative effect of shunting blood flow to the nonventilated lung. Conversely, the patients with the higher P$_a$O$_2$ presumably had a dependent lung with an adequate FRC and $\dot{V}/\dot{Q}$ ratio, and the negative effect of shunting blood flow to the nonventilated lung predominated over the positive effect of increased dependent-lung volume. Although in none of these studies was a dose (ventilated-lung PEEP)-response (P$_a$O$_2$, Q$_s$/Q$_T$ value) relationship described, it seems reasonable to postulate on the basis of these results that the therapeutic margin of using PEEP to increase P$_a$O$_2$ during one-lung ventilation is quite narrow. PEEP to just the dependent ventilated lung may be delivered by the same anesthesia machine apparatus that is ordinarily used to deliver PEEP to the whole lung. Other studies have shown that high tidal volumes,[35,36] variations in the inspiratory-to-expiratory ratio,[110] and intermittent manual hyperventilation of the lower lung are not beneficial in increasing P$_a$O$_2$ during one-lung ventilation.[110]

Selective Nondependent-Lung Continuous Positive Airway Pressure

Low levels of positive pressure can be selectively applied to just the nonventilated, nondependent lung. Since under these conditions the nonventilated lung is only slightly, but constantly, distended by oxygen, an appropriate term for this ventilatory arrangement is *nonventilated-lung continuous positive airway pressure* (CPAP). Recently, two reports, one in humans[112] and one in dogs,[113] have shown that the application of CPAP (without tidal ventilation) to only the nonventilated lung significantly increased oxygenation. The latter study was performed with the dogs in the lateral decubitus position and showed that low levels of CPAP (5 to 10 cmH$_2$O) to the nonventilated, nondependent lung greatly increased P$_a$O$_2$ and decreased shunt, while blood flow to the nonventilated lung remained unchanged; presumably, this level of CPAP does not significantly compress the small intra-alveolar vessels in the nondependent lung. Thus, it is not at all surprising to find that the institution of 10 cmH$_2$O of nondependent-lung CPAP in patients has had no significant hemodynamic effect.[114,115] In summary, low levels of CPAP simply maintain the patency of nondependent-lung airways, allowing some oxygen distention of the gas-exchanging alveolar space in the nondependent lung (Fig. 8-17C) without significantly affecting the pulmonary vasculature. In all clinical studies,[112,114–116] the application of 5 to 10 cmH$_2$O CPAP has not interfered with the performance of surgery and may, in fact, facilitate intralobar dissection; this is not surprising in view of the fact that the initial compliance of a collapsed lung is only 10 mL/cmH$_2$O, and 5 to 10 cmH$_2$O CPAP should only create a slightly distended lung that occupies a volume of 50 to 100 mL, which is hardly or not at all noticed by the surgeon.

On the other hand, in the canine study,[113] 15 cmH$_2$O of nondependent-lung CPAP caused changes in P$_a$O$_2$ and shunt similar to those of 5 to 10 cmH$_2$O nondependent-lung CPAP, while blood flow to the nonventilated, nondependent lung decreased significantly. Therefore, high levels of nonventilated-lung CPAP act by permitting oxygen uptake in the nonventilated lung as well as by causing blood flow diversion to the ventilated lung, where both oxygen and carbon dioxide exchange can take place (Fig. 8-17C). Since low levels of nonventilated-lung CPAP are as efficacious as high levels and have less surgical interference and hemodynamic implications, it is logical to first use low levels of nonventilated CPAP.

In all patients in all clinical studies to date, 5 to 10 cmH$_2$O of nondependent-lung CPAP has significantly increased P$_a$O$_2$ during one-lung ventilation.[112,114–119] It should be concluded that the single most efficacious maneuver to increase P$_a$O$_2$ during one-lung ventilation is to apply 5 to 10 cmH$_2$O CPAP to the nondependent lung. From experience, low levels of nonventilated CPAP have corrected severe hypoxemia (P$_a$O$_2$ <50 mmHg) greater than 95 percent of the time, provided the double-lumen tube was correctly positioned. *However, the nondependent-lung CPAP must be applied dur-*

ing the deflation phase of a large tidal volume so that the deflating lung can lock into a CPAP level with uniform expansion and avoid the need to overcome critical opening pressures of airway and alveoli.

In both the human[112] and canine studies,[113] oxygen insufflation at zero airway pressure did not significantly improve P_aO_2 and shunt, and this result was probably due to the inability of zero transbronchial airway pressure to maintain airway patency and overcome critical alveolar opening pressures. Although one study in patients has concluded that insufflation of O_2 at zero airway pressure does increase P_aO_2, the study is difficult to interpret, since the patients did not serve as their own control.[120]

Several selective nondependent-lung CPAP systems that are easy to assemble have recently been described.[111,117–119] All of these nondependent-lung CPAP systems have three features in common (Fig. 8-18). First, there must be a source of oxygen to flow into the nonventilated lung. Second, there must be some sort of restrictive mechanism (hand-screw valve, pop-off valve, weight-loaded valve) to retard the egress of oxygen from the nonventilated lung so that the nonventilated lung may become distended. Thus, a free-flowing pressurized source of oxygen flows into a lung, but the escape of the oxygen is restricted; the unrestricted flow in and the restricted flow out create a constant distending pressure. Third, the distending pressure must be measured by a manometer. In practice, it is often simplest to keep the restrictive mechanism constant and adjust the distending pressure with a relatively fine sensitivity by changing the oxygen flow rate. If the nondependent-lung CPAP system has a reservoir bag included (which is highly desirable), the reservoir bag will reflect the amount of CPAP (by distention) and the nondependent lung may also be ventilated with intermittent positive pressure whenever desired.

Differential Lung PEEP, CPAP

In theory, and from the above considerations, it appears that the ideal way to improve oxygenation during one-lung ventilation is the application of differential lung CPAP/PEEP (Fig. 8-17D). In this situation, the ventilated (dependent) lung is given PEEP in the usual conventional manner in an effort to improve ventilated lung volume and ventilation-to-perfusion relationships. Simultaneously, the nonventilated (nondependent) lung receives CPAP in an attempt to improve oxygenation of the blood perfusing this lung. Therefore, with differential lung PEEP/CPAP, it does not matter where the blood flow goes nearly as much as during simple one-lung ventilation, since wherever

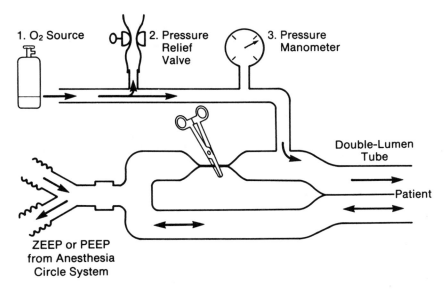

Fig. 8-18. The three essential components of a nondependent-lung continuous positive airway pressure (CPAP) system consist of (1) an oxygen source, (2) a pressure relief valve, and (3) a pressure manometer to measure the CPAP. The CPAP is created by the free flow of oxygen into the lung versus the restricted outflow of oxygen from the lung by the pressure relief valve. It is also very desirable to have a reservoir bag somewhere in-line in the CPAP system. ZEEP, zero end-expiratory pressure; PEEP, positive end-expiratory pressure. (From Benumof,[121] with permission.)

it goes (to either ventilated or nonventilated lung) it has at least some chance to participate in gas exchange with alveoli that are expanded with oxygen. In indirect support of this contention, arterial oxygenation has been increased significantly in patients during thoracotomy in the lateral decubitus position (using two-lung ventilation) when PEEP has been added to the ventilated dependent lung, while the nondependent lung was also able to participate in gas exchange by virtue of being ventilated at ZEEP.[22] In direct support of this contention, in patients undergoing thoracotomy and one-lung ventilation, arterial oxygenation was unchanged by the application of 10 cmH_2O of dependent-lung PEEP alone (consistent with an equal positive/negative effect trade-off), was significantly improved by 10 cmH_2O of nondependent-lung CPAP alone, and was further and even more significantly increased by use of 10 cmH_2O of nondependent-lung CPAP and 10 cmH_2O of dependent-lung PEEP together (differential lung PEEP/CPAP ventilation).[114,115] The use of 10 cmH_2O of nondependent-lung CPAP together with 10 cmH_2O of dependent-lung PEEP in patients caused only small, clinically insignificant hemodynamic effects.[114,115]

There are now multiple reports of significant increases in oxygenation obtained with the application of differential lung ventilation and PEEP (either PEEP/PEEP, PEEP/CPAP, or CPAP/CPAP) through double-lumen endotracheal tubes to patients in the intensive care unit with acute respiratory failure due to predominantly unilateral lung disease.[121] In all cases, conventional two-lung therapy (mechanical ventilation, PEEP, CPAP) had been administered via a standard single-lumen tube and either failed to improve or actually decreased oxygenation. In these patients, the single-lumen tube was replaced with a double-lumen tube. In most cases, the amount of PEEP initially administered to each lung was inversely proportional to the compliance of each lung; ideally, this PEEP arrangement should result in equal FRC in each lung. In some cases, the amount of PEEP that each lung received was later adjusted and titrated in an effort to find a differential lung-PEEP combination that resulted in the lowest right-to-left transpulmonary shunt.

Recommended Combined Conventional and Differential Management

Figure 8-19 summarizes the recommended plan for obtaining satisfactory arterial oxygenation during one-lung anesthesia. Two-lung ventilation is maintained for as long as possible (usually until the pleura is opened). When one-lung ventilation is commenced, a tidal volume of 10 mL/kg is used, and the respiratory rate is adjusted so that P_aCO_2 = 40 mmHg. A high inspired oxygen concentration (F_IO_2 = 0.8 to 1.0) should be used, and arterial oxygen saturation should be continuously monitored.

If severe hypoxemia is present following this initial conventional approach, the two major causes of hypoxemia (namely, malposition of the double-lumen

1. Maintain Two Lung Ventilation Until Pleura is Opened

2. Dependent Lung
   - F_IO_2 = 1.0
   - TV = 8-10 ml/kg
   - RR = So That P_aCO_2 = 40 mm Hg
   - PEEP = 0-5 mm Hg

3. If Severe Hypoxemia Occurs
   - (a) Check Position of Double-Lumen Tube With Fiberoptic Bronchoscopy
   - (b) Check Hemodynamic Status
   - (c) Nondependent Lung CPAP
   - (d) Dependent Lung PEEP
   - (e) Two Lung Ventilation
   - (f) Clamp Pulmonary Artery ASAP (For Pneumonectomy)

Fig. 8-19. An overall one-lung ventilation plan. F_IO_2, inspired oxygen concentration; TV, tidal volume; RR, respiratory rate; PEEP, positive end-expiratory pressure; CPAP, continuous positive airway pressure; ASAP, as soon as poosible. (From Benumof,[121] with permission.)

tube and poor hemodynamic status) must be ruled out. Proper tube position should be confirmed via fiberoptic bronchoscopy. If the double-lumen tube is correctly positioned and the hemodynamic status is satisfactory, simple tidal volume and respiratory rate adjustments should be made.[36] For example, if the tidal ventilation is thought to be too high, it should be decreased, and if the tidal ventilation is thought to be too low, it should be increased. If these simple maneuvers do not quickly resolve the problem, then the studies of selective nondependent-lung CPAP[112–119] and differential lung PEEP[121] dictate that the next treatment should be to apply 5 to 10 cmH$_2$O of CPAP to the nondependent lung. Nondependent-lung CPAP should be applied during the deflation phase of a large tidal volume breath in order to overcome critical opening pressures in the atelectatic lung. If oxygenation does not improve with nondependent-lung CPAP (which it does in the large majority of cases), 5 to 10 cmH$_2$O of PEEP to the ventilated dependent lung should then be applied. If dependent-lung PEEP does not improve oxygenation, nondependent-lung CPAP should be increased to 10 to 15 cmH$_2$O while the dependent lung is maintained at 5 to 10 cmH$_2$O of CPAP. If arterial oxygenation is still not satisfactory, then the nondependent-lung CPAP level should be matched with an equal amount of dependent-lung PEEP. In this way, a differential lung CPAP/PEEP search for the maximum compliance and a minimum right-to-left transpulmonary shunt is done in an attempt to find the optimal end-expiratory pressure for each lung and the patient as a whole.

If severe hypoxemia is still present following the application of differential lung CPAP/PEEP (which would be extremely rare), it should be remembered that the nondependent lung may be intermittently ventilated with positive pressure with oxygen (Fig. 8-19). Finally, most of the ventilation-perfusion imbalance is eliminated during a pneumonectomy by tightening a ligature around the nonventilated lung pulmonary artery as early as possible, which directly eliminates all shunt flow through the nonventilated lung (Fig. 8-19). Indeed, clamping the pulmonary artery to a collapsed lung functionally resects the entire lung, and the P$_a$O$_2$ is restored back to a level not significantly different from a two-lung ventilation or postpneumonectomy one-lung ventilation value.

Because nondependent-lung CPAP has been shown to consistently and reliably relieve hypoxemia during one-lung ventilation, its routine use should be considered in order to prevent hypoxemia from occurring during thoracic surgery using double-lumen endotracheal tubes.[112,114–116] Low levels of CPAP used in this situation have not compromised surgical conditions

and have occasionally improved surgical exposure by facilitating the identification of intralobar planes.[112,114–116]

REFERENCES

1. West JB, Dollery CT, Naimark A: Distribution of blood flow in isolated lung: relation to vascular and alveolar pressures. J Appl Physiol 19:713, 1964
2. Permutt S, Bromberger-Barnea B, Bane HN: Alveolar pressure, pulmonary venous pressure and the vascular waterfall. Med Thorac 19:239, 1962
3. West JB, Dollery CT, Heard BE: Increased pulmonary vascular resistance in the dependent zone of the isolated dog lung caused by perivascular edema. Circ Res 17:191–206, 1965
4. West JB (ed): Regional Differences in the Lung. Academic Press, San Diego, CA, 1977
5. Hughes JMB, Glazier JB, Maloney JE, et al: Effect of lung volume on the distribution of pulmonary blood flow in man. Respir Physiol 4:58–72, 1968
6. Hughes JM, Glazier JB, Maloney JE, et al: Effect of extra-alveolar vessels on the distribution of pulmonary blood flow in the dog. J Appl Physiol 25:701–709, 1968
7. Permutt S, Caldini P, Maseri A, et al: Recruitment versus distensibility in the pulmonary vascular bed. pp. 375–387. In Fishman AP, Hecht H (eds): The Pulmonary Circulation and Interstitial Space. University of Chicago Press, Chicago, 1969
8. Maseri A, Caldini P, Harward P, et al: Determinants of pulmonary vascular volume. Recruitment versus distensibility. Circ Res 31:218–228, 1972
9. Hoppin FG, Jr, Green ID, Mead J: Distribution of pleural surface pressure. J Appl Physiol 27:863, 1969
10. Milic-Emili J, Henderson JAM, Dolovich MB, et al: Regional distribution of inspired gas in the lung. J Appl Physiol 21:749, 1966
11. West JB: Ventilation/Blood Flow and Gas Exchange. 2nd Ed. Blackwell Scientific Publications, Oxford, 1970
12. West JB: Regional differences in gas exchange in the lung of erect man. J Appl Physiol 17:893, 1962
13. Wulff KE, Aulin I: The regional lung function in the lateral decubitus position during anesthesia and operation. Acta Anaesthesiol Scand 16:195–205, 1972
14. Rehder K, Wenthe FM, Sessler AD: Function of each lung during mechanical ventilation with ZEEP and with PEEP in man anesthetized with thiopental-meperidine. Anesthesiology 39:597–606, 1973
15. Svanberg L: Influence of posture on lung volumes, ventilation and circulation in normals. Scand J Clin Lab Invest, suppl. 25, 9:1–95, 1957
16. Rehder K, Sessler AD: Function of each lung in spontaneously breathing man anesthetized with thiopental-meperidine. Anesthesiology 38:320–327, 1973
17. Potgieter SV: Atelectasis: its evolution during upper urinary tract surgery. Br J Anaesth 31:472–483, 1959
18. Rehder K, Hatch DJ, Sessler AD, Fowler WS: The function of each lung of anesthetized and paralyzed man

during mechanical ventilation. Anesthesiology 37:16–26, 1972

19. Nunn JF: The distribution of inspired gas during thoracic surgery. Ann R Coll Surg Engl 28:223–237, 1961

20. Werner O, Malmkvist G, Beckman A, et al: Gas exchange and haemodynamics during thoracotomy. Br J Anaesth 56:1343–1349, 1984

21. Froese AB, Bryan CA: Effects of anesthesia and paralysis on diaphragmatic mechanics in man. Anesthesiology 41:242–255, 1974

22. Brown DR, Kafer ER, Roberson VO, et al: Improved oxygenation during thoracotomy with selective PEEP to the dependent lung. Anesth Analg 56:26–31, 1977

23. Benumof JL, Rogers SN, Moyce PR, et al: Hypoxic pulmonary vasoconstriction and regional and whole-lung PEEP in the dog. Anesthesiology 51:503–507, 1979

24. Tarhan S, Moffitt EA: Principles of thoracic anesthesia. Surg Clin North AM 53:813–826, 1973

25. Tarhan S, Lungborg RO: Carlens endobronchial catheter versus regular endotracheal tube during thoracic surgery: a comparison of blood gas tensions and pulmonary shunting. Can Anaesth Soc J 18:594–599, 1971

26. Casthely PA, Lear F, Cottrell JE, Lear E: Intrapulmonary shunting during induced hypotension. Anesth Analg 61:231–235, 1982

27. Benumof JL: Hypoxic pulmonary vasoconstriction and sodium nitroprusside infusion. Anesthesiology 50:481–483, 1979

28. Kerr JH, Smith AC, Prys-Roberts C, et al: Observations during endobronchial anesthesia II. Oxygenation. Br J Anaesth 46:84–92, 1974

29. Benumof JL: Mechanism of decreased blood flow to atelectatic lung. J Appl Physiol 46:1047–1048, 1978

30. Pirlo AF, Benumof JL, Trousdale FR: Atelectatic lung lobe blood flow: open vs. closed chest, positive pressure vs. spontaneous ventilation. J Appl Physiol 50:1022–1026, 1981

31. Bjertnaes LJ, Mundal R, Hauge A, et al: Vascular resistance in atelectatic lungs: effect of inhalation anesthetics. Acta Anaesthesiol Scand 24:109, 1980

32. Marshall BE, Marshall C: Continuity of response to hypoxic pulmonary vasoconstriction. J Appl Physiol 59:189–196, 1980

33. Rogers SN, Benumof JL: Halothane and isoflurane do not decrease P_aO_2 during one-lung ventilation in intravenously anesthetized patients. Anesth Analg 64:946–954, 1985

34. Torda TA, McCulloch CH, O'Brien HD, et al: Pulmonary venous admixture during one-lung anesthesia. The effect of inhaled oxygen tension and respiration rate. Anaesthesia 29:272–279, 1974

35. Khanom T, Branthwaite MA: Arterial oxygenation during one-lung anesthesia (1): a study in man. Anaesthesia 28:132–138, 1973

36. Flacke JW, Thompson DS, Read RC: Influence of tidal volume and pulmonary artery occlusion on arterial oxygenation during endobronchial anesthesia. South Med J 69:619–626,1976

37. Tarhan S, Lundborg RO: Blood gas and pH studies during use of Carlens catheter. Can Anaesth Soc J 15:458–467, 1968

38. Tarhan S, Lundborg RO: Effects of increased expiratory pressure on blood gas tensions and pulmonary shunting during thoracotomy with use of the Carlens catheter. Can Anaesth Soc J 17:4–11, 1970

39. Fiser WP, Friday CD, Read RC: Changes in arterial oxygenation and pulmonary shunt during thoracotomy with endobronchial anesthesia. J Thorac Cardiovasc Surg 83:523–531, 1982

40. Prefaut CH, Engel LA: Vertical distribution of perfusion and inspired gas in supine man. Respir Physiol 43:209–219, 1981

41. Glasser SA, Domino KB, Lindgren L, et al: Pulmonary pressure and flow during atelectasis. Anesthesiology 57:A504, 1982

42. Carlsson AJ, Bindslev L. Santesson J, et al: Hypoxic pulmonary vasoconstriction in the human lung: the effect of prolonged unilateral hypoxic challenge during anesthesia. Acta Anaesthesiol Scand 29:346–351, 1985

43. Hill NS, Antman EM, Green LH, Alpert JS: Intravenous nitroglycerin. A review of pharmacology, therapeutic effects and indications. Chest 79:69–76, 1981

44. Colley PS, Cheney FW, Hlastala MP: Pulmonary gas exchange effects of nitroglycerin in canine edematous lungs. Anesthesiology 55:114–119, 1981

45. Chick TW, Kochukoshy KN, Matsumoto S, Leach JK: The effect of nitroglycerin on gas exchange, hemodynamics and oxygen transport in patients with chronic obstructive pulmonary disease. Am J Med Sci 276:105–111, 1978

46. Kadowitz PJ, Nandiwada P, Grueter CA, et al: Pulmonary vasodilator responses to nitroprusside and nitroglycerin in the dog. J Clin Invest 67:893–902, 1981

47. Anjou-Lindskog E, Broman L, Holmgren A: Effects of nitroglycerin on central hemodynamics and V_a/Q distribution early after coronary bypass surgery. Acta Anaesthesiol Scand 26:489–497, 1982

48. Kochukoshy KN, Chick TW, Jenne JW: The effect of nitroglycerin on gas exchange in chronic obstructive pulmonary disease. Am Rev Respir Dis 111:177–183, 1975

49. Holmgren A, Anjou E, Broman L, Lundberg S: Influence of nitroglycerin on central hemodynamics and V_a/Q_c of the lungs in the postoperative period after coronary bypass surgery. Acta Med Scand S562:135–142, 1982

50. Parsons GH, Leventhal JP, Hansen MM, Goldstein JD: Effect of sodium nitroprusside on hypoxic pulmonary vasoconstriction in the dog. J Appl Physiol 51:288–292, 1981

51. Sivak ED, Gray BA, McCurdy TH, Phillips AK: Pulmonary vascular response to nitroprusside in dogs. Circ Res 45:360–365, 1979

52. Hill AB, Sykes MK, Reyes A: Hypoxic pulmonary vasoconstrictor response in dogs during and after sodium nitroprusside infusion. Anesthesiology 50:484–488, 1979

53. Colley PS, Cheney FW, Hlastala MP: Ventilation-perfusion and gas exchange effects of nitroprusside in dogs with normal and edematous lungs. Anesthesiology 50:489–495, 1979

54. Colley PS, Cheney FW: Sodium nitroprusside increases Q_s/Q_t in dogs with regional atelectasis. Anesthesiology 47:338–341, 1977

55. Wildsmith JAW, Drummond GB, Macrae WR: Blood gas changes during induced hypotension with sodium nitroprusside. Br J Anaesth 47:1205–1211, 1975

56. Veltzer JL, Doto JO, Jacoby J: Depressed arterial oxygenation during sodium nitroprusside administration for intraoperative hypertension. Anesth Analg 55:880–881, 1976

57. McFarlane PA, Mortimer AJ, Ryder WA, et al: Effects of dopamine and dobutamine on the distribution of pulmonary blood flow during lobar ventilation hypoxia and lobar collapse in dogs. Eur J Clin Invest 15:53–59, 1985

58. Furman WR, Summer WR, Kennedy PP, Silvester JT: Comparison of the effects of dobutamine, dopamine and isoproterenol on hypoxic pulmonary vasoconstriction in the pig. Crit Care Med 10:371–374, 1982

59. Bishop MJ, Cheney FW: Minoxidil and nifedipine inhibit hypoxic pulmonary vasoconstriction. J Cardiovasc Pharmacol 5:184–189, 1983

60. Tucker A, McMurtry IF, Grover RF, et al: Attenuation of hypoxic pulmonary vasoconstriction by verapamil in intact dogs. Proc Soc Exp Biol Med 151:611–614, 1976

61. Simonneau J, Escourrou P, Duroux P, Lockhart A: Inhibition of hypoxic pulmonary vasoconstriction by nifedipine. N Engl J Med 304:1582–1585, 1981

62. Redding GJ, Tuck R, Escourrou P: Nifedipine attenuates hypoxic pulmonary vasoconstriction in awake piglets. Am Rev Respir Dis 129:785–789, 1984

63. McMurtry IF, Davidson AB, Reeves TJ, Grover RF: Inhibition of hypoxic pulmonary vasoconstriction by calcium antagonists in isolated rat lungs. Circ Res 38:99–104, 1976

64. Brown SE, Linden GS, King RR, et al: Effect of verapamil on pulmonary haemodynamics during hypoxaemia at rest, and during exercise in patients with chronic obstructive pulmonary disease. Thorax 38:840–844, 1983

65. Ward CF, Benumof JL, Wahrenbrock EA: Inhibition of hypoxic pulmonary vasoconstriction by vasoactive drugs. pp. 333–334. Abstracts of Scientific Papers, 1976 Annual Meeting, American Society of Anesthesiology, 1976

66. Johansen I, Benumof JL: Reduction of hypoxia-induced pulmonary artery hypertension by vasodilator drugs. Am Rev Respir Dis 199:375, 1979

67. Conover WB, Benumof JL, Key TC: Ritodrine inhibition of hypoxic pulmonary vasoconstriction. Am J Obstet Gynecol 146:652–656, 1983

68. Marin JLB, Orchard C, Chakrabarti MK, Sykes MK: Depression of hypoxic pulmonary vasoconstriction in

the dog by dopamine and isoprenaline. Br J Anaesth 51:303–312, 1979

69. Reyes A, Sykes MK, Chakrabarti MK, et al: Effect of orciprenaline on hypoxic pulmonary vasoconstriction in dogs. Respiration 38:185–193, 1979

70. Reyes A, Sykes MK, Charkrabarti MK, et al: The effect of salbutamol on hypoxic pulmonary vasoconstriction in dogs. Bull Eur Physiopathol Respir 14:741–753, 1978

71. Rubin LJ, Lazar JD: Nonadrenergic effects of isoproterenol in dogs with hypoxic pulmonary vasoconstriction: possible role of prostaglandins. J Clin Invest 71:1366–1374, 1983

72. Benumof JL, Trousdale FR: Aminophylline does not inhibit canine hypoxic pulmonary vasoconstriction. Am Rev Respir Dis 126:1017–1019, 1982

73. Bishop MJ, Kennard S, Artman LD, Cheney FW: Hydralazine does not inhibit canine hypoxic pulmonary vasoconstriction. Am Rev Respir Dis 128:998–1001, 1983

74. Benumof JL: Choice of anesthetic drugs and techniques. pp. 209–210. In: Anesthesia for Thoracic Surgery. WB Saunders, Philadelphia, 1987

75. Domino KB, Borowec L, Alexander CM, et al: Influence of isoflurane on hypoxic pulmonary vasoconstriction in dogs. Anesthesiology 64:423–429, 1986

76. Lawler PGP, Nunn JF: A reassessment of the validity of the iso-shunt graph. Br J Anaesth 56:1325–1335, 1984

77. Benumof JL: Special physiology of the lateral decubitus position, the open chest, and one-lung ventilation. p. 113. In: Anesthesia for Thoracic Surgery. Philadelphia, WB Saunders, 1987

78. Benumof JL, Augustine SD, Gibbins J: Halothane and isoflurane only slighty impair arterial oxygenation during one-lung ventilation in patients undergoing thoracotomy. Anesthesiology 67:910–915, 1987

79. Carlsson AJ, Bindslev L, Hedenstierna G: Hypoxia pulmonary vasoconstriction in the lung. Anesthesiology 66:312–316, 1987

80. Carlsson AJ, Hedenstierna G, Bindslev L: Hypoxia-induced vasoconstriction in human lung exposed to enflurane anaesthesia. Acta Anaesthesiol Scand 31:57–62, 1987

81. Gardaz JP, McFarlane PA, Madgwick RG, et al: Effect of dopamine, increased cardiac output and increased pulmonary artery pressure on hypoxic pulmonary vasoconstriction. Br J Anaesth 55:238P–239P, 1983

82. Benumof JL, Wahrenbrock EA: Blunted hypoxic pulmonary vasoconstriction by increased lung vascular pressures. J Appl Physiol 38:846–850, 1975

83. Scanlon TS, Benumof JL, Wahrenbrock EA, Nelson WL: Hypoxic pulmonary vasoconstriction and the ratio of hypoxic lung to perfused normoxic lung. Anesthesiology 49:177–181, 1978

84. Colley PS, Cheney FW, Butler J: Mechanism of change in pulmonary shunt flow with hemorrhage. J Appl Physiol 42:196–201, 1977

85. Domino KB, Glasser SA, Wetstein L, et al: Influence of

$P_{\bar{v}}O_2$ on blood flow to atelectatic lung. Anesthesiology 57:A471, 1982

86. Benumof JL, Pirlo AF, Trousdale FR: Inhibition of hypoxic pulmonary vasoconstriction by decreased $P_{\bar{v}}O_2$: a new indirect mechanism. J Appl Physiol 51:871–874, 1981

87. Pease RD, Benumof JL: P_AO_2 and $P_{\bar{v}}O_2$ interaction on hypoxic pulmonary vasoconstriction. J Appl Physiol 53:134–139, 1982

88. Benumof JL, Mathers JM, Wahrenbrock EA: Cyclic hypoxic pulmonary vasoconstriction induced by concomitant carbon dioxide changes. J Appl Physiol 41:466–469, 1976

89. Benumof JL, Rogers SN, Moyce PR, et al: Hypoxic pulmonary vasoconstriction and regional and whole-lung PEEP in the dog. Anesthesiology 51:503–507, 1979

90. Benumof JL: One-lung ventilation and hypoxic pulmonary vasoconstriction: implications for anesthetic management. Anesth Analg 64:821–833, 1985

91. Hall SM, Chapleau M, Cairo J, et al: Effect of high-frequency positive-pressure ventilation on halothane ablation of hypoxic pulmonary vasoconstriction. Crit Care Med 13:641–645, 1985

92. Irwin RS, Martinez-Gonzalez-Rio H, Thomas HM III, Fritts HW, Jr: The effect of granulomatous pulmonary disease in dogs on the response of the pulmonary circulation to hypoxia. J Clin Invest 60:1258–1265, 1977

93. Light RB, Mink SN, Wood LDH: Pathophysiology of gas exchange and pulmonary perfusion in pneumococcal lobar pneumonia in dogs. J Appl Physiol 50:524–530, 1981

94. Craig JOC, Bromley LL, Williams R: Thoracotomy and contralateral lung. A study of the changes occurring in the dependent and contralateral lung during and after thoracotomy in the lateral decubitus position. Thorax 17:9–15, 1962

95. Benumof JL: General respiratory physiology and respiratory function during anesthesia. pp. 39–103. In: Anesthesia For Thoracic Surgery. Philadelphia, WB Saunders, 1987

96. Dantzker DR, Wagner PD, West JB: Instability of lung units with low V/Q ratios during O_2 breathing. J Appl Physiol 38:886–895, 1975

97. Ray JF III, Yost L, Moallem S, et al: Immobility, hypoxemia and pulmonary arteriovenous shunting. Arch Surg 109:537–541, 1974

98. Kerr JH: Physiological aspects of one-lung (endobronchial) anesthesia. Int Anesthesiol Clin 10:61–78, 1972

99. Johansen I, Benumof JL: Flow distribution in abnormal lung as a function of F_IO_2, abstracted. Anesthesiology 51:369, 1979

100. Benumof JL, Wahrenbrock EA: Dependency of hypoxic pulmonary vasoconstriction on temperature. J Appl Physiol 72:56–58, 1977

101. Kelman GF, Nunn JF, Prys-Roberts C, et al: The influence of the cardiac output on arterial oxygenation: a theoretical study. Br J Anaesth 39:450–458, 1967

102. Prys-Roberts C: The metabolic regulation of circulatory transport. Scientific Foundations of Anesthesia. (eds): In Scurr C, Feldman S, Chicago, Year Book Medical Publishers, 1982

103. Winter PM, Smith G: The toxicity of oxygen. Anesthesiology 37:210–241, 1972

104. Katz JA, Laverne RG, Fairley HB, Thomas AN: Pulmonary oxygen exchange during endobronchial anesthesia: effects of tidal volume and PEEP. Anesthesiology 56:164–171, 1982

105. Finley TN, Hill TR, Bonica JJ: Effect of intrapleural pressure on pulmonary shunt to atelectatic dog lung. Am J Physiol 205:1187–1192, 1963

106. Bachand RR, Audet J, Meloche R, et al: Physiological changes associated with unilateral pulmonary ventilation during operations on one lung. Can Anaesth Soc J 22:659–664, 1975

107. Kerr J, Smith AC, Prys-Roberts C, et al: Observations during endobronchial anaesthesia. I. Ventilation and carbon dioxide clearance. Br J Anaesth 45:159–267, 1973

108. Hatch D: Ventilation and arterial oxygenation during thoracic surgery. Thorax 21:310–314, 1966

109. Cohen E, Thys DM, Eisenkraft JB, Kaplan JA: PEEP during one-lung anesthesia improves oxygenation in patients with low arterial P_aO_2. Anesth Analg 64:201, 1985

110. Khanam T, Branthwaite, MA: Arterial oxygenation during one-lung anesthesia (2). Anaesthesia 23:280–290, 1973

111. Aalto-Setala M, Heinonen J, Salorinne Y: Cardiorespiratory function during thoracic anesthesia: comparison of two-lung ventilation and one-lung ventilation with and without PEEP. Acta Anaesthesiol Scand 19:287–295, 1975

112. Capan IM, Turndorf H, Chandrakant P, et al: Optimization of arterial oxygenation during one-lung anesthesia. Anesth Analg 59:847–851, 1980

113. Alfery DD, Benumof JL, Trousdale FR: Improving oxygenation during one-lung ventilation: the effects of PEEP and blood flow restriction to the nonventilated lung. Anesthesiology 55:381–385, 1981

114. Cohen E, Eisenkraft JB, Thys DM, Kaplan JA: Oxygenation and hemodynamic changes during one-lung ventilation: effects of $CPAP_{10}$, $PEEP_{10}$, and $CPAP_{10}/PEEP_{10}$. J Cardiothorac Anesth 2:34–40, 1988

115. Cohen E, Thys DM, Eisenkraft JB, et al: Effect of CPAP and PEEP during one-lung anesthesia: left versus right thoracotomies. Anesthesiology 63:A564, 1985

116. Merridew CG, Jones RDM: Nondependent lung CPAP (5 cm H_2O) with oxygen during ketamine, halothane or isoflurane anesthesia and one-lung ventilation. Anesthesiology 63:A567, 1985

117. Thiagarajah S, Job C, Rao A: A device for applying CPAP to the nonventilated upper lung during one lung ventilation. I. Anesthesiology 60:253–254, 1984

118. Hannenberg AA, Satwicz PR, Pienes RS, Jr, O'Brien JC: A device for applying CPAP to the nonventilated upper lung during one lung ventilation. II. Anesthesiology 60:254–255, 1984

119. Brown DL, Davis RS: A simple device for oxygen insuf-

flation with continuous positive airway pressure during one-lung ventilation. Anesthesiology 61:481–482, 1984

120. Rees DI, Wansbrough SR: One-lung anesthesia: percent shunt and arterial oxygen tension during continuous insufflation of oxygen to the nonventilated lung. Anesth Analg 61:507–512, 1982

121. Benumof JL: Conventional and differential lung management of one-lung ventilation. Ch. 11. In: Anesthesia for Thoracic Surgery. Philadelphia, WB Saunders, 1987

122. West JB: Ventilation/Blood Flow and Gas Exchange. 4th Ed. Blackwell Scientific Publications, Oxford, 1985

123. Benumof JL: Respiratory physiology and respiratory function during anesthesia. pp. 505–549. In Miller RD (ed): Anesthesia. 3rd Ed. Churchill Livingstone, New York, 1990

124. Benumof JL: Physiology of the open chest and one-lung ventilation. pp. 105–115. In: Anesthesia for Thoracic Surgery. WB Saunders, Philadelphia, 1987

125. Benumof JL: Anesthetic considerations (other than management of ventilation) during and at the end of thoracic surgery. pp. 272–279. In: Anesthesia for Thoracic Surgery. WB Saunders, Philadelphia, 1987

126. Benumof JL, Alfery DD: Anesthesia for thoracic surgery. pp. 1517–1603. In Miller RD (ed): Anesthesia. 3rd Ed. Churchill Livingstone, New York, 1990

127. Benumof JL: Isoflurane anesthesia and arterial oxygenation during one-lung ventilation. Anesthesiology 64:419–422, 1986

9
BRONCHODILATORS AND BRONCHOACTIVE DRUGS

Alan L. Plummer, M.D.
Linda J. Riemersma, Pharm.D.

Many patients requiring thoracic surgery have concomitant pulmonary disease. This should not be surprising, since smoking is a common risk factor for the development of lung cancer, as well as chronic bronchitis and emphysema. In addition, patients may have other airway diseases such as asthma, bronchiectasis, or cystic fibrosis; parenchymal diseases such as idiopathic pulmonary fibrosis; or combinations of obstructive and restrictive pulmonary diseases. The pre- and postoperative course in patients with pulmonary diseases will be facilitated if the pulmonary diagnosis and the severity of pulmonary dysfunction are established *before* surgery. The importance of a comprehensive history and physical examination, particularly with regard to the cardiopulmonary system, cannot be overemphasized. Those patients with pulmonary disease, or those thought to have pulmonary disease, should have preoperative measurements of lung volumes, flow rates, and arterial blood gases to ascertain the degree of functional impairment and baseline pulmonary function. *Preoperative* treatment with bronchodilator drugs as well as oxygen, antibiotics, and/or steroids may be required. It is important that airway function be optimized during this period and that aggressive therapy be continued in the postoperative period to reduce postoperative pulmonary complications[1] (see Chapters 1 and 4).

All bronchodilator agents have desirable effects, as well as undesirable dose-dependent side effects. Cautious and prudent use of these drugs requires a detailed knowledge of the pharmacology of the drug plus familiarity with the underlying pulmonary disorders and the diseases of other organ systems.

AIRWAY STRUCTURE AND FUNCTION

Gas enters the thorax from the mouth, nose, or artificial airway into the trachea, which divides into the right and left mainstem bronchi. This division and the subsequent branching of the airways occur in an ir-

This chapter is modified and updated from Plummer AL: Bronchodilator drugs and the cardiac patient. pp. 581–606. In Kaplan JA (ed): Cardiac Anesthesia. Vol. 2. Cardiovascular Pharmacology. Grune & Stratton, Orlando, FL, 1983. Reprinted with permission.

regular dichotomous fashion.[2] Each division results in two daughter branches that are unequal in diameter, length, and angle of takeoff. This is easily seen through a fiberoptic bronchoscope, as the left mainstem bronchus branches off at a more acute angle than the right, is slightly smaller, and is much longer than the right mainstem bronchus. Even though the diameter of each branch is smaller, the cross-sectional area at each division increases through bronchi, bronchioles, and terminal bronchioles.[2] The diameter of the branching in respiratory bronchioles and alveolar ducts changes little, yet the cross-sectional area continues to increase with each branching.[2] The primary function of the airway is to conduct gas through the airway to the gas-exchange area. The increasing cross-sectional area of the airway leads to a reduction in airflow resistance as gas moves to the periphery, thus facilitating mass flow of oxygen molecules. In respiratory bronchioles and alveolar ducts, gas diffusion is more important than mass gas flow and is facilitated by the large cross-sectional area present.[3]

The airway wall consists of layers of mucosa and smooth muscle and, finally, a connective tissue sleeve. Bronchi and small bronchi contain cartilage within the wall, whereas bronchioles contain no cartilage. Respiratory bronchioles contain alveoli that increase in number with each branching such that only alveoli line the alveolar ducts and sacs. In the bronchi, the mucosal layer contains tall ciliated epithelial cells as well as mucus-producing glands, goblet cells, and Clara cells.[4]

Moving peripherally, the mucosal layer thins, and ciliated cells become more cuboidal. In bronchioles, glands disappear and goblet cells decrease in number and finally disappear as the number of Clara cells increases. Clara cells decrease in number and finally disappear within respiratory bronchioles and alveolar ducts, which are lined with epithelial (type I) cells.[5]

The smooth muscle layer is continuous from the trachea to the alveolar ducts.[2] The smooth muscle bundles encircle the airways in an oblique course. Contraction results in airway narrowing as well as shortening.[2] In alveolar ducts, the muscle bundles occur in the alveolar entrance rings.[2]

The outermost layer of the airway consists of connective tissue that forms a strong sheath, particularly around large airways and bronchi, which also contain cartilage within this layer.[2]

Pulmonary arteries closely follow the pathway and branching of the airways, but provide no nutrient value, except to the bronchioles and respiratory bronchioles. The nutrient blood supply of the large and small bronchi, as well as the walls of the pulmonary arteries and veins, is supplied by the bronchial arter-

ies, two-thirds of which arise from the aorta; the remaining bronchial arteries arise from the upper intercostal arteries and, occasionally, from the internal mammary arteries. Some branches also extend to the pleura, as well as to mediastinal structures such as hilar lymph nodes, vagus nerves, and the esophagus.[6] The bronchial arteries branch, frequently forming a plexus within the peribronchial space. Small arteries arise from the bronchial arteries, which penetrate the bronchial wall to the mucosa, forming a second plexus in the submucosal region. Both plexuses extend to the terminal bronchioles. Connections between the bronchial microvasculature and the pulmonary vessels occur along the airways and beyond the terminal bronchioles. Large bronchiopulmonary connections may become prominent in disease states, particularly in bronchiectasis and lung cancer.[2] Bronchial venous drainage from the larger bronchi enters the systemic azygous and semiazygous veins, whereas the bulk (two-thirds) of the bronchial venous drainage empties into the pulmonary venous system, thereby contributing to the normal right-to-left shunt.[6]

Innervation of the airways and blood vessels originates from the autonomic nervous system. Parasympathetic, preganglionic fibers course with the vagus nerve primarily, but also with the recurrent laryngeal nerve (trachea), and end in ganglia located external to the smooth muscle and cartilage.[7] Innervation occurs down to the level of terminal bronchioles. Postganglionic cholinergic branches innervate smooth muscle and glands, causing contraction and glandular secretion, respectively. Afferent or sensory fibers originate from smooth muscle and the airway mucosa and course up the vagus nerves to the vagal nuclei. Other mucosal sensory afferents appear to enter the ganglia, which are located outside of the smooth muscle and cartilage.[7] Sympathetic, postganglionic fibers also enter these airway ganglia. However, adrenergic fibers to airway glands or smooth muscle have not been demonstrated in humans, but have been found in other mammals.[7] A third system, the nonadrenergic, noncholinergic (NANC) system of the lung, has been demonstrated in airways down to the small bronchi.[8] One component of this system appears to be the principal inhibitory system in human airways, causing bronchodilation when stimulated. The neurotransmitter involved is probably vasoactive intestinal polypeptide, which is also a bronchodilator far more potent than isoproterenol in vitro but not in vivo.[9] The exact function of this system is under investigation. There is also an excitatory component to the NANC system, probably mediated by a peptide, substance P, which, when stimulated, causes bronchoconstriction.[9]

PHARMACOLOGY OF THE AIRWAYS

In addition to the background knowledge in pulmonary anatomy and physiology, it is helpful to briefly review certain aspects of airway pharmacology in order to establish a scientific basis for the use of bronchodilator drugs.

Adrenergic Receptors

In 1948, Ahlquist advanced the theory that autonomic adrenergic receptors could be divided into two types, alpha and beta.[10] Further division of the beta-receptors into beta$_1$ and beta$_2$ was offered by Lands and colleagues.[11] Stimulation of alpha-receptors leads to arterial and venous vasoconstriction and bronchoconstriction.[12] Stimulation of beta$_1$-receptors leads to cardiac chronotropic and inotropic stimulation and an increase in free fatty acids due to lipolysis.[12] Stimulation of beta$_2$-receptors leads to vasodilatation, bronchodilation, skeletal muscle tremor, lactic acidemia,[12] and inhibition of mast cell mediator release[13] (Table 9-1). In the patient with airways disease, use of bronchodilator drugs with little or no alpha- or beta$_1$-receptor properties would be desirable.

If alpha-receptors exist on the bronchial smooth muscle membrane, they are relatively few in number and can be demonstrated only with beta-blockade[14] or under other special conditions.[14,15] The predominant airway smooth muscle receptor is the beta$_2$-receptor,[12] the stimulation of which leads to smooth muscle relaxation and bronchodilation. Stimulation of alpha-receptors leads to a reduction in cyclic adenosine 3',5'-monophosphate (cAMP) due to the inhibition of adenylate cyclase, an increase in cyclic guanosine 3',5'-monophosphate (cGMP), and subsequent bronchoconstriction.[13]

A series of complex events occurs after a beta-agonist is bound to the beta-receptor on the smooth muscle cell surface:

1. Within the cell membrane, the agonist-receptor complex couples with a guanine nucleotide regulatory protein containing bound guanosine triphosphate.[16] Two forms of the nucleotide regulatory protein exist: one stimulates and the other inhibits the production of adenylate cyclase.[17,18]
2. Next, phospholipid transmethylation is activated, which leads to a decrease in membrane viscosity and allows for a greater lateral movement of the receptor.
3. The lateral mobility of the receptor complex facilitates coupling with *membrane-bound* adenylate cyclase.[19]
4. Adenylate cyclase thus becomes activated, leading to conversion of adenosine triphosphate to cAMP *intracellularly*.
5. cAMP then activates specific protein kinases, which in turn modulate the intracellular effects of the beta agonist.[20,21]

Cyclic Nucleotides, Calcium, and Smooth Muscle Function

The cyclic nucleotides, cAMP and cGMP, and calcium are important "second messengers" to impart intracellular messages from receptor stimulation.

TABLE 9-1. Physiologic Effects of Human Adrenergic Receptor Stimulation

Alpha$_1$ and Alpha$_2$	Beta$_1$	Beta$_2$
Smooth muscle constriction of Tracheobronchial tree Veins Arteries	Cardiac stimulation Chronotropic Inotropic	Smooth muscle relaxation of Tracheobronchial tree Veins Arteries
Sphincter constriction of Gastrointestinal tract Urinary bladder trigone	Increases free fatty acids by lipolysis	Skeletal muscle tremor
Enhancement of histamine release		Lactic acidemia
Contraction of pilomotor muscles		Inhibition of histamine release
Hepatic glycogenolysis		

(From Plummer,[295] with permission.)

Beta-adrenergic stimulation leads to increases in cAMP and resultant airway smooth muscle relaxation.[22,23] The in vitro maximal smooth muscle relaxing effect, however, is achieved at submaximal levels of cAMP, indicating that beta-agonists can be administered in small doses to maximally stimulate cAMP. Increased cAMP leads to smooth muscle relaxation by the internalization of calcium into mitochondria and the sarcoplasmic reticulum, by the lowering of free calcium due to the extrusion of calcium via the calcium extrusion pump and the exchange of sodium and calcium, and by stimulating the production of protein kinases.[24]

Except for alpha-adrenergic stimulation, airway smooth muscle contraction is not generally associated with a decreased concentration of cAMP. With contraction, levels of cAMP may rise, probably secondary to prostaglandin release.[25] Prostaglandins of the E series stimulate cAMP production via a different receptor on the smooth muscle cell.[26]

cGMP also has an important function in the airway smooth muscle. Drugs that cause smooth muscle contraction, such as acetylcholine, alpha-adrenergic agonists, histamine, kinins, and prostaglandin $F_{2\alpha}$, also lead to an increase in the intracellular levels of cGMP.[27] The increased levels of cGMP appear to be secondary to the increase in intracellular calcium ion.[28,29] The exact effect of cGMP on airway smooth muscle is unknown, but it may reduce muscle excitability rather than increase muscle tension.[25] An earlier hypothesis that cGMP played a causal role in smooth muscle contraction and that cAMP and cGMP played opposite roles in smooth muscle relaxation and contraction, respectively,[30] does not appear to be correct.

As mentioned above, smooth muscle relaxation occurs when cellular levels of calcium ion are decreased. Smooth muscle contraction occurs when cellular levels of calcium ion are increased. At least two calcium channels exist in smooth muscle. One channel opens in response to cellular depolarization (termed *voltage-operated channel*) and the other channel opens in response to receptor activation (termed *receptor-operated channel*) by the activation of alpha-adrenergic, muscarinic, and other receptors (Table 9-2).[31] Calcium ions may also be released from internal stores (mitochondria and sarcoplasmic reticulum).[32] The increased calcium ions then combine with calmodulin, a specific calcium-binding protein, and this complex activates a specific kinase and enzyme cascade that leads to smooth muscle contraction.[31]

Phosphodiesterase

The cyclic nucleotides are degraded (hydrolyzed) by phosphodiesterases. cGMP phosphodiesterase appears to be chemically distinct from cAMP phosphodiesterase. They are membrane bound or soluble and require calcium ion for modulation.[33] Some studies indicate that cGMP levels may either facilitate or inhibit cAMP degradation, depending on the level of cGMP. It is possible that cGMP may influence the in-

TABLE 9-2. Airway Smooth Muscle Receptors

Type	Stimulatory Effects on Airway Smooth Muscle	Cyclic Nucleotide
Adrenergic		
Alpha$_1$ and alpha$_2$	Contraction	Decreased cAMP, increased cGMP
Beta$_2$	Relaxation	Increased cAMP
Cholinergic	Contraction	Increased cGMP
Nonadrenergic noncholinergic		
VIP/PMH	Relaxation	Increased cAMP
Substance P	Contraction	?
Mediator receptors		
Adenosine		
A$_1$	Contraction	Decreased cAMP
A$_2$	Relaxation	Increased cAMP
Histamine		
H$_1$	Contraction	Increased cGMP
H$_2$	Relaxation	Increased cAMP
Leukotrienes	Contraction	No direct effect
Prostaglandins		
PGD$_2$	Contraction	?
PGF$_2$	Contraction	?
PGE	Relaxation	Increased cAMP

tracellular levels of cAMP by its effect on cAMP phosphodiesterase.[23]

Other Receptors

Many receptors exist on airway smooth muscle (Table 9-2). As mentioned previously, receptors exist for prostaglandins of the E series, which, when stimulated, lead to increased levels of cAMP and bronchodilation. Receptors probably also exist for prostaglandins D_2 and $F_{2\alpha}$, which are potent bronchoconstrictors.[19] In animals, two histamine receptors exist: an H_1-receptor, which, when stimulated, leads to increased cGMP and bronchoconstriction, and an H_2-receptor, which, when stimulated, leads to increased levels of cAMP and smooth muscle relaxation.[33–36] In humans, a marked variability in the response to aerosolized histamine has been found.[37] In vivo, it may be that the major regulation in histamine-induced bronchoconstriction is mainly via the parasympathetic system rather than by direct stimulation of histamine receptors, since bronchoconstriction is partially or completely blocked by hexamethonium or atropine.[38,39] In vitro, histamine-induced human bronchial smooth muscle contraction is blocked by H_1-blocking agents. Leukotrienes are released during an asthmatic attack and have a profound bronchoconstrictor effect in vivo and in vitro.[13,40] Specific receptors probably exist for leukotrienes C_4, D_4, and E_4.[18] Adenosine receptors also exist on airway smooth muscle. Aerosolized adenosine causes bronchoconstriction in asthmatic subjects.[41] It has little direct effect on human airway smooth muscle, suggesting that the bronchoconstrictor response may be indirect.[42]

SYMPATHOMIMETIC BRONCHODILATORS

Sympathomimetic bronchodilators have been used widely for many years to induce bronchodilation. Recently, the development of synthetic agents has been successful in minimizing the cardiovascular (beta$_1$) effects and preserving the bronchodilator (beta$_2$) effects (Tables 9-1 and 9-3). The latter have been referred to as beta$_2$-agonists and include metaproterenol, terbutaline, albuterol (salbutamol outside the United States), bitolterol, pirbuterol, fenoterol, carbuterol, formoterol, and salmeterol. The latter four drugs have yet to be approved for use in the United States, but are in use abroad. Formoterol and salmeterol are undergoing clinical trials in the United States. Figure 9-1 displays the structures of the sympathomimetic drugs.

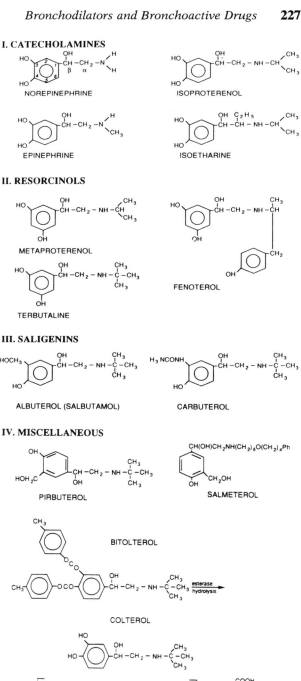

Fig. 9-1. The structures of sympathomimetic drugs.

TABLE 9-3. Beta-Agonists Used in the Treatment of Diseases with Airflow Obstruction

Drug	Mechanism of Action			Drug Dosages and Route of Administration					Duration of Action (h)
	Alpha	Beta₁	Beta₂	Subcutaneous	Metered Dose Inhaler	Aerosol	Oral	Intravenous	
Catecholamines									
Epinephrine	+	+	+	0.3–0.5 mL of 1 : 1,000 aqueous solution	160 μg/puff	2.25–12.5 mg/treatment	None	—	1–2
Isoproterenol	–	+	+	—	130–160 μg/puff	0.63–3.8 mg/treatment	None	0.04–0.225 μg/kg/min[a]	1–2
Isoetharine	–	+	++	—	340 μg/puff	1.25–7.5 mg/treatment	None	—	2–3
Resorcinols									
Metaproterenol	–	+	++	—	650 μg/puff	5–15 mg/treatment	5–20 mg qid	—	3–4
Terbutaline	–	±	++	0.25 mg	200 μg/puff	0.5–2.5 mg/treatment	1.25–5 mg qid	Up to 0.4 μg/kg/min[a]	4–6
Fenoterol	–	±	++	—	200 μg/puff[b]	0.5–2.5 mg/treatment[b]	2.5–10 mg qid[b]	μg/kg/min[c]	4–6
Saligenins									
Albuterol	–	±	++	—	90 μg/puff	1.25–2.5 mg/treatment	1–8 mg qid 4 mg bid[e]	up to 0.5 μg/kg/min[d]	4–6 12[e]
Miscellaneous									
Bitolterol	–	±	++	—	370 μg/puff	—	—	—	4–8
Pirbuterol	–	±	++	—	200 μg/puff	—	10–15 mg qid[b]	—	4–6

Abbreviation: MDI, metered dose inhaler.
[a] Not FDA approved (ref. 296).
[b] Not FDA approved.
[c] Not FDA approved. Dose not established, but probably similar to albuterol (ref. 61).
[d] Not FDA approved (refs. 61 and 297).
[e] Sustained-release preparation.

The catecholamines are characterized by a hydroxyl group located on both positions 3 and 4 of a phenolic moiety, plus a hydroxyl group on the beta carbon of an ethyl amino group located at position 1 (Fig. 9-1). Metabolism of the catecholamines occurs by catechol-O-methyltransferase (COMT), which attacks the three-position hydroxyl group, and by monamine oxidase, which attacks the terminal amino group. Weak beta-blocking compounds are formed in the metabolism of epinephrine and isoproterenol, which may have clinical significance, particularly in the rare instance when paradoxic bronchoconstriction occurs after the use of isoproterenol.[43] Catecholamines are also degraded by gut and liver sulfatases, which render them ineffective by the oral route. Catecholamines are all short-acting drugs (Table 9-3).

Selective manipulation of the ring hydroxyl groups and the N-terminal groups can reduce drug metabolism in the former and lead to a more selective beta$_2$ action in the latter. Resorcinols and saligenins are not degraded by COMT and resist action by sulfatase, resulting in compounds that have a longer duration of action. By adding larger groupings to the N-terminal site, more selective beta activity results. Reduction or loss of beta activity occurs when either of the phenolic hydroxyl units is removed or if the hydroxyl group on the beta carbon is eliminated (Fig. 9-1). The synthetic compounds thus formed by manipulation of the phenolic ring or N-terminal groups are more specific beta-receptor simulators, principally beta$_2$, and have a much longer duration of action (Table 9-3).

In vitro studies show that isoproterenol is the most potent bronchodilator, followed by albuterol, terbutaline, fenoterol, and metaproterenol.[43] Terbutaline and fenoterol are nearly equipotent. In isolated cardiac tissues, albuterol, terbutaline, and fenoterol are much less active than isoproterenol and other catecholamines, with albuterol probably having the least activity.[43]

Epinephrine

Epinephrine (adrenalin) is a naturally occurring catecholamine that is synthesized, stored, and released from the adrenal medulla and certain adrenergic nerve terminals. It stimulates all alpha- and beta-receptors (Tables 9-1 and 9-3).

Because of its broad stimulation of adrenergic receptors, epinephrine is the drug of choice in systemic hypersensitivity reactions, usually given in a subcutaneous dose of 0.3 to 1.0 mL of a 1 : 1,000 aqueous solution. Similar doses can be used to treat acute bronchospasm.

Subcutaneous epinephrine, 0.3 to 0.5 mL of a 1 : 1,000 aqueous solution, can be used for acute wheezing (Table 9-3).[44] It appears to have no more cardiovascular side effects than subcutaneous terbutaline, but has a shorter (1 to 2 hours versus 2 to 4 hours) duration of action than terbutaline.[45] Racemic epinephrine can be administered by a metered dose inhaler (MDI) or in solution delivered by a nebulizer (Table 9-3).

Norepinephrine

Norepinephrine is a weak beta$_2$ agonist and has little utility in the treatment of patients with airway diseases.

Isoproterenol

As has been mentioned previously, isoproterenol is the most potent beta$_1$ and beta$_2$ agonist. It is available in an MDI and as a solution for use in a hand-held or gas-powered nebulizer (Table 9-3). However, because of its cardiovascular effects, its use has been largely supplanted by more specific beta$_2$ agonists.

Intravenous isoproterenol has been used in asthmatic children as a final mode of therapy to obviate the need for intubation and mechanical ventilation.[46,47] The starting dose used was 0.1 μg/kg/min, which was increased by 0.1 μg/kg/min increments every 15 minutes until a heart rate of 200 beats/min was reached or the PaCO$_2$ began to fall.[47] Once improvement occurred, isoproterenol was tapered by 0.05 μg/kg/min every 1 to 2 hours, depending on the clinical improvement and favorable blood gases.[47] In adults, lower doses produced a stable tachycardia at 0.075 μg/kg/min, but bronchodilation continued up to doses of 0.225 μg/kg/min. Bronchodilation occurred or stopped within 2 to 5 minutes after starting or stopping the infusion.[48] The intravenous use of isoproterenol should be reserved as the last medication to reverse bronchospasm, and the patient must be monitored very closely in an intensive care unit.

Isoetharine

Isoetharine is a catecholamine (Fig. 9-1) originally synthesized to provide a compound with greater beta$_2$ action and fewer beta$_1$ effects than isoproterenol. It has one-tenth the potency of isoproterenol,[44] and has a duration of action of up to 3 hours. It is available as an MDI and in solution for use in a nebulizer (Table 9-3). Aerosolized doses of 0.25 to 0.5 mL diluted in 2 mL of sterile water or saline or 0.68 mg (two puffs) from an MDI can be used for wheezing; however, side effects are common. Its use also has largely been supplanted by the more selective beta$_2$ agonists.

Metaproterenol

Metaproterenol is a resorcinol (Fig. 9-1) and was the first synthetic noncatecholamine bronchodilator introduced in the United States. Its duration of action is up to 4 hours. In addition, it was the first beta$_2$ agonist to be available orally in the United States. It has less cardiovascular activity than isoproterenol, but also is a less potent bronchodilator. Oral doses of 5 to 20 mg can be used every 4 to 6 hours, depending on neuromuscular (shakiness, tremor, cramps) or cardiovascular side effects (Table 9-3). Peak effect usually occurs within 1 to 2 hours. It is also available as an MDI and as a solution for nebulization. The usual MDI dose is 1.3 mg (two puffs) given as needed up to every 3 to 4 hours for wheezing. The usual aerosolized dose is 10 to 15 mg (0.2 to 0.3 mL) diluted to 2 to 3 mL with sterile water or saline given every 3 to 4 hours. If side effects occur, 5 mg (0.1 mL) can be delivered.

Terbutaline

Terbutaline is a resorcinol (Fig. 9-1) and was the second noncatecholamine bronchodilator introduced in the United States. It is a slightly less potent bronchodilator than isoproterenol,[49] but has far fewer cardiovascular side effects than isoproterenol, with a duration of action up to 6 to 7 hours orally or by aerosol.[44,50–52] Given subcutaneously in doses of 0.25 mg, it has a duration of action of 2 to 4 hours.[45]

Cardiovascular side effects may be related to its beta$_2$ action of relaxing vascular smooth musculature, resulting in a secondary increase in cardiac rate, rather than by stimulation of beta$_1$-cardiac receptors.

Given subcutaneously, the incidence of cardiovascular side effects (mainly due to beta$_2$ effects) is similar to that of epinephrine, even though the duration of bronchodilation is longer.[45] It can be administered subcutaneously every 20 to 30 minutes for up to four doses.

Oral doses range from 1.25 to 5.0 mg every 6 hours. Peak action usually occurs within 2 hours.[50,52] Use is limited primarily by the neuromuscular side effects and less so by the cardiovascular ones.

The available MDI dose of terbutaline is 200 µg/puff, and the usual dosage is two puffs (400 µg) every 4 to 6 hours. Nebulizer use of the injectable form of terbutaline diluted to a total volume of 2 to 3 mL by sterile water or saline is rather commonplace. Side effects with doses of 1.5 mg have been infrequently experienced. The usual dose is 1 mg every 4 to 6 hours, which is supported by studies in the literature[53,54] (Table 9-3).

Albuterol (Salbutamol)

Albuterol is a saligenin (Fig. 9-1), and was the third noncatecholamine to be introduced in the United States. It has the fewest cardiovascular side effects of the sympathomimetic bronchodilators in vitro.[44] Orally or by aerosol, its peak action occurs within 2 hours and its duration of action is up to 6 hours.[51,53,55–57]

Oral doses range from 1 to 8 mg every 6 hours for the standard, short-acting preparation, to 4 to 8 mg every 12 hours for the sustained-release preparation (Table 9-3). The sustained-release preparation releases approximately one-half of its dose rapidly, similar to the short-acting preparation, then releases the remainder over several hours, thus allowing a 12-hour dosing interval (D.A. Sojka, Schering Corporation, personal communication). Food does not appear to affect the pharmacokinetics.[58] Clinical studies have shown similar improvements in pulmonary function with the sustained-release preparation given every 12 hours, as compared with the conventional tablet given four times daily.[59] Again, use is limited principally by the neuromuscular side effects rather than by cardiovascular ones.

The usual dose of the MDI is 0.18 mg (two puffs) every 4 hours. An albuterol solution for nebulizer use is available. In one study, nebulized doses up to 3.0 mg caused significant bronchodilation with no change in the pulse compared with placebo. Tremor was less with 1.5 mg than with 3.0 mg.[60] The frequency of administration of a nebulized solution depends on the severity of wheezing: every 1/2 to 1 hour for patients with acute, severe asthma to every 4 to 6 hours for aerosol maintenance therapy in patients with stable airways disease. Lower doses should be efficacious, yet safe, in patients with cardiac disease. Intravenous albuterol, 0.5 µg/kg/min, has also been shown to produce a significant general improvement in cardiac function and an improvement in the systolic and diastolic function of the left ventricle in patients with severe congestive cardiomyopathy.[61]

Bitolterol

Bitolterol is biologically inactive and considered a pro-drug. On administration, it is hydrolyzed within the lung by tissue esterases to the active compound colterol (Fig. 9-1).[62]

It was hoped that with oral administration, bitolterol would be taken up selectively by the lungs to produce prolonged bronchodilation by slow hydrolysis to colterol. However, the greatest tissue uptake following oral administration was in the liver, where subsequent methylation and glucuronide conjugation led to inconsistent bronchodilatory effects.[63,64] Tachycardia in animal models and significant frequency of musculoskeletal tremor made oral and parenteral administration of bitolterol undesirable.[63]

When administered by the aerosolized route, bitolterol is a relatively selective beta$_2$ agonist. Studies have shown a greater separation of bronchodilator and cardiovascular activities when compared with albuterol and terbutaline.[65,66] The greater tissue lung esterase concentrations and activity are probably responsible for the good bronchodilator-to-cardiovascular separation ratio.[67,68] Bitolterol has been compared with metaproterenol and albuterol aerosols.[69,70] The maximum improvement in the forced expiratory volume at 1 second (FEV$_1$) was comparable for all three drugs. Bitolterol did not have any significant effect on pulse rate in any of these studies.[69,70] In another study, bitolterol aerosol, 1,050 μg, was significantly longer in duration of action than isoproterenol, 250 μg, and albuterol, 180 μg.[71] The duration of bronchodilator action is up to 8 hours.[68,70] Onset of bronchodilation occurs within 5 minutes and peak bronchodilation occurs within 60 to 90 minutes.[72]

Bitolterol can be used to treat acute bronchospasm or can be administered on a chronic basis to prevent bronchospasm. The usual MDI dose is 2 or 3 inhalations (370 μg/puff) given up to every 8 hours. Compared with sustained-release theophylline, bitolterol appears to be inferior in controlling the symptoms, gas exchange abnormalities, and lung dysfunction in nocturnal asthma.[73]

Pirbuterol

Pirbuterol is a beta$_2$ agonist that differs structurally from albuterol in the substitution of a pyridine ring for the benzene ring (Fig. 9-1).[74] Pirbuterol is a relatively selective beta$_2$-agonist, but does demonstrate both bronchodilator and cardiovascular effects.[75,76] Pirbuterol was 9 times more selective for pulmonary tissue than was albuterol, and 1,520 times more selective than isoproterenol.[77]

The onset of pirbuterol activity occurs 5 minutes after aerosol administration and within 1 hour after oral administration. The time to peak activity (aerosol, 30 minutes; oral, 1 hour) and magnitude of activity are similar to those of equipotent doses of albuterol.[78,79] Pirbuterol is a less potent bronchodilator than albuterol on a weight basis. The lowest doses that apparently produce maximum bronchodilation are 0.4 mg of aerosolized pirbuterol and 15 mg of oral pirbuterol.[80]

The usual MDI dose is 2 inhalations (200 μg/puff)

up to every 4 hours. The oral form has yet to be approved by the Food and Drug Administration (FDA). The recommended oral dosage of pirbuterol is 10 to 15 mg 3 to 4 times per day. As with the other beta$_2$ agonists, use is limited by the neuromuscular rather than the cardiovascular side effects.

Fenoterol

Fenoterol is a resorcinol (Fig. 9-1) that has yet to be approved by the FDA. Its peak action, duration of action, and side effects are very similar to those of terbutaline and albuterol (peak action within 2 hours, duration up to 8 hours).[51,81–83]

Oral doses range from 2.5 to 10 mg every 6 hours (Table 9-3). Aerosolized doses of 0.5 to 1.0 mg are efficacious, but doses up to 2.5 mg appear to be well tolerated.[82]

Clinically, there appears to be little difference in the bronchodilator effects and cardiovascular side effects among terbutaline, bitolterol, albuterol, pirbuterol, and fenoterol.

Formoterol

Formoterol fumarate (Fig. 9-1) is a recently developed catecholamine analog (currently under clinical investigation) with distinct selective and long-acting effects on the beta$_2$-receptors of bronchial smooth muscle.[84,85] It has been shown in in vivo animal experiments to have a potency 50 times greater than albuterol, with a much longer duration of action.[86,87] Formoterol by inhalation appears to be five to 15 times more potent than inhaled albuterol, with a longer duration of action. Seventy-five percent of the maximum bronchodilator effect still remained after 8 hours.[88] The peak bronchodilator effect by aerosol occurs at around 2 hours, and a significant improvement in FEV$_1$ may last up to 12 hours.[89] The prolonged bronchodilator effect demonstrated by aerosol does not occur with oral administration, in which the duration of action is similar to albuterol.[88]

Salmeterol

Salmeterol hydroxynaphthoate (Fig. 9-1) is a new investigational inhaled beta$_2$ agonist which, in animal models, has shown a prolonged bronchodilator effect both in vitro and in vivo.[90,91] Salmeterol was designed by modifying albuterol to obtain a drug with much greater affinity for its receptors because of increased exoreceptor binding.[92,93] The plasma half-life of salmeterol appears to be similar to that of albuterol (3 hours).

A study that compared the peak bronchodilator response and duration of action of inhaled salmeterol with those of albuterol found that 50, 100, and 200 μg of salmeterol produced peak increases in FEV_1 similar to those produced by albuterol at the same doses, but the effects were more prolonged with salmeterol.[94] After albuterol, FEV_1 and peak expiratory flow had returned to baseline within 6 hours. However, after all 3 dosages of salmeterol, more than half of the bronchodilator effect remained after 12 hours.[94] The results of this study suggest that salmeterol, in dosages of 50 to 100 μg, is equipotent to 200 μg of albuterol in terms of peak bronchodilator effects, but with a significantly more prolonged bronchodilator response than albuterol. Duration of actions of formoterol and salmeterol may be of particular value in the treatment of patients with nocturnal asthma.

Prolonged Bronchodilatory Effects—Possible Mechanisms of Action

The exact mechanism behind the prolonged effect of these newer beta$_2$ agonists—salmeterol and formoterol—is not fully understood.[95] *Systemic* pharmacokinetic properties of the drugs do not seem to influence the prolonged duration of bronchodilator effect seen with inhaled formoterol and salmeterol, as the serum half-life of these two agents is comparable to albuterol ($t_{1/2}$ = 3 hours), an agent that demonstrates clinical effectiveness for only approximately 6 hours.[85] Other beta$_2$ agonists, eg, clenbuterol, have a very long plasma half-life (20 hours), with no substantial prolongation of the duration of bronchodilation with the inhaled route.[96] Perhaps the effects can be explained by *local* pharmacokinetic properties in the airways or by *general* pharmacokinetic properties of the drugs.[88]

It has been shown that there is a difference between the potency of a bronchodilator drug when administered on the serosal side, compared with intraluminal administration.[97] Most drugs show a considerably higher potency when given on the serosal side.[98] Formoterol given orally has a much shorter duration than when given by inhalation,[88] yet the oral dose would reach the airways on the serosal side. Thus, it appears that the local intraluminal pharmacokinetics are responsible for the difference in the duration of action of oral versus inhaled formoterol.

Salmeterol was designed by modifying albuterol to obtain a drug with much greater affinity for its receptors because of increased exoreceptor binding.[92] The consequence of this would be a localized persistence of salmeterol in the vicinity of the beta$_2$-receptors. Another explanation for the prolonged bronchodilator effects of salmeterol might be that the airway epithelium constitutes a diffusion barrier through which bronchodilators pass at different rates.[99] Possibly, therefore, the airway epithelium acts as a reservoir for bronchodilator drugs.[99]

A factor that might be correlated to the duration of action could be lipophilicity. Formoterol is more lipophilic than albuterol, which could increase the nonspecific binding of the drug to the cell membrane, thereby establishing a depot of the drug in the vicinity of the receptor.[89]

It appears that further investigation will be required to establish the exact mechanism(s) of the prolonged bronchodilatory effects of formoterol and salmeterol. Whatever the mechanism(s), they do hold promise for less frequent dosing, better compliance, and enhanced control in the patient with asthma.

Nonbronchodilator Actions of Sympathomimetic Drugs

The nonbronchodilator actions of beta-adrenergic drugs need to be emphasized in normal patients and in patients with airway diseases (asthma, chronic bronchitis, and cystic fibrosis) (Table 9-4). All of the drugs discussed above, except for the investigational drugs, have been shown to stimulate mucociliary clearance, although the increase in diseased airways appears to be less than in normal airways.[100] This action is independent of smooth muscle relaxation. The oral, injectable, and aerosolized routes have been shown to be effective.

Another nonbronchodilator effect of the sympathomimetic drugs is inhibition of the release of bronchoconstrictor mediators (histamine, leukotrienes, slow-reacting substance of anaphylaxis, and kinins) by mast cells.[101-103] This appears to be secondary to mast cell beta$_2$-receptor site stimulation, with subsequent generation of cAMP and reduction of available calcium ions (see above). Thus, in the patient with asthma or other diseases in which mast cell mediator release occurs, beta$_2$-adrenergic drugs are useful to promote bronchodilation and inhibit mast cell mediator release.

TABLE 9-4. Nonbronchodilator Effects of Beta$_2$-Agonists and Theophylline

Increased mucociliary clearance
Inhibition of the release of mast cell mediators
Decreased permeability edema
Decreased pulmonary hypertension and increased right ventricular ejection fraction
Increased contractility of fatigued diaphragm muscle

Beta-adrenergic agents in vitro have shown an anti-permeability effect on the venules in the lung microvascular bed.[103] However, the clinical utility of this property needs to be defined. Usual doses of beta$_2$ agonists reduce pulmonary artery pressure and increase the right ventricular ejection fraction in patients with hypoxemia.[104] These effects would be of benefit in those patients with airflow obstruction due to chronic bronchitis, emphysema, cystic fibrosis, or other airway diseases in which hypoxemia is also present. Beta$_2$ agonists have been shown to improve diaphragmatic contractility in animal studies, and this effect is additive to theophylline.[105] Whether this effect will occur in the human diaphragm needs to be elucidated.

Beta-Adrenergic Tachyphylaxis (Desensitization)

With repetitive use of beta-adrenergic agents, tachyphylaxis (drug tolerance) occurs.[83] This appears to be due to a decreased number of available beta$_2$-receptors, with a subsequent reduction in the amount of cAMP generated from adenylate cyclase stimulation,[106] although other cellular mechanisms may be responsible.[107] In the airways, tachyphylaxis results in reduced bronchodilation over time to the same dose of drug administered. With oral fenoterol, it was found that not only did the peak bronchodilator effect drop 31 percent, but the duration of a 15 percent FEV$_1$ response declined significantly from 6 hours to 4 hours.[83] All sympathomimetic drugs discussed previously, except for the newest agents, display drug tolerance, with the peak effect declining from 14 to 58 percent and the duration of a 15 percent bronchodilator response declining up to 50 percent.[108] Steroids given intravenously (200 mg of hydrocortisone or 40 mg of methylprednisolone) appear to reverse the tachyphylaxis, demonstrating an effect in 1 hour and near reversal in 6 to 8 hours.[109,110] The clinical significance of drug tolerance to the beta-adrenergic drugs has yet to be delineated fully, but it appears that the patient who has severe asthma and/or who has been receiving frequent, high doses of these drugs would be at the greatest risk for a lack of responsiveness (tachyphylaxis) to these agents when acute airway obstruction occurs. Higher bronchodilator doses (monitoring for cardiovascular side effects) and intravenous steroids should be helpful to reverse this situation.

XANTHINE BRONCHODILATORS

Xanthine bronchodilator agents (Fig. 9-2), principally theophylline, aminophylline, the ethylenedi-amine salt of theophylline, and other salts of theophylline, are potent bronchodilator drugs that have been in use for years. Naturally occurring xanthines such as caffeine and theobromine are present in coffee, tea, chocolate, and many cola beverages (Fig. 9-2). Tea leaves are the source from which theophylline is extracted.

Theophylline

The activity of aminophylline and other salts of theophylline relates to the amount of anhydrous theophylline present after degradation. Theophylline causes relaxation of bronchial smooth muscle. Theophylline has been shown to increase cellular levels of cAMP by the inhibition of phosphodiesterase, which breaks down cAMP. Previously this was thought to be the mechanism of action. However, the in vitro doses used to achieve phosphodiesterase inhibition appear to be too high to achieve clinically.[111] In guinea pig and dog tracheal muscle preparations, theophylline levels achievable in humans had no effect on cAMP or cGMP, but did increase calcium ion uptake and redistribution, consistent with a decrease of myoplasmic calcium ion and calcium ion sequestration in the mitochondrium.[111] However, the exact cellular mechanisms underlying bronchial smooth muscle relaxation remain to be clarified.[112]

Theophylline causes potent central nervous system stimulation as well as medullary center stimulation,[113] and decreases cerebral blood flow.[114] High levels can produce focal or generalized seizures. Theophylline is also a mild diuretic.

Theophylline produces a significant cardiovascular response. In normal patients, theophylline causes a chronotropic effect, a decrease in coronary artery blood flow, an increase in myocardial oxygen extraction,[115] and a decrease in left ventricular ejection time.[116] In patients with chronic obstructive pulmonary disease and cor pulmonale, increases in heart rate, stroke volume, and cardiac output and decreases in right ventricular end-diastolic pressure, left ventricular end-diastolic pressure, wedge pressure, and systemic vascular resistance can occur.[117–119]

Liquid and plain tablet forms of theophylline are rapidly and completely absorbed.[120] Slow-release preparations dominate the market, and a number of these also demonstrate complete absorption.[120,121] Absorption of theophylline solutions from the rectal mucosa is also rapid and complete,[122] although rectal suppositories are erratically and incompletely absorbed.[123] Once absorbed, theophylline is distributed rapidly throughout the body water, more in the extracellular than in the intracellular body water.[124] Theophylline binds to serum proteins, principally al-

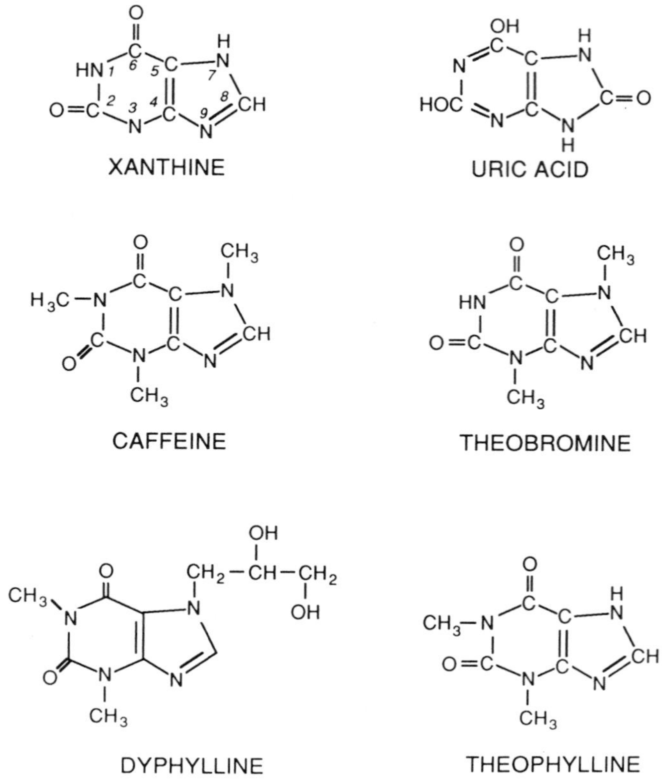

Fig. 9-2. The structures of theophylline and other methylxanthine compounds.

bumin, varying from 50 to 60 percent, which increases as serum pH increases (30 percent binding at pH 7 to 70 percent at pH 7.8).[125] Theophylline passes freely into breast milk,[126] crosses the placenta,[127] and appears in the saliva, although salivary levels are not consistent enough to allow monitoring for therapy.[128]

Theophylline is metabolized principally in the liver by the cytochrome P-450 mixed function oxidase enzyme system.[129] Approximately 10 percent is eliminated unchanged through the kidneys.[129,130] Metabolism of theophylline appears to be influenced by diet and simultaneous drug ingestion (Table 9-5). In relation to patients on normal diets, substitution of a high-protein diet reduces the half-life of theophylline, whereas substitution of a high-carbohydrate diet increases the half-life.[131] Smoking also decreases the half-life of theophylline.[132] The half-life is increased in those patients receiving erythromycin,[133] troleandomycin,[134] cimetidine,[135] ranitidine,[136] allopurinol,[137] propranolol,[138] mexiletine,[139] oral contraceptives,[132,140] verapamil,[141] diltiazem,[142] interferon,[143] ciprofloxacin,[144] and other quinolones.[145] Diseases affecting the liver directly, such as cirrhosis, or indirectly, due to heart failure or cor pulmonale, also greatly lengthen the half-life of theophylline.[146–148] In

normal patients, the half-life of theophylline varies greatly, from 3 to 9.5 hours.[149] This half-life may increase to 65 hours in the presence of liver or heart failure.[147] Several drugs decrease the half-life of theophylline, including phenytoin,[150] barbiturates,[132,151] alcohol,[132] and rifampin.[152]

Bronchodilation has been shown to increase as the levels of theophylline increase from 5 to 20 μg/mL.[149] By convention, it has been decided that the therapeutic range of serum theophylline lies between 10 and 20 μg/mL. In patients, the wide range in the half-life (liver metabolism) explains the variable serum theophylline levels found, although, in the individual patient, the half-life usually remains stable unless influenced by drugs or disease (Table 9-5). Exercise-induced asthma may also be blocked by serum theophylline levels above 10 μg/mL.[153]

Not all side effects are related to the serum theophylline level. Minor caffeine-like side effects may occur that bear no relationship to the serum level, and tolerance to these symptoms usually occurs during long-term therapy.[154] The most common side effects are nausea, vomiting, headache, insomnia, and irritability. Although the frequency of these side effects increases as the serum level approaches or exceeds 20

TABLE 9-5. Conditions and Drugs That Affect Theophylline Clearance

	Decreased	Increased
Age	Prematurity Neonate Aging	1–16 y
Diet	High carbohydrate, low protein Caffeine Theobromine	Low carbohydrate, high protein Charcoal cooking
Smoking		Cigarettes Marijuana
Diseases	Hepatic diseases Congestive heart failure (moderate-severe) Acute pulmonary edema Severe airflow obstruction Pneumonia Acute viral illness	

Drugs	Oral contraceptives
	Allopurinol
	Cimetidine
	Ranitidine
	Macrolide antibiotics
	   Erythromycin
	   Lincomycin
	   Troleandomycin
	Quinolone antibiotics
	   Ciprofloxacin
	   Enoxacin
	   Pefloxacin
	Thiabendazole
	Mexiletine
	Propranolol
	Verapamil
	Diltiazem
	Interferon
		Phenobarbital
		Phenytoin
		Alcohol
		Rifampin

μg/mL, an occasional patient will exhibit these effects at levels below 10 μg/mL. Diarrhea also occurs infrequently and may occur with serum levels that are in the therapeutic range or below. As serum levels exceed 20 μg/mL, the frequency of side effects increases, and, with levels above 35 μg/mL, cardiac dysrhythmias, seizures, and even death may occur.[156] Minor gastrointestinal or other symptoms may *not* precede the development of serious cardiac dysrhythmias or convulsions, so serum theophylline levels *must* be monitored, particularly in hospitalized patients, to avoid toxic reactions.

Theophylline may be administered via the intravenous or oral route, but is not effective in aerosolized form.[157] Rectal use is not recommended because of the large doses available in rectal solutions that could quickly elevate the serum theophylline level into a toxic range.

Given intravenously, aminophylline rather than theophylline is usually used, although an intravenous anhydrous theophylline preparation is available. A to-

tal of 70 to 85 percent of aminophylline converts to theophylline, depending on the preparation used. The intravenous dosage for aminophylline is listed in Table 9-6. If the patient has not been on theophylline, a loading dose of 6 mg/kg ideal body weight is given to all patients, since theophylline is distributed to the extra- and intracellular body water, which is related to ideal body weight. It should be given over 20 to 30 minutes to avoid toxicity. If the patient has been on theophylline, a serum theophylline level should be obtained prior to the initiation of intravenous aminophylline therapy, and a maintenance infusion should be started (Table 9-6). If the theophylline level measured is low, the patient should receive a bolus of aminophylline over 20 minutes based on the finding that, for each 0.6 mg/kg ideal body weight (IBW) increase per 24 hours in the aminophylline load (0.5 mg/kg IBW for the theophylline), the serum theophylline level should increase by 1 μg/mL.[158] A maintenance drip should then be restarted at a rate that encompasses the total dose required over 24 hours. A serum

TABLE 9-6. Intravenous Aminophylline Dosage

Group	Loading Dose[a] (Over 20–30 min)	Maintenance Dose[a]	
		Initial 12 h	Beyond 12 h
Children			
6 mo–9 yr	6 mg/kg	1.2 mg/kg/h	1.0 mg/kg/h
9–16 yr	6 mg/kg	1.0 mg/kg/h	0.8 mg/kg/h
Young adult smokers	6 mg/kg	1.0 mg/kg/h	0.8 mg/kg/h
Otherwise healthy nonsmoking adults	6 mg/kg	0.7 mg/kg/h	0.5 mg/kg/h
Older patients, patients with cor pulmonale	6 mg/kg	0.6 mg/kg/h	0.3 mg/kg/h
Patients with CHF, liver disease	6 mg/kg	0.5 mg/kg/h	0.1–0.2 mg/kg/h

Abbreviation: CHF, congestive heart failure.
[a] Based on ideal body weight: 105 + 5 lbs per inch above 5 feet (female) and 106 + 6 lbs per inch above 5 feet (male).
(Adapted from FDA Drug Bulletin.[158])

theophylline level can be drawn in 4 to 24 hours to ascertain whether a therapeutic level has been achieved. If the serum theophylline is low, another partial loading dose may be required. If side effects suggestive of theophylline toxicity occur, a serum theophylline should be drawn immediately. If the theophylline level is elevated, the infusion should be lowered by 0.6 mg/kg IBW per 24 hours for each 1 μg/mL level decrease in serum theophylline desired.

Once intravenous aminophylline is no longer required (acute bronchospasm has subsided, recovery from surgery, etc.), the patient can be switched to oral theophylline, the 24-hour theophylline dose calculated from the 24-hour aminophylline dose *reduced* by 20 percent. A slow-release theophylline preparation that is completely absorbed should be used, since dosing can be maintained on an every 12-hour basis,[121,154] which is convenient for the patient. Non-sustained-release theophylline preparations (tablets, liquid) have to be given at 6-hour intervals, which may result in uneven serum theophylline levels that may fluctuate below, within, or above the therapeutic range. Sustained-release preparations avoid these problems. Patients prefer taking medications twice a day as opposed to four times a day. If the patient develops symptoms suggestive of theophylline toxicity, a serum theophylline level should be obtained immediately and the dose adjusted if needed, according to the guidelines described previously for intravenous therapy.

Theophylline and aminophylline can be used safely in patients who have cardiovascular disease in addition to lung disease. Monitoring of serum theophylline levels needs to be more frequent, particularly after dosage changes. Once intravenous therapy has been initiated, a serum theophylline level should be obtained within 4 hours and repeated within 24 hours if no change in dosage has occurred.[120,121] Repeat levels are necessary if congestive heart failure occurs or if it has been corrected, since the dose may need to be decreased in the former case or increased in the latter (Table 9-5). Patients on oral therapy should have a peak level measured (4 hours after sustained-release preparations or 2 hours after non-sustained-release preparations) after stable levels have been reached, usually within 48 hours. Using caution and monitoring serum theophylline levels, there should be few cardiovascular side effects from theophylline use in any patient, and no convulsions or deaths. Theophylline endured a bad reputation prior to the time when rational theophylline dosage schedules and serum theophylline monitoring became available.

Nonbronchodilator Actions of Theophylline

The nonbronchodilator effects of theophylline are identical to those exhibited by beta$_2$ agonists (Table 9-4)[93]. Theophylline has been found to stimulate mucous production and to increase ciliary beat in in vitro studies.[159,160] It has been shown to increase mucociliary clearance in dogs[161] and normal humans.[162] A modest increase in mucociliary clearance occurs in patients with chronic bronchitis.[163]

Theophylline, like beta$_2$-adrenergic drugs, inhibits the release of mast cell mediators.[13] Theophylline increases diaphragmatic contractility, an effect most pronounced in the fatigued diaphragm.[163] Improvement in diaphragmatic function has been demonstrated in normal subjects[164] and in patients with airflow obstruction secondary to chronic bronchitis and emphysema.[165] The latter group was studied after 2 months of therapy. The cellular mechanism responsible is not known.

Other Xanthines

Dyphylline (7-dihydroxypropyltheophylline) is the only xanthine derivative that is marketed in the United States (Fig. 9-2). Proxyphylline and acephylline are marketed abroad. Dyphylline is one-tenth as potent as theophylline in vitro.[166] In patients with reversible airway disease, dyphylline appears to have approximately one-fifth the bronchodilator effect of theophylline.[167] Studies of the pharmacokinetics of dyphylline have shown that it is absorbed less well[168] (82 percent versus 100 percent for theophylline) and is eliminated quite rapidly (half-life, 2 hours).[168,169] The relationship among serum levels, efficacy, and toxicity has not been elucidated. Because of the short half-life, dosing would have to be less than every 4 hours, which would be difficult for patients to accept. Furthermore, the cost is considerably higher than for theophylline. Thus, there appears to be little reason to use dyphylline in the treatment of patients with airway diseases.

ANTICHOLINERGIC BRONCHODILATORS

The use of anticholinergic drugs, principally atropine, had declined after the development of the long-acting, powerful beta$_2$-adrenergic bronchodilators until a congener of atropine, ipratropium bromide, was approved for use in the United States. The latter is an effective bronchodilator agent with few or no side effects, and has revived the interest in anticholinergic bronchodilators.

Atropine

Atropine is a belladonna alkaloid that is widely dispersed throughout nature. Atropine inhibits the actions of acetylcholine on postganglionic cholinergic nerves and those of cholinergic receptors on bronchial smooth muscle (Table 9-2). The result is a reduction in bronchial gland mucous production and bronchodilation. Because of the side effects (mouth dryness, tachycardia, mydriasis, blurred vision) seen with systemic administration (intramuscular or oral), the only practical way to use atropine is in solution for nebulization, although it has never been approved for this use by the FDA. Dose-response characteristics in children or adults show that as the amount of drug delivered to the airways increases, the degree of bronchodilation, as well as the duration of the bronchodilator response, increases.[170,171] With doses of 0.025 to 0.05 mg/kg, significant bronchodilation lasts for at least 4 hours.[171] In one study, only dry mouth occurred when 0.025 mg/kg was nebulized, but tachycardia, head-

ache, and difficulties with micturition occurred at 0.05 mg/kg.[171] Thus, in adults with airflow obstruction, nebulization of 0.025 mg/kg of atropine appears to be the dose that is efficacious, yet has few side effects. Higher doses, 0.05 to 0.1 mg/kg, appear to be optimal in children with airflow obstruction.[170] Since these studies were performed with dosimeters that delivered precisely measured amounts of drug, larger doses might be needed when using current nebulizers in the hospital or at home. Side effects dictate the dose of drug that can be used in each patient. Aerosolized atropine has resulted in bronchodilation in patients with asthma as well as chronic bronchitis. However, atropine may be a more potent bronchodilator than the sympathomimetic drugs in those patients with chronic obstructive bronchitis.[172,173]

Atropine causes a decrease in mucociliary clearance in normal men and in women undergoing gynecologic surgery.[174,175] Atropine can cause a decrease in sputum volume in asthmatics without increasing sputum viscosity.[176] With aerosolized use, few episodes of tachycardia can be expected, particularly in the cardiac patient.

Ipratropium Bromide

Ipratropium bromide is available as an inhaled drug delivered via an MDI. It is available as a solution for use in a nebulizer outside the United States. Like atropine, ipratropium bromide is an anticholinergic bronchodilator with the same cellular mechanism of action. Because it is a quaternary compound (Fig. 9-3), it is much less well absorbed, less than 1 percent of a delivered dose being absorbed,[177] which helps reduce side effects.[178] Bronchodilation occurs within 30 seconds, 80 percent of the response occurs within 30 minutes, peak effect occurs in 1.5 to 2.0 hours, and the maximum duration of action is 6 hours.[179,180] Although the recommended dose is 40 μg, it appears that both the peak effect and the duration of action are prolonged by using higher doses, up to 120 μg.[181] The optimum dose delivered by nebulization appears to be between 50 and 125 μg for adults[182] and children.[183]

The virtue of ipratropium bromide lies in the fact that it has almost no side effects, even at high doses.[184,185] This is probably related to its lack of absorption. No changes in heart rate, blood pressure, or cardiac output have occurred, even with doses up to 320 μg.[185] This drug may be particularly useful in the patient with both cardiac and pulmonary diseases because of the lack of cardiovascular side effects. In some studies, bitter taste or dryness of the mouth or trachea have occurred in up to 20 to 30 percent of subjects.[178] Initial studies suggested that ipratropium

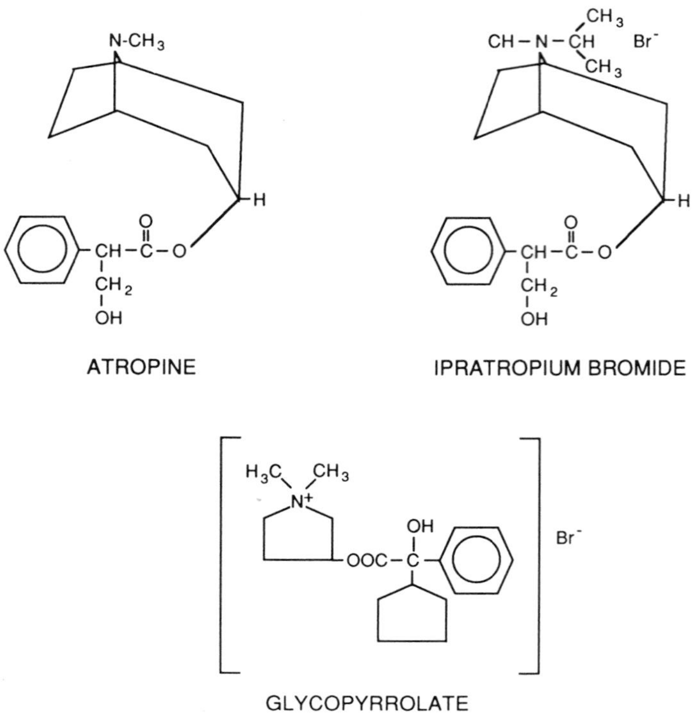

Fig. 9-3. The structures of anticholinergic drugs.

bromide was a more effective bronchodilator in patients with chronic bronchitis than was albuterol.[186] In a long-term clinical trial, ipratropium bromide was found to be a more effective bronchodilator than metaproterenol.[187] Beta agonists are more potent bronchodilators in patients with asthma than is ipratropium bromide.[188–190] Ipratropium bromide may be helpful in psychogenic asthma and asthma precipitated by beta-blocking agents.[191] In acute severe asthma (status asthmaticus), ipratropium bromide delivered by nebulizer in conjunction with a beta₂ agonist resulted in greater airflow than either agent alone.[192]

Although atropine causes a decline in mucociliary clearance, studies with ipratropium bromide have shown that it has no effect on mucociliary clearance in patients with asthma and chronic bronchitis.[193,194] No adverse effects on sputum quality appear to occur, although sputum weight declines.[193]

Glycopyrrolate

Glycopyrrolate is a quaternary ammonium anticholinergic compound, as is ipratropium bromide. Because of its quaternary structure, glycopyrrolate is poorly absorbed across biologic membranes, thus reducing the likelihood of systemic symptoms, particularly via the inhalation route.[195] Glycopyrrolate has

been shown to cause bronchodilation in normal individuals[196–198] and in patients with asthma.[199–201] In normal individuals, it appears that larger doses result in greater bronchodilation,[198] although this was not found in asthma patients.[201] The duration of action appears to be at least 8 hours and perhaps as long as 12 hours,[200,201] much longer than the duration of atropine.[196–198] The side effects were minimal after glycopyrrolate, not significantly different from placebo.[198,201]

Glycopyrrolate is not FDA approved for nebulizer use to administer as a bronchodilator. The injectable preparation (0.2 mg/mL) can be used in the nebulizer to provide 0.4 to 0.6 mg of drug per dose. Since the optimal dose is unknown and since ipratropium bromide is available, is efficacious (see above), and has minimal side effects, ipratropium bromide should be the anticholinergic bronchodilator of choice until a glycopyrrolate solution receives approval for nebulizer use.

CROMOLYN SODIUM

Cromolyn sodium (disodium cromoglycate) is a drug useful in the treatment of asthma. It has a unique structure (Fig. 9-4) and function. It is *not* a

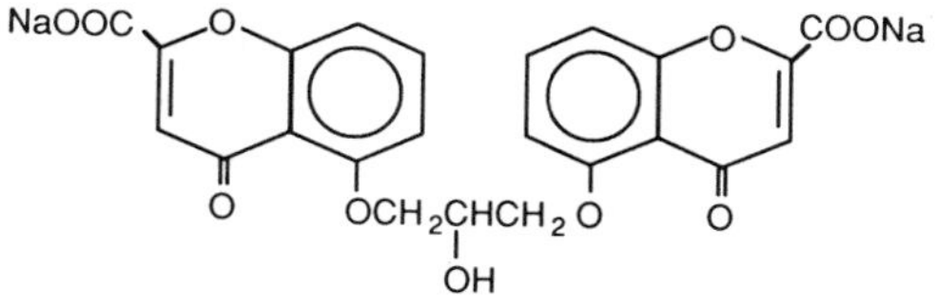

CROMOLYN SODIUM

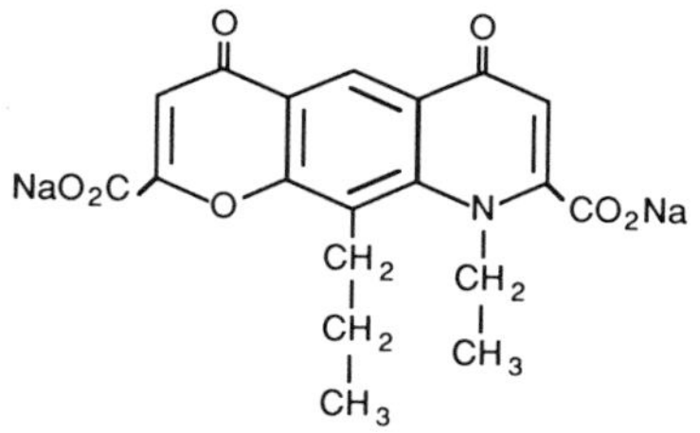

NEDOCROMIL SODIUM

Fig. 9-4. The structures of cromolyn sodium and nedocromil sodium.

bronchodilator drug, an antihistamine, an antimediator, or an anti-inflammatory agent.

Originally, cromolyn was felt to have only a single action—the inhibition of the release of mediators from immunoglobulin E-sensitized mast cells.[202] In vitro, it has no pathologic effect on the mast cell, does not interfere with the antigen-antibody reaction, and has no effect on the mediators once released. In asthmatics, it inhibits allergen-induced asthma only if taken before, not after, allergen challenge in most, but not all, patients.[203] Cromolyn sodium also blocks nonimmunologic mediator release from mast cells stimulated by compound 48/80, histamine, dextran, phospholipase-A, and polymyxin-B.[204,205] Cromolyn has also been shown to inhibit mediator release from other inflammatory cells, such as macrophages and eosinophils.[206] The cellular mechanism of action is still in question. Originally, it was felt that cromolyn sodium stabilized the mast cell membrane, preventing mediator release.[207] Cromolyn sodium also causes inhibition of intracellular phosphodiesterase, but the concentrations to effect this probably could not be achieved clinically.[208] Cromolyn sodium may stabilize the mast cell membrane by blocking calcium transport, perhaps by interfering with calcium gating at the surface[209] or by enhancing the intracellular sequestration of calcium.[210]

Recent studies indicate that cromolyn sodium has nonimmunologic actions. Many studies have shown that it may block exercise-induced bronchospasm, but it does not do so in all individuals.[211,212] Originally, mast cell mediator release was not thought to occur in exercise-induced bronchospasm.[213] With refined assay techniques, histamine and neutrophilic chemotactic factor have been shown to increase significantly with exercise-induced asthma.[214] Exercise-induced bronchospasm is related to airway heat loss, and this can be simulated in the laboratory by cold-air challenge under conditions of normocapnic hyperpnea. Mild bronchoconstriction after cold-air challenge occurs in normal patients, but is more pronounced in asthmatics. This response can be blocked by cromolyn.[215,216] Cromolyn also inhibits bronchoconstriction induced by the ultrasonic nebulization of distilled water or fog.[217] This may be due to inhibition of mediator release.[218] Sulfur dioxide can precipitate asthma by stimulating mucosal irritant receptors. This can be blocked by a dose of cromolyn sodium twice that needed to block antigen-induced bronchospasm.[219] Cromolyn sodium appears to be more effective than atropine in blocking sulfur dioxide-induced bronchospasm.[220] Exposure to sulfur dioxide and cold appears to trigger mechanisms that do not involve mast cell mediator release, yet are blocked by cromolyn sodium. Perhaps cromolyn sodium acts directly on smooth muscle or irritant receptors. The latter is suggested by experiments in dogs that have shown that intravenous chloralose-induced reflex bronchoconstriction is inhibited by cromolyn sodium, which causes a reduction in the number of impulses passing up "C" fibers from irritant receptors.[221]

The one feature that characterizes all patients with asthma is the presence of a nonspecific bronchial hyperreactivity. This can be demonstrated by bronchoprovocation challenge with histamine or mecholyl chloride, in which an exaggerated response (drop in FEV_1 or specific airway conductance) occurs in asthmatics but not in normal subjects. Cromolyn sodium has been shown to reduce this nonspecific bronchial hyperreactivity with long-term administration up to 10 years.[221–224]

Inhalation challenge with antigen may result in an early reaction causing immediate bronchoconstriction, with recovery of lung function in 1 to 2 hours. In a number of patients, a delayed or late bronchoconstrictive response occurs 4 to 12 hours after the challenge.[225,226] The late response is thought to be a manifestation of airway inflammation.[227] Cromolyn sodium blocks the early and late reactions.[228,229] The ability of cromolyn sodium to improve bronchial hyperreactivity and to inhibit the late reaction is no doubt central to the efficacy of cromolyn therapy in asthma.

Cromolyn sodium is hydrophilic but poorly absorbed orally, less than 1 percent being absorbed. To be effective, it must reach the airways by inhalation. Cromolyn sodium is available for delivery by a spinhaler, a 1 percent solution for nebulization, and in an MDI. With a spinhaler, only approximately 8 percent of the dose reaches the lower airways,[225] the rest being deposited in the upper airways, swallowed, and passed intact into the stool. The fraction that is absorbed is eliminated rapidly in bile and urine and has a half-life of 46 to 99 minutes with biotransformation.[226] The duration of action is 4 to 6 hours. The 1 percent solution comes in a vial containing 20 mg of cromolyn, which is easily added to a nebulizer for administration. The MDI produces 800 μg per puff, the usual dose being two puffs (1,600 μg). The usual frequency of dosing is initially four times a day with all preparations, which appear to be equivalent.

Cromolyn sodium is a safe drug with few side effects. Fewer than one per 10,000 patients in the United States has experienced an adverse reaction to this drug.[230] The most frequent side effects are irritative in nature and include cough, wheezing, and throat dryness. Cough and wheezing usually can be blocked by inhaling a beta$_2$ bronchodilator via an MDI 5 minutes before cromolyn sodium use. Dryness can be counteracted by drinking water after use. More serious reactions, such as dermatitis, gastroenteritis, or myositis, are very infrequent,[231] and hypersensitivity reactions are rare.[232] No cardiovascular side effects occur.

When cromolyn sodium was released in 1973, it was used enthusiastically in children and adults as a prophylactic drug. Its use then decreased in the United States, particularly in adults, because of the lack of effectiveness or, more likely, because of patient resistance to the use of the spinhaler delivery system. A trial of four 20 mg capsules inhaled per day was needed for at least 4 weeks to determine effectiveness. Many individuals would not take the medication in this fashion. A reversal of this trend occurred after the solution was introduced in 1982 and the MDI in 1986. Because of its benefit in reducing bronchial hyperreactivity and the inhibition of the late reaction, its use is on solid footing. It has been recommended that if the clinical response is minimal after 2 weeks, the dose should be increased to 40 mg four times daily and the total trial should last 8 weeks.[233] Once the clinical response has occurred, the dose should be tapered gradually, but not lower than 20 mg twice a day.[233] It should be administered 15 to 30 minutes before exercise or before an exposure to a known antigen. If used only for protection during the pollen season, it should be started 1 week before the season begins.[233] The degree to which cromolyn reaches the lungs is related to bronchial patency.[234] Airway patency can be improved by administering an inhaled beta agonist before cromolyn delivery occurs. If the patient develops acute asthma, cromolyn therapy should be maintained during exacerbation of the asthma.[230] A beta$_2$ agonist can be added to the cromolyn solution delivered by nebulization and it can be delivered before cromolyn is given by a spinhaler or MDI. If cromolyn sodium therapy is effective in controlling asthma, the daily use of bronchodilator drugs usually can be reduced or perhaps stopped, except for the occasional use of an inhaled beta agonist.

Nedocromil Sodium

Nedocromil sodium should be released in the near future for use in the United States. It is similar pharmacologically to sodium cromoglycate, but is different structurally (Fig. 9-4). Nedocromil inhibits activation and mediator release from many inflammatory cells, including eosinophils, neutrophils, macrophages, monocytes, and mast cells.[235,236] In cell preparations, nedocromil sodium was 100 times more potent than cromolyn in inhibiting mediator release from sensitized mast cells.[237,238] It has also been shown to inhibit bradykinin-induced bronchoconstriction in humans,[239] suggesting that nedocromil may inhibit axon reflexes since bradykinin stimulates axon reflexes causing release of neuropeptides.[240] The cellular mechanisms involved have yet to be elucidated.

After inhalation, the bioavailability is 6 to 7 percent, with 2.5 percent being contributed by gastrointestinal absorption.[241] Nedocromil is not metabolized and, with repeated dosing, there is no drug accumulation.[241]

No controlled trials comparing cromolyn sodium with nedocromil sodium have been reported. In placebo-controlled studies, nedocromil has been well tolerated,[242,243] has demonstrated improvement in pulmonary function, yet a decrease in concomitant bronchodilator use,[244] and has demonstrated some steroid-sparing effects.[245] Adverse reactions have been of low incidence and have been limited to a distinctive taste, headache, nausea, and vomiting.[246] Nedocromil sodium is available abroad in an MDI preparation. The recommended dose is 4 mg inhaled 2 to 4 times daily, depending on the control of asthmatic symptoms. Like cromolyn sodium, it is to be used as a preventive agent, not an active agent (such as a beta$_2$ agonist), for the relief of bronchospasm. Nedocromil sodium possesses both antiallergic and anti-inflammatory properties. Initial clinical data suggest it may be useful in the management of patients with asthma.

CORTICOSTEROIDS

After Hench et al reported the use of cortisone in patients with rheumatoid arthritis in 1949,[247] Carryer et al, in 1950, reported the efficacy of this drug in patients with asthma.[248] Since then, corticosteroids have been found to be valuable but potentially dangerous drugs in the treatment of asthma and other obstructive pulmonary diseases in which wheezing cannot be controlled effectively by bronchodilator drugs alone.

Corticosteroids are used primarily in the treatment of asthma and many of the diffuse inflammatory lung diseases. The structures of the most commonly used corticosteroids are shown in Figure 9-5. The most commonly used oral drugs are prednisone, prednisolone, and methylprednisone. Hydrocortisone, methylprednisolone, and dexamethasone are the most

commonly used intravenous agents. Beclomethasone-17,21 diproprionate, triamcinolone acetonide, flunisolide, and budesonide are used for topical (inhaled) bronchial administration. Cortisone and prednisone each have a ketone group at C^{11} (Fig. 9-5) that must be converted to a hydroxyl group, thus forming hydrocortisone and prednisolone, respectively, before the compounds are active. This ability to hydroxylate is present in many body tissues, yet a rare patient may not be able to hydroxylate prednisone to prednisolone and will exhibit steroid resistance to prednisone.

Corticosteroids possess variable glucocorticoid, mineralocorticoid, and anti-inflammatory properties,

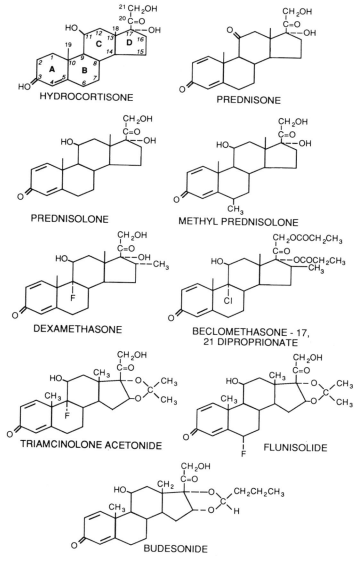

Fig. 9-5. The structures of commonly used corticosteroids.

TABLE 9-7. Comparison of the Pharmacologic Effects of Corticosteroids

Preparation	Anti-inflammatory Potency[a]	Equivalent Dose (mg)	Sodium-Retaining Potency[a]	Plasma Half-life (min)	Biologic Half-life (h)
Short-acting					
Hydrocortisone	1.0	20	2+	90	8–12
Cortisone	0.8	25	2+	30	—[b]
Intermediate-acting					
Prednisone	3.5	5	1+	60	—[b]
Prednisolone	4.0	5	1+	200	12–36
Methylprednisolone	5.0	4	0	200	12–36
Triamcinolone	5.0	4	0	200	24–48
Long-acting					
Betamethasone	30	0.60	0	300	36–54
Dexamethasone	30	0.75	0	300	36–54

[a] As determined by suppression of hypothalamic-pituitary-adrenal function.

[b] Cortisone and prednisolone first must be converted to hydrocortisone before they become active. The biologic half-lives are comparable to those of hydrocortisone and prednisolone, respectively.

(From Morris,[249] with permission.)

depending on structure. These pharmacologic properties are outlined in Table 9-7. Glucocorticoid and mineralocorticoid properties vary quite widely, but all agents produce similar anti-inflammatory effects when used in equivalent doses.

The potency and duration of action depend on the free steroid present at the tissue level, not the plasma half-life.[249] Only free, unbound steroid is active at the cellular level. Usually only 5 to 10 percent (1 to 2 μg/100 mL) of plasma hydrocortisone is free. The remaining is bound to transcortin, which is an alpha$_1$-globulin.[250] The structure of some of the synthetic analogs interferes with protein binding so that a larger proportion of free drug is present. On an equimolar basis, methylprednisolone binds to transcortin only 3 percent as well as hydrocortisone, dexamethasone binds less than 0.1 percent as well, but prednisolone binds as well as hydrocortisone.[251] After free steroid enters the cells, it combines with steroid receptors found in the cytoplasm.[252] This complex binds with DNA, leading to the synthesis of a number of messenger ribonucleic acids (mRNA), whose translations lead to the synthesis of proteins that mediate the steroid response.[252] The exact relevance of this mechanism to pulmonary diseases has not been worked out, but the delayed onset of steroid effect seen clinically is consistent with the time course of these events in vitro.

Metabolic degradation of steroids occurs in the liver, where they are rapidly inactivated, conjugated as glucuronides, and subsequently excreted in the urine.[249] Steroid analogs are also degraded in the liver, but by alternate pathways. They circulate for a longer period of time than naturally occurring ste-

roids, and a higher proportion may appear in the urine as free steroids.[249] Steroid metabolism may be increased due to liver enzyme induction by barbiturates,[253] diphenylhydantoin,[254] and rifampin.[255] Troleandomycin inhibits the clearance of methylprednisolone, thus enhancing its effects.[256] Hyperthyroidism may lead to increased steroid clearance, whereas hypothyroidism and liver disease may lead to decreased steroid clearance.[257] Some patients with asthma who are receiving steroids may have clearance rates increased by as much as three times.[258,259] The doses of steroids given may need to be lowered if clearance is inhibited by drugs or disease or increased, sometimes greatly, if steroid clearance is increased.

Thus, some steroid analogs may have an advantage over natural steroids in that the unbound level of free steroid in the blood is higher and is degraded less, and the resulting higher tissue levels exert a greater effect. Steroids have a multiplicity of effects on many organ systems. In patients with pulmonary disease, the anti-inflammatory action of steroids is probably important regardless of the specific pulmonary disease present. In addition, in patients with airway disease receiving beta$_2$ agonists, drug tolerance may occur. Steroids appear to reverse drug tolerance to the beta$_2$ agonists rather rapidly,[109,110,259] which may be one of the major positive effects of steroid therapy in these patients.

Steroids may be given orally, intramuscularly, intravenously, and topically. Most steroid preparations are water-soluble by virtue of being conjugated with various esters. Esterification has little effect on steroid effectiveness when given orally or intravenously, but it greatly influences the speed of absorption and duration of action when given topically or intramuscularly. Phosphate and hemisuccinate conjugates are rapidly absorbed, whereas acetate derivatives are slowly absorbed. Conjugation with acetonide, valerate, and proprionate enhances topical potency.[260] Generally, the absorption of oral prednisone is quite rapid and depends on tablet breakdown and dissolution. The bioavailability of some generic forms of prednisone may vary widely,[261] adversely influencing the effect of prednisone therapy.

The acute use of steroids in patients with pulmonary diseases, particularly those of the airways (such as asthma), can be lifesaving. However, the use of continuous daily doses leads to the familiar effects of hypercortisonism: cushingoid features, easy bruisability, adrenal suppression, posterior subcapsular cataracts, osteoporosis, glucose intolerance, hypertension, and growth suppression. Short-term (2 to 3 weeks) therapy with even daily high doses carries a very low risk. Long-term therapy, when needed, poses an increased risk for the development of side effects. Alternate-day therapy with a short-acting preparation such as prednisone, prednisolone, or methylprednisolone given as a single morning dose 48 hours apart will minimize side effects.[262–264] Longer-acting preparations such as dexamethasone or triamcinolone *cannot* be used since the biologic half-life persists through the 48 hours (Table 9-7), rendering the steroid therapy, in effect, daily therapy. With alternate-day therapy, the hypothalamic-pituitary-adrenal (HPA) axis is mildly depressed at 24 hours after drug administration, but returns to pretherapeutic levels by 48 hours.[265] Mild cushingoid facial features, weight gain, and easy bruisability may occur in these patients after therapy for several months, particularly if the dose is high (40 to 100 mg every other day).

Aerosolized (Topical) Steroid Therapy

A better choice than alternate-day steroid therapy for the patient with asthma is topical therapy with inhaled beclomethasone dipropionate, triamcinolone acetonide, flunisolide, or budesonide (Fig. 9-5). Steroids in general are extremely effective in the treatment of asthma, but are probably still underutilized due to the fear of the adverse side effects discussed above.[227] The exact mechanism(s) by which steroids exert their effect in asthma has not been elucidated totally, but the major effects appear to be related to the suppression of the inflammatory response, particularly in the late phase, but not in the early phase. Steroids inhibit cytokine formation and the formation of other mediators that lead to the local recruitment, proliferation, and activation of leukocytes and also inhibit the activation of cells already present.[266] Long-

term administration of steroids leads to the reduction of bronchial hyperreactivity. Inhaled steroids are more effective than oral steroids in reducing bronchial hyperreactivity.[267] Long-term therapy with topical steroids also reduces the immediate response to allergens[268] and suppresses exercise-induced asthma.[269]

Beclomethasone Dipropionate

Topical steroid therapy should be considered first-line therapy for asthma. Released in 1976, beclomethasone was the first topical steroid released in the United States. Doses up to 1,600 μg/d of beclomethasone do not cause HPA-axis suppression.[270,271] Beclomethasone is absorbed well, particularly from the gastrointestinal tract, and is rapidly metabolized in the liver such that the HPA axis remains intact until high doses are given.[260,272] Once patients are receiving oral steroids and are then gradually switched to inhaled beclomethasone, mild HPA-axis suppression may continue.[273] However, cushingoid features disappear once oral steroids are discontinued.

The dose has to be tailored for each patient. Each puff contains 50 μg. In two careful studies, optimum doses for beclomethasone ranged from 300 to 1,600 μg/d (six to 32 puffs), depending on symptom reduction, use of bronchodilator drugs, improvement in pulmonary function, and oral steroid reduction or cessation.[274–277] Particularly with regard to weaning from oral steroids, it may take 6 to 9 months to ascertain the effectiveness of beclomethasone dipropionate.[278] Even with optimal doses, the occasional use of a short course of daily steroids (20 to 40 mg/d starting dose tapered over 2 to 3 weeks) might be required. It appears that 70 to 80 percent of patients with asthma treated with aerosolized beclomethasone dipropionate can be maintained off oral steroids except for an occasional short course.[277] Side effects from beclomethasone dipropionate therapy include cough, wheezing, voice change, and oral candidiasis. Cough and wheezing are due to local irritation and usually, but not always, can be abolished by treatment 5 minutes beforehand with an inhaled beta$_2$ agonist. Voice changes are due to dyskinesia of the muscles controlling the vocal cord tension and are related to beclomethasone dipropionate and not to the propellant.[276] Voice rest rather than dose reduction appears to be required for treatment.[276] Oral candidiasis occurs in less than 10 percent of patients, and the incidence increases as the dose increases.[276] Usually, candidiasis responds to topical antifungal drugs, with only an occasional patient having to stop beclomethasone dipropionate therapy. No pathologic reactions to inhaled beclomethasone dipropionate have been noted on bronchial biopsy specimens taken from patients before therapy and 4 months, 1 year, and 3 years after therapy.[277] As has been mentioned previously, HPA-axis suppression induced by oral steroids may be maintained by inhaled beclomethasone dipropionate and may be intensified if higher doses are used.[276] However, the benefits of high doses up to 1,600 μg/d appear to outweigh the risks on careful analysis.[276] Beclomethasone dipropionate is contraindicated during an acute exacerbation of wheezing, since it may aggravate the episode due to the potential irritant effects of the aerosol.

Flunisolide

Flunisolide is a synthetic fluorinated steroid (Fig. 9-5) that was approved for use in the United States in 1984. It is absorbed rapidly and extensively from the lung and gut and is rapidly metabolized.[279,280] It is partially transformed in the lung to beclomethasone monopropionate, which is cleared more slowly than flunisolide.[281] It is very similar in safety and efficacy to beclomethasone.[276]

Each puff of the flunisolide MDI contains 250 μg of drug. The usual initial adult dosage of flunisolide is 500 μg (two puffs) twice daily (total, 1,000 μg). Up to 4 puffs twice daily can be used (2,000 μg). Unfortunately, one of the limiting features is the bad taste of flunisolide. This can be overcome to a large extent by using Chloroseptic mouthwash *before* flunisolide use. Patients will usually show improvement within 1 to 4 weeks of continuous therapy.

Triamcinolone Acetonide

Triamcinolone acetonide is a synthetic fluorinated glucocorticoid (Fig. 9-5). It was also approved for use in the United States in 1984. It is absorbed from lung and gut more slowly than the other aerosolized topical steroids. It is metabolized three times more slowly than budesonide.[282] It, too, is similar in efficacy to beclomethasone.[276]

Each puff of triamcinolone acetonide from the MDI contains 200 μg. The MDI delivery system contains a collapsible spacer device that enhances the delivery of drug to the lung while reducing drug deposition within the oral cavity.[283] In general, side effects have been minimal, and few thrush infections have been reported.[284] The usual initial dose is 600 to 800 μg/d (six to eight puffs) for milder asthma and up to 1,600 μg/d for more severe asthma. Once control of asthma has been accomplished, the dose should then be reduced to the lowest dose that is effective.

Budesonide

Budesonide is a nonhalogenated glucocorticoid (Fig. 9-5). The drug is a mixture of two epimers.[285] Budesonide, which has the greatest topical activity,[276,286] is not available in the United States. Budesonide possesses a high ratio of topical-to-systemic activity when compared with the other topical steroids reviewed above.[286] It is rapidly absorbed from the lung and gut and is rapidly metabolized, which may account for its low level of systemic activity.[282] In spite of its favorable properties, clinical trials have failed to show that budesonide is superior to beclomethasone dipropionate.[286]

Budesonide also is distributed with an MDI-spacer system. The side effects have been found to be similar to the other topical steroids.[276] Budesonide should be administered initially in doses of 400 to 1,600 μg/d, depending on the severity of the asthma, then reduced to the lowest dose that is effective.

All aerosolized topical steroids should be administered with a spacer in order to reduce oropharyngeal drug deposition and improve lung deposition.[276]

Systemic Steroid Therapy

The asthmatic who develops acute severe wheezing in spite of adequate (or excessive) bronchodilator drugs will require systemic corticosteroid therapy. With the use of intravenous hydrocortisone, plasma cortisol levels of 150 μg/dL should be reached, which can be achieved by giving 4 mg/kg of hydrocortisone (0.8 mg/kg equivalent methylprednisolone dose) intravenously every 4 hours or 8 mg/kg (1.6 mg/kg equivalent methylprednisolone dose) every 6 hours.[287] In an uncontrolled study, patients with acute, severe asthma (status asthmaticus) and respiratory failure (elevated $PaCO_2$ levels) were successfully treated with bronchodilator drugs plus up to 200 mg of hydrocortisone intravenously every 2 hours if not previously on steroids, or 400 mg every 2 hours in those previously receiving steroids.[288] In this study, none of the patients required intubation on this regimen. Equivalent doses of methylprednisone can be substituted: 40 or 80 mg intravenously up to every 2 hours. In a controlled study, hydrocortisone was given as a bolus, 2 mg/kg, and then administered at a continuous rate of 0.5 mg/kg/h (equivalent methylprednisolone dose, 0.1 mg/kg/h). There was a significant improvement in airway function in patients with acute, severe asthma, compared with a similar group who did not receive hydrocortisone.[289] A time delay of 12 hours was seen before a significant improvement in pulmonary function occurred between the treated control groups.[289] If the situation seems less severe, hydrocortisone or methylprednisolone can be administered intravenously, at 4- to 6-hour intervals, as mentioned previously. However, an insufficient dose must not be given, since the risks of unrelieved airway obstruction far outweigh the risk from steroid side effects.[249] Potassium supplementation is recommended, since urinary potassium loss can be extensive.[287]

Once the patient has improved and wheezing has cleared, oral steroid therapy can be instituted with 60 to 80 mg/d of prednisone in divided doses for several days before switching to a daily, morning dose. At this point, it must be determined whether the patient will require long-term steroid therapy.[288] If the acute attack was an isolated problem, the patient should be tapered off steroids over 2 to 3 weeks. If the patient previously has not been able to be controlled on bronchodilator drugs alone, then long-term steroid therapy should be instituted. The treatment of choice is aerosolized topical steroids (see above). If the patient's asthma does not come under optimal control with aerosolized steroids, then alternate-day prednisone should be instituted. As much as 40 to 60 mg of prednisone on alternate days may be necessary to effect control. The dose can then be tapered by 5- to 10-mg decrements every 2 to 4 weeks until the lowest dose possible (or no prednisone) is in use. Methylprednisolone for alternate-day therapy is not recommended because of its very high cost. Usually, only a small group of patients will require alternate-day steroid therapy in addition to topical steroid therapy for optimum control of asthma.[276]

The use of systemic steroids in patients with chronic bronchitis and emphysema is not as well established as in asthma. In a controlled clinical trial of patients who had chronic bronchitis and acute respiratory failure, the addition of intravenous methylprednisolone, 0.5 mg/kg every 6 hours, to bronchodilator and antibiotic therapy led to a significant improvement in pre- and postbronchodilator FEV_1 within 12 hours, as compared with a placebo group.[290] No significant changes in arterial blood gases occurred between the steroid-treated and placebo groups. Patients had been carefully screened to exclude any patients with asthma.

In patients with stable chronic bronchitis and emphysema, there appears to be a small subgroup of patients who improve their pulmonary function significantly with the addition of oral steroid therapy.[291–293] In these small studies, between 15 to 30 percent of patients showed steroid responsiveness. Most, but not all, of the responders also showed an approximately 25 percent improvement in FEV_1 to an inhaled beta agonist.[291,292] The only way to identify the group of steroid responders in patients with chronic bronchitis and emphysema is to measure pulmonary function, institute prednisone therapy of 40 mg/d (32 mg/d of methylprednisolone) for 2 weeks, then remeasure pulmonary function.[291,292] If the patient's FEV_1 value has risen by 30 percent or higher over baseline, the patient should be considered a steroid responder.[294] At this point, aerosolized steroids can be instituted and the patient tapered off oral prednisone over 2 weeks. It appears that a minority of patients will be treated effectively with aerosolized steroids,[291,292] so oral therapy will have to be restarted if the patient fails to respond to aerosolized steroids. Usually, 10 to 20 mg of prednisone given on alternate days will maintain the patient. However, some patients will not be maintained on alternate-day therapy and will require daily prednisone therapy with a dose of approximately 10 mg/d.[294] The lowest dose of prednisone needed to maintain adequate therapy should be used to avoid complications from steroid therapy (see above). If the patient on steroids develops an acute bronchitis that does not require hospitalization, prednisone can be increased to 40 mg/d for 10 to 14 days, then dropped back to the previous dose.[294]

Used judiciously, systemic steroids are beneficial and carry a reasonably low risk to the patient. The use of *daily* systemic steroids for long periods of time should be avoided if possible. If a patient receiving systemic steroids, or who has received systemic steroids within the past year, has to undergo thoracic surgery, supplemental steroids (40 mg of methylprednisolone or its equivalent) should be given on the days before and after surgery. After that, the steroids can be tapered over several days to the preoperative level.[295]

ACKNOWLEDGMENT

The authors are extremely grateful for the tireless efforts of Diane Nuckolls, who prepared the manuscript.

REFERENCES

1. Stein M, Cassara EL: Preoperative pulmonary evaluation and therapy for surgery patients. JAMA 211:787–790, 1970
2. Weibel ER, Taylor CR: Design and structure of the human lung. pp. 11–20. In Fishman AP (ed): Pulmonary Diseases and Disorders. 2nd Ed. McGraw-Hill, New York, 1988
3. Gomez OM: A physico-mathematical study of lung function in subjects and in patients with obstructive pulmonary diseases. Med Thorac 22:275–294, 1965

4. Breeze RG, Wheelden EB: The cells of the pulmonary airways. Am Rev Respir Dis 116:705–777, 1977
5. Cauldwell EW, Siebert RG, Lininger RE, et al: Anatomic study of 150 human cadavers. Surg Gynecol Obstet 86:395–412, 1948
6. Deffebach ME, Charan NB, Lakshminarayan S, Butler J: The bronchial circulation. Small, but a vital attribute of the lung. Am Rev Respir Dis 135:463–481, 1987
7. Richardson JB: Nerve supply to the lungs. Am Rev Respir Dis 119:785–802, 1979
8. Richardson JB: Non-adrenergic inhibitory innervation of the lung. Lung 159:315–322, 1981
9. Barnes PJ: Neural control of human airways in health and disease. Am Rev Respir Dis 134:1289–1314, 1986
10. Ahlquist RP: Study of adrenotropic receptors. Am J Physiol 135:586–600, 1948
11. Lands AM, Arnold A, McAulff JP, et al: Differentiation of receptor systems activated by sympathomimetic amines. Nature 214:597–598, 1967
12. Weiner N: Norepinephrine, epinephrine, and the sympathomimetic amines. pp. 138–175. In Goodman LS, Gilman A (eds): The Pharmacological Basis of Therapeutics. Macmillian, New York, 1980
13. Austen KF, Orange RP: Bronchial asthma: the possible role of the chemical mediators of immediate hypersensitivity in the pathogenesis of subacute chronic disease. Am Rev Respir Dis 112:423–436, 1975
14. Simonsson BG, Svedmyr N, Skoogh BE: In-vivo and in-vitro studies on alpha-receptors in human airway: potentiation with bacterial endotoxin. Scand J Respir Dis 53:227–236, 1972
15. Kneussl MP, Richardson JB: Alpha-adrenergic receptors in human and canine tracheal and bronchial smooth muscle. J Appl Physiol 45:307–311, 1978
16. Rodbell M: The role of nucleotide regulatory components in the coupling of hormone receptors and adenylate cyclase. pp. 1–12. In Folco G, Paolette R (eds): Molecular Biology and Pharmacology of Cyclic Nucleotides. Elsevier/North Holland, Amsterdam, 1978
17. Gilman AG: Guanine nucleotide-binding regulatory proteins and dual control of adenylate cyclase. J Clin Invest 73:1–4, 1984
18. Barnes PJ: Airway receptors. pp. 67–95. In Jenne JW, Murphy S (eds): Drug Therapy for Asthma. Marcel Dekker, New York, 1987
19. Hirata F, Axelrod J: Phospholipid methylation and biological signal transmission. Science 209:1082–1090, 1980
20. Nimmo HG, Cohen P: Hormonal control of protein phosphorylation. Adv Cyclic Nucleotide Res 8:145–266, 1977
21. Greengard P: Phosphorylated proteins as physiological effectors. Science 199:146–152, 1978
22. Bar HP: Cyclic nucleotide and smooth muscle. Adv Cyclic Nucleotide Res 4:195–237, 1974
23. Vulliemoz Y, Verosky M, Triner L: The cyclic adenosine 3′,5′-monophosphate system in bronchial tissue. pp. 293–314. In Stephens NL (ed): The Biochemistry of Smooth Muscle. University Park Press, Baltimore, 1977
24. Svedmyr N, Lofdahl CG: Physiology and pharmacodynamics of beta-adrenergic agonists. pp. 177–209. In Jenne JW, Murphy S (eds): Drug Therapy for Asthma. Marcel Dekker, New York, 1987
25. Gold WM: Role of cyclic nucleotides in airway smooth muscle. pp. 123–190. In Nadel JA (ed): Physiology and Pharmacology of the Airway. Marcel Dekker, New York, 1980
26. Stoner J, Manganiello VC, Vaughn M: Guanosine 3′,5′-monophosphate and guanylate cyclase activity in guinea pig lung: effect of acetylcholine and cholinesterase inhibitors. Mol Pharmacol 10:155–161, 1974
27. Schultz G, Hardman JG: Possible role of cyclic nucleotide in the regulation of smooth muscle tonus. pp. 667–683. In Dumont JE, Brown BL, Suria A (eds): Eukaryotic Cell Function and Growth: Regulation by Intracellular Cyclic Nucleotides. Plenum, New York, 1976
28. Hurwitz L, Suria A: The link between agonist action and response in smooth muscle. Annu Rev Pharmacol 11:303–326, 1971
29. Schultz G: Possible inter-relations between calcium and cyclic nucleotides in smooth muscle. pp. 77–91. In Lichtenstein LM, Austen KF (eds): Asthma: Physiology, Immunopharmacology, and Treatment. Academic Press, San Diego, 1977
30. Somlyo AP, Somlyo AV: Vascular smooth muscle I. Normal structure, pathology, biochemistry and biophysics. Pharmacol Rev 20:197–272, 1968
31. Barnes PJ: Calcium channel blockers. pp. 517–533. In Jenne JW, Murphy S (eds): Drug Therapy for Asthma. Marcel Dekker, New York, 1987
32. Rasmussen H, Barrett PQ: Calcium messenger system: an integrated view. Physiol Rev 64:938–984, 1984
33. Earp HS, Steiner AL: Compartmentalization of cyclic nucleotide-mediated hormone action. Annu Rev Pharmacol Toxicol 18:431–459, 1978
34. Mathe AA, Volicer L, Puri SK: Effect of anaphylaxis and histamine, pyrilamine and burimamide on levels of cyclic AMP and cyclic GMP in guinea pig lungs. Res Commun Chem Pathol Pharmacol 8:635–651, 1954
35. Chand N, Dhawan BN, Srimal RC, et al: Reactivity of trachea, bronchi, and lung strips by histamine and carbachol in rhesus monkeys. J Appl Physiol: Resp Environ Exercise Physiol 49:729–734, 1980
36. Snappes JF, Braasch BA, Ingram RH, Jr, et al: In vivo effect of cimetidine on canine pulmonary responsiveness to aerosolized histamine. J Allergy Clin Immunol 66:70–74, 1980
37. Habib MP, Pare PD, Engel LA: Variability of airway responses to inhaled histamine in normal subjects. J Appl Physiol: Resp Environ Exercise Physiol 47:51–58, 1979
38. Simonsson BG, Jacobs FM, Nadel JA: Role of autonomic nervous system and the cough reflex in the responsiveness of airways in patients with obstructive airway disease. J Clin Invest 46:1812–1818, 1967
39. Bouhuys A, Jonsson R, Lichtneckert S, et al: Effects of histamine on pulmonary ventilation in man. Clin Sci 19:79–94, 1960
40. Lewis RA, Austen KF: The biologically active leukotrienes. J Clin Invest 73:889–897, 1984

41. Cushley MJ, Tattersfield AE, Holgate ST: Inhaled adenosine and guanosine on airway resistance in normal and asthmatic subjects. Br J Clin Pharmacol 15:161–165, 1983

42. Finney MJB, Karlsson J-A, Persson CGA: Effects of bronchoconstrictors and bronchodilators on a novel human airway preparation. Br J Pharmacol 85:29–36, 1985

43. Trautlein J, Allegra J, Field J, et al: Paradoxic bronchospasm after inhalation of isoproterenol. Chest 70:711–714, 1976

44. Jack D: β-Adrenoreceptor stimulants in asthma. pp. 251–266. In Austen KF, Lichtenstein LM (eds): Asthma: Physiology, Immunopharmacology, and Treatment. Academic Press, San Diego, 1973

45. Amory DW, Burnham SC, Cheney FW, Jr: Comparison of the cardiopulmonary effects of subcutaneously administered epinephrine and terbutaline in patients with reversible airway obstruction. Chest 67:279–286, 1975

46. Wood DW, Downes JJ, Scheinkopf H, et al: Intravenous isoproterenol in the management of respiratory failure in childhood status asthmaticus. J Allergy Immunol 50:75–81, 1972

47. Hamstreet MP, Miles MV, Rutland RO: Effect of intravenous isoproterenol on theophylline kinetics. J Allergy Clin Immunol 69:360–364, 1982

48. Klaustermeyer WV, DiBernardo RL, Hale FC: Intravenous isoproterenol: Rationale for bronchial asthma. J Allergy Clin Immunol 55:325–333, 1975

49. As AA: Beta-adrenergic stimulant bronchodilators. pp. 415–432. In Stein M (ed): New Directions in Asthma. American College of Chest Physicians, Park Ridge, IL, 1975

50. Fomgren H: A clinical comparison of the effect of oral terbutaline and orciprenaline. Scand J Respir Dis 51:195–202, 1970

51. Minette A, Marcq M, Gepts L: Carbuterol, fenoterol, orciprenaline salbutamol, and terbutaline per os in reversible obstructive chronic bronchitis. Bull Eur Physiopathol Respir 12:545–553, 1976

52. Geumei A, Miller WF, Paez PN, et al: Evaluation of a new oral β₂-adrenoreceptor stimulant bronchodilator, terbutaline. Pharmacology 13:201–211, 1975

53. Trautlen JJ, Serra R: Intermittent positive-pressure breathing administration of terbutaline: a dose-response study. Ann Allergy 47:76–78, 1981

54. Haddad ZH, Stumbaugh S, Davis WR: A comparison of the bronchodilator and other responses of children to oral treatment with terbutaline tablet and solution: a bioequivalent study. Ann Allergy 44:86–90, 1980

55. Minette A: Ventilatory results and side effects of salbutamol given by different routes in coal miners with reversible bronchospasm. Postgrad Med 47:55–61, 1971

56. Brittain RT: A comparison of the pharmacology of salbutamol with that of isoprenaline, orciprenaline, and trimetoquinol. Postgrad Med 147:11–16, 1971

57. Tattersfield AE, McNicol MW: Salbutamol and isoproterenol: a double-blind trial to compare bronchodilator and cardiovascular activity. N Engl J Med 281:1323–1325, 1969

58. Bolinger AM, Young KYL, Gambertoglio JG, et al: Influence of food on the absorption of albuterol Repetabs. J Allergy Clin Immunol 83:123–126, 1989

59. Affrime M, Starkey P, Perentesis G, et al: Therapeutic efficacy and dose response of albuterol in asthmatic patients, abstracted. Acta Pharmacol Toxicol, suppl. 5. 59:228, 1986

60. Walters EH, Cockroft A, Griffiths T, et al: Optimal doses of salbutamol respiratory solution: comparison of the doses with plasma levels. Thorax 36:625–628, 1981

61. Sharma B, Goodwin JF: Beneficial effect of salbutamol on cardiac function in severe congestive cardiomyopathy. Circulation 58:449–460, 1978

62. Kass I, Mingo TS: Bitolterol mesylate (Win 32784) aerosol. A new long-acting bronchodilator with reduced chronotropic effects. Chest 78:283–287, 1980

63. Aimoto T, Ito O, Kimura R, et al: The influences of the route of administration on the metabolism and excretion of bitolterol, a new bronchodilator, in the rat. Xenobiotica 9:173–180, 1979

64. Shargel L, Dorbecker SA, Levitt M: Physiological disposition and metabolism on N-butylarterenol and its di-p-toluate ester (bitolterol) in the rat. Drug Metab Dispos 4:65–71, 1976

65. Minatoya H: Studies of bitolterol, the di-p-toluate ester of N-tert-butyl-arterenol: a new long-acting bronchodilator with reduced cardiovascular effect. J Pharmacol Exp Ther 206:515–517, 1978

66. Kelly HW: New B₂-adrenergic agonist aerosols. Clin Pharm 4:393–404, 1985

67. Kemp JP, Orgel A, Grossman J, et al: Outpatient management of asthma with regular nebulized beta-agonists: comparison of bitolterol mesylate and isoproterenol. Ann Allergy 59:17–20, 1987

68. Orgel HA, Kemp JP, Tinkelman DG, et al: Bitolterol and albuterol metered dose aerosols: comparison of two long acting beta₂-adrenergic bronchodilators for treatment of asthma. J Allergy Clin Immunol 75:55–62, 1985

69. Cockcroft W, Berscheid BA, Dosman JA, et al: Comparison of bitolterol mesylate and metaproterenol sulphate. Curr Ther Res 30:817–824, 1981

70. Tinkelman DG, Kemp J, Webb R, et al: Comparison of aerosols bitolterol mesylate (B) and albuterol (A), abstracted. J Allergy Clin Immunol 71:126, 1983

71. Webb DR, Mullarky MF, Mingo TS: Bitolterol mesylate aerosol in chronic bronchial asthma, abstract. J Allergy Clin Immunol 69:116, 1982

72. Friedel HA, Brogden RN: Bitolterol: a preliminary review. Drugs 35:22–41, 1988

73. Zwillich CW, Neagley SR, Cicutto L, et al: Nocturnal asthma therapy. Inhaled bitolterol versus sustained-release theophylline. Am Rev Respir Dis 139:470–474, 1989

74. Richards DM, Brogden RN: Pirbuterol: a preliminary review of its pharmacologic properties and therapeutic efficacy in reversible bronchospastic disease. Drugs 30:6–21, 1985

75. Moore PF, Constantine JW, Barth WE: Pirbuterol: selective beta$_2$-adrenergic bronchodilator. J Pharmacol Exp Ther 207:410–418, 1978

76. Crompton GK, Grant IW: Pirbuterol. Lancet 1:795, 1984

77. Kenakin TP, Beek D: Relative efficacy of pirbuterol for beta-1 adrenoreceptors: measurement of agonist affinity by alteration of receptor number. J Pharmacol Exp Ther 229:340–345, 1984

78. Beumer HM: Pirbuterol aerosol versus salbutamol and placebo aerosols in bronchial asthma. Drugs Exp Clin Res 2:77–83, 1980

79. Beumer HM: Long-term treatment of bronchial asthma with pirbuterol aerosol. Int J Clin Pharmacol Ther Toxicol 21:172–175, 1983

80. Littner MR, Tashkin DP, Calvarese B, Bautista M: Bronchial and cardiovascular effects of increasing doses of pirbuterol acetate aerosol in asthma. Ann Allergy 48:141–144, 1982

81. Minette A: Spirometric study of the bronchodilating effects of hydroxyphenyl orciprenaline (Th165a) in various forms in a group of 124 coal miners suffering from bronchospasm. Respiration 27:276–315, 1970

82. Watanabe S, Turner WG, Renzetti AD, et al: Bronchodilator effects of nebulized fenoterol. Chest 80:292–299, 1981

83. Plummer AL: The development of drug tolerance to B$_2$-adrenergic agents. Chest 73S:949S–956S, 1978

84. Nakajima S: Dose-response evaluation of bronchodilator effect of formoterol (BD 40) in single doses in bronchial asthma. J Med Pharmacol Sci (Jpn) 10:571–582, 1983

85. Svedmyr N, Lofdahl CG: Bronchodilators. pp. 66–70. In Wilson JW (ed): Respiratory Pharmacology. Adis Press, Sydney, 1987

86. Lawford P, Dowd DE, Palmer KNV: A comparison of the duration of action of fenoterol and salbutamol in asthma. Curr Med Res Opin 7:349–351, 1981

87. Lofdahl G, Svedmyr N: Inhaled formoterol: a new beta-2 adrenoceptor, compared to salbutamol in asthmatic patients: duration of effect and side effects. Am Rev Respir Dis 137:330–336, 1988

88. Lofdahl CG, Svedmyr N: Formoterol fumarate, a new B$_2$-adrenoceptor agonist. Allergy 44:264–271, 1989

89. Maesen FPV, Smeets JJ, Gubblemans HL: Bronchodilator effect of inhaled formoterol vs salbutamol over 12 hours. Chest 97:590–594, 1990

90. Bradshaw J, Brittain RT, Coleman RA, et al: The design of salmeterol, a long-acting B$_2$-adrenoceptor agonist, abstracted. Br J Pharmacol 92:590S, 1987

91. Ball DI, Coleman RA, Denyer LH: In vitro characterization of the B$_2$-adrenoceptor agonist salmeterol, abstracted. Br J Pharmacol 92:591P, 1987

92. Brittain RT, Dean CM, Jack D: Sympathomimetic bronchodilator drugs. Int Encyclo Pharmacol Ther 104:613–652, 1981

93. Svedmyr N, Lofdahl CG: Physiology and pharmacodynamics of beta-adrenergic agonists. pp. 177–212. In Jenne JW, Murphy S (eds): Drug Therapy for Asthma. Marcel Dekker, New York, 1987

94. Ullman A, Svedmyr N: Salmeterol, a new long-acting inhaled B$_2$-adrenoceptor agonist: comparison with salbutamol in adult asthmatic patients. Thorax 43:674–678, 1988

95. Kono O, Morita M: Evaluation of duration of action and clinical effect of formoterol (BD40) in single doses for bronchial asthma. Jpn Pharmacol Ther 11:4405–4416, 1983

96. Svedmyr N: Fenoterol: a beta-2 agonist for use in asthma. Pharmacol Ther 5:109–126, 1985

97. Widmark E, Waldeck B: Physiological and pharmacological characterization of an in vitro vagus nerve-trachea preparation from guinea pig. J Auton Pharmacol 6:187–194, 1986

98. Widmark E, Waldeck B: An experimental model for the study of transport of bronchodilating drugs through the tracheobronchial epithelium. Acta Pharmacol Toxicol, suppl. 5. 559:335–338, 1986

99. Widmark E, Waldeck B: Analysis of bronchomotor tone in anesthetized guinea pigs: a simple method for the evaluation of bronchodilator action. Methods Find Exp Clin Pharmacol 10:143–150, 1988

100. Wanner A: Clinical aspects of mucociliary transport. Am Rev Respir Dis 116:73–125, 1977

101. Church MK, Hiroi J: Inhibition of IgE-dependent histamine release from human dispersed lung mast cells by anti-allergic drugs and salbutamol. Br J Pharmacol 90:421–429, 1987

102. Howarth PH, Durham SR, Lee TH, et al: Influence of albuterol, cromolyn sodium and ipratropium bromide on the airway and circulating mediator responses to bronchial provocation in asthma. Am Rev Respir Dis 132:986–992, 1985

103. Persson CGA, Svensjo E: Airway hyperreactivity and microvascular permeability to large molecules. Eur J Respir Dis, suppl. 131. 64:183, 1983

104. Jones RM, Stockley RA, Bishop JM: Early effects of intravenous terbutaline and cardiac pulmonary function in chronic obstructive bronchitis and pulmonary hypertension. Thorax 37:746–750, 1982

105. Howell S, Roussos C: Isoproterenol and aminophylline improve contractility of fatigued canine diaphragm. Am Rev Respir Dis 129:118, 1984

106. Conolly ME, Greenacre JK: The lymphocytic β-adrenoreceptor in normal subjects and patients with bronchial asthma. J Clin Invest 58:1307–1316, 1976

107. Connolly ME, Jenne JW, Hui KK, Borst SE: Beta-adrenergic tachyphylaxis (desensitization) and functional antagonism. pp. 259–296. In Jenne JW, Murphy S (eds): Drug Therapy for Asthma. Marcel Dekker, New York, 1987

108. Nelson HS: Beta-adrenergic agonists. Chest 82S:33S–38S, 1982

109. Ellul-Micallef R, French FF: Effect of intravenous prednisolone in asthmatics with diminished adrenergic responsiveness. Lancet 2:1269–1271, 1975

110. Holgate ST, Baldwin CJ, Tattersfield AE: β-Adrenergic agonist resistance in normal human airways. Lancet 2:375–377, 1977

111. Kolbeck RC, Speir WA, Jr, Carrier GO, et al: Apparent

irrelevance of cyclic nucleotide to the relaxation of tracheal smooth muscle induced by theophylline. Lung 156:173–183, 1979

112. Persson CGA: Overview of effects of theophylline. J Allergy Clin Immunol 78:780–787, 1986

113. Rall TW: Central nervous system stimulants: the xanthines. pp. 592–607. In Goodman LS, Gilman A (eds): The Pharmacologic Basis of Therapeutics. Macmillan, New York, 1980

114. Moyer JH, Miller SI, Tashnek AB, et al: Effect of theophylline ethylenediamine (aminophylline) on cerebral hemodynamics in the presence of cardiac failure with and without Cheyne-Stokes respiration. J Clin Invest 31:267–272, 1952

115. Maxwell GM, Crumpton CW, Rowe GG, et al: The effects of theophylline ethylenediamine (aminophylline) on coronary hemodynamics of normal and diseased hearts. J Lab Clin Med 54:88–95, 1959

116. Ogilvie RI, Fernandez PG, Winsberg F: Cardiovascular response to increasing theophylline concentrations. Eur J Clin Pharmacol 12:409–414, 1977

117. Parker JO, Ashekian PB, DiGiorgi S, et al: Hemodynamic effects of aminophylline in chronic obstructive pulmonary disease. Circulation 35:365–372, 1967

118. Parker JO, Kelkar K, West RS: Hemodynamic effects of aminophylline in cor pulmonale. Circulation 33:17–25, 1966

119. Matthay RA, Berger HJ, Loke J, et al: Effects of aminophylline upon right and left ventricular performance in chronic obstructive pulmonary disease. Non-invasive assessment by radionucleotide angiocardiography. Am J Med 65:903–910, 1978

120. Weinberger M, Hendeles L, Bighley L: Relationship of product formulation to absorption of oral theophylline. N Engl J Med 299:852–857, 1978

121. Hendeles L, Weinberger M: Theophylline product and dosing interval selection for chronic asthma. J Allergy Clin Immunol 76:285–291, 1985

122. Ridolfo AS, Kohlstaedt KG: A simplified method for the rectal instillation of theophylline. Am J Med Sci 237:585–589, 1959

123. Waxler SH, Schack JA: Administration of aminophylline (theophylline ethylenediamine). JAMA 143:736–739, 1950

124. Levy G, Koysooko R: Pharmacokinetic analysis of the effect of theophylline on pulmonary function in asthmatic children. J Pediat 86:789–793, 1975

125. Vallner JJ, Speir WA, Jr, Kolbeck RC, et al: Effect of pH on the binding of theophylline to serum proteins. Am Rev Respir Dis 120:83–86, 1979

126. Yurchak AM, Jusko WJ: Theophylline secretion into breast milk. Pediatrics 57:518–520, 1976

127. Labovitz E, Spector S: Placental theophylline transfer in pregnant asthmatics. JAMA 247:786–788, 1982

128. Hendeles L, Burkey S, Bighley L, et al: Unpredictability of theophylline saliva measurements in chronic obstructive pulmonary disease. J Allergy Clin Immunol 60:335–338, 1977

129. Bukowsky M, Nakatsu K, Munt PW: Theophylline reassessed. Ann Intern Med 101:63–73, 1984

130. Levy G, Koysooko R: Renal clearance of theophylline in man. J Clin Pharmacol 16:329–332, 1976

131. Feldman CH, Hutchinson VE, Pippenger C, et al: Effects of dietary protein and carbohydrate on theophylline metabolism in children. Am Rev Respir Dis, suppl. 117:64, 1978

132. Jusko WJ, Gardner JM, Mangione A, et al: Factors affecting theophylline clearances: age, tobacco, marijuana, cirrhosis, congestive heart failure, obesity, oral contraceptives, benzodiazepines, barbiturates, and ethanol. J Pharm Sci 68:1358–1365, 1980

133. Prince R, Wing D, Hendeles L, et al: The effect of erythromycin on theophylline kinetics. Drug Intell Clin Pharm 14:637, 1980

134. Weinberger M, Hudgel D, Spector S, et al: Inhibition of theophylline clearance by troleandomycin. J Allergy Clin Immunol 59:228–231, 1977

135. Reitberg DP, Bernhard H, Schentag JJ: Alteration of theophylline clearance and half-life by cimetidine in normal volunteers. Ann Intern Med 95:582–585, 1981

136. Roy AK, Cuda MP, Levine RA: Induction of theophylline toxicity and inhibition of clearance rates by ranitidine. Am J Med 85:525–527, 1988

137. Manfred RL, Vesell ES: Inhibition of theophylline metabolism by long-term allopurinol administration. Clin Pharmacol Ther 29:224–229, 1981

138. Lombardi TP, Bertino JS, Goldberg A, Middleton E: The effects of a beta-2 selective adrenergic agonist and a beta-nonselective antagonist on theophylline clearance. J Clin Pharmacol 27:523–529, 1987

139. Stanley R, Comer T, Taylor JL, Saliba D: Mexiletine-theophylline interaction. Am J Med 86:733–734, 1989

140. Tornature KM, Kanarkowski R, McCarthy L, et al: Effect of chronic oral contraceptive steroids on theophylline disposition. Eur J Clin Pharmacol 23:29–34, 1982

141. Burnakis TG, Seldon M, Czaplicki AD: Increased serum theophylline concentration secondary to oral verapamil. Clin Pharm 2:458–461, 1983

142. Nafziger AN, May JJ, Bertino JS: Inhibition of theophylline elimination by diltiazem therapy. J Clin Pharmacol 27:862–865, 1987

143. Williams SJ, Baird-Lambert JA, Farrell GC: Inhibition of theophylline metabolism by interferon. Lancet 2:939–941, 1987

144. Schwartz J, Jauregui L, Lettieri J, Bachmann K: Impact of ciprofloxacin on theophylline clearance and steady-state concentrations in serum. Antimicrob Agents Chemother 32:75–77, 1988

145. Wijnands WJA, Vrec TB, Baars A, Van Herwaarden CLA: Steady-state kinetics of the quinolone derivatives of ofloxacin, enoxacin, ciprofloxacin, and pefloxacin during maintenance treatment with theophylline. Drugs, suppl. 1. 34:159–169, 1987

146. Mangione A, Imhoff TE, Lee RV, et al: Pharmacokinetics of theophylline in hepatic disease. Chest 73:616–622, 1978

147. Jenne JW: Rationale for methylxanthines in asthma. pp. 415–432. In Stein M (ed): New Directions in

Asthma. American College of Chest Physicians, Park Ridge, IL, 1975

148. Vicuna N, McNay JL, Ludden TM, et al: Impaired theophylline clearance in patients with cor pulmonale. Br J Clin Pharmacol 7:33–37, 1979

149. Mitenko PA, Ogilvie RI: Rational intravenous doses of theophylline. N Engl J Med 289:600–603, 1973

150. Miller M, Cosgriff J, Kuong T, Morken DA: Influence of phenytoin on theophylline clearance. Clin Pharmacol Ther 35:666–669, 1984

151. Piafsky KM, Sitar DS, Ogilvie RI: Effect of phenobarbital on the disposition of intravenous theophylline. Clin Pharmacol Ther 22:336–339, 1977

152. Boyce EG, Dukes GE, Rollins DE, Sudds TW: The effect of rifampin on theophylline kinetics. J Clin Pharmacol 26:696–701, 1986

153. Pollock J, Kiechel F, Cooper D, et al: Relationship of serum theophylline concentrations to inhibition of exercise-induced bronchospasm and comparison with cromolyn. Pediatrics 60:840–844, 1977

154. Wineberger M, Hendeles L, Ahrens R: Pharmacologic management of reversible obstructive airway disease. Med Clin North Am 65:579–613, 1981

155. Hendeles L, Bighley L, Richardson RH, et al: Frequent toxicity from IV aminophylline infusions in critically ill patients. Drug Intell Clin Pharmacol 11:12–18, 1977

156. Zwillich CW, Sutton FD, Neff TA, et al: Theophylline induced seizures in adults: correlation with serum concentrations. Ann Intern Med 82:784–787, 1975

157. Stewart BN, Block AJ: A trial of aerosolized theophylline in relieving bronchospasm. Chest 69:718–721, 1976

158. FDA dosage guidelines for theophylline products. FDA Drug Bull 10:4–6, 1980

159. Iravani J, Melville GN: Wirkung von pharmaka und Milieuanderungen auf die flimmertatigkeit der atemwege. Respiration 32:157–164, 1975

160. Nelson DJ, Wright EM: The distribution, activity and function of the cilia in the frog brain. J Physiol (Lond) 243:63–78, 1974

161. Sarafini SM, Wanner A, Michaelson ED: Mucociliary transport in central and intermediate size airways: effect of aminophylline. Bull Physiopathol Respir (Nancy) 12:415–418, 1976

162. Matthys H, Kohler D: Effect of theophylline on mucociliary clearance in man. Eur J Respir Dis, suppl. 109. 61:98–102, 1980

163. Sutton PP, Pavia D, Bateman JRM, Clark SW: The effect of oral aminophylline on lung mucociliary clearance in man. Chest 80:889S–892S, 1981

164. Aubier M, DeTroyer A, Sampson M: Aminophylline improves diaphragmatic contractility. N Engl J Med 305:249–252, 1981

165. Murciano D, Auclair MH, Pariente K, Aubier M: A randomized controlled trial of theophylline in patients with severe chronic obstructive pulmonary disease. N Engl J Med 320:1521–1525, 1989

166. Svedmyr N: The role of theophylline in asthma therapy. Scand J Respir Dis, suppl. 101:125–137, 1977

167. Hudson LD, Tyler ML, Petty TL: Oral aminophylline and dehydroxypropyl theophylline in reversible obstructive airway disease: a single-dose, double-blind, crossover comparison. Curr Ther Res 15:367–372, 1973

168. Gisclon LG, Ayres JW, Ewing GH: Pharmacokinetics of orally administered dyphylline. Am J Hosp Pharm 36:1179–1184, 1979

169. Simons FER, Simons KJ, Bierman CW: The pharmacokinetics of dihydroxypropyl theophylline: a basis for rational therapy. J Allergy Clin Immunol 56:347–355, 1975

170. Cavanaugh MJ, Cooper DM: Inhaled atropine dose-response characteristics. Am Rev Respir Dis 114:517–524, 1976

171. Pak CCF, Kradjan WA, Lakshminarayan S, et al: Inhaled atropine sulfate: dose-response characteristics in adult patients with chronic airflow obstruction. Am Rev Respir Dis 125:331–334, 1982

172. Altounyan RE: Variation of drug action on airway obstruction in man. Thorax 19:406–415, 1964

173. Crompton GK: A comparison of responses to bronchodilator drugs in chronic bronchitis and chronic asthma. Thorax 23:46–55, 1968

174. Foster WM, Bergofsky EH, Bohning De, et al: Effect of adrenergic agents and their mode of action on mucociliary clearance in man. J Appl Physiol 41:146–152, 1976

175. Annis P, Landa J, Lichtiger M: Effects of atropine on velocity of tracheal mucus in anesthetized patients. Anesthesiology 44:74–77, 1976

176. Lopez-Vidriero MT, Costello J, Clark TSH, et al: Effects of atropine on sputum production. Thorax 30:543–547, 1975

177. Deckers W: The chemistry of new derivatives of tropane alkaloids and the pharmacokinetics of a new quaternary compound. Postgrad Med J, suppl. 7. 51:76–81, 1975

178. Pakes GE, Brodgen RN, Heel RC, et al: Ipratropium bromide: a review of its pharmacological properties and therapeutic efficacy in asthma and chronic bronchitis. Drugs 20:237–266, 1980

179. Loddenkemper R: Dose- and time-response of SCH 1000 MDI on total (R_t) and expiratory (R_e) airway resistance in patients with chronic bronchitis and emphysema. Postgrad Med J, Suppl. 7. 51:97, 1975.

180. Maesen F, Buytendijk HJ: Dose- and time-response curve of SCH 1000 MDI and placebo. Differential response in asthmatics and bronchitics as measured by $FEV_{1.0}$, vital capacity, blood pressure, and heart rate. Postgrad Med J, suppl. 7. 51:97, 1975

181. Allen CJ, Campell AJ: Dose-response of ipratropium bromide assessed by two methods. Thorax 35:137–139, 1980

182. Gomm SA, Keaney NP, Hunt LP, et al: Dose-response comparison of ipratropium bromide from a metered-dose inhaler and by jet nebulization. Thorax 38:297–301, 1983

183. Davis A, Vickerson F, Worsley G, et al: Determination of

dose-response relationship for nebulized ipratropium in asthmatic children. J Pediatr 105:1002–1005, 1984

184. Simonsson BG, Jonson BV, Strom B: Bronchodilatory and circulatory effects of inhaling increasing doses of an anti-cholinergic drug, ipratropium bromide (SCH 1000). Scand J Respir Dis 56:138–149, 1975

185. Sackner MA, Friedman M, Silva G, et al: The pulmonary and hemodynamic effect of aerosols of isoproterenol and ipratropium in normal subjects and patients with reversible airway obstruction. Am Rev Respir Dis 116:1013–1022, 1977

186. Poppius H, Salorinne Y: Comparative trial of a new anticholinergic bronchodilator, SCH 1000, and salbutamol in chronic bronchitis. Br Med J 4:134–136, 1973

187. Tashkin DP, Ashutosh K, Bleecker ER, et al: Comparison of the anticholinergic bronchodilator ipratropium bromide with metaproterenol in chronic obstructive disease: a 90-day multicenter study. Am J Med, suppl. 5A. 81:81–89, 1986

188. Ruffin RE, Fitzgerald JD, Rebuck AS: A comparison of the bronchodilator activity of SCH 1000 and salbutamol. J Allergy Clin Immunol 59:139–141, 1977

189. Marlin GE, Bush DE, Berend N: Comparison of ipratropium bromide and fenoterol in asthma and chronic bronchitis. Br J Clin Pharmacol 6:547–549, 1978

190. Lefcoe NM, Toogood JH, Blennerhassett G, et al: The addition of an aerosol anticholinergic to an oral beta-agonist plus theophylline in asthma and bronchitis. Chest 82:300–305, 1982

191. Gross NJ: Ipratropium bromide. N Engl J Med 319:486–494, 1988

192. Rebuck AS, Chapman KR, Abboud R, et al: Nebulized anticholinergic and sympathomimetic treatment of asthma and chronic obstructive airways disease in the emergency room. Am J Med 82:59–64, 1987

193. Pavia D, Bateman JRM, Sheahan NF, et al: Effect of ipratropium bromide on mucociliary clearance and pulmonary function in reversible airway obstruction. Thorax 34:501–507, 1979

194. Ruffin RE, Wolff RK, Dolovich MB, et al: Aerosol therapy with SCH 1000. Short-term mucociliary clearance in normal and bronchitic subjects and toxicology in normal subjects. Chest 73:501–506, 1978

195. Gross NJ, Skorodin MS: Anticholinergic, antimuscarinic bronchodilators. Am Rev Respir Dis 129:856–870, 1984

196. Gal TJ, Suratt PM, Lu J: Bronchometer effects of glycopyrrolate and atropine aerosol inhalation. Anesthesiology 52:A479–A482, 1982

197. Gal TJ, Suratt PM: Atropine and glycopyrrolate effects on lung mechanics in normal man. Anesth Analg 60:85–90, 1981

198. Gal TJ, Suratt PM, Lu J: Glycopyrrolate and inhalation: comparative effects on normal airway function. Am Rev Respir Dis 129:871–873, 1984

199. Johnson BE, Suratt PM: Effect of inhaled glycopyrrolate and atropine in asthma. Chest 85:325–328, 1984

200. Schroeckstein DC, Bush RK, Chervinsky P, et al: Twelve hour bronchodilation in asthma with a single aerosol dose of the anticholinergic compound glycopyrrolate. J Allergy Clin Immun 82:115–119, 1988

201. Walker FB, Kaiser DL: Prolonged effect of inhaled glycopyrrolate in asthma. Chest 91:49–51, 1987

202. Cox JSG: Disodium cromoglycate: mode of action and its possible relevance to the clinical use of the drug. Br J Dis Chest 65:189–204, 1971

203. Frith PA, Ruffin RE, Juniper EF, et al: Inhibition of allergen-induced asthma by three forms of sodium cromoglycate. Clin Allergy 11:67–77, 1981

204. Marshall R: Protective effect of disodium cromoglycate on rat peritoneal mast cells. Thorax 27:38–43, 1972

205. Lichtenstein LM, Foreman JC, Conroy C, et al: Differences between histamine release from rat mast cells and human basophils and mast cells. pp. 83–96. In Pepys J, Edwards AM (eds): The Mast Cell—Its Role in Health and Disease. Pitman Medical Publishing, Tunbridge Wells, England, 1979

206. Kay AB, Walsh GM, Mogbel R, et al: Disodium cromoglycate inhibits activation of human inflammatory cells in vitro. J Allergy Clin Immunol 80:1–8, 1987

207. Orr TSC, Cox JSG: Disodium cromoglycate, an inhibitor of mast cell degranulation and histamine release induced by phospholipase A. Nature 223:197–198, 1969

208. Lavin N, Rachelefsky MD, Kaplan SA: An action of disodium cromoglycate: inhibition of cyclic 3′,5′-AMP phosphodiesterase. J Allergy Clin Immunol 57:80–88, 1976

209. Kingsley PJ, Cox JSG: Cromolyn sodium (sodium cromoglycate) and drugs with similar activities. pp. 481–498. In Middleton E, Reed CE, Ellis EF (eds): Allergy: Principles and Practice. CV Mosby, St. Louis, 1978

210. Theoharides TC, Sieghart W, Greengard P, et al: Antiallergic drug cromolyn may inhibit histamine secretion by regulating phosphorylation of a mast cell protein. Science 207:80–81, 1980

211. Corkey C, Mindorff C, Levison H, et al: Comparison of three different preparations of disodium cromoglycate in the prevention of exercise-induced bronchospasm. Am Rev Respir Dis 125:623–626, 1982

212. Ben-Dov I, Bar-Yishay E, Godfrey S: Heterogeneity in the response of asthmatic patients to pre-exercise treatment with cromolyn sodium. Am Rev Respir Dis 127:113–116, 1983

213. Deal EC, Jr, Wasserman SI, Soter NA, et al: Evaluation of role played by mediators of immediate hypersensitivity in exercise-induced asthma. J Clin Invest 65:659–664, 1980

214. Lee TH, Brown MJ, Nagy L, et al: Induced release of histamine and neutrophil chemotactic factor in atopic asthmatics. J Allergy Clin Immunol 70:73–81, 1982

215. Fanta CH, McFadden ER, Jr, Ingram RH, Jr: Effects of cromolyn sodium on the response to respiratory heat loss in normal subjects. Am Rev Respir Dis 123:161–164, 1981

216. Breslin FJ, McFadden ER, Jr, Ingram RH, Jr: The effects of cromolyn sodium on the airway response to hyperpnea and cold air in asthma. Am Rev Respir Dis 122:11–16, 1980

217. Fuller RW, Collier JG: Sodium cromoglycate and atropine block the fall in FEV_1, but not the cough induced by hypotonic mist. Thorax 39:766–770, 1984

218. Godden D, Jamieson S, Higenbottom T: "Fog"-induced bronchoconstriction is inhibited by sodium cromoglycate but not lignocaine or ipratropium. Thorax 38:226, 1983

219. Harries MG, Parkes PEG, Lessof MH, et al: Role of bronchial irritant receptors in asthma. Lancet 1:5–7, 1981

220. Harries MG: Bronchial irritant receptors and a possible new action for cromolyn sodium. Ann Allergy 46:156–158, 1981

221. Dixon M, Jackson DM, Richard IM: The action of cromoglycate on "C" fibre endings in the dog lung. Br J Pharmacol 70:11–13, 1980

222. Altounyan REC: Review of clinical activity and mode of action of sodium cromoglycate. Clin Allergy, suppl. 10:481–489, 1980

223. Dickson W, Cole M: Severe asthma in children—a 10-year follow-up. pp. 343–352. In Pepys J, Edwards AM (eds): The Mast Cell—Its Role in Health and Disease. Pitman Medical, Tunbridge Wells, England, 1979

224. Petty TL, Rollins DR, Christopher K, et al: Cromolyn sodium is effective in adult chronic asthmatics. Am Rev Respir Dis 139:694–701, 1989

225. Cox JSG, Beach JE, Blair AM, et al: Disodium cromoglycate (Intal). Adv Drug Res 5:115–196, 1970

226. Walker SR, Evans ME, Richards AJ, et al: The fate of (^{14}C) disodium cromoglycate in man. J Pharm Pharmacol 24:525–531, 1972

227. Barnes PJ: A new approach to the treatment of asthma. N Engl J Med 321:1517–1527, 1989

228. Pepys J, Hargreave FE, Chan M, McCarthy DS: Inhibitory effects of disodium cromoglycate on allergen-inhalation tests. Lancet 2:134–137, 1968

229. Hegardt B, Pauwels R, Van der Straaten M: Inhibitory effect of KWO 2131, terbutaline and DSCG on the immediate and late allergen-induced bronchoconstriction. Allergy 36:115–122, 1981

230. Murphy S: Cromolyn sodium pp. 669–717. In Jenne JW, Murphy S (eds): Drug Therapy for Asthma. Marcel Dekker, New York, 1987

231. Settipane GA, Klein DE, Boyd GK, et al: Adverse reactions to cromolyn. JAMA 241: 811–813, 1979

232. Scheffer AL, Ross EP, Goetzl EJ: Immunologic components of hypersensitivity reactors to cromolyn sodium. N Engl J Med 293:1220–1224, 1975

233. Bernstein IL: Cromolyn sodium in the treatment of asthma: coming of age in the United States. J Allergy Clin Immunol 76:381–388, 1985

234. Benson MK, Curry SH, D'A Mills GG, Hughes DTD: Uptake of sodium cromoglycate in obstructive airway disease. Clin Allergy 3:389–394, 1983

235. Autry RM: The clinical development of a new agent for the treatment of airway inflammation, nedocromil sodium (Tilade). Eur J Respir Dis, suppl. 147. 69:120–131, 1986

236. Altounyan REC, Lee TB, Rocchiccioli KMS, Shaw CL: A comparison of the inhibitory effects of nedocromil sodium and sodium cromoglycate on adenosine monophosphate-induced bronchoconstriction in atopic subjects. Eur J Respir Dis, suppl. 147. 69:277–279, 1986

237. Eady RP, Greenwood B, Jackson DM, et al: The effect of nedocromil sodium and sodium cromoglycate on antigen-induced bronchoconstriction in the Ascaris sensitive monkey. Br J Pharmacol 85:323–325, 1985

238. Pritchard DI, Eady RP, Harper ST, et al: Laboratory infection of primates with Ascaris serum to provide a model of allergic bronchoconstriction. Clin Exp Immunol 54:469–476, 1983

239. Barnes PJ: Asthma therapy: basic mechanisms. Eur J Respir Dis, suppl. 144. 68:217–265, 1986

240. Barnes PJ: Asthma as an axon reflex. Lancet 1:242–245, 1986

241. Neale MG, Brown K, Foulds RA, et al: The pharmacokinetics of nedocromil sodium, a new drug for the treatment of reversible objective airways disease in human volunteers. Br J Clin Pharmacol 87:250–252, 1987

242. Lal S, Malhotra S, Gribben D, Holder D: An open assessment study of the acceptability, tolerability and safety of nedocromil sodium in long-term clinical use in patients with perennial asthma. Eur J Respir Dis, suppl. 147. 69:136–142, 1986

243. Carrasco E, Sepulvada R: The acceptability, tolerability, and safety of nedocromil sodium in long-term clinical use. Eur J Respir Dis, suppl. 147. 69:311–313, 1986

244. Van AS, Chick TW: A group comparative study of the safety and efficacy of nedocromil sodium in reversible airways disease: a preliminary report. Eur J Respir Dis, suppl. 147. 69:143–148, 1986

245. Dorrow P: A double-blind group comparative trial of nedocromil in steroid-dependent patients. Eur J Respir Dis, suppl. 147. 69:317–319, 1986

246. Gonzalez JP, Brogden RN: Nedocromil sodium: a preliminary review of its pharmacokinetic properties and therapeutic efficacy in the treatment of reversible obstructive airways disease. Drugs 34:560–577, 1987

247. Hench PS, Kendall EC, Slocumb CH, et al: The effect of a hormone of the adrenal cortex (17-hydroxy-11-dehydrocorticosterone—compound E) and of pituitary adrenocorticotropic hormone on rheumatoid arthritis. Mayo Clin Proc 24:181–197, 1949

248. Carryer HM, Prickman LE, Maytum CK, et al: Effects of cortisone on bronchial asthma and hay fever occurring in subjects sensitive to ragweed pollen. Mayo Clin Proc 25:482–486, 1950

249. Morris HG: Pharmacology of corticosteriods in asthma. pp. 464–480. In Middleton E, Reed CE, Ellis EF (eds): Allergy: Principles and Practice. CV Mosby, St. Louis, 1978

250. Slaunwhite WR, Lockie GN, Back N, et al: Inactivity in vivo of transcortin-bound cortisol. Science 135:1062–1063, 1962

251. Morris HG, DeRoche G, Caro CM: Detection of synthetic corticosteroid analogs by the competitive protein-binding radioassay. Steroids 22:445–450, 1973

252. Munck A, Mendel DB, Smith LI, Orti E: Glucocorticoid

receptors and actions. Am Rev Respir Dis 141:S2–S10, 1990

253. Brooks SM, Werk EE, Ackerman HJ, et al: Adverse effects of phenobarbital on corticosteroid metabolism in patients with bronchial asthma. N Engl J Med 286:1125–1128, 1972

254. Jubiz W, Meikle AW, Levinson RA, et al: Effect of diphenylhydantoin on the metabolism of dexamethasone. Mechanism of the abnormal dexamethasone suppression in humans. N Engl J Med 283:11–14, 1970

255. Edwards OM, Courtnay-Evans RJ, Galley JM, et al: Changes in cortisol metabolism following rifampin therapy. Lancet 1:346–351, 1974

256. Szefler SJ, Rose JQ, Ellis EF, et al: The effect of troleandomycin on methylprednisolone elimination. J Allergy Clin Immunol 66:447–451, 1980

257. Urike M, Go VLW: Corticosteroid pharmacokinetics in liver disease. Clin Pharmacokinet 4:233–240, 1979

258. Dwyer J, Lazarus L, Hickie JB: A study of cortisol metabolism in patients with chronic asthma. Australas Ann Med 16:297–304, 1963

259. Brodde O-E, Howe U, Egerszegei S, et al: Effect of prednisolone on B₂-adrenoreceptors in asthmatic patients receiving B₂-bronchodilators. Eur J Clin Pharmacol 34:145–150, 1988

260. Harris DM: pp. 34–47. In Mygind N, Clark TJH (eds): Topical Treatment for Asthma and Rhinitis. Bailliere Tindall, London, 1980

261. Sullivan TJ, Hallmark MR, Sackman E, et al: Comparative bioavailability: eight commercial prednisone tablets. J Pharmacokinet Biopharm 4:157–172, 1976

262. Harten JG, Novitch AM: Evaluation of steroid analogs in terms of suitability for alternate day steroid therapy. J Allergy 37:108–109, 1966

263. Ackerman GL, Nolan CM: Adrenocortical responsiveness after alternate-day corticosteroid therapy. N Engl J Med 278:405–409, 1968

264. Falliers CJ, Chai H, Molk L, et al: Pulmonary and adrenal effects of alternate day corticosteroid therapy. J Allergy Clin Immunol 49:156–166, 1972

265. Morris HG, Neuman I, Ellis E: Plasma steroid concentrations during alternate day treatment with prednisone. J Allergy Clin Immunol 54:350–374, 1974

266. Schleimer RP: Effects of glucocorticoids on inflammatory cells relevant to their therapeutic applications in asthma. Am Rev Respir Dis 141:S59–S69, 1990

267. Jenkins CR, Woolcock AJ: Effect of prednisone and beclomethasone dipropionate on airway responsiveness in asthma: a comparative study. Thorax 43:378–384, 1988

268. Dah R, Johansson S-A: Importance of duration of treatment with inhaled budesonide on the immediate and late bronchial reaction. Eur J Respir Dis, suppl. 122:167–175, 1982

269. Henriksen JM: Effect of inhalation of corticosteroids on exercise-induced asthma: randomized double-blind crossover study of budesonide in asthmatic children. Br Med J 2:248–249, 1985

270. Choo-Kanag YFJ, Cooper EJ, Tribe AE, et al: Beclo-

methasone dipropionate by inhalation in the treatment of airway obstruction. Br J Dis Chest 66:101–106, 1972

271. Gaddie J, Petrie GR, Reid IW, et al: Aerosol beclomethasone dipropionate: a dose-response study in chronic bronchial asthma. Lancet 2:280–281, 1972

272. Martin LE, Tanner RJN, Clark TJH, et al: Absorption and metabolism of orally administered beclomethasone dipropionate. Clin Pharmacol Ther 15:267–275, 1974

273. Wyatt R, Waschek MS, Weinberger M, et al: Effects of inhaled beclomethasone dipropionate and alternate-day prednisone on pituitary-adrenal function in children with chronic asthma. N Engl J Med 299:1387–1392, 1978

274. Toogood JH, Lefcoe NM, Haines DSM, et al: A graded dose assessment of the efficacy of beclomethasone dipropionate aerosol for severe chronic asthma. J Allergy Clin Immunol 59:298–308, 1974

275. Toogood JH, Lefcoe NM, Haines DSM, et al: Minimum dose requirements of steroid-dependent asthmatic patients for aerosol beclomethasone and oral prednisone. J Allergy Clin Immunol 61:355–364, 1978

276. Toogood JH: Complications of topical steroid therapy for asthma. Am Rev Respir Dis 141:S89–S96, 1990

277. Cooper EJ, Grant IWB: Beclomethasone dipropionate aerosol in the treatment of chronic asthma. Q J Med 46:295–308, 1977

278. Thiringer G, Erikson N, Malmberg R, et al: Bronchoscopic biopsies of bronchial mucosa before and after beclomethasone dipropionate therapy. Scand J Respir Dis, suppl. 101:173–177, 1979

279. Chaplin MD, Rooks W II, Swenson EW, et al: Flunisolide metabolism and dynamics of a metabolite. Clin Pharmacol Ther 27:402–413, 1980

280. Chaplin MD, Cooper WC, Segre EJ, et al: Correlation of flunisolide plasma levels to eosinophilic response in humans. J Allergy Clin Immunol 65:445–453, 1980

281. Martin LE, Harrison C, Tarmer RJN: Metabolism of beclomethasone dipropionate by animals and man. Postgrad Med J, suppl. 4. 5:11–20

282. Ryrfeldt A, Anderson P, Edsbacker S, et al: Pharmacokinetics and metabolism of budesonide, a selective glucocorticoid. Eur J Respir Dis, suppl. 122. 63:62–73, 1982

283. Grieco MH, Larsen K, Petraco AJ: In vivo comparison of triamcinolone and beclomethasone inhalation delivery systems. Ann Allergy 45:231–234, 1980

284. Chervinsky P: Treatment of steroid-dependent asthma with triamcinolone acetonide aerosol. Ann Allergy 38:192–197, 1977

285. Aherne GW, Littleton P, Thalen A: A sensitive radioimmunoassay for budesonide in plasma. J Steroid Biochem 17:559–565, 1982

286. Konig P: Inhaled corticosteroids—their present and future role in the management of asthma. J Allergy Clin Immunol 82:297–306, 1988

287. Collins JV, Clark TJH, Harris PWR, et al: Intravenous corticosteroids in treatment of acute bronchial asthma. Lancet 2:1047–1050, 1970

288. Rebuck AS, Reed J: Assessment and management of severe asthma. Am J Med 51:788–798, 1971
289. Fanta CH, Rossing TH, McFadden ER: Glucocorticoids in acute asthma: a controlled clinical trial. Am J Med 74:845–851, 1983
290. Albert RK, Martin TR, Lewis SW: Controlled clinical trial of methylprednisolone in patients with chronic bronchitis and acute respiratory insufficiency. Ann Intern Med 92:753–758, 1980
291. Mendella LA, Manfreda J, Warren CPW, Anthomisen NR: Steroid response in stable chronic obstructive pulmonary disease. Ann Intern Med 96:17–21, 1982
292. Shim C, Stover DE, Williams MH, Jr: Response to corticosteroids in chronic bronchitis. J Allergy Clin Immunol 62:363–367, 1978
293. Blair GP, Light RW: Treatment of chronic obstructive pulmonary disease with corticosteroids. Comparison of daily vs alternate-day therapy. Chest 86:524–528, 1984
294. Georgopoulos D, Anthonisen NR: Are steroids useful in chronic obstructive pulmonary disease? Am Coll Chest Phys Pulm Perspect 6:6–8, 1989
295. Plummer AL: Bronchodilator drugs and the cardiac patient. pp. 581–606. In Kaplan JA (ed): Cardiac Anesthesia. Vol. 2. Cardiovascular Pharmacology. Grune & Stratton, Orland, FL, 1983
296. Laaban JP, Lung B, Chaivet JP, et al: Cardiac arrhythmias during the combined use of intravenous aminophylline and terbutaline in status asthmaticus. Chest 94:496–502, 1988
297. Bohn D, Kalloghlian A, Jenkins J, et al: Intravenous salbutamol in the treatment of status asthmaticus in children. Crit Care Med 12:392–396, 1984

10

PHARMACOLOGIC PREPARATION OF THE PATIENT FOR THORACIC SURGERY

Theodore C. Smith, M.D.

Empirical procedures firmly entrenched in the habits of good doctors seem to have a vigor and life, not to say immortality, of their own.
Henry K. Beecher, 1959

Forrest et al used these words of Beecher to introduce one of the best studies of preoperative medication ever published.[1] Their study, however, did not deal directly with premedication for thoracic surgery; there are no seminal works on the subject. Premedicant drugs, dose, route, and timing before anesthesia for chest operations are just as Beecher described: entrenched habit, empirically rather than experimentally based. Premedication need not be irrational, however, and it has changed, slowly, with the appearance of new operations and new anesthetics, as well as new premedicants. As evidence of the change, this chapter begins with a brief recounting of the historical practices of medication before anesthesia. A discussion of the problems specific or common to thoracic surgery precedes a review of anesthetic aims and techniques that bear on the choices of premedicants. The interplay of supportive psychological efforts is followed by several useful classes of pharmacologic agents, with brief notes on their benefits and side effects. A rational approach to the selection of drugs, doses, routes, and timing completes the chapter.

Agreement on certain definitions is essential. The term *sedation* is used in its proper sense, meaning induction of a relaxed, easy, calm state, without anxiety. It in no way implies a decrease in level of consciousness. It is not said that a person with a sedate personality is drowsy or depressed. "To sedate" is specifically not a synonym for "to put to sleep." For that, it is necessary "to hypnotize" or "to narcotize," meaning to provide a state of unconsciousness or unawareness. *Narcotic* drugs include barbiturates, ataractics, and some analgesics given in sufficient dose to obtund consciousness. *Narcotic analgesics* are the class of drugs typified by morphine and are referred to below as opioids; they include synthetic as well as natural products. Finally, the term *authority* simply means an investigator whose ideas have been published in a peer-reviewed journal.

The problem with the words *sedative, hypnotic,* and *narcotic* can be understood, if not corrected, with a few historical references. The early textbooks of pharmacology had chapters with titles such as "The Sedative/Hypnotic Drugs." These included the barbiturates and a few others such as paraldehyde and chloral hydrate. In small doses, these drugs had a degree of calming effect in some patients. In larger doses, they could induce sleep, a sleeplike state, or coma. Their calming property was so uncertain that when drug companies introduced the first of the post-World War II sedatives (meprobamate [Miltown, Equanil]) and the many that followed (chlorpromazine, promethazine, propiomazine, etc.), they went out of their way to avoid the descriptive term *sedative*, inventing new words instead, eg, tranquilizers, anxiolytics, ataractics.[2] Doctors knew that sedative drugs, meaning barbiturates, did not work well. Drug companies wanted to make it clear that their new psychopharmaceuticals were quite different. Popular authors of fiction also misused the term *sedative;* for example, the heroine who could not presently be interviewed by the detective because the friendly family doctor had given her a "heavy sedative." Similarly, lawyers in Congress shortened the proper but overlong term *narcotic analgesic* in the Harrison Narcotic Act of 1932, in referring to what are now called *controlled drugs* or *substances of abuse.* Seevers and Pfeiffer used the terms correctly in 1936[3]:

The difference between narcosis and analgesia can be strikingly demonstrated with a drug like scopolamine. . . . The subjects were very much depressed by 0.4 to 0.65 mg given subcutaneously, but obtained not the slightest analgesia . . . rather the development of an increased sensitivity to pain. Neither did this drug potentiate the analgesic action of morphine although the individual was obviously more subjectively and objectively depressed as a result of the combined narcosis.

Amnesia is the last term needing careful use. It refers to lack of recall at a time when a subject is observably conscious and reactive. Coma is not amnesia, nor are soporifics amnestic.

DEVELOPMENT OF PREANESTHETIC MEDICATION

Regardless of who is credited with the initial use of anesthetic drugs, no one can claim credit for introducing deliberate preanesthetic medication. The excessive salivation and stormy induction with ether, the frightening bradycardia with chloroform, and the "resistance" of patients to nitrous oxide were sufficient stimuli to legions of anesthetists to incorporate morphine and belladonna in the hours before induction. Well before McMechan introduced the term *premedication* in 1920,[4,5] it was generally understood that a preliminary, hypodermic injection could promote patient comfort and safety. The relative importance of these two objectives has tended to vary from time to time and place to place, but they were both clearly related to the anesthetic technique:

Atropine before chloroform to prevent cardiac arrest,
Atropine before ether to prevent copious salivation,
Morphine before ether to speed induction,
Morphine before nitrous oxide to potentiate the effect.

This inevitably led to the idea that the premedication was dictated by the choice of anesthetic. There was agreement that the primary objectives were (1) to minimize the dose of inhalation agent needed, and (2) to block the noxious effects of the anesthetics themselves.

The differing practices in the United States and the United Kingdom vis-a-vis choice of agent were associated with differing premedicant practice.[4,5] Between World Wars I and II, there was transoceanic agreement: some premedication was in order. Patients learned to expect it, and still do. There was agreement that a sixth of a grain of morphine and 1/100 grain of atropine were "light," and 1/4 grain of morphine, 1/150 grain of scopoline, and two grains of pentobarbital were "heavy," but acceptable, even during spontaneous respiration.[6] The introduction of cyclopropane with fast, smooth induction characteristics but imperfect abdominal muscle tone during spontaneous breathing posed a brief problem. Morphine facilitated controlled respiration, smoothed surgical access to the abdomen, and was retained. Perhaps the slow emergence, frequent emesis, and emergence delirium were stimuli for the development of the concept of recovery rooms. In a remarkably precognisant report in 1948, Comroe and Dripps showed that the high incidence of nausea, vomiting, and other undesirable effects seen in ambulatory volunteers was not seen with in-patients.[7]

After World War II, authorities began to develop both critical and scientific approaches. Numerous reports, usually reviewing how things had gone for the last few years in the practice of anesthesia, began suggesting that premedication be individualized not only for the anesthetic agent, but for the patient *and* for the proposed surgery. Clinical impression fell out of favor. Careful studies with controls and specific assessment appeared from such centers as Boston and Philadelphia.[8,9] The first of the subspecialties in anesthesiology looked at the specific goals of comfort and safety for the child.[10–12] The newly introduced ataractics were evaluated for preoperative sedation, and were largely found wanting despite initial enthusiasm for such benefits as reduced laryngospasm and hiccoughs.[13–15]

All of this happened in the absence of relevance to or input from thoracic surgery. While a few innovative surgeons breached the chest wall, aided by inventive and brave anesthesiologists, there were few cardiothoracic procedures performed anywhere. The anesthetic techniques for these occasional operations were assembled from the "empiric procedures" to which Beecher had referred. The cuffed endotracheal tube, manual control of ventilation, and nonexplosive anesthetic regimens were developed for other reasons, as were double-lumen endotracheal tubes, antibiotics, and electrocautery. "Surgical tuberculosis" (cavitary or calcified lesions in arrested mycobacterial disease) and, later, squamous cell carcinoma of the lung provided the seeds for thoracic surgery. In the same period, physiologic understanding of the heart and lungs markedly advanced.[16] Oddly enough the subject of preanesthetic medication for thoracic procedures was rarely addressed specifically, and never definitively.[17] Perhaps it was considered unimportant; more likely, thoracic patients were treated like all others.

SURGICAL AIMS AND EXPECTATIONS

Current thoracic surgical practice owes its development primarily to two diseases, tuberculosis and coronary artery disease, which provided the large number of cases on which present techniques are based. A spirit of inquiry requires asking whether the lessons from these two diseases are broadly applicable to the provision of anesthesia for thoracic surgery. Students must keep an open mind and practitioners must make up their minds, based in large part on incomplete, empiric, and noncomparable information.

In the early 1950s, the surgical decision with tuberculosis required a choice between "resting" the lung (achieved with thoracoplasty and plombage) and excision (achieved with segmental and subsegmental resection). As the severity of the presenting disease decreased, opinion largely swung from the former to the latter.[18,19] Physiologically oriented surgeons, notably, E.A. Gaensler in Boston, developed such preoperative assessment methods as the timed vital capacity

method[16] (now renamed FEV_1/FVC [forced expiratory volume in 1 second/forced vital capacity]), and established limits predicting operability.[20,21] The posterolateral thoracotomy became the standard approach for almost all thoracic procedures. Antimycobacterial therapy and double-lumen tubes helped prevent contralateral spread during surgery on the "up" lung. The postoperative expectation was for a patient willing and able to cough effectively and immediately. Carbon dioxide retention during and after surgery was recognized as a treatable problem,[17,22,23] and the pulmonary contributions to hypoxemia were recognized and treated physiologically.[24]

A score of years later, surgical tuberculosis had vanished. Instead, cardiothoracic surgeons were increasingly dealing with older patients who had cardiac disease or carcinoma of the lung (often with cardiac disease as well). Pulmonary surgery was aimed at doing a "good" cancer operation. The former limits of operability based on pulmonary function studies were breached regularly and successfully.[25] The median sternotomy became the most familiar approach and could be used successfully in most diseases, albeit with difficulty approaching the inferior pulmonary ligament. The thoracic surgeon now operates on the thoracic esophagus, parenchyma of the lung, extrapulmonary airway, four parts of the mediastinum, all of the great vessels, and the heart itself. The sternotomy appears not to affect the high end of ventilation/perfusion maldistribution,[26] and is marginally better than a lateral thoracotomy in mechanical effects on breathing.[27] The risk of bilateral pneumothorax is easily handled with chest tubes.

There is a relevant difference between the cardiac and thoracic surgical patient, in addition to the incisional approach. The former leaves the operating room with a heart about as good as was brought in, or perhaps actually improved, as is obvious in the case of valvular disease and heart transplant. However, the thoracic surgical patient will have less lung tissue and some malfunction of the remaining tissue, which may, and usually does, get worse for several days.[28,29] While the eventual pulmonary function that can be expected after lung resection can be predicted with some accuracy,[20,21] the first few postoperative days are the problem.[18,19,30] Overnight "prophylactic" ventilatory support has little or no effect on this expected course, other than ablating a day of the patient's conscious experience.[31] Patients who truly "require" prolonged ventilatory support, typically chronic obstructive pulmonary disease patients, are very likely to present weaning problems and suffer high mortality.[32] The widespread use of prolonged mechanical ventilation after cardiac surgery is dictated by the choice of anesthetic (large-dose opioid), and not a therapeutic in-tent. The pathophysiology and available therapeutic measures are reviewed by Schwieger et al.[33]

Thus, what the surgeon wants is a patient initially calm and cooperative, intraoperatively free of noxious reflexes with little or no excitement on emergence, tolerable pain, adequate ventilation and oxygenation, and effective cough or cooperation with the stirrup regimen. While copious bronchial secretions would not be wanted, neither would scant and inspissated mucous. The surgeon's hope for good intraoperative working conditions means more than simple paralysis of the patient. Even with only one twitch of the train-of-four left, the diaphragm may be capable of contracting, unexpectedly and sufficiently, to disrupt a bronchial sleeve resection or other delicate surgical maneuver. This can be prevented more reliably with depression of the respiratory drive (opioids and potent inhalation anesthetics) and reduction of chemoreceptor stimuli (hyperventilation and hyperoxia) than by partial paralysis. High-frequency jet ventilation with total paralysis may minimize motion of the surgical field, but is at best only equal to mechanical ventilation in oxygenation and CO_2 removal, and may be worse.[34,35] Similarly, the surgeon hopes to avoid dysrhythmias despite manipulation of the mediastinal structures, interference with cardiac output despite both intra- and extrapulmonary vascular obstruction, and problems with gas exchange despite the lateral position and mechanical ventilation.

Ancillary procedures and operations other than lung resection offer their own considerations. Surgical plans for preoperative fiberoptic bronchoscopy before repositioning require good blunting of adrenergic responses. The need for subsequent reintubation with a double-lumen tube also requires adequate depth to avoid deleterious vascular reflexes. Bronchoscopy and mediastinoscopy displace anesthesiologists from their accustomed position and vantage place, and may require precautions relevant to laser surgery.[36] Esophageal surgery will leave a patient with two large and painful incisions, one on either side of the diaphragm.[37] Surgery for thoracic trauma may present an already intubated and narcotized, paralyzed, or comatose patient with uncertain coexisting injury elsewhere. In all cases of trauma to the trunk, the diaphragm on one or both sides may be functionally weakened[37] and unimproved by ventilatory support.[31]

Thus, when choosing premedication and anesthetic technique, the drug effects that contribute to postoperative analgesia, gas exchange, work of breathing, and autonomic stability must be kept in mind. The use of the common opioids as part of premedication is neither justified nor condemned on analgesic and respiratory depressant grounds. In acceptable dosage (such as morphine, 0.15 to 0.20 mg/kg), none linger long enough to be a postoperative problem. Moreover, common usage tends to reduce the dose to an inconsequential amount (0.05 to 0.10 mg/kg of morphine). It is particularly irrational to avoid adequate opioid dosage if a major opioid component to anesthesia is planned. Similarly, anticholinergics in the usual antisialagogue dosage are totally benign. Thus, in general, premedication is selected for its preoperative effects, less so for its early intraoperative effects, and largely independent of postoperative expectations.

ANESTHETIC GOALS

Most anesthetic texts list a variety of goals for an ideal premedicant; these goals are as applicable to thoracic surgery as any other. The question that should concern the prescriber is whether administration of drug(s) before the patient arrives in the operating room is either the only or the best method of achieving the goals. The following goals merit consideration:

Anxiety relief
Amnestic effect
Analgesia
Antisialagogue effect
Achlorhydria
Hypnosis

If any or all of these goals are desirable, the effect should be produced before the patient is transported from the hospital room to the operating room.

Major Goals of Premedication

Relief of anxiety is usually first on the list of goals. Thoracic surgery is an anxiety-provoking procedure. The dread of cancer and incurability is much worse than the fear of cardiac surgery. Fear of pain is almost inescapable, and likely to surge with every breath, not to mention cough. There are no drugs that will ablate retrograde anxiety. While anxiety likely exists from at least as soon as the diagnosis and operation are suggested, it reaches a crescendo on the morning of surgery. A variety of pharmaceuticals have proven effective in some anxiety states and merit consideration (especially promethazine, hydroxyzine, and diazepam[38-43]), although a number of other drugs have or have had their proponents.[2,44-51] Barbiturates and opioids are ineffective or unpredictable in producing this effect and many give unintended and worrisome dysphoria,[52] as may the major tranquilizer, droperidol.[53] Preoperative anxiety is a significant predictor of recall of intraoperative events, and premedication does decrease the incidence of this undesirable effect.[54]

Sedation, properly meaning calmness, is produced by familiar or at least expected events and surroundings. Since the now classic report of Egbert et al in 1963, a supportive preoperative visit has been known to be as effective or more effective than 2 mg/kg of pentobarbital.[55] It might be argued that pentobarbital is no longer the best sedative, and that an "unstructured" visit by *an* anesthesiologist lacks the effect of a planned, structured interview by *the* anesthesiologist. Hypnotic-trance induction by standard medically qualified techniques teaches that telling the patient what will happen and then assuring that it does in fact happen in that manner is effective. Unanswered is the following question: do support and drugs add to or potentiate each other?

Amnesia is a state many patients request. There are no known drugs with retrograde amnestic properties. Lack of recall can be produced by coma or very deep narcosis, of course, but the valuable properties of patient cooperation and assessability are lost. Thus, few anesthesiologists, or none, favor basal narcosis. Drugs known to give some incidence of amnesia include scopolamine[40] (but not other anticholinergics) and several benzodiazepines, including diazepam, lorazepam, and midazolam. In all cases of demonstrable effect, some delay (which may be an hour or more) is experienced before onset of activity (Fig. 10-1).[56]

Analgesia is of minor benefit before most surgery, as there is little or no pain prior to induction. Some exceptions might be considered: surgery for the effect of trauma, reoperation for air leak or bleeding, crude technique in topical anesthesia for bronchoscopy, or the patient with existing pain from another cause, such as severe rheumatoid arthritis. Without real somatic pain of clear-cut significance, only the pain induced while establishing monitors and giving intravenous injections (which can and should be minimized with skill and local anesthetics) must be considered. Pain should be controlled when it exists and narcotic analgesics, of course, have a well-established usage; however, this utility is for their narcotic rather than analgesic property.

Antisialagogue activity is certainly less important with the present array of agents compared with diethyl ether. Aside from a minor effect of certain antihistamines (eg, diphenhydramine), only atropine, scopolamine, and glycopyrrolate are dependable drying agents. Previously expressed fear of inspissation of secretions in the airway after belladonna drugs is baseless.[57] Simple passive heat and moisture exchangers are both necessary and sufficient to abort this old worry.[58] However, timing of administration is important. Sufficient preformed saliva may be present in ducts and glands to annoy the laryngoscopist if the induction technique expresses them, as can happen with succinylcholine. After administration of antisialagogues, enough time should elapse to empty and swallow such saliva. Continued production of saliva during surgery may cause a pooling in the oropharynx or buccal pouch. This is rather more an es-

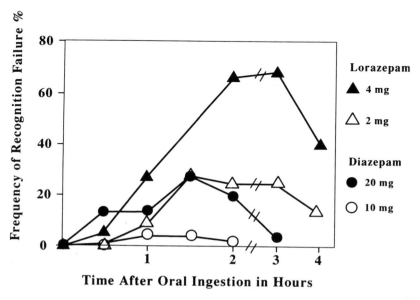

Fig. 10-1. Time course of amnesia after benzodiazepines. Given by mouth, lorazepam produced markedly more amnesia than diazepam. Note that the peak effects occur well into the second hour after ingestion. No retrograde amnesia was found. (Data from Kothary et al.[56])

thetic distraction than a practical danger, since even if this material is aspirated, effective cough will soon eliminate it.

Achlorhydria, together with a reduction of volume of gastric juice, is a desirable and eminently achievable state. While the belladonna drugs have some such beneficial effect, they are neither as efficacious nor as potent as the H_2-receptor blocking drugs. The latter, especially when combined with the gastric emptying drug, metoclopramide (which also has desirable antiemetic properties), are a more certain route to the desired state.[59] The minor worries about P-450 enzyme induction, vis-a-vis anesthetic and other drug metabolism, should not be a concern for acute administration. There are, however, no larger-scale studies of the cost/benefit nature of the increasing use of such drugs. A conservative view might limit their use to those at special risk, eg, the pregnant, the obese, those with a history of frequent heartburn, and those with an established diagnosis of symptomatic hiatal hernia. Prolonged surgical use of H_2-receptor blockers after esophageal surgery is common, and they might as well be started preoperatively.

Hypnosis is the last of the primary goals of premedication. It is confused in both incidence and terminology with sedation. The "sleepy" patient is all too easy to achieve. If the effect is overdone, it limits the desirable cooperation of the truly sedate (awake) subject. The barbiturates and, possibly, certain other classes of hypnotics are antianalgesic and (when not combined with opioids) may make starting intravenous injections and invasive monitoring more difficult. Murray et al reported that only drowsy patients had antiapprehensive effects after a variety of sedative/hypnotic drugs.[60] Unfortunately, these investigators *assumed* that all very drowsy patients were *not* anxious. In a methodologically more sound study nearly a decade later, Forrest et al used objective as well as subjective assessments of sleepiness and apprehension.[1] They found that observers reported objective, dose-related signs of calmness while patients simultaneously showed dose-related increases in anxiety (Fig. 10-2). Diazepam was ineffective in this otherwise impeccable report, perhaps because it was given intramuscularly and was studied before peak effect was likely achieved. The most telling point in this work was the demonstration that despite efforts to define and grade sedation and hypnosis, and despite double-blind, placebo-controlled, multidose design, "There was no valid assay for . . . apprehension relative to placebo as reported by the patient."[1] The search for scientific validation is further complicated by the work of Antrobus, who found that those most anxious preoperatively were most likely to withhold consent to enter a scientific double-blind study of anxiolytic agents, thus biasing studies of anxiolysis.[61]

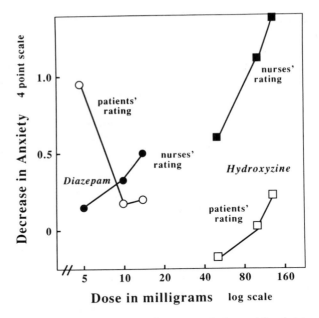

Fig. 10-2. Dose-response after two sedatives. After intramuscular injection, anxiety was separately rated by both the patient-recipient and a trained nurse-observer, and was plotted as a change in the rating on a scale of 1 to 10. Notice that patients and observers have different evaluations. In the case of diazepam, patients report more anxiety with increased dose, and for hydroxyzine, observers overrate the anxiolytic effect compared with patients. (Adapted from Forrest et al,[1] with permission.)

Minor Goals of Premedication

There are a number of minor claims for benefit from premedication, including

Decreasing cardiac vagal activity during induction
Facilitating induction of anesthesia
Blunting adrenergic response to intubation and surgery
Decreasing dose of anesthetic drug need for maintenance
Facilitating rapid emergence
Decreasing incidence of emergence delirium
Decreasing incidence of nausea and emesis
Contributing to postoperative analgesia

In general, all of these effects may be desirable, but can also be reasonably accomplished within minutes of induction by the appropriate intravenous drugs.

The vagal activity of most concern is cardiac slowing. Atropine in customary dosage does not assuredly prevent slowing in children after succinylcholine,[62] although both glycopyrrolate and atropine were effective in preventing bradycardia during abdominal surgery.[63] In most adults slowing sufficient to decrease cardiac output will not occur precipitously and will respond rapidly to atropine. The dysrhythmias formerly reported with doses of atropine between 0.05 and 0.5 mg IV were associated with now-abandoned agents and techniques.[64]

Morphine and other opioids are simply additive in producing anesthesia.[65–67] There is no absolute need to give them before induction insofar as this indication is concerned. Clinical experience suggests one caveat in this regard. If, for reasons of airway management, it is desirable to maintain spontaneous breathing, and if, for reasons of patient comfort, it is desirable to use intravenous induction with no more than brief apnea, opioids are best omitted from the premedicant and induction routine.[68–70]

The adrenergic response to laryngoscopy, intubation, incision, and other stress may be a threat to patients with coronary artery disease. No customary premedication routine alone will ablate this response, but it can help modify it.[71] It may occur repeatedly in thoracic surgery, with repetitive stimuli of initial intubation, fiberoptic bronchoscopy, double-lumen tube positioning, confirmation, and incision. Stimulation of the carina and main bronchi with double-lumen tubes is more reflexogenic than with single-lumen endotracheal tubes, although even an oral airway will stimulate some patients.[72] A variety of routes and drugs have been recommended: intravenous lidocaine, 1.5 to 2 mg/kg;[73] nasal or transdermal nitroglycerin in beta-blocked patients[74–76]; and a host of opioid and other adjuvants.[71,74,77–80] Their use is not without hazard and add to the already task-intensive workload of induction.

Facilitation of rapid emergence is a commendable goal. As increased numbers of drugs are used, with rapid beta-elimination half-lives, the emergence is more rapid. Occasional prolonged emergence is still worrisome, but, given modern agents and competent recovery room facilities, this condition, as well as emergence delirium and emergence emesis, are no longer the problems they were when the use of ether was prominent. No recent studies of the incidence of delirium or vomiting in the recovery room match the 5 to 25 percent in the 1950s,[81,82] yet the premedication techniques and even drugs may well be the same now as then.

The contribution of premedication with opioids to postoperative analgesia is real, but likely minor, more than 3 hours postinjection. If opioid analgesia is intended, it can be given during emergence, under observation, to effect. Further, alternate routes and techniques (eg, epidural, intrapleural, and intercostal block[83–88]) may be used to achieve nearly pain-free cooperation with the stirrup regimen.

PSYCHOLOGICAL PREPARATION

The nonpharmacologic preparation of a patient for anesthesia and thoracic surgery is important in view of the seminal report by Egbert et al.[55] An illuminating series of communications in the British literature clearly indicates that the much-heralded practice is poorly emulated.[89–91] Goldman et al demonstrated that even 3 minutes devoted to the cause, structured by the precedents of hypnotic induction technique, has real value.[92] The interview was specifically *not* conducted by the anesthesiologist of record, giving rise to the question, "must your anesthesiologist, or merely anyone, provide the preanesthetic support?" Then, too, an improper visit may be a source of anxiety,[93,94] as may the sterile, mechanical, inhuman decor of the preoperative areas of some hospitals.[95]

Whatever the answer to the relative merits of pharmacologic versus psychological preparation, in training programs, the additional anxiety present in trainees should be considered. Pinnock et al have begun to assess this in junior anesthesiologists in the British tradition of early, but gradual, "solo" experience.[96] Stress and anxiety in even senior residents is occasioned by a superior's terse, judgmental, and often harsh commentary about the early (preinduction) conduct of case management, even after a lengthy preoperative discussion and planning. The following questions still await proper exposition:

1. Can any anesthesiologist provide effective preoperative support?
2. Can the anesthesiologist of record provide better support than any other?
3. Can currently available drugs provide support equivalent to the best, or the least, support provided by the preanesthetic visit?

The answers are as important as advancement or mastery in the technology of ventilation, acid-base balance, and advanced monitoring. Clearly, however, these questions are harder to answer.

PHARMACOLOGIC CONSIDERATIONS

Antimuscarinic Drugs

Three antimuscarinic drugs (atropine, scopolamine, and glycopyrrolate) are commonly available, although a few others (eg, methyscopolamine, hyoscine butylbromide, methylatropine, and L-hyoscyamine) have occasionally been used.[97,98] The three primary antimuscarinic drugs differ in their kinetics and relative potency at different cholinergic receptors. Used in anesthetic practice for drying of oral secretions and reversing or blocking bradycardia, they may produce undesirable narcosis or delirium, tachycardia (although rarely over 120 beats/min), and, rarely, heat retention. All clearly have measurable but insignificant effects on dead space and bronchomotor tone, and possibly on oxygenation in the lung. Their use in thoracic surgery may, hence, be questioned because of some adverse effects:

Tachycardia in patients with coronary artery disease
Increased physiologic shunting
Increased dead space
Drying of tracheobronchial secretions

To this list might be added both acute glaucoma and dysrhythmias. The latter were undoubtedly belladonna-related and occasionally of marked hemodynamic consequence, but were only of concern during the use of now-abandoned deep anesthesia with diethyl ether and cyclopropane.[64] Reviews of these drugs by Eger[99] and Gravenstein et al,[100] dating from the 1960s, are current for all topics except bronchomotor effect, for which Gal and Suratt provided data.[101]

Atropine

The usual intramuscular dose of atropine is 8 to 10 μg/kg. Peak effect occurs in 30 to 40 minutes after injection in inactive muscles, but it may be faster when injected in better-perfused sites.[102] Intravenous atropine in doses of 0.4 to 0.6 mg raises the heart rate from 70 to approximately 110 beats/min during N_2O/thiopental or halothane anesthesia, and even higher during ether and cyclopropane anesthesia.[72] In the absence of compensatory adrenergic reflexes, Chamberlain et al found an onset of one circulation time, a peak effect in a few minutes, and a duration of less than 1 hour.[103] Doses below 10 μg/kg produce an evanescent bradycardia, presumed to be a direct effect on the sinoatrial node, and doses of up to 40 μg/kg may be necessary to achieve total vagal block (Fig. 10-3). Adrenergic mechanisms can further raise heart rate well above the 120 beats/min maximum found in beta-blocked patients. In the post-infarction syndrome of bradycardia-hypotension, the increase in heart rate is therapeutic.[104] Traction reflexes intraoperatively are blocked by intravenous atropine more effectively than by scopolamine, but are not prevented by intramuscular premedication with atropine.[105]

Dead space increases 15 percent (anatomic) and 30 percent (physiologic) after usual premedicant doses, but, in the absence of other central nervous system (CNS)-active medication and with a normal ventila-

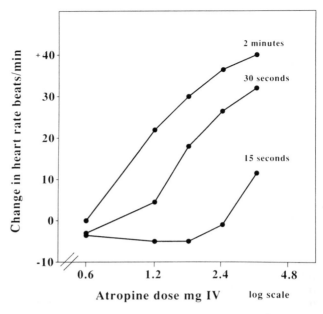

Fig. 10-3. Dose-response at different times after atropine. Intravenous injection of atropine in small-to-moderate doses causes a transient slowing of heart rate, thought to represent a direct effect on the sinoatrial node. Larger doses and longer times give an increase in heart rate plateauing at 120 beats/min. Other reflex effects were blocked by preliminary beta antagonism. (Adapted from Chamberlain et al,[103] with permission.)

tory response to CO_2, ventilation increases enough to keep arterial or end-tidal PCO_2 normal.[25,106] The work of breathing is little different since airway resistance falls as dead space increases.[101] Suggestions that atropine might have a specific deleterious effect on oxygenation[107] were not confirmed by others.[108–111] A particularly illuminating study by Nunn and Bergman found the A-aDO$_2$ unchanged by atropine during 11, 21, and 100 percent oxygen breathing, effectively eliminating any pulmonary defect in oxygen exchange.[25] One puzzling report by Rotman revealed an atropine effect on steady-state diffusing capacity for carbon monoxide, but it was a fall from above normal value to normal values.[112] The only important pulmonary effect of atropine remains a desirable one, a bronchodilation that affects moderate-to-large airways, increases airway conductance, and, on balance, reduces the work of breathing (Fig. 10-4).[113] In one report, atropine relieved isoproterenol-resistant bronchospasm during anesthesia.[114] It has also been shown to block deleterious bronchospasm after fiberoptic endoscopy in awake humans.[57] The bronchoscopist specifically looked for effects of drying and inspissation and found none, compared with control subjects receiving no atropine. Current heat and moisture ex-

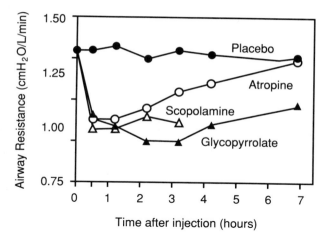

Fig. 10-4. Time course of bronchodilation after anticholinergics. Airway resistance was measured after intravenous injection of placebo, atropine, and glycopyrrolate by Gal and Suratt[101] using large doses, and after intravenous injection by Smith and DuBois[113] after normal doses. All three active drugs produce a maximal effect of approximately a one-third decrease in airway resistance within 30 minutes; this is prolonged for glycopyrrolate more than scopolamine, which in turn lasts longer than atropine.

changers can supply the water needed to prevent desiccation.[69]

A number of minor effects may be of interest to specific patients. One case of an anaphylactic reaction to atropine with demonstration of drug-specific immunoglobulin antibody, without scopolamine cross-sensitivity, has been reported.[115] A number of studies clearly show that, combined with morphine, atropine does not add to or potentiate narcosis like scopolamine,[10–12,106,116,117] but it does raise body temperature, on the order of 0.6°C in adults and possibly more in children, by postulated effects on thermoregulation and heat loss.[118] Atropine in usual premedicant doses may be given safely to patients with glaucoma.[119] General anesthesia, with intravenous or inhalation drugs, will lower intraocular pressure below normal.[120] Even if myosis develops, topical mydriatics are still rapidly effective. There is no effect on the electroencephalogram (EEG) or visual evoked response.[121] Morphine-induced nausea is only slightly decreased by atropine, while scopolamine is more effective.[10] The decision to use or to avoid atropine has been debated for decades, and is still not resolved.[105]

Scopolamine

The usual dose of scopolamine is 6 to 7 μg/kg. In humans, scopolamine raises the heart rate less than atropine.[119] Even very large doses (24 μg/kg, approxi-

mately 1.7 mg in normal subjects) did not raise the heart rate above 100 beats/min, and physostigmine, 50 μg/kg, rapidly restored normal heart rate.[122] Like atropine, a small dose produces a small decrease in heart rate, and a large dose increases heart rate.[100] Cardiac output parallels rate. The onset of effects is about as rapid as after atropine, but the duration appears to be more prolonged. Studies of arterial blood gases an hour or more after scopolamine report a decrease in oxygenation that was almost entirely accounted for by the alveolar air equation, as PCO_2 rose from 35 to 40 mmHg after the drug was administered[123,124] (Lappas et al, unpublished observation, 1971). While morphine alone had little or no effect on PCO_2, when combined with scopolamine, PCO_2 rose 4 to 6 mmHg and PO_2 fell from 72 to 60 mmHg on average.

Anatomic dead space after scopolamine, 6.6 μg/kg, increased 34 percent, an increase similar to that found after atropine.[31,125] Airway resistance fell markedly after scopolamine and remained low for 3 hours, a longer duration than either Butler et al[126] or Gal and Suratt[101] reported after atropine, but less prolonged than after glycopyrrolate.[113] The ventilatory response to CO_2 is elevated slightly by scopolamine, about enough to keep alveolar ventilation constant despite the dead space changes[117] (Fig. 10-5).

Scopolamine has a better antisialagogue effect than atropine in equimolar doses: less saliva and longer effect.[10,121] It produces no temperature elevation in adults,[118] but does have the most marked CNS effects of any antimuscarinic. Domino and Corssen found increased activity on the EEG, a decrease in primary visual-evoked response with prolonged latency, and objectively obvious drowsiness, whereas atropine had been ineffective in these measures.[121] Although not sedative, scopolamine is narcotic and adds to this effect of opioids.[10,99,117] Its widely quoted amnestic and antiemetic effects are neither very potent nor reliable.[45,121]

Glycopyrrolate

Given intramuscularly, in a dose of 3 to 5 μg/kg, glycopyrrolate is rapidly absorbed and eliminated with a 50 minute beta-half-life in plasma, but a more prolonged decay of clinical effects.[118,127] It is very slowly and incompletely absorbed after oral ingestion, but a 10-fold increase in dose will dry the mouth in the second hour and last half a day. Used intramuscularly for premedication, the heart rate rises only modestly and falls slowly after an hour, but is essentially unchanged after oral use. Bradycardia has not been reported, but the incidence of surgically related bradycardia is reduced when glycopyrrolate is incorporated in premedication.[123,128] Bronchomotor effects were slower

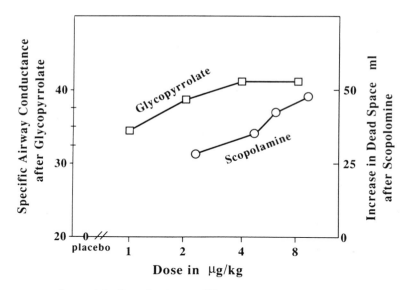

Fig. 10-5. Dose-response for anticholinergics. Two different measures of anticholinergic effect (anatomic dead space for scopolamine and airway conductance for glycopyrrolate) show a similar slope and maximal effect for approximately a three- to fourfold potency ratio: 2 μg/kg glycopyrrolate equivalent to 6 μg/kg scopolamine.[101,113]

to peak than after atropine, but there was major dilation remaining at 7 hours.[101] As with atropine and scopolamine, the arterial PCO_2 rises 3 to 4 mmHg, toward normal, and the PO_2 falls 7 to 9 mmHg, which, in elderly patients breathing air, could result in a PO_2 below 70 mmHg.[123]

Since it is a quaternary amine, fully ionized at pH 7.4, glycopyrrolate does not pass the blood-brain barrier, and no CNS effects have been reported. It is intermediate in efficacy in drying the mouth, but it lasts longer. Its kinetics make it the anticholinergic of choice for early morning oral administration when

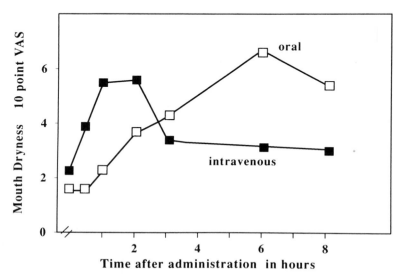

Fig. 10-6. Time course of antisialagogue effect when glycopyrrolate is given by two different routes. Ali-Melkkilä et al used a visual analog scale to assay intramuscular (8 μg/kg) and oral (4 mg/kg) glycopyrrolate. The oral dose was effective in drying saliva, but did not produce an increase in heart rate. VAS, visual analog scale. (From Ali-Melkkilä et al,[127] with permission.)

TABLE 10-1. Comparison of the Antimuscarinics[a]

Effect on				
Heart rate	A	>	G	>	S
Salivation	S	>	G	=	A
Dead space	S	=	G	=	A
Airway resistance	S	>	G	>	A
Level of consciousness	S	>	A	>>	G
Duration					
Oral	G	>>	S	>	A
Intramuscular	S	>	G	>	A
Molar potency	G	>	S	>	A

[a] The dose for the five effects are 0.2, 0.4, and 0.6 mg in the average patient for glycopyrrolate (G), scopolamine (S), and atropine (A), respectively. The symbol >> means "much greater than," while the symbol = means "about the same as."

the exact time of operation is unknown, since the oral dryness is slow in onset and not particularly distressful (Fig. 10-6). Blurred vision and tachycardia are not a cause for complaint (Table 10-1).

Opioid Drugs

A wide spectrum of opioid drugs are available, and most have been used for premedication at one time or another. There is little to choose in distinguishing them. For single small doses, morphine, fentanyl, and nalbuphine represent the choices—a longer acting, a shorter acting, and an agonist-antagonist drug, respectively. The indications usually presented for opioid premedication are primarily to relieve pain, secondarily to produce euphoria and narcosis, and, thirdly, to decrease the dose of other agents, provide cardiovascular stability, facilitate induction of anesthesia, have an antitussive effect, and blunt adrenergic stimuli.

Analgesia

Most patients are not in pain. The frequent exceptions are trauma patients, whose pain is very likely already controlled or ablated. Their established treatment needs to be continued.

A few patients have chronic pain, controlled more or less by medication and/or behavioral adaptation. In these patients, a small increase in opioid dose or a switch to opioid analgesics is humane.

A larger group of patients fear pain and suspect it will be inflicted, eg, during the starting of intravenous injections and while setting up monitors. For these patients, it would be nice if there were an analgesic that had a different dose-response curve for respiratory depression. There is not.[129–131]

Respiratory Depression

Analgesia and respiratory depression go hand in hand in the absence of pain. The opponents of opioid use say it is unnecessary to suffer any depression from opioids, and the proponents point out that even at the analgesic threshold of 0.15 mg/kg, IM, of morphine, a clinically insignificant rise in PCO_2 of 3.5 to 5 mmHg is typical[123,124] (Lappas et al, unpublished observation, 1971). A good study of the depressant effect of morphine is provided by Turnbull and Miyagishima, who used large doses, 15 mg/70 kg, to study the alveolar-arterial differences for both O_2 and CO_2 at two different oxygen tensions.[111] Slight hyperventilation before morphine was corrected toward normal; $PaCO_2$ breathing both air and oxygen rose from 34 or 35 mmHg to 38 or 39 mmHg. Dead space remained constant. The alveolar-arterial difference for oxygen fell from 22 to 18 mmHg breathing air and rose from 160 to 168 mmHg on oxygen. The most extreme interpretation that could be placed on these normal average values, devoid of statistical significance, is that somewhat frightened patients relaxed, and a few lung units changed from very low $\dot{V}/\dot{Q}$ ratios to shunts, all within normal levels.

It is important to note that morphine has very little effect on lung tissue and is no more a threat to patients with pulmonary disease than any other drug, with the exception of those few patients with chronic obstructive pulmonary disease with no remaining respiratory reserve, ablated CO_2 drive, and hypoxic-drive dependency. Opioids severely blunt hypoxic chemosensitivity, but these patients are not difficult to detect and avoid in the routine preoperative evaluation[32,132] (Rebuck et al, unpublished observation, 1982). Opioids also affect pupillary size, but do not interfere with changes associated with major cerebral deficits postoperatively (Figs. 10-7 and 10-8).[133,134]

If giving morphine preoperatively seems a good

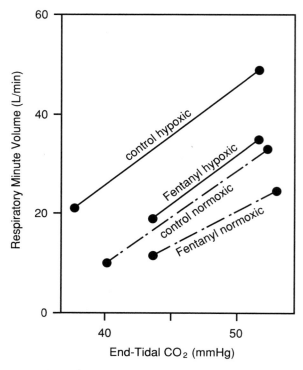

Fig. 10-7. Ventilatory response to carbon dioxide after fentanyl. The linear portion of the response is shown during hypoxia (Sat$_{ear}$, 75 percent) and normoxia (Sat$_{ear}$, 95 percent) for both control and 10 to 30 minutes after intravenous fentanyl.[132] Not only is the slope of the CO_2 response flattened, but the hypoxic response is markedly blunted by 100 μg of fentanyl.

idea, the next step is to give enough. A dose of 0.1 mg/kg has only one merit: it is easy to remember. The threshold for analgesia is higher, 0.15 mg/kg, at which dose only a 10 percent reduction in ventilation and rise in $PaCO_2$ is found. Age alone does not potentiate the action of opioids.[135]

The agonist-antagonist opioids, such as nalbuphine, offered an unfulfilled hope: that analgesia and respiratory depression could be separated. This has not been demonstrated; the work of Rutter et al is a typical report.[130] There are two minor advantages: nalbuphine is not a controlled substance, and more liberal limits can be set in self-administration.[136] There is a recent report of successful use of an agonist-antagonist opioid for a thoracic surgery-related procedure: fiberoptic bronchoscopy in awake, albeit drugged, patients.[137] Sury and Cole added nalbuphine to midazolam for intravenous sedation before and during fiberoptic bronchoscopy. They found that the opioid increased the number of patients optimally co-

operative from 30 to 65 percent at a cost of 5 percent who were overdepressed, had some delay in recovery, and had some increased emetic episodes.[137] These figures were judged acceptable in an outpatient setting.

Consideration of a recently appreciated CNS abnormality, sleep-related disorders of breathing, may be reason for decreasing opioid dose, since sleep reduces the slope of the ventilatory response to carbon dioxide.[138] Some middle-aged men and some elderly of either sex suffer periods of apnea or hypopnea during sleep, particularly rapid eye movement sleep, with marked arterial oxygen desaturation. While pre-existing airway disease does not predispose, increases in either upper or lower airway resistance increase the severity of the events.[139,140] Marked hypotension as well as hypertension may accompany the desaturation. Abnormalities of chemoreceptor drive (both O_2 and CO_2) also correlate with the magnitude of hypoxemia.[141] The important clue to this condition is a history of snoring. Neither narcotic doses of hydromorphone (4 mg/kg) in nonsnoring males nor large doses of vodka in postpartum women increased sleep-disordered breathing,[43,83] while nicotine reduced it.[142] A history of snoring should serve as a warning, perhaps triggering further study of sleep-related respiratory disorders, and suggesting nonhypnotic doses of premedicants.

Euphoria

Euphoria is a blessed state. Morphine produces it, but only in some patients. Lasagna et al found that 80 percent of normal individuals actually describe dysphoria after opioids.[52] Intravenous opioids have few advocates among patients receiving them.[143-145] Further, it takes a certain "set and setting" to yield euphoria. The patient must be expecting it ("mind set") and be in an environment with little or no distractions ("stage setting"). The drug must begin to work, and CNS catecholamine levels must begin to slowly recede. This is unlikely after "on-call" medication.

It is the last problem, slower onset of euphoria compared with analgesia and respiratory depression, that may be part of the reason that fentanyl and derivatives are rarely used for intramuscular premedication. However, to reduce the induction dose of an intravenous agent, it is practical to give the opioid intravenously just a few minutes beforehand, in or near the operating room and under better observation than on a ward.[146] The risk of chest wall spasm is more of a problem with fentanyl than other drugs, but was seen 50 years ago with meperidine above 300 mg. Midazolam may attenuate, if not prevent, this problem.[79]

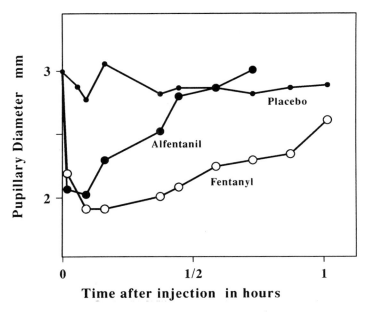

Fig. 10-8. Time course of fentanyl and alfentanil. Careful pupillary diameter measurement during general anesthesia by Asbury delineated the duration of effect of the two opioids, used intravenously in doses of 2 μg/kg (fentanyl) and 6 μg/kg (alfentanil).[133] The duration of other CNS effects would presumably be similar.

The choice between opioids depends on two factors: kinetics and cost. If the most desirable time for injection can be identified, morphine and one of the agonist-antagonist drugs can be used interchangeably. Fentanyl is probably too short-acting to permit development of euphoria before dysphoric environmental factors enter. If the exact timing is uncertain, eg, a second or later case, the prolonged action of morphine becomes an advantage. Ordered at the earliest anticipated time, the patient who has been told to expect the effects will likely feel all is going well, and will lose track of time should extraneous problems with prior cases cause delay. In the current situation of generic drugs, cost is almost the same for equieffective doses of different agents. Insistence on one-patient-use ampules adds more cost than does the choice of drug.

Classic Sedative/Hypnotics

At one time or another, more than 200 individual barbiturates or mixtures of barbiturates have been available for prescription. Pharmaceutical chemists kept looking for the right compound. They never found it. Little need be said about this class of drugs. While once a mainstay of "heavy premedication," they became less popular as doctors perceived that (1) the effect by mouth was slower and more irregular than by injection, (2) intramuscular injection hurt more than opioid-scopolamine and gave no better effect, (3) barbiturates were substances of abuse, and (4) sedation was unpredictable, but hypnosis was not a satisfactory alternative. When barbiturates were combined with scopolamine, the incidence of unpleasant side effects and dysphoric behavior increased.[117] Barbiturates also depress both hypoxic and hypercarbic drives to breathe (Fig. 10-9).[132]

There seems to be no reason for preferring one barbiturate over another, except for kinetics. However, even when the ultra-short-acting drugs used for induction, thiopental and methohexital, were given by mouth, the effects were as variable and as long-lasting as traditional short-acting drugs.[116] Diphenhydramine, an antihistamine, may be used occasionally when there is need for hypnosis and reason for avoiding other drugs, or where an H_1-blocking effect is of some value.

Ataractic Drugs

The group of ataractic drugs includes the phenothiazines, hydroxyzine, droperidol, and the benzodiazepines. The phenothiazines appeared earliest and, with the exception of promethazine, their use has generally been discontinued. Droperidol finds some use as a component of Innovar, a mixture with

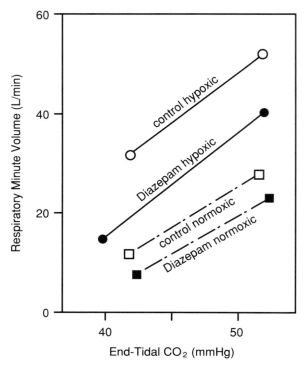

Fig. 10-9. Ventilatory response to carbon dioxide after pentobarbital. The linear portion of the response is shown during hypoxia and normoxia before and 10 to 30 minutes after intravenous injection of 100 mg of pentobarbital. Although there was no significant change in the slope of the normoxic response, the hypoxic response was markedly blunted. (Adapted from Smith and Kulp,[132] with permission.)

waning popularity. Hydroxyzine has proponents around the world, and persists.

Phenothiazines

Chlorpromazine was the first ataractic to find widespread use. Reports by Dripps et al[13] and Weiss et al[147] are typical. The expected advantages included less apprehension, less nausea and vomiting, an anti-shock feature, reduction of anesthetic dose, and reduction of laryngospasm and excitement on induction and emergence. Mild antiadrenergic and intestinal antispastic effects had been found in animals. The results of premedicant usage were not encouraging, not because the drug was ineffective, but because it was too powerful, with excessive narcosis, hypotension, and tachycardia. Chlorpromazine was largely abandoned.

As other phenothiazines with somewhat different effects were introduced, they were used in anesthesia. Some were reported to be analgesic and potentiated

opioid analgesia, enabling a dose reduction.[148] Some were said to be antihistaminic, antistress, antiadrenergic, better anxiolytics, and better sleep inducers. In an extensive series of investigations, Dundee et al studied most of the phenothiazines as premedicants and as agents influencing induction, maintenance, and emergence.[45,47–49] Conclusions include, "none of these compounds could be recommended as the main pre-anaesthetic hypnotic" and "it is obvious that an enhancement of any of the desirable effects of pethidine are generally obtained only at the expense of an increased incidence of side effects." Dundee et al did find a few compounds worth further study, but always in combination with some other agent, usually an opioid. They emphasized a need for a marked reduction in opioid dose, typically 50 percent, because of summative or potentiative properties.

Potentiation of both analgesia and respiratory depression by opioids had been reported with the earliest phenothiazine,[149] although the effect was not invariably found.[150,151] The actual difference between potentiation and simple addition was difficult to discern, and often depended on interpretation of data (Fig. 10-10). In either event, the prudent advice was that when combining phenothiazines with opioids, markedly reduce the dose of at least the opioid or, better yet, both[152,153] (Fig. 10-11).

Early reports had suggested that promethazine might be a respiratory stimulant alone or with opioids or barbiturates, although the methodology used was inadequate by current standards.[39] Nonetheless, this drug became the most frequently used phenothiazine and, except for a modest and brief competition from propiomazine,[15,38,154,155] has persisted in individual practices. As with the other compounds, most of the descriptive work appeared in the 1950s and 1960s.[70,152,156]

The major advantages documented for phenothiazines are marked narcosis and sedation when chronically used in psychiatry.[2] They certainly can depress respiration and at least add to opioid depression of breathing. They may cause orthostatic hypotension if not overt hypotension. A host of less common annoyances include oculogyric crisis, blood dyscrasia, extrapyramidal rigidity, and jaundice. Little or no reason for their use persists.

Droperidol

Brought to this country as part of the neuroleptic mixture Innovar, this butyrophenone is a very powerful antiemetic, a major tranquilizer, and a minor depressant of breathing and circulatory reflexes. A major problem lies in the inability to judge the optimal dose. There are so few objective effects, and the onset of

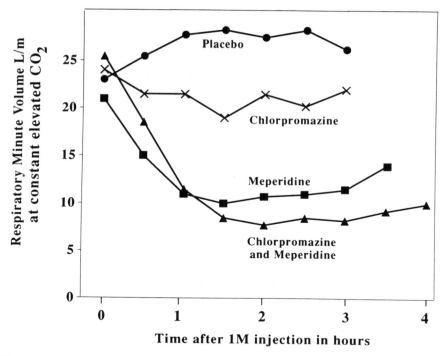

Fig. 10-10. Time course of respiratory depression after administration of opioid and ataractic drugs and a combination of the two. This figure illustrates the effect of adding two classes of drug: the result is greater than either alone. If the difference from control ventilation (●———●) is used, the statistically insignificant effect of chlorpromazine potentiates meperidine depression. However, if the difference from placebo response is used, the interaction is subadditive. (Data from Lambertsen et al.[150])

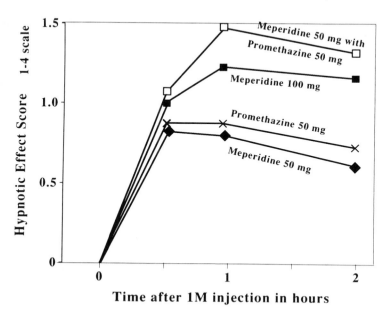

Fig. 10-11. Time course of hypnotic interaction after administration of opioid and ataractic drugs, and a combination of the two. Keats et al assayed "sleepiness" after intramuscular meperidine, 50 and 100 mg, promethazine, 50 mg, and the combination of 50 mg of each.[152] If the separate scores of meperidine and promethazine are summed, they equal a greater number than the score after the mixture at all times after administration.

action is so very slow, that "titration" is impossible. Thus, its use as a premedicant has essentially disappeared.

Hydroxyzine

By the 1970s the following claims had been made for the piperazine derivative hydroxyzine:

Anxiolytic in the young and the old[43,50]
Antiarrhythmic[157]
Antiemetic and antihistaminic[38]
Bronchodilatory[158]
Opioid-sparing[42]
Cardiovascular status-stabilizing[159]
Facilitates induction[160]

The interaction with opioids was quantitated in two reports by Gasser and Bellville.[161,162] There is a dose-related depression of respiration, manifested by a parallel rightward shift in the ventilatory response to CO_2, additive with opioids (Figs. 10-12 and 10-13). In depressing ventilation, 150 mg of hydroxyzine was equipotent with 30 mg of pentazocine and 15 mg of diazepam. However, it was not as effective at blunting adrenergic stress as pentobarbital.[159]

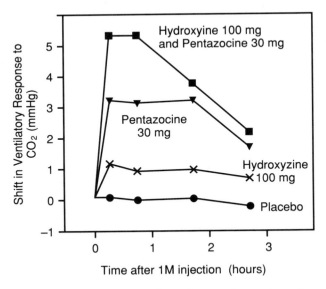

Fig. 10-12. Time course of respiratory depression after an agonist-antagonist opioid and an ataractic. A dose of pentazocine well below its ceiling effect produces a marked depression when given with a clinically nondepressing hydroxyzine dose.[161] There appears to be potentiation in the first hour after injection, but is subadditive thereafter.

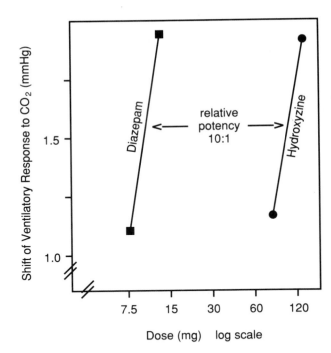

Fig. 10-13. Dose-response for two ataractics showing the potency assay. Displacement of the ventilatory response to carbon dioxide by two intramuscular premedicants, diazepam and hydroxyzine, at the time of peak effect.[162] Hydroxyzine reached peak effect in the first hour, but diazepam reached it only at 2 hours. A common-slope-log-dose assay gives a 10 : 1 ratio for potency as respiratory depressants.

Of all the ataractics mentioned previously, hydroxyzine would appear to be the most useful and the least likely to induce adverse effects. However, clinical practice seems to have resulted in a secular trend to smaller doses, as little as 25 to 50 mg per patient, for which there is no evidence of efficacy.

Benzodiazepines

If the phenothiazines were the drugs of the 1950s and 1960s, with hydroxyzine for the interlude, then the benzodiazepines are the drugs of the 1980s and 1990s. The widespread prescription and ingestion of these drugs for both sedative and hypnotic effects attest to their efficacy. In anesthesia, the benzodiazepines are increasingly used as hypnotics, preanesthetic medications, induction agents, and maintenance adjuvants. Major uses in thoracic surgery are facilitation of fiberoptic bronchoscopy,[36,137] and certain other minor but annoying procedures such as chest tube placement or removal, and reintubation of the trachea. For these, the shortest acting drug is usually the best, and the choice is usually hypnotic doses of midazolam, although propofol by infusion may supplant it. For premedication prior to major surgery, however, two other drugs merit review: diazepam and lorazepam. The premedicant use of these two drugs depends on the following: sedation, amnesia, anticonvulsant effect, and muscle relaxant (central) properties. They may have fewer deleterious effects on sleep patterns than barbiturates, less bizarre side effects than droperidol, and less respiratory depression than opioids, although rare paradoxic restlessness, anxiety, depression, and rage have been reported.[163] There is one other possible advantage over other sedative/hypnotic drugs: there is a receptor-specific antagonist for the benzodiazepine receptor on the chloride/gamma-aminobutyric acid channel, flumazenil or Ro 15-1788 (Anexate).[164] Experience with this drug as a reversal agent has shown marked, if somewhat irregular and incomplete, efficacy.[165–167] Its role in anesthetic use awaits further study in the 1990s. Its failure in some applications may reflect a multiplicity of benzodiazepine receptors, a theory supported by evidence of differing therapeutic ratios for different actions, as in sedation versus largyngeal activity, and interaction among different benzodiazepine agonists.[77,168]

A major property of diazepam and, very likely, of all benzodiazepines, is a specific right-shift of the dose-convulsant response to local anesthetics when used in sedative and not hypnotic doses. While it is true that barbiturates can protect against or abort local anesthetic convulsions, it requires a dose equivalent to induction of general anesthesia with circulatory instability in the postictal state.[169] Parenthetically, pretreatment with opioids potentiates or protracts seizures and increases mortality (Table 10-2).

Diazepam

Diazepam is a water-insoluble drug best given by mouth. The huge surface of the small intestinal microvilli provide adequate uptake of this insoluble substance. Given with metoclopramide, the onset of effect is more rapid, more predictable, and more pleasant than after intramuscular injection. The vehicle, commonly propylglycol, causes pain and often phlebitis after intravenous injection. However, dilution of 10 mg to 5 mL with 0.5 to 4 percent lidocaine forms an emulsion with the glycol (not a precipitate) and permits nearly painless and phlebitis-free intravenous use. Given by mouth, blood levels appear in the second half hour and peak approximately 2 hours after ingestion,[170] but this can be speeded up somewhat with metoclopramide. Diazepam is a widely and successfully used premedicant.[49,171]

Ventilatory depression after diazepam administration has generated some controversy, probably because the response of humans is quite variable in incidence and expression.[172,173] In smaller doses, 0.1 mg/kg and less, there may be little effect on end-tidal CO_2 and the ventilatory responses to hypoxia, and only a slight right shift of the ventilatory response to hypercarbia, provided the subject stays awake.[132,174] However, even in a respiratory laboratory, breathing dry gases with the nose clamped, such a dose may promote marked drowsiness or even sleep. Sleep causes a rightward shift and depresses the ventilatory response to CO_2 (Fig. 10-14).[138] This effect seems to be expressed in patients with obstructive pulmonary disease by a somewhat more marked depression. Catchlove and Kafer found that 0.11 mg/kg of intravenous diazepam increased the $PaCO_2$ by 3.5 mmHg on average.[175] While this was less than the increase in $PaCO_2$

TABLE 10-2. Incidence of Convulsions and Death after Local Anesthetics in Groups of 18 Pretreated Rats[a]

Pretreatment Drug	Convulsions	Death
Diazepam	0/18	0/18
Thiopental	11/18	6/18
Pentobarbital	15/18	9/18
Saline	14/18	9/18
Ketamine	13/18	11/18
Innovar	17/18	16/18

[a] In each group of rats, one-third received an LD_{50} of procaine, one-third tetracaine, and one-third lidocaine. The incidence of convulsion and death after any pretreatment did not differ significantly among the local anesthetic agents; thus the numbers have been combined.

(Data from Aldrete and Daniel.[169])

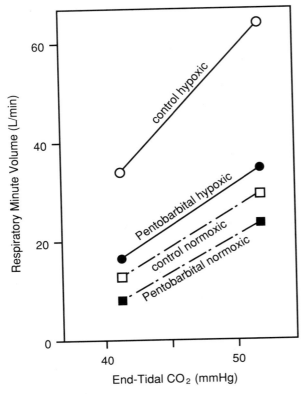

Fig. 10-14. Ventilatory response to carbon dioxide after diazepam. The linear portion of the response is shown during both hypoxic and normoxic CO_2 challenge.[132] While there is some depression during normoxia after diazepam, the slope is nearly normal. There is flattening and depression of the response during hypoxia that is both statistically and clinically more significant.

seen in their normal volunteers (6.5 mmHg), the dose was nearly 25 percent less and the increase in normal individuals was from a hyperventilated level of 34 mmHg to normal; in the obstructed patients, the level rose from normal to high normal, 38 to 41.5 mmHg. Given by mouth in premedicant dosage, 0.1 to 0.15 mg/kg, in the absence of serious CNS depression by other factors, there is no clinical problem. Diazepam has few other effects of importance in thoracic surgery. Hemodynamically, even in large doses (0.5 mg/kg), it causes no change in heart rate or pulmonary or systemic resistance, and causes tolerable falls in mean blood pressure (< 25 percent) and cardiac index (< 30 percent).[176] It does not effectively block the adrenergic response to intubation.

Diazepam has a long beta-elimination half-life. Its major metabolite, desmethyl diazepam, is nearly as effective and even longer acting. These factors are more germane to multiple doses and prolonged use than to a single premedicant dose. However, hepatic excretion of diazepam and metabolites and enterohepatic circulation partly account for the irregular blood levels and effects seen in some patients over many hours.[177]

Lorazepam

Lorazepam can be given by injection, with some local pain. Its kinetics are instructive: it has a shorter beta-decay (elimination) half-life than diazepam, but is less soluble in lipid and has a longer alpha (distribution) half-life (Fig. 10-15).[178] Thus, after a single intravenous hypnotic dose, it is longer acting than diazepam; however, after infusion or repeated doses, or when a low blood level is the end point, its effect wanes faster. Semiquantitative subjective measures of sedation showed effects at 6 hours after 2 mg orally.[179] It has been successfully used as a premedicant in a wide variety of cases,[51,180] as have many other benzodiaze-

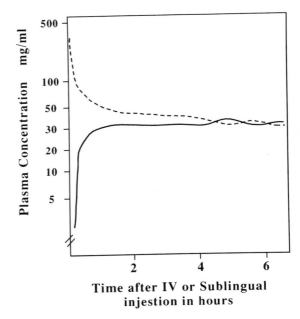

Time after IV or Sublingual injestion in hours

Fig. 10-15. Time course of blood levels of lorazepam given by different routes. The redistribution of intravenous lorezepam continues into the second hour after injection. Oral uptake has approximately the same half-life, so that by 2 hours the blood levels are nearly the same for the two different routes, and decline similarly (and slowly) thereafter. Intramuscular injection should give intermediate values. (Adapted from Cann et al,[178] with permission.)

TABLE 10-3.   Comparison of the Benzodiazepines[a]

Painful injection	D	>	L	>	M
Speed of onset	M	>	L	>	D
Duration of effect	D	>	L	>	M
Amnesia	M	>	L	>	D
Respiratory depression	D	>	M	=	L
Predictability	L	=	D	>	M

Abbreviations: D, diazepam; L, lorazepam; M, midazolam.
[a] Potency is approximately as follows: 1 mg L = 5 mg M = 10 mg D.

pines.[179,181–183] Lorazepam produces more frequent amnesia than diazepam.[56]

Midazolam

Midazolam is the newest wonder drug of the series. It exceeds even diazepam with its unpredictable dose/response behavior in groups of individuals. It is intermediate in speed of action between the barbiturates and diazepam, and has the most rapid beta decay of the three benzodiazepines discussed. Thus, it can be given to effect, albeit in a more time-consuming manner than other intravenous agents. Its metabolites are somewhat active, but have short half-lives. Because of a chemical trick (opening of a ring with mildly acidic pH), it is soluble in water and nearly painless on injection.

In approximately equipotent dosage, compared with diazepam, midazolam has approximately the same respiratory depression, but is shorter in duration.[173,184] The duration of effect was markedly prolonged in elderly emphysematous patients, however. Brief apnea may follow intravenous induction of anesthesia, but, given orally or intramuscularly for premedication, apnea has not been a problem in the absence of other narcotics.

Although not as good an anxiolytic in patients' views compared with another oral benzodiazepine (triazolam), midazolam has the most prolonged and frequent amnesic effect.[185,186] Little sedation was found at 0.1 mg/kg and a prolonged effect was found at 0.2 mg/kg when given as an oral premedicant for outpatient work.[187–189] Artru et al also found intramuscular doses below 0.1 mg/kg ineffective.[43] Thus, midazolam offered no advantage over other oral premedicants. Its major role is as an intravenous adjunct to minor procedures and anesthetic induction. A sequence of 0.15 mg/kg of midazolam, 5 μg/kg of sufentanil, and 0.1 mg/kg of pancuronium over 15 minutes gave acceptable conditions for intubation without hemodynamic response.[80] In another study of multiple drugs for induction, the adrenocortical response to stress was preserved.[190] After an opioid, intravenous midazolam facilitates endoscopy.[137]

Paradoxic response to midazolam (confusion, agitation, and uncooperativeness) have been successfully treated with physostigmine, and prolonged unconsciousness and apnea have been reversed with flumazenil.[166,167] Although benzodiazepines have a central muscle-relaxing effect, midazolam does not potentiate peripheral neuromuscular blockade with vercuronium.[191]

The three benzodiazepines are compared in Table 10-3. Side effects of the benzodiazepines include akathisia, restless agitation, rage, paradoxic anxiety, depression, convulsion, and a variation in observed effects at any given dose between patients.

GASTROINTESTINAL CONSIDERATIONS

Premedication for the gastrointestinal tract is important not only to reduce the incidence of pulmonary aspiration in the presurgical period, but also to reduce the incidence of stress-related mucosal damage (SRMD) and metabolic alkalosis, which have become evident in intensive care units. An excellent review of these topics can be found in a recent symposium.[59] While there are little data suggesting that thoracic surgery patients are at increased risk for these complications, the risk is nonetheless real.

Three Problems Affected by Gastrointestinal Premedication

Aspiration

Aspiration is the most frequent anesthesia-related problem in obstetric practice. The first description by an obstetrician was followed by identification of the role of acid in malignant aspiration syndrome.[192,193] With the major exceptions of bronchoscopy, some operations on the esophagus, and trauma surgery, the risk in thoracic surgical patients does not appear to be augmented as it is in obstetric or pediatric populations.[194] The important risk factors are obesity, increased cerebrospinal fluid pressure (but not necessarily head trauma[195]), and gastritis or ulcer disease (but not necessarily heartburn or suggestive symptoms). Other factors include abdominal surgery, especially emergency or upper abdominal procedures, pregnancy, pain, or stress, and impaired consciousness (due to drug, disease, or trauma).[196,197] Anesthesiologists have a variety of prophylactic measures at their command.[198,199] Not all need to be expended on every patient, but control of gastric acid and, perhaps, volume is increasingly popular,[200] if unnecessary.

Stress-Related Mucosal Damage

Stress-related mucosal damage leading to erosion and bleeding, and associated with significantly mortality, is increasingly evident in intensive care units.[201] With the exception of nasogastric intubation, measures anesthesiologists take for gastric acidity are part of the therapy for SRMD.[202] Importantly, these are decreasing gastric acid production and dwell time, neutralizing acid, and maintaining tissue perfusion and, hence, mucosal defense. Anesthesiologists may find their preoperative prescription for histamine blockers continued by the surgical team, and it would make sense for the same drug to be used.

Metabolic Alkalosis

Metabolic alkalosis is a problem properly receiving increased recognition postoperatively. Patients accustomed to an acid-rich diet admitted to the hospital and kept NPO continue to secrete a few hundred milliequivalents of acid before renal compensation is reset. The tendency to alkalosis is further promoted by nasogastric suction of chloride-rich fluid, administration of citrate-rich blood products, sodium bicarbonate given empirically for periods of hypoperfusion intraoperatively, and a wide variety of sodium and potassium salts of drugs that are metabolized or enter lipid solution as bases (barbiturate for induction, antibiotic prophylaxis, etc.), adding to the extracellular fluid base excess. Alkalosis is not the good side of a balance with the nemesis acidosis, but has real and profound, if somewhat arcane, effects. It is difficult for the kidney to correct, because it causes a deficit in extracellular alkali ($[K]^+$), the excretion of which is a major renal-correcting mechanism. It produces other electrolyte effects, dysrhythmias, CNS effects, respiratory effects, and metabolic effects.[203] When the observation that alkalosis increases oxygen consumption and useless heat production (by uncoupling oxidative phosphorylation) and decreases oxygen delivery (by lowering hemoglobin P_{50}) is added to this, there exists a strong argument for eliminating any possible acid loss by emesis or gastric drainage.[204]

Premedicant Drugs with Gastrointestinal Actions

Histamine₂-Blocking Drugs

Histamine₂-blocking drugs are the most widely used and effective. Cimetidine is the oldest and best known, with ranitidine and famotidine being newer drugs. All can abolish hydrogen ion excretion by the stomach, as well as other histamine manifestations expressed by the H_2-receptor.[205] A reduction in volume of gastric fluid at the time of induction is also perceived as prophylactic for aspiration, but the critical values of pH 2.5 and a volume of 25 mL seem to have been chosen by ease of recall rather than by supporting data.[206] The work of James et al suggests a predominant effect of pH over simple volume, in the absence of particulate or infectious matter.[207] Histamine₂-blockade may increase the incidence of infectious gastric juice, and oral cephazoline does not alter this risk factor.[208]

Cimetidine, 300 mg by mouth 2 to 3 hours before induction, is nearly totally effective in reducing both gastric fluid volume and its hydrogen ion concentration for 6 hours or more.[208,209] Oral ranitidine and famotidine offer protection against acid for a more prolonged time.[210] Gallagher et al found famotidine effective even when given the previous night.[211] Cimetidine is the cheapest of the H_2-blockers, even when used in equieffective regimens, which require more frequent administration compared with the other two drugs. Administration the night before operation is practiced by some, but is apparently unnecessary. Although usually given by mouth, it is compatible with most parenteral premedicants except barbiturates and some phenothiazines.[212] Two studies suggest that the volume of gastric juice may be less after cimetidine than ranitidine.[213,214]

Although all three may induce P-450 xenobiotic catabolism, it took several days of frequent dosage to promote theophylline toxicity after starting ranitidine[215] and 7 days to reach a new steady state with a cimetidine-warfarin interaction.[216] The latter interaction elevated prothrombin time only 20 to 25 percent. No difference in blood levels of lidocaine after epidural anesthesia was found after placebo, cimetidine, or ranitidine.[217] Okkonen et al found no effect on enflurane metabolism.[218] Bogod and Oh found no difference in duration of succinylcholine after cimetidine or ranitidine,[219] while Kambam et al found a prolongation that they attributed to inhibition of liver enzymes and hepatic blood flow.[220] Several reports suggest that cimetidine or ranitidine may also affect benzodiazepine kinetics.[221,222]

Metoclopramide

Metoclopramide was introduced in the mid 1960s as a centrally acting antiemetic with potent gastric emptying properties, nearly devoid of notable side effects at the usual dose of 10 mg.[171] Doubling the dose and administering it intravenously produced no more gastric effects, but extrapyramidal manifestations (ocular and facial signs responsive promptly to diphenhydramine) and some transient flushing and vertigo in 6 of 19 volunteers.[209] In the next decade, anesthetic attention focused on the gastric prokinetic action as a desirable effect in reducing gastric fluid volume and, hence, operative risk. Manchikanti et al recommended combining cimetidine with oral metoclopramide,[223] which Rao et al found effective in outpatient preparation for anesthesia.[224] Ten milligrams of metoclopramide by mouth may be insufficient, but by injection it has a marked effect on gastric volume.[208,209] The drug has no direct effect on gastric acid secretion, although in the absence of stimuli for digestion, gastric juice may be achlorhydric in some patients. However, it does not seem to be significantly more effective in reducing gastric residual volume than either cimetidine or ranitidine, and perhaps not even additive if the volume is already low.[208,209] Metoclopramide may be useful in speeding uptake of other oral premedicant drugs.

Antacids

Antacids are a proven if transient prescription for gastric acidity. Particulate suspensions of magnesium and/or aluminum silicates used in peptic ulcer disease are effective, but offer the risk of pneumonitis should aspiration ensue, and may include flavorings that decrease lower esophagal tone, eg, peppermint oil.[225] Antacid solution either locally prepared (0.3 M sodium citrate that is stable for only a few weeks) or a commercial alternate such as aspirin-free Alka Seltzer Effervescent or Bicitra are preferred.[226] The common dose of 20 mL may be insufficient if 8.4 percent sodium bicarbonate is used.[227] Repeated administration may be necessary every few hours if induction is delayed. The long-standing fear of oral intake in the preinduction period is probably not justified if intake is limited to clear fluids. Maltby et al found that up to 150 mL is almost completely emptied within 2 hours, even if opioid and atropine are given after 1 hour.[228] Even at best, however, antacids fail to inactivate pepsin secretion, so other mucosal defense factors must be promoted.[229]

ROUTES OF ADMINISTRATION

The earliest preanesthetic medication was given by mouth for reasons of practicality; the hypodermic syringe was not in common use in the 19th century. By the turn of the century, subcutaneous morphine and hyoscyamine or hyoscine were so commonly given before gas, oxygen, and/or ether, that "hypo" came to be a synonym for injection, even if an intramuscular site was specified. For reasons of pain (volume and pH effects), pentobarbital or secobarbital were given per os. However, when ordered "on call," the onset of effect was unpredictable compared with that of intramuscular morphine. As traditional premedication became "lighter," the oral barbiturates dropped from fashion. Predictably, oral use is reappearing, but so are other routes of drug administration. Enteric uptake of drug can be approached from either end of the gastrointestinal tract. Uptake is demonstrable from the oral mucosa, nasal mucosa, and even transdermally. Intravenous injection is the epitome of reliability as far as uptake is concerned. Even the choice of muscle used for intramuscular injection has a bearing on uptake kinetics.

Intramuscular Route

First studied in 1911 by Rowntree and Geraghty, who wanted rapid uptake of phenolsulfonephthalein for renal studies, paraspinous muscles were found to be the best sites in ambulatory patients.[230] More recently, Stanski et al[231] and Kirkpatrick et al[232] found deltoid uptake more rapid than gluteal in recumbent patients. This is logical, for muscles at rest have less blood flow than active ones. Intramuscular injection is convenient, nearly painless with smaller volumes for most drugs, and customary. However, with increasing use of exact dosage forms and prefilled syringes, each drug prescribed usually means a different injection. Failure to deposit the drug in muscle may be a cause for slow onset of some drugs; however, hydrophilic drugs such as atropine seem to be as rapidly absorbed subcutaneously as intramuscularly.[102]

Intravenous Route

The intravenous route may be practical for outpatient utilization to shorten the time for induction.[145] It is the rational route for very short-acting drugs with immediate effect, of which atropine and alfentanil might be examples, as well as for other adjuvants, such as antibiotics and hormones, to assure a very high blood level at induction or incision. It is not the route for achieving sedation. Drugs known to be effective intramuscularly fail to sedate short of narcosis in intravenous usage.[143,144]

Other Routes

Transdermal Route

Transdermal forms of nitroglycerin have long been available and have preoperative utility in symptomatic coronary artery disease.[76] The route has been used more recently to administer scopolamine for seasickness and nicotine for tobacco withdrawal. Clinical trials are under way with transdermal fentanyl.[233,234]

Oral Route

Oral uptake is reappearing as fashionable. Goroszeniuk et al report that patients prefer it to injection.[235] It is particularly appropriate for the relatively insoluble benzodiazepines.[178,235] In the United Kingdom, a slow-release form of morphine is available. It is as effective in premedication as intramuscular morphine[236–238] and better than oral temazepam.[239] With the demonstration that clear fluids are rapidly passed by the stomach without decrease in pH, the increas-

ing use of gastrokinetic drugs, and a more practical application of pharmacokinetic knowledge, the oral route should find increasing application.[228,240]

Buccal and Nasal Routes

Buccal and nasal mucosa provide absorptive surfaces for premedication. The mouth is a safe alternative route according to Fisher et al[241,242] and may represent an important part of the uptake from the recently proposed opioid lollypops.[243–245] A similar mucosal uptake has been shown for both nose drops and spray for sufentanil with rapid onset, short period of narcosis, and a few minor side effects.[246,247] Ketamine is also active by nasal instillation, as is nitroglycerin[75,248] (Fig. 10-16).

SYNTHESIS OF A PREMEDICANT REGIMEN

A suitable framework for discussion of a premedication regimen, individualized for patient, procedure, and practitioner can be derived from a list of potential problems organized by body systems and correlated with classes of drugs, as in Table 10-4.

Consideration of the patients' expectations and the value for hypnotic induction of an early, predictable set of events suggest that the operative morning

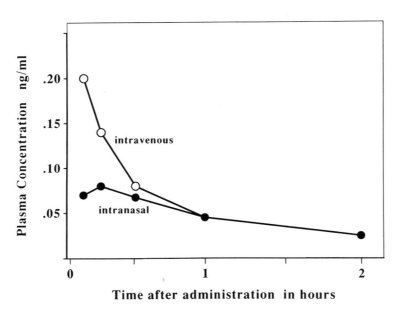

Fig. 10-16. Time course of blood levels of sufentanil by different routes. Redistribution after intravenous sufentanil is essentially complete in the first hour, as is both uptake and redistribution after nose drops. Thereafter, the elimination rate is the same, as shown by Helmers et al.[246]

TABLE 10-4. Framework for Selecting Premedicant Drugs

System	Problems	Applicable Drugs	Avoidable Drugs
Central nervous system	Pain Anxiety Recall	Opioids Sedatives Amnestics	Barbiturates Adrenergics
Respiratory system	Secretions Cough Irregularities[a]	Antisialagogues Antitussives Anesthetics	Muscarinics Barbiturates Vasopressors
Cardiovascular system	Hypertension Hypotension Rate changes Dysrhythmia	Anesthetics, vasodilators Vasopressors, inotropes Autonomics Ventilation, lidocaine, slow calcium channel blockers	Adrenergics
Gastrointestinal system	Acid secretion Gastric volume Constipation	H_2-blockers, atropine Gastrokinetics Muscarinics	Methylxanthines Drugs decreasing LES tone Opioids

Abbreviation: LES, lower esophageal sphincter.

[a] Irregularities include breath holding, hiccough, and bronchial chest wall spasm.

should start with the administration of a drug that does something, but not too much. Even if the exact hour of operation is uncertain, the replacement of coffee and breakfast with oral diazepam and clear water is well received by the patient. A dose of 10 to 15 mg is suggested for normal adults, with reduction to 5 or 2.5 mg only with overt CNS disease, marked debility, or a physiologic age well over 80 years. If a supportive visit the day before was omitted or was conducted by an anesthesiologist other than the one conducting the induction, another brief, supportive, and optimistic interview is worth the effort. If the patient has preoperative pain, an appropriate oral or intramuscular dose of morphine or other opioid should be added, and the patient should be told to expect the drug and to expect relief.

Next, the time the patient is expected to arrive in the induction area is estimated on the presumption that all is going to go optimally, especially any previous cases. Drug(s) are then selected that have sufficient duration of action so that should the start be delayed, the effect will not have waned. Recall that premedication with even those drugs known to be additive with anesthetic agents (eg, morphine) will account for less than one-tenth of the summed minimal anesthetic concentration, aid in blunting of the sympathoadrenal response to intubation, and add an advantageous lingering effect at the time of emergence. The choice of drugs offers broad leeway for individual style. What is important is that the style be consistent. The dysphoric effects of scopolamine given with barbiturates contrast with the advantages of scopolamine with opioids. The questionable advantages of opioid and ataractics in the presence of pain contrasts

with claims of potentiated sedation in the absence of pain. Some mixtures of drugs are beneficially additive, and some are problems.

The arrival of a patient in the induction area is also an important time. Some effects can be efficaciously and conveniently achieved by parenteral injection at this time. While the drying caused by atropine is not one such effect, atropine prophylaxis against bradycardia in selective cases is an application, as are the use of antitussive and other drugs to blunt the cardiac and respiratory effects of bronchoscopy and double-lumen intubation of the trachea during light anesthesia.

Practices that are not justified by data and experience include "intramuscular" injection of benzodiazepines (since oral use is effective), "on-call" injection of sedatives and hypnotics (unless the anesthesiologist makes the call in sufficient time to let anxiolysis proceed), and arbitrary reduction of dosage levels below established thresholds of efficacy (with the rationale of first doing no harm). Another presumption of dubious value is that the visit by another anesthesiologist the previous day was, in fact, supportive and resulted in informed consent; it may have been a source of anxiety.[249]

The approach to these competing decision-influencing observations is colored by local surgical practice. For example, thoracic surgical procedures may be preceded by fiberoptic bronchoscopy under general anesthesia. The desire to promote cardiovascular stability during a task-intensive induction period, before adequate inhalation anesthetic depth can be reasonably expected, in a population rich in coronary artery and bronchopulmonary disease (eg, a Veterans Hospital) most frequently leads to the following recommended orders:

1. A hypnotic such as triazolam, 0.5 to 1 mg, should be ordered to be given the night before the surgical operation, to be repeated once if needed.
2. Continue all chronic medication the morning of surgery.
3. Any oral medications may be given with sips of water or clear juice at 6:00 AM.
4. Diazepam, 0.15 mg/kg orally, should be given with a sip of water or juice at 6:00 AM.
5. The patient should be NPO after 6:00 AM.
6. Morphine, 0.15 to 0.2 mg/kg IM, should be given 1 hour before the earliest likely induction time.
7. Scopolamine, 5 μg/kg IM, should be given in the same syringe as the morphine.

The most common variations of these orders are replacement of diazepam with lorazepam; replacement of morphine with hydroxyzine, 1.25 mg/kg; replacement of scopolamine with atropine ordered "on call"; and small, frequent intravenous doses of ataractics and opioids, started on arrival in the operating room area instead of drugs given while the patient is still on the hospital floor. The most common dissatisfaction from premedication comes from either inadequately prescribed doses or inadequately prescribed timing to permit a desirable effect.

The use of H_2-blockers and metoclopramide is clearly increasing, but the author tries to limit their use to patients with some specific indication. Barbiturates have been nearly abandoned and phenothiazines have been totally abandoned. Novel routes of uptake are presently just that—novel. There is a real suspicion that opioids ought to be abandoned except in painful states, but there is concern with the alternatives. The dissatisfaction with morphine in the 1950s was, in large part, due to use with abandoned anesthetic regimens, eg, cyclopropane.[8,9] Perhaps the most useful thing to do is the hardest, identifying just how a particular patient's psyche needs to be supported, and providing that support in the truncated time allotted for the preoperative visit.

REFERENCES

1. Forrest WH, Jr, Brown CR, Brown BW: Subjective responses to six common preoperative medications. Anesthesiology 47:241–247, 1977
2. Champlin FB, Cotter CF, Moskowitz MD, et al: A comparison of chlormecanone, meprobamate and placebo. Clin Pharmacol Ther 9:11–15, 1968
3. Seevers MH, Pfeiffer CC: A study of the analgesia, subjective depression and euphoria produced by morphine, heroin, dilaudid and cocaine in the normal human subject. J Pharmacol Exp Ther 56:166–187, 1936
4. Shearer WH: The evolution of premedication. Br J Anaesth 32:554–562, 1960
5. Shearer WH: The evolution of premedication. Br J Anaesth 33:219–225, 1961
6. Bennett HA, Gray CE, Cullen SC: Effects of large doses of barbiturates and morphine and scopolamine on respiratory minute volume exchange. Anesthesiology 10:548–552, 1949
7. Comroe JH, Jr, Dripps RD: Reactions to morphine in ambulatory and bed patients. Surg Gynecol Obstet 87:221–224, 1948
8. Cohen EN, Beecher HK: Narcotics in preanesthetic medication. JAMA 147:1664–1666, 1951
9. Eckenhoff JE, Helrich M: Study of narcotics and sedatives for use in preanesthetic medication. JAMA 167:415–422, 1958
10. Buchmann G: Premedication in children. Acta Anaesthesiol Scand 9:139–144, 1965
11. Freeman A, Bachman L: Pediatric anesthesia: an evaluation of preoperative medication. Anesth Analg 38:429–437, 1959
12. Sadove MS, Frye TJ: Preoperative sedation and production of a quiescent state in children. JAMA 164:1729–1732, 1957
13. Dripps RD, Vandam LD, Pierce EC, et al: The use of chlorpromazine in anesthesia & surgery. Ann Surg 142:774–785, 1955
14. Hopkins DAB, Hurter D, Jones CM: Promethazine and pethedine in anaesthesia. Anaesthesia 12:276–284, 1957
15. Root B, Loveland JP: Premedication of children with promethazine, propiomazine and mepazine. J Clin Pharmacol 10:182–193, 1970
16. Gaensler EA: Evaluation of pulmonary function. Annu Rev Med 12:385–408, 1961
17. Swenson EW, Ställberg-Stenhagen S, Beck M: Arterial oxygen, carbon dioxide, and pH levels in patients undergoing pulmonary resection. J Thorac Cardiovasc Surg 42:179–192, 1961
18. Stead WW: Physiologic studies following thoracic surgery. II. Immediate effects of upper lobectomy combined with a five-rib thoracoplasty. J Thorac Surg 25:194–204, 1953
19. Stead WW, Soucheray PH: Physiologic studies following thoracic surgery. I. Immediate effects of thoracoplasty. J Thorac Surg 23:453–464, 1952
20. Birath G, Swenson EW, Ander L, Bergh NP: The definitive functional results after partial pulmonary resection. Am Rev Tubercul Pulm Dis 42:983–987, 1976
21. Nakahara K, Monden Y, Ohno K, et al: A method for predicting postoperative lung function and its relation to postoperative complications in patients with lung cancer. Ann Thorac Surg 39:260–265, 1985
22. Gaensler EA: Respiratory acidosis as seen following surgery. Am J Surg 103:289–301, 1962
23. Martin FE, MacDonald F, Stead WW: Bronchospirometric studies during thoracic surgery. J Thorac Surg 29:324–327, 1955

24. Ellison RG, Hall DP, Talley RE, Ellison LT: Analysis of ventilatory and respiratory function after 82 thoracic and nonthoracic operations. Am Surg 26:485–491, 1960

25. Nunn JF, Bergman NA: The effect of atropine on pulmonary gas exchange. Br J Anaesth 36:68–73, 1964

26. Fletcher R, Veintemilla F: Changes in the arterial to end-tidal PCO_2 differences during coronary artery bypass grafting. Acta Anaesthesiol Scand 33:656–659, 1989

27. Zin WA, Caldeira M, Cardoso WV, et al: Expiratory mechanics before and after uncomplicated heart surgery. Chest 95:21–28, 1989

28. Siebecker KL, Sadler PE, Mendenhall JT: Postoperative ear oximeter studies on patients who have undergone pulmonary resection. J Thorac Surg 36:88–93, 1958

29. Smith TC, Siebecker KL: Postoperative ear oximeter studies in thoracotomy patients. J Thorac Cardiovasc Surg 39:478–485, 1960

30. Craig DB: Postoperative recovery of pulmonary function. Anesth Analg 60:46–52, 1981

31. Shackford SR, Virgilio RW, Peters RM: Early extubation versus prophylactic ventilation in the high-risk patient: a comparison of postoperative management in the prevention of respiratory complications. Anesth Analg 60:76–80, 1981

32. Menzies R, Gibbons W, Goldberg P: Determinants of weaning and survival among patients with COPD who require mechanical ventilation for acute respiratory failure. Chest 95:398–405, 1989

33. Schwieger I, Gamulin Z, Suter PM: Lung function during anesthesia and respiratory insufficiency in the postoperative period: physiological and clinical implications. Acta Anaesthesiol Scand 33:527–534, 1989

34. Jenkins J, Cameron EWJ, Milne AC, Hunter AR: One-lung anaesthesia. Anaesthesia 42:938–943, 1987

35. Normandale JP, Feneck RO: Bullous cystic lung disease: its anaesthetic management using high-frequency jet ventilation. Anaesthesia 40:1182–1185, 1985

36. Conacher ID, Paes ML, Morritt GN: Carbon dioxide laser bronchoscopy. Anaesthesia 42:511–518, 1987

37. Black J, Dalloor GJ, Collis DJ: The effect of the surgical approach on respiratory function after oesophageal resection. Br J Surg 64:624–627, 1977

38. Dobkin AB, Malik K, Israel JS: Double-blind study of hydroxyzine, promethazine, secobarbital, and a placebo for preanesthetic medication. Can Anaesth Soc J 12:499–509, 1965

39. Eckenhoff JE, Helrich M, Rolph WD, Jr: The effects of promethazine upon respiration and circulation of man. Anesthesiology 18:703–710, 1957

40. Frumin MJ, Herekar VR, Jarvik ME: Amnesic actions of diazepam and scopolamine in man. Anesthesiology 45:406–412, 1976

41. Light GA, Mörch ET, Engel R, Cunningham JJ: Promethazine hydrochloride as an adjunct to anesthesia. JAMA 164:1648–1650, 1957

42. Mixon BM, Jr, Pittinger CB: Hydroxyzine as an adjunct to preanesthetic medication. Anesth Analg 47:330–333, 1968

43. Robinson HM, Jr, Robinson CV, Steahn JF: Hydroxy-zine HCL (Atarax), a new tranquilizer. South Med J 50:1282–1284, 1957

44. Artru AA, Dhamee MS, Seifen AB, Wright B: A re-evaluation of the anxiolytic properties of intramuscular midazolam. Anaesth Intensive Care 14:152–157, 1986

45. Clarke RSJ, Dundee JW, Love WJ: Studies of drugs given before anaesthesia VIII. Br J Anaesth 37:772–778, 1965

46. Davis P, Jenicek JA: Meperidine and propiomazine for preanesthetic medication. Anesthesiology 22:1013–1014, 1961

47. Dundee JW, Moore J, Love WJ, et al: Studies of drugs given before anesthesia VI. Br J Anaesth 37:332–353, 1965

48. Dundee JW, Nicholl RM, Clarke RSJ, et al: Studies of drugs given before anaesthesia VII. Br J Anaesth 37:601–612, 1965

49. Haslett WHK, Dundee JW: Studies of drugs given before anaesthesia XIV. Br J Anaesth 40:250–256, 1968

50. Nathan LA, Andelman MB: The use of a tranquilizer in private pediatric practice. IMJ 112:171–173, 1957

51. Sanders LD, Yeomans WA, Rees J, et al: A double-blind comparison between nitrazepam, forazepam, lormetazepam and placebo and pre-operative night sedatives. Eur J Anaesth 5:377–383, 1988

52. Lasagna L, von Felsinger JM, Beecher HK: Drug-induced mood changes in man. JAMA 157:1006–1020, 1955

53. Lee CM, Yeakle AE: Patient refusal of surgery following Innovar premedication. Anesth Analg 54:224–226, 1975

54. Goldmann L, Shah MV, Hebden MW: Memory of cardiac anaesthesia: psychological sequelae in cardiac patients of intra-operative suggestion and operating room conversation. Anaesthesia 42:596–603, 1987

55. Egbert LD, Battit GE, Turndorf H, Beecher HK: The value of the preoperative visit by an anesthetist. JAMA 185:553–555, 1963

56. Kothary SP, Brown ACD, Pandit UA, et al: Time course of antirecall effect of diazepam and lorazepam following oral administration. Anesthesiology 55:641–644, 1981

57. Neuhaus A, Markowitz D, Rotman HH, Weg JG: The effects of fiberoptic bronchoscopy with and without atropine premedication on pulmonary function in humans. Ann Thorac Surg 25:393–398, 1978

58. Bethume DW: Humidification in ventilated patients. Intensive and Crit Care Dig 8:37–38, 1989

59. Miller RD: The role of H_2-receptor antagonists in anesthesiology. J Drug Devel, suppl. 3. 2:1–70, 1989

60. Murray WJ, Bechtoldt AA, Berman L: Efficacy of oral psychosedative drugs for preanesthetic medication. JAMA 203:327–332, 1968

61. Antrobus JHL: Anxiety and informed consent: does anxiety influence consent for inclusion in a study of anxiolytic premedication? Anaesthesia 43:267–269, 1988

62. Janik R, Dock W, Maskos E, Kilian A: The influence of atropine, fentanyl and alfentanil on hemodynamics during induction of anesthesia. Anaesthesia 41:76, 1986

63. Coventry DM, McMenemin I, Lawrie S: Bradycardia

during intraabdominal surgery. Anaesthesia 42:835–839, 1987

64. Jones RE, Deutsch S, Turndorf H: Effects of atropine on cardiac rhythm in conscious and anesthetized man. Anesthesiology 22:67–73, 1961

65. Munson ES, Saidman J, Eger EI, Jr: Effect of nitrous oxide and morphine on the minimum anesthetic concentration of fluroxene. Anesthesiology 26:134–139, 1965

66. Saidman LV, Eger EL II: Effect of nitrous oxide and of narcotic premedication on the alveolar concentration of halothane required for anesthesia. Anesthesiology 25:302–306, 1964

67. Zinganell K: Minimale Anaesthelische Konzentration von Halothan zur Objectivierung der Working der Pramedikation. Anaesthesist 17:47–49, 1968

68. Bilaine J, Desmonts JM: Effect of premedication with atropine or hydroxyzine on induction and maintenance of anaesthesia with propofol ('Diprivan'), abstracted. Postgrad Med J, suppl. 3. 61:38–39, 1985

69. Briggs LP, White M: The effects of premedication on anaesthesia with propofol ('Diprivan'). Postgrad Med J, suppl. 3. 61:35–37, 1985

70. McCollum JSC, Dundee JW: Comparison of induction characteristics of four intravenous anaesthetic agents. Anaesthesia 41:995–1000, 1986

71. Butterworth JF, Bean VE, Royster RL: Premedication determines the circulatory responses to rapid-sequence induction with sufentanil for cardiac surgery. Br J Anaesth 63:351–353, 1989

72. Braude N, Clements EAF, Hodges UM, Andrews BP: The pressor response and laryngeal mask insertion. Anaesthesia 44:551–554, 1989

73. Grover VK, Lata K, Sharma S, et al: Effect of lignocaine in suppression of the intraocular pressure response. Anaesthesia 44:22–25, 1989

74. Achola KJ, Jones MJ, Mitchell RWD, Smith G: Effects of beta-adrenoceptor antagonism on the cardiovascular and catecholamine responses to tracheal intubation. Anaesthesia 43:433–436, 1988

75. Grover VK, Sharma S, Mahajan M, Singh H: Intranasal nitroglycerin attenuates pressor response to tracheal intubation in beta-blocker treated hypertensive patients. Anaesthesia 42:884–887, 1987

76. Kamra S, Wig J, Sapru RP: Topical nitroglycerin. Anaesthesia 41:1087–1091, 1986

77. Groves ND, Rees JL, Rosen M: Effects of benzodiazepines on laryngeal reflexes. Anaesthesia 42:808–814, 1987

78. Khan FA, Kamal RS: Effect of buprenorphine on the cardiovascular response to tracheal intubation. Anaesthesia 44:394–397, 1989

79. Neidhart P, Burgener MC, Schwieger I, Suter PM: Chest wall rigidity during fentanyl and midazolam-fentanyl induction: ventilatory and haemodynamic effects. Acta Anaesthesiol Scand 33:1–5, 1989

80. Raza SMA, Masters RW, Vasireddy AR, Zsigmond EK: Haemodynamic stability with midazolam—sufentanil analgesia in cardiac surgical patients. Can J Anaesth 35:518–525, 1988

81. Eckenhoff JE, Kneal DH, Dripps RD: The incidence and etiology of post-anesthetic excitement. Anesthesiology 22:667–673, 1961

82. Egbert LD, Norton ML, Eckenoff JE, Dripps RD: A comparison in man of the effects of promethazine, secobarbital and meperidine alone and in combination on certain respiratory functions and for use in preanesthetic medication. South Med J 51:1173–1177, 1958

83. Block AJ, Hellard DW, Slayton PC: Minimal effect of alcohol ingestion on breathing during the sleep of postmenopausal women. Chest 88:181–184, 1985

84. Hasenbos MAWM, Gielen MJM: Anaesthesia for bullectomy. Anaesthesia 40:977–980, 1985

85. Nimmo WS, Duthie DIR: Pain relief after surgery. Anaesth Intensive Care 15:68–71, 1987

86. Sabanathan S, Smith PJB, Pradhan GN, et al: Continuous intercostal nerve block for pain relief after thoracotomy. Ann Thorac Surg 46:425–426, 1988

87. Scheinin B, Lindgren L, Rosenberg PH: Treatment of post-thoracotomy pain with intermittent instillations of intrapleural bupivacaine. Acta Anaesthesiol Scand 33:156–159, 1989

88. Scott NB, Mogensen T, Bigler D, Kehlet H: Comparison of the effects of continuous intrapleural vs epidural administration of 0.5% bupivacaine on pain, metabolic response and pulmonary function following cholecystectomy. Acta Anaesthesiol Scand 33:535–539, 1989

89. Bethume DW: Preoperative visits. Anaesthesia 42:553–554, 1987

90. Curran J, Chmielewski AT, White JB, Jennings AM: Practice of preoperative assessment by anaesthetists. Br Med J 10:291, 391–393, 1985

91. Hunter AR: Preoperative visit. Anaesthesia 39:1161–1162, 1984

92. Goldman L, Ogg TW, Levey AB: Hypnosis and daycase anaesthesia: a study to reduce preoperative anxiety and intra-operative anaesthetic requirements. Anaesthesia 43:466–469, 1988

93. Birkinshaw KJ: The preoperative visit: a source of anxiety. Anaesthesia 41:1242, 1986

94. Burns THS: Informed consent. Anaesthesia 41:1242, 1986

95. Lewis R: Preoperative anxiety and anaesthetic room decor. Anaesthesia 40:1024, 1985

96. Pinnock CA, Elling AE, Eastley RJ, Smith G: Anxiety levels in junior anaesthetists during early training. Anaesthesia 41:258–262, 1986

97. Herxheimer A, Haefeli L: Human pharmacology of hyoscine butylbromide. Lancet 1:418–421, 1966

98. Pohto P, Ahtee L: Effect of atropine, methylatropine, methyscopolamine and pilocarpine on salivary secretion and heart rate in man. Ann Med Exp Fenn 44:411–414, 1966

99. Eger EI, II: Atropine, scopolamine and related compounds. Anesthesiology 23:365–383, 1962

100. Gravenstein JS, Andersen TW, De Padua CB: Effects of atropine and scopolamine on the cardiovascular system in man. Anesthesiology 25:123–130, 1964

101. Gal TJ, Suratt PM: Atropine and glycopyrrolate effects

on lung mechanics in normal man. Anesth Analg 60:85–90, 1981

102. Burchell RC, Swasdio K: Broad-ligament absorption of atropine. Obstet Gynecol 27:714–716, 1966

103. Chamberlain DA, Turner P, Sneddon JM: Effects of atropine on heart rate in healthy man. Lancet 1:12–15, 1967

104. Chadda KD, Lichstein E, Gupta PK, Choy R: Bradycardia—hypotension syndrome in acute myocardial infarction. Am J Med 59:158–164, 1975

105. Middleton MJ, Zitzer JM, Urbach KF: Is atropine always necessary before anesthesia? Anesth Analg 46:51–55, 1967

106. Smith TC, Stephen GW, Zeiger L, Wollman H: Effects of premedicant drugs on respiration and gas exchange in man. Anesthesiology 28:883–890, 1967

107. Conway CM, Payne JP: Atropine premedication and arterial oxygen tension. Acta Anaesthesiol Scand, suppl. 23. 10:538–541, 1966

108. Dobkin AB, Su JPG, Byles PH: "Normal" PaO_2 and SaO_2 in elderly patients and the effect of premedication with atropine and meperidine. Acta Anaesthesiol Scand, suppl. 23. 10:542–547, 1966

109. Knudsen J: Arterial oxygen tension during anaesthesia. Acta Anaesthesiol Scand, suppl. 23. 10:548–553, 1966

110. Medrado V, Stephen CR: Effect of premedication with atropine sulphate on arterial blood-gases and pH. Lancet 1:734–735, 1966

111. Turnbull KW, Miyagishima RT: The influence of premedication with narcotics and belladonna on oxygenation in cardiac patients. Can Anaesth Soc J 19:639–640, 1972

112. Rotman HH: Effect of atropine on pulmonary diffusing capacity in man. Br J Anaesth 36:74–76, 1964

113. Smith TC, DuBois AB: The effects of scopolamine on the airways of man. Anesthesiology 30:12–18, 1969

114. Berger JM, Stirt JA: Resolution of bronchospasm by atropine: report of a case. Acta Anaesthesiol Scand 29:856–858, 1985

115. Aguilera L, Martinez-Bourio R, Cid C, et al: Anaphylactic reaction after atropine. Anaesthesia 43:955–957, 1988

116. Bush MT, Berry G, Hume A: Ultra-short-acting barbiturates as oral hypnotics in man. Clin Pharmacol Ther 7:373–378, 1966

117. Stephen GW, Banner MP, Wollman H, Smith TC: Respiratory pharmacology of mixture of scopolamine with secobarbital and with fentanyl. Anesthesiology 31:237–242, 1969

118. Sengutpa A, Gupta PK, Pandey K: Investigation of glycopyrrolate as a premedicant drug. Br J Anaesth 52:513–516, 1980

119. Schwartz H, de Roeth A, Jr, Papper EM: Preanesthetic use of atropine and scopolamine in patients with glaucoma. JAMA 165:144–146, 1957

120. Fencek RO, Durkin MA: A comparison between the effects of fentanyl, droperidol with fentanyl, and halothane anaesthesia on intraocular pressure in adults. Anaesthesia 42:266–269, 1987

121. Domino EF, Corssen G: Central and peripheral effects of muscarinic cholinergic blocking agents in man. Anesthesiology 28:568–574, 1967

122. Crowell EB, Ketchum JS: The treatment of scopolamine—induced delirium with physostigmine. Clin Pharmacol Ther 8:409–414, 1967

123. Hetreed MA, Aps C: Hypoxaemia after premedication in cardiac patients. Glycopyrronium compared with hyoscine. Anaesthesia 43:52–53, 1988

124. Kopman EA, Ramirez-Inawat RC: Arterial hypoxaemia following premedication in patients with coronary artery disease. Can Anaesth Soc J 27:132–134, 1980

125. Severinghaus JW, Stupfel M: Respiratory dead space increase following atropine in man, and atropine, vagal, or ganglionic blockade and hypothermia in dogs. J Appl Physiol 8:81–87, 1955

126. Butler J, Caro CG, Alcala R, DuBois AB: Physiologic factors affecting airway resistance in normal subjects and in patients with obstructive respiratory disease. J Clin Invest 39:584–591, 1960

127. Ali-Melkkilä T, Kaila T, Kanto J: Glycopyrrolate: pharmacokinetics and some pharmacodynamic findings. Acta Anaesthesiol Scand 33:513–517, 1989

128. Cozanitis DA, Lindgren L, Rosenberg PH: Bradycardia in patients receiving atracurium or vecuronium in conditions of low vagal stimulation. Anaesthesia 44:303–306, 1989

129. Keats AS: Effects of drugs on respiration in man. Am Rev Pharmacol Toxicol 25:41–65, 1985

130. Rutter GGR, Aveling W, Tusiewicz K: The respiratory depressant effects of nalbuphine and papaveretum as intramuscular premedication. Anaesthesia 42:1176–1179, 1987

131. Smith TC: Pharmacology of respiratory depression. Int Anesthesiol Clin 9:125–143, 1971

132. Smith TC, Kulp RA: Blunting of the ventilatory responses to hypoxia and hypercarbia by fentanyl, diazepam and pentobarbital in man. pp. 779–780. In: Abstracts of Scientific Papers. American Society of Anesthesiologists Annual Meeting, 1977

133. Asbury AJ: Pupil response to alfentanil and fentanyl. Anaesthesia 41:717–720, 1986

134. Woodall NM, Maryniak JK, Gilston A: Pupillary signs during cardiac surgery. Anaesthesia 44:885–888, 1989

135. Daykin AP, Bowen DJ, Saunders DA, Norman J: Respiratory depression after morphine in the elderly. A comparison with younger subjects. Anaesthesia 41:910–914, 1986

136. Frank M, McAteer EJ, Cattermole R, Loughnan B, et al: Nalbuphine for obstetric analgesia. A comparison of nalbuphine with pethidine for pain relief in labour when administered by patient-controlled analgesia (PCA). Anaesthesia 42:697–703, 1987

137. Sury MRJ, Cole PV: Nalbuphine combined with midazolam for outpatient sedation. Anaesthesia 43:285–288, 1988

138. Forrest WH, Jr, Bellville JW: The effect of sleep plus morphine on the respiratory response to carbon dioxide. Anesthesiology 25:137–141, 1984

139. McGinty D, Beahm E, Stern N, et al: Nocturnal hypo-

tension in older men with sleep-related breathing disorders. Chest 94:305–311, 1988

140. Onal E, Leech JA, Lopata M: Relationship between pulmonary function and sleep-induced respiratory abnormalities. Chest 87:437–441, 1985

141. Tatsumi K, Kimura H, Kunitomo F, et al: Sleep arterial oxygen desaturation and chemical control of breathing during wakefulness in COPD. J Thorac Cardiovasc Surg 42:179–192, 1961

142. Gothe B, Strohl KP, Levin S, Cherniack NS: Nicotine: a different approach to treatment of obstructive sleep apnea. Chest 87:11–17, 1985

143. Conner JT, Bellville JW, Wender R, et al: Morphine, scopolamine and atropine as intravenous surgical premedicants. Anesth Anal 56:606–614, 1977

144. Conner JT, Bellville JW, Katz RL: Morphine and meperidine as intravenous surgical premedicants. Can Anaesth Soc J 24:559–564, 1977

145. Pandit SK, Kothary SP: Intravenous narcotics for premedication in outpatient anaesthesia. Acta Anaesthesiol Scand 33:353–358, 1989

146. Furness G, Dundee JW, Milligan KR: Low-dose sufentanil pretreatment. Anaesthesia 42:1264–1266, 1987

147. Weiss WA, McGee JP, Branford JO, Hanks EC: Value of chlorpromazine in preoperative medication. JAMA 161:812–815, 1956

148. Pearson JW, DeKornfeld TJ: Effect of methotrimeprazine on respiration. Anesthesiology 24:38–40, 1963

149. Wendel H, Lambertsen CJ, Longenhagen JB: Effect of chlorpromazine and meperidine separately and combined on respiration of man. J Pharmacol Exp Ther 119:184–188, 1957

150. Lambertsen CJ, Wendel H, Longenhagen JB: The separate and combined respiratory effects of chlorpromazine and meperidine in normal men controlled at 46 mmHg alveolar PCO_2. J Pharmacol Exp Ther 131:381–393, 1961

151. Mitchell CL: Effect of morphine and chlorpromazine alone and in combination on the reaction to noxious stimuli. Arch Int Pharmacodyn 163:387–392, 1966

152. Keats AS, Telford J, Kurosu Y: "Potentiation" of meperidine by promethazine. Anesthesiology 22:34–41, 1961

153. Steen SN, Amaha K, Weitzner SW, Martinez LR: The effect of chlordiazepoxide and pethedine alone and in combination on the respiratory response to carbon dioxide. Br J Anaesth 39:459–463, 1957

154. Holzman L, Gibbs L, Yuceoglu YZ, et al: Clinical evaluation of propiomazine for preanesthetic medication. Anesth Analg 43:433–439, 1964

155. Markello R, King BD: Effects of propiomazine on respiration and circulation. Anesthesiology 27:20–23, 1966

156. Haselhuhn DH, Brunson EG: Promethazine hydrochloride as a supplement to anesthesia. Anesth Analg 38:485–492, 1959

157. Burrell ZL, Gillenger WC, Martinez A: Treatment of cardiac arrhythmias with hydroxyzine. Am J Cardiol 1:624–626, 1958

158. Steen SN, Lyons H, Thomas JS, Crane R: The objective evaluation of hydroxyzine HCL and diazepam on airway conductances of patients with chronic broncheo-

spastic disease. Scientific Exhibit, Annual Meeting of the American Society of Anesthesiologists, 1971

159. Andersen TW, Gravenstein JS: Cardiovascular effects of sedative doses of pentobarbital and hydroxyzine. Anesthesiology 27:272–278, 1966

160. Marcus PS, Pelaez FAG: Evaluation of a premedicant. Anesth Analg 42:542–546, 1963

161. Gasser JC, Bellville JW: On human respiration. Anesthesiology 43:599–601, 1975

162. Gasser JC, Bellville JW: The respiratory effects of hydroxyzine, diazepam and pentazocine in man. Anaesthesia 31:718–723, 1976

163. Short TG, Forrest P, Galletly C: Paradoxical reactions to benzodiazepines—a genetically determined phenomenon? Anaesth Intensive Care 15:330–345, 1987

164. Pollard BJ, Masters AP, Bunting P: The use of flumazenil (Anexate, Ro 15-1788) in the management of drug overdose. Anaesthesia 44:137–138, 1989

165. Kaukinen S, Kataja J, Kaukinen L: Antagonism of benzodiazepine-fentanyl anaesthesia with flumazenil. Can J Anaesth 37:40–45, 1990

166. Knaack-Steinegger R, Schou J: Therapy of paradoxical reactions to midazolam during regional anesthesia. Anaesthesist 36:143–146, 1987

167. Zuurmond WWA, van Leeuwen L, Helmers JH: Recovery from fixed-dose midazolam-induced anaesthesia and antagonism with flumazenil for outpatient arthroscopy. Acta Anaesthesiol Scand 33:160–163, 1989

168. Boularan A, Calvet B, Rochette A, et al: Premedication with other benzodiazepines (BDZs) antagonizes sleep induced by IV Midazolam. Anaesthesia 42:72–73, 1987

169. Aldrete JA, Daniel W: Evaluation of premedicants as protective agents against convulsive (LD_{50}) doses of local anesthesia agents in rats. Anesth Analg 50:127–130, 1971

170. Fink M, Irwin P, Weinfeld RE, et al: Blood levels and electroencephalographic effects of diazepam and bromazepam. Clin Pharmacol Ther 20:184–191, 1976

171. Tornetta FJ: Clinical studies with the new antiemetic, metoclopramide. Anesth Analg 48:198–204, 1969

172. Catchlove RFH, Kafer ER: The effects of diazepam on the ventilatory response to carbon dioxide and on steady-state gas exchange. Anesthesiology 34:9–13, 1971

173. Gross JB, Smith L, Smith TC: Time course of ventilatory response to carbon dioxide after intravenous diazepam. Anesthesiology 57:18–21, 1982

174. Lakshiminarayan S, Sahn SA, Hudson LD, Weil JV: Effect of diazepam on ventilatory responses. Clin Pharmacol Ther 20:178–183, 1976

175. Catchlove RFH, Kafer ER: The effects of diazepam on respiration in patients with obstructive pulmonary disease. Anesthesiology 34:13–18, 1971

176. Kawar P, Carson IW, Clarke RSJ, et al: Haemodynamic changes during induction of anaesthesia with midazolam and diazepam (Valium) in patients undergoing coronary artery bypass surgery. Anaesthesia 40:767–771, 1985

177. Eustace PW, Hailey DM, Cox AG, Baird ES: Biliary excretion of diazepam in man. Br J Anaesth 47:983–985, 1975

178. Cann F, Maes V, Van de Velde A, Sevens C: Lorazepam fast-dissolving drug formulations (FDDF) and intravenous administrations as anaesthetic premedicants. Eur J Anesthesiology 5:261–268, 1988

179. Thomas D, Tipping T, Halifax R, et al: Triazolam premedication. A comparison with lorazepam and placebo in gynaecological patients. Anaesthesia 41:692–697, 1986

180. Ponnudurai R, Hurdley J: Bromazepam as oral premedication. A comparison with lorazepam. Anaesthesia 41:541–543, 1986

181. Irjala J, Kanto J, Irjala K, et al: Temazepam versus flunitrazepam as an oral premedication in adult surgical patients. Eur J Anaesthesiol 4:435–440, 1987

182. Padfield NL, Twohig M, Fraser ACL: Temazepam and trimeprazine compared with placebo as premedication in children. Br J Anaesth 58:487–493, 1986

183. Ratcliff A, Indalo AA, Bradshaw EG, Rye RM: Premedication with temazepam in minor surgery. Anaesthesia 33:812, 1989

184. Gross KB, Zebrowski ME, Carel WE, et al: Time course of ventilatory depression after thiopental and midazolam in normal subjects and patients with chronic obstructive pulmonary disease. Anesthesiology 58:540–544, 1983

185. Forrest P, Galletly DC, Yee P: Placebo controlled comparison of midazolam, triazolam and diazepam as oral premedicants for outpatient anaesthesia. Anaesth Intensive Care 15:296–304, 1987

186. Lanz E, Schäfer A, Brunisholz V: Midazolam for oral premedication prior to regional anaesthesia. Anaesthesist 36:197–202, 1987

187. Raybould D, Bradshaw EG: Premedication for day case surgery. Anaesthesia 42:591–595, 1987

188. Gastinne H, Venot J, Dupuy JP, Gay R: Unilateral diaphragmatic dysfunction in blunt chest trauma. Chest 93:518–521, 1988

189. Hargreaves J: Benzodiazepine premedication in minor day-case surgery: comparison of oral midazolam and temazepam with placebo. Br J Anaesth 61:611–616, 1988

190. Dawson D, Sear JW: Influence of induction of anaesthesia with midazolam on the neuro-endocrine response to surgery. Anaesthesia 41:268–271, 1986

191. Husby P, Vamnes JS, Rodt SA, et al: Midazolam does not potentiate the effect of vercuronium in patients. Acta Anaesthesiol Scand 33:280–282, 1989

192. Hall CC: Aspiration pneumonitis—an obstetric hazard. JAMA 114:728–733, 1940

193. Mendelson CL: The aspiration of stomach contents into the lungs during obstetric anesthesia. Am J Obstet Gynecol 52:191–204, 1946

194. Olsson GL, Hallon B, Hambraeus-Jonzon K: Aspiration during anesthesia: a computer-aided study of 185,358 anesthetics. Acta Anaesthesiol Scand 30:84–92, 1986

195. Powar I, Easton JC, Todd JG, Nimmo WS: Gastric emptying after head injury. Anaesthesia 44:563–566, 1989

196. Arms RA, Dines DE, Tinstman TC: Aspiration pneumonia. Chest 65:136–139, 1974

197. Bynum LU, Pierce AK: Pulmonary aspiration of gastric contents. Am Rev Respir Dis 114:1129–1136, 1976

198. Joyce TH: Prophylaxis for pulmonary acid aspiration. Am J Med, suppl. 6A. 83:46–52, 1980

199. Ostheimer GW: Pulmonary acid aspiration II: prevention of complications. J Drug Devel, suppl. 3. 2:18–32, 1989

200. Sweeney B, Wright I: The use of antacids as a prophylaxis against Mendelson's syndrome in the United Kingdom. Anaesthesia 41:419–422, 1986

201. Ostheimer GW: Stress-related mucosal damage I: clinical implications. J Drug Devel, suppl. 3. 2:33–39, 1989

202. Mazzei W: Stress related mucosal damage II: prevention and treatment. J Drug Devel, suppl. 3. 2:40–47, 1989

203. Driscol DF: Metabolic alkalosis in the perioperative period. J Drug Devel, suppl. 3. 2:48–60, 1989

204. Khambatta HJ, Sullivan SF: Effects of respiratory alkalosis on oxygen consumption and oxygenation. Anesthesiology 38:53–58, 1973

205. Tryba M, Zevounou F, Zenz M: Prevention of histamine-induced cardiovascular reactions during the induction of anaesthesia following premedication with $H_1 + H_2$ antagonists IM. Br J Anaesth 58:478–482, 1986

206. Gorback M: Pulmonary acid aspiration. J Drug Devel, suppl. 3. 2:4–17, 1989

207. James CF, Modell JH, Gibbs CP, et al: Pulmonary aspiration. Effects of pH and volume in the rat. Anesth Analg 63:665–668, 1984

208. Laws HL, Palmer MD, Donald JM, Jr, et al: Effects of preoperative medications on gastric pH, volume, and flora. Ann Surg 203:614–619, 1986

209. Pandit SK, Kothary SP, Pandit UA, Mirakhur RK: Premedication with cimetidine and metoclopramide. Anaesthesia 41:486–492, 1986

210. Escolano F, Castaño J, Paresi N, et al: Comparison of the effects of famotidine and ranitidine on gastric secretion in patients undergoing elective surgery. Anaesthesia 44:212–215, 1989.

211. Gallagher EG, White M, Ward S, et al: Prophylaxis against acid aspiration syndrome. Anaesthesia 43:1011–1014, 1988

212. Souney PF, Solomon MA, Stancher D: Visual compatibility of cimetidine hydrochloride with common preoperative injectable medications. Am J Hosp Pharm 41:1840–1841, 1984

213. Corinaldesci R, Scarpignato C, Galassi A, et al: Effect of Ranitidine and cimetidine on gastric emptying of a mixed meal in man. Int J Clin Pharmacol Ther Toxicol 22:498–501, 1984

214. Scarpignato C, Bertaccini G: Different effects of cimetidine and ranitidine on gastric emptying in rats and man. Agents Actions 12:172–173, 1982

215. Roy AK, Cuda MP, Levine PA: Induction of theophylline toxicity and inhibition of clearance rates by ranitidine. Am J Med 85:525–527, 1988

216. Sax MJ, Randolph WC, Peaceke KE: Effect of two cimetidine regimes on prothrombin time and warfarin kinetics during long-term warfarin therapy. Clin Pharm 6:492–495, 1987

217. Flynn RJ, Moore J: Lack of effect of cimetidine and ranitidine on lidocaine disposition. Anesthesiology 69:A656, 1988

218. Okkonen M, Rosenberg PH, Saarnivaara L: Cimetidine and ranitidine do not affect enflurane metabolism in surgical patients. Acta Anaesthesiol Scand 33:129–131, 1989

219. Bogod DG, Oh TE: The effect of H₂ antagonists on duration of action of suxamethonium in the parturient. Anaesthesia 44:591–593, 1989

220. Kambam JR, Dymond R, Kreslow M: Effect of cimetidine on duration of action of succinylcholine. Anesth Analg 66:191–192, 1987

221. Elwood RJ, Hildebrand PJ, Dundee JW, Collier PS: Ranitidine influences the uptake of oral midazolam. Br J Clin Pharmacol 15:743, 1983

222. Wilson CM, Robinson FP, Thompson EM, et al: Effect of pretreatment with ranitidine on the hypnotic action of single doses of midazolam, temazepam and zopiclone. Br J Anaesth 58:483–486, 1986

223. Manchikanti L, Marrero TC, Roush JR: Preanesthetic cimetidine and metoclopramide for acid aspiration prophylaxis in elective surgery. Anesthesiology 61:48–54, 1984

224. Rao TLK, Madhavareddy S, Chinthagada M, El-Etr AA: Metoclopramide and cimetidine to reduce gastric fluid pH and volume. Anesthesiology 63:1014–1016, 1984

225. Gibbs CP, Schwartz DJ, Wynne JW et al: Antacid pulmonary aspiration in the dog. Anesthesiology 51:380–385, 1979

226. Murrell GC, Rosen M: In-vivo buffering capacity of Alka Seltzer Effervescent. Anaesthesia 41:138–142, 1986

227. Mathews HML, Moore J: Sodium bicarbonate as a single-dose antacid in obstetric anaesthesia. Anaesthesia 44:590–591, 1989

228. Maltby JR, Koehli N, Shaffer EA: Gastric fluid volume, pH, and emptying in elective inpatients. Can J Anaesth 35:562–566, 1988

229. Jani K, Somaan AA: The effect of sodium citrate versus ranitidine pretreatment on gastric pepsin activity in non-obstetric patients. Br J Anaesth 60:325–326, 1988

230. Rowntree LG, Geraghty JT: An experimental and clinical study of phenolsulphonephthalein in relation to renal function in health and disease. Arch Intern Med 9:284–338, 1912

231. Stanski DR, Greenblatt DJ, Lowenstein MD: Kinetics of intravenous and intramuscular morphine. Clin Pharmacol Ther 24:52–59, 1978

232. Kirkpatrick T, Henderson PD, Nimmo WS: Plasma morphine concentrations after intramuscular injection into the deltoid or gluteal muscles. Anaesthesia 43:293–295, 1988

233. Caplan RA, Beady LB, Oden RU, et al: Transdermal fentanyl for postoperative pain management. JAMA 261:1036–1039, 1989

234. Janssen P: The past, present, and future of opioid anesthetics. J Cardiothorac Anesth 2:259–265, 1990

235. Goroszeniuk MA, Jones RM, Mohamoud O: Preoperative medication reviewed: oral temazepam compared with papaveretum and hyoscine. Eur J Anaesth 4:261–267, 1987

236. Cundy JM, Hodkinson B: Slow release morphine. Anaesthesia 41:1131, 1986

237. Pinnock CA, Derbyshire DR, Elling AE, Smith G: Comparison of oral slow release morphine (MST) with intramuscular morphine for premedication. Anaesthesia 40:1082–1085, 1985

238. Slowey HF, Reynolds AD, Mapleson WW, Vickers MD: Effect of premedication with controlled-release oral morphine on postoperative pain. Anaesthesia 40:438–440, 1985

239. Richmond MN, Dawm REO: Premedication with oral slow release morphine in dental anesthesia. Anaesthesia 43:694–696, 1988

240. Agarwal A, Chari P, Singh H: Fluid deprivation before operation. Anaesthesia 44:632–634, 1989

241. Fisher AP, Fung C, Hanna M: Absorption of buccal morphine: a comparison with slow-release morphine sulphate. Anaesthesia 43:552–553, 1988

242. Fisher AP, Vine P, Whitlock J, Hanna M: Buccal morphine premedication: a double-blind comparison with intramuscular morphine. Anaesthesia 41:1104–1111, 1986

243. Stanley TH, Hague B, Mock DL, et al: Oral transmucosal fentanyl citrate (lollipop) premedication in human volunteers. Anesth Anal 69:21–27, 1990

244. Stanley TH, Leiman BC, Rawal N, et al: The effects of oral transmucosal fentanyl citrate premedication on preoperative behavioral responses and gastric volume and acidity in children. Anesth Analg 69:328–335, 1990

245. Streisand JB, Ashburn MA, LeMaine L, et al: Bioavailability and absorption of oral transmucosal fentanyl citrate. Anesthesiology 71:A230, 1989

246. Helmers JH, Noordvin H, VanPeer A, et al: Comparison of intravenous and intranasal sufentanil absorption and sedation. Can J Anaesth 36:494–497, 1989

247. Vercauteren M, Boeckx E, Hanegreefs G, et al: Intranasal sufentanil for pre-operative sedation. Anaesthesia 43:270–273, 1986

248. Tasi SK, Wei CF, Mok HS: Intranasal ketamine vs sufentanil as premedicant in children. Anesthesiology 71:A1173, 1989

249. Pither C: The preoperative visit: a source of anxiety. Anaesthesia 401:698, 1985

11

MONITORING OF OXYGENATION AND VENTILATION

Kevin K. Tremper, Ph.D., M.D.
Steven J. Barker, Ph.D., M.D.

Ensuring the adequacy of oxygenation, ventilation, and circulation are the essentials of acute care medicine. Since the thoracic cavity contains the primary organs responsible for these vital functions, it is reasonable to expect that surgical procedures in the thoracic cavity may have deleterious effects on these dynamic processes. Although subjective signs of oxygenation and ventilation may be helpful clinically, they can also be misleading. Approximately 30 years ago, objective methods were developed for measuring blood oxygen (PO_2) and carbon dioxide (PCO_2) tensions. Over the past 20 years, techniques of in vitro blood analysis for oxygen and carbon dioxide have been adapted to invasive and noninvasive monitoring. These monitoring techniques use many of the same physical principles used in blood sample analysis, but, since they are applied at various locations in the cardiopulmonary system, each technique presents different information and has its own unique advantages and limitations. This chapter is divided into sections on oxygen, carbon dioxide, and clinical applications of monitoring in thoracic anesthesia. The oxygen and carbon dioxide sections are subdivided into discussions of gas transport physiology, specific measurement methods, and monitoring techniques. The monitoring sections are further subdivided into invasive and noninvasive techniques. The O_2 and CO_2 sections are introduced with descriptions of the basics of O_2 and CO_2 transport calculations (see Chapters 6 and 7). The data provided by each monitoring technique may be seen in the light of the entire transport system.

OXYGENATION: OXYGEN MEASUREMENT AND MONITORING

Basic Oxygen Transport Calculations

Oxygenation is adequate when oxygen is supplied to the tissues at a sufficient rate to maintain aerobic metabolism. Since blood is the transport medium, the flow rate of oxygen to the tissues can be determined by measuring or calculating both the amount of oxygen carried per unit volume of blood and flow rate of blood to the tissues. The primary oxygen transport variable is the arterial oxygen content (CaO_2).

Oxygen content is defined as the volume of oxygen (mL) carried in 100 mL of blood. It is a basic variable that is found in all oxygen transport calculations. Although oxygen content can be measured directly by the volumetric method of Van Slyke and Neills, it is usually calculated from the following equation[1]:

$$CaO_2 = Hb \times 1.34 \times SaO_2 + 0.00314 \times PaO_2 \quad (1)$$

where CaO_2 = arterial oxygen content ("a" denotes an arterial sample) in mL O_2/100 mL blood (or vol percent),

$\quad\quad$ Hb = Hemoglobin concentration (g/dL),

$\quad$ 1.34 = the volume of oxygen (mL) carried by 1 g of fully saturated hemoglobin,

$\quad$ SaO_2 = fractional hemoglobin saturation (to be discussed below),

0.00314 = the solubility coefficient of oxygen in plasma (mL of O_2/100 mL plasma/mmHg of O_2 tension), and

$\quad$ PaO_2 = the arterial oxygen tension (mmHg).

With a normal 15 g of hemoglobin and arterial PaO_2 and SaO_2 values of 95 mmHg and 95 percent, respectively, a CaO_2 of 20 vol % is obtained. This is coincidentally very similar to the oxygen content of room air at sea level. Thus, the cardiovascular system produces the same oxygen content near each cell that would exist if the cells were surrounded by room air. Methods of measuring hemoglobin saturation and oxygen tension will be discussed below. Note that in Equation 1 the oxygen content is very sensitive to the hemoglobin concentration and saturation, while it appears insensitive to the oxygen tension due to the low solubility coefficient for oxygen in plasma. However, the hemoglobin saturation itself depends nonlinearly on oxygen tension (see below). Since CaO_2 is proportional to hemoglobin concentration, if the arterial hemoglobin is fully saturated, the content can be estimated as slightly less than half the hematocrit. The hematocrit is approximately three times the hemoglobin concentration.

The overall flow rate of oxygen to the tissues is called the *oxygen delivery*, calculated by the product of arterial oxygen content and cardiac output.[1] Using a cardiac output (CO) of 5 L/min for a 70 kg adult, a normal oxygen delivery of 1,000 mL O_2/min (20 mL O_2/100 mL or 200 mL O_2/L × 5 L/min = 1,000 mL O_2/min) is obtained. Since normal cardiac output is dependent on the size of the patient, the cardiac output is usually indexed to body surface area: cardiac index (CI) equals cardiac output divided by body surface area (m²). A normal cardiac index is 3 L/min/m²; the normal range is 2.7 to 3.4 L/min/m².[2] The oxygen delivery index is defined as the arterial oxygen content times the cardiac index:

$$O_2 \text{ Del} = CaO_2 \times CI \text{ (mL } O_2/\text{min/m}^2)$$
$$\text{Normal } O_2 \text{ Del} = 20 \text{ mL/dL} \times 10 \text{ dL/L} \times 3 \text{ L/min/m}^2$$
$$= 600 \text{ mL/min/m}^2 \quad\quad (2)$$

Oxygen delivery index is an overall assessment of oxygen transport to the tissues but does not ensure adequate oxygen supply to any specific organ. The oxygen delivery to each organ can be defined as the arterial oxygen content times the blood flow to that specific organ.

The tissues consume an average of 5 mL of oxygen from every 100 mL of blood flow. Since the normal arterial oxygen content is 20 mL/100 mL of blood, 75 percent of the oxygen remains in the venous blood. The oxygen consumption of the body can be calculated by subtracting the mixed venous oxygen content from the arterial oxygen content and multiplying this difference by the cardiac output:

$$\text{Oxygen Consumption} = (CaO_2 - C\bar{v}O_2) \times CO \quad (3)$$

As with oxygen delivery, the oxygen consumption is indexed so that a normal value is independent of patient size:

$$\text{Oxygen Consumption} = \dot{V}O_2 = (CaO_2 - C\bar{v}O_2) \times CI$$
$$\text{Index}$$
$$\dot{V}O_2 = (20 \text{ mL/dL} - 15 \text{ mL/dL}) \times 3 \text{ L/min/m}^2$$
$$\times 10 \text{ dL/L}$$
$$\dot{V}O_2 = 150 \text{ mL/min/m}^2$$

The normal range of oxygen consumption index is from 115 to 165 mL/min/m². These values are for healthy patients at rest and can increase several times with exercise, shivering, hyperthermia, or sepsis. Indexed values are also significantly greater in infants and children. $\dot{V}O_2$ can be reduced by anesthetics and hypothermia.

Mixed venous blood is sampled from the pulmonary artery to ensure proper mixing, and it does not reflect the oxygen returned to the heart from any specific organ. The normal mixed venous oxygen content of 15 mL/dL corresponds to a mixed venous oxygen saturation ($S\bar{v}O_2$) of 75 percent and an oxygen tension ($P\bar{v}O_2$) of 40 mmHg. Mixed venous blood should reflect tissue PO_2. Although there is great variability in tissue PO_2 values, the mean PO_2 of interstitial fluid is the same as the mixed venous PO_2, ie, 40 mmHg.[3]

The oxygen extraction ratio is a supply-demand balance for oxygenation, given by the ratio of oxygen consumption to oxygen delivery:

$$O_2 \text{ Ext} = \frac{CO(CaO_2 - C\bar{v}O_2)}{CO \times CaO_2} \times 100\%$$
$$= \frac{CaO_2 - C\bar{v}O_2}{CaO_2} \times 100\% \quad (4)$$
$$\text{Normal } O_2 \text{ Ext} = 25\%$$

O_2 Ext is thus independent of cardiac output, which made it an especially useful variable prior to the availability of routine clinical methods for measuring cardiac output. Since the normal extraction ratio is only 25 percent, there is a wide margin of safety for oxygen transport. In fact, the body can easily extract up to 50 percent of the delivered oxygen without obligatory tissue hypoxia. When the extraction ratio exceeds 50 percent, there is an increasing likelihood of tissue hypoxia because of the low oxygen tension corresponding to a 50 percent hemoglobin saturation (P_{50} of adult hemoglobin is normally 26.7 mmHg).

Hypoxia is defined as inadequate tissue oxygenation. From the definition of oxygen delivery, it can be seen that hypoxia can be due to either inadequate blood flow or low arterial oxygen content. Hypoxia due to inadequate blood flow is called *ischemic hypoxia*. Hypoxia due to low oxygen content is called *hypoxemic hypoxia*. Arterial oxygen content can be decreased as a result of low hemoglobin (anemic hypoxemia), low PaO_2 (hypoxemic hypoxemia), or low SaO_2 (toxic hypoxemia). Toxic hypoxemia (decreased fractional hemoglobin saturation) can be the result of increasing methemoglobin or carboxyhemoglobin. This will be discussed further in the section on hemoglobin saturation.

OXYGEN TENSION MEASUREMENT

Clark PO$_2$ Electrode

In 1956, Leland Clark developed the polarographic oxygen electrode for measuring oxygen tension.[4] Before this invention, blood oxygen tension was not routinely measured. With the addition of the Severinghaus-Stowe carbon dioxide electrode in 1958, the blood gas machine was developed and critical patient care was revolutionized.[5]

The Clark electrode is an electrical cell composed of a platinum cathode and a silver anode (Fig. 11-1). As in any resistive circuit, as the voltage is increased, the current will also increase. In this electrochemical cell there is a plateau voltage range over which the current does not increase with voltage but does increase with oxygen tension in the cell. An oxygen-consuming electrochemical reaction takes place at the cathode, and the electric current in the circuit is directly proportional to the oxygen consumed. Clark's polarographic oxygen electrode has been used for more than 30 years to measure oxygen tension in gases and liquids in both medicine and industry. Other methods to measure oxygen in the gas phase are used clinically to measure inspired and expired oxygen concentration. These methods include paramagnetic oxygen analysis and the oxygen fuel cell.[6]

PO$_2$ Optode

Recently, a new technique, called *photoluminescence quenching*, has been used experimentally to measure arterial blood oxygen tension in vivo.[7,8]

When light shines on a luminescent dye, specific light frequencies are absorbed, exciting electrons to a higher energy state (Fig. 11-2). These electrons then fall into a lower energy state by emitting photons of a frequency different from the original light. In some luminescent dyes, this light emission is "quenched" by the presence of oxygen. When an excited electron falls into a lower energy state in these dyes, the excess energy can be either emitted as a photon (luminescence) or absorbed by an oxygen molecule, thereby increasing the vibrational and rotational energy of the latter (Fig. 11-2). The oxygen tension in the dye can be related to the luminescent intensity by an empiric relationship known as the Stern-Volmer equation[7]:

$$\frac{1}{I} = \frac{1}{I_0} + K \times PO_2 \qquad (5)$$

where I = the intensity of the luminescent signal at the PO_2 being measured,

I_0 = the intensity of the luminescent signal in the absence of oxygen,

PO_2 = the oxygen tension, and

K = quenching constant.

The advantages of the photoluminescence quenching sensor, or "optode," as a PO_2 measuring device are its simplicity and size. The sensor consists of a thin fiberoptic strand with dye encapsulated at the tip, and it can be easily miniaturized. Figure 11-3 shows an optode that can fit through a 22-gauge intravenous cannula.[8] Another advantage of optode technology is that pH- and PCO_2-sensitive dyes are also available, and, therefore, a three-fiber optode can simultaneously measure PO_2, PCO_2, and pH.[9]

CONTINUOUS OXYGEN TENSION MONITORING

Invasive PO$_2$ Monitoring: Clark Electrode

The initial problem in continuous invasive PaO_2 monitoring is miniaturization of a Clark electrode to fit through an arterial cannula. There are two approaches to this, the first of which is to insert only the platinum cathode into the cannula and place the reference anode on the skin surface. The cathode is surrounded by a thin layer of electrolyte and covered with an oxygen-permeable membrane.[10,11] The second approach involves miniaturization of the entire anode-cathode electrode for intra-arterial insertion.[12,13]

There have been several studies of intra-arterial PO_2 monitoring using Clark electrodes, and the results are somewhat conflicting with respect to accuracy. It is often difficult to compare such studies because the

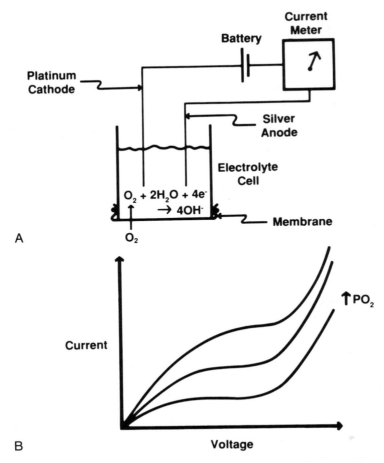

Fig. 11-1. (A) Schematic of a Clark polarographic oxygen electrode. The circuit consists of a voltage source (battery) and a current meter connecting the platinum and silver electrodes. The electrodes are immersed in an electrolyte cell. A membrane permeable to oxygen, but not to the electrolyte, covers one surface of the cell. Oxygen diffuses through the membrane and reacts at the platinum cathode with water to produce hydroxyl ions. The ammeter measures the current produced by the electrons consumed in this reaction at the cathode. **(B)** A plot of current produced as a function of the voltage between the two electrodes (polarizing voltage). This plot is called a *polarogram*. In the range near 660 mV there is a plateau in the polarogram. The plateau occurs at higher currents as the PO_2 in the cell is increased. Most polarographic oxygen electrodes use 600 to 800 mV polarizing voltage to obtain a stable current at each PO_2.

data are usually analyzed by linear regression and correlation coefficients. Altman and colleagues have shown that this may be inappropriate and often misleading in methods-comparison studies.[14–16] The correlation coefficient is extremely sensitive to the x and y range over which the data are collected. Furthermore, a high correlation coefficient (an *r* value close to 1.0) implies a high degree of association between the methods (ie, when one measurement increases, the other will also increase), but it does not imply that one method can replace the other. As an alternative,

Altman recommends using the mean and standard deviation of the difference between the two methods of measurement as an assessment of agreement. The mean difference is called the *bias* and the standard deviation is referred to as the *precision*. The bias indicates a consistent over- or underestimate of one method relative to the other (a systematic error). The precision represents the scatter or random error.[14–16] As an example, Figure 11-4 is a "scattergram" plot of data from an intra-arterial Clark electrode used in neonatal patients.[13] The abscissa of this plot is PaO_2

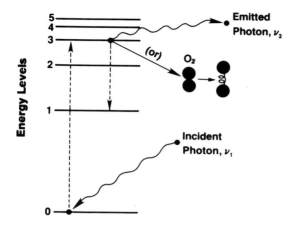

Fig. 11-2. The fluorescence-quenching phenomenon. An electron of the fluorescent dye is excited to a higher energy level by an incident photon (ν_1). This excited electron can return to a lower energy level either by emitting a photon (ν_2) or by interacting with an oxygen molecule and raising the latter to a higher vibrational energy level. (From Barker et al,[8] with permission.)

determined in vitro on arterial samples by a blood gas analyzer, and the ordinate is the intra-arterial electrode PaO_2. Although these data yield a correlation coefficient of 0.88, a large amount of variation of y on x over the entire range of PaO_2 is seen. For example, at

an in vitro PaO_2 of 40 mmHg, the intra-arterial probe PO_2 values vary from the mid 20s to 70 mmHg, with one data point as high as 100 mmHg.

The size of the electrode has caused problems with blood pressure monitoring and arterial blood sampling.[11] Early electrodes required an 18 gauge or larger arterial cannula, but difficulties in pressure monitoring and blood sampling still occurred.[17,18] More recently, the electrodes have been miniaturized to fit through 20 gauge arterial cannulae[12] (personal communication, Stanley Frank, Ph.D., Biomedical Sensors, Inc., Kansas City, MO). Damping of the arterial pressure waveform and inaccurate blood pressure measurements are commonly reported.[12,17] It is unclear whether this phenomenon results from the Clark electrode itself or from the formation of blood clot around the sensor. Reported problems in accuracy include calibration drift and systematic underestimation of PaO_2. The causes of these errors are not understood, but may involve decreased blood flow around the electrode tip or clot formation on the electrode surface. The most recently developed electrodes may have reduced these problems, but there are no studies to confirm this (personal communication, Stanley Frank).

Because of the difficulties of miniaturizing both the Clark electrode and the glass components required for electrochemical CO_2 and pH measurement, it is unlikely than an electrochemical blood gas monitoring

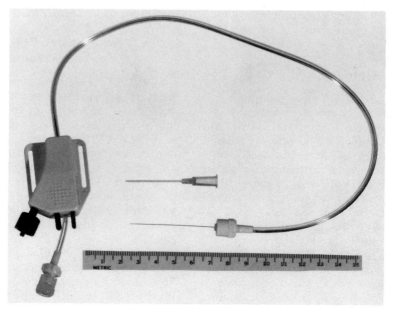

Fig. 11-3. An optode probe and the 20-gauge cannula through which it is inserted. (From Barker et al,[8] with permission.)

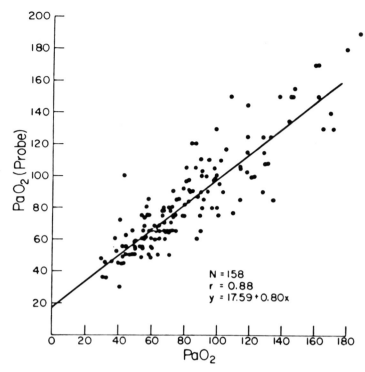

Fig. 11-4. Relationship between arterial oxygen tension (PaO_2) and intravascular oxygen tension (probe) measurements. (From Malalis et al,[13] with permission.)

system using current technology will be developed for intra-arterial use. The fluorescence quenching optode technology is much more promising for this application.

Optode

From the previous discussion on optode theory, it would be expected that this method of measuring oxygen tension can be more easily miniaturized. Several recent studies have examined the accuracy of 0.5 mm diameter PO_2 optodes.[19] These fiberoptic sensors will fit through a 22 gauge catheter, although the studies cited have reported results only with 20 gauge catheters. Figure 11-5 is a scattergram plot of intra-arterial optode PO_2 versus arterial sampled PaO_2 in 12 patients during surgery. The bias and precision over the range from 0 to 700 mmHg are -1.1 ± 19 mmHg.[19] For data in the range from 0 to 150 mmHg, the bias and precision are 3.74 ± 11.7 mmHg. Because of the small diameter of these optode sensors, problems with arterial pressure monitoring and blood sampling have been reduced. Studies of long duration to evaluate drift are yet to be published, but it is anticipated that optode sensors may have problems similar to

those noted with the Clark electrodes, ie, thrombus formation and underestimation of PaO_2.

Noninvasive PO_2 Monitoring: Transcutaneous PO_2

In 1972, two European researchers reported that when a Clark electrode was heated and placed on the skin surface of a newborn infant, the PO_2 values obtained were very similar to arterial PO_2.[20,21] Over the next decade, this technique, known as *transcutaneous oxygen monitoring*, became routine in the care of premature infants, who are at risk of both hypoxia and hyperoxia.[22,23] In the late 1970s, it was found that transcutaneous PO_2 ($PtcO_2$) values were significantly lower than PaO_2 values during conditions of hemodynamic instability.[24,25] Although this discovery lessened the usefulness of $PtcO_2$ as an arterial oxygen tension monitor, it provided the user with a valuable indicator of peripheral perfusion (ischemic hypoxia). This blood flow dependence of $PtcO_2$ has also been illustrated in several animal studies of shock and resuscitation.[26,27]

$PtcO_2$ is the oxygen tension of heated skin. To obtain a measurable PO_2 at the skin surface with a fast re-

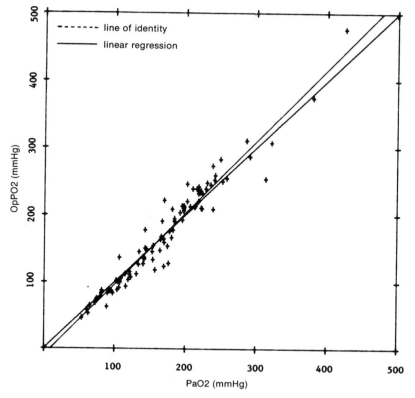

Fig. 11-5. Arterial oxygen tension determined by optode (OpPO₂) versus arterial oxygen tension determined by blood gas analysis (PaO₂). There are 96 data points. (From Barker and Tremper,[19] with permission.)

sponse time, the skin temperature must be at least 43°C. This heating causes several changes in the various layers of the skin. The stratum corneum, composed of lipid in a protein matrix, is normally a very efficient barrier to gas transport. When heated above 41°C, the structural characteristics of this layer change, allowing gases to readily diffuse through it.[28,29] In the epidermis, heating causes vasodilation of the dermal capillaries, which tends to "arterialize" the capillary blood. The perfusion of this hyperemic epidermal capillary bed is also dependent on adequate blood flow to the dermal vasculature. Consequently, a decrease in cardiac output will lead to a decrease in skin blood flow and, hence, in oxygen delivery to the transcutaneous sensor. Figure 11-6 illustrates the relationship between PaO_2 and $PtcO_2$ during induced hypoxemia (hypoxemic hypoxia) followed by hemorrhagic shock (ischemic hypoxia) in an animal study.[26] During the shock state, $PtcO_2$ fell with decreasing cardiac output even though PaO_2 was relatively unchanged (Fig. 11-6). This effect of cardiac output on the $PtcO_2$-PaO_2 relationship can be quantitated

in terms of the transcutaneous oxygen index:

$$PtcO_2 \text{ Index} = PtcO_2/PaO_2 \qquad (6)$$

$PtcO_2$ index has been used as an indicator of peripheral oxygen delivery, analogous to the alveolar-to-arterial PO_2 ratio for the assessment of pulmonary function.[30] Table 11-1 lists the mean values of the $PtcO_2$ index as a function of cardiac index found in adult intensive care unit patients. Under stable hemodynamic conditions, the normal $PtcO_2$ index for adult patients in this study was 0.8, but it fell to 0.49 when the cardiac index dropped to less than 2.2 L/min/m².[31] In the early work on newborn infants, $PtcO_2$ was found to be similar to PaO_2; ie, the $PtcO_2$ index was approximately 1.0.[20,21] A review of the published $PtcO_2$ values on hemodynamically stable patients in various age groups reveals that $PtcO_2$ index decreases progressively with age from premature infants to elderly patients (Table 11-1). Glenski and Cucchiara found that $PtcO_2$ index is relatively independent of probe location as long as the probe is on the central body rather than the extremities.[31] $PtcO_2$ index may

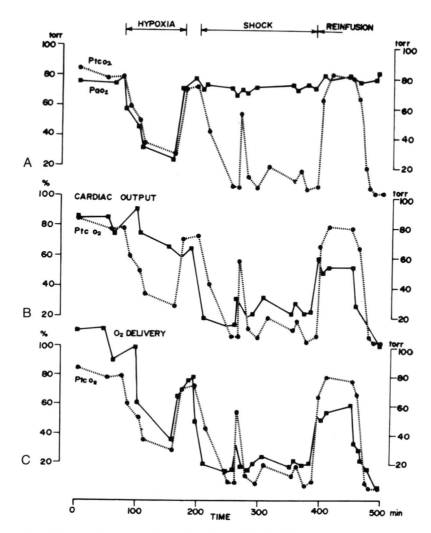

Fig. 11-6. Hypoxia and hypovolemic shock study in dogs. **(A)** Serial transcutaneous oxygen tension (PTcO₂) and arterial oxygen tension (PaO₂); **(B)** PTcO₂ and cardiac output; **(C)** PTcO₂ and oxygen delivery throughout a representative experiment. Note that PTcO₂ values follow the PaO₂ values during hypoxia, but not during shock, and that PTcO₂ values follow cardiac output during shock, but not during hypoxia. However, PTcO₂ values most closely follow oxygen delivery throughout the entire experiment. (From Tremper et al,[26] with permission.)

be slightly higher in female adult patients.[31] PTcO₂ is, therefore, a continuous, noninvasive measure of peripheral tissue oxygen tension. It will follow changes in PaO₂ under conditions of hemodynamic stability, and it will decrease relative to PaO₂ as cardiac output falls below the normal range.

There are several practical considerations and limitations that must be kept in mind when monitoring PTcO₂. Since the PTcO₂ electrode is heated above body temperature, there is a possibility of producing electrode-sized skin burns. Every time a PTcO₂ sensor is

applied to the skin, it will produce a red, hyperemic area that usually disappears within 24 hours after electrode removal. No study has reported the incidence of burns from transcutaneous electrodes as a function of probe temperature and duration of application. From the experience of frequent users of the technique, the following guidelines are suggested. For premature infants, an electrode temperature of 43.0° to 43.5°C is used and the electrode location is changed every 2 to 4 hours. For older children and adults, an electrode temperature of 44°C is used and the site is

TABLE 11-1. **Changes in P$_{TC}$O$_2$ Index with Age and Cardiac Output**

	P$_{TC}$O$_2$ Index (P$_{TC}$O$_2$/P$_a$O$_2$)
Age group	
Premature infants	1.14[a]
Newborn	1.0 [a]
Pediatric	0.84[a]
Adult	0.8 [a]
Older adult (65 years or older)	0.7 [a]
Cardiac index (L/min/m²)	
>2.2	0.8 [b]
1.5 to 2.2	0.5 [b]
<1.5	0.1 [b]

[a] These values have a standard deviation of approximately 0.1.

[b] These data are from adult patients.

changed every 4 to 6 hours. From personal intraoperative experience on adult patients, a 44°C electrode may be left in one location for as long as 8 hours with a very low incidence (<0.1 percent) of blister formation. Although 45°C has been used in the past, this higher electrode temperature is not needed for adequate function and it significantly increases the incidence of burns.

As with any Clark electrode, the P$_{TC}$O$_2$ sensor must be properly calibrated and maintained. The zero point on the P$_{TC}$O$_2$ electrode (PO$_2$ = 0 mmHg) is usually extremely stable and requires calibration only on a monthly basis. The high PO$_2$ calibration usually employs room air, and this should be rechecked prior to each application on the skin. Current P$_{TC}$O$_2$ electrodes have miniaturized electrolyte reservoirs to bathe the electrode, and 12 to 25 μm-thick membranes covering them. These small electrolyte reservoirs carry about one drop (0.05 mL) of electrolyte. Since the electrode is heated to 44°C, the electrolyte will evaporate more quickly than in the 37°C Clark electrode found in a blood gas analyzer. The electrolyte and membrane should, therefore, be checked daily and usually require replacement at least once a week. If the high PO$_2$ calibration point drifts more than 1 percent per hour, the membrane should be replaced.

In 1971, Severinghaus et al reported that halothane was reduced at the cathode of the Clark electrode, producing a dramatic upward drift of the PO$_2$ reading.[32] Since the halothane exposure of the Clark electrode in a blood gas analyzer is very small, little calibration drift is noted during intermittent blood gas analysis. On the other hand, the P$_{TC}$O$_2$ sensor is applied directly and continuously to the skin surface, where there is an opportunity for significant halothane interference. This problem was investigated in vitro by Muravchick, who reported that direct exposure of a transcutaneous electrode to 3 percent halothane caused an upward drift of 50 mmHg.[33] This problem was investigated in the operating room by measuring P$_{TC}$O$_2$ calibration drift after anesthetics involving halothane, enflurane, isoflurane, nitrous oxide, and local anesthesia. A statistically significant drift of 0.7 mmHg/h was noted in the zero-point calibration for the patients who had halothane anesthesia.[34] This drift is clinically insignificant, and is within the manufacturer's specifications for the electrode. These data were collected with an electrode covered by a 25 μm Teflon membrane. There has been more recent clinical experience with combination transcutaneous O$_2$ and CO$_2$ electrodes, in which the membrane is 12.5 μm Teflon. In these probes, the P$_{TC}$O$_2$ value exhibits a clinically significant upward drift in the presence of halothane anesthesia.

Most of the P$_{TC}$O$_2$ clinical data have been collected using a sensor on the chest or abdomen. There is a significant site-to-site variation of P$_{TC}$O$_2$ values; approximately 10 percent variation occurs even with adjacent locations. Lower values are found on the extremities even in the absence of peripheral vascular disease. After being placed on the skin surface, a P$_{TC}$O$_2$ sensor requires at least 8 to 10 minutes to equilibrate before yielding a steady value. In some circumstances, it may take as long as 20 minutes for complete equilibration. This may present a problem for intraoperative monitoring, especially in cases of short duration or when the sensor site must be changed during the procedure. Another limitation to intraoperative use is that the sensor should be placed in a location visible to the user. If the sensor becomes dislodged from the skin surface, it will indicate room air PO$_2$ (approximately 159 mmHg at sea level). Furthermore, if the sensor is beneath the surgical drapes, it may be under external pressure, which produces falsely low P$_{TC}$O$_2$ values due to compression of the dermal capillaries.

Noninvasive PO$_2$ Monitoring: Conjunctival PO$_2$

When the eyes are closed, the cornea receives its oxygen supply from the palpebral conjunctiva. This inner layer of the eyelid is well vascularized and has few cell layers between the capillaries and the mucous surface. The blood supply to the palpebral conjunctiva is derived from a branch of the ophthalmic artery, which in turn is a branch of the ipsilateral internal carotid artery. To measure PO$_2$ on this well-perfused surface, miniaturized Clark electrodes have been made to fit inside a polymethylmethacrylate ocular conformer ring. This conformer directly applies the Clark electrode to the inner surface of the palpebral conjunctiva. The electrode is not heated and, therefore, measures the surface oxygen directly from the tissue. This device is a true tissue oxygen monitor; unlike PtcO$_2$, its values are not perturbed by heating.

There are several advantages to this technique. First, since the probe is not heated, it requires only 60 seconds to equilibrate with the local tissue PO$_2$. Second, since the blood supply is from the carotid artery, this monitor may detect changes in carotid blood flow.[35] Conjunctival PO$_2$ (PcjO$_2$) is another measurement of tissue oxygenation, and its values will depend on both PaO$_2$ and cardiac output in the same manner that was described above for PtcO$_2$.[36-38] Therefore, PcjO$_2$ values are also divided by PaO$_2$ to yield an index analogous to the transcutaneous O$_2$ index. The PcjO$_2$ index is then a measurement of perfusion of conjunctival tissue. The normal PcjO$_2$ index is reported to be 0.6 to 0.7, with lower values in elderly patients.[39,40] The index progressively decreases with decreasing blood volume or cardiac output in a manner similar to PtcO$_2$.[36] Clinical studies have demonstrated that a PcjO$_2$ index of less than 0.5 is associated with a blood volume deficit of at least 15 percent.[41]

The practical limitations of conjunctival oxygen monitoring are also the same as transcutaneous monitoring: electrode maintenance, calibration, and anesthetic (halothane) interference. The PcjO$_2$ sensor does not produce burns or require a 10 minute warm-up time, but, since the monitor is placed on the eye, there is a potential for injury to this sensitive tissue. To date, clinical studies have not reported serious problems with eye damage.

HEMOGLOBIN SATURATION MEASUREMENTS

Hemoglobin Saturation Versus Oxygen Saturation

Oxygen saturation is defined as the blood oxygen content divided by the oxygen capacity times 100 percent. As discussed earlier, oxygen content was originally measured volumetrically by the method of Van Slyke and Neills.[1] The oxygen capacity is defined as the oxygen content of the blood after equilibration with room air (PO$_2$ = 159 mmHg). At the time of this definition, the maximum blood oxygen content achieved clinically occurred while breathing room air, because supplemental oxygen was not available. From the oxygen content formula (Eq. 1), it is seen that this definition of oxygen saturation includes contributions from both hemoglobin-bound and dissolved oxygen. Adult blood usually contains four species of hemoglobin: oxyhemoglobin (O$_2$Hb), reduced

hemoglobin (Hb), methemoglobin (MetHb), and carboxyhemoglobin (COHb). COHb and MetHb are found in low concentrations except in pathologic states. Because these dyshemoglobins do not transport oxygen, they do not contribute to the oxygen content or to the above definition of oxygen saturation.

When spectrophotometric methods for measuring hemoglobin species concentrations became available, hemoglobin saturation could be more easily determined. The term *functional hemoglobin saturation* is defined as

$$\text{Functional SaO}_2 = \frac{\text{O}_2\text{Hb}}{\text{O}_2\text{Hb} + \text{Hb}} \times 100\% \qquad (7)$$

This definition of hemoglobin saturation does not include MetHb or COHb because they do not contribute to oxygen transport. Fractional hemoglobin saturation, also called *oxyhemoglobin fraction*, is defined as

$$\text{Fractional SaO}_2 = \frac{\text{O}_2\text{Hb}}{\text{O}_2\text{Hb} + \text{Hb} + \text{COHb} + \text{MetHb}} \qquad (8)$$

This ratio of oxyhemoglobin to total hemoglobin is the saturation used in the calculation of oxygen content and delivery (Eq. 2). It is important to remember these definitions when evaluating the clinical applications and limitations of hemoglobin saturation monitors.

Hemoglobin Saturation Measurement: Beer's Law

Spectrophotometry was first used to determine the hemoglobin concentration of blood in the 1930s.[42] This method is based on the Lambert-Beer law, which relates the concentration of a solute to the intensity of light transmitted through the solution (Fig. 11-7):

$$I_{trans} = I_{in}e^{-DC}\,\alpha_\lambda \qquad (9)$$

where I_{trans} = intensity of transmitted light,
I_{in} = intensity of incident light,
D = distance light is transmitted through the liquid,
C = concentration of the solute (hemoglobin), and
α_λ = extinction coefficient of the solute (a constant for a given solute at a specific light wavelength α_λ).*

Thus, if a known solute is dissolved in a clear solvent in a transparent cuvette of known dimensions, the sol-

---

* This law further states that the exponent DC represents multiple solutes in solution and is the sum of the absorbances of the various solutes times their respective concentrations, eg, $D(C_1\,\alpha_1 + C_2\,\alpha_2 + C_3\,\alpha_3)$.

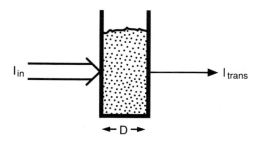

$$I_{trans} = I_{in}e^{-(D \times C \times \alpha_\lambda)}$$

I_{trans} = intensity of light transmitted

I_{in} = intensity of incident light

D = distance light is transmitted through the liquid

C = concentration of solute (oxyhemoglobin)

α_λ = extinction coefficient of the solute (a constant)

Fig. 11-7. The concentration of a solute dissolved in a solvent can be calculated from the logarithmic relationship between the incident and transmitted light intensity and the solute concentration (Beer's law). (From Tremper and Barker,[131] with permission.)

ute concentration can be calculated if the incident and transmitted light intensity are measured (Fig. 11-8). The extinction coefficient α_λ is independent of the concentration, but is a function of the light wavelength used (Fig. 11-9).

Laboratory oximeters use this principle to determine hemoglobin concentration by measuring the intensity of light transmitted through a hemoglobin dispersion produced from lysed red blood cells.[43] For each wavelength of light used, an independent Lambert-Beer equation (Eq. 9) can be written. If the number of equations is equal to the number of solutes (ie, hemoglobin species), then the concentration of each can be determined. Therefore, to determine the concentrations of four species of hemoglobin, at least four wavelengths of light are required. For the Lambert-Beer equation to be valid, both the solvent and cuvette must be transparent at the light wavelengths used, the light path length must be known exactly, and no other absorbers can be present in the solution. It is difficult to fulfill all of these requirements in clinical devices. Consequently, although these devices are theoretically based on the Lambert-Beer law, they also require empiric corrections to improve their accuracy.

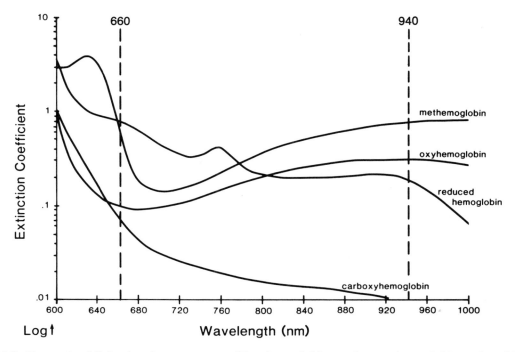

Fig. 11-8. Transmitted light absorbance spectra of four hemoglobin species: oxyhemoglobin, reduced hemoglobin, carboxyhemoglobin, and methemoglobin. (From Barker and Tremper,[132] with permission.)

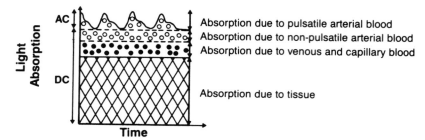

Fig. 11-9. Schematic illustration of the light absorption through living tissue. The AC signal is due to the pulsatile component off the arterial blood, while the DC signal comprises all the nonpulsatile absorbers in the tissue: nonpulsatile arterial blood, nonpulsatile venous and capillary blood, and all other tissues. (Adapted from Ohmeda Pulse Oximeter Model 3700 Service Manual,[133] with permission.)

Invasive Hemoglobin Saturation Monitoring

Mixed venous oxygen tension ($P\bar{v}O_2$) and hemoglobin saturation ($S\bar{v}O_2$) reflect global tissue oxygenation and the ability of the cardiopulmonary system to transport sufficient oxygen to meet body needs (Eq. 3). This physiologic principle implies that continuous mixed venous oxygen monitoring should have great clinical utility. In 1973, a fiberoptic system was reported to accurately monitor mixed venous hemoglobin saturation in humans.[44] This device used optical fibers incorporated into a pulmonary artery catheter to estimate the hemoglobin saturation by measuring reflected light. Light at red and infrared wavelengths was transmitted down one set of fibers, while the reflected light from intact circulating red blood cells was transmitted back via other fibers to an external photodetector.[44] Although this first system appeared to work, it was not commercially produced due to the technical difficulty of inserting a pulmonary artery catheter made relatively stiff by the inclusion of fiberoptic bundles. In the late 1970s, Oximetrix, Inc. (a division of Abbott Laboratories) developed two fiberoptic reflectance systems for measuring hemoglobin saturation. The first system, introduced in 1977, employed a 7-Fr, double-lumen umbilical artery catheter to be used in monitoring critically ill neonates.[45] The second sysetm, introduced in 1981, used a 7.5-Fr pulmonary artery catheter capable of thermodilution cardiac output measurements as well as continuous mixed venous saturation monitoring.[46] These new systems used three wavelengths of light (670, 700, and 800 nm) to calculate saturation. It was stated that a minimum of four wavelengths are required to calculate hemoglobin saturation from Beer's law in the presence of MetHb and COHb. The Oximetrix mixed venous saturation monitor can accurately measure functional hemoglobin saturation in the absence of

significant dyshemoglobin concentrations.[46] However, a recent experimental study has shown that methemoglobinemia produces large errors in the saturation measurement.[47] American Edwards Corporation has also produced a mixed venous saturation pulmonary artery catheter that uses two wavelengths of light. This device requires manual entry of the total hemoglobin to improve accuracy, whereas the Oximetrix system accurately measures mixed venous saturation over a wide range of hematocrits.[48,49]

Continuous $S\bar{v}O_2$ monitoring can detect any acute changes in the relationship of oxygen delivery to oxygen consumption. Therefore, $S\bar{v}O_2$ monitors have been recommended for cardiac surgery and in other critically ill patients at risk of acute cardiopulmonary decompensation.[50–52] $S\bar{v}O_2$ monitoring will not determine the source of an imbalance between oxygen delivery and consumption, nor will it detect regional ischemia. $S\bar{v}O_2$ monitoring also requires the insertion of a pulmonary artery catheter and, hence, will be inappropriate for many patients.

Noninvasive Hemoglobin Saturation Monitoring: Pulse Oximetry

In only a few years since its introduction to the operating room, the pulse oximeter has become a standard of care.[53,54] This technique has been rapidly accepted by the anesthesia community because it continuously and noninvasively monitors arterial oxygenation with little user effort.

Technical Development of Pulse Oximetry

The term *oximeter* was coined by Glen Millikan who, in the 1940s, developed a lightweight device for noninvasively monitoring hemoglobin saturation.[55] This device estimated saturation by transilluminating the ear with the light of two wavelengths, one in the red and one in the infrared range. The transmitted light was measured by a photodetector. This Beer's law device effectively used the earlobe as a cuvette containing hemoglobin (Fig. 11-7). Two primary technical problems with in vivo oximetry involve estimating arterial hemoglobin saturation in living tissue rather than in vitro. First, there are many light absorbers in the tissues other than hemoglobin. Second, the tissues contain not only arterial blood, but also venous and capillary blood. Millikan approached these problems by first measuring the absorbance of the ear while it was compressed to eliminate the blood. After this bloodless baseline measurement, the ear was heated to cause hyperemia and, thus, "arterialize" the blood. The difference between this absorbance signal and the baseline value was thus related to the arterial blood. This device was shown to accurately detect intraoperative desaturations in the early 1950s, but, because of technical difficulties with its use, it was never adopted as a routine clinical monitor.[56]

In the mid 1970s, a Japanese engineer named Takuo Aoyagi made an ingenious discovery. He noted that the pulsatile components of the absorbances of red and infrared light transmitted through tissue were related to arterial hemoglobin saturation.[55] This eliminated the need to heat the tissue to obtain an arterial estimate. He used two wavelengths of light, one red (660 nm), the other infrared (940 nm). Since this device relies on the detection of a pulsatile absorbance signal, it is referred to as a *pulse oximeter*. Figure 11-9 schematically illustrates the absorbers in the living tissue. At the top of the figure is the pulsatile or AC component, which is attributed to the pulsating arterial blood. The baseline or DC component represents the absorbance of the tissue bed including venous blood, capillary blood, and nonpulsatile arterial blood. All pulse oximeters assume that the only pulsatile absorbance between the light source and the photodetector is that of arterial blood. The pulse oximeter first determines the AC component of the absorbance at each wavelength and then divides this by the corresponding DC component to obtain a "pulse-added" absorbance that is independent of the incident light intensity. It then calculates the ratio of the pulse-added absorbances at the two wavelengths, which is empirically related to SaO_2:

$$R = \frac{AC_{660}/DC_{660}}{AC_{940}/DC_{940}} \qquad (10)$$

Figure 11-10 is an example of a pulse oximeter calibration curve. These curves are developed by measuring the pulse oximeter absorbance ratio R in human volunteers and simultaneously sampling arterial blood for in vitro saturation measurements. The ratio of absorbances R varies from 0.4 to 3.4 over the satu-

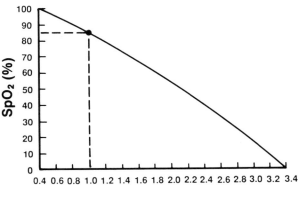

$$R = \frac{AC_{660}/DC_{660}}{AC_{940}/DC_{940}}$$

Fig. 11-10. A typical oximeter calibration curve. Note that arterial oxygen saturation (SaO_2) is estimated from the ratio (R) of the pulse-added red absorbance at 660 nm (AC_{660}/DC_{660}) to the pulse-added infrared absorbance at 940 nm (AC_{940}/DC_{940}). The ratios of red-to-infrared absorbances vary from approximately 0.4 at 100 percent saturation to 3.4 at 0 percent saturation. Note also that the ratio of red-to-infrared absorbance is 1.0 at a saturation of approximately 85 percent. Although approximate determinations of this curve can be made on a theoretic basis, accurate predictions of saturation by the oximeter (SpO_2) require experimental data. (From Tremper and Barker,[134] with permission.)

ration range of 0 to 100 percent. All values of R for saturation less than 70 percent are the result of extrapolation of experimental data. Note that an absorbance ratio of 1 : 0 corresponds to a pulse oximeter saturation (SpO_2) of approximately 85 percent.

Although the theory of the pulse oximeter is straightforward, the application of this theory to a clinically useful device engenders technical problems and physiologic limitations. One of these limitations is a consequence of Beer's law and the definitions of functional and fractional hemoglobin saturation. Being a two-wavelength device, the pulse oximeter assumes that there are only two absorbing hemoglobin species in the blood: O_2Hb and Hb. If $MetHb$ or $COHb$ are present, they will contribute to the pulse-added absorbance signal and be interpreted as either O_2Hb or Hb, or some combination of the two. Some insight into the effects of dyshemoglobins on the pulse oximeter can be gained by examining their absorbance spectra (Fig. 11-8). Note that $COHb$ absorbs very little light at 940 nm (infrared), while at 660 nm (red light), it absorbs as much as does O_2Hb. This is clinically illustrated by the fact that patients with toxicity appear red. The effects of COHb on pulse oximeter SpO_2 values have been evaluated experimentally in animals.[57] It was found that SpO_2 was roughly given by $[(O_2Hb + 0.9 \times COHb)/\text{total Hb}] \times 100$ percent.

In the case of MetHb, the extinction coefficient is high at both the red and infrared wavelengths (Fig. 11-8). Consequently, MetHb will produce a large pulse-added absorbance at both wavelengths used by the pulse oximeter. Adding a large absorbance to both the numerator and denominator of the ratio R in Equation 10 tends to force this ratio toward unity. On the pulse oximeter calibration curve (Fig. 11-10), an R of 1 corresponds to an SpO_2 of 85 percent, as noted above. The effects of MetHb have also been evaluated experimentally confirming the hypothesis that high MetHb levels will drive SpO_2 toward 85 percent regardless of the actual PaO_2 and SaO_2 values.[47]

Any substance that absorbs light at the red or infrared pulse oximeter wavelengths and is present in the arterial blood may cause errors. This effect is clinically illustrated by intravenously injected dyes. Scheller et al evaluated the effects of bolus injections of methylene blue, indigo carmine, and indocyanine green on pulse oximeter SpO_2 values in volunteers.[58] They found that methylene blue caused a fall in SpO_2 to approximately 65 percent for 1 to 2 minutes, while indigo carmine produced a very slight decrease. Indocyanine green had an intermediate effect.

With the adoption of pulse oximetry in the neonatal intensive care unit, its accuracy must be considered in the presence of fetal hemoglobin (HbF), which has a greater affinity for oxygen (ie, a lower P_{50}) than adult hemoglobin (HbA). Thus, it will become fully saturated at a lower PaO_2. In other words, the O_2Hb dissociation curve of HbF is shifted to the left from that of HbA, and the PaO_2 at a given SaO_2 will be lower for HbF. However, the extinction coefficients for HbF are similar to those of HbA, so the presence of HbF should not cause an error in SpO_2.[59,60]

Since the photodiode detectors in the pulse oximeter sensor will respond to light of any wavelength, ambient light can contaminate the light-emitting diode (LED) signal.[61–63] Most pulse oximeter designers reduce this light interference by alternately turning on the red LED and the infrared LED, then turning both LEDs off. The photodiode detects first a signal from the red LED plus room light, followed by the infrared LED plus room light, and finally the ambient room light alone when both LEDs are turned off. This sequence is repeated up to 480 times a second in an effort to subtract the room light signal in a quickly changing light background. Unfortunately, despite this clever design, room light interference can cause erroneous SpO_2 values or prevent the pulse oximeter from obtaining any SpO_2 value. This problem is alle-

viated by covering the sensor with an opaque shield, such as a dark towel.[64]

The most difficult problem in the engineering design of the pulse oximeter is the management of low signal-to-noise ratios, which arise from two sources. First, when there is a small absorbance signal due to a weak pulse, the device will automatically increase signal amplification so that it can calculate the pulse-added absorbance. Unfortunately, as the signal is amplified, the background noise is also amplified. In situations of a very weak or nonexistent pulse signal, the noise may be amplified until it is interpreted as a pulse-added absorbance. Newer pulse oximeters have signal strength lower limits, below which they will display a "low signal-strength" error message. Some devices also display an analog pulse waveform as a visual indicator of signal quality.

Because of its automatic gain control, the pulse oximeter can deal with large or small pulse signals and is relatively insensitive to changes in peripheral pulse amplitude and flow. Lawson et al objectively assessed the blood flow limits of pulse oximeter SpO_2 estimation by performing the following experiment.[65] The peripheral blood flow at the finger was measured by a laser Doppler flow probe that follows changes in red blood cell velocity. A pulse oximeter was placed on the finger adjacent to the flow probe while a blood pressure cuff was progressively inflated on the upper arm. The oximeter stopped estimating saturation and gave a "low perfusion" warning when the peripheral blood flow decreased to a mean of 8.6 percent of the control value. As the blood pressure cuff was slowly deflated from full occlusion, the pulse oximeter began to display a pulse and saturation estimate when the blood flow was only 4 percent of baseline. This study demonstrates the pulse oximeter's ability to estimate saturation over a wide range of peripheral blood flow. Clinical and experimental studies have also found that the pulse oximeter can function over a wide range of cardiac output as long as an adequate pulse is detected.[66,67]

The second major source of low signal-to-noise ratios is patient motion artifact. For recovery room and intensive care unit applications, this may be the most troublesome design problem. Most pulse oximeters use a variety of signal averaging techniques to minimize motion effects. That is, the device averages multiple pulses to obtain its SpO_2 value, thereby diminishing the effect of spurious motion signals. However, increasing the signal averaging time has a deleterious effect on the time response to acute changes in saturation. The manufacturers can also incorporate more sophisticated algorithms to discriminate motion signals from arterial pulse signals by using the rate of change of SpO_2. For example, if the calculated SpO_2 changes from 95 to 50 percent in one-tenth of a second, this new and presumably spurious saturation estimate will either be dropped from the averaging or given a lower weighting factor. As with amplified background noise, motion artifact is probably detected best by direct observation of the plethysmograph waveform.

A final limitation on pulse oximeter accuracy involves the variability of the wavelengths of light emitted by the LEDs. Although these diodes nominally emit monochromatic light at either 660 nm or 940 nm, in reality, each diode emits a slightly different wavelength spectrum. The peak or center emission wavelength can vary ± 10 nm from the specified value. As can be seen from the extinction coefficients in Figure 11-8, a shift in the source wavelength will change the measured absorbance. Since the oximeter software assumes an extinction coefficient at a specified wavelength, an unknown change in that wavelength will cause a systematic error in the saturation estimate. This results in a probe-to-probe variability in accuracy. Some manufacturers minimize this error by narrowing the acceptable wavelength tolerance on the LEDs used in their sensors. Others compensate for the error by designing the sensor to identify its specific LED wavelengths to the instrument, which then electronically corrects for shifted center wavelengths.

Accuracy and Response

Most pulse oximeters have a specified accuracy of ± 2 percent from 100 percent down to 70 percent saturation, ± 3 percent from 70 percent to 50 percent saturation, and accuracy is unspecified below 50 percent saturation.[68] This implies that the displayed SpO_2 is within 2 percent above or below the actual SaO_2 68 percent of the time (± 1 SD around the mean). This corresponds to a 99 percent confidence interval (ie, 3 SD) of ± 6 percent from 100 percent to 70 percent saturation and ± 9 percent from 70 percent to 50 percent saturation. Although these specifications are based on volunteer data collected under optimal conditions, the accuracies found in clinical studies are comparable. Studies on adult, pediatric, and neonatal patients indicate that under steady-state conditions, the pulse oximeter SpO_2 value is generally within ± 2 to 3 saturation points (± 1 SD) of actual SaO_2.[69–74]

Two recent experiments in adult volunteers evaluated the response times of pulse oximeters to sudden desaturation and resaturation.[73,74] Kagle et al measured the time for 50 percent recovery of resaturation from a hypoxic state. They used a fast (3 seconds) time averaging mode and found a 50 percent recovery time ($T_{1/2}$) of 6 seconds for the ear probe and 24 seconds for the finger probe.[73] Severinghaus and Naifeh also found that the ear probe responded to changing SaO_2 more quickly than the finger probe.[73] Their $T_{1/2}$ values

for ear probes ranged from 9.6 to 19.8 seconds, while the $T_{1/2}$ for finger probes ranged from 24 to 35.1 seconds.

Clinical Applications and Limitations of Pulse Oximetry

In 1947, Comroe and Botelho published a classic study that revealed the unreliability of direct observation for the detection of cyanosis.[75] This finding was confirmed for patients under general anesthesia in 1951.[56] With the advent of pulse oximetry, several perioperative studies have again confirmed this fact during even routine anesthetics in healthy patients.[76–81] Coté et al conducted a randomized, controlled study of 152 pediatric surgical patients who were continuously monitored with pulse oximeters.[76] In half of these patients, the pulse oximeter data were unavailable to the anesthesia team. A major desaturation event was defined to be an SpO_2 value of less than 85 percent for 30 seconds or longer. The study revealed 24 major desaturation events in the patients for whom the SpO_2 values were unavailable to the anesthesiologists, and only 11 in the patients for whom SpO_2 values were available. Most of these major events occurred in patients 2 years of age or less.[76] Raemer et al conducted a similar study on healthy outpatients during gynecologic surgery.[77] They noted severe desaturations (pulse oximeter values < 85 percent) in 5 percent of their cases.

Two studies have evaluated oxygenation by pulse oximetry during transport from the operating room to the recovery room.[78,79] Pullerits et al monitored 71 healthy pediatric patients during transport without supplemental oxygen and found that 28.1 percent had SpO_2 values ≤ 90 percent, while in only 45 percent of these patients was cyanosis clinically observed.[79] In a similar study of adults, Tyler et al found that 12 percent of the patients experienced saturation values ≤ 85 percent during transport.[79] Both studies concluded that all patients should receive supplemental oxygen during transport to the recovery room.

Two studies of recovery room patients have again emphasized the fact that clinical abilities to detect hypoxemia are poor. Soliman et al compared pulse oximeter SpO_2 values with postanesthesia recovery (PAR) scores in children.[80] These PAR scores are based on motor activity, respiratory effort, blood pressure, level of consciousness, and skin color. They found no correlation between PAR scores and SpO_2 values in these healthy pediatric patients. Morris et al evaluated adult patients in the recovery room by measuring SpO_2 on admission, 5 minutes after admission, 30 minutes after admission, and, finally, just before discharge.[81] Of the 149 patients studied, 14 percent had episodes of desaturation (SpO_2 < 90 percent). Curiously, the highest incidence of desaturation was at the time of discharge from the recovery room. Both of these studies concluded that patients in the recovery room should be continuously monitored with pulse oximeters or at least tested as part of routine discharge criteria.

There are two general categories of limitations of pulse oximetry. First, the hemoglobin saturation provides limited information on oxygen transport status. Saturation does not imply oxygen content unless the total hemoglobin is known. Furthermore, saturation values do not reveal the trends in arterial oxygen tension until the latter drops below 75 to 80 mmHg. Thus, there may be large intraoperative changes in PaO_2 that are not detected by pulse oximetry. Furthermore, the pulse oximeter detects a pulse but not peripheral perfusion. The pulse oximeter is designed to be insensitive to changes in perfusion via its automatic gain control. The presence or absence of a pulse will be quickly detected, but a pulse does not ensure adequate blood flow.

The second set of limitations of pulse oximetry are the technical problems discussed above, which involve errors in the saturation estimates or the inability to obtain an adequate signal. Sources of error in SpO_2 include intravenous dyes, dyshemoglobins, motion artifact, ambient light artifact, and probe wavelength variability. Inadequate signal strength may be due to low cardiac output, cold extremities, or severe peripheral vascular disease. A recent study found that the overall incidence of failure to generate an SpO_2 in clinical use was approximately 1.2 percent.[82] In older patients with a higher incidence of peripheral vascular disease, the failure rate rose to 4.25 percent.[82]

Pulse oximetry has already been adopted as a standard in monitoring during anesthesia. It is now being adopted as routine monitoring in the recovery room, the intensive care unit, and other settings where supplemental oxygen is required or the possibility of cardiopulmonary compromise is significant. As the pulse oximeter is so easy to use and provides data continuously and noninvasively, it is difficult to find an argument not to use one in any acute care setting.

VENTILATION: CARBON DIOXIDE MEASUREMENT AND MONITORING

Basic Carbon Dioxide Transport: Dead Space and the Capnogram

Although auscultation and observation may detect the presence or absence of ventilation, its adequacy must be confirmed by a normal arterial blood carbon dioxide tension ($PaCO_2$). CO_2 transport differs from oxygen transport in that the net transport of CO_2 is in the opposite direction, ie, from the tissues to the lungs and hence to the atmosphere. The normal arterial carbon dioxide content ($CaCO_2$) is 48 vol % (48 mL CO_2/100 mL blood). CO_2 is carried in the blood by three basic mechanisms: dissolved in plasma, bound to protein (hemoglobin), and transported as bicarbonate ion. CO_2 attaches to the terminal amino group on the globulin portion of the hemoglobin molecule, forming carbamino hemoglobin. Since carbamino hemoglobin contributes only a small portion of the total CO_2 content of blood (approximately 1.5 vol % of the total 50 vol %), hemoglobin CO_2 saturation does not have the same significance as hemoglobin O_2 saturation. The majority of carbon dioxide is carried in the form of bicarbonate ion. The usual venous CO_2 content ($C\bar{v}CO_2$) is 52 vol %, corresponding to a $P\bar{v}CO_2$ of 44 mmHg. Arterial blood thus picks up approximately 4 mL of carbon dioxide/100 mL of blood perfusing the tissue. The ratio of 4 vol % CO_2 picked up in the tissue to the 5 vol % of oxygen released to the tissue results in the accepted respiratory quotient value of 0.8. To remain at equilibrium with respect to CO_2, the lungs must ventilate 4 mL of CO_2 to the atmosphere for every 100 mL of blood flow. Due to the greater solubility of CO_2 in water (approximately 20 times that of oxygen) and the body's ability to store CO_2 in the form of bicarbonate ion, the total amount of carbon dioxide in the body is approximately 100 times that of oxygen.[83]

The rate at which CO_2 is removed from the body is dependent on the ventilation of well-perfused alveoli. To understand CO_2 removal, the concept of dead space must first be understood. Physiologic dead space is defined as that portion of the tidal volume that does not participate in CO_2 exchange.

$$V_T = V_D + V_A \qquad (11)$$

where V_T = tidal volume,

V_D = physiologic dead space volume, and

V_A = alveolar volume.

V_A is assumed to be ideal alveolar gas from well-perfused alveoli. The CO_2 tension in this alveolar gas ($PACO_2$) is nearly equal to $PaCO_2$. At the turn of the century, Bohr derived an equation for the ratio of the V_D to the V_T, based on the simple assumption that the total CO_2 leaving the mouth equals the CO_2 leaving the alveolar volume. Using the fact that CO_2 concentration in the gas phase is proportional to CO_2 tension,

$$V_T \times P_{ME}CO_2 = V_A \times PACO_2 \qquad (12)$$

$P_{ME}CO_2$ is the mixed expired carbon dioxide tension in a tidal volume. That is, if a patient expires one V_T into a bag, $P_{ME}CO_2$ is the CO_2 tension in that bag. Equation 11 can be solved for V_A and substituted into Equation 12, producing

$$V_T \times P_{ME}CO_2 = (V_T - V_D) \times P_ACO_2 \qquad (13)$$

If it is assumed that $P_ACO_2 = PaCO_2$, Equation 13 can be solved for $\frac{V_D}{V_T}$:

$$\frac{V_D}{V_T} = \frac{PaCO_2 - P_{ME}CO_2}{PaCO_2} \qquad (14)$$

Using Equation 14, clinicians can determine the "wasted ventilation" (V_D) by measuring $P_{ME}CO_2$ and analyzing an arterial blood sample for $PaCO_2$. This derivation assumes there is no CO_2 in the inspired gas.

In the 1920s, Ailken and Clark-Kennedy measured the concentration of CO_2 in the expired gas during the respiratory cycle.[84] Analysis of this expired CO_2 waveform (capnogram) requires a more detailed understanding of dead space. Physiologic dead space is divided into three components: apparatus dead space (V_{app}), anatomical dead space (V_{an}), and alveolar dead space (V_{AD}).[83]

$$V_D = V_{app} + V_{an} + V_{AD} \qquad (15)$$

Apparatus dead space is that part of the V_T contained within the breathing apparatus. For a circular anesthetic circuit, this is any part of the apparatus on the patient's side of the "Y" connector. Anatomic dead space is the volume within the trachea and all the conducting airways. Alveolar dead space consists of those alveoli that are ventilated but not perfused. Figure 11-11 illustrates the effect of each of these components of dead space on the capnogram. The first gas to

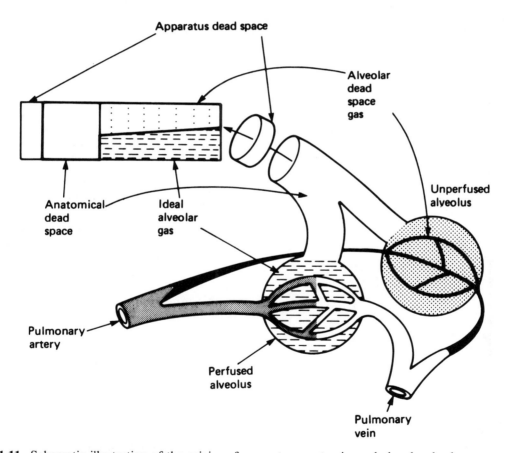

Fig. 11-11. Schematic illustration of the origins of apparatus, anatomic, and alveolar dead space and how they affect the capnogram. The apparatus and anatomic dead space are expired sequentially at the beginning of expiration and are referred to as *series dead space*. When alveolar gas reaches the detector, there is an abrupt rise to a plateau. Note that this plateau is composed of gas from the alveolar dead space (nonperfused alveoli) and "ideal" alveolar gas. The proportions of each will produce the resultant alveolar plateau value of the capnogram. (From Nunn,[83] with permission.)

be expired is the gas left within the breathing apparatus at the end of inspiration (V_{app}). This gas has the same CO_2 tension as that of the inspired gas, which is usually zero. Following the V_{app}, the V_{an} is expired, which also should contain no CO_2. Finally, the gas from the alveoli is expired, which contains both V_{AD} and V_A. These two alveolar gases mix and the resulting PCO_2 are a function of the relative volume of each and the $PaCO_2$. As this alveolar gas reaches the airway, the expired CO_2 abruptly rises to this mixed value, forming the alveolar plateau.[83] On inspiration, the PCO_2 in the airway drops to zero (assuming the inspired PCO_2 is zero). If there were no alveolar dead space, then the end-expired PCO_2 value would approximately equal $PaCO_2$. If half of the alveolar volume were alveolar dead space and the other half were well-perfused alveoli, the end-expired value should equal approximately one-half the $PaCO_2$. The difference between $PaCO_2$ and the end-expired plateau PCO_2 value (end-tidal PCO_2 [$PetCO_2$]) is thus proportional to the alveolar dead space.

Figure 11-12 shows a normal capnogram, ie, expired CO_2 tension as a function of time. During early expiration, which is referred to as phase I, the PCO_2 value is zero (as V_{app} and V_{an} are expired). As alveolar gas begins to reach the CO_2 detector at the mouth, the PCO_2 value quickly rises to reach the alveolar plateau. This quickly rising portion is referred to as phase II of the capnogram, and results from a mixture of V_{AD}, V_A, and V_{an}. The final plateau (phase III) is achieved when only alveolar gas is being expired.

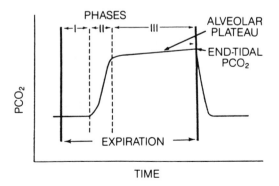

Fig. 11-12. The three phases of a normal capnogram. Phase I is series dead space, the length of which depends on the amount of apparatus and anatomic dead space. Phase II is a mixture of anatomic series and alveolar parallel dead space gas. Phase III (the alveolar plateau) is produced by a mixture of ideal alveolar gas from well-perfused alveoli and alveolar dead space gas from unperfused alveoli.

Alveolar dead space implies a ventilation-to-perfusion ratio ($\dot{V}/\dot{Q}$) of infinity, ie, no perfusion. In this model, it is assumed that all alveoli are either well perfused (ideal alveoli with a PCO_2 equal to $PaCO_2$) or unperfused (alveolar dead space with no CO_2 exchange). In reality, the lung is composed of many units having various $\dot{V}/\dot{Q}$ ratios. The apparatus and anatomic dead spaces are "series" dead spaces because they are sequentially expired before the alveolar gas, while the alveolar dead space is "parallel" dead space because it is expired at the same time as the ideal alveolar gas (Fig. 11-11).

From the above discussion, it can be concluded that to obtain a normal capnogram, there must be metabolism to produce CO_2, circulation to transport CO_2 from the tissues to the lungs, and ventilation. Because continuous capnography noninvasively monitors these vital functions, it is an extremely useful clinical tool in the care of anesthetized patients. Deviations from the normal size or shape of the capnogram should be immediately investigated. A depressed or absent capnogram may be a sign of disconnection of the ventilator circuit, cardiac arrest, pulmonary embolism, or a dislodged, misplaced, or obstructed endotracheal tube. The presence of a capnogram is the quickest and most certain way of preventing undiagnosed esophageal intubation. Although there may be CO_2 in the stomach, it will produce a very low amplitude capnogram, which disappears after several breaths. A normal capnogram may be absent after a proper endotracheal intubation if there is no circulation, an obstructed endotracheal tube, or a disconnect in the capnometer itself. A depressed alveolar plateau and $PetCO_2$ value can be caused by any increase in the alveolar dead space. During anesthesia, this is frequently due to hypotension, which produces more high $\dot{V}/\dot{Q}$ units (West's zone I) of the lung. Increases in the height of the capnogram can reflect either increases in metabolism relative to ventilation (malignant hyperthermia or fever) or the addition of CO_2 to the circulation (bicarbonate injection, CO_2 insufflation for laparoscopy, or release of a tourniquet). CO_2 rebreathing is detected as a non-zero baseline during the inspiratory phase. Because capnometers can detect serious airway and circulatory complications on a breath-to-breath basis, they have become a standard of care during anesthesia.

Measurement of CO_2 Tension in Blood

The polio epidemic of the 1950s spurred the development of the rapid measurement of arterial blood carbon dioxide tension. In 1958, John Severinghaus presented the first blood gas analyzer, using a Clarke PO_2 electrode and a new PCO_2 electrode of his own

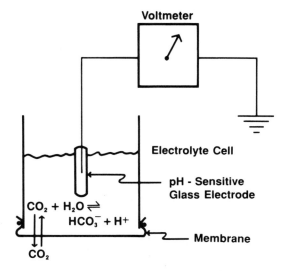

Fig. 11-13. Schematic of a Severinghaus PCO_2 electrode. (From Tremper and Waxman,[135] with permission.)

design.[86] The Severinghaus-Stowe PCO_2 electrode consists of a pH-sensitive glass electrode in an electrolyte cell surrounded by a CO_2-permeable membrane (Fig. 11-13). CO_2 diffuses through the membrane into the cell and reacts with water, producing carbonic acid, which lowers the pH within the cell. The pH electrode is then calibrated to indicate PCO_2. This "secondary sensing" PCO_2 electrode is currently used in all blood gas analyzers. Like the oxygen electrode, the Severinghaus-Stowe CO_2 electrode has also been used to continuously monitor carbon dioxide tension on heated skin: $PTcCO_2$.

Because the PCO_2 electrode is a membrane-covered glass pH electrode, it is fragile and has, therefore, never been clinically applied to continuous invasive CO_2 monitoring. On the other hand, photoluminescent dyes, which are pH sensitive, are available. These dyes can be used to construct pH-sensitive optodes, employing the same design principles as the oxygen optodes discussed earlier. The pH optode can also be adapted to measure PCO_2 by the secondary sensing technique used in the Severinghaus CO_2 electrode. CO_2 as well as O_2 optodes have been inserted in the extracorporeal circuit for continuous monitoring during cardiopulmonary bypass.[87,88] The continuous PCO_2 values were found to accurately follow trends of $PaCO_2$, with a 2- to 3-minute 90 percent response time, although the absolute accuracy was less than that of in vitro laboratory blood gas analysis. Initial studies of intra-arterial PCO_2 optodes have found similar results.[90–92]

CO₂ Measurement in the Gas Phase: Mass Spectrometry, Raman Scattering, and Infrared Absorption

Although CO_2 optodes and the Severinghaus-Stowe electrode will measure PCO_2 in either the liquid or gas phase, their response time is relatively slow (2- to 3-minute 90 percent response time). To obtain an accurate real-time tracing of PCO_2 from the airway (a capnogram), the measurement must have a response time of 50 to 100 ms or better. Three technologies have been used in clinical capnometers: mass spectrometry, Raman scattering, and infrared absorption.

Mass Spectrometry

A mass spectrometer measures the concentrations of various constituents in a gas mixture by first ionizing the components then separating them on the basis of charge-to-mass ratio.[92] Ionizing is accomplished by aspirating a sample of gas into a high-vacuum chamber and bombarding it with a stream of electrons. The high-energy electrons form ionized fragments of the gas molecules, which are then accelerated by an electric field. A magnetic field oriented perpendicular to the ion trajectories will deflect the particles by an amount proportional to their charge-to-mass ratio. An ion collector then measures the current produced by the stream of separated ions, thereby determining the relative proportion of each type of particle (Fig. 11-14).

The magnetic field in a clinical mass spectrometer can be applied to the ion stream in one of two ways. The quadrapole spectrometer produces an oscillating magnetic field whose frequency is continuously varied through a range of interest. This allows the use of only one ion detector, which collects particles of various charge-to-mass ratios as a function of magnetic field frequency. In contrast, the magnetic sector spectrometer varies the intensity of the magnetic field, again allowing the use of one ion collector to measure the current of particles with various charge-to-mass ratios. Whichever method is used to apply the magnetic field, all mass spectrometers have several properties in common. First, they use high-vacuum chambers (internal pressure $< 10^{-10}$ atmospheres). Second, they are able to identify and measure a wide variety of substances within the gas stream, ie, all respiratory gases, including inert gases (such as helium), and anesthetic vapors and gases. Third, mass spectrometers are relatively large, expensive devices, and, therefore, have been, until recently, used to simultaneously monitor multiple operating rooms in a time-sharing mode (Fig. 11-14).[92,93] While time sharing allows one mass spectrometer to serve multiple patients, it also

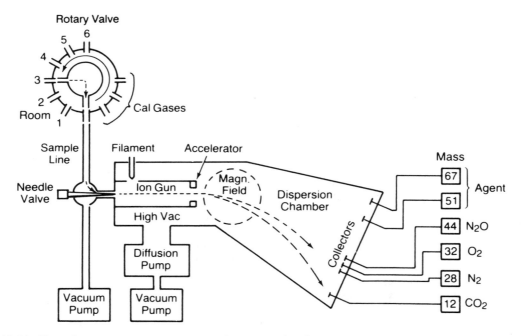

Fig. 11-14. Shared mass spectrometer-magnetic sector with fixed detectors. Patient gases and calibration gases are sequentially sampled by means of a rotary valve. A low flow into the mass spectrometer is controlled by a needle valve or molecular leak. Here the gas molecules are charged and fragmented by an electron beam, accelerated in an electric field, and dispersed in a magnetic field. Discrete detectors in the focal plane (collectors) measure the component gases. Carbon dioxide is measured as C^+, and nitrous oxide as N_2O^+. Anesthetic agents are identified by the ratio of fragments with masses 67/51. (From Gravenstein et al,[92] with permission.)

creates a problem with respect to continuous capnogaphy. For example, if eight rooms are monitored, each room will have a continuous capnogram only one-eighth of the time. Less expensive portable "mini" mass spectrometers that can be dedicated to individual rooms are now available.[94]

Raman Spectrometry

Raman spectrometry is an analytic technique that has recently been applied to clinical medicine.[95] Raman scattering is a light absorption and reemission phenomenon that occurs when photons from a high-energy laser beam strike gas molecules. In a small percentage of the photon-molecule interactions, the molecules are energized into an unstable state. These molecules emit a spectrum of photons as they relax into a more stable state. The majority of the laser light passes through the gas sample without producing Raman scattering. The Raman-scattered light spectrum is usually measured at right angles to the laser beam, as illustrated in Figure 11-15. In theory, Raman scattering can be used to identify nearly all types of molecules in a gas stream. However, it cannot identify

monatomic gases because it requires the presence of a bond between two atoms. For practical purposes, Raman spectrometry can identify anything of clinical interest except helium. Probably the most costly and troublesome aspect of a Raman-scattering spectrometer is the necessity of a high-energy laser light source. This laser not only has a limited lifetime, but also consumes a lot of electrical power (20 A at 120 VAC) and generates significant heat that is dissipated to the room. The current cost of the available clinical device is similar to that of the "mini" mass spectrometer, which makes it feasible for use as a dedicated monitor in each operating room.

Infrared Absorption Spectrometry

Although mass spectrometers and Raman-scattering spectrometers are often used as capnometers, the infrared absorption technique is most commonly used in clinical practice. CO_2 absorbs infrared light at approximately 4.3 μm, as seen in Figure 11-16.[92] As with other absorption spectrophotometers, the infrared CO_2 analyzer is based on the Lambert-Beer law (Eq. 9). Figure 11-17 schematically illustrates a double-

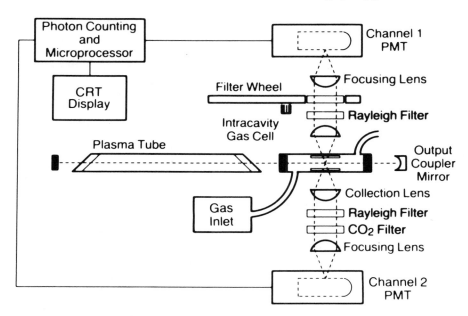

Fig. 11-15. Block diagram of the Raman spectrometer. Note that the Raman signal is collected at right angles to the laser beam. (From Westenskow et al,[95] with permission.)

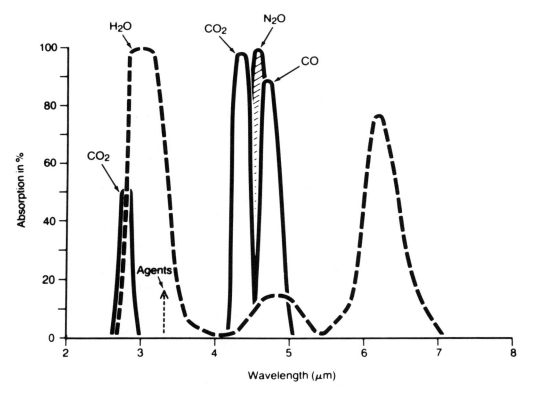

Fig. 11-16. Absorption spectra of anesthetic and respiratory gases in the red and infrared range. (From Gravenstein et al,[92] with permission.)

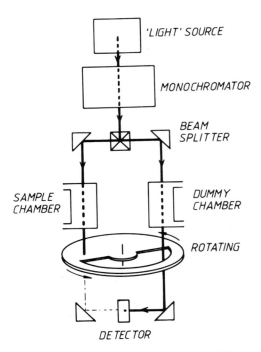

Fig. 11-17. Schematic of a parallel beam CO_2 analyzer. (From Mushin and Jones,[136] with permission.)

beam CO_2 analyzer. The light source is a broad spectrum emitter that includes light at the absorption wavelength of interest for CO_2 (4.3 μm).[96] This is followed by a filter that transmits only the wavelength of interest. Next, the light is split into two parallel beams, one passing through a sample chamber containing the unknown CO_2 concentration while the other passes through a reference chamber. The chambers have the same optical characteristics, and their windows are made of sapphire because glass absorbs infrared light. The beams then pass through a rotating disk or "chopper wheel," which alternately allows the light from one beam and then the other to reach the detector. Early CO_2 analyzers were constructed in this fashion so that a single light source and a single detector could be used. Variations in the light source or detector system affect both parallel beams equally and, therefore, do not change the relative intensity of the transmitted light. The gas to be analyzed is continuously circulated through the sample chamber to give a continuous measurement of carbon dioxide.

Two practical problems must be solved when designing a clinical capnometer. First, the instrument must obtain a respiratory gas sample without contaminating the analyzer with water vapor while achieving a fast response time. The second problem is interference with the CO_2 measurement by other gases.

Gas Sampling Design

Most clinical capnometers aspirate a sample from an adapter in the patient's airway through a capillary tube into the measurement chamber using a low-pressure vacuum pump (Fig. 11-18). In this configuration, two factors affect response time: the time delay due to the gas sampling system and the response time of the infrared analyzer.[92] The sampling delay time is a function of the volume of the tubing (ie, tubing length × internal diameter) and the gas sampling volume flow rate. Practical considerations dictate that the length of the sampling tube be at least 2 to 3 m for dedicated capnometers. The delay time for the sample to reach the infrared analyzer must, therefore, be minimized by using small-caliber tubing. Unfortunately, if the tubing is too small, it may be easily clogged by condensed water droplets. Most clinical capnometers use a sampling flow rate of 150 mL/min and a sampling tube diameter near 1 mm, resulting in a delay time of approximately 1 s. Higher sampling flow rates reduce delay time but may cause errors by aspirating a portion of fresh gas in addition to expired gas during the expiratory cycle. The sampling site in the ventilator circuit, patient size, and respiratory rate also may affect sampling errors.[92,97–99] The response time of the infrared analyzer is a function of the sample cell volume, the flow rate, and the time required to process the data. This response time (or rise time) is usually 50 to 150 ms. Monitors of this design are referred to as *sidestream* or *aspiration-type capnometers*.

The second configuration for monitoring expired CO_2 consists of an infrared detector placed directly in the patient's breathing circuit. This type of device is called a *mainstream capnometer*. Hewlett-Packard developed a mainstream capnometer in the late 1970s by modifying and miniaturizing the standard infrared detection system (Fig. 11-19).[100] With a mainstream capnometer, the patient is actually breathing through the CO_2 measurement chamber, which eliminates the aspiration system with its time delay. Mainstream capnometers have their own problems, however. The entire optical system must be small and light enough to be placed directly in the airway circuit. To accomplish this, a single-beam detection system was developed by using alternating light of two wavelengths. The two alternating light beams are produced by a rotating disk with optical filters. Sealed cells of CO_2 and nitrogen are used as optical filters in the Hewlett-Packard system.

Recently, a solid-state mainstream detection system has been developed by Novametrix.[101] This device accomplishes the same result as the Hewlett-Packard system without a rotating disk. The light is from a flashing thermal source that produces a broad-band

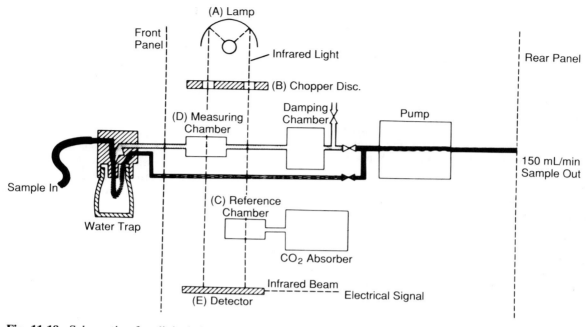

Fig. 11-18. Schematic of a clinical sidestream capnometer. (From Mogue and Rantala,[96] with permission.)

emission in pulses. The light passes through the airway sample cell, then impinges on dual photodetectors. Each detector is coated with a thin filter that allows only the wavelengths of interest to be transmitted to the photoconductor beneath. The ratio of these two filtered signals is calibrated to CO_2 concentration (personal communication, Mark Tuccillo, Project Manager, Novametrix Medical Systems, Inc., Wallingford, CT).

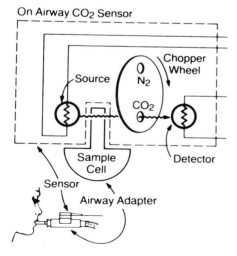

Fig. 11-19. Schematic of the Hewlett-Packard mainstream capnometer. (From Carver,[138] with permission.)

Infrared Absorption Interference

Infrared radiation may be absorbed by a molecule only if it is both polyatomic and asymmetric. The molecule must also have allowable vibrational energy levels that will alter its dipole moment. Monatomic molecules, such as helium and argon, and symmetric diatomic molecules, such as oxygen and nitrogen, will not absorb infrared radiation. Asymmetric gas molecules such as carbon dioxide, water vapor, nitrous oxide, and halogenated anesthetic agents will absorb infrared radiation. As illustrated in Figure 11-16, the absorption peaks for nitrous oxide overlap with those of carbon dioxide. There are two methods to correct for this nitrous oxide interference. By using one additional wavelength of light, the capnometer can independently measure nitrous oxide concentration. Corrections for nitrous oxide interference can then be automatically programmed into the capnometer. This is possible in a sidestream capnometer, where the size of the infrared detection system is not limited. For mainstream capnometers, independent measurement of nitrous oxide is not feasible with present technology. Mainstream capnometers, therefore, have manual correction switches activated by the user when nitrous oxide is present.

Another phenomenon, called *collision* or *pressure broadening*, causes absorption interference by molecules that do not in themselves absorb infrared light.[93] When a CO_2 molecule absorbs light, it increases its vibrational energy level. These vibrational states depend on forces acting both internally and externally to the molecule. Internal forces are a function of the atoms within the molecule, their atomic weights and bond energies. External intermolecular forces and collisions with other molecules can also influence vibrational energy levels. High concentrations of gases that do not absorb infrared light (such as nitrogen and oxygen) can thereby influence the absorption bands of carbon dioxide. For clinical purposes, this collision-broadening interference is most significant for nitrous oxide, oxygen, and nitrogen. Because of the almost certain presence of nitrous oxide and oxygen in the gas mixture, clinical capnometers incorporate corrections for both gases.

Infrared capnometers are spectrophotometers that have been adapted to clinical use for the specific detection of carbon dioxide. They are calibrated in vitro using known concentrations of carbon dioxide, or with calibrated sample cells in the case of mainstream capnometers. There are many practical design considerations that will ultimately affect the accuracy of the displayed CO_2 waveform. On the other hand, as opposed to a pulse oximeter, there is relatively little signal processing involved in the analysis of the absorption data.

CONTINUOUS CO_2 MONITORING: CO_2 OPTODE, TRANSCUTANEOUS CO_2, AND CAPNOGRAPHY

CO_2 Optode

As mentioned earlier in the discussion of oxygen, the technique of photoluminescence quenching (the optode) has been applied to the measurement of CO_2 in a manner analogous to the Severinghaus-Stowe CO_2 electrode. A photoluminescent dye, which is sensitive to changes in pH, is used within a cell to measure CO_2 partial pressure. CO_2 diffuses through a membrane and reacts with water in the cell, producing carbonic acid, and the optode measures the pH change. This secondary sensing cell has a relatively slow response time (approximately 2- to 3-minute 90 percent response), and, therefore, cannot be used to measure CO_2 in a capnometer. The CO_2 optode has been applied to invasive monitoring in the form of an extracorporeal continuous blood gas analyzer that continuously measures arterial and venous PCO_2 during cardiopulmonary bypass.[87,88] More recently, small fiberoptic probes have been developed for continuous intra-arterial measurement of $PaCO_2$.[89-91] Although this technique shows promise of clinical utility during thoracic anesthesia, it is currently only investigational.

Transcutaneous CO_2

Transcutaneous CO_2 ($PtcCO_2$) was introduced shortly after $PtcO_2$ in the early 1970s. It was demonstrated that if a Severinghaus-Stowe CO_2 electrode was heated and placed on the skin surface, continuous PCO_2 values that followed changes in $PaCO_2$ were measured. It is reasonable to expect that the PCO_2 of heated skin will be higher than $PaCO_2$, because tissue PCO_2 is higher than venous PCO_2 and heated tissue should produce more carbon dioxide. Indeed, the original $PtcCO_2$ values on awake volunteers were approximately 60 mmHg. Over the next decade, several methods were proposed to adjust $PtcCO_2$ values to closely approximate $PaCO_2$ values, so that clinicians could more easily interpret these data.[102,103] The most commonly used correction is that proposed by Severinghaus et al, which divides the $PtcCO_2$ value by 1.33 and then subtracts 3.0 mmHg.[102] The Severinghaus adjustment is physiologically justified by the fact that heating the blood increases the PCO_2 by approximately 33 percent and there is a tissue to blood metabolic gradient of 3 mmHg. $PtcCO_2$ with the Severinghaus adjustment has been shown to predict $PaCO_2$ within ± 10 percent.[104] As with $PtcO_2$, $PtcCO_2$ has been most extensively used in the care of neonatal patients. In contrast to $PtcO_2$, $PtcCO_2$ values are relatively insensitive to perfusion and do not change significantly with age. For this reason, it is much easier to interpret $PtcCO_2$ than its oxygen counterpart. Like $PtcO_2$, the $PtcCO_2$ sensor also requires calibration (in this case, a two-point gas calibration) and maintenance.

Capnography

Many early capnometers presented data in the form of an analog PCO_2 meter and a digital value of the peak PCO_2 measured during expiration. For this reason, the technique became known clinically as end-tidal CO_2 monitoring. Although this peak PCO_2 value provides useful information regarding the presence of ventilation and a minimum expected value for the $PaCO_2$, inspection of the capnogram can provide additional valuable information. In 1975, Smalhout and Kalenda published the first atlas of capnography, which described the clinical conditions that resulted in various capnographic patterns.[105] The earlier section discussing CO_2 transport describes a normal capnogram illustrated in Figure 11-12. The phase I portion, produced by expiration of the apparatus and anatomic dead space, should be a straight line near $PCO_2 = 0$ (the inspired CO_2 concentration). The phase II (quickly rising) portion of the capnogram will exhibit a decreased slope in the presence of either acute or chronic problems affecting expiratory flow, eg,

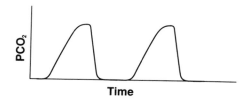

Fig. 11-20. Capnogram usually seen in patients with increased expiratory resistance, such as in asthma and chronic obstructive pulmonary disease. Note the phase II portion of the capnogram has a decreased slope due to mixing of anatomic and alveolar dead space with alveolar gas caused by abnormal emptying of various lung segments. If the mixing is severe enough, there may be no alveolar plateau or phase III portion of the capnogram. In such an instance, it would be expected to have an increased arterial-end-tidal gradient in excess of that, due to increases in purely alveolar dead space.

bronchospasm or emphysema. This reduced slope in the phase II portion is due to a mixing of both parallel and series dead space gas with ideal alveolar gas (Fig. 11-20). If the expiratory resistance is very high, the capnogram may never reach an alveolar plateau (phase III) and the peak expired PCO_2 value may be substantially lower than the alveolar PCO_2.

Figure 11-21 illustrates what has been called the "camel" capnogram. It can be produced by either physiologic or technical problems. If a patient is placed in the lateral position during general anesthesia, the nondependent lung will receive more ventilation and less perfusion (have a higher $\dot{V}/\dot{Q}$), and will thus contain more alveolar dead space. The nondependent lung empties first and, when it empties, it produces a lower phase III plateau in the capnogram. A second, higher plateau follows as the dependent

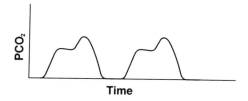

Fig. 11-21. The "camel" capnogram, so called because of the hump. This capnogram may occur when patients are placed in the lateral position, causing the upper lung to have a higher $\dot{V}/\dot{Q}$ and, consequently, more alveolar dead space. The upper lung empties first, forming a lower plateau, because of the increased alveolar dead space. As the alveolar gas with lower lung (with lower $\dot{V}/\dot{Q}$) reaches the detector, there is an increase in CO_2, causing the hump. A late phase III peak or hump may also be produced when a sidestream capnometer has a leak in the sampling tube.

lung empties, because this lung has a lower $\dot{V}/\dot{Q}$ ratio and less alveolar dead space. A similar capnographic pattern can occur when there is a leak in the aspiration tubing of a sidestream analyzer. The initial phase III plateau value will be reduced in proportion to the size of the leak because of the aspiration of room air into the sampling tube and the resulting dilution of the alveolar gas sample. The abrupt rise at the end of expiration (Fig. 11-21) is caused by the beginning of a positive-pressure breath, which increases the pressure in the aspiration tubing above ambient. This causes the leak to flow in the opposite direction, allowing the gas contained in the segment of aspiration tubing between the patient and the leak to reach the capnometer without dilution.[106] This undiluted alveolar gas causes the second phase III plateau in this case.

As a patient regains neuromuscular function following paralysis by muscle relaxants, there is a lack of coordination between the diaphragm and intercostal muscles. For this reason, the capnogram illustrated in Figure 11-22 has been called the *curare capnogram*. In anesthetized, paralyzed patients, it is an early clinical sign that the diaphragm is regaining neuromuscular function. A regular plateau with multiple irregular peaks and valleys can also be produced by surgeons pressing on the chest or abdominal contents. These fluctuations in intrathoracic pressure will cause a small amount of gas to move in and out of the lungs. A similar pattern may occur when a patient fights the ventilator.

Normally, phase IV begins with an abrupt drop to the baseline zero value with the start of inspiration. During anesthesia, it is common to see an undulating, gradual reduction, which has been called *cardiogenic oscillations* (Fig. 11-23). The peaks, which are in sequence with the heart rate, are produced when the right heart pumps a stroke volume of blood into the lungs, thus causing a small amount of alveolar gas to be expelled. As that blood volume drains from the pulmonary bed into the left heart, there is a "mini"

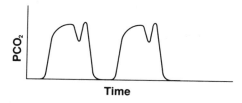

Fig. 11-22. The "curare" capnogram, so called because it is often seen when patients are recovering from neuromuscular blockade. Since the diaphragm regains neuromuscular function prior to the chest wall muscles, it may contract slightly during the end of expiration, causing a mini-inspiration and producing the notch in the end of the expiratory cycle.

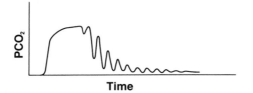

Fig. 11-23. A frequently seen capnographic pattern, especially during slow respiratory rates. The oscillations during the end of the phase III and phase IV portions of the capnogram are known as *cardiogenic oscillations*. The peaks are produced during systole as blood is pumped into the pulmonary bed producing a mini-expiration. During cardiac contraction, the right heart pumps more blood into the lungs, producing less alveolar dead space and, therefore, higher expired CO_2 values. During diastole, as blood drains from the pulmonary bed to the left heart, there is a mini-inspiration, producing a dip between each peak.

inspiration that yields the valleys in the oscillations.[107] The phase IV portion of the capnogram may also exhibit a decreased negative slope with a sidestream capnometer due to aspiration of fresh gas at the end of expiration. This is commonly seen in pediatric patients, when the expired minute volume is

small relative to the aspiration flow rate of the capnometer. The problem is aggravated when the sampling site is located near the fresh gas flow (Fig. 11-24).[97] In very small pediatric patients with high respiratory rates, the tracing produced by a sidestream capnometer can be distorted to the point of a sinusoidal oscillation, never achieving a plateau or a flat, zero phase I baseline (Fig. 11-25). A slowly down-sloping phase IV can also be caused by an incompetent inspiratory valve in a circle system.

If the phase I portion of the capnogram (inspiration) fails to return to a baseline value of zero, either there is CO_2 in the inspired gas or the capnometer has not been properly "zeroed." When using a partial rebreathing or semiopen system (eg, a Bain circuit), a non-zero baseline implies that there is an inadequate fresh gas flow rate. In a circle system, a non-zero baseline implies that either the CO_2 absorber is not removing carbon dioxide from the system or one of the valves is incompetent. A malfunctioning absorber may result from exhausted soda lime or channeling of gas through the absorber. A non-zero baseline may also be produced by water vapor condensation on the cuvette windows of a mainstream capnometer (note in Fig. 11-16 that water absorbs infrared light at 4.3 nm). Since mainstream capnometers heat their cuvette windows to 44°C to "defrost" them, vapor con-

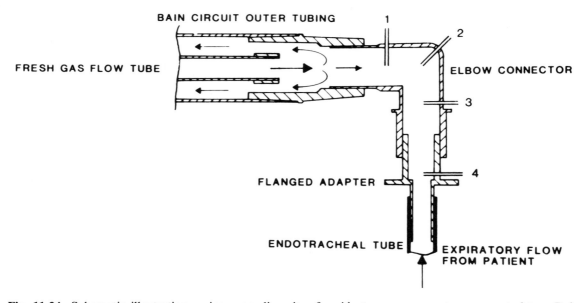

Fig. 11-24. Schematic illustrating various sampling sites for sidestream capnometers connected to a Bain circuit. If the sidestream port is connected at the site labeled *1*, the aspirated sample gas can be contaminated with fresh gas flow, especially during increased fresh gas flow rates. This is aggravated in smaller patients, with small expiratory flows and volumes relative to the sample rate of the aspiration-type capnometer. If the expired gas is sampled at site *4*, the degree of contamination with fresh gas is substantially reduced. (From Gravenstein et al,[137] with permission.)

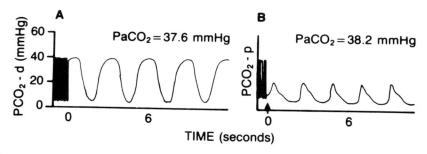

Fig. 11-25. Capnographic waveforms obtained from **(A)** distal and **(B)** proximal ends of the endotracheal tube in a 6.9-kg, 9-month-old infant. The change from distal to proximal sampling is indicated by the arrow. Fresh gas flow was 1.8 L/min, respiratory rate was 34 breaths/min, and peak airway pressure/positive expiratory pressure was 24/2. (From Badgwell et al,[97] with permission.)

densation implies either excessive humidification of the breathing circuit or contamination of the cuvette windows by secretions.

As stated in the section discussing CO_2 transport, a high capnogram plateau level or end-tidal PCO_2 ($PETCO_2$) value implies hypoventilation, whereas a low $PETCO_2$ implies either hyperventilation or increased alveolar dead space. Complete absence of a capnogram implies either no ventilation, no circulation, or a disconnected capnometer. A cardiac arrest will not actually produce a zero capnogram until all of the CO_2 has been removed from the lungs. It has been shown in experimental and clinical studies that a cardiac arrest will produce an abrupt drop in $PETCO_2$, which will increase with effective cardiopulmonary resuscitation (CPR), but will remain at a low value with ineffective CPR.[108,109] Unfortunately, an esophageal intubation may temporarily produce a similar depressed capnographic pattern.[110] The depressed capnogram seen with esophageal intubation will decrease in height with each breath until the CO_2 is removed from the stomach. However, in an emergency involving a cardiac arrest and a difficult intubation, initial observation of the capnogram may not indicate whether the trachea has been intubated properly or not.

Whether to manage patients with temperature-corrected or noncorrected (37°C) $PaCO_2$ values remains a controversy. Most anesthesiologists today treat patients using noncorrected or 37°C values (alpha-stat); that is, it is assumed for any patient temperature that a $PaCO_2$ of 40 mmHg is normal when measured at 37°C in the blood gas machine.[111] Although an in-depth discussion of the rationale for this is beyond the scope of this chapter, it can be shown that the use of alpha-stat blood gas values will maintain constant ionic charge on active proteins. Changing patient temperature also affects the relationship between noninvasively monitored carbon dioxide and $PaCO_2$.

Expired PCO_2 should more closely follow temperature-corrected $PaCO_2$ values, since expired CO_2 is in equilibrium with the patient's blood at that temperature. On the other hand, $PTCCO_2$ is measured from skin heated to a constant temperature (usually 44°C) and, therefore, is expected to maintain a constant relationship with $PaCO_2$ measured at 37°C. This hypothesis is supported by clinical studies, although no reported study has compared all three CO_2 variables over a wide range of patient temperature.[112] Since cardiopulmonary bypass is the most frequent clinical setting in which patient temperature is dramatically reduced, this is the focus of much of the discussion. A recent randomized clinical study has found no difference in clinical outcome of cardiopulmonary bypass patients whether they were treated with temperature-corrected or noncorrected $PaCO_2$ values.[113]

APPLICATIONS OF O_2 AND CO_2 MONITORING IN THORACIC ANESTHESIA

Due to the inevitable intrapulmonary shunt occurring during one-lung anesthesia, close monitoring of oxygenation is a primary concern.[114–116] Arterial oxygenation is a dynamic variable that may depend on many factors, including blood flow to the nonventilated lung, cardiac output, oxygen consumption, anesthetic effects on hypoxic pulmonary vasoconstriction, and pre-existing disease of both lungs. Consequently, the potential for arterial hypoxemia is high, providing a need for continuous monitoring. Although the ear oximeter has been available since the early 1950s, there are no reports of its use during anesthesia for thoracic surgery. It was not until the early 1980s that either $PTCO_2$ or noninvasive oximetry was studied during thoracic anesthesia.[117–123] $PTCO_2$ was the first of

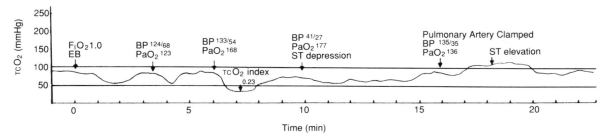

Fig. 11-26. Continuous transcutaneous oxygen (PtcO₂) recording from a patient who sustained intraoperative myocardial infarction. Comparative arterial oxygen tensions (PaO₂) are given. The drop in PtcO₂ to 38 mmHg (corresponding to the PtcO₂ index of 0.23) occurred 3 minutes before any changes in heart rate or blood pressure were noted. (From Cubra-Smith et al,[120] with permission.)

these techniques applied to monitoring these patients, and it was found extremely useful in providing a continuous trend of arterial oxygenation. PtcO₂ values ranged between 70 percent and 80 percent of PaO₂ values, but, because of its dependence on cardiac output, PtcO₂ could not be used alone to estimate PaO₂. Cubra-Smith et al noted that a decreasing PtcO₂ value during one-lung ventilation was the earliest indicator of myocardial ischemia (Fig. 11-26).[120] It was suggested that a PtcO₂ index value (PtcO₂/PaO₂) be established for each patient, and that changing values of PtcO₂ then be used to determine when it would be appropriate to obtain an arterial blood gas sample.[117–120] It was also reported that oxygenation not only decreased dramatically at the initiation of one-lung ventilation, but that it continued to fall for at least 10 to 20 minutes thereafter.[119,123] The time at which the PtcO₂ and, presumably, PaO₂ values reached a minimum showed substantial patient-to-patient variability, pointing out the necessity for continuous monitoring as opposed to random, intermittent blood gas sampling of arterial blood.

In 1985, Brodsky et al reported data from 19 patients undergoing one-lung ventilation while continuously monitored by pulse oximetry.[122] Arterial blood samples were drawn prior to the initiation of one-lung ventilation and every 5 minutes during one-lung ventilation. The pulse oximeter SpO₂ values were found to be in good agreement with the SaO₂ values, although several data points showed discrepancies as great as ± 6 percent. These investigators concluded that the reliability of pulse oximetry in detecting changes in oxygenation was sufficient enough that frequent arterial blood gas determinations of PaO₂ were no longer required. Viitanen et al studied 10 patients undergoing one-lung ventilation using continuous monitoring by both pulse oximetry and PtcO₂.[123] They found both techniques to correlate well with their cor-

responding arterial blood values. However, the pulse oximeter responded rapidly to changes in oxygenation, while PtcO₂ values lagged behind rapid changes in PaO₂ (Figs. 11-27 and 11-28).[123] They also found that the nadir in oxygenation occurred an average of 12 minutes after the initiation of one-lung ventilation. These researchers concluded that pulse oximetry was a simpler, more reliable, and more quickly responding monitor of changes in oxygenation during one-lung anesthesia.[123]

All of these studies document large changes in PaO₂ during one-lung ventilation. If the patient was ventilated with 100 percent oxygen, the PaO₂ would usually fall from the 400 to 500 mmHg range to less than 100 mmHg during one-lung ventilation and return to near baseline after resumption of two-lung ventilation. The PtcO₂ followed this trend, decreasing from the 200 to 300 mmHg range to below 75 mmHg and again rising to near baseline after resumption of two-lung ventilation.[119,123] Since normal hemoglobin does not desaturate measurably until the PaO₂ decreases to less than 90 mmHg, the pulse oximeter will not detect large changes in PaO₂ until it drops into the 80s. As was demonstrated by Brodsky et al and Viitanen et al, once arterial desaturation occurs, the pulse oximeter quickly detects changes in oxygenation with less time lag than PtcO₂ monitoring.[122,123] Although no serious harm can come to a patient from arterial hypoxemia without desaturation occurring first, PaO₂ data are still needed to assess oxygenation during two-lung ventilation before and after one-lung ventilation. Barker et al demonstrated in an experimental study that endobronchial intubation may not be detected by pulse oximetry for F₁O₂ values greater than 0.3 (Figs. 11-29 and 11-30).[124] Consequently, continuous monitoring of PaO₂ during thoracic anesthesia would be very helpful. Although intra-arterial Clark electrodes have been available for at least 15 years, they have not

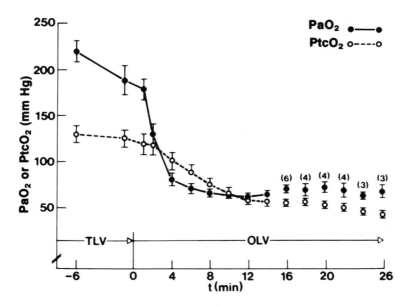

Fig. 11-27. Mean arterial oxygen tension (PaO_2) and transcutaneous oxygen tension ($PtcO_2$) values ($\pm$ SEM) in 10 patients who became hypoxemic during one-lung ventilation (OLV). Numbers in parentheses are numbers of patients studied. TLV, two-lung ventilation. (From Viitanen et al,[123] with permission.)

been applied to thoracic anesthesia. The PO_2 optode described above has recently been used in an experimental study of the detection of endobronchial intubation.[124] Figure 11-29 presents data obtained from a dog undergoing endobronchial intubation at $F_IO_2 = 0.5$ while being monitored by pulse oximetry, $PtcO_2$,

PO_2 optode, and intermittent arterial blood samples. The optode followed rapid changes in PaO_2 during this endobronchial intubation with no apparent delay, while $PtcO_2$ lagged slightly. Both optode PO_2 and $PtcO_2$ values underestimated the PaO_2 in this study. Note that the pulse oximeter SpO_2 values showed neg-

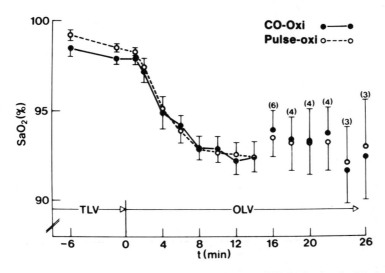

Fig. 11-28. Mean arterial blood oxygen saturation (SaO_2) values ($\pm$ SEM) obtained with the co-oximeter (Co-Oxi) or the pulse oximeter (Pulse-oxi) in 10 patients who became hypoxemic during one-lung ventilation (OLV). Numbers in parentheses are numbers of patients studied. TLV, two-lung ventilation. (From Viitanen et al,[123] with permission.)

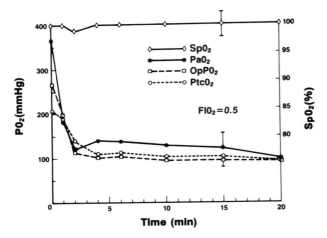

Fig. 11-29. Oxygenation variables versus time from onset of endobronchial intubation. Inspired oxygen fraction (F$_I$O$_2$) = 0.5. Arterial oxygen tension (PaO$_2$), optode arterial oxygen tension (OpPO$_2$), and transcutaneous oxygen tension (P$_{TC}$O$_2$) fell rapidly in the first 2 minutes, while pulse oximeter saturation (SpO$_2$) did not change significantly. Error bars represent standard deviations at 15 minutes. PO$_2$, oxygen tension. (From Barker et al,[124] with permission.)

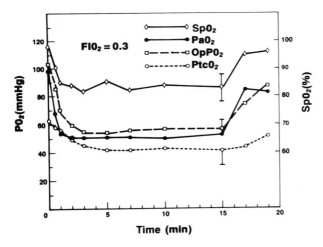

Fig. 11-30. Oxygenation variables versus time from onset of endobronchial intubation. Inspired oxygen fraction (F$_I$O$_2$) = 0.3. In this case, all four variables fell significantly within 2 minutes. Error bars represent standard deviations at 15 minutes. SpO$_2$, pulse oximeter saturation; PaO$_2$, arterial oxygen tension; OpPO$_2$, optode arterial oxygen tension; P$_{TC}$O$_2$ = transcutaneous oxygen tension; PO$_2$, oxygen tension. (From Barker et al,[124] with permission.)

ligible change throughout the procedure because the dog's PaO$_2$ never decreased to the point of desaturation. Figure 11-30 represents an animal ventilated with F$_I$O$_2$ = 0.3 during the same protocol. In this case, all oxygen monitors, including the pulse oximeter, showed immediate changes with the initiation of endobronchial ventilation because the PaO$_2$ decreased to the 50s, resulting in SpO$_2$ values in the 80s. The P$_{TC}$O$_2$ changes in Figure 11-30 lagged slightly behind the other monitors of oxygenation and, as would be expected, P$_{TC}$O$_2$ was significantly less than the corresponding PaO$_2$ value.

The maintenance of adequate ventilation (ie, normal PaCO$_2$) during one-lung ventilation has usually not been a problem.[125,126] If the same tidal volume can be maintained when switching from two-lung to one-lung ventilation, a stable PaCO$_2$ value usually results. The increased tidal volume to the single ventilated lung removes more CO$_2$ from the blood leaving that lung, thereby compensating for the higher CO$_2$ content of the blood perfusing the nonventilated lung. Because most of the oxygen content is carried by hemoglobin, which is normally saturated by both lungs, the ventilated lung cannot increase the oxygen content of its blood sufficiently to compensate for the desaturated blood leaving the nonventilated lung. For this reason, one-lung ventilation is usually associated with dramatic decreases in PaO$_2$.

Since the adequacy of ventilation during one-lung anesthesia is considered a less serious problem than oxygenation, little has been published on monitoring of ventilation during these anesthetics. Capnography has recently been shown to be useful in detecting endobronchial intubation and improper placement of double-lumen endotracheal tubes.[127,128] Monitoring of both lumens of a double-lumen tube with two capnometers provides continuous assessment of ventilation in both lungs during positioning of the patient, and can verify isolation of each lung during the procedure (Fig. 11-31).[127] Neither of these studies addresses the accuracy of P$_{ET}$CO$_2$ values in predicting PaCO$_2$ during one-lung ventilation, which should depend on changes in alveolar dead space as described earlier. Recently, Fletcher has shown that the PaCO$_2$ − P$_{ET}$CO$_2$ difference increases during thoractomy and single-lung ventilation.[129] There is one recently published report of P$_{TC}$CO$_2$ monitoring during one-lung anesthesia.[130] The authors found P$_{TC}$CO$_2$ values to be useful trend monitors of PaCO$_2$, but noted some significant discrepancies. This single report presents insufficient data to draw conclusions regarding the usefulness of P$_{TC}$CO$_2$ monitoring during one-lung ventilation. More recent work on P$_{TC}$CO$_2$ referred to earlier in this chapter suggests that the technique can

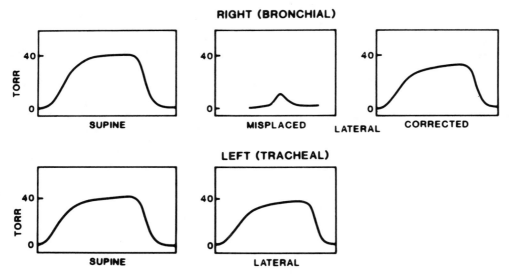

Fig. 11-31. Drawings of capnographs in a patient in the lateral decubitus position who has developed moderate obstruction of the right (bronchial) side, which was later relieved. (From Shafieha et al,[127] with permission.)

predict $PaCO_2$ with an accuracy of approximately $\pm$ 5 mmHg. More research on continuous monitoring of carbon dioxide during endobronchial anesthesia is clearly warranted.

REFERENCES

1. Van Slyke DD, Neills JM: The determination of gases in blood and other solutions by vacuum extraction and manometric measurement. Int J Biol Chem 61:523–557, 1924

2. Shoemaker WC, Appel PL, Bland R, et al: Clinical trial of an algorithm for outcome prediction in acute circulatory failure. Crit Care Med 10:390–397, 1982

3. Guyton AC: Transport of oxygen and carbon dioxide in the blood and body fluids. Ch. 41. In: Textbook of Medical Physiology. WB Saunders, Philadelphia, 1981

4. Clark LC: Monitor and control of tissue O_2 tensions. Trans Am Soc Artif Internal Organs 2:41–48, 1956

5. Severinghaus JW, Bradley AF: Electrodes for blood PO_2 and PCO_2 determination. J Appl Physiol 13:515–520, 1958

6. Parbrook GD, David PD, Parbrook EO: Basic Physics and Measurement in Anesthesia. 2nd Ed. Appleton-Century-Crofts, Norwalk, CT, 1986

7. Gehrich JL, Lubbers DW, Opitz N, et al: Optical fluorescence and its application to an intravascular blood gas monitoring system. IEEE Trans Biomed Eng 33:117–132, 1986

8. Barker SJ, Tremper KK, Hyatt J, et al: Continuous fiberoptic arterial oxygen tension measurements in dogs. J Clin Monit 3:48–52, 1987

9. Shapiro BA, Cane RD, Chomka CM, et al: Evaluation of a new intra-arterial blood gas system in dogs. Crit Care Med 15:361, 1987

10. Kollmeyer KR, Tsang RC: Complications of umbilical oxygen electrodes. J Pediatr 84:894–897, 1974

11. Harris TR, Nugent M: Continuous arterial oxygen tension monitoring in the newborn infant. J Pediatr 82:929–939, 1973

12. Bratanow N, Polk K, Bland R, et al: Continuous polarographic monitoring of intra-arterial oxygen in the perioperative period. Crit Care Med 13:859–860, 1985

13. Malalis L, Bhat R, Vidyasagar D: Comparison of intravascular PO_2 with transcutaneous and PaO_2 values. Crit Care Med 11:110–113, 1983

14. Altman DG, Bland JM: Measurement in medicine: the analysis of method comparison studies. Statistician 32:307–317, 1983

15. Bland JM, Altman DG: Statistical methods for assessing agreement between two methods of clinical measurement. Lancet 1:307–310, 1986

16. Altman DG: Statistics and ethics in medical research. Vol. 6. Presentation of results. Br Med J 2:1542–1544, 1980

17. Rithalia SVS, Bennett PJ, Tinker J: The performance characteristics of an intra-arterial oxygen electrode. Intensive Care Med 7:305–307, 1981

18. Arai T, Hatano Y, Komatsu K, et al: Real-time analysis of the change in arterial oxygen tension during endotracheal suction with a fiberoptic bronchoscope. Crit Care Med 13:855–858, 1985

19. Barker SJ, Tremper KK: Intra-arterial PO_2 monitoring. Int Anesthesiol Clin 25:206, 1987

20. Eberhard P, Hammacher K, Mindt W: Perkutane

messung des sauerstoffpartialdruckes: methodik und anwendugen, abstracted. Stuttgart Proc Medizin-Technik 26, 1972

21. Huch A, Huch R, Meinzer K, et al: Eine schuelle, behitze Ptoberflachenelektrode zur kontinuierlichen Uberwachung des PO_2 beim Menschen: Elektrodenaufbau und Eigenschaften, abstracted. Stuttgart Proc Medizin-Technik xx:26, 1972

22. Huch R, Huch A, Albani M, et al: Transcutaneous PO_2 monitoring in routine management of infants and children with cardiorespiratory problems. Pediatrics 57:681–688, 1976

23. Peabody JL, Willis MM, Gregory GA, et al: Clinical limitations and advantages of transcutaneous oxygen electrodes. Acta Anaethesiol Scand, Suppl. 68:76–81, 1978

24. Marshall TA, Kattwinkel J, Bery FA, Shaw A: Transcutaneous oxygen monitoring of neonates during surgery. J Pediatr Surg 15:797–803, 1980

25. Versmold HT, Linderkamp O, Holzman M, et al: Transcutaneous monitoring of PO_2 in newborn infants. Where are the limits? Influences of blood pressure, blood volume, blood flow, viscosity, and acid base state. Birth Defects 4:286–294, 1979

26. Tremper KK, Waxman K, Shoemaker WC: Effects of hypoxia and shock on transcutaneous PO_2 values in dogs. Crit Care Med 7:526–531, 1979

27. Rowe MI, Weinberg G: Transcutaneous oxygen monitoring in shock and resuscitation. J Pediatr Surg 14:773–778, 1979

28. Baumgardner JE, Graves DJ, Neufeld GR, Quinn JA: Gas flux through human skin: effects of temperature, stripping and inspired tension. J Appl Physiol 5:1536–1545, 1985

29. Van Duzee BF: Thermal analysis of human stratum corneum. J Invest Dermatol 65:404–408, 1975

30. Tremper KK, Shoemaker WC: Transcutaneous oxygen monitoring of critically ill adults, with and without low flow shock. Crit Care Med 9:706–709, 1981

31. Glenski JA, Cucchiara RF: Transcutaneous O_2 and CO_2 monitoring of neurosurgical patient: detection of air embolism. Anesthesiology 64:546–550, 1986

32. Severinghaus JW, Weiskopf RB, Nishimura M, Bradley AF: Oxygen electrode errors due to polarographic reduction of halothane. J Appl Physiol 31:640–642, 1971

33. Muravchick S: Teflon membranes do not eliminate halothane interference with transcutaneous oxygen electrodes. Anesthesiology 57:A168, 1982

34. Tremper KK, Barker SJ, Blatt DH, Wender RH: Effects of anesthetic agents on the drift of a transcutaneous PO_2 sensor. J Clin Monit 2:234–236, 1986

35. Shoemaker WC, Lawner P: Method for continuous conjunctival oxygen monitoring during carotid artery surgery. Crit Care Med 11:946–949, 1983

36. Smith M, Abraham E: Conjunctival oxygen monitoring during hemorrhage. J Trauma 26:217–224, 1986

37. Abraham E, Fink S: Conjunctival and cardiorespiratory monitoring during resuscitation from hemorrhage. Crit Care Med 12:1004–1009, 1986

38. Abraham E: Continuous conjunctival and transcutaneous oxygen tension monitoring during resuscitation in a patient. Resuscitation 12:207–211, 1984

39. Hess D, Evans C, Thomas K, et al: The relationship between conjunctival PO_2 and arterial PO_2 in 16 normal persons. Respir Care 31:191–198, 1986

40. Chapman KR, Liu FLW, Watson RM, Rebuck AS: Conjunctival oxygen tension and its relationship to arterial oxygen tension. J Clin Monit 2:100–104, 1986

41. Abraham E, Oye RK, Smith M: Detection of blood volume deficits through conjunctival oxygen tension monitoring. Crit Care Med 12:931–934, 1985

42. Severinghaus JW: Historical development of oxygenation monitoring. In Payne JP, Severinghaus JW (eds): Pulse oximetry. Springer-Verlag, Berlin, 1986

43. Brown LJ: A new instrument for the simultaneous measurement of total hemoglobin, % oxyhemoglobin, % carboxyhemoglobin, % methemoglobin, and oxygen content in whole blood. IEEE Trans Biomed Eng 27:132–138, 1980

44. Martin WE, Cheung PW, Johnson CC, Wong KC: Continuous monitoring of mixed venous oxygen saturation in man. Anesth Analg 52:784–793, 1973

45. Wilkinson AR, Phibbs RH, Gregory GA: Continuous measurement of oxygen saturation in sick newborn infants. J Pediatr 93:1016–1019, 1978

46. Baele PL, McMichan JC, Marsh HM, et al: Continuous monitoring of mixed venous oxygen saturation in critically ill patients. Anesth Analg 61:513–517, 1982

47. Barker SJ, Tremper KK, Hyatt J, Zaccari J: Effects of methemoglobinemia on pulse oximetry and mixed venous oximetry. Anesthesiology 70:112–117, 1989

48. Gettinger A, Detraglia MC, Glass DD: In vivo comparison of two mixed venous saturation catheters. Anesthesiology 66:373–375, 1987

49. Lee SE, Tremper KK, Barker SJ: Effects of anemia on pulse oximetry and continuous mixed venous oxygen saturation monitoring in dogs. Anesthesiology 1991 (in press)

50. Jamieson WRE, Turnbull KW, Larrieu AJ, et al: Continuous monitoring of mixed venous oxygen saturation in cardiac surgery. Can J Surg 25:538–543, 1982

51. Schmidt CR, Frank LP, Forsythe MJ, Estafanous FG: Continuous measure and oxygen transport patterns in cardiac surgery patients. Crit Care Med 12:523–527, 1984

52. Waller JL, Kaplan JA, Bauman DI, et al: Clinical evaluation of a new fiberoptic catheter oximeter during cardiac surgery. Anesth Analg 61:676–679, 1982

53. Eichorn JH, Cooper JB, Cullen BF, et al: Standards for patient monitoring during anesthesia at Harvard Medical School. JAMA 1256:1017–1020, 1986

54. American Society of Anesthesiologists: Standards for basic intra-operative monitoring. APSF March:3, 1987

55. Severinghaus JW, Astrup PB: History of blood gas analysis. Int Anesthesiol Clin 25:xx–xx, 1987

56. Stephen CR, Slater HM, Johnson AL, Sekelj P: The oximeter—a technical aid for the anesthesiologist. Anesthesiology 12:541–555, 1951

57. Barker SJ, Tremper KK: The effect of carbon monoxide

inhalation on pulse oximeter signal detection. Anesthesiology 67:599–603, 1987

58. Scheller MS, Unger RJ, Kelner MJ: Effects of intravenously administered dyes on pulse oximetry readings. Anesthesiology 65:550–552, 1986

59. Pologe JA, Raley DM: Effects of fetal hemoglobin on pulse oximetry. J Perinatol 7:324–326, 1987

60. Anderson JV: The accuracy of pulse oximetry in neonates: effects of fetal hemoglobin and bilirubin. J Perinatol 7:323, 1987

61. Brooks TD, Paulus DA, Winkle WE: Infrared heat lamps interfere with pulse oximeters, letter. Anesthesiology 61:630, 1984

62. Costarino AT, Davis DA, Keon T: Falsely normal saturation reading with the pulse oximeter. Anesthesiology 67:830–831, 1987

63. Eisele JH, Downs D: Ambient light affects pulse oximeters. Anesthesiology 67:864–865, 1987

64. Siegel MN, Gravenstein N: Preventing ambient light from affecting pulse oximetry. Anesthesiology 67:280, 1987

65. Lawson D, Norley I, Korbon G, et al: Blood flow limits and pulse oximeter signal detection. Anesthesiology 67:599–603, 1987

66. Tremper KK, Barker SJ, Hufstedler S, Weiss M: Transcutaneous and liver surface PO_2 during hemorrhagic hypotension and treatment with phenylephrine. Crit Care Med 17:537–540, 1989

67. Tremper KK, Hufstedler S, Barker SJ, et al: Accuracy of a pulse oximeter in the critically ill adult: effect of temperature and hemodynamics. Anesthesiology 63:A175, 1985

68. Nellcor N100 Technical Manual. Nellcor Corporation, Hayward, CA

69. Mihm FG, Halperin DH: Noninvasive detection of profound arterial desaturations using pulse oximetry device. Anesthesiology 62:85–87, 1985

70. Cecil WT, Thorpe KJ, Fibuch EE, Tuohy GF: A clinical evaluation of the accuracy of the Nellcor N100 and the Ohmeda 3700 pulse oximeters. J Clin Monit 4:31–36, 1988

71. Boxer RA, Gottesfeld I, Singh S, et al: Noninvasive pulse oximetry in children with cyanotic congenital heart disease. Crit Care Med 15:1062–1064, 1987

72. Fait CD, Wetzel RC, Dean JM, et al: Pulse oximetry in critically ill children. J Clin Monit 1:232–235, 1985

73. Kagle DM, Alexander CM, Berko RS, et al: Evaluation of the Ohmeda 3700 pulse oximeter: steady-state and transient response characteristics. Anesthesiology 66:376–380, 1987

74. Severinghaus JW, Naifeh KH: Accuracy of response of six pulse oximeters to profound hypoxia. Anesthesiology 67:551–558, 1987

75. Comroe JH, Jr, Botelho S: The reliability of cyanosis in the recognition of arterial anoxemia. Am J Med Sci 214:1–6, 1947

76. Coté CJ, Goldstein EA, Coté MA, et al: A single blind study of pulse oximetry in children. Anesthesiology 68:184–188, 1988

77. Raemer DB, Warren DL, Morris R, et al: Hypoxemia during ambulatory gynecologic surgery as evaluated by the pulse oximeter. J Clin Monit 3:244–248, 1987

78. Pullerits J, Burrows FA, Roy WL: Arterial desaturation in healthy children during transfer to the recovery room. Can J Anesth 34:470–473, 1987

79. Tyler IL, Tantisira B, Winter PM, Motoyama EK: Continuous monitoring of arterial oxygen saturation with pulse oximetry during transfer to the recovery room. Anesth Analg 64:1108–1112, 1985

80. Soliman IE, Patel RI, Ehrenpreis MB, Hannallah RS: Recovery scores do not correlate with postoperative hypoxemia in children. Anesth Analg 67:53–56, 1988

81. Morris RW, Buxchman A, Warren DI, et al: The prevalence of hypoxemia detected by pulse oximetry during recovery from anesthesia. J Clin Monit 4:16–20, 1988

82. Overand PT, Freund PR, Cooper JO, et al: Failure rate of pulse oximetry in clinical practice. Anesth Analg 70:S289, 1990

83. Nunn JF: Respiratory deadspace and distribution of the inspired gas. pp. 213–245. In: Applied Respiratory Physiology. 2nd Ed. Butterworth, London, 1977

84. Ailken RS, Clark-Kennedy AE: On the fluctuations in the composition of the alveolar air during the respiratory cycle in muscular exercise. J Physiol 65:389–411, 1928

85. Severinghaus JW, Bradley AF: Electrodes for blood PO_2 and PCO_2 determination. J Appl Physiol 13:515, 1958

86. Severinghaus JW: A combined transcutaneous PO_2-PCO_2 electrode with electrochemical HCO_3 stabilization. J Appl Physiol 51:1027, 1981

87. Pino JH, Bashein G, Kenny MA: In vitro assessment of a flow-through fluorometric blood gas monitor. J Clin Monit 4:186–194, 1988

88. Bashein G, Pino JA, Nessly ML, et al: Clinical assessment of a flow-through fluorometric blood gas monitor. J Clin Monit 4:195–203, 1988

89. Gehrich JL, Lubbers DW, Opitz N, et al: Optical fluorescence and its application to an intervascular blood gas monitoring system. IEEE Trans Biomed Eng 33:117–132, 1986

90. Shapiro BA, Cane RD, Chomka CM, et al: Preliminary evaluation of an intra-arterial blood gas system in dogs and humans. Crit Care Med 17:455–460, 1989

91. Barker SJ, Hyatt J, Tremper KK, Gehrich JL: Continuous fiberoptic blood-gas monitoring: a comparison of 18 and 20 gauge arterial cannulas. Anesthesiology 71:A376, 1989

92. Gravenstein JS, Paulus DA, Hayes TJ: Capnography in Clinical Practice. Butterworth, Boston, 1989

93. Ozanne GM, Young WF, Mazzei WJ, Severinghaus JW: Multipatient anesthetic mass spectrometry: rapid analysis of data stored in long catheters. Anesth 55:62–70, 1981

94. Ohmeda 6000 Multi-Gas Monitor Operation and Maintenance Manual. Ohmeda, Madison, WI

95. Westenskow DR, Smith KW, Coleman DL, et al: Clinical evaluation of Raman-scattering multiple gas ana-

lyzer for the operating room. Anesthesiology 70:350, 1989

96. Mogue LR, Rantala B: Capnometers. J Clin Monit 4:115, 1988

97. Badgwell JM, McLeoud ME, Lerman J, Creighton RE: End-tidal PCO₂ measurement sampled at the distal and proximal ends of the endotracheal tube in infants and children. Anesth Analg 66:959, 1987

98. Schieber RA, Namnoum A, Sugden A, et al: Accuracy of expiratory carbon dioxide measurement using the co-axial and circle breathing circuits in small subjects. J Clin Monit 1:149, 1985

99. From RP, Scamman FL: Ventilatory frequency influences accuracy of end-tidal CO_2 measurements. Anesth Analg 67:884, 1988

100. Soloman RJ: A reliable, accurate CO_2 analyzer for medical use. Hewlett Packard J September 1981

101. Scammon FL, Fron RP: High frequency response of six capnometers, Anesthesiology 71:A360, 1989

102. Severinghaus JW, Stafford M, Bradley AF: TCPCO₂ electrode design calibration and temperature gradient problem. Acta Anaesthesiol Scand 68:188–122, 1978

103. Monaco F, Nickerson BG, Mcquitty JC: Continuous transcutaneous oxygen and carbon dioxide monitoring in the pediatric ICU. Crit Care Med 10:765–766, 1982

104. Palmirano B, Severinghaus JW: Transcutaneous PCO₂ and PO₂: a multi-centered study of accuracy. J Clin Monit 1990 (in press)

105. Smalhout D, Kalenda Z: An Atlas of Capnography. Institute of Anesthesiology. University Hospital, Utrecht, The Netherlands, 1975

106. Zupan J, Martin M, Bennett J: End-tidal CO_2 excretion waveform and error with gas sampling line leak. Anesth Analg 67:579–881, 1988

107. Fowler KT, Read J: Cardiac oscillation in expired gas tensions and regional pulmonary blood flow. J Appl Physiol 16:863–868, 1961

108. Trevino RP, Bisera J, Weil MH, et al: End-tidal CO_2 as a guide to successful cardiopulmonary resuscitation; a preliminary report. Crit Care Med 13:910–911, 1985

109. Weil MH, Bisera J, Trevino RP, Rackow EC: Cardiac output and end-tidal carbon dioxide. Crit Care Med 13:907–909, 1985

110. Ping STS: Letter to the editor. Anesth Analg 66:483, 1987

111. Williams JJ, Marshall BE: A fresh look at an old question. Anesthesiology 56:1–2, 1982

112. Phan CQ, Tremper KK, Lee SE, Barker SJ: Noninvasive monitoring of carbon dioxide: a comparison of the partial pressure of transcutaneous and end-tidal carbon dioxide with the partial pressure of arterial carbon dioxide. J Clin Monit 3:149–154, 1987

113. Bashein G, Towns BD, Nessly ML, et al: A randomized study of carbon dioxide management during hypothermic cardiopulmonary bypass. Anesthesiology 72:7–15, 1990

114. Kerr JH, Smith C, Prys-Roberts C, et al: Observations during endobronchial anesthesia II: oxygenation. Br J Anesth 46:84–92, 1974

115. Flacke JW, Thompson DS, Read RC: Influence of tidal volume and pulmonary artery occlusion on arterial oxygenation during endobronchial anesthesia. South Med J 69:619–626, 1976

116. Slinger P, Triolel W, Wilson J: Improving arterial oxygenation during one-lung ventilation. Anesthesia 69:291–295, 1988

117. Goltyer I, Jackson E, Rasmusson JP: Transcutaneous oxygen measurement during thoracic anesthesia. Acta Anaesthesiol Scand 24:491–494, 1980

118. Chung M, Lichtor JL, Ragachari K: Transcutaneous monitoring of PO₂ and PCO₂ during one-lung anesthesia: Are they reliable? J Cardiothorac Anesth 2:313–319, 1988

119. Tremper KK, Konchigeri HN, Cullen BF, et al: Transcutaneous monitoring of oxygen tension during one-lung anesthesia. J Thorac Cardiovasc Surg 88:22–25, 1984

120. Cubra-Smith N, Grant RP, Jenkins LC: Perioperative transcutaneous oxygen monitoring in thoracic anesthesia. Can Anesth Soc J 33:745–753, 1986

121. Salmenpera M, Heinonen J: Transcutaneous oxygen measurement during one-lung anesthesia. Acta Anaesthesiol Scand 28:241–244, 1984

122. Brodsky JB, Shulman MS, Suran M, Mark JB: Pulse oximetry during one-lung ventilation. Anesthesiology 63:212–214, 1985

123. Viitanen A, Salmenpera M, Heinonen J: Noninvasive monitoring of oxygenation during one-lung ventilation: a comparison of transcutaneous oxygen tension measurement and pulse oximetry. J Clin Monit 3:90–95, 1987

124. Barker SJ, Tremper KK, Hyatt J, Heitzman H: Comparison of three oxygen monitors in detecting endobronchial intubation. J Clin Monit 4:240–243, 1988

125. Kerr JH, Smith C, Prys-Roberts C, Meloche R: Observations during endobronchial anesthesia I: ventilation and carbon dioxide clearance. Br J Anaesth 45:159–166, 1973

126. Flacke JW, Thompson DS, Read R: Influence of tidal volume and pulmonary artery occlusion on arterial oxygenation during endobronchial anesthesia. South Med J 69:619–626, 1976

127. Shafieha MJ, Sit J, Kartha R, et al: End-tidal CO_2 analyzers in proper positioning of the double-lumen tubes. Anesthesiology 64:844–845, 1986

128. Riley RH, Marcy JH: Unsuspected endobronchial intubation detected by continuous mass spectrometry. Anesthesiology 63:203–204, 1985

129. Fletcher R: The arterial-end-tidal CO_2 difference during cardiothoracic surgery. J Cardiothorac Anesth 4:105–117, 1990

130. Chung MR, Lichtor JL, Rangachari K, Roizen MF: Transcutaneous monitors during one-lung ventilation: are they reliable? J Cardiothorac Anesth 2:313–319, 1988

131. Tremper KK, Barker SJ: Pulse oximetry and oxygen transport. pp. 19–27. In Payne JP, Severinghaus JW (eds): Pulse Oximetry. Springer-Verlag, Berlin, 1986

132. Barker SJ, Tremper KK: Pulse oximetry: applications and limitations. Int Anesthesiol Clin 25:155–175, 1987

133. Ohmeda Pulse Oximeter Model 3700 Service Manual. Ohmeda, Madison, WI

134. Tremper KK, Barker SJ: Pulse oximetry. Anesthesiology 70:98–108, 1989

135. Tremper KK, Waxman KS: Transcutaneous monitoring of respiratory gases. pp. 1–28. In Nochomovitz ML, Cherniak NS (eds): Noninvasive Respiratory Monitoring. Churchill Livingstone, New York, 1986

136. Mushin WW, Jones PL: Physics for the Anesthetist. Blackwell Scientific Publications, London, 1987

137. Gravenstein J, Lampotang S, Benekin JE: Factors influencing capnography in Bain's circuit. J Clin Monit 1:6–10, 1985

138. Carver CD: A Special Collection of Infrared Spectra from The Coblenz Society, Inc. The Coblenz Society, Kirkwood, MO, 1980

12

ANESTHESIA FOR THORACIC DIAGNOSTIC PROCEDURES

Jan Ehrenwerth, M.D.
Sorin J. Brull, M.D.

Although thoracic diagnostic procedures have been considered to be relatively minor operations, they present a unique challenge to the anesthesiologist. Frequently, it is necessary to anesthetize a patient who is debilitated, has multisystem disease, and possesses only marginal respiratory reserve. Each of the diagnostic procedures requires special consideration. For example, during bronchoscopy the airway has to be shared with the surgeon and delivery of predictable levels of inhalational anesthetics may be difficult, while mediastinoscopy may cause compression of major intrathoracic blood vessels and is occasionally associated with sudden catastrophic hemorrhage. Likewise, thoracoscopy may lead to tension pneumothorax, and esophageal tears may occur during endoscopy.

While it is theoretically possible to perform any of these diagnostic procedures under either regional or general anesthesia, there is no clear-cut advantage of one technique over the other for all patients. Rather, the anesthetic technique must be individualized. The anesthesiologist should consider the patient's preoperative condition and preferences, the indications for the procedure and its anticipated duration, as well as the anesthesiologist's familiarity with the various surgical techniques.

PREOPERATIVE EVALUATION

A careful and detailed preoperative evaluation of the patient presenting for a thoracic diagnostic procedure is essential. Not only do patients undergoing these procedures often present with problems of oxygenation and ventilation, but they may also have disease processes involving several other organ systems. To most effectively minimize perioperative problems, the clinician must assess the patients' risk factors. Conditions that have been associated with increased risk of perioperative pulmonary complications include advanced age, pre-existing pulmonary disease, obesity, history of smoking, cardiac dysfunction, kyphoscoliosis, neuromuscular disease, pulmonary infections, history of postoperative pulmonary complications, and poor preoperative physical condition[1] (see Chapter 3).

Warner et al showed that a smoking history of more than 20 pack-years is associated with an increased risk of developing postoperative pulmonary complications, and that cessation of smoking for 8 weeks prior to surgery results in decreased postoperative respiratory compromise.[2] However, even short-term smoking cessation has been shown to be beneficial. Kambam et al demonstrated that P_{50} values return toward normal and that carboxyhemoglobin levels decrease if smoking cessation is undertaken at least 12 hours preoperatively.[3] Likewise, Smith and Landaw showed that elevated red blood cell volume and reduced plasma volume will both return toward normal in heavy smokers within a week after stopping smoking.[4] Thus, encouraging the patient to refrain from smoking preoperatively produces both long- and short-term benefits.

The examination of the airway is of paramount importance. Assessment of neck and jaw mobility and visualization of oropharyngeal structures give important clues as to the ability to manage the airway and to instrument the trachea. Mallampati et al have described three airway classifications based on physical examination of the oropharynx.[5] Although this may serve as a guide, it is by no means an absolute predictor of airway adequacy or ease of intubation. Patients who are difficult to intubate because of physical characteristics or previous history may be candidates for awake intubation or fiberoptic techniques.

Examination of the lungs may reveal wheezing, stridor, rales, or rhonchi. The presence of wheezing often indicates disease of the small airways, and may be reversible. Wheezing can also be caused by a foreign body obstructing the large airways. Rales are associated with excess interstitial lung water from transudation of fluid. This is associated with decreased plasma oncotic pressure or increased amounts of interstitial fluid from left-sided congestive heart failure. Rhonchi are heard in patients with chronic obstructive lung disease, particularly in heavy smokers. These patients are prone to having a productive cough with thick secretions, and they are at higher risk for developing perioperative atelectasis.

The presence of stridor is an extremely important clinical finding, as it may indicate a significant obstruction of the airway. Furthermore, stridor can be helpful in pinpointing the area of obstruction. Inspiratory stridor is associated with *extrathoracic* lesions, because negative pressure is generated inside the trachea during inspiration. This negative pressure allows the extrathoracic lesion to further compress the airway and worsen the obstruction. Conversely, stridor that occurs during exhalation is associated with variable *intrathoracic* lesions. The increase in intrathoracic pressure that occurs during exhalation further compromises the already narrowed intrathoracic segment (Figs. 12-1 to 12-3). The use of accessory muscles of respiration, substernal retractions, and tracheal tug are also indicative of an obstructive process.

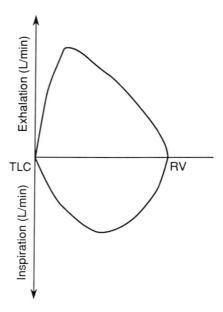

Fig. 12-1. Schematic representation of normal flow-volume curves generated during inhalation (bottom curve) and exhalation (top curve). TLC, total lung capacity; RV, residual volume.

Other physical signs such as cyanosis, clubbing of the fingers, and increased anterior to posterior chest diameter are usually associated with severe chronic hypoxemia and chronic pulmonary disease. Absence of breath sounds may represent long-standing disease processes such as atelectasis, consolidation from pneumonia, or loss of parenchymal tissue. On the other hand, it may also indicate an acute process such as aspiration, pneumothorax, or obstruction of a main bronchus by a foreign body. Fever, leukocytosis, and sputum production should alert the anesthesiologist to the presence of an intrapulmonary infectious process.

Examination of old medical records often provides important clues as to previous problems. Frequently, patients have had multiple diagnostic procedures, and the anesthesia record can serve as a guide to the difficulty of intubation as well as to any problems encountered during the procedure. Current diagnostic tests can be compared with previous ones to assess the progression of the disease process. Communication with the endoscopist may reveal other previously obtained information about the airway (ie, indirect laryngoscopy), which can help the anesthesiologist in formulating the anesthetic plan.

In addition to the history and physical assessment of the patient, laboratory data and diagnostic tests will shed further light on the extent of the disease process. Analysis of room air arterial blood gases pro-

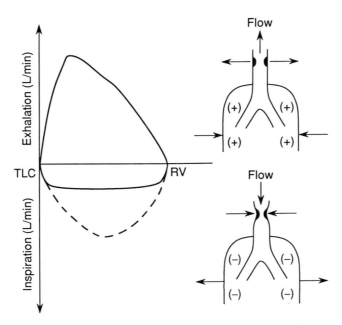

Fig. 12-2. Schematic representation of an *extrathoracic* variable obstruction. The solid lines represent actual flow-volume curves, while the dashed line represents a normal inspiratory pattern. Note that with the extrathoracic variable obstruction, exhalation induces a positive (+) intratracheal pressure, which in turn results in little or no resistance to flow past the narrowed segment (*top figure*). Conversely, inhalation generates negative (−) intrathoracic pressure, which in turn induces negative pressure in the trachea below the point of obstruction. This negative pressure will induce further obstruction and increase resistance to flow (*bottom figure*).

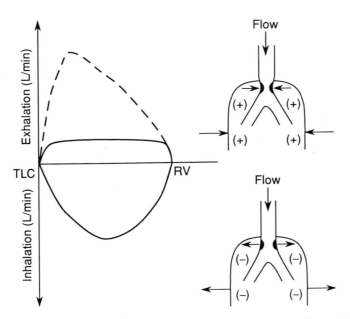

Fig. 12-3. Schematic representation of an *intrathoracic* variable obstruction. The solid lines represent actual flow-volume curves, while the dashed line represents the normal expiratory pattern. During exhalation, the transthoracic positive (+) pressure is transmitted to the intrathoracic narrowed segment, which results in an increased resistance to flow (*top figure*). Conversely, during inhalation, the negative (−) intrathoracic pressure will distend the narrowed segment, resulting in little or no resistance to flow (*bottom figure*).

vides important information as to the status of the patient's oxygenation and ventilation. The presence of hypoxemia and hypercarbia indicates a severe disease process and, probably, decreased pulmonary reserve. It should also warn the anesthesiologist of potential perioperative complications.

Preoperative electrocardiographic (ECG) examination may also reveal current processes usually associated with chronic pulmonary disease, such as right atrial and right ventricular hypertrophy. Comparison of a recent ECG to previous tracings will help delineate the progression of the disease, and can signal development of myocardial ischemia.

Pulmonary function tests can be helpful in assessing the degree of impairment. Forced expiratory volume in 1 second (FEV_1) and forced vital capacity (FVC) done both with and without bronchodilators can demonstrate whether there is a reversible component of airway obstruction. If there is significant reversibility, initiation of preoperative bronchodilator therapy is indicated. Flow-volume loops may also give important clues as to the degree and location of airway obstructions (Figs. 12-1 to 12-3).

Patients undergoing thoracic diagnostic procedures are more likely to develop postoperative pulmonary complications. Tisi recommended that preoperative spirometry be done in patients who are undergoing thoracotomy or upper abdominal operations, in those who are over 70 years of age, obese, or heavy smokers, and in those with previous pulmonary disease.[6] Stein and Cassara found that a maximum expiratory flow rate of less than 200 L/min was predictive of patients at risk for pulmonary complications[7] (see Chapter 1).

A myriad of radiologic diagnostic procedures is currently available. These range from simple anteroposterior and lateral chest x-rays to sophisticated procedures such as tomography, computed tomography scans, magnetic resonance imaging, and arteriograms. These tests may provide invaluable information to the anesthesiologist as to the location and degree of airway compromise (see Chapter 2). The failure to detect significant preoperative pulmonary compromise does not guarantee an uncomplicated intraoperative course. Induction of anesthesia or manipulation of the airway may unmask problems that were previously well compensated.

BRONCHOSCOPY

Indications

Bronchoscopy evolved about 100 years ago, when the first translaryngeal intubation of the trachea with a tube was recorded.[8] At first, this procedure was performed mainly to recover inhaled foreign bodies, although it was later used by Jackson for removal of excessive secretions from the pulmonary tree and for resection of endobronchial tumors.[9] New advances in technology have permitted the broadening of the use of bronchoscopy after the introduction by Ikeda et al of the fiberoptic bronchoscope.[10] Today, bronchoscopy is a common procedure, and both fiberoptic as well as rigid bronchoscopies have their own indications and involve specialized techniques. Indications for bronchoscopy can be divided into one of three categories: diagnostic, therapeutic, and preoperative evaluation of pathology.

Diagnostic Indications

The most common indication for bronchoscopy is when patients present with signs and symptoms causing suspicion of bronchial neoplasm. The presenting complaints may include cough, hemoptysis, wheezing, or stridor. Cough is most often due to chronic bronchitis and is frequently associated with cigarette smoking. Sometimes a change in either the frequency or the character of the cough may be the only subtle hint of the presence of bronchogenic neoplasm. When cough is associated with other symptoms, such as stridor, it may suggest the presence of upper airway compromise from tumor. When cough is associated with wheezing, or when it leads to acute bronchospasm, it may indicate a tracheal or mediastinal tumor causing obstruction. Hemoptysis must also be regarded as an ominous sign until the presence of neoplasm is excluded. Although patients with chronic bronchitis from cigarette smoking may expectorate blood-stained sputum, hemoptysis can also be the first sign of a bronchogenic neoplasm.

Other diagnostic indications for bronchoscopy include localized wheezing, atelectasis, persistent pneumonia, positive sputum cytology, and assessment of the airway. Localized wheezing or atelectasis may indicate partial endobronchial obstruction from neoplasm or from an aspirated foreign body. Bronchoscopy is useful after prolonged intubation in order to rule out the presence of subglottic stenosis, tracheomalacia, or, rarely, tracheoesophageal fistula. Examination of the tracheobronchial tree should also be performed after exposure to chemical fumes or smoke inhalation in order to assess the level and severity of the injury. Bronchoscopy can also be performed when it is difficult to ascertain the correct placement of an endotracheal tube, such as in a difficult intubation, or to document proper positioning of a double-lumen endotracheal tube. Recently, bronchoscopy and alveolar lavage have provided better diagnostic yields than both transbronchial and open-lung biopsy procedures in patients with the acquired immunodeficiency syndrome (AIDS).[11]

Therapeutic Indications

Bronchoscopy is performed for therapeutic purposes such as removal of aspirated foreign objects or suctioning of copious secretions, which could result in atelectasis and worsening of ventilation-to-perfusion matching. When therapeutic bronchoscopy is performed after aspiration of particulate gastric contents, the removal of the particulate matter may lessen the degree and severity of the resulting Mendelson's syndrome. Other therapeutic indications include endoscopy for instillation of vasoconstrictors to decrease edema. Drainage of a lung abscess with the aid of a bronchoscope can facilitate obtaining cultures and biopsy specimens and has been used in the diagnosis and treatment of bronchial stump suture granulomas.[12]

Indications for Preoperative Assessment of Pathology

Most patients undergoing thoracotomy for lobe resection or pneumonectomy will require a preoperative bronchoscopic examination. These patients present for lung resection because of carcinoma, and preoperative bronchoscopy will allow the surgeon to evaluate the extent of the tumor and to rule out malignancy of the contralateral lung.

Indications for Rigid Versus Fiberoptic Bronchoscopy

Rigid Bronchoscopy

The rigid or open-tube endoscopic examination of the airway has been used extensively for removal of foreign bodies. It is easier to remove large foreign bodies in toto with the rigid bronchoscope, whereas the fiberoptic bronchoscope may require fragmentation of the object. Moderate or massive hemoptysis is also an indication for rigid bronchoscopy, as it will provide the operator with a better opportunity to suction the airway and improve the visualization of the bleeding site. In the case of a vascular tumor, the use of the rigid bronchoscope will enable the endoscopist to pack the airway should massive bleeding occur during resection. In infants and small children, the rigid bronchoscope is the instrument of choice, since it allows better ventilation and control of the airway. When the patency of the airway is compromised by granulation tissue or tumor, the rigid bronchoscope may be the only instrument that can be inserted past the point of obstruction. Other advantages of the rigid technique include direct visualization of the tracheobronchial tree without the optical distortion associated with fiberoptic bronchoscopy. The rigid broncho-scope also allows the endoscopist to obtain a relatively larger biopsy specimen, thus enhancing the diagnostic yield. Finally, the rigid bronchoscope is preferred for visualization of the carina and for the assessment of its mobility and sharpness, since these observations provide diagnostic clues about bronchial involvement and carcinogenic infiltration.

Fiberoptic Bronchoscopy

Flexible fiberoptic bronchoscopy provides a better yield in diagnosing bronchogenic carcinoma than rigid bronchoscopy. The advantages of the flexible technique include improved optical resolution, which allows detailed visualization of the tracheobronchial tree. In contrast to the rigid bronchoscope, the fiberoptic bronchoscope has a flexible tip and can be maneuvered into peripheral zones of the lung (ie, fifth division bronchi), thus improving the diagnostic and therapeutic yields of biopsy procedures and exploration. Other advantages of the fiberoptic bronchoscope include facilitation of intubation in patients who have difficult airway anatomy, facial trauma, neck injury, and an edematous airway from inhalation injury.

Fiberoptic bronchoscopy affords improved patient comfort when compared with rigid bronchoscopy. Thus, the need for heavy premedication in order to allay fears is lessened. In patients at risk for developing hypoxia, fiberoptic bronchoscopy may be performed with the patient in a sitting or semisitting position, which improves their ventilatory capacity. Other indications for fiberoptic bronchoscopy include patients with vertebral artery insufficiency in whom extension of the neck may induce cerebral ischemia, and in patients who are at risk for dental damage. Finally, video imaging (ie, closed-circuit television) allows closer cooperation between the endoscopist and the anesthesiologist when fiberoptic bronchoscopy is performed.

Although there are numerous reports that attest to the usefulness of the fiberoptic bronchoscope for removing aspirated foreign bodies, a disadvantage of this technique includes the need to fragment the object before removal. This could lead to aspiration of small fragments distally. Another limitation of the fiberoptic bronchoscope is the relatively small size (2 mm) of the aspirating channel. This limits its usefulness in patients with hemoptysis and copious secretions.

Complications and Physiologic Changes

Many complications of bronchoscopy have been reported.[13–17] These are generally divided into two categories: complications associated with anesthesia and complications arising from the procedure itself. Hypoventilation and hypoxemia are two complications that can have potentially disastrous effects.[18-22] Both of these conditions can occur either as a result of excessive premedication or inadequate ventilation during the procedure. Since many bronchoscopies are performed under topical anesthesia, quantitative assessment of ventilation is more difficult than with general anesthesia. The use of volume monitoring and capnography is impractical during regional anesthesia. Even under general anesthesia, oxygenation and ventilation may be impaired depending on the type of bronchoscopy being performed and the method of ventilation used during the bronchoscopy. Other complications related to anesthesia include hypertension, hypotension, and tachycardia, all of which can result in myocardial ischemia.[23,24] Dysrhythmias are also possible, and are frequently related to hypoxia and hypercarbia.[23-25]

Another potentially serious complication associated with bronchoscopy is toxic reactions to local anesthetics. In two large retrospective studies, 73,000 bronchoscopies were reported by Credle et al[13] and Suratt et al.[14] Both groups reported major complications related to local anesthetic toxicity. In both studies, tetracaine was the agent most often implicated. In Credle et al's report of over 24,000 bronchoscopies, there were seven major complications related to topical anesthesia.[13] Excessive tetracaine was responsible for six of the seven toxic reactions, which included three cases of respiratory arrest, two seizures, one case of methemoglobinemia, and the only mortality in a patient who was not seriously ill at the time of bronchoscopy. Excessive lidocaine was responsible for a seizure and two other unspecified minor complications. Although highly effective as a topical anesthetic, tetracaine is toxic and has a low therapeutic index. The maximum recommended dose is 1.0 to 1.5 mg/kg, to a total dose of 100 mg/70 kg.[26] Weisel and Tella[27] and Adriani and Campbell[28] have reported complications related to tetracaine administration. One of the most difficult problems is that tetracaine toxicity may manifest itself without any warning. Indeed, the first sign of tetracaine toxicity may be a seizure or cardiovascular collapse. In contrast, lidocaine offers a much wider margin of safety than tetracaine. Toxicity from lidocaine is likely to include recognizable and reversible central nervous system symptoms prior to cardiovascular collapse.

The other group of complications relates to the bronchoscopic procedure itself. Severe hemorrhage following a biopsy, pneumothorax, and laceration of a bronchial wall are the most frequent problems. In addition, laryngospasm and bronchospasm can occur with manipulation of the airway or in conjunction with inadequate levels of anesthesia. Complication

rates are significantly higher in asthmatics who undergo bronchoscopy, probably as a result of their increased airway reactivity.[16,29-31]

Although there are many potentially life-threatening complications related to bronchoscopy, the overall rates of morbidity and mortality are quite low. Several large-scale studies have been undertaken to assess the rate of complications with bronchoscopy.[13,14,16,17] Overall, the highest rate of complications was 8.2 percent, while the highest death rate was 0.1 percent.

The physiologic changes associated with bronchoscopy relate mainly to the cardiovascular and respiratory systems. Prys-Roberts et al noted a significant increase in sympathetic activity during laryngoscopy, which was most often manifested by tachycardia and hypertension.[23] This sympathetic response can be attenuated by a number of maneuvers. Stoelting demonstrated that intravenous lidocaine reduces the hypertensive response to laryngoscopy.[32] Similarly, other agents, including narcotics, beta-blocking drugs, and sodium nitroprusside, have been used to decrease the sympathetic response.[33-36] Recently, use of calcium channel blockers has been reported in patients at risk for developing bronchospasm related to the administration of beta-blockers.[37,38] Roizen et al have demonstrated that very deep levels of inhalation anesthesia (two to three minimum alveolar concentrations) are required to suppress the adrenergic responses.[39] Treatment with fentanyl or alfentanil prior to bronchoscopy has also been shown to attenuate the hypertensive response seen in the control group, but ST segment changes suggestive of myocardial ischemia were present in both the control and narcotic-treated groups.[40]

Bronchoscopy is frequently associated with changes in cardiac rhythm. Minor rhythm disturbances have been reported in up to 73 percent of the patients undergoing bronchoscopy, although major dysrhythmias occur in only 4 to 11 percent of patients.[41,42] The dysrhythmias tended to be self-limited and did not cause major hemodynamic instability. Systemic absorption of topically applied anesthesics, particularly lidocaine, may have a salutary effect on cardiac dysrhythmias during bronchoscopy.

Bronchoscopy can also cause impairment of the respiratory system. Several studies have demonstrated that fiberoptic bronchoscopy induces hypoxia in awake, spontaneously breathing patients.[18,19] Salisbury et al demonstrated that fiberoptic bronchoscopy induced a decline in PO_2 in both normal volunteers and in patients with chronic airway obstruction.[43] This decline in PO_2 occurred without significant changes in PCO_2 or pH. The change in PO_2 is transient and may last from 15 minutes to 4 hours.[18,43] The decline in PO_2 can be avoided by administering supplemental oxygen to the patient via a face mask or nasal cannula, or by insufflating oxygen through the suction port of the fiberoptic bronchoscope or through a nasopharyngeal airway.[44,45] Increasing the inspired oxygen concentration is more easily accomplished during general anesthesia.

Fiberoptic bronchoscopy can also affect pulmonary mechanics. Forced vital capacity and FEV_1 have been reported to decrease 13 to 30 percent.[46] The proposed mechanisms for the deterioration in pulmonary mechanics during fiberoptic bronchoscopy include bronchoconstriction and airway edema. These deleterious effects of fiberoptic bronchoscopy can be eliminated by pretreating the patient with anticholinergic agents such as atropine or glycopyrrolate.[27,47,48]

Awareness during bronchoscopy is still a potentially significant problem. Moore and Seymour reported an overall 7 percent incidence of awareness during bronchoscopy.[49] These patients frequently receive "light" general anesthesia with a short-acting barbiturate and muscle relaxant. It is important for the anesthesiologist to remember that with this technique, patients undergoing bronchoscopy are capable of auditory awareness. Use of headphones with random noise or music may be helpful in reducing this problem.

Not infrequently, critically ill patients undergo fiberoptic bronchoscopy in the intensive care unit. They often have decreased or absent pulmonary reserve and have been mechanically ventilated for significant periods of time. Since many of these patients are awake, bronchoscopy can result in significant increases in blood pressure and heart rate with subsequent myocardial ischemia. Lindholm et al have reviewed the potential problems of performing fiberoptic bronchoscopy in an intubated patient.[50,51] The introduction of a fiberoptic bronchoscope into an endotracheal tube may create a significant increase in airway resistance (Fig. 12-4). Unless the endotracheal tube is of sufficient size, the patient will not be adequately ventilated. The increased resistance within the endotracheal tube can cause the ventilator to exceed its pressure limit and not deliver the preset tidal volume. A 5.7 mm external diameter adult bronchoscope inserted into a 7.0 mm inside diameter (ID) endotracheal tube causes an increase in the peak airway pressure of up to 60 cmH$_2$O, while up to 35 cmH$_2$O of positive end-expiratory pressure (PEEP) has been reported[50] (Table 12-1). Vigorous suctioning of the airway in an intubated patient can be responsible for withdrawing as much as 300 mL of delivered tidal volume.[51] This decrease in delivered tidal volume may result in hypercarbia and hypoxemia. Therefore,

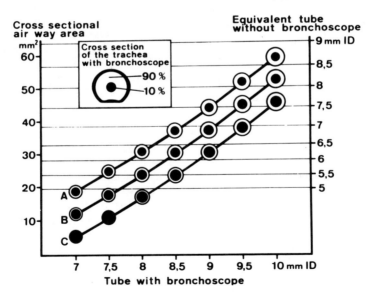

Fig. 12-4. Schematic representation of the cross-sectional areas of different-size endotracheal tubes in which a fiberoptic bronchoscope has been inserted. The outer circle represents the internal diameter of the endotracheal tube, while the solid inner circle represents the external diameter (ED) of the bronchoscope. The different-size bronchoscopes represented are (*A*) 5 mm ED, (*B*) 5.7 mm ED, and (*C*) 6.0 mm ED. The white portion inside each circle represents the area inside the endotracheal tube that remains available for air exchange. The insert at the top left of the figure illustrates the relative relationship between a normal airway and a bronchoscope inserted in a nonintubated airway. (From Lindholm et al,[50] with permission.)

**TABLE 12-1.   Relationship of Endotracheal Tube Size and
PEEP Produced by Insertion of a 5.7 mm FOB**

Endotracheal Tube Size (mm ID)	Cross-sectional Area (% Occupied by the 5.7 mm FOB)	Maximum Measured PEEP in Patients (cmH$_2$O)
7	66	35
8	51	20
9	40	—

Abbreviations: PEEP, positive end-expiratory pressure; FOB, fiberoptic bronchoscope.
(From Lindholm et al,[50] with permission.)

when intensive care unit patients require fiberoptic
bronchoscopy, the following guidelines are recommended:

1. Endoscopists should ensure that the endotracheal
   tube is of adequate size to accommodate the bronchoscope being used. Generally, an 8.5 to 9.0 mm
   endotracheal tube is necessary for most adult fiberoptic bronchoscopes.
2. Mechanically ventilated patients should be hand-
   ventilated with a non-rebreathing anesthesia circuit and 100 percent oxygen. In this manner, adequacy of ventilation and the amount of resistance
   generated by the bronchoscope can be readily assessed.
3. Only intermittent suctioning should be performed
   for short periods of time.
4. The patient's mental status should be considered
   and appropriate sedation administered as the
   physical condition permits.
5. Any mechanical PEEP should be removed from the
   circuit, as bronchoscopy may itself induce PEEP.
6. The patient's cardiovascular status should be carefully monitored, and continuous assessment of oxygen saturation with a pulse oximeter in this setting
   is mandatory.

Methods of Ventilation During Bronchoscopy

Rigid Bronchoscopy

The original bronchoscopes were merely an open tube
through which the endoscopist could operate. If general anesthesia was required, one of three methods of
ventilation was possible: (1) spontaneous ventilation
by the patient; (2) positive-pressure ventilation with
oxygen delivered through the side port while the open
end of the bronchoscope was occluded; or (3) apneic
oxygenation. Apneic oxygenation was first described
in the anesthesia literature by Frumin et al.[52] In this
technique, the patient is denitrogenated with 100 percent oxygen then relaxed with neuromuscular block-

ers, and oxygen is continuously delivered into the trachea through a catheter or via the bronchoscope. This
allows the bronchoscopist to work uninterrupted for
significant periods of time. Since there is no ventilation, levels of carbon dioxide will continuously rise. In
their article, Frumin et al reported PaCO$_2$ levels of up
to 250 mmHg after 53 minutes of apneic oxygenation,
with uneventful patient recovery.[52] Fraioli et al described a group of patients with low functional residual capacity-to-body weight ratios, in whom significant decreases in oxygenation occurred after
4 minutes and in whom apneic oxygenation could not
be continued beyond 15 minutes.[53] In addition,
awareness during general anesthesia with apneic oxygenation has been reported.[54]

The ventilating bronchoscope (Fig. 12-5) provides a
significant improvement in the care of patients undergoing bronchoscopy. This technique uses an anesthesia circuit that is attached directly to the side port of
the bronchoscope. A glass window is then placed over
the proximal end of the bronchoscope, and general
anesthesia and positive-pressure ventilation can be
administered to the patient. This system has the advantage of allowing both inhalation and intravenous
anesthesia to be administered to the patient. All anesthetic gases are easily scavenged from the circuit, and
leaks around the bronchoscope can usually be managed by applying manual pressure over the larynx.
Alternatively, leaks around the bronchoscope can be
prevented by fitting an inflatable cuff around the
bronchoscope or by packing the pharynx with moist
sponges. Adequacy of ventilation can be assessed by
using a respirometer or an end-tidal carbon dioxide
monitor. As with any bronchoscopic procedure, continuous monitoring of arterial oxygen saturation with
a pulse oximeter should be done. The disadvantage of
this system is that the occluding window must be removed in order for the endoscopist to obtain biopsy
specimens or to suction the airway. The removal of
the window results in an open-ended bronchoscope
through which positive-pressure ventilation is not
possible, while anesthetic gases may escape from the
open end and pollute the room. Finally, an estimation

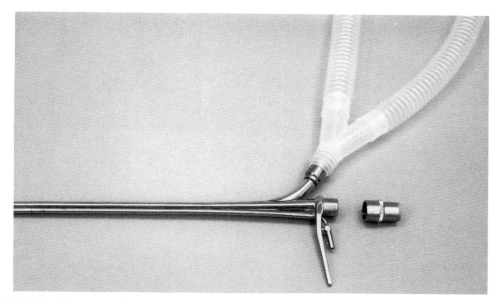

Fig. 12-5. Rigid side-arm ventilating bronchoscope with an attached anesthesia circuit. Note that the viewing window that seals the open end of the bronchoscope has been removed for illustration purposes.

of the patient's compliance can be obtained by the anesthesiologist from the "feel" of the reservoir bag and by observing peak inspiratory pressures within the circuit.

This system was further improved by the introduction of the Hopkins lens telescope (Fig. 12-6). When inserted in a side-arm ventilating bronchoscope, the telescope gives the endoscopist an improved view of the tracheobronchial tree. In addition, this instrument has special side ports through which suction catheters and biopsy instruments can be introduced without having to open the proximal end of the bronchoscope to the atmosphere.

Another method of ventilating the patient while providing general anesthesia for bronchoscopy is to place a small endotracheal tube (5.0 to 6.0 mm ID) alongside the bronchoscope. This technique allows administration and scavenging of inhalational anesthetics as long as the proximal end of the bronchoscope remains covered. When the window of the bronchoscope is removed, anesthetic gases will escape into the atmosphere. Anesthesiologists must ensure that the endotracheal tube is large enough to allow for passive exhalation. If the tube is not large enough, then the end of the bronchoscope must be opened to allow for this. Most adults have a trachea that is able to accommodate both an endotracheal tube and a bronchoscope. However, in cases of tracheal narrowing or external compression, this technique would not be advisable.

A major addition to the anesthetic care of the patient undergoing bronchoscopy occurred in 1967 when Sanders introduced the ventilating attachment for the bronchoscope.[55] This consisted of a source of high-pressure oxygen (50 psi) that was intermittently jetted through a 16-gauge cannula attached to the proximal end of the bronchoscope (Figs. 12-7 and 12-8). To understand how the Sanders attachment works, it is necessary to understand Bernoulli's law.[56] Bernoulli's law states that the velocity of a fluid flowing through a pipe is inversely proportional to the cross-sectional area. In addition, Bernoulli demonstrated that the pressure a fluid exerts is least in the area where the speed is greatest (Fig. 12-9). Thus, when the fluid is forced to flow through a constriction, the speed of the fluid increases, but the lateral wall pressure is decreased. Venturi used this information to develop his injector (Fig. 12-10). By passing a high-pressure gas through a narrow orifice, there is a marked decrease in the pressure surrounding the injector. This decrease in pressure entrains surrounding gas and markedly increases the total flow. This is frequently referred to as the Sanders Venturi principle.

The oxygen jet entrains large volumes of room air, which enables the patient to receive adequate ventilation. With this technique, the endoscopist could work uninterrupted through the open bronchoscope. A number of studies attest to the efficacy of this technique.[57–62] Giesecke et al compared the injector to the side-arm ventilating methods for bronchoscopy and

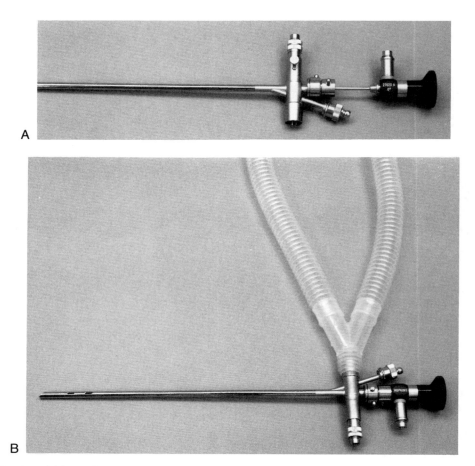

Fig. 12-6. **(A)** Rigid ventilating bronchoscope with a Hopkins lens being inserted. **(B)** Rigid side-arm bronchoscope containing the Hopkins lens and an attached anesthesia circuit.

found essentially similar results.[63] Both groups of patients could be adequately ventilated and oxygenated with minimal side effects.

Although the Sanders technique had the advantage of providing adequate ventilation to the patient by entraining room air, it had the disadvantage of lowering the F_IO_2 delivered to the patient to approximately 30 percent. Another disadvantage of the Sanders Venturi technique is the inability to adequately ventilate the patient who has decreased lung compliance. The

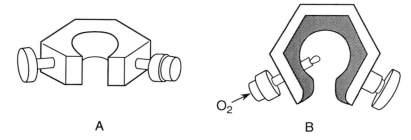

Fig. 12-7. A diagrammatic representation of the Sanders injector: **(A)** side view; **(B)** top view. The oxygen is jetted into the side port after fitting the Sanders injector over the open end of the rigid bronchoscope.

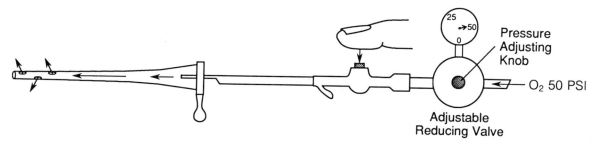

Fig. 12-8. The Sanders attachment fitted to the open end of the bronchoscope and connected to a valve that will allow intermittent jetting of the high-pressure oxygen via the Venturi injector. The wall oxygen at 50 psi pressure is connected to a reducing valve, which allows the pressure to be adjusted from 0 to 50 psi.

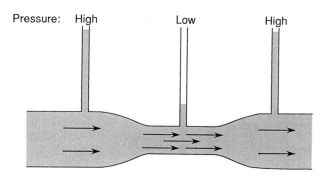

Fig. 12-9. A schematic illustration of Bernoulli's principle. As the diameter of the pipe narrows, the speed of the fluid flowing through it increases. At the same time, the lateral wall pressure generated by the fluid flowing through the narrowed pipe segment is decreased when compared with the wall pressure of the fluid flowing through the unobstructed segment of the tube.

Sanders system is capable of generating a maximum pressure of 22 cmH₂O. Carden et al modified the Sanders technique by using the side-arm of the bronchoscope as the injector site,[57,64] enabling them to deliver an airway pressure of up to 55 cmH₂O with a driving pressure of only 30 psi (Fig. 12-11). Thus, they were able to more efficiently ventilate patients with decreased pulmonary compliance, while markedly lowering the amount of room air entrained. This significantly increased the F_1O_2 delivered to the patient. Various other modifications of this technique include placing a chest tube or nasogastric tube into the trachea beside the bronchoscope, then attaching it to the jet ventilating device.[65] Nitrous oxide could also be mixed with the oxygen and jetted into the trachea for enhanced levels of anesthesia.[66,67]

These systems worked well, but required the anesthesiologist to be extremely vigilant. The best indicator of adequate ventilation is obtained by observing the patient's chest movement with inflation. Quantitative assessment of ventilation by spirometry and end-tidal CO_2 cannot be obtained. Use of pulse oximetry is highly recommended with this technique. Newer technology, such as a transcutaneous PCO_2

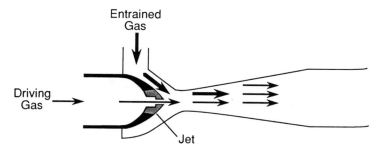

Fig. 12-10. A diagrammatic representation of the Venturi principle. The high-pressure driving gas (oxygen) jetted through the narrow orifice creates a negative pressure around the jet orifice and entrains large amounts of surrounding gas (room air).

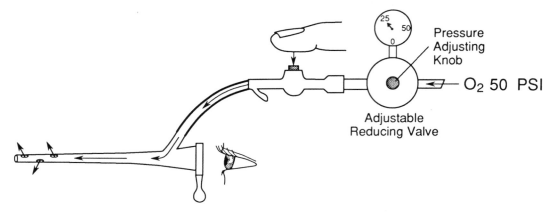

Fig. 12-11. A schematic of the Carden modification of the Venturi injector. This modification uses the side port of the bronchoscope as the injector site, allowing reduced driving pressures and increased oxygen concentration delivery to the patient. This also allows the endoscopist to operate via an open-ended rigid bronchoscope.

monitor, would also be useful to assess ventilation. A hazard of using a Venturi system is that exhalation is passive, and it must occur either through the bronchoscope or through the open glottis. If muscle relaxation is inadequate and the vocal cords are closed, the exhaled gas may be trapped, causing barotrauma and pneumothorax.

Several studies have demonstrated that high-frequency jet ventilation can also be a useful technique for ventilation during bronchoscopy.[68-71] This technique is particularly beneficial in patients who have bronchopleural fistulae because mean airway pressure is minimal with this mode of ventilation. In addition, this technique results in no air entrainment through the proximal end of the bronchoscope, thus allowing consistent and predictable inhalational anesthetic concentrations to be delivered to the patient.[71] The high-frequency ventilation technique can also be used with the fiberoptic bronchoscope.[72]

Fiberoptic Bronchoscopy

The introduction of the fiberoptic bronchoscope has increased the comfort and safety of the patient undergoing bronchoscopy. The awake patient can easily ventilate around the bronchoscope as it occupies only approximately 10 percent of the cross-sectional area of the trachea. If general anesthesia is used, fiberoptic bronchoscopy usually involves passing the bronchoscope through an endotracheal tube fitted with a special adaptor (Fig. 12-12). In this manner, the patient can be continuously ventilated and end-tidal CO_2 and ventilatory volumes can be easily monitored (Fig. 12-13). Since fiberoptic bronchoscopy involves the introduction of the fiberscope through the endotracheal tube, the relationship of the diameter of the bronchoscope to the diameter of the endotracheal tube becomes critical. Poiseuille's law states that flow is directly proportional to the fourth power of the radius;

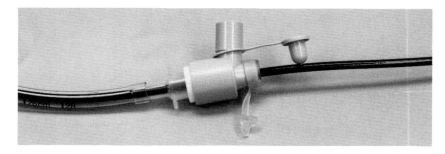

Fig. 12-12. An endotracheal tube fitted with an elbow adapter that allows passage of the fiberoptic bronchoscope. The bronchoscope is passed through a rubber diaphragm located at the top of the elbow. The tight fit of the diaphragm around the bronchoscope allows continued ventilation during bronchoscopy.

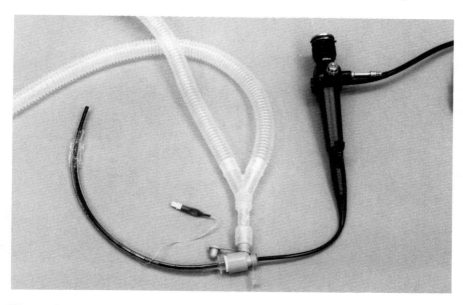

Fig. 12-13. Fiberoptic bronchoscope inserted through an elbow (right angle) adapter into the endotracheal tube. The anesthesia circuit is attached.

thus, minimal changes in the diameter of the endotracheal tube will have a great impact on the tidal volume delivered. For this reason, it has been shown that even the minimal kinking associated with a nasotracheally placed tube will affect the tidal volume and the airway pressure generated during ventilation more than orotracheal intubation.[73] Carden and Raj's modification of the endotracheal tube also takes advantage of the fact that flow is directly proportional to the diameter and inversely proportional to the length of the tube.[74] The Carden endotracheal tube is tapered and has a wide supraglottic portion (thus decreasing the resistance to flow), while the subglottic portion (where most of the resistance occurs) is effectively shortened to one-fourth of the normal length of 30 cm.

Lindholm et al delineated these relationships and showed that a 5.7 mm bronchoscope will occupy 40 percent of the cross-sectional area of a 9.0 mm ID endotracheal tube, whereas the same bronchoscope will occupy nearly 70 percent of a 7.0 mm ID endotracheal tube.[50,51] Fiberoptic bronchoscopes are available in several different sizes. It is important for the anesthesiologist to select an endotracheal tube of sufficient diameter to accommodate the bronchoscope without producing a significant increase in airway pressure. This will also prevent production of PEEP, and will allow passive exhalation around the bronchoscope. Use of a 9.0 mm endotracheal tube for fiberoptic bronchoscopy is recommended whenever possible (Fig. 12-14). Although positive-pressure ventilation using a standard anesthesia circle system is the most commonly used method, other modes of ventilation have been described. Smith et al used the technique of jet ventilation through a small chest tube that was placed in the trachea beside the fiberoptic bronchoscope.[75] A modification of this technique involves using jet ventilation through the suction channel of the fiberscope.[76]

Laser therapy for endobronchial tumors has become quite popular. The carbon dioxide and argon lasers have been used successfully and require a rigid bronchoscope. The Nd-YAG laser can transmit its energy along a fiberoptic cable. Therefore, it is suitable for use with either a rigid or a fiberoptic bronchoscope. More detailed discussion of lasers can be found in Chapter 16.

Anesthetic Technique

Premedication for the patient scheduled to undergo bronchoscopy depends not only on the physical status of the patient, but also on the proposed surgical technique. If fiberoptic bronchoscopy under local anesthesia is planned, patients require relatively less sedation preoperatively than if they were to undergo rigid bronchoscopy. Also, patients who are at greater risk of pulmonary complications or who have very limited pulmonary reserve should not be heavily premedicated, as this might further compromise gas exchange. For these patients, a good rapport established

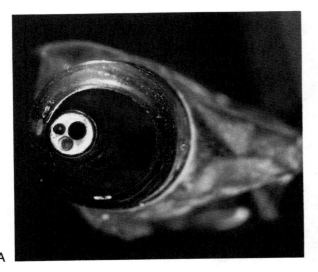
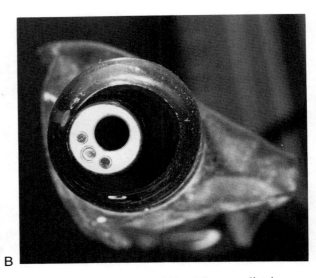

A   B

Fig. 12-14. A 9.0 mm endotracheal tube containing two different-size bronchoscopes: **(A)** a 4.0 mm pediatric scope, and **(B)** a 6.2 mm adult bronchoscope. Note that even with a 9.0 mm endotracheal tube, a significant portion of the lumen is occupied by the adult bronchoscope.

with the anesthesiologist during the preoperative visit may be the most valuable premedication (see Chapter 10).

Three classes of medication are given preoperatively:

1. Narcotics are administered for analgesia, to decrease the cough reflex, and to provide euphoria. Morphine has been shown to have salutary effects in mild asthmatics because of its inhibition of vagally mediated bronchoconstriction.[77] Because of its ability to induce release of histamine by the mast cells, however, morphine must be used cautiously in severe asthmatics. Alternatively, other narcotics, such as meperidine, fentanyl, or hydromorphone, are effective premedications.

2. Anticholinergics such as atropine (0.4 to 0.6 mg/70 kg) and glycopyrrolate (0.1 to 0.2 mg/70 kg) given intramuscularly will minimize the vasovagal reflexes and diminish oral and bronchial secretions. Although not recommended in the outpatient setting, scopolamine is an excellent adjuvant to narcotic premedication, as it has superior sedative, amnesic, and antisialagogue properties. Atropine and glycopyrrolate are equally effective in producing bronchodilation, while both atropine and scopolamine reduce the incidence of laryngospasm during induction of anesthesia.[78]

3. Benzodiazepines, such as diazepam or midazolam, can be administered as a premedication because of their anxiolytic effects. Benzodiazepines are useful because of their amnesic properties, and because they protect against the central nervous system toxicity of local anesthetics by increasing the seizure threshold.

The preoperative use of one other medication needs to be mentioned, if only because of its controversial role. Steroids have been suggested for the prevention of postoperative airway edema. Although several studies have attested to the usefulness of this premedication technique, most of the studies have dealt with the reduction of postoperative facial and oral edema following facial surgery.[79,80] The role of steroids in preventing airway edema postoperatively remains unclear.

Flexible Fiberoptic Bronchoscopy

The use of the fiberoptic bronchoscope allows for greater versatility on the part of the endoscopist in tailoring the anesthetic approach to the particular patient's needs and comfort. Fiberoptic bronchoscopies are frequently performed under local or topical anesthesia. The most commonly used local anesthetics for topical anesthesia include lidocaine, tetracaine, and cocaine. Of these, tetracaine is known to have a low therapeutic index, with a maximum safe dose of 1 to 1.5 mg/kg (100 mg/70 kg), while cocaine is less frequently used because of its potential for abuse. Topicalization of the pharynx and tracheobronchial tree is, therefore, most easily accomplished by inhaled, nebulized lidocaine. For this purpose, 4 to 6 mL of 4 percent lidocaine is placed in an ultrasonic nebulizer that is attached to a face mask. This method of anesthetizing the tracheobronchial tree probably causes the least amount of discomfort to the patient, and it is also technically very easy to accomplish. Furthermore, nebulized lidocaine was shown to be of sufficiently small size (average, 6.3 μm) to be distributed over the entire mucosa of the upper and lower respiratory tracts.[81] This distribution of local anesthetic into the distal bronchioles will greatly facilitate the fiberoptic examination.

The drawbacks of this method include the inability to properly anesthetize areas of the tracheobronchial tree that do not come in direct contact with the inhaled local anesthetic, such as the area immediately below the vocal cords. The other disadvantage is that the amount of local anesthetic that is being absorbed is unknown, but, for safety purposes, it must be assumed to be equal to the amount of local anesthetic that is being nebulized. Other means of anesthetizing the posterior pharynx include sprays, droppers, and anesthetic-soaked applicators such as cotton-tipped swabs, which may be placed in the posterior pharynx.

It is important to remember that topical anesthesia will only obtund the tactile receptors of the airway, leaving intact the more deeply situated pressure receptors that are found in the posterior pharynx. Blocking the pressure receptors is very important in order to ablate the gag reflex. In general, the abolition of the gag reflex can be accomplished by blocking the afferent pathways, including glossopharyngeal and superior laryngeal nerves, or by attenuating the hemodynamic responses by use of intravenous narcotics or local anesthetics[82] (Fig. 12-15).

Glossopharyngeal nerve blockade may be accomplished by injection of local anesthetic into the lateral pharyngeal wall at the root of the tongue, as the lingual branch of the glossopharyngeal nerve is relatively superficial when it traverses the posterior aspect of the palatoglossal arch (Fig. 12-16). A 26- or 27-gauge, short (1/2- to 5/8-inch) needle is used, and a negative aspiration test must be performed to ensure that injection is not made into the carotid artery. A total dose of 40 mg of lidocaine (2 mL of 1 percent lidocaine on each side) will provide 10 to 15 minutes of anesthesia. If a longer duration is desired, then the block is performed with an epinephrine-containing solution (1 : 200,000). The superior laryngeal nerve block may be accomplished by injecting local anesthetic (2 to 3 mL of 2 percent lidocaine) at the tip of each superior thyroid cornu. The superior laryngeal nerve may also be blocked topically by applying local anesthetic-soaked pledgets to the pyriform sinuses bilaterally (Fig. 12-17).

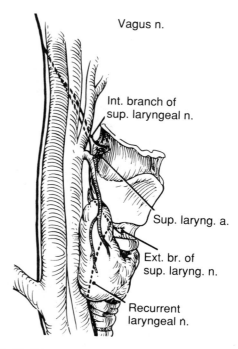

Fig. 12-15. Diagram of the nerve supply of the larynx. (From Gaskill and Gillies,[85] with permission.)

Finally, anesthetizing areas immediately underneath the vocal cords may be accomplished by injecting local anesthetic directly into the trachea through the cricothyroid membrane (ie, transtracheal injection of 2 to 3 mL of 4 percent lidocaine). Injection of the local anesthetic should be performed very rapidly while the patient is taking a vital capacity breath, as this is usually followed by a forceful cough. To prevent the needle from puncturing and injuring the

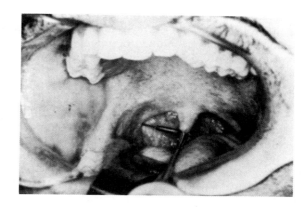

Fig. 12-16. Glossopharyngeal nerve block using an angled peroral tonsillar needle. (From Cooper and Watson,[84] with permission.)

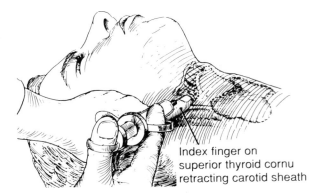

Index finger on
superior thyroid cornu
retracting carotid sheath

Fig. 12-17. Percutaneous block of the internal branch of the superior laryngeal nerve. (From Gaskill and Gillies,[85] with permission.)

structures posterior to the trachea as the patient coughs and lunges forward, a surgical clamp can be snapped onto the needle at the level of its skin entry before injecting the local anesthetic. Alternatively, a 22-gauge Teflon intravenous catheter may be introduced percutaneously into the trachea, and the needle withdrawn before injecting the local anesthetic.[83] This Teflon catheter is malleable, so the tissues are not injured when the patient coughs.

Before performing any topical anesthesia, it must be remembered that anesthesia of the larynx and trachea is relatively contraindicated in patients with a full stomach because obtundation of protective airway reflexes may place them at increased risk for aspiration of gastric contents. Furthermore, local anesthetic toxicity is enhanced in the face of hypercarbia and acidosis. Therefore, the anesthesiologist must be very vigilant to ensure proper ventilation and oxygenation of the patient during the entire perioperative period.

A safe and technically easy fiberoptic bronchoscopic examination may be performed during general anesthesia. For this technique, maintenance may be provided by intermittent boluses or by continuous infusion of intravenous agents, such as narcotics (fentanyl, sufentanil, or alfentanil), ketamine, etomidate, sodium thiopental, or, more recently, propofol.

Fiberoptic bronchoscopy may also be performed with general anesthesia using potent inhalation agents. For this technique, several options are possible. The first involves passing the fiberoptic bronchoscope through the patient's endotracheal tube, which has been fitted with an adaptor (Fig. 12-12). This method will allow continuous ventilation of the patient while the bronchoscopic examination is being performed, and will also have the benefit of scavenging exhaled gases.

The second option involves passing the fiberscope into the trachea, beside an existing, smaller-sized endotracheal tube. This technique has the disadvantage of not scavenging the anesthetic gases, since inflating the endotracheal cuff will not allow further maneuvering of the fiberoptic bronchoscope. A third method involves jet ventilation with oxygen via a catheter placed perorally into the trachea. Anesthesia and muscle relaxation are then accomplished with intravenous agents.[75] Alternatively, oxygen may be delivered via the suction channel of the fiberscope.[75,76] Topicalization of the airway is beneficial in patients undergoing general anesthesia for bronchoscopy, as it will reduce the anesthetic requirements, attenuate the cough reflex, and allow for more rapid emergence.

Rigid Bronchoscopy

Although the literature describes the use of local anesthesia for performance of rigid bronchoscopy, since the introduction of the flexible bronchoscope, most of the techniques involving topical or local anesthesia have been performed with the fiberoptic bronchoscope.[84–86] Thus, rigid bronchoscopy is most often performed with a general anesthetic technique.

Depending on the preoperative evaluation of the patient, the airway may first need to be secured by an awake fiberoptic intubation. Alternatively, an adequate airway may allow induction of anesthesia with a barbiturate/relaxant technique, followed by intubation with either an endotracheal tube or directly with the rigid bronchoscope.

After induction of anesthesia, the specific anesthetic technique depends on the type of rigid bronchoscope used. When using an open-ended bronchoscope with the mass apneic oxygenation, jet ventilation, or Sanders Venturi techniques, anesthesia must consist of intravenous agents plus muscle relaxation. Although it is technically possible to deliver a nitrous oxide/oxygen mixture via the Sanders attachment, this is not recommended because of operating room pollution.[65]

Modification of the open-end to a closed-end bronchoscope by the addition of a window or a Hopkins telescope to the proximal end allows the use of a semiclosed anesthesia circle system. This facilitates an inhalational anesthetic technique, while allowing waste anesthetic gases to be properly scavenged. If the closed system is opened by frequent removal of the window, then the primary anesthetic technique should be converted to an intravenous general anesthetic.

Whether performed with a rigid or fiberoptic instrument, bronchoscopy is a very stimulating procedure that requires an adequate depth of anesthesia. This

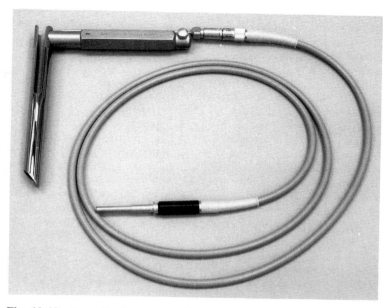

Fig. 12-18. A mediastinoscope with an attached fiberoptic light cable.

level of anesthesia must be maintained until the end of the procedure. Rapid emergence and recovery of protective airway reflexes is desirable. The introduction of newer, short-acting agents such as propofol, atracurium, vecuronium and, potentially, desflurane can facilitate these goals.[87]

MEDIASTINOSCOPY

In 1954, Harken et al reported a new procedure for the tissue diagnosis of mediastinal disease using a modified laryngoscope[88] (Figs. 12-18 and 12-19). This approach (cervical mediastinal exploration) was re-

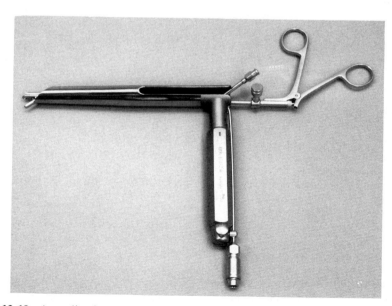

Fig. 12-19. A mediastinoscope through which a biopsy forceps has been inserted.

fined in 1959 by Carlens, who reported the technique of anterior cervical mediastinoscopy.[89] The anatomic basis for development of this procedure for tissue diagnosis of mediastinal tumors rests on the lymphatic drainage of the lungs that proceeds from the hilar nodes to the subcarinal, paratracheal, and, finally, supraclavicular lymph nodes. The major indications for performance of mediastinoscopy are evaluation of lymph node involvement in patients with carcinoma of the lung and obtaining a tissue biopsy of suspected tumors. Patients with bilateral lymph node involvement are an absolute contraindication for thoracotomy, while unilateral involvement does not constitute a contraindication to definitive surgery.[90]

Contraindications to mediastinoscopy can be classified as either absolute or relative. The absolute contraindications include (1) anterior mediastinal tumors, (b) inoperable tumor, (3) previous recurrent laryngeal nerve injury, (4) extremely debilitated patients, (5) ascending aortic aneurysm, and (6) previous mediastinoscopy.[91,92] The relative contraindications to mediastinoscopy include thoracic inlet obstruction and the presence of a superior vena cava syndrome.

The tumors that can be identified during mediastinoscopy include primary malignant tumors, such as lymphoma, as well as bone, vascular, or connective tissue tumors. Secondary malignant mediastinal tumors may originate from lung and pericardium. Mediastinoscopy has also proved to be a valuable tool in the diagnosis of benign tumors such as thymic, tracheal, and bronchial cysts, thymic lymphomas or hyperplasia, nervous system tumors, thyroid masses (ie, goiter), or aneurysms of the ascending aorta, as well as enlarged nodes associated with sarcoidosis. Less common mass lesions present in the mediastinum include pheochromocytoma, teratoma, myxoma, lipoma, and hiatal hernia.[93]

Four approaches to mediastinoscopy have been described. In the early 1990s, von Hacker described the method of reaching the retroesophageal space by introducing the mediastinoscope along the anterior border of the sternocleidomastoid muscle and passing medial to the vessels within the carotid sheath.[94] In 1954, Harken et al described a technique of entering the mediastinum by introducing a laryngoscope through a lateral supraclavicular incision.[88] The anterior mediastinotomy, first described by McNeil and Chamberlain in 1966,[95] involves a vertical incision on either the right or left side of the chest, over the lateral sternal border, through which the mediastinum can be entered.[96] The disadvantage of all these techniques is that they allow only for unilateral exploration and biopsy. If bilateral exploration is necessary the same procedure must be repeated on the contralateral side. In 1959, Carlens introduced a midline approach for mediastinoscopy via a suprasternal incision.[89] This approach allows for safe bilateral exploration and biopsy of tissue from both the paratracheal and the subcarinal areas.

Preoperative Evaluation

Preoperative evaluation of the patient scheduled to undergo mediastinoscopy is extremely important in decreasing or preventing the incidence of perioperative morbidity and mortality. As with all preoperative patients, a complete history and physical examination should be performed. Particular attention should be paid to respiratory symptoms such as wheezing, dyspnea, and orthopnea. It is also important to ascertain whether the respiratory symptoms are exacerbated by exercise or by assuming the supine position. Presence of these respiratory changes should raise the suspicion of major airway obstruction secondary to a mediastinal mass. Dyspnea has been reported to be an important indicator of airway obstruction. In one study, 9 percent of patients with a mediastinal mass compressing the trachea had dyspnea as their presenting complaint.[97] Dysphagia as a preoperative finding may indicate the presence of a large mediastinal mass impinging on both the trachea and the esophagus.

If the preoperative evaluation reveals a potentially serious airway obstruction due to a mediastinal mass, a preoperative course of chemotherapy or radiation has been suggested in order to shrink the size of the tumor and decrease the likelihood of respiratory compromise during induction and maintenance of anesthesia.[98] Although this course of therapy can be effective in patients with mediastinal tumors, it is of no value in patients with airway obstruction secondary to a substernal goiter.[99]

Preoperative workup should include chest x-rays with posteroanterior and lateral views, tomograms, computed tomography scan of the chest and neck, and pulmonary function tests such as flow-volume loops. If tracheal deviation is suspected, then specific studies (neck films and/or tomograms) should be obtained to evaluate the location and extension of the mass as well as the degree of airway compromise. Flow-volume loops in both the upright and supine position are particularly useful in determining whether the obstruction is fixed and if it is intra- or extrathoracic (Fig. 12-1 to Fig. 12-3). Patients with oat cell carcinoma of the lung may have the Eaton-Lambert syndrome, which is associated with prolonged recovery from nondepolarizing muscle relaxants.

Mediastinal tumors have been associated with development of superior vena cava obstruction.[100] Mediastinoscopy in these patients is particularly hazardous, because of the increased risk of major venous bleeding. Presenting symptoms in patients with caval obstruction (superior vena cava syndrome) include shortness of breath (83 percent of cases), cough (70 percent), and orthopnea (64 percent).[101,102]

Anesthetic Technique

Patients undergoing mediastinoscopy may already be at increased risk of pulmonary complications because of airway obstruction, so premedication is probably best avoided. However, thorough preoperative discussion of plans and proposed techniques will allow the anesthesiologist to form a good rapport with the patient. In the majority of cases, this will be sufficient to allay most patients' fears.

Anesthetic management of patients for mediastinoscopy can involve either local or general anesthesia. Advocates of mediastinoscopy under local anesthesia consider this a safer technique in the very debilitated patient.[92,94,103–105] They report superior results and numerous advantages, such as shortened operating time, decreased patient discomfort after the procedure, and early detection and correction of pneumothorax or bilateral recurrent laryngeal nerve paralysis.[103]

Today, however, general anesthesia is the technique of choice in most centers, if the patient scheduled for mediastinoscopy has no preoperative signs or symptoms of airway obstruction.[106–110] In these patients, the general anesthetic technique may involve inhalational or intravenous agents, or, most commonly, a combination of the two. The occurrence of a pneumothorax during mediastinoscopy must be anticipated. It is, therefore, prudent to avoid the use of nitrous oxide, which may increase the size of the pneumothorax and lead to tension pneumothorax.

Other intraoperative considerations include the possibility of innominate artery compression by the mediastinoscope. To detect this complication, several measures have been advocated. They include constant palpation of the right radial or carotid pulse, placement of a right indwelling radial artery catheter, or monitoring of the continuous plethysmographic tracing of a pulse oximeter.[110,111] The danger of innominate artery compression is that falsely low blood pressure readings will be obtained. Simultaneous measurement of blood pressure in the left arm will ensure that therapeutic decisions will not be based on erroneous readings.[112]

The possibility of sudden and massive hemorrhage as a complication of mediastinoscopy exists. For this reason, typed and cross-matched blood must be available. Preoperative placement of at least two large-bore intravenous catheters is advised. In the particular case of superior vena caval obstruction, placement of an intravenous catheter in the lower extremity will ensure venous access below the level of obstruction.

Following intubation, the use of muscle relaxants will provide the endoscopist with an operative field that is safe from sudden movements, which might lead to injury of the adjacent organs by the mediastinoscope. Nondepolarizing muscle relaxants must be used judiciously in patients undergoing mediastinoscopy, because airway collapse from loss of muscle tone has been reported.[98,113–116] In addition, the existence of the myasthenic syndrome must be kept in mind when using nondepolarizing muscle relaxants.

If the preoperative workup is indicative of airway compromise secondary to compression, the anesthetic management is more controversial and depends on whether a tissue diagnosis exists. If it does, the most prudent course of action would be to proceed with preoperative chemotherapy or radiotherapy in order to shrink the tumor size and, thus, decrease the degree of obstruction. In a series of 98 cases, Piro et al reported a 7 percent (5 of 74) incidence of airway complications in patients not receiving preoperative radiation therapy.[117] In contrast, there were no reported cases of airway complications in the 24 patients who underwent preoperative radiotherapy.

If tissue diagnosis of the mediastinal mass does not exist and the patient has signs and symptoms of airway compromise, the most prudent management would be to obtain percutaneous needle biopsy under local anesthesia, followed by radiation and then general anesthesia for mediastinoscopy.[98]

When airway obstruction is present preoperatively, general anesthesia is fraught with problems. Acute tracheal collapse, inability to ventilate the patient, and subsequent death have been reported in patients with mediastinal masses.[98,115,118–120] In the event that circumstances do not permit preoperative shrinkage of the obstructive tumor by radiotherapy,[121] special precautions must be taken when inducing general anesthesia. First, the location of the obstruction should be defined, if possible. Second, a variety of different-sized rigid bronchoscopes, endotracheal tubes (including wire-reinforced), and a fiberoptic bronchoscope should be available. Third, in patients with large mediastinal masses that compress the distal trachea and the mainstem bronchi, the ability to quickly institute cardiopulmonary bypass is preferable.

In the case of *extrathoracic* variable obstruction, fiberoptic intubation under topical anesthesia should be performed in the awake patient. This allows the anesthesiologist to inspect the tracheobronchial tree and to ensure placement of the endotracheal tube below the level of obstruction. If fiberoptic intubation cannot be accomplished, an endotracheal tube can be inserted through a tracheotomy or cricothyroidotomy performed under local anesthesia. General anesthesia, muscle relaxation, and positive-pressure ventilation can then be safely undertaken in most circumstances.

Intrathoracic obstructing masses create the most challenging management dilemmas. First, the extent of airway compromise may be difficult to ascertain preoperatively. Second, the tumor may compress the distal trachea and both mainstem bronchi, so that introduction of an endotracheal tube distal to the compromised area is not feasible. Third, positive-pressure ventilation and muscle relaxation will worsen the intrathoracic obstruction because the distending, negative intrathoracic pressure generated by spontaneous inspiration is lost.

Endotracheal intubation should, therefore, be performed in the spontaneously ventilating patient. Anesthesia maintenance should likewise consist of a technique that permits spontaneous ventilation by the patient. If muscle relaxation and/or positive-pressure ventilation become unavoidable, collapse of the airway may ensue. In this situation, the only recourse would be rapid institution of partial cardiopulmonary bypass.[122,123] In the case of an intrathoracic obstructing mass involving the trachea and only one of the mainstem bronchi, the use of a double-lumen endotracheal tube may provide a patent airway.

Complications

When performed by an experienced endoscopist, mediastinoscopy has a lower morbidity and mortality than exploratory thoracotomy.[107] The incidence of major respiratory complications is directly related to the size of the preoperative mediastinal mass and to the extent of the disease within the mediastinum and the thoracic cage.[106,107]

In a collective series of 9,543 cases, there were nine deaths directly attributable to mediastinoscopy or the anesthetic technique.[109] The mortality rate was 0.09 percent, and the morbidity rate was 1.5 percent. In this literature review, the most common complication was hemorrhage, followed by pneumothorax, recurrent nerve injury, infection, tumor spread, phrenic nerve injury, esophageal injury, chylothorax, air embolism, and hemiparesis. Failure to achieve hemostasis from the inferior thyroid venous plexus will make mediastinoscopy technically more complicated, and it may produce a significant wound hematoma. In up to 10 percent of patients, the right bronchial artery may pass anteriorly across the trachea and down the anterior aspect of the right bronchus. This anatomy may render the bronchial artery particularly susceptible to injury by the mediastinoscope. Esophageal perforation may also occur during paratracheal lymph node dissection and biopsy, particularly if tracheal deviation is present preoperatively.[94] Other reports of complications during mediastinoscopy include laceration of the left pulmonary artery, compression of the innominate artery simulating cardiac arrest, acute tracheal collapse following mediastinoscopy, right bronchial artery hemorrhage, and transient hemiparesis.[109,112,118,124,125]

Mediastinoscopy is a procedure that has very well-defined indications and contraindications, and has proven to be a procedure that can be performed safely under either local or general anesthesia. Preoperative evaluation of the patient with particular emphasis on the degree of airway compromise due to obstruction is crucial. If the safety caveats are followed, mediastinoscopy is a relatively safe procedure with a mortality rate of less than 1:1,000 and a morbidity rate of less than 2 percent. Depending on the indications, the diagnostic yield with mediastinoscopy varies from 38 percent in patients with carcinoma to nearly 100 percent in patients with sarcoidosis.[109]

There are several unique postoperative concerns in patients who have had a mediastinoscopy. Vocal cord paralysis, as a result of injury to the recurrent laryngeal nerve, may lead to stridor and airway compromise. Furthermore, diaphragmatic weakness or paralysis may be the result of intraoperative injury to the phrenic nerves. Finally, hemorrhage into the mediastinum may lead to cardiovascular collapse from cardiac tamponade.

THORACOSCOPY

Thoracoscopy is a procedure that was first introduced in 1910 by Jacobaeus for the diagnosis and treatment of effusions secondary to tuberculosis. Today, thoracoscopy is used for the diagnosis of pleural effusions and for biopsy and preoperative evaluation of primary malignant lesions of the lung and pleura.[126–132] Other indications for thoracoscopy include the diagnosis of cardiac herniation after a pneumonectomy and the identification of the origin of a bronchopleural fistula.[126,133] More recently, thoracoscopy has been used for therapeutic maneuvers. Retrieval of intrathoracic foreign bodies, such as a sheared catheter or a surgical sponge, has been reported.[134] Other therapeutic uses of thoracoscopy include chemical pleurodesis for recurrent pneu-

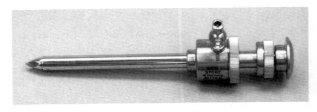

Fig. 12-20. A thoracoscope with the trocar in place.

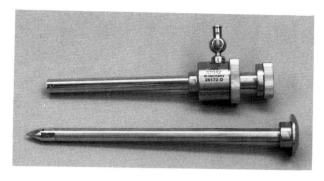

Fig. 12-21. A thoracoscope with the trocar removed and ready to accept viewing or surgical biopsy instruments.

mothorax and drainage of pleural effusions or empyemas. Thoracoscopy has also been used in trauma patients to assess the degree of injury and sometimes to coagulate bleeding vessels. Jones et al reported that emergency thoracoscopy prevented an unnecessary thoracotomy in 16 of 36 (44 percent) patients who had sustained thoracic trauma.[135]

Thoracoscopy is generally regarded as a safe procedure. Reported complications include postoperative bleeding, intrapleural hemorrhage, subcutaneous emphysema, and postoperative pneumothorax. Overall, the procedure is extremely well tolerated, even in debilitated patients.[134,136]

Thoracoscopy is usually performed by introducing a sheath with a trocar into the pleural space (Fig. 12-20). The trocar is then removed, and any number of viewing instruments can be placed into the pleural space via the sheath (Fig. 12-21). Commonly, a rigid

telescope with various viewing angles is used. In addition, use of a fiberoptic bronchoscope (Fig. 12-22) has been reported to be extremely useful for examination of the lung and pleural space, as well as rigid bronchoscopes, laparoscopes, and mediastinoscopes.[137-140] An additional sheath sometimes can be introduced, thus allowing the endoscopist to have an unobstructed view to suction or take biopsy specimens of the operative site. Some surgeons prefer the rigid thoracoscope, while others prefer the fiberoptic. The rigid thoracoscope is reported to provide a better field of vision and better overall lighting, while the fiberoptic is more maneuverable.[126] Once the thoracoscope is introduced, the operative lung is selectively deflated to allow a complete inspection of the pleura and adjacent organs.

Preoperative assessment of patients undergoing thoracoscopy should include the same considerations as the patients undergoing bronchoscopy. Thoracoscopy can be done under either general or regional anesthesia without difficulty.[127,141] Regional anesthesia for thoracoscopy consists of performing intercostal nerve blocks at least two segments above and below the anticipated operative site. This, however, does not anesthetize the visceral pleura, which requires the application of topical local anesthetics. It is also advisable to perform a stellate ganglion block to obtund the cough reflex and prevent injury to adjacent viscera. Alternatively, intravenous narcotics can be used to depress the cough reflex.

Regional anesthesia has the advantage of improving the patient's ability to cough postoperatively compared with general anesthesia, and provides postoperative analgesia secondary to intercostal nerve

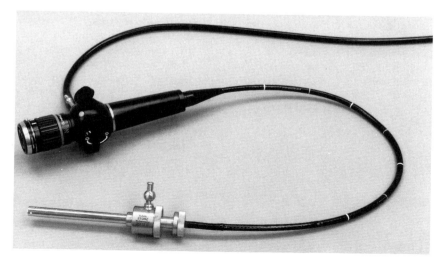

Fig. 12-22. The thoracoscope sheath through which a fiberoptic bronchoscope has been inserted.

blockade. Regional anesthesia may also be better tolerated by debilitated patients. The major disadvantage of regional anesthesia is that the patient has to breathe spontaneously while the operative lung is collapsed. Although this may be tolerated for short periods of time, it is probably not advisable for longer procedures. Finally, the placement of talc or other sclerosing agents into the pleura is frequently uncomfortable in the awake patient.

When general anesthesia is selected for thoracoscopy, a double-lumen endotracheal tube is recommended so that ventilation and oxygenation can be carefully controlled and monitored. This also allows deflation of the operative lung during the procedure. In some instances, bilateral thoracoscopy is performed, and each lung can be successively collapsed and ventilated as needed by the surgeon. Furthermore, the double-lumen tube allows the lung to be re-expanded under the direct vision of the surgeon, which is helpful in the case of a lung trapped by adhesions or in the case of a bronchopleural fistula. The patient's oxygenation and ventilation are more easily monitored with capnography and pulse oximetry during general anesthesia.

General anesthesia for thoracoscopy can be accomplished with either intravenous or potent inhalational agents. As with bronchoscopy, the use of short-acting intravenous agents is important to allow rapid emergence and prompt recovery of airway reflexes. The same goal may be achieved by using potent inhalational anesthetics, with the additional advantage of being able to deliver high concentrations of inspired oxygen during one-lung anesthesia.

At the end of the surgical procedure, the patient should be monitored in a postoperative recovery room setting regardless of the type of anesthetic used. Because of the surgically induced pneumothorax, these patients should be transported from the operating room to the recovery room while supplemental oxygen is being administered. Postoperative thoracoscopy patients are at higher risk of sudden pulmonary decompensation, as well as postoperative bleeding. Therefore, recovery room personnel must keep a high

index of suspicion when caring for these patients. Continuous pulse oximetry, along with all other routine monitoring, should be used.

ESOPHAGOSCOPY

Indications for esophagoscopy include removal of a foreign body, dilatation for strictures, evaluation and biopsy of esophageal lesions, and sclerotherapy for bleeding esophageal varices.[142–144] Since many of the patients undergoing esophagoscopy cannot eat, preoperative assessment should include evaluation of fluid balance and nutritional status, serum albumin, and serum electrolytes.

Patients undergoing esophagoscopy present a unique challenge to the anesthesiologist. Routine measures taken to prevent aspiration of gastric contents on induction of anesthesia may be inadequate or even contraindicated. For instance, oral antacids and H_2-receptor blockers may be ineffective in the patient with achalasia. Patients with esophageal diverticula or strictures may not be able to completely empty the esophagus. Therefore, food retained above the level of the lesion can be aspirated during induction. Furthermore, when performing Sellick's maneuver, the application of cricoid pressure may actually dislodge retained food from the esophagus, with resulting tracheal aspiration. Foreign bodies in the esophagus may also constitute a contraindication to rapid-sequence induction. A large foreign body such as a chicken bone could cause an esophageal perforation during application of cricoid pressure. Similarly, a sharp foreign body, such as an open safety pin, could also lead to an esophageal perforation.

Esophageal perforation during endoscopy is of particular concern, since it is associated with a high incidence of morbidity and mortality.[145,146] Esophagoscopy can be performed either with a rigid or a flexible fiberoptic esophagoscope. Both of these procedures can be performed with topical anesthesia plus sedation or with general anesthesia. General anesthesia is usually preferred for rigid esophagoscopy, par-

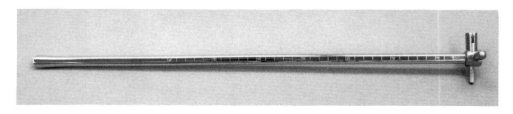

Fig. 12-23. A rigid esophagoscope.

ticularly when a foreign body is present, since coughing and bucking during the procedure can lead to esophageal perforation (Fig. 12-23).

Awake intubation should be performed in any situation in which cricoid pressure is contraindicated. A small-sized or wire-reinforced endotracheal tube may be necessary when a large rigid foreign body impinges on or obstructs the trachea. An awake fiberoptic intubation allows identification of any tracheal narrowing and enables the anesthesiologist to precisely place the endotracheal tube below the level of obstruction. This is particularly important in the case of a tracheo-esophageal fistula, in order to ensure that the endotracheal tube is placed below the level of the communication. It is important to remember that during emergence from anesthesia following esophagoscopy, patients are still at significant risk for aspiration of gastric contents. Thus, the anesthesiologist must be certain that the patients are fully awake and are able to protect their airway prior to extubation.

REFERENCES

1. Vaughn GC, Downs JB: Perioperative pulmonary function. Assessment and intervention. Anesthesiol Rev 17:19, 1990
2. Warner MA, Divertie MB, Tinker JH: Postoperative cessation of smoking and pulmonary complications in coronary artery bypass patients. Anesthesiology 60:380, 1984
3. Kambam JR, Chen LH, Hyman SA: Effect of short-term smoking halt on carboxyhemoglobin levels and P_{50} values. Anesth Analg 65:1186, 1986
4. Smith RJ, Landaw SA: Smokers polycythemia. N Engl J Med 298:6, 1978
5. Mallampati SR, Gatt SP, Gugino LD, et al: A clinical sign to predict difficult tracheal intubation: a prospective study. Can Anaesth Soc J 32:429, 1985
6. Tisi GM: Preoperative evaluation of pulmonary function: validity, indications and benefits. Am Rev Respir Dis 119:293, 1979
7. Stein M, Cassara EL: Preoperative pulmonary evaluation and therapy for surgery patients. JAMA 211:787, 1970
8. Sackner MA: Bronchofiberoscopy: state of the art. Am Rev Respir Dis 111:62, 1975
9. Jackson C: Bronchoscopy; past, present and future. N Engl J Med 199:759, 1928
10. Ikeda S, Yanai N, Ishikawa S: Flexible bronchofiberscope. Keio J Med 17:1, 1968
11. McKenna RJ, Campbell A, McMurtrey MJ, Mountain CF: Diagnosis for interstitial lung disease in patients with acquired immunodeficiency syndrome (AIDS): a prospective comparison of bronchial washing, alveolar lavage, transbronchial lung biopsy, and open-lung biopsy. Ann Thorac Surg 41:318, 1986
12. Baumgartner WA, Mark JBD: Bronchoscopic diagnosis and treatment of bronchial stump suture granulomas. J Thorac Cardiovasc Surg 81:553, 1981
13. Credle WF, Jr, Smiddy JF, Elliott RC: Complications of fiberoptic bronchoscopy. Am Rev Respir Dis 109:67, 1974
14. Suratt PM, Smiddy JF, Gruber B: Deaths and complications associated with fiberoptic bronchoscopy. Chest 69:747, 1976
15. Zavala DC: Complications following fiberoptic bronchoscopy: the "good news" and the "bad news." Chest 73:783, 1978
16. Lukomsky GI, Ovchinnikov AA, Bilal A: Complications of bronchoscopy: comparison of rigid bronchoscopy under general anesthesia and flexible fiberoptic bronchoscopy under topical anesthesia. Chest 79:316, 1981
17. Pereira W, Kounat DM, Snider GL: A prospective cooperative study of complications following flexible fiberoptic bronchoscopy. Chest 73:813, 1978
18. Albertini RE, Harrell JH, Kurihara N, Moser KM: Arterial hypoxemia induced by fiberoptic bronchoscopy. JAMA 230:1666, 1974
19. Dubrawsky C, Awe RJ, Jenkins DE: The effect of bronchofiberscopic examination on oxygenation status. Chest 67:137, 1975
20. Kleinholtz EJ, Fussel J: Arterial blood gas studies during fiberoptic bronchoscopy. Am Rev Respir Dis 108:1014, 1973
21. Hoffman S, Bruderman I: Blood-pressure and blood gas changes during anesthesia for bronchoscopy using a modified method of ventilation. Anesthesiology 37:95, 1972
22. Miller EJ: Hypoxemia during fiberoptic bronchoscopy, letter. Chest 75:103, 1979
23. Prys-Roberts C, Greene LT, Meloche R, Foex P: Studies of anaesthesia in relation to hypertension II: Haemodynamic consequences of induction and endotracheal intubation. Br J Anaesth 43:531, 1971
24. Prys-Roberts C, Foex P, Biro GP, Roberts JG: Studies of anaesthesia in relation to hyertension V: adrenergic beta-receptor blockade. Br J Anaesth 45:671, 1973
25. Luck JC, Messeder OH, Rubenstein MJ, et al: Arrhythmias from fiberoptic bronchoscopy. Chest 74:139, 1978
26. Wood M: Local anesthetic agents. p. 340. In Wood M, Wood AJJ (eds): Drugs and anesthesia. 2nd Ed. Williams & Wilkins, Baltimore, 1990
27. Weisel W, Tella RA: Reaction to tetracaine (Pontocaine) used as topical anesthetic in bronchoscopy. JAMA 147:218, 1951
28. Adriani J, Campbell D: Fatalities following topical application of local anesthesia to mucous membranes. JAMA 162:1527, 1956
29. Poe RH, Dass T, Celebic A: Small airway testing and smoking in predicting risk in surgical patients. Am J Med Sci 283:57, 1982
30. Olsson GL: Bronchospasm during anaesthesia. A computer-aided incidence study of 136,929 patients. Acta Anaesthesiol Scan 31:244, 1987
31. Gass GD, Olsen GN: Preoperative pulmonary function

testing to predict postoperative morbidity and mortality. Chest 89:127, 1986

32. Stoelting RK: Circulatory changes during direct laryngoscopy and tracheal intubation: influence of duration of laryngoscopy with or without prior lidocaine. Anesthesiology 47:381, 1977

33. Martin DE, Rosenberg H, Aukburg SJ, et al: Low-dose fentanyl blunts circulatory responses to tracheal intubation. Anesth Analg 61:680, 1982

34. Inada E, Cullen DJ, Nemeskal R, et al: Effect of labetalol on the hemodynamic response to intubation: a controlled randomized double-blind study. Anesthesiology 67:A31, 1987

35. Maharaj RJ, Thompson M, Brock-Utne JG, et al: Treatment of hypertension following endotracheal intubation: a study comparing the efficacy of labetalol, practolol and placebo. S Afr Med J 63:691, 1983

36. Stoelting RK: Attenuation of blood pressure response to laryngoscopy and tracheal intubation with sodium nitroprusside. Anesth Analg 58:116, 1979

37. Townley RG: Calcium channel antagonists in coronary artery spasm and bronchial spasm. Chest 82:401, 1982

38. Russi EW, Marchette B, Yerger L, et al: Modification of allergic bronchoconstriction by a calcium antagonist: mode of action. Am Rev Respir Dis 127:675, 1983

39. Roizen MR, Horrigan RW, Frazer BM: Anesthetic doses blocking adrenergic (stress) and cardiovascular responses to incision—MAC BAR. Anesthesiology 54:390, 1981

40. Wark KJ, Lyons J, Feneck RO: The haemodynamic effects of bronchoscopy. Anaesthesia 41:162, 1986

41. Elguindi AS, Harrison GN, Abdulla AM, et al: Cardiac rhythm disturbances during fiberoptic bronchoscopy: a prospective study. J Thorac Cardiovasc Surg 77:557, 1979

42. Shrader DL, Lakshminarayan S: The effect of fiberoptic bronchoscopy on cardiac rhythm. Chest 73:821, 1978

43. Salisbury BG, Metzger LF, Altose MD, et al: Effect of fiberoptic bronchoscopy on respiratory performance in patients with chronic airways obstruction. Thorax 30:441, 1975

44. Harless KW, Scheinhorn DJ, Tannen RC, et al: Administration of oxygen with mouth-held nasal prongs during fiberoptic bronchoscopy, letter. Chest 74:237, 1978

45. Britton RM, Nelson KG: Improper oxygenation during bronchofiberscopy. Anesthesiology 40:87, 1974

46. Neuhaus A, Markowitz D, Rotman HH, Weg JG: The effects of fiberoptic bronchoscopy with and without atropine premedication on pulmonary function in humans. Ann Thorac Surg 25:393, 1978

47. Belen J, Neuhaus A, Markowitz D, Rotman HH: Modification of the effect of fiberoptic bronchoscopy on pulmonary mechanics. Chest 79:516, 1981

48. Thorburn JR, James MFM, Feldman C, et al: Comparison of the effects of atropine and glycopyrrolate on pulmonary mechanics in patients undergoing fiberoptic bronchoscopy. Anesth Analg 65:1285, 1986

49. Moore JK, Seymour AH: Awareness during bronchoscopy. Ann R Coll Surg Engl 69:45, 1987

50. Lindholm CE, Ollman B, Snyder JV, et al: Cardiorespiratory effects of flexible fiberoptic bronchoscopy in critically ill patients. Chest 74:362, 1978

51. Lindholm CE: Flexible fiberoptic bronchoscopy in the critically ill patient. Ann Otol 83:786, 1974

52. Frumin MJ, Epstein RM, Cohen G: Apneic oxygenation in man. Anesthesiology 20:789, 1959

53. Fraioli RL, Sheffer LA, Steffenson JL: Pulmonary and cardiovascular effects of apneic oxygenation in man. Anesthesiology 39:588, 1973

54. Barr AM, Wong RM: Awareness during general anaesthesia for bronchoscopy and laryngoscopy using the apnoeic oxygenation technique. Br J Anaesth 45:894, 1973

55. Sanders RD: Two ventilating attachments for bronchoscopes. Del Med J 39:170, 1967

56. MacIntosh R, Mushin WW, Epstein HG: Physics for the anaesthetist. FA Davis, Philadelphia, 1963

57. Carden E: Positive-pressure ventilation during anesthesia for bronchoscopy: a laboratory evaluation of two recent advances. Anesth Analg 52:402, 1973

58. Sullivan MT, Neff WB: A modified Sanders ventilating system for rigid-wall bronchoscopy. Anesthesiology 50:473, 1979

59. Morales GA, Epstein BS, Cinco B, et al: Ventilation during general anesthesia for bronchoscopy. J Thorac Cardiovasc Surg 57:873, 1969

60. Spoerel WE: Ventilation through an open bronchoscope (preliminary report). Can Anaesth Soc J 16:61, 1969

61. Duvall AJ, Johnsen AF, Buckley J: Bronchoscopy under general anesthesia using the Sanders ventilating attachment. Ann Otol Rhinol Laryngol 78:490, 1969

62. Carden E: Recent improvements in techniques for general anesthesia for bronchoscopy. Chest 73:697, 1978

63. Giesecke AH, Gerbershagen HU, Dortman C, Lee D: Comparison of the ventilating and injection bronchoscopes. Anesthesiology 38:298, 1973

64. Carden E, Trapp WG, Oulton J: A new and simple method for ventilating patients undergoing bronchoscopy. Anesthesiology 33:454, 1970

65. Gillick JS: The inflation-catheter technique for ventilation during bronchoscopy. Anesthesiology 40:503, 1974

66. El-Naggar M: The use of a small endotracheal tube in bronchoscopy. Br J Anaesth 47:390, 1975

67. Carden E, Schwesinger WB: The use of nitrous oxide during ventilation with the open bronchoscope. Anesthesiology 39:551, 1973

68. Vourc'h G, Fischler M, Michon F, et al: High-frequency jet ventilation v. manual jet ventilation during bronchoscopy in patients with tracheo-bronchial stenosis. Br J Anaesth 55:969, 1983

69. Rouby JJ, Viars P: Clinical use of high-frequency ventilation. Acta Anaesthesiol Scand 33:134, 1989

70. Eriksson I, Sjostrand U: Effects of high-frequency positive pressure ventilation (HFPPV) and general anesthesia on intrapulmonary gas distribution in patients undergoing diagnostic bronchoscopy. Anesth Analg 59:585, 1980

71. Bor U, Eriksson I, Sjostrand U: High-frequency positive-pressure ventilation (HFPPV): a review based upon

its use during bronchoscopy and for laryngoscopy and microlaryngeal surgery under general anesthesia. Anesth Analg 59:594, 1980

72. Schlenkhoff D, Droste H, Scieszka S, Vogt H: The use of high-frequency jet ventilation in operative bronchoscopy. Endoscopy 18:192, 1986

73. Wright PE, Marini JJ, Bernard GR: In vitro versus in vivo comparison of endotracheal tube airflow resistance. Am Rev Respir Dis 140:10, 1989

74. Carden E, Raj PP: Special new low resistance to flow tube and endotracheal tube adapter for use during fiberoptic bronchoscopy. Ann Otol 84:631, 1975

75. Smith RB, Lindholm CE, Klain M: Jet ventilation for fiberoptic bronchoscopy under general anesthesia. Acta Anaesth Scand 20:111, 1976

76. Satyanarayana T, Capan L, Ramanathan S, et al: Bronchofiberscopic jet ventilation. Anesth Analg 59:350, 1980

77. Eschenbacher WL, Bethel RA, Baushay HA, Shepard D: Morphine sulfate inhibits bronchoconstriction in subjects with mild asthma whose responses are inhibited by atropine. Am Rev Respir Dis 130:363, 1984

78. Wood M: Local anesthetic agents. p. 115. In Wood M, Wood AJJ (eds): Drugs and anesthesia. 2nd Ed. Williams & Wilkins, Baltimore, 1990

79. Schaberg SJ, Stuller CB, Edwards SM: Effect of methylprednisolone on swelling after orthognathic surgery. J Oral Maxillofac Surg 42:356, 1984

80. Shieh HL, Hutton CE, Kafrawy AH, et al: Comparison of meclofenamate sodium and hydrocortisone for controlling the postsurgical inflammatory response in rats. J Oral Maxillofac Surg 46:777, 1988

81. Christoforidis AJ, Tomashefski JF, Mitchell RI: Use of an ultrasonic nebulizer for the application of oropharyngeal, laryngeal and tracheobronchial anesthesia. Chest 59:629, 1971

82. Steinhaus JE, Gaskin L: A study of intravenous lidocaine as a suppressant of cough reflex. Anesthesiology 24:285, 1963

83. Stiffel P, Hameroff SR: A modified technique for transtracheal anesthesia. Anesthesiology 51:274, 1979

84. Cooper M, Watson RL: An improved regional anesthetic technique for peroral endoscopy. Anesthesiology 43:372, 1975

85. Gaskill JR, Gillies DR: Local anesthesia for peroral endoscopy. Arch Otolaryngol 84:654, 1966

86. Kandt D, Schlegel M: Bronchologic examinations under topical ultrasonic aerosol inhalation anesthesia. Scand J Respir Dis 54:65, 1973

87. Steegers PA, Foster PA: The use of propofol in a group of older patients undergoing oesophagoscopy. S Afr Med J 73:279, 1988

88. Harken DE, Black H, Clauss R, Farrand RE: A simple cervicomediastinal exploration for tissue diagnosis of intrathoracic disease. N Engl J Med 251:1041, 1954

89. Carlens E: A method for inspection and tissue biopsy in the superior mediastinum. Dis Chest 36:343, 1959

90. Pearson FG: Lung cancer: the past 25 years. Chest 89:200S, 1986

91. Weissberg D, Herczeg E: Perforation of thoracic aortic aneurysm: a complication of mediastinoscopy, letter. Chest 78:119, 1980

92. Vaughan RS: Anaesthesia for mediastinoscopy. Anaesthesia 33:195, 1978

93. Burkell CC, Cross JM, Kent HP, Nanson EM: Mass lesions of the mediastinum. Curr Probl Surg 100:1, 1969

94. Foster ED, Munro DD, Dobell ARC: Mediastinoscopy: a review of anatomical relationships and complications. Ann Thorac Surg 13:273, 1972

95. McNeill TM, Chamberlain JM: Diagnostic anterior mediastinotomy. Ann Thorac Surg 2:532, 1966

96. Stemmer EA, Calvin JW, Steedman RA, Connolly JE: Parasternal mediastinal exploration to evaluate resectability of thoracic neoplasms. Ann Thorac Surg 12:375, 1971

97. Oldham HN, Jr: Mediastinal tumors and cysts. Ann Thorac Surg 11:246, 1971

98. Neuman GG, Weingarten AE, Abramowitz RM, et al: The anesthetic management of the patient with an anterior mediastinal mass. Anesthesiology 60:144, 1984

99. Shambaugh GE, Seed R, Korn A: Airway obstruction in substernal goiter: clinical and therapeutic implications. J Chronic Dis 26:737, 1973

100. Tonnesen AS, Davis FG: Superior vena caval and bronchial obstruction during anesthesia. Anesthesiology 45:91, 1976

101. Mackie AM, Watson CB: Anaesthesia and mediastinal masses. A case report and review of the literature. Anaesthesia 39:899, 1984

102. Lochridge SK, Knibble WP, Doty DB: Obstruction of the superior vena cava. Surgery 85:14, 1979

103. Ward PH, Stephenson SE, Jr, Harris PF: Exploration of the mediastinum under local anesthesia. Ann Otol Rhinol Laryngol 75:368, 1966

104. Selby JH, Jr, Leach CL, Heath BJ, Neely WA: Local anesthesia for mediastinoscopy: experience with 450 consecutive cases. Am Surg 44:679, 1978

105. Morton JR, Guinn GA: Mediastinoscopy using local anesthesia. Am J Surg 122:696, 1971

106. Prakash UBS, Abel MD, Hubmayr RD: Mediastinal mass and tracheal obstruction during general anesthesia. Mayo Clin Proc 63:1004, 1988

107. Philips PA, Van De Water JM: Mediastinoscopy vs exploratory thoracotomy. Arch Surg 105:48, 1972

108. Flynn JR, Rossi NP, Lawton RL: Significance of mediastinoscopy in carcinoma of the lung. Arch Surg 94:243, 1967

109. Ashbaugh DG: Mediastinoscopy. Arch Surg 100:568, 1970

110. Petty C: Right radial artery pressure during mediastinoscopy. Anesth Analg 58:428, 1979

111. Trinkle JK, Bryant LR, Hiller AJ, Playforth RH: Mediastinoscopy—experience with 300 consecutive cases. J Thorac Cardiovasc Surg 60:297, 1970

112. Lee JH, Salvatore A: Innominate artery compression simulating cardiac arrest during mediastinoscopy: a case report. Anesth Analg 55:748, 1976

113. Sibert KS, Biondi JW, Hirsch NP: Spontaneous respiration during thoracotomy in a patient with a mediastinal mass. Anesth Analg 66:904, 1987

114. Bittar D: Respiratory obstruction associated with induction of general anesthesia in a patient with mediastinal Hodgkin's disease. Anesth Analg 54:399, 1975

115. Bray RJ, Fernandes FJ: Mediastinal tumour causing airway obstruction in anaesthetized children. Anaesthesia 37:571, 1982

116. Levin MB, Bursztein S, Heifetz M: Cardiac arrest in a child with an anterior mediastinal mass. Anesth Analg 64:1129, 1985

117. Piro AJ, Weiss DR, Hellman S: Mediastinal Hodgkin's disease: a possible danger for intubation anesthesia. Int J Radiat Oncol Biol Phys 1:415, 1976

118. Barash PG, Tsai B, Kitahata LM: Acute tracheal collapse following mediastinoscopy. Anesthesiology 44:67, 1976

119. Keon TP: Death on induction of anesthesia for cervical node biopsy. Anesthesiology 55:471, 1981

120. Todres ID, Reppert SM, Walker PF, Grillo HC: Management of critical airway obstruction in a child with a mediastinal tumor. Anesthesiology 45:100, 1976

121. Younker D, Clark R, Coveler L: Fiberoptic endobronchial intubation for resection of an anterior mediastinal mass. Anesthesiology 70:144, 1989

122. Wilson RF, Steiger Z, Jacobs J, et al: Temporary partial cardiopulmonary bypass during emergency operative management of near total tracheal occlusion. Anesthesiology 61:103, 1984

123. Hall KD, Friedman M: Extracorporeal oxygenation for induction of anesthesia in a patient with an intrathoracic tumor. Anesthesiology 42:493, 1975

124. Lee CM, Grossman LB: Laceration of left pulmonary artery during mediastinoscopy. Anesth Analg 56:226, 1977

125. Dalton ML, Gerken MV, Neely WA: Right bronchial artery hemorrhage complicating mediastinoscopy. Contemp Surg 24:75, 1984

126. Bloomberg AE: Thoracoscopy in perspective. Surg Gynecol Obstet 147:433, 1978

127. Baumgartner WA, Mark JBD: The use of thoracoscopy in the diagnosis of pleural disease. Arch Surg 115:420, 1980

128. Rodgers BM, Ryckman FC, Moazam F, Talbert JL: Thoracoscopy for intrathoracic tumors. Ann Thorac Surg 31:414, 1981

129. Miller JI, Hatcher CR, Jr: Thoracoscopy: a useful tool in the diagnosis of thoracic disease. Ann Thorac Surg 26:68, 1978

130. Boutin C, Viallat JR, Cargnino P, Rey F: Thoracoscopic lung biopsy: experimental and clinical preliminary study. Chest 82:44, 1982

131. Poulos C, Ponn R, Tranquilli M, et al: Thoracoscopy for diagnosis of chest disease. Conn Med 52:201, 1988

132. Canto A, Blasco E, Casillas M, et al: Thoracoscopy in the diagnosis of pleural effusion. Thorax 32:550, 1977

133. Rodgers BM, Moulder PV, DeLaney A: Thoracoscopy: new method of early diagnosis of cardiac herniation. J Thorac Cardiovasc Surg 78:623, 1979

134. Oakes DD, Sherck JP, Brodsky JB, Mark JBD: Therapeutic thoracoscopy. J Thorac Cardiovasc Surg 87:269, 1984

135. Jones JW, Kitahama A, Webb WR, McSwain N: Emergency thoracoscopy: a logical approach to chest trauma management. J Trauma 21:280, 1981

136. Weissberg D, Kaufman M, Zurkowski Z: Pleuroscopy in patients with pleural effusion and pleural masses. Ann Thorac Surg 29:205, 1980

137. Ben-Isaac FE, Simmons DH: Flexible fiberoptic pleuroscopy: pleural and lung biopsy. Chest 67:573, 1975

138. Senno A, Moallem S, Quijano ER, et al: Thoracoscopy with the fiberoptic bronchoscope. J Thorac Cardiovasc Surg 67:606, 1974

139. Gwin E, Pierce G, Boggan M, et al: Pleuroscopy and pleural biopsy with the flexible fiberoptic bronchoscope. Chest 67:527, 1975

140. Kaiser LR: Diagnostic and therapeutic uses of pleuroscopy (thoracoscopy) in lung cancer. Surg Clin North Am 67:1081, 1987

141. Rusch VW, Mountain C: Thoracoscopy under regional anesthesia for the diagnosis and management of pleural disease. Am J Surg 154:274, 1987

142. Wilson RH, Campbell WJ, Spencer A, Johnston GW: Rigid endoscopy under general anaesthesia is safe for chronic injection sclerotherapy. Br J Surg 76:719, 1989

143. Bornman PC, Kahn D, Terblanche J, et al: Rigid versus fiberoptic endoscopic injection sclerotherapy. Ann Surg 208:175, 1988

144. Bendig DW: Removal of blunt esophageal foreign bodies by flexible endoscopy without general anesthesia. Am J Dis Child 140:789, 1986

145. Wolloch Y, Zer M, Dintsman M, Tiqva P: Iatrogenic perforations of the esophagus. Arch Surg 108:357, 1974

146. Steyn JH, Brunnen PL: Perforation of cervical oesophagus at oesophagoscopy. Scott Med J 7:494, 1962

13

CHOICE OF ANESTHETIC AGENTS FOR INTRATHORACIC SURGERY

Lawrence C. Siegel, M.D.
Jay B. Brodsky, M.D.

The practice of anesthesiology, particularly the subspecialties like thoracic anesthesia, is rapidly evolving and changing. Today, complex and extensive intrathoracic operations are routinely performed on increasingly ill patients, some of whom less than 20 years ago would not even have been considered surgical candidates. The anesthetic management of the patient undergoing thoracic surgery is often especially challenging since adequate oxygenation and hemodynamic stability must be maintained while providing satisfactory operating conditions.

The choice of anesthetic agent for intrathoracic surgery is determined by many factors. Each individual patient's specific needs must be considered. The nature and extent of pre-existing pulmonary, cardiovascular, and other physiologic impairment must be fully appreciated before surgery in order to plan and deliver a safe anesthetic during surgery. Furthermore, any potential postoperative effects of drugs used intraoperatively must be recognized, since these can have considerable impact on overall recovery.

This chapter provides a background to use in choosing anesthetic agents for intrathoracic procedures. It will consider the effects of anesthetics on pulmonary mechanics, airway resistance, pulmonary blood flow, and the control of ventilation. Each of these responses may be altered by the presence or absence of lung disease, by changes in body position, by the mode of ventilation used, especially if selective lung ventilation is used, and by surgical manipulation. For the same operation, no single agent or technique is always indicated, but the choice of agents remains an individual one based on the patient's condition, the surgeon's needs, and the anesthesologist's clinical judgment.

EFFECTS OF ANESTHESIA ON LUNG VOLUMES

Functional residual capacity (FRC) is reduced during anesthesia by an increase in lung elastic recoil and a decrease in chest recoil.[1-3] In humans, the reduction of FRC occurs during the first few minutes of anesthesia and does not seem to depend on the specific anesthetic agent.[4] Reduction of FRC is important because airway closure and absorption atelectasis may occur when the closing capacity (CC) exceeds the end-expiratory lung volume. However, in addition to reducing FRC, anesthetics also reduce closing capacity, and the relationship between FRC and CC, on average, is unchanged by anesthesia.[5] Patients whose FRC was greater than the CC when awake had less decrease in CC than FRC when anesthetized and paralyzed. In contrast, patients whose FRC was less than CC when awake had a greater decrease in CC than FRC with anesthesia[6] (Fig. 13-1). The major effect on respiratory

system compliance of isoflurane in humans, for example, is a decrease in chest recoil,[7] whereas anesthesia with meperidine and thiopental produces a large increase in lung elastic recoil.[3]

AIRWAY RESISTANCE

Airway resistance varies inversely with lung volume; thus, the reduction of FRC that occurs with anesthesia produces an increase in airway resistance. The autonomic nervous system and chemical mediators control bronchomotor tone.[8] Parasympathetic afferents transmit from irritant receptors of the airway epithelial cells via the vagus nerve. This pathway may be blocked with a local anesthetic aerosol[9]; however, aerosols may irritate the mucosa and transiently stimulate receptors.[10] Vagal efferents produce bronchial smooth muscle constriction through stimulation of cholinergic receptors, which may be blocked with anticholinergic agents.[11] Adrenergic receptors modu-

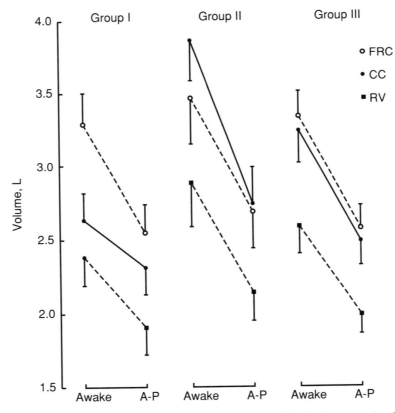

Fig. 13-1. Values (mean ± SE) of functional residual capacity (FRC), closing capacity (CC), and residual volume (RV) for group I (12 patients whose FRC was greater than CC while awake) and for group II (11 patients whose FRC was less than CC while awake). FRC and CC were reduced when the patients were anesthetized and paralyzed (A-P). In group I, FRC decreased more than CC; in group II, CC decreased more than FRC. (From Juno et al,[6] with permission.)

late smooth muscle tone when stimulated by cate-cholamines that are released from sympathetic nerve endings and the adrenal medulla. Alpha-receptor stimulation produces bronchoconstriction, especially in asthmatic patients who have an excess of alpha-receptors. Mediators of bronchoconstriction include histamine, prostaglandin $F_{2\alpha}$, bradykinin, and leuko-trienes (see Chapter 9).

Patients undergoing thoracic surgery are at risk for increased airway resistance for several reasons. Frequently, these patients have excess pulmonary mucous, blood, and tumor cell production, which cause airway plugging. Many patients have chronic obstructive pulmonary disease, asthma, cystic fibrosis, or other lung diseases that affect airway caliber and reactivity. Surgical trauma to the lung may produce hemorrhage and bronchospasm. Furthermore, surgical retraction of the lung and trachea may induce reflex bronchospasm. Endotracheal intubation, especially with a double-lumen tube for endobronchial intubation, may produce bronchospasm from direct mucosal stimulation. An appreciation of the effects of anesthetics on airway resistance is useful in selecting agents for thoracic anesthesia.

Anesthetic Effects on Airway Resistance

The effects of anesthetics on the airway vary from bronchoconstriction to bronchodilation. In general, little bronchodilation occurs without pre-existing constriction, and bronchoconstriction is more common and occurs to a greater degree in patients who are predisposed to bronchoconstriction.

Halothane appears to produce direct smooth muscle bronchomotor relaxation regardless of the mechanism of bronchoconstriction.[12–14] Isolated tracheal smooth muscle is relaxed by halothane.[15] Interpretation of clinical studies on the effect of halothane on airway resistance is complicated by the failure of many investigators to measure lung volume. General anesthesia reduces lung volume and thereby increases airway resistance; however, bronchodilation by halothane offsets this effect.[8] In addition to direct action on smooth muscle, halothane may also affect bronchomotor tone by altering the release or effect of mediators of bronchoconstriction. These interactions may be difficult to interpret. For example, the role of histamine in clinical bronchoconstriction during anesthesia is controversial. Halothane, unlike thiopental, was effective in preventing the increase in pulmonary resistance associated with ascaris antigen aerosol administration in a canine model. Plasma histamine levels were the same with both anesthetics; thus, inhibition of histamine release did not appear to be important.[16] Study of in vitro human tissue suggests that halothane impairs the release of histamine

prompted by *d*-tubocurarine.[17] Furthermore, halothane attenuates the bronchoconstriction produced by administration of histamine; however, this effect may be due to blockade of vagal reflexes because the same results were obtained using atropine.[18] Isoflurane and enflurane are also potent bronchodilators, although they have not been studied as thoroughly as halothane.[19,20]

Isoflurane and halothane were equally effective in preventing the increase in pulmonary resistance produced by aerosol administration of ascaris antigen in greyhounds.[19] Isoflurane may be chosen in preference to halothane because isoflurane produces less myocardial depression and fewer ventricular dysrhythmias than halothane.[21] Patients treated with aminophylline and beta-adrenergic agonists are especially susceptible to ventricular dysrhythmias and may benefit from receiving isoflurane rather than halothane.

Intravenous drugs can release histamine with potentially undesirable effects on bronchomotor tone. In vitro mast cell studies show that thiopental and thiamylal produce dose-related histamine release, whereas pentobarbital and methohexital do not.[22] Propanidid and thiopental produce histamine release in human subjects, and bronchospasm has occurred in patients having anaphylactoid reactions to propanidid.[23] Etomidate rarely causes histamine release, even in asthmatic patients.[24] Etomidate has been advocated for patients at risk for bronchoconstriction[25]; however, anaphylaxis and severe bronchospasm attributable to etomidate administration have been reported.[26] Ketamine has bronchodilating properties, probably through direct and adrenergic mechanisms, and has been quite popular for induction of anesthesia in the patient with increased airway reactivity.[27,28] Preliminary work with propofol reveals that histamine release is probably uncommon with this agent[29]; however, basophils taken from anesthesiologists using propofol in clinical practice released histamine when exposed to propofol.[30]

A narcotic that produces little release of histamine may be of particular clinical utility. Fentanyl and oxymorphone do not cause histamine release from skin mast cells; however, histamine release occurs with morphine. Naloxone neither promotes nor inhibits histamine release.[31] Despite the propensity for morphine to produce histamine release, vagally mediated bronchospasm in subjects with mild asthma is inhibited by morphine[32]; this effect is reversed by naloxone. Meperidine may produce histamine release[32] and bronchoconstriction.[34]

Neuromuscular blocking drugs differ in their ability to release histamine. Administration of 0.6 mg/kg of *d*-tubocurarine over 30 seconds increases human serum histamine concentration by a factor of five.[35] At equipotent doses for neuromuscular junction blockade, metocurine releases histamine approximately one-third as readily as curare, and atracurium releases approximately one-tenth as much histamine as curare.[36,37] Vecuronium and pancuronium do not cause histamine release.[38] Reversal of neuromuscular blockade is accomplished by inhibiting acetylcholinesterase with neostigmine, pyridostigmine, or edrophonium. These drugs increase airway resistance by increasing cholinergic tone unless atropine or glycopyrrolate are concomitantly administered. Atropine also increases dead space ventilation.[39]

Histamine H_2-receptor blockade is used to reduce gastric secretion volume and acidity to lower the risk of pulmonary aspiration of gastric contents. Selective H_2 blockade may result in greater airway reactivity to histamine, with cimetidine being more problematic than ranitidine.[40,41]

In summary, proper selection of anesthetics will minimize the risk of bronchoconstriction in the patient undergoing thoracic surgery. Ketamine may be particularly useful for intravenous induction of anesthesia, although etomidate and thiopental may be used effectively if sufficient attention is paid to assuring adequate anesthetic depth. The notion that inadequate anesthetic depth is more frequently a contributor to clinical bronchospasm than is the particular choice of anesthetic agent has merit; however, clinical studies in this area are limited by the difficulties of quantifying anesthetic depth. Propofol and midazolam may prove useful; however, further investigation is necessary to clarify the role of these agents in patients at risk for bronchospasm. Halothane, enflurane, and isoflurane are useful because of the bronchodilation they produce. For inhalational induction, halothane may be preferred because of differences in pungency; however, any of these three inhalation anesthetics are useful for the maintenance phase. Because of fewer cardiovascular effects, isoflurane is frequently preferred to halothane. Fentanyl is preferable to morphine or meperidine; further investigation is necessary to evaluate sufentanil and alfentanil. It is wise to avoid curare for muscle relaxation; vecuronium and pancuronium are preferred, although atracurium is satisfactory.

PULMONARY BLOOD FLOW DURING ANESTHESIA

Hypoxemia

Hypoxemia may be a troublesome problem during anesthesia for thoracic surgical procedures requiring one-lung anesthesia. An arterial oxygen tension (PaO_2) of less than 70 mmHg occurs in 15 to 25 percent of

cases using one-lung anesthesia with inhalational anesthetics.[42,43] While many patients tolerate thoracic surgery with clinically acceptable reductions of PaO_2, the causes of a decreased PaO_2 must be understood to permit effective diagnosis and therapy. Proper selection of anesthetic agents and techniques is one aspect of this issue. Hypoxemia may result from an inadequate inspired oxygen tension, inadequate alveolar ventilation, or an abnormally large alveolar-to-arterial oxygen tension gradient [$P(A - a)O_2$].

During thoracic operations, an abnormally large $P(A - a)O_2$ may result from venous admixture due to a ventilation-perfusion ($\dot{V}/\dot{Q}$) mismatch and shunting. The use of 100 percent inspired oxygen and mechanical ventilation minimizes the effect of a ventilation-perfusion mismatch on PaO_2, but shunting is particularly prominent during one-lung ventilation. The mixed venous oxygen tension ($P\bar{v}O_2$), the inspired oxygen concentration, and the shunt fraction combine to determine $P(A - a)O_2$. $P\bar{v}O_2$ may be abnormally low during conditions of a low cardiac output or high oxygen consumption. Thus, the proper selection of anesthetic agents requires an understanding of their effects on shunt, cardiac output, and oxygen consumption (see Chapters 6 and 8).

General anesthesia produces an increased pulmonary venous admixture and $P(A - a)O_2$.[44] This phenomenon may result from changes in lung mechanics and pulmonary blood flow distribution. Anesthesia increases shunting and ventilation-perfusion mismatch; however, there is considerable individual variability to the extent and distribution of these effects.[45] In Figure 13-2, pulmonary ventilation and perfusion are shown for two patients before and during halothane-oxygen anesthesia, demonstrating the differences in shunt and $\dot{V}/\dot{Q}$ abnormality associated with anesthesia. Inhalational anesthesia produces greater venous admixture than does barbiturate anesthesia. The reduction of FRC with anesthesia may produce increased shunt, and differences in lung volume may partially explain differences in shunt with inhalational versus intravenous anesthetics.[46] However, it is most likely that changes in venous admixture related to anesthesia are produced by changes of pulmonary blood flow distribution and not changes in lung volume.

Hypoxic Pulmonary Vasoconstriction

In the 44 years since the observations of Euler and Liljestrand, considerable investigation has been undertaken to understand the mechanism by which alveolar hypoxia produces arteriolar constriction.[47] Hypoxic pulmonary vasoconstriction (HPV) has attracted great interest as a vital homeostatic mecha-

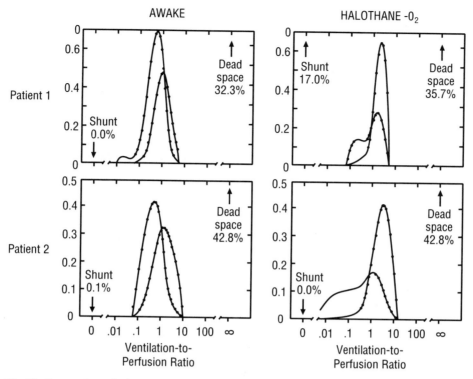

Fig. 13-2. Ventilation and perfusion are plotted against the ventilation-to-perfusion ratio for two subjects awake and during halothane anesthesia. Distinct patterns of shunt and ventilation-perfusion distribution occurred with anesthesia, demonstrating the variability in the human response to anesthesia. (From Dueck et al,[46] with permission.)

nism for maintaining normal ventilation-perfusion relationships and achieving efficient oxygenation.

Mechanical effects on the pulmonary circulation have been considered as potentially important determinants of pulmonary blood flow and shunt. The suggestion that mechanical factors might be important in reducing blood flow to atelectatic lung was prompted by the observation that the large pulmonary arteries of atelectatic lung are "kinked and gnarly."[48] However, several studies have shown that the flow diversion is the result of HPV and not mechanical factors.[49] In a canine study, flow to the left lower lobe was markedly reduced by lobar atelectasis (Fig. 13-3). The re-expansion of the atelectatic lobe by ventilation with nitrogen to restore lung volume and mechanics did not restore flow; however, flow was restored by ventilation with oxygen. Thus, in the open-chest preparation, HPV was the major cause of reduced blood flow to the atelectatic lobe.[50,51] The possibility that mechanical factors created further vasoconstriction for periods of atelectasis in excess of 1 hour has not been excluded[52]; however, in animal studies, HPV is of greater importance.[53]

Hypoxic pulmonary vasoconstriction is a local phenomenon; however, the overall increase of pulmonary vascular resistance may be appreciable if a large portion of the lung is hypoxic. In experimental models, HPV may be quantified by measurement of the increase in pulmonary artery pressure and by measurement of the reduction of blood flow to the hypoxic lung segment. The smaller the hypoxic segment, the more readily flow is diverted to nonhypoxic lung. The larger the hypoxic segment, the greater the increase in pulmonary artery pressure.[54,55] Thus, the extent of the HPV response must be evaluated in regard to the size of the hypoxic segment. Flow diversion is prominent with a small hypoxic segment, while increased pulmonary artery pressure is prominent with a large hypoxic segment. For example, under normal conditions, left lung blood flow is reduced by 50 percent when the lung becomes atelectatic.[50] Hypoxic pulmonary vasoconstriction acts primarily on the pulmonary arterioles. Although it is widely appreciated that alveolar hypoxia produces precapillary vasoconstriction,[56] the importance of the mixed venous oxygen tension ($P\bar{v}O_2$) must not be overlooked. The pressor

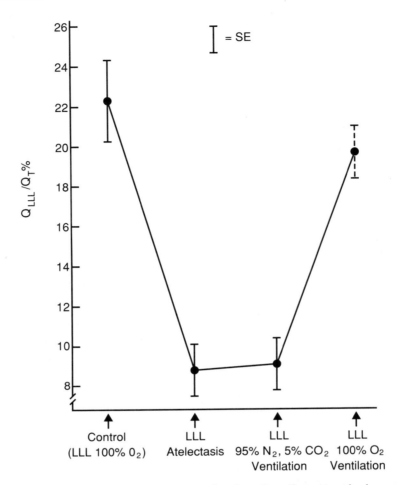

Fig. 13-3. Flow to the left lower lobe test segment as a fraction of cardiac output is shown for six dogs. Left lower lobe atelectasis and left lower lobe hypoxic ventilation each produced a similar reduction in test segment perfusion, suggesting that HPV rather than mechanical factors is largely responsible for decreasing blood flow to an atelectatic lung. (From Benumof,[51] with permission.)

response depends on alveolar oxygen tension (P_AO_2) and $P\bar{v}O_2$.[57] In a study of left lung atelectasis, increasing $P\bar{v}O_2$ above 100 mmHg with venovenous bypass completely eliminated the diversion of flow from the left lung.[50] Hypoxic pulmonary vasoconstriction is the most important regulator of the distribution of blood flow to the atelectactic lung, and $P\bar{v}O_2$ is the primary stimulus for this response.[50]

Although the intensity of the HPV response is a function of P_AO_2 and $P\bar{v}O_2$, this response may be modified by other factors. For example, pharmacologic direct smooth muscle relaxation with sodium nitroprusside or nitroglycerin will blunt the efficacy of HPV and increase shunt[58–60]; thus, vasodilators must be used with care during one-lung anesthesia. Surgical manipulation of the lung may transiently blunt HPV,

perhaps due to thromboxane and prostacyclin mediation.[61–63] This effect may be quite variable and species dependent. The effects of anesthetics on HPV have been extensively studied, and an understanding of these effects is useful in selecting anesthetic agents and techniques.

Anesthetics and Hypoxic Pulmonary Vasoconstriction

In Vitro Studies

In vitro studies of HPV show no effect of intravenous anesthetics. Pentobarbital, thiopental, hexobarbital, diazepam, droperidol, ketamine, fentanyl, and pentazocine did not alter the HPV response in isolated blood-perfused rat lungs.[64] There was no attenuation of the HPV response by fentanyl either when administered via the blood stream or when administered in a nebulized form via the airway.[65] Morphine and buprenorphine also did not modify the HPV response in an isolated perfused cat lung.[66]

In contrast, volatile inhaled anesthetics inhibit HPV dose dependently in vitro. Studies of the isolated rat lung and the perfused cat lung have shown blunting of HPV by halothane[64,67–70] and methoxyflurane.[67,71] Enflurane[70,72] and isoflurane[70] also inhibit HPV in rat lungs in vitro. The inhibition of HPV is dose dependent and the potency of this effect is a function of the minimal alveolar concentration (MAC) for halothane, enflurane, and isoflurane (Fig. 13-4).

In Vivo Studies

Studies of intact animals consistently reveal no inhibition of HPV by intravenous anesthetics.[73,74] Ketamine, thiopental, pentobarbital, fentanyl, meperidine, lidocaine, and chlorpromazine did not inhibit HPV in the left lower lobe of open-chest dogs.[74] Animal and patient studies of HPV, pulmonary shunt,

and oxygenation have demonstrated a wide range of effects of the inhalational anesthetics. These seemingly conflicting results may be explained by the complex interactions of anesthetics, cardiac output, oxygen consumption, shunt, and $P\bar{v}O_2$ (see Chapter 8). In addition, surgical manipulation of the lung, the use of positive end-expiratory pressure, global versus lobar administration of anesthetics, and the duration, dose, and sequence of anesthetic use also complicate the observations. For example, $P\bar{v}O_2$ is an important determinant of HPV, especially in the atelectatic lung. Anesthetics that decrease cardiac output more than they decrease oxygen consumption will lower $P\bar{v}O_2$, thereby producing a more potent stimulus for HPV. This situation was present in a clinical study comparing one-lung anesthesia with ketamine versus enflurane.[75] PaO_2 was not affected by the choice of anesthetic; however, $P\bar{v}O_2$ and cardiac output were lower for patients receiving enflurane than for patients receiving ketamine. This example illustrates the important concept that inhalational anesthetics may directly inhibit, but indirectly augment, HPV. An anesthetic that lowers $P\bar{v}O_2$ through an effect on cardiac output may thereby indirectly affect HPV. The

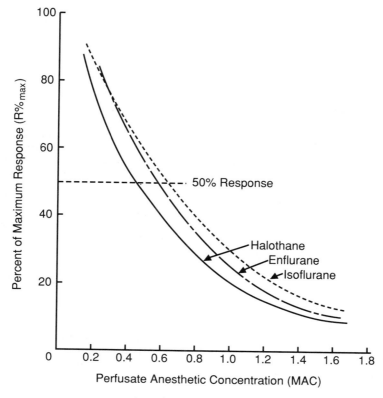

Fig. 13-4. The dose-response curves for inhibition of HPV by halothane, enflurane, and isoflurane are similar in the perfused rat lung. (From Marshall et al,[70] with permission.)

manifestation of this phenomenon depends on the size of the hypoxic lung segment and the manner in which the HPV response is quantified. HPV causes diversion of flow away from the hypoxic segment and increases pulmonary artery pressure. A reduction of $P\bar{v}O_2$ will affect HPV in the entire lung, not only the test segment. This effect may require rather subtle interpretation of experimental results since the test segment interacts with the control segment. The relationship between cardiac output and shunt is complex. Studies of normal or diffusely abnormal lungs in humans and animals reveal that pulmonary shunt fraction is decreased with an acute decrease of cardiac output.[76] This relationship appears to result from augmentation of HPV by the reduced $P\bar{v}O_2$ that accompanies a decreased cardiac output.[77]

In clinical situations, volatile anesthetics reach the atelectatic lung during one-lung ventilation via mixed venous blood. In animal studies, the anesthetic may be administered to a test lobe that is ventilated with a hypoxic gas, or to the entire lung. Figure 13-5 shows a summary of studies using these two techniques in dogs. Isoflurane and fluroxene inhibited HPV dose dependently, and nitrous oxide moderately diminished HPV. Halothane and enflurane had little effect on HPV.[78] These observations were not substantially affected by the administration of anesthetics to the test lobe versus the entire lung.

HPV was studied in dogs using hemorrhage and surgically produced arteriovenous fistulae to control cardiac output and $P\bar{v}O_2$ during isoflurane administration.[79] In this study, isoflurane was administered to the left lung in 0, 1, and 2.5 MAC concentrations. The left lung was ventilated with either 100 percent oxygen or a mixture of 4 percent oxygen, 3 percent carbon dioxide, and 93 percent nitrogen. Figure 13-6 shows venous admixture and cardiac output at the three anesthetic doses. Comparing points a, b, and c, a dose-dependent increase in venous admixture produced by isoflurane when cardiac output and $P\bar{v}O_2$ are constant can be seen. This study shows that isoflurane produces dose-dependent inhibition of HPV independent of effects on cardiac output or $P\bar{v}O_2$. These results are consistent with the inhibition of HPV observed in vitro. Thus, inhalational anesthetics have the potential to inhibit HPV, increase shunt, and decrease arterial oxygenation during clinical application. However, clinical studies encompass all of the effects of the anesthetics, and, in general, the inhalation anesthetics are clinically well tolerated.

Clinical Studies

A comparison of ketamine and enflurane in 24 patients undergoing lung resection found no difference in shunt or PaO2 attributable to anesthetic selection.[75]

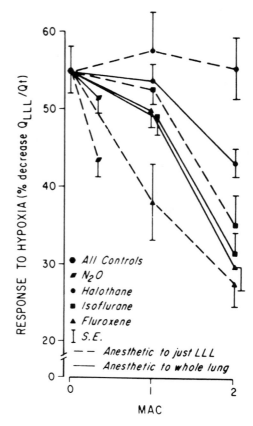

Fig. 13-5. The fraction of cardiac output perfusing the left lower lobe was reduced by left lower lobe hypoxia. This HPV response is shown with administration of the anesthetic to either the whole lung or the left lower lobe. Exclusive lobar administration reduced systemic effects that did not appear to substantially affect the measured HPV response. (From Mathers et al,[78] with permission.)

Unilateral lung ventilation with 100 percent nitrogen in supine volunteers produced blood flow diversion from the hypoxic lung that was diminished by halothane compared with intravenous anesthesia.[80] Propofol did not affect venous admixture, PaO2, or cardiac output in subjects during one-lung ventilation in the lateral position.[81] A study of 20 adults undergoing thoracotomy in the lateral position was conducted with a period of unilateral lung atelectasis during which an inhaled anesthetic (isoflurane or halothane) and an intravenous anesthetic (ketamine or methohexital) were sequentially administered. This study showed no difference in PaO2 or shunt when comparing inhaled and intravenous anesthesia during one-lung atelectasis.[82] Unfortunately, the results of this study are not readily clinically applicable because the duration of the exposure to the inhaled anesthetic was very brief. A study using more appropriate durations

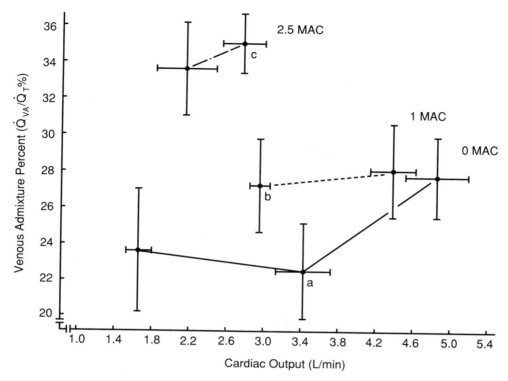

Fig. 13-6. Venous admixture is shown during left-lung hypoxia at three doses of isoflurane with a range of cardiac outputs produced using an arteriovenous fistulae. Examination of points *a*, *b*, and *c* reveals that with a constant cardiac output and $P\bar{v}O_2$, isoflurane produced dose-dependent increases in venous admixture. (From Domino et al,[79] with permission.)

of inhalation anesthesia was conducted in 12 patients undergoing thoracic surgery.[83] Patients received either halothane or isoflurane in 100 percent oxygen for at least 1 hour before nondependent one-lung atelectasis was produced. After 40 minutes of one-lung ventilation with the inhaled anesthetic, intravenous anesthesia with fentanyl, diazepam, and thiopental was instituted, and 40 to 60 minutes were allowed for elimination of the inhaled anesthetic to a measured end-tidal value of less than 0.1 percent. The study concluded with a period of two-lung ventilation during intravenous anesthesia. In Figure 13-7, the mean and individual patient values for PaO_2 and shunt are shown for the two inhaled anesthetic study groups. Shunt was significantly greater during halothane anesthesia than during intravenous anesthesia and PaO_2 was significantly less. Interpretation of this study is complicated by the thoracic surgery and lung trauma that occurred contemporaneously with the anesthetic protocol. Transient inhibition of HPV is associated with manipulation of the lung and should not be misconstrued as an anesthetic effect. Nonetheless, the results of this study suggest there is blunting of HPV by inhaled anesthetics, but the clinical effect is small.

However, examination of the individual patient data reveals that substantial variability occurs; hence, inhibition of HPV by inhaled anesthetics may be of greater clinical significance in select individual cases.

A study of eight subjects exposed to unilateral hypoxic ventilation supports the concept that the clinical effect of isoflurane inhibition of HPV is small.[84] Intravenous anesthesia was induced, and the lungs were ventilated separately and synchronously in the supine position. After 30 minutes of ventilation with an F_IO_2 of 1.0 bilaterally, the right (test) lung was ventilated with an F_IO_2 of 0.08 while the left (control) lung was ventilated with an F_IO_2 of 1.0. Measurements were obtained after 15 minutes; isoflurane was then administered to both lungs at an end-tidal concentration of 1 percent for 15 minutes, followed by 1.5 percent for 15 minutes. The study concluded with the termination of isoflurane administration and a 15-minute period of an F_IO_2 of 1.0 bilaterally. The distribution of blood flow to the two lungs was measured using the inert gas technique. The right (test) lung received 54 percent of the total blood flow during the control condition. Hypoxia reduced this fraction to 41 percent and the addition of isoflurane at 1 percent or

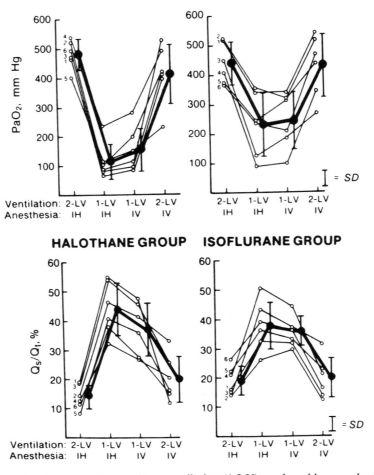

Fig. 13-7. During inhalational anesthesia, one-lung ventilation (1-LV) produced large reductions in PaO$_2$ and increases in shunt. Elimination of halothane (IH) and use of intravenous (IV) anesthesia during one-lung ventilation produced an increase in PaO$_2$ of 39 mmHg and a decrease in shunt by 7 percent of cardiac output. These effects were smaller when switching from isoflurane to intravenous anesthesia. Individual patient data are shown to demonstrate the considerable variability encountered clinically. 2-LV, two-lung ventilation. (From Benumof et al,[83] with permission.)

1.5 percent end-tidal concentration had minimal effect, with fractional flows of 41 percent and 43 percent, respectively. The moderate hypoxic stimulus of this study produced the expected changes in regional blood flow and vascular resistance. Higher-dose isoflurane and a more potent hypoxic stimulus might have demonstrated a larger effect of isoflurane; nonetheless, this study suggests that the magnitude of reduction of HPV by isoflurane in clinical situations may frequently be small.

Clinically, inhalational anesthetics may produce modest reductions in PaO$_2$ and increases in shunt through partial inhibition of HPV. At the same time, application of continuous positive airway pressure to the nondependent lung may substantially increase PaO$_2$ during one-lung ventilation.[85] This maneuver

and one-lung ventilation with 100 percent oxygen may be of greater clinical importance than the effects of inhaled anesthetics on HPV. Nonetheless, clinical variability is large, and the potentially deleterious effects of HPV inhibition by inhaled anesthetics should be considered in evaluating hypoxia during thoracic surgery. Measurement of cardiac output and P$\bar{v}$O$_2$ may provide clues to interpreting the changes produced by therapeutic maneuvers.

Vasodilators and Hypoxic Pulmonary Vasoconstriction

Vasodilators may be valuable for hemodynamic control during thoracic surgery; however, they may interfere with HPV and thereby worsen oxygenation.

For example, while receiving 40 percent oxygen, a patient with an inadvertent intubation of the right mainstem bronchus had a decrease of PaO_2 from 105 to 50 mmHg when nitroprusside was administered. In pentobarbital-anesthetized dogs with left lung atelectasis, the infusion of sodium nitroprusside to achieve a reduction of mean arterial pressure by 25 percent reduced PaO_2 from 134 to 75 mmHg and increased $\dot{Q}_s/\dot{Q}_T$ from 30 to 39 percent.[58] The effect of sodium nitroprusside on HPV was studied in 10 dogs using unilateral hypoxia with an F_IO_2 of 0.7 and 0.0. Blood flow as measured by ^{133}Xe showed attenuation of the redistribution due to hypoxia during infusion of nitroprusside.[86]

Hydralazine did not inhibit HPV in a canine study using global hypoxia with an F_IO_2 of 0.1. Hydralazine produced an increased cardiac output, but HPV was not affected, even when the cardiac output was reduced to the predrug level by adjustment of intravascular volume.[87] Administration of 0.4 mg of sublingual nitroglycerin in 19 unanesthetized men undergoing cardiac catheterization produced a significant increase of venous admixture from 8.8 to 12.6 percent and a decrease of mean PaO_2 from 80 to 72 mmHg. Cardiac output and $P\bar{v}O_2$ did not change significantly.[60] Nicardipine produced a dose-dependent attenuation of HPV in a study of 14 dogs using ventilation of the left lower lobe with 100 percent nitrogen,[88] and verapamil attenuated HPV in a canine study using global hypoxia.[89] Before treatment with nifedipine, ventilation for 5 minutes with an F_IO_2 of 0.1 instead of an F_IO_2 of 0.3 produced an 87 percent increase in pulmonary vascular resistance. After administration of nifedipine, 0.5 mg/kg, the hypoxic challenge produced only a 38 percent increase in PVR. The same experimental protocol was used to demonstrate the inhibition of HPV by sodium nitroprusside. Aminophylline did not inhibit acute in vivo lobar HPV in dogs.[90]

Prostaglandin $F_{2\alpha}$ ($PGF_{2\alpha}$) is a potent pulmonary vasoconstrictor. In a canine study, exogenous $PGF_{2\alpha}$ infused into the pulmonary artery of an atelectatic lung potentiated vasoconstriction and improved oxygenation by redistribution of blood flow to the ventilated lung.[91] Venous admixture was 11 percent during two-lung ventilation, and increased to 40 percent with one-lung atelectasis. Doses of $PGF_{2\alpha}$ of 0.4, 0.6, and 1.2 μg/kg/min produced reduction of venous admixture to 35, 27, and 25 percent, respectively. This study suggests that $PGF_{2\alpha}$ infusion into the pulmonary artery of an acutely atelectactic lung may be useful for improving the distribution of blood flow during one-lung ventilation. Peripheral intravenous infusion of $PGF_{2\alpha}$ did not enhance HPV and is probably not of use in the management of one-lung ventilation.[92] Prostaglandin E_1 (PGE_1) attenuated hypoxia-induced increases of pulmonary artery pressure in a canine study using global hypoxia.[93] Similarly, PGE_1 attenuated pulmonary vasoconstriction in conscious sheep while the F_IO_2 was 0.1.[94]

The effects on HPV of the inotropes, dopamine and dobutamine, have been studied in a canine model using global hypoxia. When cardiac output was held constant using balloon occlusion of the inferior vena cava, HPV was not inhibited by dopamine or dobutamine at doses of 10 and 20 μg/kg/min.[95] Studies of dopamine and dobutamine using lobar hypoxia and atelectasis demonstrated reduced flow diversion with these drugs, which may in part be explained by increases in cardiac output and $P\bar{v}O_2$.[96,97]

EFFECTS OF ANESTHETICS ON CONTROL OF VENTILATION

The inhalational anesthetics, opioids, and sedatives act on the central nervous system to produce a loss of awareness and analgesia. A side effect common to each of these is depression of breathing. Normally, spontaneous ventilation increases linearly as arterial or alveolar CO_2 concentration rises (Fig. 13-8). Although not routinely used as a test of pulmonary function, a CO_2 challenge can give useful information on the integrity of the respiratory center and ventilatory drive (see Chapter 7).

Respiratory sensitivity to CO_2 can be measured several ways. The *steady-state method* requires the simultaneous measurement of minute ventilation and arterial CO_2 tension ($PaCO_2$) or end-tidal CO_2 at intervals as $PaCO_2$ is raised by increasing the concentration of inspired CO_2. This technique is time consuming since several points are needed to define a curve. The slope of the CO_2 response curve can be determined with the *rebreathing method*, in which the patient breathes from a bag filled with 7 percent CO_2, 50 percent O_2 and N_2.[98] The CO_2 concentration in the bag rises steadily during rebreathing while the high O_2 concentration eliminates any chance of hypoxia contributing to the ventilatory stimulus. Ventilation is measured and plotted against the CO_2 tension in the bag, which reflects $PaCO_2$. Although the CO_2 response curve, as measured by the rebreathing technique, is displaced slightly to the right when compared with the steady-state method, the slope of the curve is essentially the same with either method. Introducing an airway obstruction for 0.1 second at the beginning of inspiration can be used to eliminate any effect due to increased airway resistance or reduced compliance; this response curve is felt to be a better indicator of central sensitivity to CO_2. The ventilatory response to CO_2 can also be separated into rib cage and abdominal components.

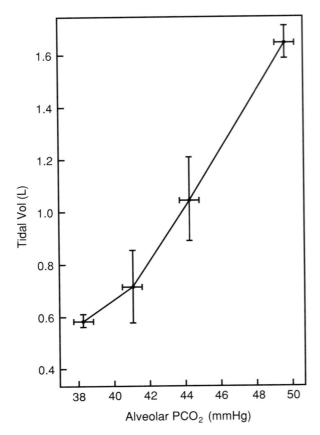

Fig. 13-8. Spontaneous ventilation, depicted here as tidal volume, increases linearly as alveolar CO_2 rises when healthy, nonanesthetized subjects breathe increasing amounts of CO_2. (From Lambertsen,[207] with permission.)

These tests all demonstrate that increasing the depth of anesthesia results in an elevation of $PaCO_2$ and a diminished ventilatory response to added CO_2, reflected as a decrease in the slope and a shift to the right of the CO_2 response curve. At deep levels of anesthesia, there may be no response to CO_2 at all.

There is some reluctance to measure ventilatory response to hypoxia because patients must be exposed to reduced concentrations of O_2. The ventilatory response to moderately low O_2 levels is less sensitive than to increases in CO_2 (Fig. 13-9). Several methods are used to test ventilatory response to hypoxia. The *steady-state method* requires that several CO_2 response curves be determined at different levels of inspired O_2 (Fig. 13-10). The *rebreathing method* that is used for CO_2 testing can be modified to measure the response to hypoxia. While CO_2 is held constant, the O_2 concentration in the bag is reduced by consumption by the subjects. Ventilation is plotted against oxyhemoglobin saturation as determined by noninvasive pulse

oximetry. At critically low O_2 concentrations, hypoxia stimulates peripheral chemoreceptors which, in turn, stimulate the respiratory center.[99] The hypoxic ventilatory response is also impaired in a dose-related manner by anesthetic agents.

The effects of drugs on ventilatory control are of little concern when ventilation is mechanically controlled, the usual situation *during* intrathoracic procedures. However, unimpaired control of ventilation is of paramount importance in the postoperative period when the decision to extubate an otherwise stable patient is often determined by the degree of respiratory depression present.

The discussion that follows does not describe which of the different study methodologies were used, but summarizes the results of the effects of various anesthetic agents and sedatives on ventilatory response to CO_2 or O_2 (see Chapter 7).

Opioids

The newer short-acting, potent opioids (fentanyl, sufentanil, alfentanil) have replaced morphine and meperidine in clinical practice. They are used with nitrous oxide or in combination with an inhalational agent. During surgery, they have minimal hemodynamic depressive effects when compared with equivalent amounts of morphine or meperidine or to the halogenated anesthetics when the latter are used alone.[100,101] In studies of cardiac patients that compare equivalent high doses of morphine, fentanyl, and sufentanil, patients receiving sufentanil demonstrated earlier emergence from anesthesia and time to extubation.[102]

All opioids are potent respiratory depressants.[103–105] Respiratory depression after parenteral opioids appears related to serum concentration and is present soon after administration. For example, morphine, 10 mg IV, given to healthy volunteers, maximally depressed the ventilatory response to CO_2 within 30 minutes of administration.[104] Since the newer drugs are shorter acting and multiple doses may be required during long procedures, a prolonged cumulative effect on ventilation may be observed.[106] An equivalent degree of intraoperative anesthesia with opioids renders the patient at greater risk for hypoventilation in the immediate postoperative period when compared with a pure inhalational anesthetic technique. Concomitant intraoperative use of parenteral opioids with intrathecal or epidural opioids further increases the risk of respiratory depression in the postoperative period.

Volatile Anesthetics

The halogenated inhalational agents (halothane, enflurane, isoflurane) are popular for thoracic surgery because of their dose-related direct bronchodilatory

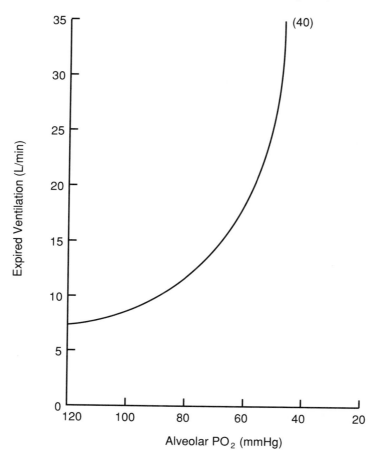

Fig. 13-9. The ventilatory response to low levels of O_2 is less sensitive than to rises in CO_2. With alveolar CO_2 tension held constant at 40 mmHg, the effect of changing alveolar O_2 concentration on expired ventilation is shown.

effects and because they obtund bronchoconstrictive airway reflexes in patients with reactive airways.[107] Nitrous oxide need not be used, so a high inspired F_IO_2 can be maintained both during two-lung and one-lung ventilation. The inhalational agents depress ventilation in a dose-dependent manner in spontaneously breathing volunteers.[108–110] Tidal volume is reduced and respiratory rate is increased, with an overall decrease in minute ventilation.[111] At a similar MAC, $PaCO_2$ levels are highest and alveolar ventilation most depressed with enflurane and isoflurane, followed by sevoflurane and halothane[108,112–115] (Fig. 13-11).

Since the volatile anesthetics are rapidly eliminated, they usually do not contribute significantly to ventilatory depression in the immediate postoperative period. Although both the hypercapnic ventilatory response and the hypoxic ventilatory drive are depressed at clinical concentrations, subanesthetic concentrations of halothane and enflurane have *no* effect on the ventilatory response to hypercarbia.[116]

However, at levels as low as 0.1 MAC, depression of the ventilatory response to hypoxemia occurs with all halogenated anesthetics (Fig. 13-12).[112,117,118] As little as 0.05 MAC of halothane can depress the hypoxic ventilatory response by as much as 50 percent. The obtundation of the hypoxic drive by subanesthetic concentrations of inhalational anesthetics persists into the early postoperative period after the patient has regained consciousness and may appear to be recovering. This may be particularly important for patients with advanced pulmonary disease who are normally dependent on their hypoxic drive to breathe.[112,113,117]

Recovery from inhalation anesthesia is often marked by the occurrence of postoperative shivering, which causes a significant increase in oxygen consumption and CO_2 production.[119] Rapid elimination of an inhalational agent resulting in a fast awakening time theoretically should reduce this increased metabolic demand. Sevoflurane, a potent, nonexplosive ha-

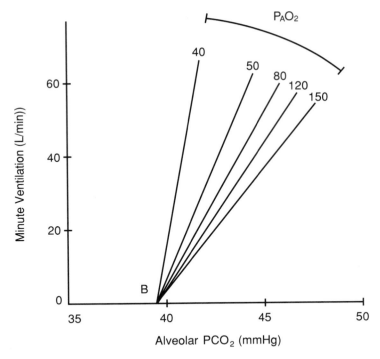

Fig. 13-10. The minute ventilation response to changes in alveolar CO_2 concentration increases at lower O_2 concentrations. (From Forster et al,[208] with permission.)

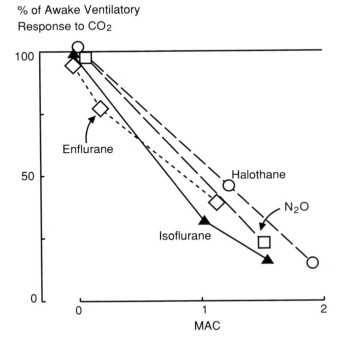

Fig. 13-11. The ventilatory response to CO_2 was measured in awake volunteers breathing enflurane, halothane, isoflurane, and nitrous oxide. All inhalational anesthetics depress the ventilatory response to increases in CO_2 in a dose-dependent manner. (From Eger,[209] with permission.)

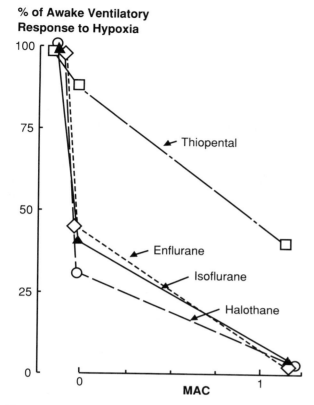

% of Awake Ventilatory Response to Hypoxia

Thiopental

Enflurane

Isoflurane

Halothane

MAC

Fig. 13-12. In humans, even subclinical concentrations of isoflurane, halothane, and enflurane decrease the ventilatory response to hypoxia when $PaCO_2$ is kept constant. As little as 0.1 MAC will depress the awake ventilatory response to hypoxia by as much as 50 percent. (From Eger,[209] with permission.)

logenated ether, has a low blood/gas partition coefficient (0.69) relative to halothane (2.5) and isoflurane (1.4). Its excretion from the body is quite rapid.[120,121] Hemodynamic stability and lack of sensitization to catecholamines, coupled with the low blood solubility allowing faster awakening, may make sevoflurane a useful agent for thoracic anesthesia.[115]

Nitrous Oxide

Nitrous oxide is a weak anesthetic and is never used alone, but always in combination with inhalational agents or opioids. During pulmonary surgery, high inspired oxygen concentrations are often needed, and nitrous oxide is used in relatively low concentrations or avoided completely. The response to hypercapnia is not depressed by nitrous oxide, and respiration may actually be increased.[122] However, in the immediate postoperative period, nitrous oxide in concentrations

below 50 percent depresses the respiratory response to hypoxia.[123] This blunted hypoxic response may aggravate "diffusion hypoxia," the phenomenon that occurs when nitrous oxide is discontinued and the sudden outflow of gas from the blood into the lungs dilutes other gases present in the alveoli.[124] If the patient is allowed to breathe room air, arterial desaturation occurs, which may be significant in critically ill patients.[125]

Ketamine

Ketamine, with its rapid onset and stimulatory cardiovascular effects, is mainly used for induction of anesthesia in unstable patients or for an emergency thoracotomy,[126] but it has been used as the sole anesthetic during thoracic surgery.[127,128] Other than direct bronchodilation and antagonism of bronchoconstriction from histamine release, the respiratory effects of ketamine are minimal and transient.[129] Respiratory stimulation is generally seen,[130] although a decrease in tidal volume associated with CO_2 elevation and decreased PaO_2 can occur.[131] Unpleasant emergence reactions have limited its use, although patients undergoing thoracotomy with a continuous ketamine infusion did not demonstrate emergence phenomena.[75,132,133]

Local Anesthetics

Subarachnoid or epidural local anesthetics are often combined with general anesthesia for thoracic operations.[134,135] The potential benefits of this technique are suppression of the neuroendocrine stress response during and after surgery,[136–138] a positive effect on postoperative nitrogen balance,[139] and a reduction in cardiac pre- and afterload with improvement in myocardial oxygen supply relative to demand during ischemia.[140–143] Despite the increasing popularity of these techniques, a paucity of information exists on the effects of local anesthetics on pulmonary function.

Local anesthetics are believed to interfere with the control of ventilation in two ways: by direct blockade of spinal nerves and by central effects. Intravenous infusion of lidocaine stimulates respiration in healthy, unpremedicated subjects.[144,145] In volunteers, epidural lidocaine either had minimal effects on ventilation[146] or increased the ventilatory response to CO_2.[145] Increased responsiveness to CO_2 was also seen with intrathecal bupivacaine and tetracaine in unpremedicated surgical patients.[147,148] Such increased sensitivity to CO_2 may be due to a drug effect on the brain from systemic absorption.[145] The initial effect of lidocaine and other local anesthetics on the central nervous system (CNS) is selective depression of inhibitory pathways leading to unopposed excitatory activity.[149,150] It is postulated that this excitation in patients is reflected as an increased ventilatory response to CO_2.[144] At higher concentrations, generalized CNS depression occurs.

Although epidural anesthesia alone was once used for thoracic operations on spontaneously breathing patients,[151] in current practice, ventilation is always controlled during thoracic surgery. Thus, effects on ventilatory drive by local anesthetics are masked. For the patient undergoing thoracotomy, uncomplicated regional anesthesia usually has no clinical effect on ventilation unless the level of anesthesia involves paralysis of the intercostal and phrenic nerves.[152–154] High thoracic epidural anesthesia causing mechanical impairment of rib cage movement may decrease the ventilatory response to CO_2 as a result of blockade of the efferent and afferent pathways of the intercostal nerve roots.[155] Residual motor block as a cause of postoperative ventilatory depression must always be considered.

Patients with CO_2 retention whose resting ventilation depends on hypoxic drive could be at risk of ventilatory failure when lidocaine is administered for dysrhythmia control or for regional anesthesia. In a study of the effect of a lidocaine infusion in healthy volunteers, at a serum concentration of 3.6 $\mu g/mL$, the ventilatory response to isocapnic hypoxia was significantly depressed in 8 of 9 subjects.[156]

Spinal Opioids

Intraoperatively, all the commonly used opioids have been given either intrathecally or epidurally to reduce pain and improve the quality of recovery following thoracic surgery.[157–172] Other than potentiation of analgesia, they have no known intraoperative effects.[169,173] Unlike local anesthetics, epidural morphine and diamorphine do not prevent intraoperative changes in plasma cortisol or glucose concentrations.[137,174–176] Since the spinal effects of the opioids are "selective" for pain, the side effects (muscle paralysis, sympathectomy) and complications (convulsions, cardiovascular collapse) of local anesthetics administered at the same site do not occur.[173] The complications of intraoperatively administered spinal opioids occur in the postoperative period. The frequency and occurrence of minor complications (pruritus, urinary retention, nausea and vomiting) vary with the specific agent used (see Chapter 21).

All spinally administered opioids have been associated with hypoventilation following thoracotomy, but significant respiratory depression and apnea are rare.[173,177] Hypoventilation may be noted shortly after surgery or may be delayed for hours. In general, the lipophilic drugs (fentanyl, sufentanil) cause an early onset of respiratory depression,[169,178–180] probably due to central effects from systemic absorption.[181] However, decreased response to CO_2 can be present for up to 20 hours after the epidural administration of lipid-soluble opioids.[182] The hydrophilic opioids like morphine are associated with delayed respiratory depression occurring hours after administration, presumably due to the rostral spread of the drug in the cerebrospinal fluid to the brain.[177,179,183]

In healthy volunteers[104,183,184] and surgical patients,[183,185] epidural morphine reduces minute ventilation and increases end-tidal CO_2 progressively with time. The slope of the ventilatory response to exogenous CO_2 is reduced and the depressive effects persist for up to 24 hours.[104,183,186] Increasing amounts of epidural morphine depress the ventilatory response to a standardized CO_2 challenge in a dose-related manner.[183] In healthy volunteers, the slope of the CO_2 response curve and its position for a fixed stimulus ($P_{ET}CO_2$ = 54 mmHg) were depressed to a greater degree at 3 and 22 hours following 10 mg of epidural morphine than with an identical dose of intravenous morphine.[104] Additional administration of parenteral opioids or sedatives increases these respiratory effects.

The ventilatory depression seen in volunteers may be exaggerated compared with postoperative patients since the latter may have respiratory stimulation from postoperative pain.[173] The situation is complex since, by alleviating pain, lumbar epidural morphine improves pulmonary function as measured by spirometry following thoracotomy.[162] However, hypoventilation with CO_2 retention occurs in the majority of these patients.[179] Because patients undergoing thoracotomy often have poor pulmonary function and the effect of spinal opioids on respiration is unpredictable, continuous monitoring or close observation in the postoperative period is advised.

The factors predisposing to significant respiratory depression after spinal opioid administration include concomitant administration of opioids or CNS depressant drugs by other routes prior to or during surgery, high spinal doses, the hydrophilicity of the specific agent, advanced age, site of administration (intrathecal > thoracic epidural > lumbar epidural), and increased intra-abdominal or intrathoracic pressure.[173]

Sedatives

Drugs used in the perioperative period to provide sedation, allay anxiety, reduce anesthetic requirements, and produce amnesia can all contribute to potential postoperative respiratory problems. The benzodiazepine derivatives (diazepam, lorazepam, and midazolam) are used as sedatives and in larger doses for induction of general anesthesia. Conflicting data concerning the ventilatory effects of the benzodiazepines may be due to the large variability in investigational conditions. Whereas some investigators have failed to demonstrate significant effects on the ventilatory response to CO_2 in volunteers and patients given intravenous diazepam and midazolam[187] or oral midazolam,[188] the majority of investigations implicate the benzodiazepines as respiratory depressants.[189] In healthy volunteers, intravenous diazepam, 0.15 mg/kg, and midazolam, 0.05 mg/kg, produce similar decreases in tidal volume associated with an increased respiratory rate, but with little overall change in minute ventilation.[190–192] These alterations in breathing pattern result in CO_2 retention and arterial oxygen desaturation. Hypnotic doses of intravenous diazepam caused a significant (50 percent) decrease in the slope of the CO_2 response curve that required 30 minutes to return to baseline in normal healthy volunteers.[193] Diazepam, 10 mg orally, in healthy subjects also produced a significant reduction in ventilatory response to CO_2 that was not associated with any effect on respiratory muscle power.[194,195] Combining meperidine with midazolam or diazepam caused a profound decrease in the diaphragmatic component of breathing, which was not seen with the benzodiazepines alone.[191]

The effect of midazolam on the hypoxic ventilatory response in healthy volunteers has been examined. With a sedative dose, 0.1 mg/kg IV, the slope of the ventilatory response to hypoxia was depressed by more than 50 percent, while the normal hyperpnea and tachycardia associated with hypoxemia were attenuated.[196] Diazepam also depresses hypoxic ventilatory drive, and the benzodiazepine antagonist flumazenil is only partially effective in reversing this depression.[197]

Some investigators have reported that lorazepam stimulates ventilation,[198] while others have reported that it depresses ventilation.[199] Lorazepam, 0.05 mg/kg IV, produced a decrease in the slope and a shift to the right of the CO_2 response curve.[200] End-expiratory CO_2 was elevated in healthy adult men treated before elective surgery. A unique potentially dangerous ventilatory effect, periodic breathing, occurred in 9 of 10 patients following small (2 mg IV) doses of lorazepam.[201]

Although the respiratory effects of these agents are thought to be relatively mild and short-lived, severe respiratory depression has been reported in elderly or debilitated patients following both oral and intravenous administration.[202,203] The ventilatory effects of induction doses (0.2 mg/kg IV) of midazolam in nor-

mal volunteers and in subjects with chronic obstructive pulmonary disease (COPD) have been studied. In the healthy volunteers, the slope of the CO_2 response curve was markedly depressed, but returned to 75 percent of control value within 15 minutes. In contrast, in subjects with clinical COPD, the slope of the curve returned to only 33 percent of baseline control 15 minutes after injection. As Gross et al reported, the ventilatory response to midazolam differs between normal and COPD patients, with a profound depressant effect seen in the latter.[204] These investigators postulated that if midazolam is used in doses of 0.2 mg/kg IV for the induction of anesthesia or for sedation and the patient is maintained on inhalational anesthetics, emergence from general anesthesia could be delayed.

Unlike the benzodiazepines, the butyrophenone droperidol in moderate doses caused only a minimal reduction in tidal volume and minute ventilation, with no significant changes in respiratory rate or blood gas parameters.[205]

When used in usual clinical doses, sedatives and hypnotics have mild-to-moderate respiratory effects. However, their depressant effects on ventilation in both healthy volunteers and surgical patients are greatest in the absence of stimulation. Thus, a patient who is breathing adequately in the immediate postoperative period might hypoventilate if left unattended in a quiet environment.[195] Patients receiving sedative agents and/or opioids intraoperatively should be observed closely in the postanesthetic period for signs of respiratory insufficiency.[204] When those agents are used in combination with "spinal" opioids, the incidence of significant respiratory depression is greatly increased.[206]

CONCLUSION

Selection of anesthetic agents for thoracic surgery requires consideration of the multiple, sometimes conflicting, effects of the drugs used (Table 13-1). Drug effects, the presence of underlying disease, and the effects of surgery all complicate the anesthetic management. The importance of each issue and interaction must be thoroughly evaluated and interpreted in the context of the properties of the specific agents chosen. Avoiding intraoperative hypoxemia and postoperative respiratory failure requires the proper use of anesthetic agents. No single agent or technique is always recommended; rather, many factors must be considered and the choice of agent determined in context. Clinical judgment of individual anesthesiologists and their past experiences are important in the proper

TABLE 13-1. Properties of Anesthetics

Anesthetic	Desirable	Undesirable
Volatile	Permits use of high F_IO_2 Bronchodilation Diminishes airway reflexes Readily eliminated	Inhibits HPV Myocardial depression

Narcotics	Do not inhibit HPV
	No myocardial depression
	  when used alone
	Provide postoperative analgesia
		Not general anesthetics
		May depress ventilation in immediate
		  postoperative period

Nitrous oxide	Readily eliminated Probably no effect on HPV	Reduces F_IO_2
Ketamine	Diminishes airway irritability Does not inhibit HPV Cardiovascular stability during hypovolemia	Myocardial ischemia Emergence delirium
Thiopental	Does not inhibit HPV	Minor potential for histamine release and bronchospasm

Muscle relaxants	Facilitate mechanical ventilation
	Enhance surgical exposure
	
	Minimize doses of general
	  anesthetics
		Potential for postoperative weakness
		Possible histamine release
		  and bronchospasm
		Need for use of reversal agent

Cholinesterase
  inhibitors
	Reverse neuromuscular
	  blockade
		May produce acetylcholine-mediated
		  bronchospasm

Abbreviation: HPV, hypoxic pulmonary vasoconstriction.

selection and use of anesthetics for intrathoracic surgical procedures.

ACKNOWLEDGMENT

Excellent secretarial assistance by Roz Mandell in the preparation of the manuscript was greatly appreciated.

REFERENCES

1. Don HF, Wahba M, Cuadrado L, Kelkar K: The effects of anesthesia and 100 percent oxygen on the functional residual capacity of the lungs. Anesthesiology 32:521, 1970
2. Hewlett AM, Hulands GH, Nunn JF, Heath JR: Functional residual capacity during anaesthesia: II. Spontaneous respiration. Br J Anaesth 46:486, 1974
3. Westbrook PR, Stubbs SE, Sessler AD, et al: Effects of anesthesia and muscle paralysis on respiratory mechanics in normal man. J Appl Physiol 34:81, 1973
4. Bergman NA: Reduction in resting end-expiratory position of the respiratory system with induction of anesthesia and neuromuscular paralysis. Anesthesiology 57:14, 1982
5. Bergman NA, Tien YK: Contribution of the closure of

pulmonary units to imposed oxygenation during anesthesia. Anesthesiology 59:395, 1983
6. Juno P, Marsh HM, Knopp TJ, Rehder K: Closing capacity in awake and anesthesized-paralyzed man. J Appl Physiol 44:238, 1978
7. Rehder K, Mallow JE, Fibuch EE, et al: Effects of isoflurane anesthesia and muscle paralysis on respiratory mechanics in normal man. Anesthesiology 41:477, 1974
8. Hirshman CA: Airway reactivity in humans. Anesthesiology 58:170, 1983
9. Mue S, Ishihara T, Tamura G, et al: The participation of the subepithelial airway receptor in the bronchoconstriction of monkeys. Tohoku J Exp Med 145:465, 1985
10. Ruffles SP, Gayres JG: Fatal bronchospasm after topical lignocaine before bronchoscopy. Br Med J 294:1658, 1987
11. Berger JM, Stirt JA: Resolution of bronchospasm by atropine: report of a case. Acta Anaesthesiol Scand 29:856, 1985
12. Waltemath CL, Bergman NA: Effect of ketamine and halothane on increased respiratory resistance provoked by ultrasonic aerosols. Anesthesiology 41:473, 1974
13. Patterson RW, Sullivan SF, Malm JR, et al: The effects of halothane on human airway mechanics. Anesthesiology 29:900, 1968
14. Lehane JR, Jordan C, Jones JG: Influence of halothane and enflurane on respiratory airflow resistance and specific conductance in anaesthetized man. Br J Anaesth 52:773, 1980

15. Fletcher SW, Flacke W, Alper MH: The action of general anesthetic agents on tracheal smooth muscle. Anesthesiology 29:517, 1968

16. Hermens JM, Edelstein G, Hanifin JM, et al: Inhalational anesthesia and histamine release during bronchospasm. Anesthesiology 61:69, 1984

17. Kettlekamp NS, Austin DR, Downes H, et al: Inhibition of *d*-tubocurarine-induced histamine release by halothane. Anesthesiology 66:666, 1987

18. Shah MV, Hirshman CA: Mode of action of halothane on histamine-induced airway constriction in dogs with reactive airways. Anesthesiology 65:170, 1986

19. Hirshman CA, Edelstein G, Peetz S, et al: Mechanisms of action of inhalational anesthesia on airways. Anesthesiology 56:107, 1982

20. Gold MI, Schwam SJ, Goldberg M: Chronic obstructive pulmonary disease and respiratory complications. Anesth Analg 62:975, 1983

21. Johnston RR, Eger EI, Wilson C: A comparative interaction of epinephrine with enflurane, isoflurane, and halothane in man. Anesth Analg 55:709, 1976

22. Hirshman CA, Edelstein RA, Ebertz JM, Hanifin JM: Thiobarbiturate-induced histamine release in human skin mast cells. Anesthesiology 63:353, 1985

23. Lorenz W, Doenicke A, Meger R, et al: Histamine release in man by propanidid and thiopentone: pharmacological effects and clinical consequences. Br J Anaesth 44:355, 1972

24. Guldager H, Sondergaard I, Jensen FM, Cold G: Basophil histamine release in asthma patients after in vitro provocation with althesin and etomidate. Acta Anaesthesiol Scand 29:352, 1985

25. Watkins J: Etomidate: an "immunologically safe" anesthetic agent. Anaesthesia, Suppl. 38:34–38, 1983

26. Fazackerley EJ, Martin AJ, Tolhurst-Cleaver CL, Watkins J: Anaphylactoid reaction following the use of etomidate. Anaesthesia 43:953, 1988

27. Vitkun SA, Foster WM, Chane H, et al: Bronchodilating effects of the anesthetic ketamine in an in vitro guinea pig preparation. Lung 165:101, 1987

28. Hirshman CA, Downes H, Farbood A, Bergman NA: Ketamine block of bronchospasm in experimental canine asthma. Br J Anaesth 51:713, 1979

29. Doenicke A, Lorenz W, Stamwerth D, et al: Effects of propofol ("Diprivan") on histamine release, immunoglobulin levels and activation of complement in healthy volunteers. Postgrad Med J, Suppl. 3, 61:15–20, 1986

30. Withington DE: Basophil histamine release studies in the evaluation of a new anesthetic agent. Agents Actions 23:337, 1988

31. Hermens JM, Ebertz JM, Hanifin JM, Hirshman CA: Comparison of histamine release in human skin mast cells induced by morphine, fentanyl, and oxymorphone. Anesthesiology 62:124, 1985

32. Eschenbacher WL, Bethel RA, Baushay HA, Sheppard D: Morphine sulfate inhibits bronchoconstriction in subjects with mild asthma whose responses are inhibited by atropine. Am Rev Respir Dis 130:363, 1984

33. Finer BL, Partington MW: Pethidine and the triple response. Br Med J 1:431, 1953

34. Shemano I, Wendel H: Effects of meperidine hydrochloride and morphine sulfate on the lung capacity of intact dogs. J Pharmacol Exp Ther 149:379, 1965

35. Moss J, Rosow CE, Savarese JJ, et al: Role of histamine in the hypotensive action of *d*-tubocurarine in humans. Anesthesiology 55:19, 1981

36. Stoelting RK: Hemodynamic effects of dimethyl-tubocurarine during nitrous oxide-halothane anesthesia. Anesth Analg 53:513, 1974

37. Basta SJ, Ali HH, Savarese JJ, et al: Clinical pharmacology of atracurium besylate (BW 33A): a new nondepolarizing muscle relaxant. Anesth Analg 61:723, 1982

38. Booij LH, Edwards RP, Sohn YJ, Miller RD: Cardiovascular and neuromuscular effects of Org NC 45, pancuronium, metocurine, and *d*-tubocurarine in dogs. Anesth Analg 59:26, 1980

39. Severinghaus JW, Stupfel M: Respiratory dead space increases following atropine in man and atropine, vagal or ganglionic blockade and hypothermia in dogs. J Appl Physiol 8:81, 1955

40. Jackson PJ, Manning PJ, O'Byrne PM: A new role for histamine H_2-receptors in asthmatic airways. Am Rev Respir Dis 138:784, 1988

41. Hofman J, Michalska I, Rutkowski R, Chyrek-Borowska S: The role of H_2 receptors in bronchial reactivity in atopic asthma. Agents Actions 23:370, 1988

42. Torda TA, McColloch CH, O'Brien HD, et al: Pulmonary venous admixture during one-lung anaesthesia. Anaesthesia 20:272, 1974

43. Kerr JH, Smith AC, Prys-Roberts C, et al: Observations during endobronchial anaesthesia II: oxygenation. Br J Anaesth 46:84, 1974

44. Marshall BF, Cohen PJ, Klingenmaier CH, Aukberg S: Pulmonary venous admixture before, during, and after halothane oxygen anesthesia in man. J Appl Physiol 27:653, 1969

45. Dueck R, Young I, Clausen J, Wagner PD: Altered distribution of pulmonary ventilation and blood flow following induction of inhalational anethesia. Anesthesiology 52:113, 1980

46. Dueck R, Rathbun M, Greenburg AG: Lung volume and $\dot{V}_A/\dot{Q}$ distribution response to intravenous versus inhalation anesthetics in sheep. Anesthesiology 61:55, 1984

47. Euler USV, Liljestrand G: Observations on the pulmonary arterial blood pressure in the cat. Acta Physiol Scand 12:301, 1946

48. Burton AC, Patel DJ: Effect on pulmonary vascular resistance of inflation of the rabbit lungs. J Appl Physiol 12:239, 1958

49. Bjertnaes L, Mundal R, Hauge A, Nicolaysen A: Vascular resistance in atelectatic lungs: effects of inhalation anesthetics. Acta Anaesthesiol Scand 24:109, 1980

50. Domino KB, Wetstein L, Glosser SA, et al: Influence of mixed venous oxygen tension ($P\bar{v}O_2$) on blood flow to atelectatic lung. Anesthesiology 59:428, 1983

51. Benumof JL: Mechanism of decreased blood flow to atelectatic lung. J Appl Physiol 46:1047, 1979

52. Glasser SA, Domino KB, Lindgren L, et al: Pulmonary blood pressure and flow during atelectasis in the dog. Anesthesiology 58:225, 1983

53. Miller FL, Chen L, Malmkvist G, et al: Mechanical factors do not influence blood flow distribution in atelectasis. Anesthesiology 70:481, 1989

54. Marshall BF, Marshall C, Benumof J, Saidman LJ: Hypoxic pulmonary vasoconstriction in dogs: effects of lung segment size and oxygen tension. J Appl Physiol 51:1543, 1981

55. Zasslow MA, Benumof JL, Trousdale FR: Hypoxic pulmonary vasoconstriction and the size of the hypoxic compartment. J Appl Physiol 53:626, 1982

56. Siegel LC, Pearl RG, Shafer SL, et al: The longitudinal distribution of pulmonary vascular resistance during unilateral hypoxia. Anesthesiology 70:527, 1989

57. Marshall C, Marshall B: Site and sensitivity for stimulation of hypoxic pulmonary vasoconstriction. J Appl Physiol 55:711, 1983

58. Colley PS, Cheney FW: Sodium nitroprusside increases $\dot{Q}_S/\dot{Q}_T$ in dogs in regional atelectasis. Anesthesiology 47:338, 1977

59. Castely PA, Lear S, Cotrell JE, Lear F: Intrapulmonary shunting during induced hypotension. Anesth Analg 61:231, 1982

60. Mookherjee S, Fuleihan D, Warner RA, et al: Effects of sublingual nitroglycerin on resting pulmonary gas exchange and hemodynamics in man. Circulation 57:106, 1978

61. Benumof JL: Intermittent hypoxia increases lobar hypoxic pulmonary vasoconstriction. Anesthesiology 58:399, 1983

62. Chen L, Miller FL, Williams JJ, et al: Hypoxic pulmonary vasoconstriction is not potentiated by repeated intermittent hypoxia in closed chest dogs. Anesthesiology 63:608, 1985

63. Amira T, Matsuura M, Shiramatso T, et al: Synthesis of prostaglandins TXA_2 and PGI_2 during one-lung anesthesia. Prostaglandins 34:668, 1987

64. Bjertnaes LJ: Hypoxia-induced vasoconstriction in isolated perfused lungs exposed to injectable or inhalation anesthetics. Acta Anaesthesiol Scand 21:133, 1977

65. Bjertnaes L, Hauge A, Kriz M: Hypoxia-induced pulmonary vasoconstriction: effects of fentanyl following different routes of administration. Acta Anaesthesiol Scand 24:53, 1980

66. Gibbs JM, Johnson H: Lack of effect of morphine and buprenorphine on hypoxic pulmonary vasoconstriction in the isolated perfused cat lung and the perfused lobe of the dog lung. Br J Anaesth 50:1197, 1978

67. Bjertnaes LJ, Hauge A, Torgrimsen T: The pulmonary vasoconstriction response to hypoxia. The hypoxic-sensitive site studied with a volatile inhibitor. Acta Physiol Scand 109:447, 1980

68. Loh L, Sykes MK, Chakrabarti MK: The effects of halothane and ether on the pulmonary circulation in the innervated perfused cat lung. Br J Anaesth 49:309, 1977

69. Gibbs JM, Sykes MK, Tait AR: Effects of halothane and hydrogen ion concentration on the alteration of pulmonary vascular resistance induced by graded alveolar hypoxia in the isolated perfused cat lung. Anaesth Intensive Care 2:231, 1974

70. Marshall C, Lindgren L, Marshall BF: Effects of halothane, enflurane, and isoflurane on hypoxic pulmonary vasoconstriction in rat lungs in vitro. Anesthesiology 60:304, 1984

71. Sykes MK, Davies DM, Loh L, et al: The effect of methoxyflurane on pulmonary vascular resistance and hypoxic pulmonary vasoconstriction in the isolated perfused cat lung. Br J Anaesth 48:191, 1976

72. Bjertnaes LJ, Mundal R: The pulmonary vasoconstrictor response to hypoxia during enflurane anesthesia. Acta Anaesth Scand 24:252, 1980

73. Lumb PD, Silvay G, Weinreich AI, Shiang H: A comparison of the effects of continuous ketamine infusion and halothane on oxygenation during one-lung anaesthesia in dogs. Can Anaesth Soc J 26:394, 1979

74. Benumof JL, Wahrenbrock EA: Local effects of anesthetics on regional hypoxic pulmonary vasoconstriction. Anesthesiology 43:525, 1975

75. Rees DI, Gaines GY: One-lung anesthesia—a comparison of pulmonary gas exchange during anesthesia with ketamine or enflurane. Anesth Analg 63:521, 1984

76. Cheney FW, Colley PS: The effect of cardiac output on arterial blood oxygenation. Anesthesiology 52:496, 1980

77. Smith G, Cheney FW, Winter PM: The effect of change in cardiac output on intrapulmonary shunting. Br J Anaesth 46:337, 1974

78. Mathers J, Benumof JL, Wahrenbrock EA: General anesthetics and regional hypoxic pulmonary vasoconstriction. Anesthesiology 46:111, 1977

79. Domino KB, Borowec L, Alexander CM, et al: Influence of isoflurane on hypoxic pulmonary vasoconstriction in dogs. Anesthesiology 64:423, 1986

80. Bjertnaes LJ: Hypoxia-induced pulmonary vasoconstriction in man: Inhibition due to diethyl ether and halothane anesthesia. Acta Anaesthesiol Scand 22:570, 1978

81. Van Keer L, Van Aken H, Vandermeersch E, et al: Propofol does not inhibit hypoxic pulmonary vasoconstriction in humans. J Clin Anesth 1:284–288, 1989

82. Rogers SN, Benumof JL: Halothane and isoflurane do not decrease PaO_2 during one-lung ventilation in intravenously anesthetized patients. Anesth Analg 64:946, 1985

83. Benumof JL, Augustine SD, Gibbons JA: Halothane and isoflurane only slightly impair arterial oxygenation during one-lung ventilation in patients undergoing thoracotomy. Anesthesiology 67:910, 1987

84. Carlsson AJ, Bindslev L, Hedenstierna G: Hypoxia-induced pulmonary vasoconstriction in the human lung—the effect of isoflurane anesthesia. Anesthesiology 66:312, 1987

85. Capan LM, Turndorf H, Chandrakant P, et al: Optimization of arterial oxygenation during one-lung anesthesia. Anesth Analg 59:847, 1980

86. Hill AB, Sykes MK, Reyes A: A hypoxic pulmonary vasoconstriction response in dogs during and after infusion of sodium nitroprusside. Anesthesiology 50:484, 1979.

87. Bishop MJ, Kennard S, Artman LD, Cheney FW: Hy-

dralazine does not inhibit canine hypoxic pulmonary vasoconstriction. Am Rev Respir Dis 128:998, 1983

88. Nakatawa K, Amaha K: Effect of nicardipine hydrochloride on regional hypoxic pulmonary vasoconstriction. Br J Anaesth 60:547, 1988

89. Tucker A, McMurtry IF, Grover RF, Reeves JT: Attenuation of hypoxic pulmonary vasoconstriction by verapamil in intact dogs. Proc Soc Exp Biol Med 151:611, 1976

90. Benumof JL, Trousdale FR: Aminophylline does not inhibit canine hypoxic pulmonary vasoconstriction. Am Rev Respir Dis 126:1017, 1982

91. Scherer RW, Vigfusson G, Hultsch E, et al: Prostaglandin $E_{2\alpha}$ improves oxygen tension and reduces venous admixture during one-lung ventilation in anesthetized paralyzed dogs. Anesthesiology 62:23, 1985

92. Chen L, Miller FL, Malmkvist G, et al: Intravenous $PGE_{2\alpha}$ infusion does not enhance hypoxic pulmonary vasoconstriction during canine one-lung hypoxia. Anesthesiology 68:226, 1988

93. Leeman M, Lejeune P, Melot C, Naeije R: Pulmonary artery pressure-flow plots in hyperoxic and in hypoxic dogs: effects of prostaglandin E_1. Eur Respir J 1:711, 1988

94. Yoshimura K: Effects of prostaglandin E_1 and isosorbide dinitrate on acute hypoxic pulmonary vasoconstriction in conscious sheep. Jpn Circ J 49:1081, 1985

95. Lejeune P, Leeman M, Delout T, Naeije R: Pulmonary hemodynamic response to dopamine and dobutamine in hyperoxic and in hypoxic dogs. Anesthesiology 66:49, 1987

96. McFarlane PA, Mortimer AJ, Ryder WA, et al: Effects of dopamine and dobutamine on the distribution of pulmonary blood flow during lobar ventilation hypoxia and lobar collapse in dogs. Eur J Clin Invest 15:53, 1985

97. Gardaz JP, McFarlane PA, Sykes MK: Mechanisms by which dopamine alters blood flow distribution during lobar collapse in dogs. J Appl Physiol 60:959, 1986

98. Read DJC: A clinical method for assessing the ventilatory response to carbon dioxide. Australas Ann Med 16:20, 1967

99. Comroe JH, Jr: The peripheral chemoreceptors. p. 557. In Fenn WO, Rahn H (eds): Handbook of Physiology. Section 3. Respiration. Vol. 1. American Physiological Society, Washington, DC, 1964

100. Prys-Roberts C, Kelman GR: The influence of drugs used in neurolept-analgesia on cardiovascular and respiratory function. Br J Anaesth 39:134, 1967

101. Clark NJ, Meuleman T, Liu WS, et al: Comparison of sufentanil-N_2O and fentanyl-N_2O in patients without cardiac disease undergoing general surgery. Anesthesiology 66:130, 1987

102. Sanford TJ, Jr, Smith NT, Dec-Silver H, Harrison WK: A comparison of morphine, fentanyl, and sufentanil anesthesia for cardiac surgery: induction, emergence, and extubation. Anesth Analg 65:259, 1986

103. Grell FL, Koons RA, Denson US: Fentanyl in anesthesia. Anesth Analg 51:16, 1972

104. Camporesi EM, Nielsen CH, Bromage PR, Durant PA: Ventilatory CO_2 sensitivity after intravenous and epidural morphine in volunteers. Anesth Analg 62:633, 1983

105. Hasenbos M, Simon M, van Egmond J, et al: Postoperative analgesia by nicomorphine intramuscularly versus high thoracic epidural administration. Effects on ventilatory and airway occlusion pressure responses to CO_2. Acta Anaesthesiol Scand 30:426, 1986

106. Adams AP, Pybus DA: Delayed respiratory depression after use of fentanyl during anesthesia. Br J Anaesth 1:278, 1978

107. Coon RL, Kampine JP: Hypocapnic bronchoconstriction and inhalation anesthetics. Anesthesiology 43:635, 1975

108. Bahlman SH, Eger EI, Halsey MJ, et al: The cardiovascular effects of halothane in man during spontaneous ventilation. Anesthesiology 36:494, 1972

109. Fourcade HE, Stevens WC, Larson CP, Jr, et al: Ventilatory effects of Forane—a new inhaled anesthetic. Anesthesiology 35:26, 1971

110. Doi M, Ikeda K: Respiratory effects of sevoflurane. Anesth Analg 66:241, 1987

111. Munsson ES, Larson CP, Babad AA, et al: The effects of halothane, fluroxene and cyclopropane on ventilation: a comparative study in man. Anesthesiology 27:716, 1966

112. Gelb AW, Knill RL: Subanaesthetic halothane: its effect on regulation of ventilation and relevance to the recovery room. Can Anaesth Soc J 25:488, 1978

113. Calverley RK, Smith NT, Jones CW, et al: Ventilatory and cardiovascular effects of enflurane anesthesia during spontaneous ventilation in man. Anesth Analg 57:610, 1978

114. Cromwell TH, Stevens WC, Eger EI, et al: The cardiovascular effects of compound 469 (Forane) during spontaneous ventilation and CO_2 challenge in man. Anesthesiology 35:17, 1971

115. Wallin RF, Regan BM, Napoli MD, Stern IJ: Sevoflurane: a new inhalational anesthetic agent. Anesth Analg 54:758, 1975

116. Hickey RF, Fourcade HE, Eger EI, et al: The effects of ether, halothane and Forane on apneic thresholds in man. Anesthesiology 35:32, 1971

117. Hirshman CA, McCullough RH, Cohen PJ: Depression of hypoxic ventilatory response by halothane, enflurane and isoflurane in dogs. Br J Anaesth 49:957, 1977

118. Knill RL, Manninen PH, Clement J: Ventilation and chemoreflexes during enflurane sedation and anesthesia in man. Can Anaesth Soc J 26:353, 1979

119. Ciofolo MJ, Clergue F, Devilliers C, et al: Changes in ventilation, oxygen uptake, and carbon dioxide output during recovery from isoflurane anesthesia. Anesthesiology 70:737, 1989

120. Eger EI, Johnson BH: Rates of awakening from anesthesia with I-653, halothane, isoflurane, and sevoflurane: a test of the effect of anesthetic concentration and duration in rats. Anesth Analog 66:977, 1987

121. Dale O, Brown BR, Jr: Clinical pharmacokinetics of the inhalational anesthetics. Clin Pharmacokinet 12:145, 1987

122. Eckenhoff JE, Helrich M: The effect of narcotics,

thiopental, and nitrous oxide on respiratory response to hypercapnea. Anesthesiology 19:240, 1958

123. Yacoub O, Doell D, Kryger MH, et al: Depression of hypoxic ventilatory response by nitrous oxide. Anesthesiology 45:385, 1976

124. Fink BR: Diffusion anoxia. Anesthesiology 16:511, 1955

125. Brodsky JB, McKlveen RE, Zelcer J, Margary JJ: Diffusion hypoxia: a reappraisal using pulse oximetry. J Clin Monit 4:244, 1988

126. Tween TW, Minuck M, Mymin D: Circulation responses to ketamine anesthesia. Anesthesiology 37:613, 1972

127. Vaughan RW, Stephen CR: Abdominal and thoracic surgery in adults with ketamine, nitrous oxide, and d-tubocurarine. Anesth Analg 53:271, 1974

128. Weinreich AI, Silvay G, Lumb PD: Continuous ketamine infusion for one-lung anesthesia. Can Anaesth Soc J 27:485, 1980

129. Corssen G, Gutierrez J, Reves JG, et al: Ketamine in the anesthetic management of asthmatic patients. Anesth Analg 51:588, 1972

130. Coppel DL, Dundee JW: Ketamine anesthesia for cardiac catheterization. Anaesthesia 27:25, 1972

131. Savege TM, Blogg CE, Foley EI, et al: The cardiorespiratory effects of althesin and ketamine. Anaesthesia 28:391, 1973

132. McCarthy G, Coppel DL, Gibbons JF, Cosgrove J: High-frequency jet ventilation for bilateral bullectomy. Anaesthesia 42:411, 1987

133. Rees DI, Howell ML: Ketamine-atracurium by continuous infusion as the sole anesthetic for pulmonary surgery. Anesth Analg 65:860, 1986

134. Brodsky JB, Shulman MS, Mark JBD: Management of postoperative thoracotomy pain: lumbar epidural narcotics. p. 288. In Kettle CF (ed): Current Controversies in Thoracic Surgery. WB Saunders, Philadelphia, 1986

135. Temeck BK, Scafer PW, Park WY, Harmon JW: Epidural anesthesia in patients undergoing thoracic surgery. Arch Surg 124:415, 1989

136. Enquist A, Brandt MR, Fernandes A, Kehlet H: The blocking effect of epidural anesthesia on the adrenocortical and hyperglycaemic response to surgery. Acta Anaesthesiol Scand 21:330, 1977

137. Scheinin B, Scheinin R, Asantila R, et al: Sympathoadrenal and pituitary hormone responses during and immediately after thoracic surgery—modulation by four different pain treatments. Acta Anaesthesiol Scand 31:762, 1987

138. Kehlet H: The modifying effect of general and regional anaesthesia on the endocrine metabolic response to surgery. Reg Anaesth 7:4538, 1982

139. Kehlet H, Brandt MR, Prangehansen H, Albert GMM: Effect of epidural analgesia on metabolic profiles during and after surgery. Br J Surg 66:543, 1979

140. Wattwil M, Sundberg A, Arvill A, Lennquist C: Circulatory changes during high thoracic epidural anesthesia—influence of sympathetic block and of systemic effect of local anaesthetic. Acta Anaesthesiol Scand 29:849, 1985

141. Vik-Mo H, Ottesen S, Renck H: Cardiac effects of thoracic epidural analgesia before and during acute coronary artery occlusion in open-chest dogs. Scand J Clin Lab Invest 38:737, 1978

142. Davis RF, DeBoer LWV, Maroko PR: Thoracic epidural anesthesia reduces myocardial infarct size after coronary artery occlusion in dogs. Anesth Analg 65:711, 1986

143. Blomberg S, Emanuelsson H, Ricksten SE: Thoracic epidural anesthesia and central hemodynamics in patients with unstable angina pectoris. Anesthesiology 69:558, 1989

144. Gross JB, Caldwell CB, Shaw LM, Laucks SO: The effect of lidocaine on the ventilatory response to carbon dioxide. Anesthesiology 59:521, 1983

145. Labaille T, Clergue F, Samii K, et al: Ventilatory response to CO_2 following intravenous and epidural lidocaine. Anesthesiology 63:179, 1985

146. Dohi S, Takeshima R, Naito H: Ventilatory and circulatory responses to carbon dioxide and high levels of sympathectomy induced by epidural blockade in awake humans. Anesth Analg 65:9, 1986

147. Steinbrook RA, Concepcion M, Topulos GP: Ventilatory responses to hypercapnia during bupivacaine spinal anesthesia. Anesth Analg 67:247, 1988

148. Steinbrook RA, Topulos GP, Concepcion M: Ventilatory responses to hypercapnia during tetracaine spinal anesthesia. J Clin Anesth 1:75, 1988

149. Mori J, Fukuda T: Effects of thalamic stimulation on the reticular neuron activities and their modifications by lidocaine and pentobarbital. Jpn J Pharmacol 21:641, 1971

150. Steen P, Michenfelder J: Neurotoxicity of anesthetics. Anesthesiology 50:437, 1979

151. Crawford OB, Ottosen P, Buckingham WW, Bradsher CA: Peridural anesthesia in thoracic surgery: a review of 677 cases. Anesthesiology 12:73, 1951

152. Takasaki M, Takahashi T: Respiratory function during cervical and thoracic extradural analgesia in patients with normal lungs. Br J Anaesth 52:1271, 1980

153. Moir DD: Ventilatory function during epidural analgesia. Br J Anaesth 35:3, 1963

154. Sjogren S, Weight B: Respiratory changes during continuous epidural blockade. Acta Anaesthesiol Scand 16:27, 1972

155. Kochi T, Sako S, Nishino T, Mizuguchi T: Effect of high thoracic extradural anaesthesia on ventilatory response to hypercapnia in normal volunteers. Br J Anaesth 62:362, 1989

156. Gross JB, Caldwell CB, Shaw LM, Apfelbaum JL: The effect of lidocaine infusion on the ventilatory response to hypoxia. Anesthesiology 61:662, 1984

157. Stenseth R, Sellevold O, Breivik H: Epidural morphine for postoperative pain: experience with 1085 patients. Acta Anaesthesiol Scand 29:148, 1985

158. Rawal N, Sjostrand U, Dahlstrom B: Postoperative pain relief by epidural morphine. Anesth Analg 60:726, 1981

159. Welch DB, Hrynaszkiewicz A: Postoperative analgesia using epidural methadone. Administration by the lumbar route for thoracic pain relief. Anaesthesia 36:1051, 1981

160. Jacobson L, Phillips PD, Hull CJ, Conacher ID: Extradural versus intramuscular diamorphine. A controlled study of analgesic and adverse effects in the postoperative period. Anaesthesia 38:10, 1983

161. El-Baz NM, Faber LP, Jensik RJ: Continuous epidural infusion of morphine for treatment of pain after thoracic surgery: a new technique. Anesth Analg 63:757, 1984

162. Shulman M, Sandler AN, Bradley JW, et al: Postthoracotomy pain and pulmonary function following epidural and systemic morphine. Anesthesiology 61:569, 1984

163. Horan CT, Beeby DG, Brodsky JB, Oberhelman HA: Segmental effect of lumbar epidural hydromorphone. A case report. Anesthesiology 62:84, 1985

164. Fromme GA, Steidl LJ, Danielson DR: Comparison of lumbar and thoracic epidural morphine for relief of postthoracotomy pain. Anesth Analg 64:454, 1985

165. Hasenbos M, van Egmond J, Gielen M, Crul JF: Postoperative analgesia by epidural versus intramuscular nicomorphine after thoracotomy. Part I. Acta Anaesthesiol Scand 29:572, 1985

166. Larsen VH, Christensen P, Brinklov MM, Axelsen F: Postoperative pain relief and respiratory performance after thoracotomy: a controlled trial comparing the effect of epidural morphine and subcutaneous nicomorphine. Dan Med Bull 33:161, 1986

167. Gray JR, Fromme GA, Nauss LA, et al: Intrathecal morphine for postthoracotomy pain. Anesth Analg 65:873, 1986

168. Asantila R, Rosenber PH, Scheinin B: Comparison of different methods of postoperative analgesia after thoracotomy. Acta Anaesthesiol Scand 30:421, 1986

169. Rosseel PM, van den Broek WG, Boer EC, Prakash O: Epidural sufentanil for intra- and postoperative analgesia in thoracic surgery: a comparative study with intravenous sufentanil. Acta Anaesthesiol Scand 32:193, 1988

170. Shulman MS, Wakerlin G, Yamaguchi L, Brodksy JB: Experience with epidural hydromorphone for postthoracotomy pain relief. Anesth Analg 66:1331, 1987

171. Brodsky JB, Kretzschmar KM, Mark JBD: Caudal epidural morphine for post-thoracotomy pain. Anesth Analg 67:409, 1988

172. Gough JD, Williams AB, Vaughan RS, et al: The control of post-thoracotomy pain. A comparative evaluation of thoracic epidural fentanyl infusions and cryo-analgesia. Anaesthesia 43:780, 1988

173. Cousins MJ, Mather LE: Intrathecal and epidural administration of opioids. Anesthesiology 61:276, 1984

174. Christensen P, Brandt MR, Rem J, Kehlet H: Influence of extradural morphine on the adrenocortical and hyperglycaemic response to surgery. Br J Anaesth 54:23, 1980

175. Cowen MJ, Bullingham RES, Paterson GMC, et al: A controlled comparison of the effects of extradural diamorphine and bupivacaine on plasma glucose and plasma cortisol in postoperative patients. Anesth Analg 61:15, 1982

176. Jorgensen BC, Andersen HB, Engquist A: Influence of epidural morphine on postoperative pain, endocrine-metabolic, and renal responses to surgery. A controlled study. Acta Anaesthesiol Scand 26:63, 1982

177. Bromage PR, Camporesi EM, Durant PAC, Nielsen CH: Rostral spread of epidural morphine. Anesthesiology 56:431, 1982

178. Ahuja BR, Strunin L: Respiratory effects of epidural fentanyl. Changes in end-tidal CO_2 and respiratory rate following single doses and continuous infusions of epidural fentanyl. Anaesthesia 40:949, 1985

179. Sandler AN, Chovaz P, Whiting W: Respiratory depression following epidural morphine: a clinical study. Can Anaesth Soc J 33:542, 1986

180. Renaud B, Brichant JF, Clergue F, et al: Ventilatory effects of continuous epidural infusion of fentanyl. Anesth Analg 67:971, 1988

181. Whiting WC, Sandler AN, Lau LC, et al: Analgesic and respiratory effects of epidural sufentanil in patients following thoracotomy. Anesthesiology 69:36, 1988

182. Molke Jensen F, Jensen NH, Holk IK, Ravborg M: Prolonged and biphasic respiratory depression following epidural buphrenorphine. Anaesthesia 42:470, 1987

183. Rawal N, Wattwil M: Respiratory depression after epidural morphine—an experimental and clinical study. Anesth Analg 63:8, 1984

184. Knill RL, Clement JL, Thompson WR: Epidural morphine causes delayed and prolonged ventilatory depression. Can Anaesth Soc J 28:537, 1981

185. Doblar DB, Muldoon SM, Abbrecht PH, et al: Epidural morphine following epidural local anesthetic: effect of ventilatory and airway occlusion pressure response to CO_2. Anesthesiology 55:423, 1981

186. Attia J, Ecoffey C, Sandouk P, et al: Epidural morphine in children: pharmacokinetics and CO_2 sensitivity. Anesthesiology 65:590, 1986

187. Power SJ, Chakrabarti MK, Whitwam JG: Response to carbon dioxide after oral midazolam and pentobarbitone. Anaesthesia 39:1183, 1984

188. Power SJ, Morgan M, Chakrabarti MK: Carbon dioxide response curves following midazolam and diazepam. Br J Anaesth 55:837, 1983

189. Bell GD, Morden A, Coady T, et al: A comparison of diazepam and midazolam as endoscopy premedication assessing changes in ventilation and oxygen saturation. Br J Clin Pharmacol 26:595, 1988

190. Berggren L, Ericksson I, Mollenholt P, Sunzel M: Changes in respiratory pattern after repeated doses of diazepam and midazolam in healthy subjects. Acta Anaesthesiol Scand 31:667, 1987

191. Berggren L, Ericksson I, Mollenholt P: Changes in breathing pattern and chest wall mechanics after benzodiazepines in combination with meperidine. Acta Anaesthesiol Scand 31:381, 1987

192. Forster A, Morel D, Bachmann M, Gemperle M: Respiratory depressant effects of different doses of midazolam and lack of reversal with naloxone—a double-blind randomized study. Anesth Analg 62:920, 1983

193. Gross JB, Smith L, Smith TC: Time course of ventilatory response to carbon dioxide after intravenous diazepam. Anesthesiology 57:18, 1982

194. Gilmartin JJ, Corris PA, Stone TN, et al: Effects of diazepam and chlormethiazole on ventilatory control in normal subjects. Br J Clin Pharmacol 25:766, 1988

195. Ranlov PJ, Nielsen SP: Effect of zopiclone and diazepam on ventilatory response in normal human subjects. Sleep, Suppl. 1, 10:40, 1987

196. Alexander CM, Gross JB: Sedative doses of midazolam depress hypoxic ventilatory responses in humans. Anesth Analg 67:377, 1988

197. Mora CT, Torjman M, White PF: Effects of diazepam and flumazenil on sedation and hypoxic ventilatory drive. Anesth Analg 68:473, 1989

198. Cormack RS, Milledge JS, Hanning CD: Respiratory effects of amnesia after premedication with morphine or lorazepam. Br J Anaesth 49:351, 1977

199. Denaut M, Yernault JC, De Coster A: Double-blind comparison of the respiratory effects of parenteral lorazepam and diazepam in patients with chronic obstructive lung disease. Curr Med Res Opin 2:611, 1975

200. Paulson BA, Becker LD, Way WL: The effects of intravenous lorazepam alone and with meperidine on ventilation in man. Acta Anaesthesiol Scand 27:400, 1983

201. Adeoshun IO, Healy TEJ, Patrick JM: Ventilatory pattern following diazepam and lorazepam. Anaesthesia 34:450, 1979

202. Utting JH, Pleuvry BJ: Benzoctamine—a study of the respiratory effects of oral doses in human volunteers and interactions with morphine in mice. Br J Anaesth 47:987, 1975

203. Dalen JE, Evans GL, Banas JR, et al: The hemodynamic and respiratory effects of diazepam. Anesthesiology 30:259, 1969

204. Gross JB, Zebrowski ME, Carel WD, et al: Time course of ventilatory depression after thiopental and midazolam in normal subjects and in patients with chronic obstructive pulmonary disease. Anesthesiology 58:540, 1983

205. Soroker D, Barzilay E, Konickzky S, et al: Respiratory function following premedication with droperidol or diazepam. Anesth Analg 57:695, 1978

206. Van den Hoogen RH, Bervoets KJ, Colpaert FC: Respiratory effects of epidural morphine and sufentanil in the absence and presence of chlordiazepoxide. Pain 37:103, 1989

207. Lambertson CJ: Carbon dioxide and respiration in acid-base homeostasis. Anesthesiology 21:642, 1960

208. Forster RE II, DuBois AB, Briscoe WA, Fisher AB (eds): The Lung—Physiologic Basis of Pulmonary Function Tests. 2nd Ed. Year Book Medical Publishers, Chicago, 1986

209. Eger EI II: Isoflurane (Forane)—A Compendium and Reference. 2nd Ed. Anaquest, Madison, WI, 1985

14

ENDOBRONCHIAL INTUBATION

Roger S. Wilson, M.D

Endobronchial (one-lung) intubation has been widely used in the setting of thoracic surgery, in the management of critically ill patients requiring differential lung ventilation, and during specialty procedures such as pulmonary lavage. The primary objective of this technique is to selectively eliminate ventilation to one lung or a portion of a lung and, thus, produce distal parenchymal collapse. This chapter will consider the indications for endobronchial intubation, review the spectrum of available methods, and discuss potential complications.

Although the need for use of one-lung anesthesia during thoracic surgery has been recognized for several decades, relative and absolute indications for its use have changed and techniques have improved.[1-3] These changes have been necessitated by the nature of the lung pathology requiring surgery and the increased complexity of surgical procedures. Through the years, there has been a reduction in the number of patients with pulmonary pathology resulting from infection, requiring surgical drainage or resection, and an increase in the number of operations performed for malignancy. There are several well-recognized indications for the use of one-lung anesthesia (Table 14-1). A specific indication is the need to prevent spillover of secretions or blood from one area of the lung to the other. When patients are in the lateral position, there is potential risk of contamination of the dependent (nonoperative) lung with material from the nondependent (operative) side. Although the advent of antibiotic therapy has dramatically diminished the existence of the "wet" (bronchiectatic) lung and the incidence

of patients requiring surgery, there is still need to operate in the presence of significant regional bronchiectasis. Thus, the need for isolation of an infected lung still exists today. Lung abscess, requiring surgical excision or drainage, always poses a major problem with potential for intraoperative spillage and contamination of the contralateral lung. In addition, the patient with existing hemoptysis requiring pulmonary resection is frequently a candidate for use of an isolation technique. There is increased potential for tube obstruction with the presence of blood when isolation techniques are used. This will be considered in a later section.

A second indication is a need to maintain airway continuity to ensure the ability to provide positive-pressure ventilation. This occurs in the presence of acute or chronic bronchopleural fistula or during operative techniques necessitating interruption of the airway to a lung segment, notably, during lobectomy with sleeve resection.

A third, and perhaps the most common, current indication for the use of this technique is the ability to provide better surgical exposure and operating conditions; the so-called "quiet" lung. Collapse of the operative lung improves surgical exposure and optimizes conditions in a wide variety of pulmonary resections and esophageal procedures. In addition to these major indications during surgery, several nonsurgical applications have been described. Endobronchial intubation has been used to provide selective positive-pressure ventilation during acute respiratory failure.[4] This technique is useful in intensive care unit pa-

TABLE 14-1. Indications for One-Lung Anesthesia

Control of secretions
  Abscess
  Bronchiectasis
  Hemoptysis

Airway control
  Bronchopleural fistula
    Chronic
    Acute
  Sleeve resection

Quiet surgical field/improved exposure

Teaching

tients, especially when large chronic bronchopleural fistula or acute pulmonary disease create major differences in airway resistance and compliance between right and left lungs. In addition, the technique of bronchopulmonary lavage performed for alveolar proteinosis, bronchiectasis, asthma, and other pulmonary diseases requires the use of endobronchial intubation.[5]

ISOLATION TECHNIQUES

Several approaches to isolating a portion of or an entire lung have proved effective (Table 14-2). The choice of technique is dictated by several considerations, including the nature of the operative procedure, pre-existing pulmonary pathology, urgency of the situation, anatomic considerations, and knowledge/experience of the user. The methods and equipment, including advantages and disadvantages of each, are discussed below.

TABLE 14-2. Tube Types for Various Isolation Techniques

Bronchial blockers
  Magill blocker
  Fogarty (venous occlusion) catheter
  Foley catheter
  Univent tube

Single-lumen endobronchial tubes
  Macintosh-Leatherdale (left)
  Gordon-Green (right)

Double-lumen endobronchial tubes
  Carlens (left)
  White (right)
  Robertshaw (left and right)
  Disposable-polyvinylchloride (left and right)

Bronchial Blockers

Intraluminal obstruction of the main bronchi or lobar divisions of the airway can be achieved with several devices, including gauze tampons or specially designed balloon-tipped catheters. Such approaches have been described by several investigators.[6-11] Although such devices are simple and generally inexpensive, several inherent problems have limited their use in favor of other methods.

Crafoord's tampon, described in 1938, consisted of ribbon gauze that was packed into the main or lobar bronchus of the operative lung and visualized with rigid bronchoscopy.[6] Endotracheal intubation was performed with a standard endotracheal tube, with resultant absorption atelectasis distal to the site of airway occlusion. The gauze was eventually removed as part of the surgical specimen. In 1936, Magill described a similar technique using a balloon-tipped bronchial blocker (Fig. 14-1).[7] The Magill blocker, a long, double-lumen rubber catheter, provided a methodologic improvement. One lumen is used to inflate a cuff on the distal end of the catheter; the second, to accommodate a stylet during placement and to allow suctioning and degassing of the lung distal to the catheter tip. A bronchoscope, passed with the aid of local or general anesthesia, is used to identify the bronchial segment to be blocked. The blocker is passed into position through the bronchoscope and the balloon is inflated to a volume sufficient to hold the catheter firmly in place. The stylet is removed and a standard-cuffed endotracheal tube placed, with the cuff inflated to provide additional stability for the blocker. The position and function of the blocker can be confirmed by chest auscultation if a sufficient portion of the lung is nonventilated. Prior to surgical division of the bronchus, the cuff is deflated and the blocker removed from the airway. Refinements of this technique included a larger lumen for suctioning and the addition of a woven net on the cuff to provide a firmer grip in the airway and prevent overdistention of the cuff.[8] Stephen further modified the Magill blocker with a short cuff for use in blocking the right and left upper lobe bronchi.[9]

There are several reasons why these techniques are now seldom used in the practice of thoracic anesthesia. Positioning of the obstructing device in the desired portion of the airway requires use of the rigid bronchoscope. Thus, an additional procedure with its attendant risks and complications has to be performed. Once the blocker is placed and endotracheal intubation done, it is difficult to reconfirm the existence of the original position. Slippage of the blocker with a change in position of the patient, coughing, or

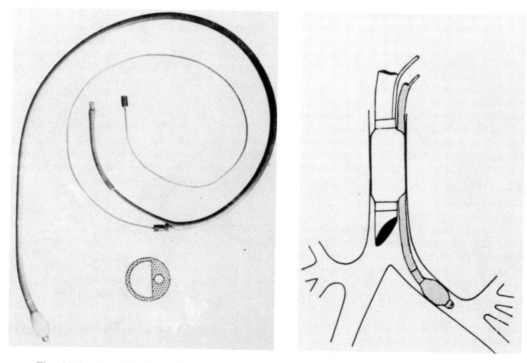

Fig. 14-1. Magill balloon-tipped bronchial blocker. (From Mushin,[38] with permission.)

surgical manipulation is common; when the blocker inadvertently slips into the trachea, it can be associated with life-threatening obstruction. Inability to effectively suction the airway distal to the blocker is an additional disadvantage.

A simplified version of the bronchial blocker technique has been described.[10,11] This approach uses a standard single-lumen endotracheal tube, a fiberoptic bronchoscope, and a vascular catheter to occlude the airway. The most commonly used device is a venous-occlusion Fogarty catheter with a 10 mL balloon. This technique is useful in a number of clinical settings, such as massive hemoptysis with the potential for occlusion of double-lumen tubes due to their small cross-sectional internal diameter and in patients in whom altered anatomy of the upper airway, secondary to natural anatomic variation or disease, makes intubation with a double-lumen tube impossible. In addition, this technique can be used in patients in whom previous surgery has altered the geometry of the distal airway such that standard double-lumen tubes do not conform to the anatomy. Although placement of the Fogarty catheter was originally described through the suction port of the fiberoptic bronchoscope, a more contemporary approach is to place the catheter either through the vocal cords external to the single-lumen endotracheal tube or through the endotracheal tube itself. Choice of approach is dictated by the timing of intubation relative to the placement of the catheter, anatomic considerations, and experience of the anesthesiologist. The standard approach when using this technique is to place the fiberoptic bronchoscope through the endotracheal tube, visualizing the airway distal to the tip of the tube. The Fogarty catheter is then advanced into the airway until the tip comes into view. The catheter is then manipulated under direct vision using the fiberoptic scope so that it is positioned into the section of the airway to be occluded. Once in position, the balloon is inflated with a sufficient volume of air to provide isolation. Chest auscultation is generally used to confirm adequacy of airway obstruction. The bronchoscope is then withdrawn and the endotracheal tube and catheter are secured in appropriate fashion. In the author's experience, the catheter appears to be more stable when it is passed external to the endotracheal tube and affixed separately from the tube. The alternative is to thread the catheter through the lumen of the endotracheal tube, using a device such as a disposable bronchoscopy adapter, with placement of the catheter through the membrane on the adapter. It is useful to keep the fiberoptic bronchoscope readily available in the operating room since repositioning of the Fogarty catheter following alteration in patient position, surgical manipulation, or movement with ventilation may be required. This technique, as previously described, is useful during thoracotomy and also as an emergency life-saving maneuver in the critical care setting when acute bronchopleural fistula and/or hemoptysis exists. Disadvantages of the technique are similar to those described for other blockers.

A more recent innovation is the availability of a combined endotracheal tube/bronchial blocker (Univent tube).[12–14] As shown in Figure 14-2, the device consists of a silastic single-lumen endotracheal tube with a smaller internal lumen used to incorporate a small semirigid catheter with a balloon tip. Prior to intubation, the bronchial cuff on the catheter is deflated and the catheter tip is retracted into the body of the endotracheal tube. Intubation is accomplished with direct laryngoscopy, with confirmation of tube position in the trachea using standard visual, auscultatory, and capnographic methods. Placement of the bronchial blocker into the desired airway can be accomplished in either blind fashion or with use of fiberoptic bronchoscopy. For insertion with a blind technique, it is suggested that the endotracheal tube be rotated 90 degrees toward the side to be occluded and the bronchial blocker advanced an adequate distance to facilitate entrance into the desired bronchus. The distal balloon is inflated through the side arm on the blocker. Adequacy of the blocker position is then confirmed with visual inspection of chest wall motion and auscultation of breath sounds. The fiberoptic bronchoscope can be used as previously described for the Fogarty catheter technique. With this method, the catheter is advanced into the appropriate bronchus under direct vision and the balloon inflated as previously described. Advantages of this particular approach include the benefit of a large single-lumen endotracheal tube, again of potential importance when significant quantities of blood exist within the airway, and the versatility with respect to the ability to isolate various portions of the respiratory system during the same procedure. This is a particular benefit in procedures such as a median sternotomy, in which bilateral, multiple wedge resections are being performed for metastatic disease. Another potential use for this approach is during lung isolation for esophageal surgery. In this particular setting, especially when postoperative intubation and ventilation are deemed necessary, a single endotracheal tube may suffice rather than the use of multiple intubations. The ultimate utility of this device remains to be defined.

Single-Lumen Endobronchial Tubes

Although single-lumen tubes are still theoretically useful, they are described briefly due to historic significance.

Endobronchial anesthesia, pioneered with the design of an endobronchial tube by Gale and Waters in 1932, was intended to offer improved protection during thoracotomy by isolation of the diseased or opera-

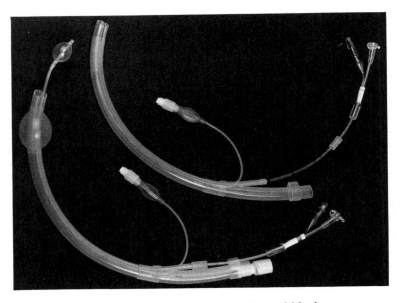

Fig. 14-2. Univent endotracheal tube and blocker.

tive lung from the contralateral lung. Numerous tubes have subsequently been designed and later improved in an attempt to make endobronchial anesthesia simpler and more efficient. In a survey conducted in the United Kingdom, only a very small percentage of the anesthesiologists questioned used single-lumen endobronchial techniques for one-lung anesthesia.[15]

In 1936, Magill introduced both a right and left endobronchial tube equipped with a single endobronchial (no tracheal) cuff.[7] This tube was later modified by Machray using a left-sided tube similar to the Magill, but with a shorter bronchial cuff. Endobronchial tubes of this design required placement using an intubating bronchoscope of the Magill or modified Magill type. Intraoperative slippage from its original position, particularly with right-sided types, posed a significant risk when these tubes were used, and, hence, when combined with the need for rigid bronchoscopy for intubation, this technique has fallen into disuse.

Two existing single-lumen tubes of improved design are the Macintosh-Leatherdale (left-sided) and the Gordon-Green (right-sided), shown in Figures 14-3 and 14-4.[16] The Macintosh-Leatherdale endobronchial tube, described in 1955, was designed to be used when operative procedures were performed on the right

lung.[8] The advantages of this tube are that it can be passed "blindly" (without need for bronchoscopy), its shape conforms to that of the trachea and left mainstem bronchus and, therefore, is not easily dislodged, and the double-cuff system allows bilateral lung ventilation. The tube is equipped with both endobronchial and tracheal cuffs; a small pilot tube opens distally between the cuffs, near the level of the carina, and enables suctioning of the right lung or provides a means for delivery of low-flow oxygen to the right lung.

Tube insertion requires direct laryngoscopy. Tubes are available in sizes 7.5, 8.0, 9.0, and 9.5 mm internal diameter (ID). Once the tip of the tube is passed through the cords, the laryngoscope is removed and the tube is advanced until the angle impinges on the carina, with the distal tip situated in the left mainstem bronchus just proximal to the left upper lobe bronchus. The endobronchial cuff is inflated and the position confirmed by the presence of breath sounds throughout the left chest and their absence on the right. The tracheal cuff is inflated to secure the tube in place. If ventilation to the right lung is desired, the endobronchial cuff is deflated and air entry into the right side (often limited) is confirmed by auscultation.

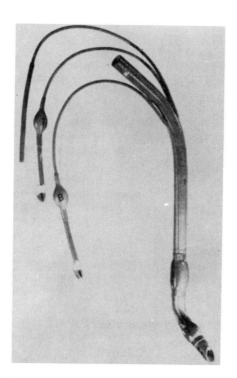
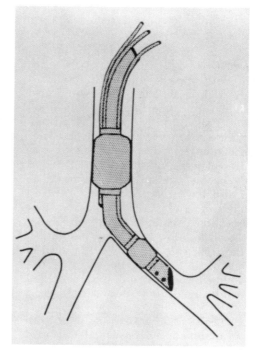

Fig. 14-3. The Macintosh-Leatherdale left-sided single-lumen endobronchial tube. (From Mushin,[38] with permission.)

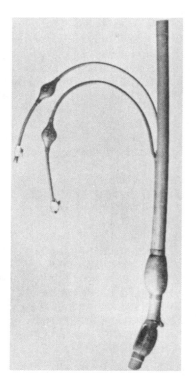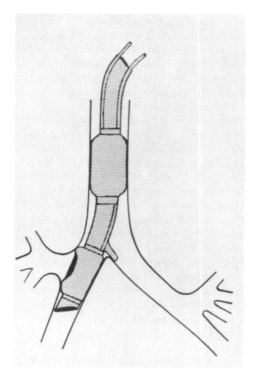

Fig. 14-4. The Gordon-Green right-sided single-lumen endobronchial tube. (From Mushin,[38] with permission.)

Right lung ventilation, if not present or if limited, may be improved by slowly withdrawing the tube, which not infrequently impacts into the left bronchus, resulting in an airtight seal. The tube is withdrawn until right-sided air entry is satisfactory. Reinflation of the bronchial cuff should still permit left lung ventilation without air entry into the right side. Inadvertent intubation of the right bronchus is easily corrected by withdrawal of the tube into the trachea and attempted readvancement. A specially designed "reinforced rubber director" or stylet is available to aid in the redirection from right to left bronchus. Once the surgical dissection is completed, the endobronchial cuff is deflated to allow right lung ventilation. Suctioning of the right side requires withdrawal of the tube until the distal tip is positioned in the trachea; the suction line incorporated in the side wall of the tube is generally inadequate due to its limited diameter.

Macintosh and Leatherdale are also credited with the design of a combined endobronchial tube and bronchial blocker (Fig. 14-5) used for left thoracic surgery.[8] Available in four sizes (7.5, 8.0, 9.0, and 9.5 mm ID), this tube is introduced in the same manner as the single-lumen tube previously described. The angula-

ted distal tip, which is a cuffed blocker with a central suction channel, enters the left bronchus. When in proper position, with bronchial and tracheal cuffs inflated, right lung ventilation is achieved through the air channel opening into the trachea just proximal to the carina. The blocker, which is hollow, can be used to supply oxygen or to suction the left lung.

Although right endobronchial intubation (for left thoracotomy) is technically easier than left due to angulation of the bronchi, positioning of the right tubes is more difficult than the left due to the close proximity of the right upper lobe bronchus to the carina. It is, therefore, not generally possible to use a standard cuff on the bronchial limb without producing obstruction to the right upper lobe. Green and Gordon developed a right endobronchial tube with a 20 × 5 mm slot in the lateral wall for the right upper lobe.[16] As shown in Figure 14-4, this tube is designed with both bronchial and tracheal cuffs and, in addition, has a carinal hook to stabilize it once it is in position. This tube, available in 8.0 and 9.0 mm ID sizes, is introduced by direct laryngoscopy. The tube is advanced until the hook impinges on the carina. The tracheal cuff is inflated to produce an airtight seal and to stabilize the tube. The bronchial cuff is inflated next until sounds

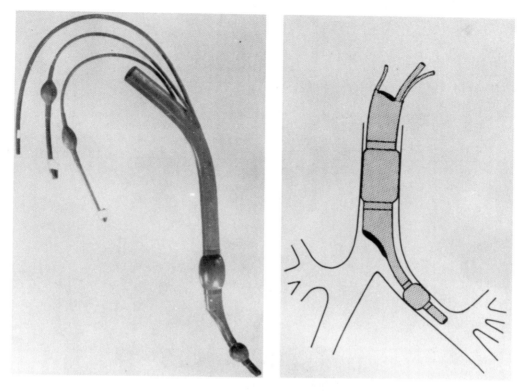

Fig. 14-5. The Macintosh-Leatherdale combined endobronchial tube and bronchial blocker used for left-sided thoracic surgery. (From Mushin,[38] with permission.)

are no longer present on the left. Inadvertent left endobronchial intubation is rarely encountered because of the angulation of the distal tip of the tube.

Double-Lumen Endobronchial Tubes

The third and most popular technique involves use of double-lumen tubes, available in several designs.[15] There are several advantages of this method when compared with those previously discussed. The ability to selectively ventilate and suction either lung and the stability of the tube, once positioned, are notable features. The large cross-sectional diameter of these tubes often makes intubation and positioning more difficult, a minor disadvantage of the technique. As listed in Table 14-2, four types of double-lumen tubes are currently available, designed for right or left lung surgery. Included are the Carlens (left-sided intubation, right thoracotomy), White (right-sided), Bryce-Smith (right- and left-sided), Robertshaw (right- and left-sided), and a variety of disposable polyvinylchloride (PVC) types.[17-20] The general design of all such tubes is similar, with a few notable differences (Table 14-3). One lumen is long enough and appropriately

angulated to reach into one mainstem bronchus (usually the nonoperative dependent lung); the second shorter lumen is designed to terminate in the distal trachea. Separation of gas flow and isolation of foreign material from the nonoperative (dependent) lung are achieved with use of an inflatable cuff on the endobronchial limb. An airtight seal for the operative (nondependent) lung, ventilated through the tracheal lumen, is achieved with inflation of a tracheal cuff. This cuff is located in a position proximal to the endobronchial opening. Tubes designed for intubation of the right bronchus (for left thoracotomy) must incorporate a slitlike opening in the endobronchial cuff to permit ventilation of the right upper lobe. The proximal end of these tubes must be fitted with a special connector between the tube and the anesthesia system to allow diversion of gas from bilateral to unilateral ventilation, to enable each lumen and lung to be opened to atmospheric or continuous positive airway pressure, and to permit passage of suction catheters and fiberoptic bronchoscopes. Reusable (Cobbs) and disposable connectors are shown in Figure 14-6.

Although there is not unanimous agreement, in general, it is advisable to attempt to intubate the bron-

TABLE 14-3. Endobronchial Tubes

Type	Side	Material	Size	Carinal Spur	Comments
Carlens	Left	Reb rubber	French 35, 37, 39, 41	Yes	Reusable, low compliant cuff
White	Right	Red rubber	French 37, 39, 41	Yes	Similar to above; (?) difficult to position
Robertshaw	Left and right	Red rubber	Small, medium, large	No	Low compliant cuff; large upper lobe eye
Disposable multiple manu-facturers[a]	Left and right	Polyvinyl-chloride	French 28, 35, 37, 39, 41	Yes, on specific types	Expensive; (?) more easily malpositioned; designs of right-sided endotracheal cuffs vary

[a] Rusch, New York, NY; Sheridan, Argyle, NY; Mallinckrodt, Glens Falls, NY; Concord Portex, Keene, NH.

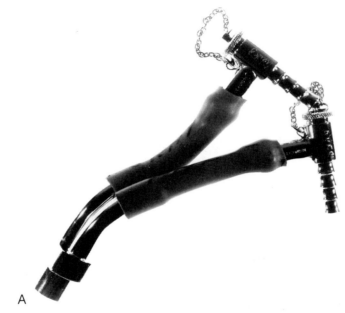

A

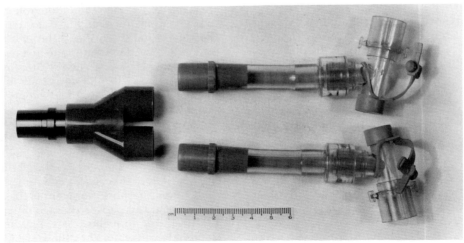

B

Fig. 14-6. (A) Reusable Cobb connector; **(B)** disposable connectors for double-lumen tubes.

chus of the nonoperative or dependent lung. Bronchial intubation of the operative lung, especially in the lateral position when the lung is in the nondependent position, can create situations in which tubes will fail to function correctly. Compression of the mediastinum or surgical manipulation can displace the bronchial limb and interrupt the isolation of the operative lung. Intermittent occlusion of the tracheal lumen against the most dependent lateral tracheal wall can create a ball-valve obstruction to gas flow. The latter situation is most common during expiration, resulting in wheezing, prolonged expiratory flow, and, if severe enough, hypercarbia. The ability to correctly place and position right-sided tubes, discussed below, must be weighed against such potential complications when tube type is selected.

Double-lumen endobronchial tubes, although used for bronchospirometry since 1949, were not used for thoracic surgery until 1951. Carlens[17] and Bjork and Carlens[18] are credited with both improvement of tube design and stimulation of interest in their application during thoracic surgery.

The Carlens tube is still manufactured of molded rubber with a latex covering (Fig. 14-7). The two lumina are D-shaped on cross section, with the endobronchial limb (left) extended as a round tube. The tip is at a 45 degree angle in relation to the shaft of the tube in order to enter the left bronchus. A hook is incorporated to position the tube by impinging it on the carina. Four sizes are available: 35, 37, 39, and 41 French (F). The two smaller sizes generally are adequate for females and adolescents, and the larger two are used for adult males.

The carinal hook, although beneficial for tube placement and stability, is a source of difficulty during intubation. In the past, techniques such as use of slip-knot silk ties to approximate the hook to the tube, or removal of the hook, have been advocated. Intubation is generally performed following induction of general anesthesia and use of muscle relaxants and topical anesthesia to the larynx and trachea. The endobronchial tip is advanced through the vocal cords following direct laryngoscopy. A Macintosh laryngoscope blade generally provides better working conditions than does a straight blade. The tube is rotated 180 degrees to the left to allow the carinal hook to pass through the anterior commissure of the cords. Once the hook has entered the trachea, the tube is rotated 90 degrees back to the right; the endobronchial tip is now positioned to the left and the carinal hook on the right lateral tracheal wall. The tube is slowly and gently advanced until resistance is felt as the hook en-

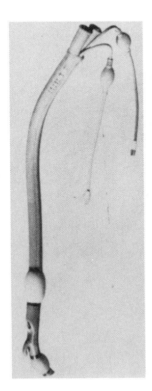
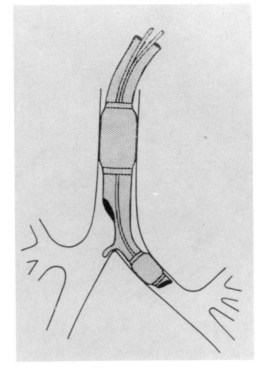

Fig. 14-7. Carlens double-lumen endobronchial tube. (From Mushin,[38] with permission.)

gages the carina. An alternate technique is to rotate the tube 180 degrees to the right to allow the hook to pass the cords and then to rotate it another 90 degrees to the right (clockwise) to position the tube at the carina (Fig. 14-8). Cuff inflation techniques, although not described by Carlens, should follow a logical sequence. Inflation of the lungs with one or two positive-pressure breaths is necessary to confirm (with visual inspection of chest motion) an endotracheal position. Gas flow to the tracheal lumen is occluded and the bronchial cuff inflated until left lung inflation (with manual compression of the bag) is achieved in the absence of right-sided ventilation; the latter is confirmed by visual inspection and chest auscultation. Release of the clamp on the tracheal lumen limb should permit bilateral lung ventilation. The endobronchial limb is occluded and, with positive pressure being applied, the tracheal cuff is inflated until an airtight seal is obtained. Bilateral lung ventilation is generally maintained until the pleura is opened and exposure within the thorax is required.

White has modified the Carlens tube for use in the right bronchus (Fig. 14-9).[19] This tube is also designed for blind endobronchial intubation. Made of rubber, it is molded to the shape conforming to the right mainstem bronchus, with the tip at a 30 degree angle from the tracheal portion of the tube. As in the Carlens tube, the lumina are D-shaped at the tracheal portion, with the left lumen terminating just above the carina. A small rubber hook is designed to engage the carina.

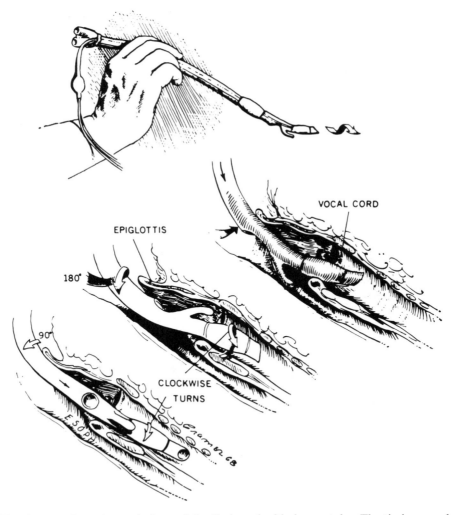

Fig. 14-8. The alternate insertion technique of the Carlens double-lumen tube. The tip is passed through the vocal cords and then rotated 180 degrees to the right. When the hook passes through the larynx, the tube is rotated an additional 90 degrees to the right for placement on the carina. (From El-Etr,[39] with permission.)

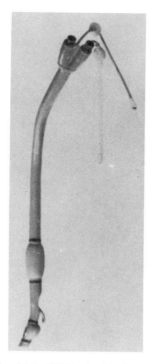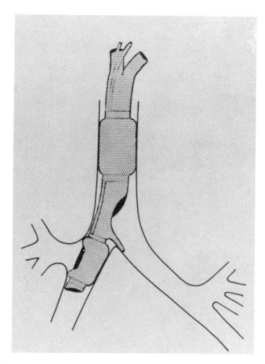

Fig. 14-9. White double-lumen endobronchial tube. (From Mushin,[38] with permission.)

The bronchial cuff is designed with a lateral slit opening to the right upper lobe bronchus. Three sizes are available: 37, 39, and 41 F.

Intubation is accomplished by a technique similar to that described for the Carlens tube, differing only in tube manipulation. The endobronchial portion of the tube is advanced through the cords; the tube is rotated 180 degrees to position the carinal hook so it will pass through the anterior commissure. Once the hook is within the trachea, the tube is rotated 90 degrees to the left (counterclockwise). The endobronchial tip should now point toward the right and the carinal hook toward the left. The tube is advanced until the hook engages the carina. The cuff inflation sequence is similar to that previously described, with bronchial cuff inflation first. Auscultation confirms tube position, but cannot guarantee ideal position for right upper lobe ventilation.

In 1962, Robertshaw described a double-lumen endobronchial tube especially designed for thoracic surgery.[20] This tube is designed in both left- and right-sided versions (Fig. 14-10), and in three sizes suitable for adults and adolescents.[21] These tubes provide independent control of each lung through a double-lumen system with a larger internal cross-sectional diameter that is ovoid in shape. They are equipped with inflatable cuffs on the distal endobronchial portion

and the tracheal portion. Inflating tubes for these cuffs are positioned in an anterioposterior configuration to minimize the external cross-sectional diameter of the tubes. The advantages of this design over previous designs is that it offers a larger internal cross-sectional diameter and, hence, lower resistance to gas flow at equivalent external diameters.

The left-sided tube is designed to enter the left mainstem bronchus with the distal tip at an angle of 45 degrees. The right lumen terminates in the trachea just above the carina. When the left bronchial and tracheal cuffs are inflated, the right lumen communicates only with the right mainstem bronchus.

The right-sided version of this tube has a tip that is angled at 20 degrees to enter the right mainstem bronchus. This tube follows principles described in the design incorporated by Green and Gordon.[16] A slotted endobronchial cuff, designed to open wider with cuff inflation, allows for ventilation of the right upper lobe. The cuff is designed so that it inflates above the upper edge of the slot to seal it from the trachea and the left mainstem bronchus. The tube is inserted into the larynx under direct vision by the laryngoscope techniques already described. The absence of a carinal hook makes manipulation during intubation less cumbersome than that experienced with tubes equipped with a hook. Once the double-lumen portion

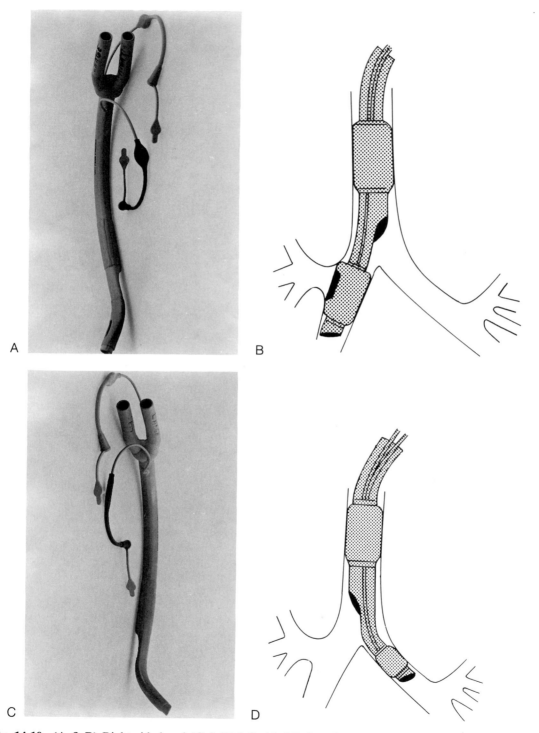

Fig. 14-10. **(A & B)** Right-sided and **(C & D)** left-sided Robertshaw double-lumen endobronchial tubes.

of the tube has passed the cords and reaches the larynx, it is advisable to withdraw the laryngoscope blade, support the jaw with the left hand, and, with the right hand, slowly advance the tube with the endobronchial portion directed toward the bronchus to be intubated. The appropriate position is confirmed by a firm but secure sense of impingement within the bronchus and location of the bite-block positioned between the incisors. In general, intubation with the left-sided tube, with the bronchial tip angled at 45 degrees, is aided with the use of a stylet carefully placed within the left lumen. The right-sided tube, on the other hand, with an endobronchial portion directed at a 30 degree angle off-center, is easily passed without the use of a stylet. Once the tube is in appropriate position, the sequence for cuff inflation should be undertaken as described by Robertshaw.[20] One or two positive-pressure breaths are required to confirm endotracheal position and adequate expansion of both lungs, generally observed with visual inspection. The tracheal lumen is clamped to eliminate fresh gas flow, and the bronchial cuff is slowly inflated (with a syringe containing a maximum of 5 mL of air) until no discernible air leak is detected coming from the open port on the tracheal lumen. Visual inspection of the endobronchial side should confirm adequacy of ventilation, and proper ventilation may be reconfirmed with chest auscultation. Bilateral lung ventilation with the clamp removed ensures that overinflation of the bronchial cuff and herniation occluding the nonintubated bronchus have not occurred. Once bilateral lung ventilation is confirmed, the endobronchial limb is clamped and the tracheal cuff inflated until air is no longer detected leaking around the tracheal cuff and exiting through the oropharynx. Bilateral lung ventilation is again reconfirmed.

Selection of appropriate tube size is facilitated by the careful design and limited number of options available. This tube is manufactured in three sizes, small, medium, and large, with both large and medium sizes being used for adults and the small size generally reserved for adolescents. As described by Zeitlin et al, the majority of male patients will accept the large size, while most female patients will require the medium size.[21] Simpson has even shown that, when needed, a standard Robertshaw tube can be passed successfully via a tracheostomy stoma.[22]

The advantages of the Robertshaw over other double-lumen tubes relate to the design characteristics of a large lumen, which facilitates the ease of passage of suction catheters and offers minimum resistance to gas flow. Occasionally, the tube may not be readily passed through the glottis due to the bulk of the double-lumen portion, even though the endobronchial portion is of appropriate size. Under such circumstances, it is advisable to select either a single-lumen endobronchial tube, a bronchial blocker, or an ordinary endotracheal tube, depending on the type of surgical operation and the indications for lung isolation.

Double-lumen endobronchial tubes (right-sided) have also been designed by Bryce-Smith and Salt.[23,24] Their design features are similar to those of the right- and left-sided Robertshaw tubes, but, in general, these tubes are infrequently used.

A variety of disposable double-lumen tubes are currently available from several tube manufacturers. Current practice appears to favor use of the disposable tubes rather than the previously described nondisposable red rubber variety. As described in Table 14-3, these tubes are available in both right- and left-sided versions and in a variety of sizes. They are manufactured of clear PVC, with thin-walled tracheal and endobronchial cuffs (Fig. 14-11). Radiopaque markers are provided at the bottom of the tracheal cuff and at the distal end of the tube just below the bronchial cuff. Most are supplied with appropriate connectors to facilitate connection to the anesthesia circuit, and are equipped with an appropriate stylet within the endobronchial lumen. Distinct lettering and color coding identify pilot balloon and endobronchial/tracheal lumina to reduce confusion during utilization. Due to the low-pressure characteristics of the cuff when compared with the higher pressure cuffs found in the nondisposable types, these tubes are well-suited for use during prolonged intubation in the intensive care unit setting.

Selection of a given technique and type of tube is governed by a variety of factors. Cost, availability, preference for single-use disposable tubes, and experience of the user are obvious and important issues. Advantages of the double-lumen endobronchial tube when compared with other techniques include the following: (1) wide lumina to allow passage of adequate suction catheters; (2) wide lumina to provide low resistance to gas flow; and (3) stability and versatility once placed. Obvious anatomic differences in the conducting airway on the right when compared with the left mainstem bronchus create potential problems in selection of right- versus left-sided endobronchial tubes. Design of the distal end of the left endobronchial tube offers little problem due to the length of bronchus between the carina and take-off of the left mainstem bronchus.[25] Right-sided tubes need to incorporate specially designed endobronchial cuffs to facilitate ventilation of the right upper lobe. As shown in Figure 14-12, a wide variety of designs have been incorporated into right-sided endotracheal tubes to facilitate adequacy of ventilation when the right

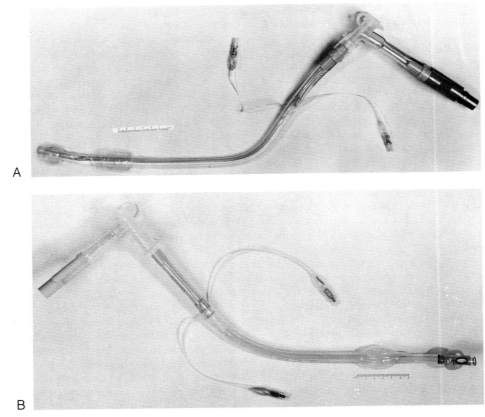

Fig. 14-11. (A & B) The Bronchocath double-lumen disposable endobronchial tube with attached Cobb adapter.

mainstem bronchus is intubated. This issue is considered in detail in a latter portion of this chapter. In general, development of adequate cuff designs for PVC tubes has evolved slowly during the past several years and, to a greater extent, has limited use of right-sided PVC tubes when compared with the left-sided versions.

Complications of Use

Complications of isolation techniques include trauma, malposition, and hypoxemia. Direct laryngeal trauma (including soft tissue injury), arytenoid dislocation, and similar injuries are potentially more prone to develop, due to the increased bulk of the double-lumen tubes, than when endotracheal tubes are used. No true incidence of such injury has been reported to date. Tracheobronchial rupture has been reported as a rare complication following intubation with all types of double-lumen tubes.[26–30] The site of laceration is usually the membranous wall of the distal trachea or the mainstem bronchus, generally a few

centimeters from the carina. Factors leading to such complications could include use of an inappropriately small tube, requiring overinflation of the bronchial cuff, malposition of the tip of the tube, or too-rapid inflation of the distal cuff. Intraoperative detection of such injury usually coincides with development of a large air leak during positive-pressure ventilation, visualization of air within mediastinal tissues, and direct visualization of the endobronchial tube tip in the surgical field. Surgical repair of the tracheal laceration is essential and should, as supported by the sparse data available, produce a favorable outcome.

Malpositioning of the tube in the airway with impaired gas exchange is a common problem with all types of endobronchial tubes.[31,32] Abnormalities of ventilation include (1) the inability to isolate one lung so that both lungs are ventilated in spite of clamping; (2) conditions in which neither lung is ventilated or "ball-valving" occurs, with or without air leakage around the bronchial cuff; and (3) inability to deflate the nonintubated lung. A variety of factors are responsible for inadequacy of endobronchial tube position.

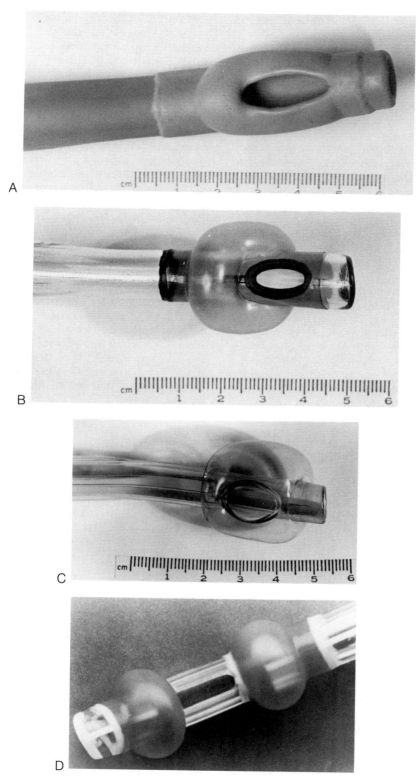

Fig. 14-12. (A–D) Various right-sided double-lumen tube cuff designs.

As discussed by Benumof et al, the margin of safety in positioning double-lumen endotracheal tubes is a function of several variables.[25] Included are the differences in anatomy of the left and right mainstem bronchi, individual variation in bronchial diameter and length from subject to subject, and tube design. These issues give rise to questions such as: (1) Should right-sided endobronchial tubes be avoided in preference to left-sided tubes? (2) Is there an ideal double-lumen endobronchial tube available? and (3) How should tube position be confirmed once it is placed? Several compelling arguments can be made in favor of selecting a right-sided endobronchial tube when left thoracotomy is performed. Dislodgment of the endobronchial portion of the tube when it rests within the surgical (nondependent) lung occurs, albeit with unknown frequency. There is also potential for less than adequate ventilation to the dependent lung through the tracheal port secondary to secretion and soft tissue obstruction. This produces potential for a ball-valving effect, with limitation during expiration resulting in overinflation of the lung. Although the author has experienced this, there is no reported incidence to cite. Another argument is to avoid intubation of the operative bronchus when there is the potential for a pneumonectomy requiring withdrawal of the double-lumen tube into a more proximal position. The latter maneuver is potentially fraught with hazards secondary to mechanical problems with tube manipulation in the lateral position. A final argument for continued use of right-sided tubes is improvement in design and function of these tubes, a heightened awareness for potential problems, and an alternative (namely, fiberoptic bronchoscopy) to determine position. In answer to the second question, it is unlikely, given the multitude of variables, that any single tube design will incorporate features such that it will be ideal in all circumstances. Again, appreciation for potential problems and awareness of the solutions make this question somewhat moot. The third, and perhaps most debatable, issue is whether fiberoptic bronchoscopy needs to be carried out under all circumstances of double-lumen tube use or only on a selective basis.[33,34]

A number of predictable circumstances should lead to inevitable malpositioning of endobronchial tubes. A most common cause for malposition appears to be the selection of a tube that is inappropriately small and, thus, too short, such that it fails to advance far enough into the bronchus. Several factors could lead to inappropriate selection of a small tube, including the inability to pass the desired size because of limitations in diameter of the upper airway, either at the laryngeal aperture or at the level of the cricoid. In addition, the inability to advance the distal tip of the appropriate-sized tube into the bronchus, due to bronchial narrowing, extrinsic compression, or endobronchial pathology, may lead to intubation with a tube of smaller size. The result is that the endobronchial tip does not advance far enough into the bronchus. Thus, when the bronchial cuff inflates, it does so at or above the level of the carina, producing partial obstruction to the nonintubated bronchus. This creates a situation in which it is possible to ventilate both lungs through the endobronchial portion and impossible to ventilate with the tracheal lumen. A bronchial cuff, inflated at the carina with herniation to the nonintubated bronchus, often produces gas trapping and inability to deflate the nonintubated or operative lung. Abnormalities arising from such malpositioning may be detected if a carefully designed program for cuff inflation, visual inspection of chest movement, and chest auscultation is carried out. As described above, once the tube is in position, bilateral ventilation is usually possible without inflation of either cuff. Slow inflation of the endobronchial cuff with the tracheal limb clamped should confirm appropriate tube position in the desired bronchus. The ability to inflate both lungs when the tracheal limb is unclamped and positive pressure delivered should be confirmed with auscultation and visual inspection of both lung fields. If, during this maneuver, either poor or no breath sounds are heard over the nonintubated lung, malposition of the cuff at or near the level of the carina should be suspected. Under such circumstances, the endobronchial cuff is deflated and the tube either advanced or withdrawn. Repositioning is then attempted and the sequence of cuff inflation is repeated. Inadvertent intubation of the opposite bronchus is detected during the second maneuver, when the endobronchial cuff is inflated. Under such circumstances, the tube is withdrawn and rotated slightly in the desired direction to obtain appropriate endobronchial intubation. Causes for intubating the opposite or wrong bronchus are generally associated with the continued use of the laryngoscope during the process of tube insertion, or with an attempt by the intubator to twist or turn the tube in an overzealous manner as it is advanced down the airway. Occasionally, anatomic abnormalities within the trachea or mainstem bronchus may deviate the tube into the inappropriate lung.

Another predictable complication relating to malpositioning may be the advancement of the tube too far down into the tracheobronchial tree. When right endobronchial tubes are used, this may produce abnormal positioning of the cuff at the takeoff of the right upper lobe bronchus, resulting in insufficient ventilation and atelectasis of the lobe. With left-sided tubes, it is more difficult, due to the length of the left mainstem bronchus, to produce left upper lobe collapse.

Fiberoptic bronchoscopy is a useful adjunct to visual inspection and chest auscultation to determine the position of double-lumen tubes.[35] Smith et al have described the use of fiberoptic bronchoscopy to confirm the position of double-lumen endobronchial tubes in 23 patients undergoing thoracotomy.[36] Double-lumen tubes were placed with the conventional technique and the position was ascertained with chest expansion and auscultation. Subsequent fiberoptic bronchoscopy revealed a 48 percent (11 of 23 patients) incidence of less than satisfactory position. In four instances (17 percent), there was herniation of the bronchial cuff over the carina; in six patients (26 percent), the bronchial cuff could not be visualized with the fiberoptic scope introduced in the tracheal port and, hence, the tube was assumed to be in a too distal position. In all cases, a PVC disposable-type tube was used: one right endobronchial tube and 22 left-sided tubes. In an additional study, McKenna et al used fiberoptic bronchoscopy to compare adequacies of position with right-sided red rubber Robertshaw and PVC tubes.[37] In this study, patients were randomized into two groups, one receiving the Robertshaw and the second receiving the PVC type. Tubes were placed under controlled conditions prior to surgery, and the position was confirmed with visual inspection and auscultation. Subsequent fiberoptic bronchoscopy through tracheal and endobronchial ports confirmed adequacy of tube position. In a group of 20 patients intubated with the right-sided Robertshaw tube, adequacy of position was confirmed in 90 percent (18 of 20 cases) using conventional visual and auscultatory techniques. In comparison, 89 percent (eight of nine patients) intubated with the PVC tube were inadequately positioned when assessed with the fiberoptic technique. The study was terminated at nine patients due to the high incidence of malposition. It is likely, due to the variables previously cited, that PVC tubes, when compared with the older Robertshaw type of tube or with those equipped with a carinal spur, are more easily and more likely to be malpositioned. Although routine bronchoscopic evaluation of tube position is one alternative, it must be considered to be time consuming, requires special equipment and operator experience, and potentially introduces an additional source of airway trauma. Existing data support the fact that when nondisposable tubes are utilized, use of fiberoptic confirmation is unnecessary in the absence of specific airway-related problems, while use of visual confirmation is highly desirable when right-sided endobronchial tubes of current design are utilized. Although left PVC endobronchial tubes do carry an appreciable incidence of malposition, the greater margin of error afforded by left-sided bronchial anatomy makes fiberoptic positioning more elective than mandatory.

The most common abnormality associated with the use of endobronchial intubation is undoubtedly hypoxemia. This subject is considered in detail in Chapter 8, which discusses the physiology of one-lung anesthesia.

REFERENCES

1. Bjork VO, Carlens E, Frieberg O: Endobronchial anesthesia. J Thorac Cardiovasc Surg 14:60–72, 1953
2. Newman RW, Finer GE, Downs JE: Routine use of the Carlens' double-lumen endobronchial catheter. J Thorac Cardiovasc Surg 42:327–333, 1961
3. Edwards EM, Hatch DJ: Experiences with double-lumen tubes. Anesthesia 20:461–467, 1965
4. Carlon GC, Ray C, Jr, Klein R, et al: Criteria for selective positive end-expiratory pressure and independent synchronized ventilation of each lung. Chest 74:501–507, 1978
5. Rogers RM, Tantum KR: Bronchopulmonary lavage, a "new" approach to old problems. Med Clin North Am 54:755–771, 1970
6. Crafoord C: On technique of pneumonectomy in man. Acta Chir Scand 81:1–142, 1938
7. Magill IW: Anesthetics in thoracic surgery with special reference to lobectomy. Proc Soc Med 29:643–653, 1936
8. Macintosh R, Leatherdale RAL: Bronchus tube and bronchus blocker. Br J Anaesth 27:556–557, 1955
9. Stephen EDS: Problems of "blocking" in upper lobectomies. Curr Res Anesth 31:175, 1952
10. Gottlieb LS, Hillberg R: Endobronchial tamponade therapy for intractable hemoptysis. Chest 67:482–483, 1975
11. Gourin A, Garzon AA: Control of hemorrhage in emergency pulmonary resection for massive hemoptysis. Chest 68:120–121, 1975
12. Inoue H, Shohtsu A, Ogawa J, et al: Endotracheal tube with movable blocker to prevent aspiration of intratracheal bleeding. Ann Thorac Surg 37:497–499, 1984
13. Kamaya H, Krishna PR: New endotracheal tube (Univent tube) for selective blockade of one lung. Anesthesiology 63:342–343, 1985
14. Herenstein R, Russo JR, Moonka N, Capan LV: Management of one-lung anesthesia in an anticoagulated patient. Anesth Analg 67:1120–1122, 1988
15. Pappin JC: The current practice of endobronchial intubation. Anesthesia 34:57–64, 1979
16. Green R, Gordon W: Right-lung anesthesia. Anesthesia for left lung surgery using a new right endobronchial tube. Anesthesia 12:86–87, 1957
17. Carlens E: A new flexible double-lumen catheter for broncho-spirometry. J Thorac Cardiovasc Surg 18:742–746, 1949
18. Bjork VO, Carlens E: The prevention of spread during pulmonary resection by the use of a double-lumen catheter. J Thorac Cardiovasc Surg 20:151–157, 1951

19. White GMJ: A new double-lumen tube. Br J Anaesth 32:232–234, 1960

20. Robertshaw FL: Low-resistance double-lumen endobronchial tubes. Br J Anaesth 34:576–579, 1962

21. Zeitlin GL, Short DH, Rider GH: An assessment of the Robertshaw double-lumen tube. Br J Anaesth 37:858–860, 1965

22. Simpson PM: Tracheal intubation with a Robertshaw tube via a tracheostomy. Br J Anaesth 48:373–374, 1976

23. Bryce-Smith R, Salt R: A right-sided double-lumen tube. Br J Anaesth 32:230–231, 1960

24. Bryce-Smith R: A double-lumen endobronchial tube. Br J Anaesth 31:274–275, 1959

25. Benumof JL, Partridge NL, Salvaiterra C, et al: Margin of safety in positioning modern double-lumen endotracheal tubes. Anesthesiology 67:729–738, 1987

26. Guernelli N, Bragaglia RB, Briccoli A, et al: Tracheobronchial ruptures due to cuffed Carlens tubes. Ann Thorac Surg 28:66–68, 1979

27. Heiser M, Steinberg JJ, Macvaugh H, et al: Bronchial rupture, a complication of use of the Robertshaw double-lumen tube. Anesthesia 51:88, 1979

28. Burton NA, Fall SM, Lyons T, et al: Rupture of the left main-stem bronchus with a polyvinylchloride double-lumen tube. Chest 83:928–929, 1983

29. Wagner DL, Gammage GW, Wong ML: Tracheal rupture following the insertion of a disposable double-lumen endotracheal tube. Anesthesiology 63:698–700, 1985

30. Hannallah M, Gomes M: Bronchial rupture associated with the use of a double-lumen tube in a small adult. Anesthesiology 71:457–459, 1989

31. Black AMS, Harrison GA: Difficulties with positioning Robertshaw double-lumen tubes. Anaesth Intensive Care 3:299–304, 1975

32. Brodsky JB, Shulman MS, Mark JB: Malposition of left-sided double-lumen endobronchial tubes. Anesthesiology 62:667–669, 1985

33. Ehrenwerth J: Pro: Proper positioning of a double-lumen endobronchial tube can only be accomplished with endoscopy. J Cardiothorac Anesth 2:101–104, 1988

34. Brodsky JB: Con: Proper positioning of a double-lumen endobronchial tube can only be accomplished with endoscopy. J Cardiothorac Anesth 2:105–109, 1988

35. Slinger PD: Fiberoptic bronchoscopic positioning of double-lumen tubes. J Cardiothorac Anesth 3:486–496, 1989

36. Smith GB, Hirsch NP, Ehrenwerth J: Placement of double-lumen endobronchial tubes: correlation between clinical impressions and bronchoscopic findings. Br J Anaesth 58:1317–1320, 1986

37. McKenna MJ, Wilson RS, Botelho RJ: Right upper lobe obstruction with right-sided double-lumen endobronchial tubes: a comparison of two tube types. J Cardiothorac Anesth 2:734–740, 1988

38. Mushin WW: Thoracic Anesthesia. Blackwell Scientific Publications, Oxford, 1963

39. El-Etr AA: Improved technique for insertion of the Carlens catheter. Anesth Analg 48:738, 1969

15

ANESTHESIA FOR ESOPHAGEAL AND MEDIASTINAL SURGERY

James B. Eisenkraft, M.D.
Steven M. Neustein, M.D.

ESOPHAGEAL SURGERY

The development of anesthetic techniques to manage patients during thoracic surgery has permitted the development of a variety of surgical treatments for esophageal disease. These anesthetic techniques include the use of double-lumen endobronchial tubes to provide one-lung anesthesia and collapse of the lung on the ipsilateral side to the thoracotomy incision. The surgical diseases discussed in this section include tumors, hiatus hernia, rupture and perforation, achalasia, stricture, and esophagorespiratory tract fistula. It is essential to understand the pathophysiology of these lesions to safely anesthetize patients presenting for surgical treatment.

The esophagus is a muscular tube that extends from the pharynx, through the neck and thorax, to the abdomen. In adults, it averages 23 to 25 cm in length. The esophagus enters the superior mediastinum posterior to the trachea and the left recurrent laryngeal nerve and anterior to the vertebral bodies. It traverses to the posterior mediastinum and slightly to the left, passing posterior to the left mainstem bronchus (Fig. 15-1). It continues posterior to the pericardium and

left atrium and anterior to the descending aorta. Throughout the entire thoracic cavity, the right side of the esophagus is adjacent to the right mediastinal pleura and lung. On the left side at the level of T_{5-7}, interposed between the left mediastinal pleura and esophagus, are the aortic arch, common carotid artery, subclavian artery, and descending aorta. The esophagus continues a short distance in the abdomen until it joins the stomach at the cardia.

The blood supply to the esophagus is from the inferior thyroid arteries in the neck, the bronchial and intercostal arteries and the aorta in the thorax, and the left gastric artery in the abdomen. Venous drainage from the upper esophagus is to the inferior thyroid veins, from the middle esophagus to the azygos veins, and from the lower esophagus to the gastric veins. These venous systems anastomose with one another, and the azygos and gastric veins form connections between the systemic and portal venous systems.

The esophagus receives both vagal and sympathetic innervation. The vagus nerves lie on either side of the esophagus and form a plexus around it. The esophageal wall consists of two muscular layers, an inner circular and an outer longitudinal. The outer layer in

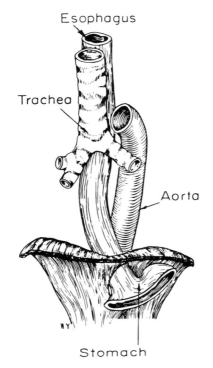

Esophagus

Trachea

Aorta

Stomach

Fig. 15-1. The esophagus and its anatomic relations. (From Orringer,[186] with permission.)

the proximal esophagus is primarily striated muscle; distally, it is mainly smooth muscle.

The peristaltic wave, which normally takes 5 to 10 seconds to pass from the pharynx to the stomach, is predominantly under vagal control.[1] There is a sphincter at both the proximal and distal ends of the esophagus. The lower esophageal sphincter, which forms a barrier between the stomach and esophagus, has a normal resting pressure of 15 to 20 mmHg.[1] A rise in intra-abdominal pressure results in an increase in the lower esophageal pressure such that the barrier pressure (difference in pressures between the stomach and esophagus) remains unchanged.[2] Drugs that decrease lower esophageal sphincter pressure include anticholinergics, sodium nitroprusside, dopamine, beta-adrenergic agonists, tricyclic antidepressants, and opioids.[2] Drugs that increase lower esophageal sphincter pressure include anticholinesterases, metoclopramide, prochlorperazine, and metoprolol (Table 15-1).[2]

In the following sections, the anesthetic management of patients with hiatus hernia, esophageal cancer, intrathoracic esophageal rupture and perforation, achalasia, and esophagorespiratory tract fistula is discussed.

Surgical Diseases and Treatment

Hiatus Hernia

Although most patients with gastroesophageal reflux have a sliding hiatus hernia, most patients with a hiatus hernia do not have significant reflux.[3] Patients with heartburn have a lowered barrier pressure and may be at increased risk for regurgitation of gastric contents. Two types of hiatus hernia have been described. Type I hernias, also called *sliding hernias*, make up approximately 90 percent of esophageal hiatal hernias. In this type, the esophagogastric junction and fundus of the stomach have herniated axially through the esophageal hiatus into the thorax.[3] Although the hernia may move cephalad and caudad in response to pressure changes in the chest and abdomen, the term *sliding* refers not to this movement, but to the presence of a partial sac of parietal peritoneum. The lower esophageal sphincter is cephalad to the diaphragm and may not respond appropriately to in-

TABLE 15-1. Effects of Drugs on Lower Esophageal Sphincter Pressure

Increase	Decrease	No Change
Metoclopramide	Atropine	Propranolol
Domperidone	Glycopyrrolate	
Prochlorperazine	Dopamine	Cimetidine
Cyclizine	Sodium nitroprusside	Ranitidine
Edrophonium	Ganglion blockers	Atracurium
Neostigmine	Thiopental	?Nitrous oxide
Histamine	Tricyclic antidepressants	
Succinylcholine	Beta-adrenergic agonists	
Pancuronium	Halothane	
Metoprolol	Enflurane	
Alpha-adrenergic	Opioids	
stimulants		
Antacids	?Nitrous oxide	

(From Aitkenhead,[2] with permission.)

creased abdominal pressure. Thus, a reduced barrier pressure during coughing or breathing leads to regurgitation. The type II, or *paraesophageal hiatus hernia*, is characterized by portions of the stomach herniating into the thorax next to the esophagus. In the presence of a type II hernia, the esophagogastric junction is still located in the abdomen. The most common complications from type II hernias are blood loss, anemia, and gastric volvulus.

Obese patients with a hiatus hernia usually have impaired respiratory function due to both the obesity (when present) and the presence of the stomach in the thorax.[4] The total lung volume and the maximum breathing capacity are reduced and the residual volume is increased.[4,5]

Patients presenting for esophageal surgery should have a preoperative chest x-ray, which may reveal evidence of aspiration or reduced lung volume. Patients with aspiration pneumonia should be treated with chest physiotherapy and antibiotics, and bronchospasm should be treated if present. Coexisting lung disease and obesity are indications for pulmonary function testing in any patient scheduled to undergo thoracotomy.

Patients with an incompetent lower esophageal sphincter are at risk for reflux and aspiration and should receive preoperative treatment to raise the pH of the gastric juice. One choice is the administration of an H_2-blocker, such as ranitidine or cimetidine. The oral or intravenous dose of cimetidine is 300 mg, four times a day. Alternative oral dosing regimens are 400 mg twice a day or 800 mg once a day. When given intravenously, cimetidine should be given slowly since rapid intravenous administration over two minutes may cause hypotension.[6] Bradycardia and heart block may also occur.[7,8] With continued administration, there may be central nervous system effects that can include confusion, agitation, seizures, and coma.[9] Cimetidine can also lead to delayed awakening from anesthesia.[10] Metabolism of drugs with a high hepatic extraction, such as lidocaine, propranolol, and diazepam, may be delayed. This may be due to reduced liver blood flow and inhibition of the mixed function oxidase system.[11]

Ranitidine is a more potent inhibitor of gastric parietal cell hydrogen ion secretion than cimetidine. There are fewer side effects from ranitidine.[12] Central nervous system effects are less likely, probably due to a decreased ability to cross the blood-brain barrier. Although cardiac effects are unusual, bradycardia has been reported in association with intravenous administration.[13] Both ranitidine and cimetidine decrease liver blood flow. The oral dose of ranitidine is 150 mg twice a day, but the intravenous dose is 50 mg every 6 to 8 hours. The intravenous route is preferred over the oral since esophageal emptying is likely to be delayed

in the presence of esophageal dysfunction. The medication should be administered both the night before and on the morning of surgery.

An alternative to an H_2-blocker is sodium citrate (Bicitra), a nonparticulate antacid. Particulate antacids are harmful if aspirated and should be avoided. Also, the whitish color of most antacids will obscure the surgeon's view if esophagoscopy is planned.

Metoclopramide, 10 to 20 mg IV over 3 to 5 minutes, can be given to increase lower esophageal sphincter tone. Anticholinergics can be administered if necessary, but will lower the sphincter tone (Table 15-1).

The goal of surgical repair of a sliding hernia is to obtain gastroesophageal competence. Since restoration of the normal anatomy is not always successful in preventing subsequent reflux, several antireflux operations have been developed, the so-called *wrap-around procedures*. For example, Nissen fundoplication, which can be performed via an abdominal or thoracic incision, entails wrapping the distal esophagus with the fundus of the stomach.[3]

Esophageal Cancer

Due to its distensibility, the esophagus proximal to an obstruction can be dilated and filled with food (Fig. 15-2). This material is not exposed to the acid milieu of the stomach and becomes infected with bacterial growth. Regurgitated liquid may lead to aspiration pneumonitis and atelectasis in patients with poor laryngeal reflexes. Even with prolonged fasting, the esophagus may not be empty above the obstruction and the patient will be at risk for aspiration of infected material on induction of general anesthesia. In the presence of esophageal obstruction, suctioning of the esophagus proximal to the obstruction using a large-bore nasogastric tube may reduce, but not totally eliminate, the risk of aspiration.

Although chemotherapy alone is ineffective for either squamous cell carcinoma or adenocarcinoma, combined therapy with radiation and surgery is often undertaken since the disease is likely to be systemic by the time of diagnosis. The chemotherapeutic agents used most often are antibiotic derivatives, such as doxorubicin and bleomycin.[14] In addition to myelosuppression, doxorubicin may lead to a dose-related cardiomyopathy in either an acute or slowly progressive manner. Ten percent of patients may develop the acute form, in which the ECG shows nonspecific ST-T wave changes and decreased QRS voltage, and there may be premature ventricular contractions, supraventricular tachyarrhythmias, cardiac conduction abnormalities, and left-axis deviation.[15] With the exception of decreased QRS voltage, these changes resolve within 1 to 2 months of discontinuing treatment. The slowly progressive form of cardiomyopathy is charac-

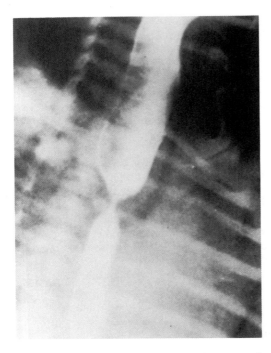

Fig. 15-2. Cancer in the upper third of the esophagus. The esophageal lumen is almost occluded by the tumor and the proximal esophagus is distended, forming a pouch. (From Rao and El-Etr,[14] with permission.)

terized by the slow onset of symptoms and is then followed by rapidly progressive heart failure. Cardiomyopathy is unlikely if the total dose of doxorubicin has been less than 500 mg/m^2 of surface area.[15] A preoperative echocardiogram or nuclear scan to evaluate cardiac function is recommended following treatment with doxorubicin.

Bleomycin is used to treat esophageal squamous cell carcinoma. This agent causes only minimal myelosuppression, but pulmonary toxicity occurs in 5 to 10 percent of patients, with death resulting in 2 percent of patients taking bleomycin.[16] The presence of pulmonary toxicity is initially manifested by cough, dyspnea, and basilar rales that can then develop into a mild or severe form.[15] While there may be exertional dyspnea and a normal resting PaO_2 with the mild form, in the severe form there is resting hypoxemia and interstitial pneumonia and fibrosis appearing on the chest x-ray.[17] There may be an increased alveolar-arterial gradient for oxygen and reduced diffusion capacity.[15] These patients are at increased risk for developing adult respiratory distress syndrome postoperatively.[18] It has been hypothesized that exposure to an increased F_IO_2, leading to superoxide and other free radicals, may be responsible; however, there are data to contradict this.[19] The de-

velopment of interstitial fluid in the lungs may be due to impaired lymphatic drainage secondary to the fibrotic changes. Patients over the age of 70 years who have received radiation treatment and more than 400 U of bleomycin were found to be at increased risk for toxicity.[15] The use of bleomycin has fallen out of favor in recent years due to its pulmonary toxicity. Other drugs that may be used include cisplatinum, vinblastine, or 5-fluorouracil.[20]

Radiation is another treatment used for esophageal cancer. It is much more effective for squamous cell carcinoma than adenocarcinoma. Complications of this form of treatment include pneumonitis, pericarditis, bleeding, myelitis, and tracheoesophageal fistula.[1]

The three types of surgical treatment of esophageal carcinoma are esophagectomy with gastric replacement, esophagogastrectomy, and replacement of the esophagus with the colon. For esophagectomy with gastric replacement (Ivor Lewis procedure), the stomach is first mobilized via an abdominal incision. Following a right thoracotomy, tumor resection is performed, which may lead to surgical compression of the vena cava and heart, causing hypotension. The stomach is pulled up into the chest and anastomosed to the proximal esophagus. For esophageal tumors involving the stomach, an esophagogastrectomy is performed via a left thoracoabdominal incision. Following the resection, the jejunum is anastomosed to the proximal esophagus.

Colon replacement of the esophagus, which can be used to treat lesions throughout the esophagus, keeps the stomach intact. It is usually performed for tumors within 20 cm of the cricopharyngeus.[2] The approach can vary depending on the level of the lesion, a left thoracoabdominal approach being used for low thoracic lesions, and separate upper abdominal and right thoracic incisions for higher thoracic lesions.[2]

In the presence of an unresectable tumor, the placement of a wide-bore tube, such as Celestin's tube, can provide palliation of dysphagia. For insertion of such a tube, a gastrostomy is first performed. A catheter is passed from the stomach retrograde past the lesion and into the pharynx. The wide-bore tube to be used for palliation is sutured to the catheter and pulled past the lesion into the stomach. A risk of this procedure is esophageal perforation.

Benign Esophageal Stricture

Chronic reflux of acidic gastric contents leads to ulceration, inflammation, and, eventually, esophageal stricture. Reflux is the most common cause of benign stricture formation in the lower esophagus.[2] The pathologic changes are reversible if the acidic gastric contents cease contact with the esophageal mucosa.[2]

Surgery may be necessary if medical treatment and dilatations are inadequate (Fig. 15-3). There are two types of surgical repair, both of which are usually approached via a left thoracoabdominal incision. Gastroplasty after esophageal dilatation interposes the fundus of the stomach between esophageal mucosa and the acidic milieu of the stomach. The remaining fundus may be sewn to the lower esophagus to create a valvelike effect.[2] The second type of repair is resection of the stricture and the creation of a thoracic end-to-side esophagogastrostomy. Vagotomy and antrectomy are performed to eliminate stomach acidity, and a Roux-en-Y gastric drainage procedure is performed to prevent alkaline intestinal reflux.

Intrathoracic Esophageal Rupture and Perforation

A rupture is a bursting injury often due to uncoordinated vomiting, straining associated with weight lifting, childbirth, defecation, and crush injuries to the chest and abdomen. The rupture is usually located within 2 cm of the gastroesophageal junction, and is usually on the left side.[2] The rupture is due to a sudden increase in abdominal pressure with a relaxed

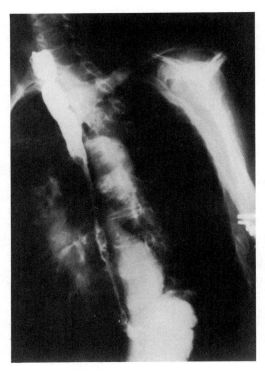

Fig. 15-3. Esophageal stricture. Twenty-four hours following a barium swallow, contrast material can still be seen in the esophagus. (From Rao and El-Etr,[14] with permission.)

lower esophageal sphincter and an obstructed esophageal inlet. In contrast to a perforation, in the presence of a rupture, the stomach contents enter the mediastinum under high pressure and the patient becomes symptomatic much more abruptly.

There are multiple causes of esophageal perforation, including foreign bodies, endoscopy, bougienage, traumatic tracheal intubation, and oropharyngeal suctioning at birth.[1,21–24] Iatrogenic causes are most common, with upper gastrointestinal endoscopy being the most frequent cause.[23] Other etiologies of iatrogenic esophageal perforation include endoesophageal intubation, esophageal obturator airways, esophageal balloon tamponade, and nasogastric tubes.[23] An endoscope will most likely cause a perforation at the upper esophageal sphincter, which is the narrowest point in the esophagus.[1] Perforations resulting from bougienage are most often at the level of the lesion. A perforation from traumatic endotracheal intubation usually occurs near the cricopharyngeus muscle.[1] At this level, the cricopharyngeus muscle and the cervical vertebrae may compress the esophageal lumen.[21] Hyperextension of the neck may increase the chances of perforation during instrumentation.

In addition to pain, patients with intrathoracic esophageal perforation or rupture may develop hypotension, diaphoresis, tachypnea, cyanosis, emphysema, and hydrothorax or hydropneumothorax.[2,21] Radiologic studies may reveal subcutaneous emphysema, pneumomediastinum, widening of the mediastinum, pleural effusion, and pneumoperitoneum.[25] An esophagogram with either barium or iodinated water-soluble contrast material may localize the injury.[23] Air may be seen in the mediastinum on a computed tomography (CT) scan of the chest.[23] These patients should receive antibiotics, and require intravascular volume repletion as determined by central venous pressure monitoring. The patients may also require supplementary oxygen and even inotropic support of the circulation if arterial pressure remains low despite the administration of fluids. A large hydrothorax or hydropneumothorax, if present, should be drained preoperatively to improve circulatory and respiratory function.[2]

Important principles of treatment for a perforation of the thoracic portion of the esophagus include drainage and prevention of further contamination.[25] Esophagoscopy may first be needed to localize the rupture or perforation.[2] A right-sided thoracotomy is used for a rupture or perforation of the upper half of the thoracic esophagus, and a left-sided thoracotomy is used when the injury is in the lower third of the esophagus.[1] In the presence of a healthy esophageal wall and unobstructed esophagus, a primary closure can be done. When the injury is at the lower end of the esophagus, it can be repaired with a portion of the stomach.

Esophagectomy is performed if there is an operable esophageal carcinoma present. If the patient's medical condition is very poor, it may be more prudent to avoid a thoracotomy by isolating the esophagus. The esophagus is divided in the neck and a cervical esophagostomy is done. The distal esophagus is divided from an abdominal incision and a feeding gastrostomy is placed.[2]

Achalasia

Achalasia is a disorder in which there is a lack of peristalsis of the esophagus and a failure of the lower esophageal sphincter to relax in response to swallowing. It is thought to have a neurogenic etiology, and many patients are either missing or have degeneration of the ganglion cells of Auerbach's plexus. This plexus, the plexus myentericus, is a nerve plexus consisting of unmyelinated fibers and postganglionic autonomic cell bodies in the esophageal wall. Clinically, the patients have esophageal distention that may lead to chronic regurgitation and aspiration.

Since it is not currently possible to correct the motility disorder, the goal of treatment is to alleviate the distal obstruction. This can be done by either esophageal dilatation or by surgery. Dilatation, which carries with it the risk of perforation, can be achieved by mechanical, hydrostatic, or pneumatic means. The surgical repair consists of a Heller's myotomy, which is an incision through the circular muscle of the esophagogastric junction. The myotomy is often combined with a hiatus hernia repair to prevent subsequent reflux.[26-28] However, this is controversial and some investigators have reported that myotomy without a fundoplication relieves dysphagia without causing reflux.[29-31] The procedure is usually performed via a thoracic incision, but an abdominal approach is also possible. A thoracic approach is required for extension of the myotomy more proximally, which may be continued by some to the level of the aortic arch.[26] The esophagomyotomy provides the best results and is the preferred treatment unless the patient is a poor surgical risk or refuses surgery, in which case an esophageal dilatation can be performed.[3] Failure to provide initial relief of dysphagia reflects an inadequate myotomy, whereas later recurrence may be due to either reapposition of severed muscle or stricture from postmyotomy gastroesophageal reflux and esophagitis.[32] The Dor operation is a modification of the procedure in which a stent is inserted into the muscular defect created by the myotomy in order to prevent muscular reapposition and, thus, recurrent dysphagia.[32,33] Good results following the Dor operation were recently reported in 16 of 17 patients, with only one patient experiencing mild persistent dysphagia.[32]

Esophagorespiratory Tract Fistula

Esophagorespiratory tract fistula in an adult is most often due to malignancy.[34,35] Occasionally, the fistula is benign, and may be due to endotracheal tube injury, trauma, or inflammation.[34] Rarely, an adult may present with congenital benign tracheoesophageal fistula without esophageal atresia. Of the malignant fistulae, approximately 85 percent are secondary to esophageal cancer.[36] The incidence of fistula formation in the presence of esophageal cancer ranges from 5 to 18 percent.[37,38] Palliation is the usual treatment since there is often local tumor extension, the patients have received radiation, and long-term survival is poor.[36-38] It is controversial as to whether the palliation should take the form of endoesophageal intubation or esophageal bypass and exclusion.[34] There is a higher perioperative morbidity and mortality (25 to 40 percent)[39,40] from esophageal bypass than from esophageal intubation (20 to 30 percent),[41] but the palliation afforded by esophageal bypass surgery is better and survival may be slightly longer.[36,42,43] The goal of palliation is to eliminate the passage of esophageal contents into the respiratory tract and to restore the continuity to the alimentary tract. Regardless of the technique used for esophageal bypass or exclusion, the fistula still exists at the end of the operation, but has effectively been removed from the alimentary tract. In this procedure, the esophagus is divided in two places, the cardia of the stomach and proximally in the neck. The fundus of the stomach is connected to the proximal portion of the divided esophagus. Either stomach, jejunum, or colon may be used as the connection, which may be placed in either a presternal or a retrosternal position. The isolated portion of esophagus may be drained, either internally or externally. Drainage of the isolated esophagus has been recommended in patients with poor pulmonary function since these patients may not be able to tolerate the additional secretions that would accumulate without such drainage.[34] Preoperatively, these patients are likely to experience dysphagia, abdominal or substernal pain, and severe coughing associated with eating or drinking. Chronic aspiration will lead to hypoxemia, pneumonia, fever, sepsis, dyspnea, and sputum production.

In addition to the fistula, aspiration may also be due to recurrent laryngeal nerve dysfunction secondary to tumor extension. Due to the juxtaposition of the esophagus and aorta, there may be a connection between these two structures. If present, such a communication could be disrupted by any manipulation of the fistula, leading to severe hemorrhage.[44] Aortography may not identify the fistula since it is clotted, but the aortic lumen may be altered in appearance due to invasion by tumor.[45] Esophageal bypass and exclusion is very hazardous in the presence of an esophago-aortic fistula and is more likely to result in death than in palliation.[34]

Localization of the fistula preoperatively is part of the preoperative evaluation. In contrast to the pediatric patient with esophagorespiratory tract fistulae, which usually connect the distal esophagus to the posterior tracheal wall, these fistulae may connect to any part of the respiratory tract.[34] In most cases, the fistula can be seen on esophagography,[46–48] but aspiration of barium is a complication of this study. Bronchoscopy has been recommended as the best method for fistula identification, but success rates of only 50 to 75 percent have been reported.[46,48]

Anesthetic Considerations

Preoperative Evaluation and Preparation

A thorough preoperative evaluation is essential. Patients with esophageal obstruction have dysphagia to solids and, subsequently, to liquids, and frequently develop poor nutritional status. Improving the nutritional status prior to surgery can lead to lowered morbidity and mortality.[49,50] Chapter 25 of this book is devoted to nutritional status, which will not, therefore, be further discussed here. In addition to a poor nutritional status, patients with esophageal disease may suffer from chronic aspiration, leading to a poor preoperative respiratory status.

During and following thoracotomy for esophageal surgery, there is a high incidence of supraventricular tachyarrhythmias due to manipulation of the heart and lungs. Although preoperative digitalization may decrease the incidence of dysrhythmias, there is a possibility of digitalis toxicity.[51] When digitalization is done preoperatively, it is not possible to titrate the dose to clinical effect, making the possibility of toxicity more likely.[52,53] Preoperative digitalization is controversial. Many of the patients with esophageal cancer are elderly, further increasing the chances of coexisting cardiopulmonary dysfunction. Other preoperative considerations include chemotherapeutic treatment for cancer, and the use of antacids, H_2-blockers, and metoclopramide in patients with hiatus hernia. These treatments have been discussed in the preceding sections.

Monitoring

In addition to the routine monitors, an arterial catheter is needed for continuous blood pressure monitoring and intermittent arterial blood sampling. Continuous blood pressure monitoring is indicated, as there may be dysrhythmias with resulting hypotension due to surgical intrathoracic manipulation and blood loss. Central venous access is indicated to allow central delivery of medications that may be needed to treat dysrhythmias and hypotension, and for measurement of central venous pressure to guide fluid administration. If indicated by the patient's preoperative cardiac status, a pulmonary arterial catheter may be needed. Continuous pulse oximetry is particularly important since there may be periods of hypoxemia during one-lung anesthesia.

Induction of Anesthesia

Since patients presenting for esophageal surgery may be at risk for aspiration, either an awake intubation or a rapid-sequence induction with cricoid pressure is indicated. Additionally, a patient with mediastinal lymphadenopathy may have tracheal compression and collapse of the airway with the onset of muscle relaxation. Ventilation may only be possible by passage of an endotracheal tube beyond the obstruction (see the section *Mediastinal Mass*).

Choice of Endotracheal Tube

For lower esophageal resections via a left thoraco-abdominal incision, it is not necessary to collapse the left lung using a double-lumen endobronchial tube. A single-lumen endotracheal tube can be placed, and surgical exposure can be obtained by retraction of the left lung. For esophageal surgery via a thoracotomy, it is usually necessary to place a double-lumen endobronchial tube to collapse the ipsilateral lung. Although some investigators have advocated placing a left-sided double-lumen tube irrespective of the side of the thoracotomy,[2] a right-sided double-lumen tube offers some advantages for a right-sided thoracotomy for esophageal surgery. The major risk of a right-sided double-lumen tube is collapse of the right upper lobe. This is unlikely to be significant during a right thoracotomy, however, since the right lung will be collapsed in any case. On the other hand, obstruction of the left upper lobe, which may occur during use of a left-sided double-lumen tube, is likely to cause hypoxemia during a right thoracotomy with collapse of the right lung. Additionally, a right-sided double-lumen tube is technically easier to place in the correct bronchus, an important consideration in a patient at risk for aspiration.

Intraoperative Considerations and Management

Hypotension may occur, which may be due to hypovolemia from blood loss, inferior vena caval compression, or surgical manipulation of the heart. Should hypotension occur, the surgeon should be notified to determine if it is due to surgical compression. Another potential complication is surgical trauma to the trachea, which can be managed by ventilating only via the bronchial lumen of the double-lumen endobronchial tube if present in the bronchus of the lung being ventilated, or by advancing the single-lumen endobronchial tube beyond the tracheal rupture into the bronchus.

High concentrations of nitrous oxide are contraindicated with bowel present in the chest due to bowel distention resulting in respiratory impairment and possible interference with surgical exposure. In addition, one-lung anesthesia should be conducted using a high inspired concentration of oxygen. A patient with relatively normal lungs undergoing esophageal surgery may be more likely to experience hypoxemia during one-lung ventilation than a patient presenting for lung resection. This is because the patient presenting for lung surgery may already have limitation of blood flow to the diseased lung and, thus, less ventilation/perfusion mismatching during one-lung anesthesia. Also, during lung resection, the surgeon ligates the pulmonary artery or a branch thereof, which decreases the shunt.

The surgeon may request the anesthesiologist to pass an oropharyngeal bougie to facilitate the surgical repair. The bougie is then removed. To test the integrity of the anastomosis or repair, methylene blue is injected via a naso- or oroesophageal tube, the lower end of which has been carefully positioned by the surgeon in relation to the anastomosis. If the patient is to remain intubated at the end of a procedure in which a double-lumen endobronchial tube has been used, reintubation with a single-lumen endobronchial tube must be done very carefully and checked immediately since unrecognized esophageal intubation and ventilation may acutely disrupt the suture line.

Anesthetic Management for Esophageal Dilatation

Indications for esophageal dilatation include achalasia, stricture, and collagen diseases involving the esophagus, such as scleroderma, myopathies, and spasm.[54] If an esophageal dilatation is to be performed, the patient will require a general anesthetic. Prior to induction, the esophagus should be suctioned using wide-bore tubing. A rapid-sequence induction with cricoid pressure applied, or an awake intubation if a difficult airway is suspected, should be done. Retching and bucking can increase the possibility of esophageal perforation and subsequent mediastinitis and should, therefore, be avoided. Agents such as atropine, which decrease the tone of the esophageal body, should be avoided since the tone is necessary for suc-

cessful rupture of muscle fibers produced by the dilatation.[54] One technique that has been described uses neuroleptanesthesia (droperidol and fentanyl) and a succinylcholine infusion.[54] The trachea should not be extubated until the patient is fully awake and able to protect the airway, since aspiration remains a risk postoperatively.

Anesthetic Management for Esophagorespiratory Tract Fistula Surgery

Anesthetizing the patient with an esophagorespiratory tract fistula carries with it unique considerations, distinguishing it from other types of esophageal surgery. Since positive-pressure ventilation may result in loss of inspired gas through the fistula and inadequate ventilation, spontaneous ventilation should be maintained during induction until gentle ventilation by mask has been shown to provide effective ventilation. The lung on the same side as the fistula is likely to be less compliant due to chronic aspiration, allowing the contralateral lung to receive most of the ventilation. Some researchers have recommended avoidance of positive-pressure ventilation prior to endotracheal intubation due to the possibility of gas flow through the fistula causing abdominal distention, secondary respiratory insufficiency, and even hypotension and cardiac arrest.[55-57] This can be accomplished either as an awake intubation or following an inhalation induction, which is likely to be slow and stormy due to poor respiratory function and the presence of secretions. Routine gastrostomy under local anesthesia has been recommended prior to induction to serve as a vent if positive-pressure ventilation by mask becomes necessary.[57,58] However, due to the risk of leakage and mediastinitis, gastrostomy is not available as an option if the stomach is to be moved into the thorax. High-frequency jet ventilation is another alternative that can reduce gas loss through the fistula.[59]

Unless the fistula is located high enough in the trachea such that the cuff of a single-lumen tube can make a seal distal to the fistula, which is rare, a double-lumen endobronchial tube will be needed. Such a tube will protect the contralateral lung from contamination and provide the ability to ventilate it without applying positive pressure to the fistula.[60] Since a double-lumen tube may not always pass to the intended side when placed blindly, it may be useful to use a flexible fiberoptic bronchoscope to position the tube under direct vision so as to minimize the possibility of disrupting the fistula. A right-sided double-lumen tube should be used for a fistula in the distal trachea, left mainstem bronchus, or left lung, and a left-sided double-lumen tube should be used for a fistula in the right mainstem bronchus or right lung. If the site of the fistula cannot be determined preoperatively, a right-sided double-lumen tube should be placed since statistically, the fistula is most likely to communicate with the trachea or left mainstem bronchus.[34] Right-sided ventilation should be attempted first. Either gastric distention or loss of delivered tidal volume indicates presence of a right-sided fistula, and left-lung ventilation should then be used instead. If two-lung ventilation becomes necessary, a nasogastric tube can be passed to vent the stomach, but there may be loss of tidal volume through the vent. If two-lung ventilation is used, the excluded esophageal portion must be drained to protect against suture line disruption.[34]

At the conclusion of the procedure, resumption of spontaneous ventilation is preferred.[34] Postoperatively, positive-pressure ventilation can be harmful in a number of different ways. It can disrupt the esophageal suture lines if the excluded esophageal segment is not drained. It can also lead to loss of tidal volume if the fistula is externally drained and to abdominal distention if the fistula is internally drained.[34] Another potential complication of continued positive-pressure ventilation is disruption of the fistula. It is, therefore, important to optimize the patient's respiratory function intraoperatively by suctioning secretions, avoiding excessive intravenous sedation, and providing good postoperative analgesia with either intrathecal or epidural narcotics. In one series, 9 of 18 patients had postoperative ventilation, which was required from 3 days to 3 weeks.[40] High-frequency jet ventilation is an attractive alternative if postoperative ventilation is required, since minimal pressure is applied to the airway.

Postoperative Considerations

Postoperative complications include hypotension, which is most likely due to hypovolemia or hemorrhage. Patients who have been receiving total parenteral nutrition may be at risk for delayed awakening due to hypoglycemia or hyperosmolar coma. The rate of administration of parenteral nutrition should be either reduced or stopped and substituted with 10 percent dextrose.

Respiratory complications are frequent following thoracic esophageal surgery, especially in the presence of obesity and coexisting lung disease, such as aspiration pneumonia. Incisional pain can lead to hypoventilation, hypoxemia, and atelectasis. Administration of intrathecal or epidural narcotics provides analgesia with minimal sedation and may improve respiratory function. The patient may have received subcutaneous heparin to prevent deep venous thrombosis; the use of intrathecal or epidural narcotics is controversial in such cases due to the possibility of epidural hematoma.

There is a high incidence of postoperative complications following thoracotomy for esophageal perforation or rupture. If present, mediastinitis often leads to severe septicemia with anaerobic or gram-negative organisms. The chance of primary repair dehiscence is greater than 50 percent.[2] Patients should remain intubated at the conclusion of a thoracic repair of an esophageal perforation or trauma due to the likelihood of infection, respiratory impairment, hypotension from blood loss, hypothermia, dysrhythmias, and fluid transudation.

Additional complications following esophageal bypass and exclusion for esophageal respiratory tract fistula include pneumothorax if either pleural cavity is inadvertently entered from a retrosternal approach. Aspiration may occur due to recurrent laryngeal nerve injury from cervical dissection.

MEDIASTINAL MASS

Patients with a mediastinal mass pose special problems for the anesthesiologist. While some mediastinal masses may produce obvious superior vena caval obstruction, they may also cause compression of the major airways and/or heart, which may be less obvious and become apparent only following induction of or emergence from general anesthesia.

The most likely complication from such a mass in relation to anesthesia is tracheobronchial obstruction, although the mechanical (compression) complications produced by such tumors depend on the part of the mediastinum in which they occur. Patients presenting with mediastinal masses often need anesthesia for diagnostic procedures, such as node biopsy or bronchoscopy, as well as therapeutic surgery, such as thoracotomy or laparotomy. Numerous case reports attest to serious potential problems that may develop during these cases. These complications will be briefly considered.

Tracheal and Bronchial Compression

Complete airway obstruction has been reported and may develop acutely during induction of anesthesia, intubation, patient positioning, maintenance, or recovery. In a review of 22 case reports, this complication was found in 20.[61] Five of these 20 had respiratory symptoms or signs preoperatively and, in three cases, the symptomatology varied with posture.

In three cases, inhalation induction of anesthesia precipitated airway obstruction, which was not completely alleviated by intubation. Indeed, in some cases, intubation made an incomplete obstruction complete until a longer, thinner tube was passed beyond the obstruction. It has been suggested that loss of chest wall muscle tone and loss of the expansile forces of spontaneous inspiration following the administration of muscle relaxants may abolish the extrinsic support of a bronchus (or trachea) that has been critically narrowed. This mechanism also explains tracheobronchial obstruction occurring in a patient in the supine position, which is relieved by a change in position or by return of spontaneous respiration.[62]

If tracheobronchial compression or distortion is present, tracheal intubation may cause complete airway obstruction if the distal orifice of the tube abuts the tracheal wall or is occluded by a narrowed section or acute angle in the airway. Such obstruction has been relieved by passage of a long thin tube or a bronchoscope beyond the stenotic region.[61–64] In some cases, respiratory obstruction due to edema developed during recovery, requiring reintubation.[65] Large negative airway pressures developed by vigorously attempted spontaneous inspirations can cause distal airway collapse and/or pulmonary edema.[66]

Anesthetic Management

The anesthetic management of the patient with tracheobronchial obstruction due to mediastinal tumor is based on an appreciation of the potential for total airway obstruction and the chemosensitivity and/or radiosensitivity of most mediastinal tumors. An algorithm for the anesthetic management of these patients has been proposed (Fig. 15-4).[67] If, during the preoperative evaluation, the patient has dyspnea or positional dyspnea and is scheduled for biopsy, the procedure should be performed under local anesthesia. If the tumor is believed to be radio- or chemosensitive, these treatments should be instituted and their benefits assessed (by x-ray, CT, or magnetic resonance imaging [MRI]) before any surgical procedure is undertaken. If the patient is not dyspneic, a flow-volume loop test of pulmonary function should be performed in both the sitting and supine positions. This test is helpful in assessing potentially obstructing lesions of the airway and will distinguish between intra- and extrathoracic obstructions (see Chapters 1 and 12). Figures 15-5 and 15-6 show how radiation therapy to an anterior mediastinal mass can improve vital capacity and expiratory flow rate. The effects of a large mediastinal tumor on gas exchange have been described in detail by Fletcher and Nordstrom.[68] Other useful studies include a chest CT scan, which may reveal anatomic airway obstruction, and echocardio-

graphy (in the upright and supine positions), which will show the effect of the tumor on the heart. If the results of the flow-volume, CT, and echocardiography studies are negative, the patient can receive general anesthesia if indicated. Local anesthesia would still be considered the ideal method of management in case the normal studies represented false-negative results. In one case, flow-volume loops demonstrated marked decreases in forced expiratory volume at 1 second and peak expiratory flow rate in the supine position, suggesting the potential for airway obstruction. Following radiotherapy, repeat studies showed improved function and the planned procedure was then performed under local anesthesia.[67]

Preoperative radiation therapy may, however, distort tissue histology and prevent an accurate histologic diagnosis. Furthermore, in pediatric patients it may be difficult to obtain tissue under local anesthesia. Ferrari and Bedford have reported a series of 44 patients, 18 years of age or younger, with anterior mediastinal mass who underwent general anesthesia prior to treatment with radiation or chemotherapy even in the presence of cardiovascular and respiratory symptoms.[67a] Although none of their patients died as a result of the anesthetic or operative experience, seven did develop airway compromise. The authors concluded that "in the absence of life-threatening preoperative airway obstruction and severe clinical symptoms, general anesthesia may be safely induced prior to radiation therapy," and that "the benefit of obtaining an accurate tissue diagnosis and initiating an appropriate therapeutic regimen outweigh the possible risks inherent in anesthetizing children with anterior mediastinal masses."[67a] Others have disagreed with the conclusion that general anesthesia is "safe" when the reported rate of life-threatening complications is 16 to 20 percent.[67b,c]

When the patient is to receive general anesthesia, a careful evaluation of the airway using a fiberoptic bronchoscope should first be performed.[67] Indeed, the fiberoptic bronchoscope may be used as a means to intubate the trachea. Some have recommended that general anesthesia then be induced with the patient in the lateral decubitus position so that the tumor falls away from the airway. One advantage of spontaneous ventilation is that during spontaneous inspiration, the normal transpulmonary pressure gradient tends to distend the airways and maintains their patency, even in the presence of extrinsic compression.[69] Neuromuscular blockers should not be used. If airway obstruction occurs during general anesthesia, it may be relieved by passage of a rigid ventilating bronchoscope or anode tube beyond the obstruction. In some cases, obstruction may be relieved by direct laryngoscopy, allowing the laryngoscopist to lift up the laryngeal

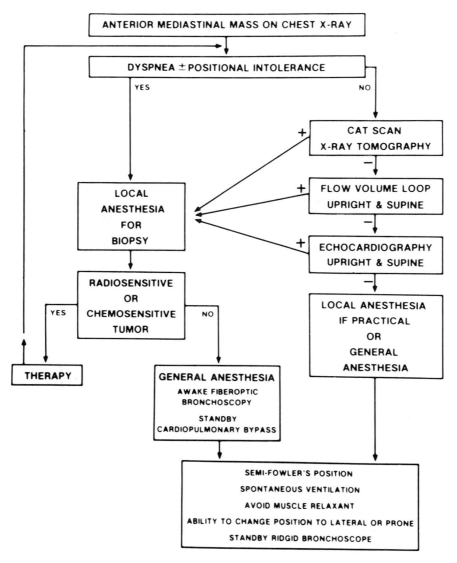

Fig. 15-4. Flow chart depicting the preoperative evaluation of the patient with an anterior mediastinal mass. A plus sign (+) indicates a positive finding; a minus sign (−) indicates a negative workup. (From Neuman et al,[67] with permission.)

structures, thus replacing the lost muscle tone caused by any muscle relaxation.[70] Relief of obstruction may also be achieved by changing the position of a supine patient to lateral or prone.[71] If the surgical procedure undertaken is via a median sternotomy, the extramural pressure on the airway is relieved when the chest is opened, thus decreasing the degree of obstruction. In one reported case, following opening of the chest, the inspiratory and expiratory flows were normalized, although the inspiratory pressure pattern remained abnormal.[68] When the chest was closed following a biopsy, the flows again became abnormal.

Airway obstruction and pulmonary edema are potential complications in the postoperative period. Obstruction may be due to expansion of the tumor caused by edema secondary to surgical manipulation and may necessitate reintubation of the airway.[66] Vigorous attempts at inspiration against an obstructed airway may lead to negative pressure pulmonary edema following relief of the obstruction.

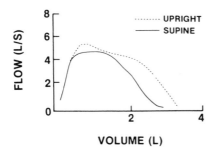

Fig. 15-5. Flow-volume loop before radiation therapy in the upright and supine positions. Note marked reduction in vital capacity and expiratory flow rates. The expiratory flow rate plateaus, which is indicative of an intrathoracic airway obstruction. (From Neuman et al,[67] with permission.)

Superior Vena Caval, Pulmonary Arterial, and Cardiac Involvement

Obstruction of the superior vena cava (SVC) is most often due to a malignant tumor, usually on the right side. Etiologies include bronchial carcinoma, malignant lymphoma, and benign causes such as SVC-induced thrombosis by a pulmonary arterial catheter. The syndrome is most severe if the tumor is rapidly growing, because a collateral circulation does not have adequate time to develop (Fig. 15-7).[72]

The SVC syndrome is characterized by engorged veins in the upper part of the body caused by an increased peripheral venous pressure; edema of the head, neck, and arms; dilated veins over the chest wall, which represent anastomotic pathways; and cyanosis. Respiratory symptoms include dyspnea, cough, and orthopnea, possibly due to venous engorgement in the airway. Changes in mental status may occur due to an increase in cerebral venous pres-

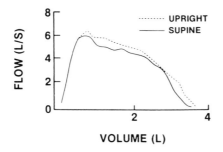

Fig. 15-6. Flow-volume loop after radiation therapy in the upright and supine positions. There is improvement in expiratory flow rates and vital capacity, with minimal change when supine. (From Neuman et al,[67] with permission.)

sure. The SVC syndrome may be exacerbated or first noted during anesthesia, and the combination of decreased venous return from the upper part of the body coupled with pharmacologic vasodilatation can result in severe hypotension.[73]

Mediastinal tumors may compress the pulmonary artery, causing a flow murmur, decrease in cardiac output, and decrease in pulmonary perfusion. This situation has been fatal.[74] In another case in which tumor enveloped the pulmonary artery, the patient became severely cyanosed after induction of anesthesia, but subsequently was safely anesthesized after establishment of extracorporeal oxygenation by femoro-femoral bypass under local anesthesia.[75]

Large mediastinal lymphomas have been associated with dysrhythmias under anesthesia due to pericardial or myocardial involvement.[76] In addition, a large thymoma was reported to have compressed the heart, simulating cardiac tamponade.[77]

Anesthesia Considerations

In general, anesthesia considerations are similar to those for patients with tracheobronchial compression. All diagnostic procedures should ideally be performed under local anesthesia. If general anesthesia is required, the same positional considerations should be taken into account. When severe and potentially untreatable airway obstruction seems likely, an extracorporeal oxygenator and support team should be immediately available.

If a SVC obstruction is present, a preoperative course of mediastinal irradiation is a priority unless the syndrome is mild.[69,72] Such patients should be brought to the operating room in an upright position so as to reduce airway edema. It has been recommended that a radial arterial catheter be inserted in all patients and that, depending on the patient's medical condition, a central venous catheter be placed via the femoral vein.[78] A wide-bore intravenous cannula should be inserted in a lower extremity. The veins of the SVC drainage region (arms and neck) should be avoided because of the obstruction and unpredictable effects of drugs administered via these routes. No attempts at central venous cannulation via the SVC should be made because the risk of perforation and major hemorrhage is high and any pressure readings obtained would likely be erroneous. If an awake fiberoptic intubation in the sitting position is planned, the patient should first receive a drying agent. Extreme care should be taken to avoid airway trauma during intubation since the increased venous pressure and congestion make hemorrhage more likely. Topical anesthesia of the airway in these patients may best be achieved by inhalation of nebulized local anes-

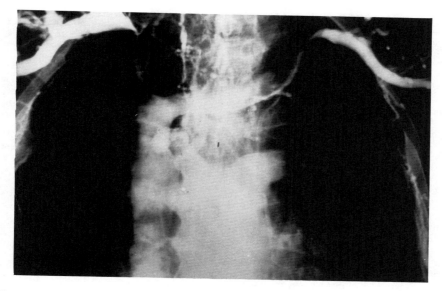

Fig. 15-7. Venogram showing superior vena cava obstruction. Note bilateral obstruction to venous return from innominate veins due, in this case, to a large anterior mediastinal tumor.

thetic (lidocaine 4 mL of 4 percent with or without 10 mg of phenylephrine). This will provide anesthesia for the trachea and avoid the necessity of a transtracheal injection of local anesthetic. The latter is usually associated with coughing, which may exacerbate any hemorrhage.

During surgery, massive hemorrhage, respiratory obstruction, or fatal exacerbation of the SVC obstruction may occur. Compatible blood should be kept available in the operating room in the event of severe hemorrhage. If SVC obstruction develops during anesthesia, diuretics and steroids may be of benefit.[73] No information is available as to whether spontaneous or controlled ventilation is preferable, although it should be remembered that coughing, straining, and the supine or Trendelenburg positions exacerbate the syndrome.[79]

Following diagnostic procedures in patients with SVC obstruction in whom the obstruction has not been relieved, acute respiratory failure may develop, necessitating reintubation and ventilatory support.[80] These patients, therefore, require intense observation during the recovery period.

MYASTHENIA GRAVIS AND THYMIC SURGERY

Myasthenia gravis (MG) is an uncommon condition, but one of particular interest to the thoracic anesthesiologist because of the relationship between the thymus gland and the disease mechanism. Thymectomy is now considered to be the treatment of choice for most patients with MG.

Clinical Aspects

The worldwide prevalence of MG is 1 per 20,000 to 30,000 population, and the incidence is two to five new cases per million per year. The disorder affects females more than males (6 : 4 ratio) and there appear to be two peak ages for incidence, the third decade for females and the fifth for males.[81,82] While several different types of MG have been described (congenital, neonatal, D-penicillamine-induced, and acquired autoimmune MG), only acquired autoimmune MG will be discussed here, as it is the type most likely encountered by the thoracic anesthesiologist. The reader is referred to a number of excellent reviews for more information on the other varieties.[83,84]

Acquired autoimmune MG is a chronic neuromuscular disorder characterized by weakness and fatigability of voluntary muscles with improvement following inactivity. The onset of MG is often slow, insidious, and difficult to pinpoint. Any muscle or muscle group may be affected and the condition is characteristically associated with periods of relapse and remission. Most commonly, onset is ocular (diplopia, ptosis) and, if the disease remains localized to the eyes for 2 to 3 years, progression to generalized MG becomes less likely.

In some patients, the condition may be generalized

TABLE 15-2. Clinical Classification of Myasthenia Gravis (MG)

I. *Ocular*—involvement of ocular muscles only. Mild with ptosis and diplopia. Electrophysiologic (EMG) testing of other musculature is negative for MG.

    1A. *Ocular*—peripheral muscles showing no clinical symptoms, but showing a positive EMG for MG.

II. *Generalized*

    A. *Mild*—slow onset, usually ocular, spreading to skeletal and bulbar muscles. No respiratory involvement. Good response to drug therapy. Low mortality rate.

    B. *Moderate*—same as group IIA, but progressing to more severe involvement of skeletal and bulbar muscles. Dysarthria, dysphagia, difficulty chewing. No respiratory involvement. Patient's activities limited. Fair response to drug therapy.

III.

    Acute fulminating—rapid onset of severe bulbar and skeletal weakness with involvement of muscle respiration. Progression usually within 6 months. Poor response to therapy. Patient's activities limited. Low mortality rate.

IV.

    Late severe—severe MG developing at least 2 years after onset of group I or group II symptoms. Progression of disease may be gradual or rapid. Poor response to therapy and poor prognosis.

Abbreviation: EMG, electromyogram.
(Adapted from Osserman and Genkins,[81] with permission.)

and may even involve the bulbar musculature, resulting in difficulties in breathing, chewing, swallowing, and speech. Peripheral neuromuscular involvement may result in difficulty walking or using the arms and hands. Vague complaints are not uncommon and emotional overlay has resulted in substantial delays in diagnosis. The disease may also present as an unexpected response to certain drugs.[85–87]

A classification of severity of MG is difficult as the clinical spectrum is so broad; therefore, a number of systems have been described. The classification most commonly used is shown in Table 15-2.

Pathophysiology

The fundamental abnormality in MG is a decrease by 70 to 90 percent in the number of postsynaptic acetylcholine receptors (AchRs) at the end-plates of affected neuromuscular junctions,[88,89] which causes a decrease in the margin of safety of neuromuscular transmission. When the number of AchRs is normal, 75 percent of receptors must be occupied or *occluded* (by an antagonist, eg, curare) to produce a threshold clinical decrease in neuromuscular function; for an almost complete block, 92 percent of receptors must be occupied by an antagonist.[90] Patients with MG, who may be lacking 70 to 90 percent of their receptors, are therefore on or close to the steep part of the receptor occlusion-transmission decrement relationship curve and are especially sensitive to anything that may adversely affect neuromuscular transmission.

Autoimmune Aspects

Anti-AchR antibodies have been detected in some 90 percent of patients with MG. The actual titer of antibodies is not always directly related to disease severity and, in some patients with MG, no antibodies are detectable.[91] The antibodies produce their effects by causing a complement-mediated lysis of the postsynaptic membrane, by directly blocking the AchRs, and by modulating the turnover rate of AchRs such that the degradation rate exceeds the rate of synthesis and incorporation into the postsynaptic membrane. Electron-micrographic studies of the motor-end plate area in affected muscles show a loss of synaptic folds (thus decreasing the area), a widening of the synaptic cleft, and decreased numbers of AchRs, as assessed by binding of alpha-bungarotoxin.[92]

Diagnosis of Myasthenia Gravis

The diagnosis should be suspected from the patient's history and confirmation sought using pharmacologic, electrophysiologic and immunologic testing. Since fatigue is the most characteristic feature, the patient cannot sustain or repeat muscular contraction. The electrical counterpart of this is the progressive decline or decrement (fade) of the muscle action potentials evoked by repetitive stimulation of a motor nerve. Both the mechanical and electrical fades characteristically improve with edrophonium, 2 to 10 mg IV (the Tensilon test).

Electromyography (EMG) is commonly used to confirm the diagnosis. The median, ulnar, or nerve to the deltoid is stimulated at 3 Hz for 3 seconds while muscle action potentials are recorded via surface electrodes. A positive test for MG is characterized by a decrement of more than 10 percent when comparing the amplitude of the fifth with that of the first response (T_5/T_1). This fade is found in more than 95 percent of MG patients if three or more muscle groups are tested.[93]

Myasthenic patients are characteristically sensitive to curare and, when the EMG is equivocal, a regional curare test may be performed in a limb that has been isolated by a tourniquet.[94,95] If the symptoms are limited to the bulbar musculature, a generalized curare test may be needed and requires the presence of an anesthesiologist in the event severe respiratory distress ensues.[95]

In equivocal cases, a positive result of a test for anti-AchR antibodies is diagnostic. A negative result of this test in a patient with generalized weakness virtually excludes MG as the diagnosis.

Medical Treatment

Anticholinesterases represent the most common initial therapy in the medical management of MG. These drugs (Table 15-3) prolong the action of acetylcholine at the neuromuscular junction and may also exert a nicotinic agonist effect of their own on the AchRs. Pyridostigmine (Mestinon) is used most commonly and is administered orally (60 mg tablets; 12 mg/mL solution) every 3 to 4 hours. Being quaternary amines, anticholinesterases are highly ionized in, and therefore poorly absorbed from, the gastrointestinal tract. If the patient is unable to accept oral preparations, pyridostigmine may be given parenterally in 1/30 of the usual oral dose. Serum concentration of pyridostigmine is related to the clinical response, which peaks at 1.5 to 2.0 hours following an oral dose and wanes by 4 hours.[96] For those patients who are extremely weak on awakening in the morning, pyridostigmine is available in slow-release capsules (180 mg) for a prolonged overnight effect. Neostigmine (Prostigmin) has a shorter onset and duration of action and may be given orally, subcutaneously, or intravenously.

Patients with MG learn to regulate their anticholinesterase medications and to titrate dosage against optimum effect in those muscles most severely affected by the condition. This may result in certain nonessential muscle groups being either over- or underdosed while the most important (eg, respiratory, bulbar) are adequately controlled. Some patients may develop a psychological dependence on their anticholinesterase therapy and be reluctant to decrease or stop it preoperatively.[84]

Overdosage of anticholinesterase can lead to the muscarinic effects of acetylcholine, manifested by colic, diarrhea, miosis, lacrimation, and salivation. Atropine (an antimuscarinic) is not routinely administered to patients receiving pyridostigmine as it would mask the above signs of overdosage. Atropine is used, however, in cases of severe muscarinic side effects.

Myasthenic Emergencies (Crises)

Myasthenic Crisis

In untreated cases, a myasthenic crisis may represent the onset of the condition. In treated cases, it is manifested as gradually increasing weakness and, perhaps, the involvement of previously unaffected muscles. Myasthenic crisis may be due to omission or underdosage with anticholinesterase.

Cholinergic Crisis

Cholinergic crisis is rare and due to overdosage with anticholinesterase, which causes a depolarization block of neuromuscular transmission. Symptoms may include salivation, sweating, abdominal cramps, urinary frequency and urgency, fasciculations, and weakness. It is treated by ventilatory support, antimuscarinic agents (atropine), and cessation of all anticholinesterase therapy until the crisis is resolved.

Distinction between a myasthenic and cholinergic crisis may be made using an edrophonium (Tensilon) test. Edrophonium, 2 to 10 mg IV, is administered and will cause transient improvement in the case of a my-

TABLE 15-3. Anticholinesterase Drugs Used to Treat Myasthenia Gravis

Drug	Dosage (mg)			Efficacy
	Oral	IV	IM	
Pyridostigmine (Mestinon)	60	2.0	2.0–4.0	1
Neostigmine (Prostigmin)	15	0.5	0.7–1.0	1
Ambenonium (Mytelase)	6	NA	NA	2.5

Abbreviation: NA, not available.

asthenic crisis, but exacerbation or no improvement in a cholinergic crisis. Crises may also be distinguished by examining the pupils, which will be dilated (mydriatic) in a myasthenic crisis, but constricted (miotic) in a cholinergic crisis.

Desensitization Crisis

The third and rarest type of crisis, desensitization crisis, is associated with inefficacy of anticholinesterase medication and has been attributed to end-plate desensitization.[97] Supportive measures and immunotherapy are the required treatments.

Immunosuppressive Therapy

Since MG is now known to have an immunologic basis, glucocorticoids and azathioprine have been used to suppress the immune response. Indications for steroid therapy vary widely among different centers and include patients with ocular MG as well as patients with severe disease who are unsuitable for, or respond poorly to, thymectomy.[84] Steroids may exert a direct therapeutic effect at the neuromuscular junction in addition to having a thymolytic and/or lympholytic effect. Patients commonly show a clinical deterioration when steroid therapy (usually prednisone, 1 mg/kg on alternate days) is begun, and improvement usually takes several weeks. High-dose methylprednisolone has been suggested for the perioperative management of patients undergoing thymectomy and in the medical management of MG.[98,99]

Azathioprine (1 to 2 mg/kg/d) has been effective in producing clinical improvement and reducing antibody titers.[100] Cyclophosphamide (1 to 2 mg/d) has also been used effectively. A recent trial of cyclosporine therapy in MG suggests that this drug may similarly have a place in the medical management of these patients.[101]

Plasmapheresis

Plasma exchange can produce transient improvement in muscle strength and decreases in anti-AchR antibody titers. It is used in severe cases of MG and, prior to thymectomy, has been reported to improve postoperative respiratory function.[102–104] Anesthetic implications of preoperative plasmapheresis include decreases in plasma pseudocholinesterase levels and prolonged paralysis following succinylcholine.[105]

Role of the Thymus Gland

Blalock pioneered thymectomy as a treatment for MG, when, following removal of a cyst from the thymic region of a patient with severe MG, dramatic improvement ensued.[106] Abnormalities are found in 75 percent of thymus glands removed from patients with MG. Of these, 85 percent show hyperplasia of germinal centers and proliferation of B cells, while 15 percent show thymoma, a frequently invasive tumor of the thymus. Only 30 percent of patients with thymoma, however, have symptomatic MG.

Following thymectomy, 80 percent of MG patients will be improved or go into remission,[82,107] and it is believed that cells of the thymus gland are related in some way to the production of the antibodies responsible for the condition. Recent evidence suggests that the thymus produces a chemotactic factor that attracts the appropriate white blood cells that form the anti-AchR antibodies. The myasthenic patients who improved after thymectomy had greater chemotactic activity than those who showed no improvement. It was postulated that stromal cells within the thymus gland of MG patients selectively attract peripheral helper T cells and potentially facilitate activation of these T cells. Activated T cells, in turn, activate B cells to produce anti-AchR antibody.[108]

Medical Versus Surgical Management

A retrospective study of 80 MG patients treated medically matched with 80 patients treated surgically (groups similar in terms of age, sex, severity, and duration of MG) showed that the surgically treated patients lived longer and had more clinical improvement than the group treated medically.[109] The difference was most marked among the female patients. Early thymectomy is now considered the treatment of choice for most patients with MG,[110] exceptions being those in Osserman group I (Table 15-2).[81]

Thymectomy

The thymus gland lies behind the sternum in the anterior mediastinum. The traditional surgical approach is via a sternal splitting incision (median sternotomy), which permits total exposure but may be associated with some morbidity in terms of postoperative ventilatory need. An alternative surgical approach is via the transcervical route, an approach similar to that used for suprasternal mediastinoscopy.[110] Controversy surrounds the question of which is the best surgical approach. While a more radical procedure can be achieved via the transsternal route,[111] the morbidity is greater, and equally good outcome results have been claimed following transcervical thymectomy.[112] Performance of a transcervical thymectomy does not preclude subsequent exploration by a median sternotomy or anterior thoracotomy (Chamberlain approach) in the event that the MG is not improved by transcervical thymectomy. The converse also holds true. In the presence of a large mediastinal mass or suspected thymoma, however, a transsternal approach is usually preferred.[113]

Anesthetic Management for Thymectomy

Preoperative Evaluation

Ideally, patients with MG should undergo elective surgery while in remission. However, since early thymectomy is now the treatment of choice for MG, most patients have active disease when admitted for thymectomy. Patients should have their physical and emotional states optimized as much as possible. Those with severe disease are admitted several days prior to surgery; milder cases are admitted the day before surgery. A physical examination should include assessment of the airway and evaluation of muscle power and the ability to chew and swallow. Ideally, lung function studies and arterial blood gas analysis should be obtained preoperatively, especially if postoperative respiratory difficulties are anticipated. The chest x-ray and CT scans (or MRI) should be examined to determine the presence of a tumor. In those patients with bulbar symptoms, nutritional status can be evaluated by measuring serum protein, electrolyte, and hemoglobin concentrations.

Optimizing the Physical Condition

If found, nutritional, fluid balance, or other deficiencies should be corrected. Patients with dysphagia may require nasogastric feeding via a tube. Any infections should be treated, bearing in mind that certain antibiotics may exacerbate muscle weakness. Other (autoimmune) diseases sometimes associated with MG (eg, thyroid, rheumatoid) should be sought, ruled out, or adequately treated. In cases with severe bulbar involvement, the tracheobronchial tree may need to be cleared of secretions. This may occasionally require bronchoscopy.

Management of Drug Therapy

The perioperative management of anticholinesterase therapy varies among institutions. One effective practice is that on admission, the daily dosage of pyridostigmine is decreased by 20 percent by reducing the size of each dose and/or increasing the interval between successive doses. The rationale for this is to prevent possible overdosing because the patient is less active in the hospital and because, following thymectomy, the anticholinesterase requirement is usually decreased.

The surgical, anesthetic, and perioperative procedures should be fully explained to the patient, including the possible need for postoperative ventilation. Education in breathing exercises and use of an incentive spirometer are also helpful.

Thymectomy is usually scheduled to be the first case of the day, particularly if the usual morning dose of pyridostigmine is to be withheld. Premedication should be with agents that do not cause respiratory depression, and narcotics should, therefore, generally be avoided. Oral diazepam to reduce anxiety and intramuscular atropine to decrease secretions are usually satisfactory. Unless the patient is physically or psychologically dependent on it, pyridostigmine is not administered on the morning of surgery. The patient, therefore, will tend to be weak on arrival to the operating room and requires less drug to produce relaxation, whether potent inhaled agents or neuromuscular blocking drugs. If, however, it should be indicated, 1/30 of the usual dose is given intramuscularly. Those patients receiving chronic steroid therapy require additional parenteral coverage during the perioperative period.

Monitoring

Standard monitoring should be used in all MG patients for thymectomy. Invasive hemodynamic monitoring is used if indicated by other existing cardiovascular conditions. Neuromuscular transmission should be monitored using a peripheral nerve stimulator (blockade monitor) and, ideally, a recording device to quantify the response to supramaximal peripheral nerve stimulation. Mechanical (mechanomyographic [MMG]) responses may be recorded and displayed using a force transducer and recording system. More recently introduced modalities for clinical monitoring of neuromuscular function in the operating room include an integrated EMG monitoring system[114] (Datex 221 Neuromuscular Transmission Monitor [NTM], Puritan Bennett Co., Wilmington, MA) and the Accelograph acceleration monitor[115] (Biometer, Inc., Copenhagen, Denmark). Both systems have been used to quantitatively assess neuromuscular function in patients with MG.[31] Both devices provide digital readouts of the T_1/control and T_4/T_1 ratios as well as an optional hard copy printout.[115,116]

Induction and Maintenance of General Anesthesia

Induction of anesthesia is easily achieved using thiamylal or thiopental sodium. With the patient breathing N_2O and O_2, baseline MMG, EMG, or accelographic recordings should be obtained to establish baseline neuromuscular responses in the nerve-muscle group being monitored (usually the ulnar nerve and the adductor pollicis if using MMG or accelography, or the ulnar nerve and first dorsal interosseous, adductor pollicis, or hypothenar muscles if using the EMG monitor). Anesthesia may be deepened using a potent inhaled volatile agent (halothane, enflurane, isoflurane) until direct laryngoscopy is possible, when the larynx is sprayed with lidocaine, 4 mL of 4 percent (in adults), and the trachea is intubated without the use of muscle relaxants. The lungs are then mechanically ventilated according to end-tidal or arterial blood gas CO_2 tensions. Temperature and breath sounds are monitored using an esophageal stethoscope and temperature probe.

Transcervical thymectomy is performed via a suprasternal incision (similar to that used for mediastinoscopy); therefore, the patient is positioned with the neck extended as much as possible using a folded sheet(s) under the shoulders and a donut to support the occiput. The transcervical approach to the thymus is anterior to the innominate vessels, whereas for mediastinoscopy an instrument is passed *behind* the vessels. Since retraction is only anteriorly (upward) on the sternum, innominate vessel compression and pseudo-cardiac arrest are not usually problems. Dissection in the anterior mediastinum via a small ("keyhole") incision is not without risk or complications, which include hemorrhage and pneumothorax. Hemorrhage is uncommon but it is important to preoperatively identify suitable venous access sites in the lower limbs so that if hemorrhage does occur in structures draining to the SVC, blood and fluids administered may reach the right atrium via the inferior vena cava. This has been lifesaving in patients who have suffered major hemorrhage during mediastinoscopic procedures.

Pneumothorax, if it occurs, is usually right-sided and due to adherence of the thymus to the pleura. It is usually identifiable at the time of surgery and can be drained. The transcervical thymectomy procedure usually lasts approximately 80 minutes.

During the surgical procedure, the potent inhaled agent is titrated according to hemodynamic response and depth of anesthesia required. It is discontinued when closure is begun. Nitrous oxide is discontinued on skin closure and extubation is performed when the patient is awake, responsive, and able to generate negative inspiratory pressures of more than 20 cmH_2O.

Following tracheal extubation, all patients are carefully monitored in the recovery room. Once able to swallow soft food (custard, Jello) they are given their usual oral dose of pyridostigmine. In cases of mild respiratory distress, nausea, or difficulty swallowing, pyridostigmine in 1/30 of the oral dose is administered intravenously or intramuscularly.

A chest x-ray is obtained routinely in the recovery room to rule out the presence of significant pneumothorax. Once the patient has been stable for 2 to 3 hours following oral pyridostigmine, they are discharged to the floor. Following transcervical thymectomy, most patients may be discharged on the third postoperative day. Those patients with more severe myasthenia who require postoperative ventilation and admission to the intensive care unit have a more prolonged hospital stay.

The transcervical approach to thymectomy has several advantages over the transsternal approach. The thoracic cage is not disrupted, so vital capacity is not decreased.[113] Thus, the need for postoperative mechanical ventilation is less likely following transcervical rather than transsternal thymectomy.

The management of anesthesia for transsternal thymectomy is essentially similar to that for transcervical except that the requirement for postoperative ventilation may be more likely. The latter approach is used most commonly for patients with large thymic tumors and thymomas and for re-exploration following transcervical thymectomy. Because these represent more extensive surgical procedures, arterial and central venous cannulae are generally indicated for hemodynamic monitoring purposes.

Choice of Anesthetic Technique

Potent Inhaled Volatile Anesthetics

Inhalation anesthesia, avoiding the use of neuromuscular blocking drugs, probably represents the most popular technique because the effects of the inhaled agents are considered to be readily controllable and reversible. However, myasthenic patients appear to be more sensitive than normal individuals to the neuromuscular depressant effects of these agents.[117,118] In normal patients, low concentrations of inhaled agents are known to potentiate the effects of nondepolarizing muscle relaxants, but, when given alone, produce neuromuscular depression only at high concentrations (eg, > 3 percent enflurane).[119] In myasthenic patients, 1 percent enflurane caused a 37 percent decrease in the T_4/T_1 ratio, and higher concentrations further decreased the T_1/control and T_4/T_1 ratios.[117] In a group of eight Chinese myasthenic patients, 1.5 percent isoflurane in 60 percent N_2O caused a 40 percent decrement in the train-of-four ratio, demonstrating that myasthenics are also more sensitive to the relaxant effects of isoflurane.[118] The sensitivity to potent inhaled agents varies widely among myasthenics; the responses to enflurane and isoflurane in two such patients are shown in Figures 15-8 and 15-9.

Of the potent inhaled anesthetics, the ethers, isoflurane and enflurane, seem to have greater neuromuscular depressant effects compared with the alkane, halothane. Indeed, one myasthenic patient who

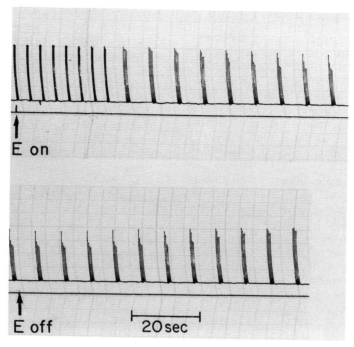

Fig. 15-8. Continuous mechanomyogram (force-transducer) of responses to train-of-four stimulation (2 Hz) in a sensitive myasthenic patient. At *E on*, enflurane 1 percent inspired concentration was begun. Note the rapid onset of the decrease in first twitch height compared with control (T_1/C), and the decrease in fade ratio (T_4/T_1). At *E off*, enflurane was discontinued, and the recovery of T_1/C and T_4/T_1 ratios is observed after this brief ($1\frac{1}{4}$ minute) exposure to enflurane. (From Eisenkraft,[133] with permission.)

was receiving 3 percent halothane was reported to show little or no relaxation.[120] Another study found that isoflurane possesses approximately twice as strong a neuromuscular blocking effect as halothane in myasthenic patients. To date, use of the new potent inhaled agents desflurane and sevoflurane in myasthenic patients has not been reported.

Muscle Relaxants

Certain myasthenic patients may show inadequate relaxation with or be unable to tolerate (hemodynamically) potent inhaled agents, in which case a balanced technique involving muscle relaxants may be selected.

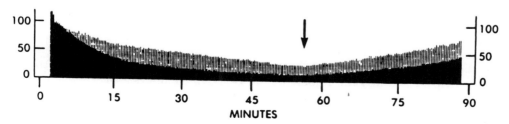

Fig. 15-9. Integrated electromyographic (EMG) recording (Datex 221 Neuromuscular Transmission Monitor) demonstrating the effect of isoflurane on the T_4/T_1 (fade) ratio. The EMG monitor tracing shows the responses to T_1 and T_4. At time 0, isoflurane administration was commenced; at the arrow, it was discontinued. Note the slow recovery of both T_1/controls and T_4/T_1 ratios after a prolonged (approximately 55 minute) exposure as compared with Figure 15-8. (From Eisenkraft,[133] with permission.)

Depolarizing Relaxants (Succinylcholine)

Based on several clinical case reports and studies, myasthenic patients demonstrate resistance to succinylcholine.[122–127] Clinically, the use of succinylcholine has been generally without incident,[125–128] despite the occasional earlier onset of phase II block.[129] The ED_{50} and ED_{95} (the effective doses producing 50 and 95 percent decreases in twitch response) for succinylcholine in normal patients are 0.17 and 0.31 mg/kg, respectively. In myasthenic patients, these values are 0.33 and 0.82 mg/kg, or 2.0 and 2.6 times the normal values. However, because the doses of succinylcholine in common clinical use (1.0 to 1.5 mg/kg) represent three to five times the ED_{95} in normal individuals, adequate intubating conditions should be achieved in MG patients when these doses are used. If a rapid-sequence tracheal intubation is required, however, the data suggest that a dose of at least 1.5 to 2.0 mg/kg may be needed to produce rapid onset of excellent intubating conditions.[125] The mechanism whereby myasthenic patients are resistant to succinylcholine is unknown, but is probably related to the decreased number of AchRs at the motor endplate.

It should also be recognized that if the patient has received anticholinesterase therapy prior to succinylcholine, while the potency in terms of relaxation produced may not be affected, the duration of action will be prolonged.[130]

Nondepolarizing Relaxants

Patients with MG are characteristically sensitive to the effects of the nondepolarizing muscle relaxants. Pancuronium and *d*-tubocurarine have been used without complications, but careful titration of small doses against quantified effect is essential if uncontrolled prolonged paralysis is to be avoided.[126]

In myasthenic patients, the regional curare test shows both an increased response and a prolonged effect, suggesting an increased affinity between AchR and relaxant.[94] Because *d*-tubocurarine and pancuronium have long elimination half-lives, most anesthesiologists now prefer to avoid these agents in patients with MG. The intermediate duration relaxants, atracurium and vecuronium, offer significant advantages over their long-acting predecessors and have been safely used in patients with MG.

Atracurium has been used in at least 18 patients with MG.[131,132] The potency data reported are very much a function of methodology used, but suggest that the ED_{95} in MG patients is approximately one-fifth that of normal patients.[133] The time course of the blockade was normal.

An advantage of atracurium is that with an elimination half-life of only 20 minutes, even if an overdose were to be given, the prolongation of relaxation would be relatively short. Rapid breakdown may also make reversal of residual blockade unnecessary, which might be advantageous in a patient who was sensitive to anticholinesterases.[133]

Vecuronium has also been successfully used in MG patients. It has a slightly longer elimination half-life than atracurium (55 minutes versus 20 minutes), but possesses other potential advantages. The ED_{95} for vecuronium in MG patients was reported to be 40 to 50 percent of that in controls, and duration of action may also be prolonged.[134–136a]

Whichever nondepolarizing relaxant is chosen for use in a myasthenic patient, it is strongly recommended that all patients be considered sensitive and that small (1/10 normal) incremental doses be titrated against quantified effect using MMG, EMG, or accelographic monitoring. In this way, excessive doses can be avoided while providing adequate relaxation and the potential for reversal of residual blockade.

A prospective study of the effect of preoperative administration of pyridostigmine on the sensitivity of subsequently administered nondepolarizing relaxant has not been reported. However, in one pharmacodynamic study of vecuronium in MG patients, there did not appear to be a significant difference between the ED_{50} and ED_{95} values in four patients who did receive preoperative pyridostigmine compared with six who did not.[135]

Reversal of Residual Neuromuscular Blockade

There are numerous reports of the uneventful reversal of residual neuromuscular blockade produced by nondepolarizing relaxants in patients with MG. Use of pyridostigmine in 1.0 to 2.0 mg increments intravenously with atropine, 0.4 mg, added to the first dose and additional 0.2 mg increments being given as needed to prevent muscarinic side effects has been advocated,[126] although small incremental doses of neostigmine may also be used. Because atracurium and vecuronium are associated with a rapid spontaneous recovery of neuromuscular function, reversal may not always be necessary following these agents. Although the potential for cholinergic crisis exists when anticholinesterases are used for reversal, crisis seems to be rare. One group reversed residual relaxation due to atracurium using two doses of neostigmine, 2.5 mg IV, given 5 minutes apart,[131] and used a similar technique following vecuronium in MG patients.[134] Reference to Table 15-3 indicates that neostigmine, 5 mg IV, is equivalent to pyridostigmine, 600 mg PO, much greater than the 320 mg average total oral daily pyridostigmine doses in these patients, yet no instance of cholinergic crisis was reported.[131,134]

Edrophonium might be the drug of choice for reversing residual relaxation, because the time from administration to peak onset of effect is the least of all the anticholinesterase agents, making titration of dose against monitored effect that much easier.

Responses of Patients in Remission

Some MG patients become asymptomatic when receiving steroid therapy. Such patients have been reported both as sensitive[137] and showing normal response[138] to curare. In one patient who was studied both during relapse and remission using the regional curare test, little difference in sensitivity was noted between each occasion.[94]

Patients in true remission, ie, asymptomatic when off all therapy, are reported to demonstrate increased sensitivity to vecuronium[139] and atracurium.[133] The one report of responses to succinylcholine during true remission suggests that the patient showed a normal response to this drug (ie, no resistance).[140]

Other Techniques

Since muscle relaxation (due to inhaled agents or muscle relaxant drugs) is not absolutely necessary to most cases of thymectomy (transsternal or transcervical), anesthetic techniques avoiding these agents have been used. Anesthesia for transcervical thymectomy has been satisfactorily provided using fentanyl/etomidate or fentanyl/Althesin (alphaxolone/alphadolone) infusions together with N_2O (50 percent) in oxygen.[141] Bradycardia occurred during induction of anesthesia and most of the patients required naloxone postoperatively. All patients were extubated in the operating room and none required reintubation.[141]

Combined regional and general anesthesia techniques have also been used to provide good surgical conditions and improved postoperative analgesia in patients undergoing transsternal thymectomy. The use of thoracic[142] or lumbar[143] epidural anesthesia in combination with light general anesthesia has been reported to provide excellent intra- and postoperative conditions for surgeon and patient.

In an alternative technique, subarachnoid morphine (5.0 to 7.5 $\mu g/kg$) was administered immediately following induction of general anesthesia. The opioid resulted in a decreased requirement for inhaled anesthetic, early extubation, excellent postoperative analgesia, and improved respiratory function in the early postoperative period (unpublished data).

Sensitivities to Other Medications

Medications that possess neuromuscular blocking properties should be avoided or used with caution in myasthenic patients. Such drugs include antiarrhyth-

mics (quinidine, procainamide, and calcium channel blockers), diuretics, or other drugs causing hypokalemia, such as nitrogen mustards (thiotepa), quinine, and aminoglycoside antibiotics (gentamicin, neomycin, and colistin). Dantrolene sodium has been reported as not increasing the neuromuscular deficit in one patient with MG who had a strongly positive family history for malignant hyperthermia and was scheduled for thymectomy.[144]

Postoperative Ventilatory Requirement

Patients with MG are more likely to develop postoperative respiratory failure; indeed, it has been reported that surgery is the leading cause of respiratory failure among these patients, the most common type of procedure undergone being thymectomy.[145]

When thymectomy was originally introduced as a treatment for myasthenia, a tracheostomy was routine since all patients were electively ventilated in the postoperative period. At The Mount Sinai Medical Center, New York, elective tracheostomy was performed in all patients scheduled for thymectomy until 1967. Since that time, the earlier diagnosis and performance of surgery, together with improved medical, surgical, and anesthesia management, have resulted in tracheostomy being the exception rather than the rule for myasthenic patients.

A number of studies have attempted to preoperatively identify those myasthenic patients who are most likely to develop postoperative ventilatory failure and, therefore, need prolonged ventilatory support. Most of these studies have addressed transsternal thymectomy since as many as 50 percent of patients undergoing this procedure may require a prolonged period of ventilation afterward.

In 1974, Mulder et al suggested that a tracheotomy was indicated if bulbar muscle weakness, a past history of respiratory or myasthenic crisis, or a vital capacity of < 2 L was present.[146] In 1975, Loach et al reported that ventilation was required if vital capacity was < 2 L and that further risk factors were the presence of thymoma, bulbar symptoms (particularly dysphagia), and an age > 50 years.[147] In the latter study of 28 patients, 14 needed postoperative ventilation, usually for 12 days or longer.

Leventhal et al reported a retrospective analysis of experience with 24 myasthenic patients who had undergone transsternal thymectomy at the Hospital of the University of Pennsylvania.[148] Of these 24 patients, 8 required prolonged ventilation (defined as > 3 hours, but was in general > 18 hours) and were compared with 16 who did not. Four risk factors were identified and a predictive scoring system was developed to identify those patients who would need ventilation postoperatively. The risk factors and point weighting were (1) a duration of MG > 6 years (12 points), (2) a history of chronic respiratory disease other than respiratory disease or failure directly due to MG (10 points), (3) a daily pyridostigmine dose requirement > 750 mg 48 hours before surgery (8 points), and (4) a preoperative vital capacity < 2.9 L (4 points). It was found that those patients with a score ≥ 10 points were more likely to need prolonged ventilation.[148] When applied to the 24 patients on whom it was based, this predictive model was correct in 22 of the 24 cases (91 percent), with no false-negatives (ie, no patients incorrectly predicted to be ready for extubation) and two false-positives (2 of 16 patients were incorrectly predicted to need ventilation when they did not). When tested in an additional 18 patients at the same institution, the predictions were 78 percent correct, with no false-negatives.[149]

The predictive scoring system was tested in 27 patients who had undergone thymectomy (4 transcervical, 23 transsternal) in Vancouver and was found to be of limited value, with a sensitivity of only 43 percent.[150] These investigators reported the scoring system to be of even less value in myasthenic patients undergoing other forms of surgery.[150]

Others have also failed to validate the scoring system.[151,152] Gracey et al stated that, "the most important preoperative observation signifying need for postoperative mechanical ventilation was the severity of bulbar involvement (Osserman groups III and IV), usually indicated by significant dysarthria and dysphagia along with borderline respiratory function."[151]

Expiratory weakness, by reducing cough efficacy and the ability to remove secretions, has been suggested as the main predictive determinant. Younger et al studied expiratory function in 32 patients with MG who underwent transsternal thymectomy.[153] Preoperative clinical lung function and expiratory muscle pressure data were analyzed in an attempt to identify preoperative factors that correlated with duration of postoperative ventilatory support. Ten of the 32 patients (31 percent) needed support for > 3 days, and duration of ventilation correlated best with maximal static expiratory pressure. This observation is significant since anesthesiologists usually use peak *negative* inspiratory pressure (−25 mmHg) as one of the criteria for evaluating the adequacy of spontaneous ventilation and when mechanical ventilation may be discontinued. In addition, Pavlin et al studied the recovery of airway protection in normal conscious volunteers who received intravenous *d*-tubocurarine.[154] They reported that although ventilation may be adequate at a maximum inspiratory pressure of −25 mmHg, the muscles of airway protection are still nonfunctional although all patients who could accomplish a head lift for 5 seconds could perform airway-protective maneuvers. Thus, both adequacy of ventilation as well as ability to protect the airway and clear secretions are essential prerequisites before considering withdrawal of ventilatory support and tracheal extubation.

Ringqvist and Ringqvist measured respiratory mechanics in a group of 9 patients with untreated myasthenia and found that maximum inspiratory force was decreased less than the maximum expiratory pressure.[155] It therefore seems desirable to assess both inspiratory and expiratory forces, especially in those patients thought to be at greatest risk for postoperative respiratory failure.

Postoperative respiratory failure appears to be less common following transcervical rather than transsternal thymectomy. This is most likely because there is no disruption of the thoracic cage with its associated decrease in vital capacity. It may also be argued that the transsternal thymectomy series has included patients with more severe myasthenia than the transcervical series, hence the apparently lower morbidity with the latter approach. In one study of 22 patients who underwent transcervical thymectomy, none required postoperative ventilation.[156] A review of transcervical thymectomy patients at The Mount Sinai Medical Center indicated that only 8 of 92 (8.7 percent) needed postoperative ventilation for > 3 hours.[152] The predictive scoring system of Leventhal et al[148] was also tested in these 92 patients and found to be of no value, having a sensitivity of only 37.5 percent.[152] Analysis of The Mount Sinai Medical Center MG patient data indicates that the risk factors associated with the need for postoperative ventilation following transcervical thymectomy are severity of disease (Osserman groups III and IV), a previous history of respiratory failure due to myasthenia, and concurrent corticosteroid therapy for myasthenia.[157]

Redfern et al reported their experience of anesthesia for 30 myasthenic patients who underwent transsternal thymectomy in the United Kingdom.[158] Of these, only 3 (10 percent) developed postoperative respiratory failure in relation to myasthenia. A fourth patient required reintubation for severe stridor due to prolapse of an arytenoid cartilage. The requirement for postoperative ventilation in the other three patients may have been related to cholinergic crisis caused by a relative overdose of neostigmine.[158,159]

It is evident that the accurate preoperative prediction of postoperative respiratory failure in MG is not completely elaborated. Such a project is made difficult by the small numbers of patients available for study, analysis of data obtained retrospectively, wide variety of patient disease states, and management techniques used. Meanwhile, each case should be treated on its individual merits and controlled ventilation discontinued only when clinically indicated. Those patients with the most severe myasthenia are at greatest risk for ventilatory failure and should be carefully monitored. Short-term ventilation via a soft cuff (low pressure) oro- or nasotracheal tube is suitable for most patients requiring ventilatory assistance. Tracheostomy is now usually performed only in those patients likely to need long-term (> 10 days) ventilation.

Techniques to Decrease the Need for Postoperative Ventilation

Preoperative Plasmapheresis

Patients with severe myasthenia have been successfully treated with plasmapheresis, and it has been suggested that plasmapheresis be performed preoperatively in high-risk groups (Osserman groups III and IV).[160] In one study of 37 myasthenic patients undergoing thymectomy, it was found that those patients with respiratory weakness who had received preoperative plasmapheresis required significantly less time on mechanical ventilation and in the intensive care unit than a similarly weak group who did not receive this treatment preoperatively.[161] Others have also found plasmapheresis to be a worthwhile adjuvant in the preparation of myasthenics (Osserman group IV) for thymectomy.[162] The anesthetic implications of plasmapheresis have been mentioned previously.[105]

Large-Dose Steroids

It has been reported that the perioperative administration of methylprednisolone, 1 g, significantly reduced the morbidity (in terms of neuromuscular function and respiratory complications) of transsternal thymectomy.[163] Of 32 patients who underwent transsternal thymectomy, all were extubated within 2 hours of surgery and none required postoperative ventilatory support.

Preoperative Administration of Anticholinesterase

Anticholinesterase therapy is generally withheld on the day of surgery. However, if muscle relaxants are to be avoided altogether and if profound relaxation is not essential, a case can be made for giving the usual morning dose of anticholinesterase. One study has compared two groups of myasthenic patients undergoing transsternal thymectomy.[164] In one group, the usual dose of pyridostigmine was administered preoperatively; in the other, it was withheld. The requirement for postoperative ventilatory support was found to be higher in the group that had not received pyridostigmine preoperatively. By administering oral pyridostigmine preoperatively, the peak effect would occur approximately 3 hours later, when it would be

expected that the operation would be complete and the patient prepared for extubation.

Postoperative Considerations

During the postoperative period, pain relief is commonly provided by narcotic analgesics, traditionally meperidine, but in reduced dosages. The analgesic effects of morphine have been reported to be increased by anticholinesterases,[165] which prompted the recommendation that the dose of narcotic analgesics be reduced by one-third in patients receiving anticholinesterase agents.[126] The mechanism for any potentiation, if it exists, is not elaborated.

As mentioned previously, spinal opioids have been used successfully to provide intra- and postoperative analgesia. In one report, a thoracic (T_6-T_7) epidural catheter was placed in each of two patients undergoing transsternal thymectomy.[142] Postoperative analgesia was achieved in one patient with 100 μg of fentanyl in 10 mL of 0.9 percent sodium chloride, followed by a continuous epidural infusion of fentanyl, 4 μg/mL in 0.9 percent sodium chloride. Following extubation, the patient remained pain-free overnight in the intensive care unit, receiving epidural fentanyl, 48 μg/h (12 mL/h). In a second patient, postoperative analgesia was achieved with epidural fentanyl, 75 μg in 10 mL of 0.9 percent sodium chloride. In the intensive care unit, the patient received epidural fentanyl by infusion at 10 mL/h (4 μg/mL). Satisfactory analgesia and no complications were reported with this technique, which clearly warrants further study in this patient population. In another report, anesthesia for transsternal thymectomy was provided by a combination of 2 percent epidural lidocaine (15 mL injected at L_1/L_2) and light general anesthesia (N_2O/O_2, 3L/2L; isoflurane, 0.4 to 1.2 percent).[143] The patient received 0.8 mg of epidural hydromorphone in the operating room and again in the postanesthesia care unit. After extubation on the following day, patient-controlled analgesia with morphine was instituted. When the latter proved unsatisfactory, a further dose of 1 mg of hydromorphone was administered epidurally, this was effective in improving respiratory parameters. The following day, the patient was discharged to the floor with a reduced patient-controlled analgesia maintenance dose.[141]

An alternative technique is the use of subarachnoid morphine. As mentioned previously, this has been used in doses of 5.0 to 7.5 μg/kg prior to the start of transsternal thymectomy, and provided satisfactory analgesia for 24 to 30 hours postoperatively (unpublished data).

Following tracheal extubation, myasthenic patients should be carefully observed for signs of respiratory distress or choking on secretions. Avoidance of infections and attention to clearing secretions are essential.

Effects of Thymectomy

Often, in the immediate postoperative period, patients show a dramatic improvement in their clinical condition.[167,168] For this reason, the dosage of anticholinesterase is routinely reduced preoperatively. However, the immediate improvement is usually short-lived and lasting improvement or a remission may take months or years to occur. In general, it is reported that within 1 year following thymectomy, 30 percent of patients go into remission and 80 percent are clinically improved.[76] While the natural history of all MG patients is to eventually go into remission, the prevention of disease progression and earlier onset of remission are both enhanced by thymectomy.[76,77] It has also been reported that there is an increased incidence of extrathymic neoplasia among patients with MG,[168] but that the incidence reverts to normal following thymectomy.[169]

MYASTHENIC SYNDROME

Myasthenic syndrome may represent a nonmetastatic effect of bronchial carcinoma and may be humorally mediated. However, in a recent review of 50 cases of Lambert-Eaton myasthenic syndrome (LEMS), carcinoma was detected in only 25 patients (50 percent), of whom 21 had small-cell lung cancer.[170] The latter carcinoma was evident within 2 years of onset of LEMS symptoms in 20 of 21 cases. In the patients in whom no carcinoma was detected, 14 of 25 had a history of LEMS for more than 5 years. The main neurologic features of the syndrome are proximal lower limb weakness (100 percent), depressed tendon reflexes (92 percent) with posttetanic potentiation (78 percent), and autonomic features, particularly dry mouth (74 percent) and ptosis (54 percent).[170] Analysis indicated that a patient who presented with LEMS had a 62 percent chance of an underlying small-cell carcinoma of the lung and that this risk declined sharply after 2 years, becoming very low by 5 years. It was suggested that in cases associated with small-cell carcinoma of the lung, antigenic determinants on tumor cells initiated the autoimmune response.[170]

The LEMS is more common in males than females. The main symptoms are weakness and easy fatigability of the proximal muscles of the extremities (especially the thighs). Involvement of muscle innervated by cranial nerves occurs in 70 percent of cases. In contrast to MG, in which there is fatigue on exercise,

in LEMS, there is a transient increase in strength on activity that precedes weakness and muscle pain is common. There is increased sensitivity to all muscle relaxants, both depolarizing and nondepolarizing.[171] The neuromuscular transmission defect in LEMS is presynaptic and similar to that produced by an excess of magnesium ions, botulinum toxin, or neomycin, all of which decrease the number of quanta of acetylcholine released by a nerve impulse from the motor nerve terminal.[172] This is secondary to destruction of the active release zones in the nerve terminal[173] and is believed to be of autoimmune etiology.[174]

The electrophysiologic characteristics of LEMS are (1) an abnormally low amplitude of muscle action potential in response to a single supramaximal stimulus, (2) a decremental response at low rates (1 to 3 Hz) of nerve stimulation, (3) marked facilitation of the response at high rates of stimulation (50 Hz) and after 10 seconds of maximum contraction of the muscle, and (4) posttetanic facilitation.[175] Differences between MG and myasthenic syndrome are shown in Table 15-4.

Treatment of LEMS differs from that of classic MG. Although both conditions improve with local cooling, LEMS patients respond poorly to anticholinesterase drugs.[175] The most successful treatment has been with so-called facilitatory agents, which act to increase the release of acetylcholine from the motor nerve terminal by selectively blocking potassium channels.[176,177] These agents include guanidine in doses of 10 to 35 mg/kg/d. This drug may cause renal failure, hypotension, and bone marrow depression.[178] Other agents that have been used are caffeine, calcium, germine, and 4-aminopyridine.[179–181] Treatment is not uniformly successful and is often limited by drug side effects, particularly central nervous system stimulation. In this rare condition, 3,4-diaminopyridine causes less central nervous system depression and may be the drug of choice.[183] The maximum daily dose is 100 mg, given in divided doses.

The possible coexistence of LEMS should always be considered when evaluating a patient with bronchial carcinoma for anesthesia, since affected patients are reported to be extremely sensitive to all muscle relaxants.[94,183] One patient with a 6-month history of LEMS who was being treated with 3,4-diaminopyridine, 30 mg PO every 6 hours, demonstrated normal response to succinylcholine, but a marked sensitivity to vecuronium as well as a slow recovery time.[184] Reversal of residual neuromuscular blockade with neostigmine was largely ineffective, but was improved by oral 3,4-diaminopyridine. This patient received nitrous oxide (70 percent) and isoflurane (0.5 percent) in oxygen for anesthesia maintenance. These researchers[184] concluded that if such a patient requires anes-

TABLE 15-4.   Differences Between Myasthenia Gravis and the Myasthenic (Lambert-Eaton) Syndromes

	Myasthenia Gravis	Myasthenic Syndrome
Sex	Female > Male	Male > Female
Presenting symptoms	External ocular muscle bulbar and facial weakness	Proximal limb weakness (legs > arms)
Other symptoms	Fatigue on activity	Increased strength on activity precedes fatigue
	Muscle pains uncommon Reflexes normal	Muscle pains common Reflexes reduced or absent
EMG	Initial muscle action potential relatively normal Decremental response on high-frequency stimulation ("fade")	Initial muscle action potential abnormally small Decremental response at low rates of stimulation, incremental response on high-frequency stimulation
Response to blocking drugs	Sensitivity to nondepolarizing blockers Resistance to depolarizing blockers	Sensitivity to both nondepolarizing and depolarizing blockers
	Good response to anticholinesterases	Poor response to anticholinesterases
Pathologic state	Thymoma present in 20–25% of patients	Small-cell bronchogenic carcinoma usually present

(Adapted from Telford and Hollway,[184] with permission.)

thesia, the 3,4-diaminopyridine should be continued up to the time of surgery and that, if possible, neuromuscular blockers should be avoided or used sparingly with close monitoring.

In patients with LEMS, use of a potent inhaled anesthetic may represent the most conservative course of management. If a muscle relaxant is needed, atracurium may represent the most appropriate choice. Should the condition be suspected clinically preoperatively, the diagnosis may be confirmed by EMG.

PANCOAST'S SYNDROME

A Pancoast tumor is an apical carcinoma of the bronchus that invades the brachial plexus, resulting in pain in the arm by invasion and compression of the lower roots of the plexus. It is recognized that muscles that are partially or totally denervated demonstrate increased sensitivity to cholinergic nicotinic agonists. These muscles respond to succinylcholine by developing a contracture instead of the paralysis observed in normally innervated striated muscle. Reports of the development of contracture in such a denervated muscle during anesthesia are rare. However, it is reported that a patient with a right-sided Pancoast tumor, in response to succinylcholine, developed fasciculations over most of the body except for the right arm, which became rigid as the rest of the body re-

laxed.[185] The rigidity gradually wore off within 3 to 4 minutes, at which time muscle power returned to the rest of the body. If such a tumor is present or suspected, use of a nondepolarizing relaxant may be preferable since it should produce relaxation without contractures.

REFERENCES

1. Greenhow DE: Esophageal surgery. pp. 451–470. In Marshall BE, Longnecker DE, Fairley HB (eds): Anesthesia for Thoracic Procedures. Blackwell Scientific Publications, Boston, 1988
2. Aitkenhead AR: Anesthesia for esophageal surgery. pp. 181–206. In Gothard JW (ed): Thoracic Anesthesia. Bailliere-Tindall, London, 1987
3. Pairolero PC, Trastek VF, Payne WS: Esophagus and diaphragmatic hernias. pp. 1103–1156. In Schwartz SI, Shires GI, Spencer FL (eds): Principles of Surgery. McGraw-Hill, New York, 1989
4. Semyk J, Arborelius M, Jr, Lilja B: Respiratory function in esophageal hiatus hernia I. Spirometry, gas distribution and arterial blood gases. Respiration 32:93–102, 1975
5. Semyk J, Arborelius M, Jr, Lilja B: Respiratory function in esophageal hiatus hernia II. Regional lung function. Respiration 32:103–111, 1975
6. Iberti TJ, Paluch TA, Helmer L, et al: The hemodynamic effects of intravenous cimetidine in intensive

care patients; a double-blind, prospective study. Anesthesiology 64:87–89, 1986

7. Cohen J, Weetman AP, Dargie HJ, Krikler DM: Life-threatening arrhythmias and intravenous injection of cimetidine. Br Med J 2:768, 1979

8. Shaw RG, Mashford ML, Desmond PV: Cardiac arrest after intravenous injection of cimetidine. Med J Aust 2:629–630, 1980

9. Schentag JJ, Cerra FB, Calleri G, et al: Pharmacokinetic and clinical studies in patients with cimetidine-associated mental confusion. Lancet 1:177–181, 1979

10. Viegas OJ, Stoops CA, Ravindran RS: Reversal of cimetidine-induced postoperative somnolence. Anesthesiol Rev 9:30–31, 1982

11. Feely J, Wilkinson GR, Wood AJ: Reduction of liver blood flow and propranolol metabolism by cimetidine. N Engl J Med 304:692–695, 1981

12. Zeldis JB, Friedman LS, Isselbacher KJ: Ranitidine: a new H_2-receptor antagonist. N Engl J Med 309:1368–1373, 1983

13. Camarri E, Chirone E, Fanteria G, Zoahi M: Ranitidine-induced bradycardia. Lancet 2:100, 1982

14. Rao TLK, El-Etr AA: Esophageal and mediastinal surgery. pp. 447–471. In Kaplan JA (ed): Thoracic Anesthesia. Churchill Livingstone, New York, 1983

15. Stoelting RK: Pharmacology and Physiology in Anesthetic Practice. pp. 490–493. JB Lippincott, Philadelphia, 1987

16. Crooke ST, Bradner WT: Bleomycin: a review. J Med 7:333–428, 1976

17. Luna MA, Bedrossian CW, Lichtiger B, et al: Interstitial pneumonitis associated with bleomycin therapy. Am J Clin Pathol 58:501–510, 1972

18. Goldiner PL, Carlon G, Cuitkovic E, et al: Factors influencing postoperative morbidity and mortality in patients treated with bleomycin. Br Med J 1:1664–1667, 1978

19. Lamantia KR, Glick JH, Marshall BE: Supplemental oxygen does not cause respiratory failure in bleomycin-treated surgical patients. Anesthesiology 60:65–67, 1984

20. DeVita VT: Principles of cancer therapy. pp. 431–446. In Braunwald E, Isselbacher KJ, Petersdorf RG, et al (eds): Harrison's Principles of Internal Medicine. McGraw-Hill, New York, 1987

21. Topsis J, Kinas H, Kandall S: Esophageal perforation—a complication of neonatal resuscitation. Anesth Analg 69:532–534, 1989

22. Krasna I, Rosenfeld D, Benjamin B, et al: Esophageal perforation in the neonate: an emerging problem in the newborn nursery. J Pediatr Surg 22:784–790, 1987

23. Sakurai H, McElhinney J: Perforation of the esophagus: experience at Bronx VA Hospital 1969–1984. Mt Sinai J Med (NY) 54:487–494, 1987

24. O'Neill JE, Giffin JP, Cottrell JE: Pharyngeal and esophageal perforation following endotracheal intubation. Anesthesiology 60:487–488, 1984

25. Sarr MG, Pemberton JH, Payne WS: Management of instrumental perforations of the esophagus. J Thorac Cardiovasc Surg 84:211, 1982

26. Little AG, Soriano A, Ferguson MK, et al: Surgical treatment of achalasia: results with esophagomyotomy and Belsey repair. Ann Thorac Surg 45:489–494, 1988

27. Murray GF, Battaglini JW, Keagy BA, et al: Selective application of fundoplication in achalasia. Ann Thorac Surg 37:285–188, 1984

28. Belsey R: Functional disease of the esophagus. J Thorac Cardiovasc Surg 52:164–188, 1966

29. Ellis FH, Jr, Gibb SP, Crozier RE: Esophagomyotomy for achalasia of the esophagus. Ann Surg 192:157–161, 1980

30. Thompson D, Shoenut JP, Thenholm BG, Teskey JM: Reflux patterns following limited myotomy without fundoplication for achalasia. Ann Thorac Surg 43:550–553, 1987

31. Pai GP, Ellison RG, Rubin JW, Moore HV: Two decades of experience with modified Heller's myotomy for achalasia. Ann Thorac Surg 38:201–206, 1984

32. Desa LA, Spencer J, McPherson S: Surgery for achalasia cardiae: the Dor operation. Ann R Coll Surg Engl 72:128–131, 1990

33. Dor J, Humbert P, Paoli JM, et al: Traitment du reflux par la technique dite de Heller-Nissen modifie. Presse Med 50:2563–2565, 1967

34. Hindman B, Bert A: Malignant esophago-respiratory tract fistulas: anesthetic considerations for exclusion procedures using esophageal bypass. J Cardiothorac Anesth 1:438–447, 1987

35. Wesselhoeft C, Keshishian J: Acquired non-malignant esophagotracheal and esophagobronchial fistulas. Ann Thorac Surg 6:187–195, 1968

36. Duranceau A, Jamieson C: Malignant tracheoesophageal fistula. Ann Thorac Surg 37:346–354, 1984

37. Little AG, Fergisson M, Demeester TR, et al: Esophageal carcinoma with respiratory tract fistula. Cancer 15:1322–1328, 1984

38. Schuchmann GF, Heydorn WH, Hall RV, et al: Treatment of esophageal carcinoma: a retrospective review. J Thorac Cardiovasc Surg 79:67–73, 1980

39. Angorn I: Intubation in the treatment of carcinoma of the esophagus. World J Surg 18:417–430, 1974

40. Conlan A, Nicolaou N, Delikaris P, Dool R: Pessimism concerning palliative bypass procedures for established malignant esophagorespiratory fistulas: a report of 18 patients. Ann Thorac Surg 37:108–110, 1984

41. Girardet R, Rensdell H, Jr, Wheat M, Jr: Palliative intubation in the management of esophageal carcinoma. Ann Thorac Surg 18:417–430, 1974

42. Symbas P, McKeown P, Hatcher C, Jr, et al: Tracheoesophageal fistula from carcinoma of the esophagus. Ann Thorac Surg 38:382–386, 1984

43. Weaver R, Matthews H: Palliation and survival in malignant esophago-respiratory fistula. Br J Surg 67:539–542, 1980

44. Bryant LR, Bowlin J, Malette W, et al: Thoracic aneurysms with aortico-bronchial fistula. Ann Surg 168:79–84, 1968

45. Graeber G, Farrell B, Neville J, Jr, Parker F, Jr: Successful diagnosis and management of fistulas between

the aorta and the tracheobronchial tree. Ann Thorac Surg 29:555–561, 1980

46. One G, Kwong K: Management of malignant esophagobronchial fistula. Surgery 67:293–301, 1970

47. Steiger Z, Wilson R, Leichman L, et al: Management of malignant bronchoesophageal fistulas. Surg Gynecol Obstet 157:201–204, 1983

48. Campion J, Bourdelat D, Launois B: Surgical treatment of malignant bronchoesophageal fistulas. Am J Surg 146:641–646, 1983

49. Moghissi K, Hornshaw J, Teasdale PR: Parenteral nutrition in carcinoma of the esophagus treated by surgery: nitrogen balance and clinical studies. Br J Surg 64:125–128, 1977

50. Heatley RV, Williams RHP, Lewis MH: Preoperative intravenous feeding—a controlled trial. Postgrad Med J 55:541–545, 1979

51. Juler GL, Stemmer EA, Connolly JE: Complications of prophylactic digitalization in thoracic surgical patients. J Thorac Cardiovasc Surg 68:352–358, 1969

52. Shields TW, Unik GT: Digitalization for prevention of arrhythmias following pulmonary surgery. Surg Gynecol Obstet 126:743–746, 1968

53. Burman SO: The prophylactic use of digitalis before thoracotomy. Ann Thorac Surg 14:359–368, 1972

54. Owitz S, Pratilas V, Pratilas M, Sampson IH: Anesthetic and pharmacologic considerations in esophageal dilatation. Anesthesiol Rev 8:21–25, 1981

55. Calverley RK, Johnson AE: The anesthetic management of tracheo-esophageal fistula: a review of ten years' experience. Can Anaesth Soc J 19:270–282, 1972

56. Grant D, Thompson G: Diagnosis of congenital tracheoesophageal fistula in the adolescent and adult. Anesthesiology 49:139–140, 1978

57. Baraka A, Slim M: Cardiac arrest during IPPV in a newborn with tracheo-esophageal fistula. Anesthesiology 32:564–565, 1970

58. Myers CR, Love JW: Gastrostomy as a gas vent in repair of tracheoesophageal fistula. Anesth Analg 47:119–121, 1968

59. Turnball AD, Carlon G, Howland WS, et al: High-frequency jet ventilation in major airway or pulmonary disruption. Ann Thorac Surg 32:468–474, 1981

60. Grebenik C: Anaesthetic management of malignant tracheo-esophageal fistula. Br J Anaesth 63:492–496, 1989

61. Mackie AM, Watson CB: Anaesthesia and mediastinal masses. Anaesthesia 39:899–903, 1984

62. Bray RJ, Fernandes FJ: Mediastinal tumour causing airway obstruction in anaesthetized children. Anaesthesia 37:571–575, 1982

63. Amaha K, Okutsu Y, Nakamuru Y: Major airway obstruction by mediastinal tumour. A case report. Br J Anaesth 45:1082–1084, 1973

63. Shambaugh BE, Seed R, Korn A: Airway obstruction in a substernal goiter. Clinical and therapeutic implications. J Chronic Dis 26:737–743, 1973

65. Piro AJ, Weiss DR, Hellman S: Mediastinal Hodgkin's disease: a possible danger for intubation anesthesia. Int J Radiat Oncol Biol Phys 1:415–419, 1976

66. Price SL, Hecker BR: Pulmonary oedema following airway obstruction in Hodgkin's disease. Br J Anaesth 59:518–521, 1987

67. Neuman GG, Weingarten AE, Abramowitz RM, et al: The anesthetic management of the patient with an anterior mediastinal mass. Anesthesiology 60:144–147, 1984

67a. Ferrari LR, Bedford RF: General anesthesia prior to treatment of anterior mediastinal masses in pediatric cancer patients. Anesthesiology 72:991–995, 1990

67b. Tinker TD, Crane DL: Safety of anesthesia for patients with anterior mediastinal masses: I (correspondence). Anesthesiology 73:1060, 1990

67c. Zornow MH, Benumof JL: Safety of anesthesia for patients with anterior mediastinal masses: II (correspondence). Anesthesiology 73:1061, 1990

68. Fletcher R, Nordstrom L: The effects on gas exchange of a large mediastinal tumor. Anaesthesia 41:1135–1138, 1986

69. Silbert KS, Biondi JW, Hirsch NP: Spontaneous respiration during thoracotomy in a patient with mediastinal mass. Anesth Analg 66:904–907, 1987

70. DeSoto H: Direct laryngoscopy as an aid to relieve airway obstruction in a patient with a mediastinal mass. Anesthesiology 67:116–118, 1987

71. Prakash UBS, Abel MD, Hubmay RD: Mediastinal mass and tracheal obstruction during general anesthesia. Mayo Clin Proc 63:1004–1007, 1988

72. Lokich JJ, Goodman R: Superior vena cava syndrome. Clinical management. JAMA 231:58–61, 1975

73. Tonnesen AS, Davis FG: Superior vena caval obstruction during anesthesia. Anesthesiology 45:912, 1976

74. Gutman JA, Haft JI: Mediastinal tumor presenting as a heart murmur: diagnosis and treatment. J Med Soc NJ 76:364–366, 1979

75. Hall DK, Friedman M: Extracorporeal oxygenation for induction of anesthesia in a patient with an intrathoracic tumor. Anesthesiology 42:493–495, 1975

76. Keon TP: Death on induction of anesthesia for cervical node biopsy. Anesthesiology 55:471–472, 1981

77. Canedo MI, Otken L, Stefadouros MA: Echocardiographic features of cardiac compression by a thymoma simulating cardiac tamponade and obstruction of the superior vena cava. Br Heart J 39:1038–1042, 1977

78. Benumof JL: Anesthesia for special elective therapeutic procedures. p. 366. In: Anesthesia for Thoracic Surgery. WB Saunders, Philadelphia, 1987

79. Steen SN: Superior vena cava obstruction during anesthesia. NY State J Med 69:2906–2907, 1969

80. Quong GG, Brigham BA: Anaesthetic complications of mediastinal masses and superior vena caval obstruction. Med J Aust 2:487–488, 1980

81. Osserman KE, Genkins G: Studies in myasthenia gravis—review of a 20-year experience in over 1200 patients. Mt Sinai J Med (NY) 38:862–863, 1971

82. Herrmann C, Lindstrom JM, Kessey JC, et al: Myasthenia gravis—current concepts. West J Med 142:797–809, 1985

83. Engel AG: Myasthenia gravis and myasthenic syndromes. Ann Neurol 16:516–534, 1984

84. Havard CWH, Scadding GK: Myasthenia gravis: pathogenesis and current concepts in management. Drugs 26:174–184, 1983

85. Kornfeld P, Horowitz SH, Genkins G, Papatestas AE: Myasthenia gravis unmasked by antiarrhythmic agents. Mt Sinai J Med (NY) 43:10–14, 1976

86. Elder BF, Beal H, DeWald W, Cobb S: Exacerbation of subclinical myasthenia by occupational exposure to an anesthetic. Anesth Analg 50:363–367, 1971

87. Wojciechowski APJ, Hanning CD, Pohl JEF: Postoperative apnoea and latent myasthenia gravis. Anaesthesia 39:51–53, 1985

88. Fambrough DM, Drachman DB, Satyamurti S: Neuromuscular junction in myasthenia gravis: decreased acetylcholine receptors. Science 182:293–295, 1973

89. Albuquerque EX, Rash JE, Meyer RF, Satterfield JR: An electrophysiological and morphological study of the neuromuscular junction in patients with myasthenia gravis. Exp Neurol 51:536–563, 1976

90. Paton WDM, Waud DR: The margin of safety of neuromuscular transmission. J Physiol 191:59–90, 1967

91. Lindstrom JM, Seybold ME, Lennon VA, et al: Antibody to acetylcholine receptor in myasthenia gravis: prevalence, clinical correlates and diagnostic value. Neurology 26:1054–1059, 1976

92. Tsujihata M, Hazama R, Ishii N, et al: Ultrastructural localization of acetylcholine receptor at the motor endplate: myasthenia gravis and other neuromuscular diseases. Neurology 30:1203–1211, 1980

93. Ozdemir C, Young RR: The results to be expected from electrical testing in the diagnosis of myasthenia gravis. Ann NY Acad Sci 274:203–222, 1976

94. Brown JC, Charlton JE: A study of sensitivity to curare in myasthenic disorders using a regional technique. J Neurol Neurosurg Psychiatry 38:27–33, 1975

95. Balestrieri FJ, Prough DS: Diagnostic value of systemic curare testing. Anesthesiology 57:226–227, 1982

96. Cohan SL, Pohlmann JLW, Mikszewski J, et al: The pharmacokinetics of pyridostigmine. Neurology 26:536–539, 1976

97. Glaser G: Crisis, precrisis and drug resistance in myasthenia gravis. Ann NY Acad Sci 135:335–345, 1966

98. Bolooki H, Schwartzman RJ: High-dose steroids for the perioperative management of patients with myasthenia gravis undergoing thymectomy. A preliminary report. J Thorac Cardiovasc Surg 75:754–757, 1978

99. Arsura E, Brunner NG, Namba T, Grob D: High-dose intravenous methylprednisolone in myasthenia gravis. Arch Neurol 42:1149–1153, 1985

100. Niakan E, Harati Y, Rolak LA: Immunosuppressive drug therapy in myasthenia gravis. Arch Neurol 43:155–156, 1986

101. Tindall RSA, Rollins JA, Phillips JT, et al: Preliminary results of a double-blind, randomized placebo-controlled trial of cyclosporine in myasthenia gravis. N Engl J Med 316:719–724, 1987

102. d'Empaire G, Hoaglin DC, Perlo VP, Pontoppidan H: Effect of prethymectomy plasma exchange on postoperative respiratory function in myasthenia gravis. J Thorac Cardiovasc Surg 89:592–596, 1985

103. Gracey DR, Howard FM, Divertie MB: Plasmapheresis in the treatment of ventilator-dependent myasthenia gravis patients. Report of four cases. Chest 85:739–743, 1984

104. Spence PA, Morin JE, Katz M: Role of plasmapheresis in preparing myasthenic patients for thymectomy: initial results. Can J Surg 27:303–305, 1984

105. Lumley J: Prolongation of suxamethonium following plasma exchange. Br J Anaesth 52:1149–1150, 1980

106. Blalock A, Mason MG, Morgan HJ, Riven SS: Myasthenia gravis and tumors of the thymic region. Ann Surg 110:544–561, 1939

107. Mulder DG, Graves M, Herrmann C: Thymectomy for myasthenia gravis: recent observations and comparisons with past experience. Ann Thorac Surg 48:551–555, 1989

108. Annoh T, Torisu M: Immunologic studies of myasthenia gravis II: a new chemotactic factor for lymphocytes found in patients with myasthenia gravis. Surgery 105:615–624, 1989

109. Buckingham JM, Howard FM, Bernatz PE, et al: The value of thymectomy in myasthenia gravis. A computer-assisted matched study. Ann Surg 184:453–458, 1976

110. Heiser JC, Rutherford RB, Fingel SP: Thymectomy for myasthenia gravis. A changing perspective. Arch Surg 117:533–537, 1982

111. Jaretski A, Bethea M, Wolff M, et al: A rational approach to total thymectomy in the treatment of myasthenia gravis. Ann Thorac Surg 24:120–130, 1977

112. Papatestas AE, Genkins G, Kornfeld P: Comparison of the results of transcervical and transsternal thymectomy in myasthenia gravis. Ann NY Acad Sci 377:766–778, 1981

113. Donnelly RJ, LaQuaglia MP, Fabir B, et al: Cervical thymectomy in the treatment of myasthenia gravis. Ann R Coll Surg Engl 66:305–308, 1984

114. Nilsson E, Meretoja DA: Force and EMG responses of vecuronium in myasthenia gravis. Anesthesiology 71:A812, 1989

115. Viby-Mogensen J, Jensen E, Werner M, et al: Measurement of acceleration: a new method of monitoring neuromuscular function. Acta Anaesth Scand 32:45–48, 1987

116. Weber S: Integrated electromyography: is it the new standard for clinical monitoring of neuromuscular blockade? Int J Clin Monit Comput 4:53–57, 1987

117. Eisenkraft JB, Papatestas AE, Sivak M: Neuromuscular effects of halogenated agents in patients with myasthenia gravis. Anesthesiology, suppl. 61:A307, 1984

118. Rowbottom SJ: Isoflurane for thymectomy in myasthenia gravis. Anaesth Intensive Care 17:444–447, 1989

119. Lebowitz MH, Blitt CD, Walts LF: Depression of twitch response to stimulation of the ulnar nerve during Ethrane anesthesia in man. Anesthesiology 33:52–57, 1970

120. Ward S, Wright DJ: Neuromuscular blockade in myasthenia gravis with atracurium besylate. Anaesthesia 62:692–694, 1984

121. Nilsson E, Muller K: Neuromuscular effects of isoflurane in patients with myasthenia gravis. Acta Anaesthesiol Scand 34:126–131, 1990

122. Baraka A, Afifi A, Muallem M, et al: Neuromuscular effects of halothane, suxamethonium and tubocurarine in a myasthenic undergoing thymectomy. Br J Anaesth 43:91–94, 1971

123. Stanski DR, Lee RF, MacCannell KL, et al: Atypical cholinesterase in a patient with myasthenia gravis. Anesthesiology 46:298–301, 1977

124. Wainwright AP, Brodrick PM: Suxamethonium in myasthenia gravis. Anaesthesia 42:950–957, 1987

125. Eisenkraft JB, Book WJ, Mann SM, et al: Resistance to succinylcholine in myasthenia gravis. A dose-response study. Anesthesiology 69:760–763, 1988

126. Foldes FF, Nagashima H: Myasthenia gravis and anesthesia. pp. 171–203. In Oyama T (ed): Endocrinology and the Anaesthetist. Monographs in Anaesthesiology. Vol. 2. Elsevier Science Publishing, New York, 1984

127. Ginsberg H, Varejes L: The use of a relaxant in myasthenia gravis. Anaesthesia 10:177–178, 1955

128. Miller JD, Lee C: Muscle diseases. p. 619. In Katz J, Benumof JL, Kadis LB (eds): Anesthesia and Uncommon Diseases. WB Saunders, Philadelphia, 1990

129. Azar I: The response of patients with neuromuscular disorders to muscle relaxants: a review. Anesthesiology 61:173–187, 1984

130. Foldes FF, McNall PG: Myasthenia gravis: a guide for anesthesiologists. Anesthesiology 23:837–872, 1962

131. Bell CF, Florence AM, Hunter JM, et al: Atracurium in the myasthenic patient. Anaesthesia 39:961–968, 1984

132. Smith CE, Donati F, Bevan DR: Cumulative dose-response curves for atracurium in patients with myasthenia gravis. Can J Anaesth 36:402–406, 1989

133. Eisenkraft JB: Myasthenia gravis and thymic surgery—anaesthetic considerations. pp. 133–162. In Gothard JW (ed): Thoracic Anaesthesia. Bailliere-Tindall, London, 1987

134. Hunter JM, Bell CF, Florence AM, et al: Vecuronium in the myasthenic patient. Anaesthesia 40:848–853, 1985

135. Eisenkraft JB, Book WJ, Papatestas AE: Sensitivity to vecuronium in myasthenia gravis—a dose-response study. Can J Anaesth 37:301–306, 1990

136. Buzello W, Noeldge G, Krieg N, et al: Vecuronium for muscle relaxation in patients with myasthenia gravis. Anesthesiology 64:507–509, 1986

136a. Nilsson E, Meretoja OA: Vecuronium dose-response and maintenance requirements in patients with myasthenia gravis. Anesthesiology 73:28–32, 1990

137. Lake CL: Curare sensitivity in steroid-treated myasthenia gravis. Anesth Analg 57:132–134, 1978

138. Fillmore RB, Herren AL, Perlo AF: Curare sensitivity in myasthenia gravis. Anesth Analg 57:515–516, 1978

139. Lumb AR, Calder I: 'Cured' myasthenia gravis and neuromuscular blockade. Anaesthesia 44:828–830, 1989

140. Abel M, Eisenkraft JB, Patel N: Sensitivity to succinylcholine in myasthenia gravis during true remission: a dose-effect study. Anaesthesia 43:30–32, 1991

141. Florence AM: Anaesthesia for transcervical thymectomy in myasthenia gravis. Ann R Coll Surg Engl 66:309–312, 1984

142. Burgess FW, Wilcosky B: Thoracic epidural anesthesia for transsternal thymectomy in myasthenia gravis. Anesth Analg 69:529–531, 1989

143. Gorback MS: Analgesic management after thymectomy. Anesthesiol Rep 2:262–266, 1990

144. Mora CT, Eisenkraft JB, Papatestas AE: Intravenous dantrolene in a patient with myasthenia gravis. Anesthesiology 64:371–373, 1986

145. Gracey DR, Divertie MB, Howard FM: Mechanical ventilation for respiratory failure in myasthenia gravis. Two years' experience with 22 patients. Mayo Clin Proc 85:739–743, 1983

146. Mulder DG, Herrmann C, Buckberg GB: Effect of thymectomy in patients with myasthenia gravis. Am J Surg 128:202–206, 1974

147. Loach AB, Young AC, Spalding JMK, et al: Postoperative management after thymectomy. Br Med J 1:309–312, 1975

148. Leventhal R, Orkin FK, Hirsch RA: Prediction of the need for postoperative mechanical ventilation in myasthenia gravis. Anesthesiology 53:26–30, 1980

149. Orkin FK, Leventhal SR, Hirsch RA: Predicting respiratory failure following thymectomy. Ann NY Acad Sci 377:862–863, 1981

150. Grant RP, Jenkins LC: Prediction of the need for postoperative mechanical ventilation in myasthenia gravis. Can Anaesth Soc J 29:112–116, 1982

151. Gracey DR, Divertie MB, Howard FM, Payne WS: Postoperative respiratory care after transsternal thymectomy in myasthenia gravis. A three-year experience in 53 patients. Chest 86:67–71, 1984

152. Eisenkraft JB, Papatestas AE, Kahn CH, et al: Predicting the need for postoperative mechanical ventilation in myasthenia gravis. Anesthesiology 65:79–82, 1986

153. Younger DS, Braun NMT, Jaretzki A, et al: Myasthenia gravis: determinants for independent ventilation after transsternal thymectomy. Neurology 34:336–340, 1984

154. Pavlin EG, Holle RH, Schoene RB: Recovery of airway protection compared with ventilation in humans after paralysis with curare. Anesthesiology 70:381–385, 1989

155. Ringqvist I, Ringqvist T: Respiratory mechanics in untreated myasthenia gravis with special reference to the respiratory forces. Acta Med Scand 190:499–508, 1971

156. Donnelly RH, LaQuaglia MP, Fabri B, et al: Cervical thymectomy in the treatment of myasthenia gravis. Ann R Coll Surg Engl 66:305–308, 1984

157. Eisenkraft JB, Papatestas AE, Pozner JN, et al: Prediction of ventilatory failure following transcervical thymectomy in myasthenia gravis. Ann NY Acad Sci 505:888–890, 1987

158. Redfern N, McQuillan PJ, Conacher I, Pearson DT: Anaesthesia for transsternal thymectomy in myasthenia gravis. Ann R Coll Surg Engl 68:289–292, 1987

159. Eisenkraft JB, Papatestas AE: Anaesthesia for trans-

sternal thymectomy in myasthenia gravis. Ann R Coll Surg Engl 70:257–258, 1988

160. Gracey DR, Howard FM, Divertie MB: Plasmapheresis in the treatment of ventilator-dependent myasthenia gravis patients. Report of four cases. Chest 85:739–743

161. d'Empaire G, Hoaglin DC, Perlo VP, Pontoppidan H: Effect of prethymectomy plasma exchange on postoperative respiratory function in myasthenia gravis. J Thorac Cardiovasc Surg 89:592–596, 1985

162. Spence PA, Morin JE, Katz M: Role of plasmapheresis in preparing myasthenic patients for thymectomy. Initial results. Can J Surg 27:303–305, 1984

163. Bolooki H, Schwartzman RJ: High-dose steroids for the perioperative management of patients with myasthenia gravis undergoing thymectomy. A preliminary report. J Thorac Cardiovasc Surg 75:754–757, 1978

164. Pandit SK, Kothary S, Orringer M: Preoperative anticholinesterase therapy in myasthenic patients for thymectomy, abstracted. Anaesthesia, suppl. 1982

165. Slaughter D: Neostigmine and opiate analgesia. Arch Int Pharmacodyn Ther 83:143–148, 1950

166. Mulder DG, Graves M, Herrmann C: Thymectomy for myasthenia gravis. Observations and comparisons with past experience. Ann Thorac Surg 48:551–555, 1989

167. Oosterhuis HJ: Observations of the natural history of myasthenia gravis and the effect of thymectomy. Ann NY Acad Sci 377:679–690, 1981

168. Papatestas AE, Genkins G, Kornfeld P: The relationship between the thymus and oncogenesis. A study of the incidence of non-thymic malignancy in myasthenia gravis. Br J Cancer 24:635–645, 1971

169. Vessey MP, Doll R: Thymectomy and cancer. Br J Cancer 26:53–58, 1972

170. O'Neill JH, Murray NMF, Newsom-Davis J: The Lambert-Eaton myasthenic syndrome. A review of 50 cases. Brain 111:577–596, 1988

171. Anderson HJ, Churchill-Davidson HC, Richardson AT: Bronchial neoplasm with myasthenia; prolonged apnoea after administration of succinylcholine. Lancet 2:1291–1292, 1953

172. Lambert EH, Eaton LM, Rooke ED: Defect of neuromuscular transmission associated with malignant neoplasm. Am J Physiol 178:612–613, 1956

173. Fukunaga H, Engel AG, Osame M, Lambert EH: Paucity and disorganization of presynaptic membrane active zones in the Lambert-Eaton myasthenic syndrome. Muscle Nerve 5:686–697, 1982

174. Lang B, Newson-Davis J, Wray D, Vincent A: Autoimmune aetiology for myasthenic syndrome. Lancet 2:224–226, 1981

175. Elmquist D, Lambert EH: Detailed analysis of neuromuscular transmission in a patient with the myasthenic syndrome sometimes associated with bronchogenic carcinoma. Mayo Clin Proc 43:689–713, 1968

176. Vizi ES, van Dijk, Foldes FF: The effect of 4-aminopyridine on acetylcholine release. J Neural Transm 41:265–274, 1975

177. Lundh H: Effects of 4-aminopyridines on neuromuscular transmission. Brain Res 153:307–318, 1978

178. Norris FH, Eaton JM, Nielke CH: Depression of bone marrow by guanidine. Arch Neurol 30:184–185, 1974

179. Takamori M: Calcium, caffeine and Eaton-Lambert syndrome. Arch Neurol 27:285–291, 1972

180. Cherington M: Guanidine and germine in Eaton-Lambert syndrome. Neurology 26:944–946, 1976

181. Agoston S, VanWeeden T, Westra P, et al: Effects of 4-aminopyridine in Eaton-Lambert syndrome. Br J Anaesth 50:383–385, 1978

182. Lundh H, Nilsson D, Rosen I: Novel drug of choice in Eaton-Lambert syndrome. J Neurol Neurosurg Psychiatry 46:684–685, 1983

183. Wise RP: A myasthenic syndrome complicating bronchial carcinoma. Anaesthesia 17:488–504, 1962

184. Telford RJ, Hollway TE: The myasthenic syndrome: anaesthesia in a patient treated with 3.4 diaminopyridine. Br J Anaesth 64:363–366, 1990

185. Brim JD: Denervation supersensitivity. The response to depolarizing muscle relaxants. Br J Anaesth 45:222–226, 1973

186. Orringer MB: Historical aspects and anatomy. pp. 698–773. In Sabiston D, Jr (ed): Textbook of Surgery. WB Saunders, Philadelphia, 1986

16

ANESTHETIC MANAGEMENT OF THERAPEUTIC PROCEDURES OF THE LUNGS AND AIRWAY

James B. Eisenkraft, M.D.
Steven M. Neustein, M.D.

The anesthetic considerations for and the management of therapeutic procedures involving the lungs and airway are reviewed in this chapter. These procedures include pulmonary resection (lobectomy, pneumonectomy); management of bronchopleural fistula and empyema, lung cysts, and bullae; bronchopulmonary lavage; airway hemorrhage; and laser surgery of airway tumors.

PULMONARY RESECTION

The number of noncardiac thoracic operations performed annually in the United States has been estimated to be 120,000 to 130,000 cases per year in the 1980s, and is expected to be even greater in the 1990s.[1] Pulmonary resection is the most commonly performed of all of the major thoracic procedures done today. Due to a higher morbidity and mortality associated with pneumonectomy and a similar prognosis following either pneumonectomy or lobectomy, this parenchyma-saving resection has replaced pneumonectomy as the operation of choice when the primary tumor can be removed without a pneumonectomy. Due to advances in both thoracic surgical and anesthetic techniques, pulmonary resections are now being performed on high-risk patients who were previously considered inoperable.

Perioperative Considerations

Dysrhythmias

Cardiac dysrhythmias occur frequently in the perioperative period of pulmonary resections. The incidence of dysrhythmias is increased in patients over 50 years of age who have had pulmonary resections, and is greater following right pneumonectomy as com-

419

pared with left pneumonectomy. One retrospective review of 236 patients who had undergone pneumonectomy indicated a 22 percent incidence of perioperative dysrhythmias, with atrial fibrillation being the most common (64 percent).[2] Fifty-five percent of the dysrhythmias became recurrent or persistent, and 31 percent of these patients died during hospitalization. Tachyarrhythmias occurred more often in patients who had undergone pericardial dissection or who developed pulmonary edema. In this study, none of the patients had received prophylactic digitalis prior to undergoing surgery.[2]

Routine preoperative digitalization has been reported to reduce the incidence of cardiac dysrhythmias.[3,4] If atrial fibrillation does occur in this setting, it will probably be at a slower rate. If digitalis is administered prophylactically, the patient should ideally be underdigitalized since if a dysrhythmia does occur, it may be difficult to distinguish from digitalis toxicity. Esmolol can be useful for treatment of a tachyarrhythmia that occurs intraoperatively in the digitalized patient. In a recent controlled prospective randomized study of 140 consecutive patients for thoracic surgery, the authors reported no benefit from preoperative digitalization.[4a] Preoperative prophylactic digitalization remains a controversial issue (see Chapter 3).

Monitoring

Patients scheduled to undergo a lobectomy or pneumonectomy for neoplasm should have an arterial catheter placed for continuous measurement of blood pressure and intermittent arterial blood sampling. A pulse oximeter is essential for continuous monitoring of oxygen saturation during one-lung anesthesia, during which hypoxemia may occur. A central venous catheter will provide central access for rapid delivery of medications should dysrhythmias or hypotension occur. The central venous pressure will also serve as a guide to fluid administration. A pulmonary arterial catheter may also be beneficial during a pneumonectomy to measure the pulmonary arterial pressure following ligation of one pulmonary artery, to guide fluid therapy, and to measure cardiac output. The decision as to whether to place a central venous catheter or a pulmonary arterial catheter should be based on the cardiac status of the patient and the likelihood of pneumonectomy, and is an individualized decision.

Choice of Endotracheal Tube

A double-lumen endobronchial tube will facilitate surgical exposure by allowing collapse of the ipsilateral lung. The presence of this tube will also permit suctioning of secretions and blood. There are different approaches regarding the choice of a right- or left-sided tube. Since, in adults, the distance from the left upper lobe bronchus to the carina (4 to 5 cm) is greater than the distance from the carina to the right upper lobe bronchus (2 to 3 cm), some clinicians prefer to always place a left-sided double-lumen tube unless there is disease of the left mainstem bronchus. This will decrease the chances of obstructing the upper lobe bronchus. If a left pneumonectomy is to be performed, the bronchial catheter must be withdrawn into the trachea prior to division of the bronchus.

Another option is to place the endobronchial tube into the nonoperative side. This will avoid the possibility of placing the tube into a potentially diseased bronchus, and will eliminate the need to withdraw the tube if a pneumonectomy is to be performed. However, if the tube obstructs the upper lobe bronchial orifice, there is likely to be hypoxemia during one-lung ventilation since this is the lung being ventilated during one-lung anesthesia. This is most likely to occur during use of a right-sided tube for a left thoracotomy (see Chapter 14).

Yet a third approach is to place the endobronchial tube into the operated side. Following positioning of the patient for the surgery in the lateral decubitus position with the diseased lung uppermost, the tube will be in the nondependent lung. In this case, even if the tube is too distal and obstructs the upper lobe, this lung will be collapsed in any case during one-lung anesthesia and is less likely to cause hypoxemia. With the chest open, direct visual inspection of lung movement can facilitate endobronchial tube positioning.

Intraoperative Considerations and Management

Most pulmonary resections are performed with the patient in the lateral decubitus position, using a posterolateral incision that extends from the anterior axillary line at the point where the surgeon plans to enter the chest, usually in the fifth intercostal space. The incision continues posteriorly and inferiorly to the angle of the scapula, and then superiorly midway between the medial edge of the scapula and the vertebral column. After transecting the muscle layers of the chest wall, the surgeon enters the pleural space by either resecting a rib or entering through an intercostal space. Prior to surgical entry into the pleura, the anesthesiologist should deflate the lung to prevent injury and bleeding. Lung resection or pneumonectomy involves ligation of the arterial supply, venous drainage, and the bronchus of the affected lobe or lung. The upper lobes are those most commonly resected, the right more frequently than the left. If a pulmonary arterial catheter has been placed in a patient undergoing a pneumonectomy, it is essential that the catheter not be in the artery when it is ligated. Unless the catheter is known to lie in the contralateral artery (most often, it floats into the right pulmonary artery), it must be withdrawn prior to ligation of the artery, after which it can be floated back into position. It is also necessary to withdraw the distal tip of an ipsilateral endobronchial tube into the trachea. This must be done very carefully so that the trachea does not become extubated. Urgent need for reintubation with the patient in the lateral decubitus position is highly undesirable.

It is usually not necessary to administer blood for a lobectomy or pneumonectomy, but blood should be cross-matched and available. Blood loss may be extensive during pleuropneumonectomy, pleurectomy, or decortication for mesothelioma, and the patient is likely to require transfusion of blood for these procedures. Assessment of blood loss and measurement of central venous pressure and hematocrit provide a guide to fluid and blood administration. The fluids should be warmed since the temperature of the patient will tend to decrease during thoracic surgery. Patients are at increased risk of developing pulmonary edema following lung resection due to a decreased pulmonary vascular reserve.[5] Fluids should, therefore, be administered cautiously, especially during and following a pneumonectomy. Fluid overload in the presence of a decreased pulmonary vascular reserve may also lead to right atrial distention and tachyarrhythmias.

General anesthesia can be maintained with oxygen, a potent inhaled agent, and muscle paralysis to prevent patient movement. The addition of nitrous oxide following one-lung anesthesia may expedite extubation by allowing the use of lesser amounts of a potent inhaled agent. If possible, the patient should receive intrathecal or epidural narcotics to provide postoperative analgesia and also improve postoperative pulmonary function. If this is done just prior to the surgical incision, there may also be a decreased anesthetic requirement,[6] which may facilitate earlier extubation. In addition, prior to chest closure, the surgeon can place intercostal nerve blocks or an interpleural catheter under direct vision for delivery of local anesthetic into the interpleural space to supplement postoperative pain management. Interpleural bupivacaine administration has been reported to provide analgesia following nonthoracic surgery, such as cholecystectomy, unilateral breast surgery, and renal surgery.[7–11] Following thoracic surgery, the results have been mixed.[12,13] The catheter should be placed posteriorly for better pain relief,[9] and the chest tube clamped for 20 minutes following the injection of lo-

cal anesthetic to limit loss via the chest tube(s). The addition of epinephrine to the bupivacaine may have the beneficial effect of delaying absorption and minimizing plasma levels of bupivacaine[9] (see Chapter 21).

Prior to reinflation of any remaining lung tissue, the appropriate lumen of the endobronchial tube should be suctioned clear of secretions and blood. Following division of the bronchus, the suture line is tested by applying 20 to 40 cmH$_2$O pressure to the airway by compressing the anesthesia reservoir bag.

Before closing the chest of a patient who has undergone a lobectomy, thoracostomy tubes are placed for drainage of air and fluid. Two tubes are usually placed, one anteriorly in the apex for drainage of air and one posteriorly at the base for drainage of fluid. The chest tubes are connected to underwater seals with negative 15 to 20 cmH$_2$O pressure of suction. After placement of sutures in the chest, but before the chest is closed, the remaining lung is re-expanded under direct vision to assure adequate re-expansion.

Following a pneumonectomy, thoracostomy tubes are usually not placed since there is no remaining lung tissue to re-expand. The use of nitrous oxide once the chest is closed may lead to a tension pneumothorax since the remaining intrathoracic space is closed without the presence of chest tubes. Immediately following the procedure, air is aspirated from the pleural cavity percutaneously to apply negative 4 to 8 cmH$_2$O of subatmospheric pressure to the postpneumonectomy thoracic cavity space. The mediastinum should then be midline or slightly shifted toward the operated side. If a small catheter has been left in the postpneumonectomy space, the position of the mediastinum can be adjusted by either aspiration or injection of air into this space prior to removal of the catheter.

The decision as to whether to extubate the trachea immediately following surgery or to delay extubation is individualized, depending on the patient's temperature, duration of surgery, hemodynamic stability, extent of surgery, and severity of pulmonary dysfunction. Return to spontaneous ventilation will lessen an air leak from the lung and allow for less stress on the bronchial suture line. If the patient is to remain intubated at the end of the procedure, reintubation with a single-lumen tube is necessary to replace the double-lumen tube. Since the tissue may now be edematous, this may be difficult. If the trachea was difficult to intubate at the beginning of the procedure, being that it may now be even more difficult, it may be advisable to change the tube over a guide or a flexible fiberoptic bronchoscope, or not change the tube at all. Ventilator pressure limits and tidal volume should be set to avoid suture line dehiscence.

BRONCHOPLEURAL FISTULA AND EMPYEMA

A bronchopleural fistula (BPF) is an abnormal communication between the bronchial tree and the pleural cavity. A bronchopleural-cutaneous fistula is present when there is additional communication to the skin on the surface of the chest. Bronchopleural fistulae arise most often following lung resection for carcinoma. Other etiologies include traumatic rupture of a bronchus or a bulla, sometimes due to barotrauma, penetrating wounds, or spontaneous drainage into the bronchial tree of an empyema cavity or a lung cyst. The incidence of fistula is greater following pneumonectomy than following other types of lung resection.

The anesthetic considerations associated with BPF and empyema are that positive-pressure ventilation may result in contamination of healthy lung, loss of gas, decreased alveolar ventilation resulting in hypoventilation and increased $PaCO_2$, and the possible development of a tension pneumothorax.

Anesthesia Considerations

An empyema (a collection of pus in the pleural space), if present, should be drained first under local anesthesia before any surgery is undertaken close to the BPF. Drainage is performed with the patient in the sitting position and leaning toward the affected side. Drainage to an underwater seal system is inserted into the empyema cavity prior to the induction of anesthesia for surgery to the fistula, although it should be recognized that the fluid collections are loculated and complete drainage may not always be possible. Following drainage, an x-ray of the chest should be obtained to assess the efficacy of the procedure.

The primary consideration in the anesthetic management of a patient with a BPF is the isolation of the affected side in terms of contamination and ventilation. The ideal approach is an awake intubation using a double-lumen tube while the patient breathes spontaneously. Supplemental oxygen should be given and the patient constantly reassured. Neuroleptanalgesia provides a suitably cooperative patient and the airway is then treated with local anesthetic. The double-lumen tube selected should be such that the bronchial lumen is on the side opposite to the fistula. The largest possible tube size should be used to permit a close fit in the trachea, which helps to stabilize the tube. Once the tube is adequately positioned and the healthy lung isolated by inflation of the bronchial cuff, there may be a massive outpouring of pus from the tracheal lumen if an empyema is present; therefore, the tracheal lumen should be immediately suctioned using a wide-bore catheter. The healthy lung and, possibly, the affected lung may then be ventilated. Adequacy of oxygenation is assessed by pulse oximetry and ventilation by capnometry, and both should be checked by arterial blood gas analysis.

An alternative technique is to insert the double-lumen tube with the patient under general anesthesia and breathing spontaneously to avoid development of a tension pneumothorax. With either of the two techniques described, awake or asleep, the chest drainage tube should be left unclamped to avoid any bouts of coughing and the development of a tension pneumothorax if a predisposing valvular mechanism exists. In the absence of an empyema, a single-lumen tube may be adequate if the fistula and its air leak are small.

Bronchopleural fistula may also be treated conservatively using various techniques of specialized ventilation. The bronchus of the normal lung may be intubated and ventilated with a single-lumen tube, permitting the fistula to rest and heal. This approach, however, may result in intolerable venous admixture and hypoxemia, and positive end-expiratory pressure (PEEP) may be necessary to maintain adequate oxygenation. Differential lung ventilation using a double-lumen tube has also been used, the healthy lung being ventilated with normal tidal volumes, while the affected side was ventilated with smaller volumes or continuous positive airway pressure (CPAP) with oxygen using pressures just below the critical opening pressure of the fistula.[14] The critical opening pressure may be estimated by determining the level of CPAP at which continuous bubbling appears in the underwater seal chest drainage system. If a single-lumen endotracheal tube has been used and, following opening of the chest, an excessive air leak is found from the fistula, the patient's ventilation may be increased by packing the lung and manually controlling the leak.[15]

In those patients with large BPF, high-frequency jet ventilation (HFJV) may be the nonsurgical treatment of choice.[16] The use of small ventilatory volumes and low pressures results in minimal loss of gas through the fistula, which may, therefore, heal more quickly. The hemodynamics of HFJV are usually minimal and the patient's spontaneous ventilatory efforts are usually abolished, thereby decreasing the work of breathing and avoiding the requirement for muscle relaxants or heavy sedation.

High-frequency jet ventilation may not always be superior to conventional ventilation in the conservative management of patients with a BPF.[17] It has been reported that HFJV was less effective in reducing the ventilatory leak through a BPF when the peripheral leak was combined with severe injury and decreased compliance in the remainder of the lung than when only the airway had been disrupted.[17] In the seven patients reported, HFJV was compared with conventional intermittent positive-pressure ventilation (IPPV), and it was found that adequate gas exchange could not be achieved at comparable mean airway pressures using HFJV, although peak airway pressures were decreased. In some cases, gas flow through the fistula actually increased during HFJV. The investigators concluded that HFJV should be used selectively in patients with bronchopleural fistula.[17]

Whichever mode of ventilation and tube drainage system is being used, it is recommended that the therapeutic approach be evaluated continuously, monitoring the flow of gas passing through the chest drainage system. This may be accomplished by placing a flow sensor into the drainage system.[18] Such measurement permits the on-line titration of ventilatory tidal volume and PEEP.[19]

LUNG CYSTS AND BULLAE

Air-containing cysts of the lung are usually categorized as bronchogenic, postinfective, infantile, or emphysematous.[20–22] They can occur in association with chronic obstructive pulmonary disease (COPD), or may represent an isolated finding. A bulla is a thin-walled space, filled with air, that results from the destruction of alveolar tissue. The walls of the space are composed of visceral pleura, connective tissue septa, or compressed lung parenchyma. In general, bullae represent an area of end-stage emphysematous destruction of the lung. In most patients, the bullae expand with age. Due to a one-way valve-like mechanism, more and more air becomes trapped within the cavity. The bullae can inflate, but, because distention compresses their opening, they are unable to deflate. Expansion of cysts or bullae causes progressively decreasing exercise tolerance as the healthy lung parenchyma is compressed (Figure 16-1). Other complications include infections and recurrent pneumothoraxes.

Indications for surgical bullectomy include incapacitating dyspnea, when the bullae are expanding (giant bullae), when there are repeated pneumothoraxes due to rupture of bullae, or when the bullae compress a significant amount of normal lung ("disappearing lung"). Functional impairment of compressed lung tissue can be assumed if radioisotope studies show that the compressed lung tissue has good perfusion but reduced ventilation.[23,24]

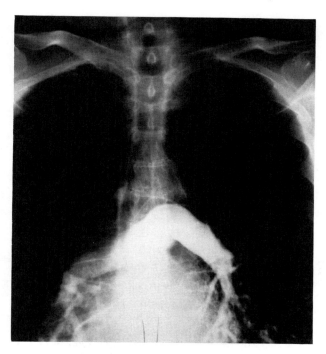

Fig. 16-1. Chest x-ray showing bilateral giant bullous disease. Note hyperlucency of lung fields bilaterally.

Anesthesia Considerations

Most of the affected patients have severe COPD and carbon dioxide retention with little functional reserve. They should receive a high F_IO_2, and, when the bulla or cyst is known to communicate with the bronchial tree, positive-pressure ventilation should be used cautiously since the bulla will expand if it is compliant, compressing normal lung tissue, and it may even rupture. The latter event would produce a situation analogous to a tension pneumothorax. The larger the bulla, the more compliant it becomes, which is an illustration of the law of Laplace: the distending pressure inside a bulla is given as $P = 2T/R$, where T is the surface tension and R is the radius.[25] When the air space communicates with the bronchial tree, much of the tidal volume delivered by IPPV may enter the space, representing wasted ventilation and an increase in alveolar dead space. Nitrous oxide should be avoided because this gas causes expansion of all air spaces, including bullae.[26] Once the patient's chest has been opened, even more of the delivered tidal volume may enter the compliant bulla, whose expansion is no longer limited by the integrity of the chest wall. An increase in minute ventilation is, therefore, needed until surgical control of the bulla has been obtained.

The ideal anesthetic management of the patient presenting for bullectomy involves insertion of a double-lumen endobronchial tube while the patient is awake or under general anesthesia and breathing spontaneously. Avoidance of positive-pressure ventilation decreases the likelihood of the problem cited above, although it must be remembered that oxygenation may be somewhat precarious during spontaneous ventilation. Once the double-lumen tube has been inserted and placed correctly, each lung may be controlled separately and adequate ventilation can be delivered to the healthy lung provided that the bullous disease is not bilateral. Positive-pressure ventilation with small tidal volume delivered at a rapid rate and pressures < 10 cmH$_2$O may be used during the induction and maintenance of anesthesia, especially if a preoperative ventilation scan has shown that the bullae have little or no bronchial communication. When positive-pressure ventilation is used, the anesthesiologist must be prepared to identify and treat any pneumothorax if it should arise. Signs of a pneumothorax may be decreased or absent breath sounds (often decreased already on the side affected by bullae), increase in airway pressure, wheezing, tracheal shift, cyanosis, and hemodynamic deterioration due to mediastinal shift and kinking of the great vessels. While a chest-tube insertion kit should be immediately available, dangers of insertion should be considered. The most important is that if the bulla communicates with the bronchial tree, a large bronchopleural cutaneous fistula would be created, resulting in problems with positive-pressure ventilation. In addition, if the pneumothorax is localized, it may be difficult to drain.

An alternative approach to management in the patient with bilateral bullae is that general anesthesia is induced only after the surgeon has prepared the operative field and draped the patient. If the patient's condition should deteriorate acutely during the induction, the surgeon can make an immediate median sternotomy. In either case, the time from induction of anesthesia to sternotomy should be kept to a minimum.

To avoid the problems associated with conventional positive-pressure ventilation, HFJV has been used in a patient with a large bulla scheduled to undergo coronary artery bypass grafting[20] and in another patient undergoing bilateral bullectomy.[27] Indeed, with a double-lumen tube in place, any combination of differential ventilatory modes can be applied to each lung, as indicated. Also, during the course of surgery, as each bulla is resected, the operated lung can be separately ventilated to check for air leaks and the coexistence of additional bullae.

In patients undergoing bilateral bullectomy, a median sternotomy is generally used, together with the use of sequential one-lung ventilation via a double-lumen tube.[28] The side with the largest bulla and least lung function should be assessed preoperatively by V/Q scanning, and this side should be operated on first. In this way, the lung with the better function supports gas exchange first. If hypoxemia should develop during one-lung ventilation, CPAP may be applied to the nonventilated lung during the deflation phase of a tidal breath to improve PaO$_2$.

When no respiratory reserve exists, PaO$_2$ may not be adequately maintained during one-lung ventilation. In such a situation, the use of an extracorporeal oxygenator with femoro-femoral bypass may be required. In such a case, the required heparinization would represent an additional surgical problem. Another approach to such a severe situation might be the use of a hyperbaric operating chamber where oxygenation could be assured and where the cyst or bulla would decrease in size under the conditions of increased ambient pressure.

Unlike most patients who have undergone pulmonary resection, after bullectomy, patients are left with a greater amount of functional lung tissue than was available to them preoperatively, and the mechanics of respiration should be improved. On completion of the surgery, the double-lumen tube is replaced by a single-lumen tube and patients generally require several days to be weaned from the respirator.[29] During this recovery period, the positive airway pressures used should be kept to a minimum to avoid causing a pneumothorax due to rupture of suture or staple lines or any residual bullae. The prognosis for patients who have undergone bullectomy for bullous emphysema is generally favorable.[25] The postoperative improvement in lung function depends on the type of bullae. In cases in which there was communication between the air space and a bronchus or bronchiole, a decrease in airways resistance (ie, increase in the ratio of forced expiratory volume at 1 second to forced vital capacity [FEV$_1$/FVC ratio]) resulted. In those patients who had resection of closed air spaces, bullectomy resulted in an increase in lung capacity.[30]

In another study, the most consistent changes in lung function following bullectomy were an increase in PaO$_2$ and a decrease in functional residual capacity because the patient's tidal volume was no longer entering the alveolar dead space of bullae but was now actively participating in gas exchange.[31]

The prognosis after surgery depends on the patient's age, history of smoking, condition of the nonbullous lung (in the case of unilateral bullectomy), cardiac status (cor pulmonale, coronary artery disease), extent of bronchitis and lung infection, and postoperative complications.[32] In spite of these problems, many patients have demonstrated marked improvement in their exercise tolerance following surgery,[33] in some cases for many years.[34]

ANESTHESIA FOR BRONCHOPULMONARY LAVAGE

Bronchopulmonary lavage is a therapeutic procedure involving irrigation of the lung and bronchial tree. It is used as a treatment for alveolar proteinosis, inhalation of radioactive dust, cystic fibrosis, bronchiectasis, and asthmatic bronchitis. The procedure is performed under general anesthesia using a double-lumen tube so that one lung can be ventilated while the other is being treated with lavage fluid.[35]

Lavage improves patients with alveolar proteinosis by removing lipoproteinaceous material (thought to be surfactant), which accumulates in abnormal amounts due to failure of clearance mechanisms.[36,37] The diagnosis of alveolar proteinosis is made by a history of dyspnea, chest x-ray appearance of consolidation, and results of lung biopsy. Indications for therapeutic lung lavage include a $PaO_2 < 60$ mmHg while resting or limited activity due to hypoxemia.[38]

Anesthetic Management

The preoperative assessment of patients scheduled for lavage should include $\dot{V}/\dot{Q}$ scans to identify the more severely affected lung. Lavage is performed first on the more severely affected side, while the healthier lung is used to provide oxygenation and ventilation. If both lungs are assessed to be equally involved, the left lung should be lavaged first because gas exchange should be better through the larger right lung. Measurements of diffusing capacity may also be helpful in terms of establishing a baseline and following subsequent progress. The patients are usually premedicated lightly if there is evidence of respiratory compromise, and they should be provided with supplementary oxygen during transit to the operating room.

General anesthesia is usually induced using an intravenous agent, and is maintained with a potent inhaled agent in oxygen to maximize the F_IO_2. Insertion and placement of a double-lumen endobronchial tube is facilitated by muscle relaxation; once the tube is positioned, it should be checked, ideally using a fiberoptic bronchoscope (Fig. 16-2). The cuff seal on the bronchial catheter should be tested to ensure perfect separation of the lungs at a pressure of 50 cmH$_2$O to prevent leakage of lavage fluid around the cuff (Fig. 16-3). The position of the tube, cuff seal, and adequacy

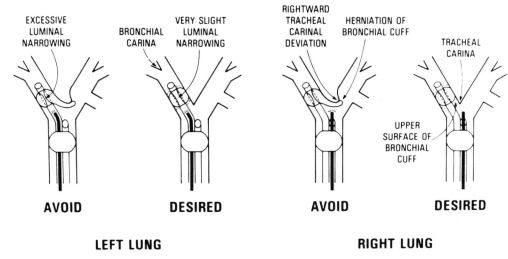

Fig. 16-2. Use of fiberoptic bronchoscopy to determine double-lumen tube position and adequacy of cuff seal. When the bronchoscope is passed down the right lumen, a clear straight-ahead view of the tracheal carina is seen, and the upper surface of the bronchial cuff just below the tracheal carina should be apparent. Excessive pressure in the bronchial cuff as manifested by tracheal carinal deviation to the right and herniation of the bronchial cuff over the carina should be avoided. When the bronchoscope is passed down the left lumen, a very slight left luminal narrowing and a clear straight-ahead view of the bronchial carina are seen. Excessive left luminal narrowing should be avoided. (From Alfery et al,[112] with permission.)

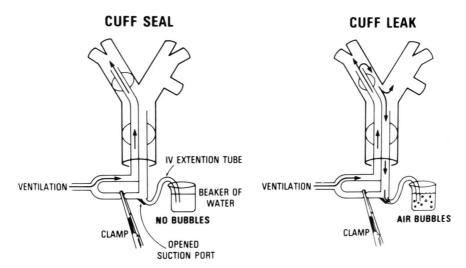

Fig. 16-3. Air bubble detection method for adequacy of cuff seal. **(A)** When the left endobronchial cuff is sealed and the left lung is selectively ventilated, no air bubbles should emerge from the right open suction port (no air bubbles are observed passing through the beaker of water). **(B)** When the left endobronchial cuff is not sealed (ie, leaks) and the left lung is ventilated, air bubbles will escape from the right suction port and bubble through the beaker of water. (From Alfery et al,[112] with permission.)

of lung separation should be reconfirmed after the patient has been turned to the lateral position. An arterial catheter should be placed for sampling of arterial blood and continuous monitoring of blood pressure, and oxygenation should be continuously monitored using a pulse oximeter. A stethoscope should be placed over the ventilated lung to monitor breath sounds, particularly to listen for rales, which, if new, may indicate leakage of lavage fluid into the ventilated lung.

An F_IO_2 of 1.0 should be maintained throughout the procedure. Prior to lavage, this will denitrogenate the lungs so that only oxygen and carbon dioxide will be present. Instillation of lavage fluid will permit the oxygen and carbon dioxide to be absorbed and will result in greater accessibility of the alveolar spaces to the lavage fluid than if the more soluble gas, nitrogen, had remained. Following intubation, the patient is turned to the lateral position, placing the lung to be lavaged lowermost; the tube positions and lung separation are rechecked. With the patient in a head-up position, warmed heparinized isotonic saline (0.9 percent NaCl with 1,000 U of heparin and 7 mEq of sodium bicarbonate buffer, pH 7.8, added to each liter) is infused by gravity from a reservoir 30 to 40 cm above the level of the sternum into the bronchial catheter in the dependent lung. This arrangement results in a hydrostatic infusion pressure of approximately 30 mmHg (Fig. 16-4). The nondependent lung, meanwhile, is ventilated with oxygen and a potent inhaled agent. Once the lavage fluid ceases to flow in (usually after 1,000 mL in an adult), the patient is placed in a

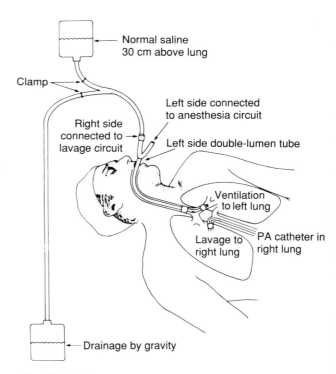

Fig. 16-4. Schematic diagram of double-lumen endotracheal tube and fluid filling and drainage set up in a patient undergoing unilateral right lung lavage for treatment of pulmonary alveolar proteinosis. A pulmonary artery catheter is located in the right main pulmonary artery. (From Alfery et al,[112] with permission.)

head-down position and the lavage fluid is permitted to drain out passively to a collecting system. The lavage procedure is repeated until the drainage fluid is clear, in contrast to the milky fluid that first drains when a lung is being lavaged for alveolar proteinosis. The procedure usually needs to be repeated approximately seven times before the drainage is clear, following which the lung is suctioned and ventilation is re-established using large tidal volumes and pressures because compliance is reduced due to loss of surfactant. During each lavage cycle, the inflow and outflow fluid volumes are carefully monitored so that the patient is not "drowned" in fluid and excessive absorption of fluid or leakage to the ventilated side does not occur. Following the lavage procedure, two-lung ventilation is reinstituted with large tidal volumes, and, as compliance improves, a mixture of air and oxygen may be used to help maintain alveolar patency. Once the compliance of the lavaged hemithorax has returned to its prelavage level, neuromuscular blockade is reversed. In most cases, the trachea may be extubated in the operating room. Postlavage, patients should be encouraged to cough and to perform breathing exercises to fully expand the treated lung. After 3 to 7 days, following satisfactory recovery from lavage of the first lung, the patient may return for lavage of the contralateral lung.

Certain complications occasionally occur during lavage. These include spillage of fluid from the treated to the untreated side. This situation is managed by stopping the lavage and ensuring functional separation of the two lungs before the procedure is continued. Correct position of the double-lumen tube is critical, as is the efficacy of the cuff seal in the bronchus. Any spillage of lavage fluid may result in profound decreases in oxygenation, which, if severe, may necessitate termination of the procedure and institution of two-lung ventilation with an F_IO_2 of 1.0 and PEEP.

Changes in hemodynamics and oxygenation that occur during bronchopulmonary lavage have been reported by a number of investigators.[39–41] When lavage fluid is being instilled into the dependent lung, oxygenation generally improves. This is because the increased intra-alveolar pressure due to the fluid increases the pulmonary vascular resistance in the lavaged lung and causes diversion of pulmonary blood flow to the nondependent, ventilated lung, thereby reducing venous admixture. When lavage fluid is drained from the dependent lung, hypoxemia may occur as pulmonary blood flow increases to the dependent, nonventilated lung, resulting in a significant increase in venous admixture.

In one report of right lung lavage, left lung ventilation with an F_IO_2 of 1.0 prior to lavage resulted in a PaO_2 of 81 mmHg.[41] Instillation of lavage fluid into the right lung caused the PaO_2 to increase to 195 mmHg, and fluid drainage was associated with a decrease in PaO_2 to 74 mmHg. In this report, fluid instillation caused no change in heart rate, but was associated with decreases in cardiac output and venous admixture. Following drainage of fluid, cardiac output and shunt both increased. Mixed venous oxygen saturation, continuously monitored via an oximetric pulmonary arterial catheter, showed no change between fluid instillation and drainage.[41]

Because drainage of lavage fluid may be associated with severe hypoxemia for the reasons discussed above, the use of a balloon-tipped, flow-directed pulmonary arterial catheter has been studied to manipulate unilateral lung blood flow in dogs undergoing bronchopulmonary lavage of the right lung.[42] Using nonocclusive inflation of the balloon in the right main pulmonary artery, it was possible to decrease venous admixture and increase oxygenation (PaO_2) during periods of fluid drainage from the right lung. This technique is not without risk of pulmonary artery rupture, however, and should be reserved for those patients who are considered to be at increased risk of hypoxemia during lavage, although the investigators[42] speculated that the increase in PaO_2 would be less in humans than in dogs because the degree of vascular obstruction by the balloon would be less in the larger human pulmonary artery.

Although, as classically described, bronchopulmonary lavage involves instillation of fluid into the dependent lung, from a pulmonary blood flow and venous admixture aspect it might seem more logical to lavage the nondependent lung. In this way, the dependent lung would always be optimally ventilated and perfused. A potential disadvantage of this approach is, however, that the uppermost alveoli may not be effectively lavaged. In addition, if the bronchial cuff should leak, the dependent lung would become flooded with lavage fluid. As a compromise, bronchopulmonary lavage may be performed with the patient supine.[43]

If the patient has recently undergone a diagnostic open-lung biopsy, the possibility of a BPF must be considered. If such a possibility exists, a chest drain should be inserted into the side with the fistula and this lung should be lavaged first. The chest drain is removed several days later.

Hydropneumothorax has been reported as a complication of bronchopulmonary lavage in a patient with asthma.[44] In this case, the hydropneumothorax presented as hypoxemia in the recovery room with high airway pressures (up to 60 cmH2O) and tachycardia. Following a chest x-ray, a chest tube was inserted, through which was drained more than 500 mL of fluid, as well as air. Following drainage of the chest cavity, the patient's condition rapidly improved.[44]

Bronchopulmonary lavage may not be feasible in small patients (weighing less than 40 kg) using the above-described technique because of limitations in the sizes of available double-lumen tubes. Adequate lung isolation and controlled ventilation have been accomplished in a 7-year-old, 25-kg patient undergoing lavage via a bronchoscopically positioned endobronchial tube, while the contralateral lung was ventilated via a modified nasal airway.[45] Techniques for selective blind endobronchial intubation in children (and adults) have been reported.[46] In other cases, extracorporeal oxygenation techniques may be necessary during bronchopulmonary lavage.[47]

AIRWAY HEMORRHAGE

Chronic infection is the underlying etiology in over 90 percent of cases of massive hemoptysis. The most common infectious etiologies are tuberculosis and bronchiectasis, with neoplasms making up most of the noninfectious causes of bronchial hemorrhage. The bleeding is due to erosion or perforation of vascularized high-pressure bronchial arteries with inflammation, or erosion into the bronchial arteries by tumor.[48]

Cardiovascular etiologies include mitral stenosis, arteriovenous malformations, pulmonary embolism, and pulmonary artery perforation or rupture due to a pulmonary arterial catheter.[49] The risk of pulmonary artery perforation by a pulmonary artery catheter is increased by heparinization and pulmonary hypertension. Catheter-related pulmonary artery rupture has been reported in 0.1 to 0.2 percent of catheterizations.[50,51] This event may present as either hemoptysis or hemothorax. Of 4,684 patients studied in one report, 4 experienced rupture of the pulmonary artery.[50] Three of these events occurred during cardiac surgery with the patients fully heparinized. The bleeding in these 3 cases was severe, but was controlled by 20 cmH_2O of PEEP. The fourth episode was caused by inflating the balloon with 5 mL of air; this patient died. Successful termination of massive hemoptysis following pulmonary arterial catheter balloon inflation has been reported with the use of PEEP.[52] Postmortem studies have indicated that the perforation in such cases may be caused by tip perforation, eccentric balloon inflation, and balloon disruption of the vessel due to high intraballoon pressures of 250 mmHg or more.[53,54] Mortality from hemoptysis is usually due to hypoxia rather than exanguination, and is more likely if the patient is heparinized. Swallowing of blood that has been coughed up can lead to an underestimation of the blood loss. The differential diagnosis of airway hemorrhage is shown in Table 16-1.

Management

A chest x-ray may help to localize the site of bleeding, but this may be obscured by aspiration of blood

TABLE 16-1. Causes of Massive Hemoptysis

I. Infection
  Tuberculosis
  Bronchiectasis
  Bronchitis
  Lung abscess
  Necrotizing pneumonia

II. Neoplasm
  Bronchogenic carcinoma
  Metastatic carcinoma
  Mediastinal tumor
  Endobronchial polyp

III. Cardiovascular disease
  Mitral stenosis
  Pulmonary arteriovenous malformation
  Pulmonary embolus
  Pulmonary vasculitis

IV. Miscellaneous causes
  Pulmonary artery catheterization
  Exploratory needling
  Cystic fibrosis
  Pulmonary contusion, laceration
  Reperfusion of pulmonary vasculature
    after pulmonary embolectomy and
    cardiopulmonary bypass

(From Benumof,[55] with permission.)

into other areas of the lung. Bronchoscopy during active bleeding is important for localizing the source of the bleeding. Insertion of a rigid bronchoscope facilitates improved ventilation and suctioning. However, if the patient is not actively bleeding or is bleeding from the upper lobes or periphery, flexible fiberoptic bronchoscopy may be preferred. Applications of cold saline and vasoconstrictors through the bronchoscope may be sufficient to stop the bleeding in some cases (Fig. 16-5).

Surgery is indicated in the patient who has required multiple blood transfusions, persistent hemoptysis, or deterioration of pulmonary function.[55] The presence of inoperable cancer, an unknown bleeding site, and severe bilateral lung disease represent contraindications to surgery. In patients with a contraindication to surgery or those who refuse surgery, selective bronchial arterial embolization can be performed. The latter procedure is associated with the risk of spinal cord embolization and spinal cord injury in the presence of arterial collaterals to the cord.

In addition to locating the source of the airway bleeding, important principles of anesthesia include fluid resuscitation, isolation of the bleeding lung, and maintenance of normal blood gases. The patient should be volume-repleted through large-bore intravenous catheters. Supplemental oxygen will be needed, and, until intubated, the patient should be positioned in the lateral decubitus position with the

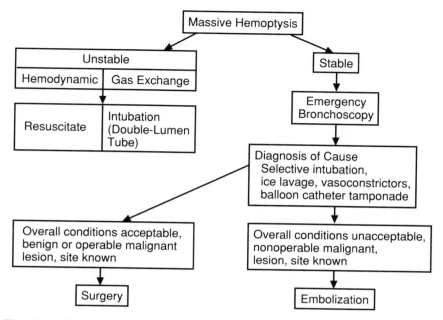

Fig. 16-5. Managent of massive hemoptysis. (From Benumof,[55] with permission.)

bleeding side lowermost to decrease spillage and contamination of the other lung. Although coughing may increase bleeding, it may be essential in the unintubated patient and should not be suppressed. Coughing should be suppressed in the intubated patient, since suctioning is effective as a means to clear the airway.

The patient should be intubated with a double-lumen tube for isolation of the lung into which the bleeding is occurring. The presence of a double-lumen tube will, in addition, facilitate surgical exposure. As compared with merely advancing a single-lumen tube into the bronchus of the nonbleeding lung, the double-lumen tube will also facilitate suctioning and the application of CPAP to the bleeding lung.

If the patient presents for surgery without an endotracheal tube already in place, either an awake intubation or a rapid-sequence intubation with cricoid pressure may be performed. Only a small dose of barbiturate, ketamine, or etomidate should be used for induction if there are any signs of hypovolemia. Intubation may be very difficult in a patient with a bleeding airway who is then paralyzed. If the patient presents with a single-lumen tube in place, either a bronchial blocker (balloon-tipped Fogarty catheter) can be placed by the side of the endotracheal tube with the aid of a bronchoscope, or the tube can be changed to a double-lumen tube. Following resection of the bleeding lung segment, the patient should remain intubated and mechanically ventilated.

ANESTHESIA FOR LASER SURGERY OF AIRWAY TUMORS

The term *laser* is an acronym for light amplification by stimulated emission of radiation. A gaseous medium, such as argon (Ar) or carbon dioxide (CO_2), when stimulated by an energy source (electricity), emits energy in the form of light. By repeated reflections, the emitted light obtains the characteristics of a laser. These characteristics are coherence (light waves in phase with respect to time and space), collimation (same direction), and monochromaticity (same wavelength). Characteristics of lasers used for medical purposes are shown in Table 16-2.

The effects of a laser on tissue depend on both its wavelength (measured in nanometers, ie, 10^{-9} m) and its power density (W/cm²). The excited medium, from which the laser derives it name (eg, Ar, CO_2), determines the emitted wavelength. Longer wavelengths are more strongly absorbed by tissues and, therefore, are converted into heat energy within a more shallow depth of tissue penetration. This is in contrast to laser light of shorter wavelength, which tends to be more scattered. The CO_2 laser emits a long wavelength (10,600 nm) which is, therefore, absorbed at the tissue surface and allows for precise cutting. The neodymium-yttrium-aluminum-garnet (Nd-YAG) laser, which has a shorter wavelength (1,064 nm), penetrates tissue and is used for tumor debulking.[56]

TABLE 16-2. Characteristics of Common Medical Lasers

Laser Type	Wavelength (nm)	Absorber	Principal Use/Remarks
Carbon dioxide	10,600 (far infrared)	All tissues	By vaporization, coagulation, sealing, cauterization
Nd-YAG	1,060 (near infrared)	Darkly pigmented tissue	Photocoagulation (gastrointestinal bleeding), deep thermal necrosis for tumor debulking (bronchial carcinoma)
Ruby	694 (red)	Melanin, cytochrome	Photoablation of pigmented tissue (dermatology, plastic surgery, ophthalmology)
Argon	488/514 (blue/green)	Melanin, hemoglobin	Photocoagulation (ophthalmology, dermatology)

Abbreviation: Nd-YAG, neodymium-yttrium-aluminum-garnet.
(From Pashayan,[56] with permission.)

The extinction length (EL) of a laser is defined as that distance or depth of tissue within which 90 percent of the laser beam energy is absorbed. The EL for the CO_2 laser in most tissues and in water is 0.03 mm.[57] The EL for the Nd-YAG laser is 60 mm in water and 1 to 3 mm in soft tissue.[57] Since only the surface of the affected tissue is visibly changed by the Nd-YAG laser and there is underlying edema formation, complications such as hemorrhage or luminal obstruction may be delayed for up to 2 days.[57]

The power density of a laser is defined as the amount of energy per unit area. It is usually expressed as watts per square centimeter. The absorption by tissue of most medical lasers leads to heating but not to ionization. The heating resulting from those lasers with a low flux (rate of energy delivery) causes coagulation of proteins followed by intracellular water vaporization and cell lysis. While the flux of the Nd-YAG laser mainly causes coagulation of proteins and carbonization over a large area, the flux of the CO_2 laser beam is high and yields almost immediate cellular vaporization, with carbonization only at the tissue edge.

An inhomogeneous tissue substance and a low absorption tend to increase scattering, which increases the cross-sectional area of the laser beam. Thus, the critical volume, defined as the volume in which 90 percent of the interaction with the material occurs, is increased.[2] The critical volume for the Nd-YAG laser is 300 to 900 times greater than that for the CO_2 laser, accounting for a wider range of heating and more edema formation than occurs with the CO_2 laser. Van der Spek et al have likened the effects on tissue of the Nd-YAG laser to an iceberg in that only the tip of the affected tissue is visible.[57] They stated that, "when a high flux is used the center of the 'iceberg' may undergo vaporization, with rapid expansion of the tissues, resulting in a limited explosion of the overlying tissue—the 'popcorn' effect."[57]

Applications of Lasers in Airway Procedures

The laser has become a useful tool for the resection of airway tumors and other lesions, such as laryngeal papillomata, subglottic stenoses, and vascular anomalies.[58] The first use of the CO_2 laser during bronchoscopy was reported in 1974.[59] The most common lesion treated is squamous cell carcinoma, but metastatic lesions also respond.[60] Cancer tissue has been reported to be more vulnerable to destruction by laser than normal tissue.[61] Criteria for laser resection have been reported by McDougall and Cortest,[62] and include the lesion extending into the bronchial wall, but not beyond the cartilage, and an axial length of less than 4 cm. Most bronchoscopists use these criteria in selecting patients.[63]

The laser is the most effective treatment for recurrent respiratory papillomata, which are benign tumors occurring in the larynx and trachea in patients of all ages and may cause airway obstruction.[64] It has been recommended that the laser not be used for carcinoid, if resectable, since there may be bleeding and there may be only a limited resection possible.[65] The best treatment for granulation tissue and tracheal webs due to tracheostomies and prolonged intubation is resection with tracheal reconstruction[60]; the laser may lead to improvement, but only temporarily. Other lesions that have been reported to be resectable using the laser include lipomata, hemartochondromas, schwannomas, histiocytofibroma, sclerosing hemangioma, squamous metaplasia, and amyloid.[66]

The laser provides a palliative treatment of malignant lesions, with success based on relief of symptoms. When treatments such as external radiation and chemotherapy are used, it may take several weeks for tumor shrinkage to occur and for obstructive symptoms to be relieved. These methods also have the disadvantages of systemic toxicity and dosage limits. The laser can be used either to tunnel through a totally obstructing lesion or to widen an existing but narrowed airway lumen. Complete or partial relief of symptoms is immediate and is associated with improvements in blood gas status.[67–70]

From a technical aspect, a totally obstructing lesion of the airway must be blindly "bored" axially, with the associated increased risk of perforation or hemorrhage. A partially obstructing tumor may be approached tangentially. This may explain why the best results of laser therapy are generally obtained with partially obstructing lesions (85 percent success rate) as compared with a more limited improvement (30 to 50 percent success rate) with masses that are totally obstructing.[69,70] The greatest clinical improvement is seen when obstructions of the trachea and mainstem bronchi are relieved, since all or most of the lung tissue, respectively, is distal to the lesion. The Nd-YAG laser is useful for treating lesions lying beyond the range of a rigid bronchoscope since it can be transmitted through a flexible fiber.

Hazards

Dangers associated with the use of lasers include damage to the eyes. Since the CO_2 laser has minimal tissue penetrability, it can damage and opacify the cornea. The Nd-YAG laser, on the other hand, passes through the cornea and can cause retinal damage. Protective measures are, therefore, essential. Either plastic or glass eyewear of any color will afford protection against the CO_2 laser, which is absorbed by almost any material. Contact lenses do not provide adequate protection for the eyes.[57] Special eyewear, designed for the particular wavelength in use, must be worn for protection against other lasers, such as the Nd-YAG. Even proper eyewear may not protect completely against a direct laser "hit." The patient's eyes must also be protected and can be covered with moist pads.[57] The windows of the operating room should be covered and there must be a clearly visible sign on the outside of the room door warning personnel not to enter while the laser is in use. Other dangers include burns from a direct laser "hit" and ignition of flammable material, which includes the endotracheal tube.

The Dermacare Laser Safety System (PSC Corp, Louisville, KY) has been recently developed to protect the patient, operating room personnel, and equipment from the laser. The surface is nonflammable and has a matte finish to diffuse an incident laser beam, thereby decreasing the danger from a reflected beam. The eye shields contain gauze inner pads that must be moistened before use to provide additional protection. There is a personnel/anesthetic shield that serves as the ether screen and contains an inner layer that is heat resistant. There is also an anesthetic circuit shield that can be fitted around the circuit tubing and endotracheal tube. A recent study reported excellent protection by this system against both the CO_2 and the Nd-YAG laser, although the eye shields reflected the laser, which could be potentially dangerous.

Smoke and plume (products of combustion) are released during laser resection and may be harmful,[72] possibly mutagenic, and may transmit infectious disease.[73] Concern exists that live DNA particles in smoke might cause viral disease, including the acquired immunodeficiency syndrome.[74] Additionally, smoke and plume impair the surgeon's vision and are a source of ignition.[74] Smoke may cause bronchospasm, alveolar edema, and atelectasis.[75] McLeskey has recommended suctioning the smoke with special filters to avoid obstruction of the suction line.[74] Masks are now manufactured specifically for use with the laser to filter small particles (≥ 0.3 μm) of plume (eg, Lazer surgical mask, Technol, Fort Worth, TX). Complications caused by the laser's effect on tissue in the airway include perforation, hemorrhage, pneumothorax, and pneumomediastinum. Bleeding into the airway may cause hypoxemia and hypoventilation. Bleeding occurs most often when a mainstem bronchus is totally occluded since the lumen direction is masked and perforation of the bronchus may occur with subsequent perforation of vessels.[60,76] A mapping technique, which consists of piercing the lesion and then injecting Renografin to locate the postobstructive bronchus, has been developed to minimize the chance of hemorrhage.[77] Perforation of the trachea may occur, which can result in tracheoesophageal fistula and pneumothorax.[78] There may be endotracheal tube, cuff, or cottonoid ignition creating an airway fire, which is further discussed later in this section. Another complication is airway obstruction due to edema[76,79]; some investigators have, therefore, advocated prophylactic dexamethasone or methylprednisolone.[80–82]

Mortality associated with airway laser surgery is usually related to hypoxemia and perforation.[79] Although hemorrhage rarely leads to exsanguination, it may cause death secondary to hypoxemia.[79] In addition, secretions and debris may cause obstruction and concomitant hypoxemia. Electrocution resulting from the servicing of high-voltage laser equipment has been reported.[56] There should be a laser safety committee that provides standard operating procedures and certifies personnel using the laser.[74]

General Considerations: Choice of Laser and Methods of Use

The Nd-YAG laser destroys tissue by a coagulation-vaporization sequence such that there is minimal edema and bleeding.[83] The Nd-YAG laser, unlike the CO_2 laser, can be transmitted through a flexible quartz fiber. For transmission of the laser beam to its target, this filament can be introduced into the airway either through a rigid bronchoscope or via the suction channel of a fiberoptic instrument. Use of the latter for Nd-YAG laser surgery of the airway facilitates the resection of upper lobe and peripheral tumors, which would otherwise be beyond the reach of a rigid bronchoscope. The flexible fiberoptic bronchoscope can be passed directly into the airway following the application of local anesthesia, or through an endotracheal tube after the induction of general anesthesia and endotracheal intubation. In the latter case, it is critical that the laser be fired only when the tip of the bronchoscope is *beyond* the end of the endotracheal tube, otherwise, the tube may be ignited by a misaimed laser beam (see Chapter 12).

Since the Nd-YAG laser beam is invisible, a coaxial light source is needed for aiming. The helium-neon laser, which is visible, may be used as the aiming beam for both the CO_2 and Nd-YAG lasers. The aiming beam has a very low power output (1 to 2 mW), and is produced by splitting the original beam.[57] A xenon pilot beam, which appears red, can also be used.[76] The alignment of the aiming beam should be checked prior to each usage.[75] Malalignment of the aiming beam may lead to damage of normal tissue. The aiming guide allows a fiber-to-target beam distance of 5 to 10 mm, with a laser beam divergence of less than 10 degrees and a photovaporization area of 1 to 2 mm in diameter.[76] There is also a Teflon sheath through which a cooling gas must flow (eg, air at 3 L/min) to keep the fiber tip clear and cool.[57,76] Any collection of debris at the tip of the fiber conducting the laser beam may melt and flare.[57]

The CO_2 laser is used to excise lesions that can be directly visualized in, or proximal to, the larynx. The CO_2 laser is preferred if minimal penetration and edema formation are desirable, such as in the pediatric airway.[84,85] If the lesion to be treated is subglottic, passage of a rigid bronchoscope is required and the anesthesia technique and considerations are similar to those associated with use of the Nd-YAG laser with rigid bronchoscopy (see below). If the lesion is supraglottic, an endotracheal tube can be used to permit ventilation of the patient, but the tube must be protected from the laser beam to prevent a fire from occurring. A flexible fiberoptic system, which is a combination of metallic halides, has been developed for the CO_2 laser but is not yet in clinical use.[85] The potassium-titanyl-phosphate (KTP) laser is being used with increasing frequency for laryngeal and upper airway procedures.[86] The laser beam is green and has a wavelength of 532 nm.[86] Unlike the CO_2 laser, it can be transmitted via a fiberoptic bundle.

General Anesthesia

During laser use, it is imperative that the field be stationary to avoid tissue damage by a misdirected laser beam. Another consideration is that in the event of hemorrhage, the flexible bronchoscope will not allow for both suctioning and laser coagulation, both of which are needed. General anesthesia is usually preferred for rigid bronchoscopy and has been recommended for fiberoptic bronchoscopy.[87] Either an awake intubation or slow induction maintaining spontaneous ventilation may be necessary, since induction of general anesthesia may convert a partially obstructing lesion to a total airway obstruction due to loss of muscle tone with onset of paralysis.

General anesthesia for bronchoscopic laser resection is often combined with topical anesthesia of the larynx. In this way, less general anesthesia is needed. A balanced anesthesia technique uses nitrogen/oxygen, incremental doses of an intravenous agent (such as thiopental or thiamylal), a narcotic (such as fentanyl or alfentanil), and a muscle relaxant (such as succinylcholine, atracurium, or vecuronium). A potent inhaled agent technique (such as nitrous oxide/oxygen/enflurane or nitrogen/oxygen/isoflurane) is also satisfactory. The use of a potent inhaled agent may cause an operating room pollution problem with regard to waste anesthesia gases. Limited scavenging is possible by placing a suction catheter into the patient's oropharynx (see Chapter 12).

The use of rigid bronchoscopy provides visibility and suction and allows for easier retrieval of debris. The rigid bronchoscope itself maintains the airway and substantially decreases the risk of fire since the metal is nonignitable and nonflammable. The metal can, however, reflect the laser beam and thereby produce indirect tissue damage. The use of a pulse oximeter is essential and, if there is an indication of desaturation, the anesthesiologist must have the surgeon interrupt the use of the laser so that the patient may be ventilated with a high F_IO_2 to improve arterial saturation. Desaturation may be due to distal aspiration of resected material, so that any debris in the airway resulting from tumor resection must be suctioned. Although the steel bronchoscope will not burn, carbonized tissue may flare.[75] Some researchers recommend limiting the F_IO_2 to 0.50, with nitrogen making up the remainder during periods of laser resection.[76] It is important that the oxygen not be diluted with nitrous oxide as the latter supports combustion. Dilution of oxygen may be more safely achieved using nitrogen (air) or helium.

Unless there is a contraindication, the patient is paralyzed and ventilation during bronchoscopy is controlled. The maintenance of a patient breathing spontaneously under general anesthesia during laser resection would be difficult. The patient would be likely either to move due to inadequate anesthesia or to hypoventilate due to deep anesthesia. Controlled ventilation reduces the risk of trauma that might occur if the patient moved with a rigid bronchoscope in place. In any patient scheduled for a thoracic procedure for a suspected malignancy, the possibility of the myasthenic (Eaton-Lambert) syndrome should be considered. This syndrome is associated with an increased sensitivity to nondepolarizing muscle relaxants; therefore, these agents should be given in incremental doses and titrated to effect using a blockade monitor (see Chapter 15).

A contemporary rigid ventilating bronchoscope is essentially a hollow tube with a blunted, bevelled tip at the distal (patient) end and an eyepiece at the proximal (operator) end. Side holes must be present at the distal end of the instrument for ventilation of lung segments proximal to the tip of the bronchoscope. Several sizes and designs of bronchoscopes are available, but all have a side arm for connection to an anesthesia delivery system. Modern bronchoscopes (eg, Wolfe-Dumon) especially designed for laser resection have two proximal entrances for passage of a laser fiber and a suction catheter. Use of the suction channel can reduce operating room pollution.

Ventilation During Rigid Bronchoscopy

A number of techniques have been described for maintaining ventilation and oxygenation during rigid bronchoscopy, including intermittent positive-pressure ventilation, the Sanders injection system, and high-frequency positive-pressure ventilation. In one study using general anesthesia and rigid bronchoscopy for Nd-YAG laser resection of obstructing endobronchial tumors, a total of 15 patients received 20 treatments.[88] All patients were premedicated with only an anticholinergic. An air/oxygen blender with a high-pressure outlet connected to the Sanders injector was used to ventilate a group of patients during 12 treatments with an F_IO_2 of 0.3 to 0.4. Anesthesia was

maintained with intravenous thiopental and fentanyl. In the other group, which received 8 treatments, a circle system was attached to the side arm of the ventilating bronchoscope. These patients were ventilated with air/oxygen (F_IO_2 = 0.3 to 0.4) and a potent inhaled agent by manually squeezing the reservoir bag. Hypoxemia was managed by temporarily discontinuing laser usage, repositioning the bronchoscope if beyond the carina, and increasing the F_IO_2. Following the tumor resection and reversal of neuromuscular blockade, the tracheas of patients with respiratory insufficiency were intubated with an endotracheal tube, treated with humidified oxygen and steroids, and observed overnight in the intensive care unit. Intraoperative hypoxemia was noted in both groups, and may have been related to one-lung ventilation during passage of the bronchoscope tip beyond the carina. The Sanders-ventilated group (no potent inhaled agent) had improved ventilation as reflected by lower $PaCO_2$ levels, but some patients in this group displayed recall. It is possible to use potent inhaled agents with the Sanders technique, but this would cause operating room contamination, as previously mentioned. Also, there may be greater somnolence following anesthesia with intravenous as compared with potent inhaled agents[76] (see Chapter 12).

Dumon et al reported a series of 1,503 Nd-YAG laser treatments in 839 patients, performed via a rigid bronchoscope under general anesthesia in 1,156 cases.[79] Based on experimental data suggesting that a continuous laser output of 40 W produces massive coagulation and uncontrolled penetration,[89] laser power was restricted to 45 W, with intermittent durations of 0.5 to 1.0 seconds. The laser was only fired parallel to the airway wall, and F_IO_2 was limited to 0.5. There were no intraoperative mortalities and no fires in this series. There were, however, six postoperative deaths (0.4 percent), all of which were related to hypoxemia.

Manual jet ventilation has been compared with HFJV through the rigid bronchoscope during laser resection of tracheobronchial stenosis.[90] There was moderate hypercarbia only in the group receiving HFJV. The investigators hypothesized that since the tip of the bronchoscope was in a bronchus, the high pressure from manual jet ventilation allowed ventilation through the side vents, but this was not achieved using the low pressure during high-frequency ventilation. These researchers recommended manual jet ventilation during resections of bronchial stenosis despite the fact that high inflation pressures caused the tracheobronchial wall to move and blood and secretions to be sprayed, thereby worsening visibility. This did not happen with HFJV. In addition to moving the tracheal wall, turbulent gas movement can also deflect the laser beam.[75] One method that has been described is to alternate ventilation and laser resection to provide the surgeon with an immobile field.[91]

Use of the Nd-YAG Laser Through an Endotracheal Tube

An alternative technique is to pass the Nd-YAG laser through the working channel of a fiberoptic bronchoscope, which has been inserted into the airway through an endotracheal tube, under general anesthesia. In one study using this method, 22 adult patients with bronchial obstruction were treated.[76] General anesthesia was achieved using intravenous agents and/or enflurane and muscle paralysis. The F_1O_2 was limited to 0.5. Laser resection was performed using 50 to 90 W for 0.5- to 2.0-second bursts. The investigators reported hypercarbia during 30 of 32 procedures ($PaCO_2$ 45 to 60 mmHg). Dyspnea, which was universally present preoperatively, improved immediately following 29 of the procedures. There were 2 intraoperative deaths (9.1 percent) due to uncontrolled hemorrhage during resection through totally obstructing lesions. Two patients required reintubation within 24 hours postoperatively, the indications being airway edema following prolonged resections. As compared with none of 12 patients receiving potent inhaled agents, five patients anesthetized with intravenous agents had prolonged somnolence and respiratory depression necessitating postoperative mechanical ventilation.

Local Versus General Anesthesia

In a retrospective study of the use of the Nd-YAG laser for resection of tracheobronchial tumors, local anesthesia and flexible fiberoptic bronchoscopy in 51 patients was compared with general anesthesia and rigid bronchoscopy in 46 patients.[87] The patients under general anesthesia were ventilated using a Sanders injector system with 100 percent oxygen entraining room air. In these patients, the fiberoptic bronchoscope was passed through a rigid bronchoscope to facilitate laser resection of the tumor, extending the range of resection to that provided under local anesthesia. The amount of improvement in response to treatment, number of patients improved, and the intervals between treatment courses were similar in both groups. Under general anesthesia, there was improved airway control and better removal of blood and debris by allowing the use of a larger suction catheter. The mean number of treatment sessions during each treatment course was decreased in this group (the patients under local anesthesia could not tolerate the procedure as long). No deaths occurred under general anesthesia, but there were two operative deaths under local anesthesia. These were due to obstruction secondary to bleeding into an already narrowed airway. Bleeding in both groups was controlled by the application of topical epinephrine followed by laser photocoagulation. Although myocardial infarction did occur in one patient who received general anesthesia, the investigators recommended the use of general anesthesia unless there was severe coexisting cardiovascular or pulmonary disease.[87]

Endotracheal Tube Protection

External ignition of an endotracheal tube is due to transfer of heat between the laser and tube, whereas internal ignition is due to laser perforation of the tube with support of combustion by the gases inside the tube. When endotracheal intubation is indicated, the endotracheal tube may be protected by wrapping it with metallic tape along its entire length with the exceptions of the cuff and the tip of the tube distal to the cuff. The taping must be done in an overlapping manner so that even when the tube is flexed none of the surface of the endotracheal tube is left exposed. Copper foil tape (Venture Tape Corp., Rockland, MA) and 3M #425 tape (St. Paul, MN) have been reported to provide excellent protection against the hazards of CO_2 laser use.[92] Aluminum tape is also protective, but copper tape is better since it has a higher coefficient of reflectivity for light of the infrared wavelength and is also more malleable.[93] In another study, 3M #65 tape was also reported to provide excellent protection.[94] Wrapping the tube itself has been associated with complications such as aspiration of the wrapping and kinking of the tube, causing airway obstruction. If not done properly with the edges of the tape overlapping, the tube may be inadequately protected. An overlap of half the tape width has been recommended to provide good protection as well as a smooth surface.[95] There are many tapes available that appear to be metallic but which, in fact, are not; these do not reflect the laser. Tapes should, therefore, be tested prior to use by firing the laser at the tape. The reflected beam from reflective tape may cause an airway burn; therefore, a tape with a matte finish, which results in a more diffuse reflected beam, is preferred. Wet muslin can also be used as an effective protective wrapping, but is bulky and can ignite if it dries out.

Laser-Guard (American Corp., Mystic, CT) has an adhesive corrugated silver foil bonded to a thin absorbent sponge layer that is to be saturated with water. Silver is used because it has a high thermal conductivity. The Laser-Guard endotracheal tube wrapping decreases potential damage from the reflected beam by absorbing the laser beam with less reflection, as compared with aluminum- and copper foil-wrapped tubes.[96] The Laser-Flex stainless steel metallic tube (Mallinckrodt, St. Louis, MO) was even better than the Laser-Guard wrapped tube in this regard.[96]

Endotracheal tube cuffs should be inflated with saline so that if they rupture the saline will help to extinguish a fire. In a recent study, inflating the endotracheal tube cuffs with saline prevented endotracheal tube explosion in most cases of testing.[97] The liquid in the cuff can be colored with methylene blue to indicate if the cuff has ruptured. Packing the cuff of an endotracheal tube with saline-soaked pledgets has been shown to prevent CO_2 laser-induced cuff ignition, but the pledgets must be carefully retrieved after surgery.[98] Even with the exterior surface of the endotracheal tube protected, the tube can still be ignited by tissue debris blown inside the tube.[99] Also, an oil-based ointment should not be used to lubricate the tube since it may be combustible and can be ignited. Recently, 3M #425 and Venture copper foil tapes were reported to provide protection from the Nd-YAG laser set at 110 W for 1 minute of exposure in an atmosphere of 98 percent O_2.[100]

Choice of Endotracheal Tube

The Rusch red rubber endotracheal tubes have been reported to be less flammable than polyvinylchloride (PVC) tubes. Also, if ignited, they release fewer combustible toxic products that, in turn, would require additional laser energy to ignite. Gupta et al[94] reported that the PVC tube burned like a blowtorch compared with the red rubber tube, which tended only to smolder when ignited. Pashayan,[56] however, reported that PVC tubes were less flammable, but melted at lower temperatures.

Patel and Hicks,[101] in an in vitro study of flammability using a CO_2 laser, found that PVC tubes were more easily penetrated or ignited than red rubber tubes. At 0.5 seconds' exposure to 30 W of laser energy, all PVC tubes were ignited or penetrated, as compared to only one red rubber tube. The PVC tubes also burned and produced much more smoke.

Wolf and Simpson[102] studied the O_2 and N_2O indices of flammability of PVC, silicone, and red rubber endotracheal tubes. The index of flammability is defined as the minimum concentration of O_2 and N_2O, respectively, that supports a candlelike flame with a standard ignition source. The results indicated that both these indices (O_2 and N_2O), which are additive if O_2 and N_2O are used together, were higher for PVC tubes than for silicone or red rubber tubes. In this study of flammability, ignition was accomplished using a propane torch. When tested with CO_2 laser exposure, the red rubber was found to be less flammable than PVC.[101–103] The tubes flared at 10 W at even the

shortest exposure time (0.1 seconds). None of the red rubber tubes flared, even with 100 percent oxygen, although testing was only performed up to 20 W for 1 second. In another study, 15 W for 0.5 seconds in an environment of 30 percent oxygen diluted in air allowed the combustion of red rubber tubes.[104]

In a dog study, the most severe tracheal burns occurred with the use of PVC tubes, as compared with red rubber or silicone tubes.[105] Silica ash was found in the airway after silicone tube fires, and the investigators were concerned about the possible future development of silicosis. These researchers recommended the Rusch red rubber tube as being the safest for use with the CO_2 laser.[105]

The Nd-YAG laser is absorbed by pigmented tissues, but not by clear plastic, water, or glass.[106] The Sheridan YAG Tracheal Tube (Sheridan Corp., Argyle, NY) is a clear PVC endotracheal tube designed for use with the Nd-YAG laser. However, in a recent study, small amounts of blood, saliva, or mucus on the tube greatly increased the risk of endotracheal tube explosion and was not recommended.[106] Despite the controversy, red rubber tubes are generally considered to be safer than the PVC variety for use with both the Nd-YAG and the CO_2 lasers.[57]

There are now available endotracheal tubes designed specifically for use during airway laser surgery. The Laser Shield tube (Xomed, Jacksonville, FL) contains metallic particles in a silicone base and is designed to reflect the laser beam. However, it is expensive and designed for single use only. It can be perforated after a number of direct laser "hits" and is most vulnerable in the area of the cuff. It provides no resistance to the Nd-YAG laser.[101] The Fome-Cuff tube (Bivona, Gary, IN) has a sponge contained in the cuff. The latter is inflated with water or saline and offers the advantage of remaining in position even if ruptured. Another option is the flexible metal tube, which is cuffless.[107] If ventilation is inadequate, a cuff can be added over the tube, but this also adds the risk of ignition. Soaked sponges or cottonoids can also be used to create a seal around the tube.

The special tubes described above (Laser Shield, Fome-Cuff) have been tested with the CO_2 laser and compared with other tubes in use.[108] In this study, the laser was operated continuously and at high power, but the resistance to ignition of the cuff was not tested. A red rubber tube, wrapped with 3M #4 aluminum foil tape, provided excellent protection.[80] An unwrapped red rubber tube was perforated immediately, but did not burn. Although the Bivona Fome-Cuff and the Xomed Laser Shield tubes are designed for use with the laser, both ignited very quickly and burst into flames. The Mallinckrodt tube (St. Louis, MO), which contains a metal shaft and two PVC cuffs, provided excellent protection against the CO_2

laser and against the KTP laser.[86] A metal tube, like reflective tape, can still cause an airway burn by a reflected beam.

Choice of Anesthesia Gases

The use of a helium/oxygen (60/40 percent) mixture with the CO_2 laser has been reported to prevent the ignition and fires of nonwrapped unmarked PVC tubes.[109] The barium stripe in the wall of the PVC tube lowers the ignition threshold, making unmarked tubes preferable. The advantage of using helium is that, compared with nitrogen, it has a much higher thermal diffusivity, which leads to decreased heating of matter. Only one flash fire has been reported with the use of this helium protocol in 523 cases, and that was due to improper procedure.[109] In this particular case, following endotracheal tube cuff perforation by the laser, the anesthesiologist ventilated the patient using the O_2 flush valve on the anesthesia machine without first notifying the surgeon, who continued to use the laser. In all of the other cases in which no fire occurred, the maximum F_IO_2 was limited to 0.4. Subsequently, Pashayan et al reported the use of a premixed helium/oxygen gas (Heliox) composed of 30 percent oxygen and 70 percent helium that allows an increase in the flow of gas without altering the F_IO_2 should a cuff leak develop.[109]

In addition to protecting against fire, helium may improve ventilation beyond an obstructing airway lesion because its density is less than that of nitrogen, and orificial (turbulent) flow is inversely proportional to the square root of the density of a gas.[110] The use of helium, however, prevents an accurate measurement of anesthesia gases by most mass spectrometry units, which have no collector plates for helium, and erroneously high values for other gases (O_2, CO_2, N_2, N_2O, potent agents) will be obtained. Another consideration when using helium is that the proportioning systems for O_2 and N_2O on contemporary anesthesia machines (Dräger Oxygen Ratio Monitor Controller; Ohmeda Link-25 Proportion Limiting System), which ensure an O_2 concentration of at least 25 percent at the flowmeter level, are only functional between O_2 and N_2O. The use of helium would eliminate this safety feature and, thus, potentially allow for the delivery of a hypoxic ($F_IO_2 < 0.25$) mixture. The use of an O_2 analyzer in the anesthesia circuit, therefore, takes on an even greater importance when helium is being used. The helium protocol is summarized in Table 16-3.

For laser surgery of the larynx, a small-size endotracheal tube can be used but it needs to be protected, as discussed. The presence of this tube in the airway, however, may interfere with the surgery. An alternative is to ventilate the patient using a Venturi jet attached to an operating laryngoscope. This does not involve the use of an endotracheal tube and affords the surgeon complete visibility. Anesthesia can be maintained intravenously with barbiturates and muscle relaxants. Complications of this technique include pneumomediastinum, pneumothorax, gastric distention, and hypoventilation. Prolonged laryngoscopy often causes hypertension and tachycardia from the prolonged stimulation. This can be effectively controlled by the administration of a short-acting beta-adrenergic blocker, such as esmolol, either as a bolus or by continuous infusion.

Airway Fires

Endotracheal ignition of a fiberoptic bronchoscope during Nd-YAG laser resection has been reported.[109] In this case report, the patient was inadvertently being given 80 percent oxygen instead of the intended 40 percent. Snow et al reported that during 700 uses of the CO_2 laser, there were four instances of endotracheal tube ignition that led to tracheal burns.[111]

TABLE 16-3. Helium Protocol for Laryngotracheal Carbon Dioxide Laser Operations

Protocol Consideration	Limitation
Gases	
Helium	60%
Oxygen	F_IO_2-0.40
Inhalational anesthetics	Enflurane, halothane, or isoflurane
Nitrous oxide	Cannot be used for anesthetic maintenance
Endotracheal tube	Unmarked, unwrapped PVC
Carbon dioxide laser power density	10 W at 0.8-mm spot size (1,992 W/cm²), repeated bursts (10 seconds of 0.5-second pulsed beam)
Monitoring	Standard monitors, oxygen analyzer, and pulse oximeter

(From Pashayan et al,[109] with permission.)

TABLE 16-4. Measures, in Order of Importance, in Managing an Airway Fire

Stop ventilation
Disconnect oxygen source, douse with water if needed
Remove burned tracheal tube/endoscope
Mask ventilate, reintubate
Diagnose injury, provide therapy by bronchoscopy
Monitor patient for at least 24 hours
Administer short-term steroids
Administer antibiotics, ventilatory support as needed

(Modified from Pashayan et al,[109] with permission.)

In the case of an airway fire occurring during laser surgery, the first step in management is to discontinue use of the laser, stop ventilation, remove the oxygen source, and extubate the trachea. This will decrease inhalation of the toxic products of combustion and decrease the amount of oxidizing agents and fuel present to perpetuate the fire. Any debris should be suctioned from the airway. The patient can then be ventilated by face mask and bag and the trachea reintubated. Prior to emergence from anesthesia, bronchoscopy should be performed, both for evaluation of airway damage and for further removal of debris. After first removing the tube, McLeskey[74] has recommended flooding the field with saline to extinguish the fire, then following the sequence described here. Postoperatively, the patient should be closely monitored in general and by continuous pulse oximetry in particular. Steroids may help to decrease airway edema. Antibiotics are indicated only in the presence of infection. The management of an airway fire is outlined in Table 16-4.[56]

REFERENCES

1. Rutkow IM: Thoracic and cardiovascular operations in the United States, 1979 to 1984. J Thorac Cardiovasc Surg 92:181–1985, 1986
2. Krowke MJ, Pairolero PC, Trustek VF, et al: Cardiac dysrhythmia following pneumonectomy: clinical correlates and prognostic significance. Chest 91:490–495, 1987
3. Shields TW, Unik GT: Digitalization for prevention of arrhythmias following pulmonary surgery. Surg Gynecol Obstet 126:743–746, 1968
4. Burman SO: The prophylactic use of digitalis before thoracotomy. Ann Thorac Surg 14:359–368, 1972
4a. Ritchie AJ, Bowe P, Gibbons JRP: Prophylactic digitalization for thoracotomy: a reassessment. Ann Thorac Surg 50:86–88, 1990
5. Hutchin P, Terzi RG, Hollandsworth LA, et al: Pulmonary congestion following infusion of large fluid loads in thoracic surgical patients. Ann Thorac Surg 8:339–347, 1969
6. Grant GJ, Ramanathan S, Turndorf H: Epidural fentanyl reduces isoflurane requirement during thoracotomy. Anesthesiology 71:A668, 1989
7. Kvalheim L, Ristad F: Intrapleural catheter in the management of postoperative pain. Anesthesiology 61:A231, 1984
8. Seltzer JL, Larijani GE, Goldberg ME, et al: A kinetic and dynamic evaluation of intrapleural bupivacaine for subcostal incision pain. Anesthesiology 65:A213, 1986
9. Reistad F, Tromskag KE, Holmquist E: Intrapleural administration of bupivacaine in postoperative management of pain. Anesthesiology 65:A204, 1986
10. Reistad F, Stromskag KE: Intrapleural catheter management of postoperative pain. A preliminary report. Reg Anaesth 11:89–91, 1986
11. Stromskag KE, Reistad F, Holmquist EL, Ogenstad S: Intrapleural administration of 0.25%, 0.375%, and 0.5% bupivacaine with epinephrine after cholecystectomy. Anesth Analg 67:430–434, 1988
12. Rosenberg PH, Scheninin BMA, Lepantalo MJ, Linfors O: Continuous intrapleural infusion of bupivacaine for analgesia after thoracotomy. Anesthesiology 67:811–813, 1987
13. Kambam JR, Handte RE, Flanagan J, et al: Intrapleural analgesia for post-thoracotomy pain relief. Anesth Analg 66:590, 1987
14. Rafferty TD, Palma J, Motoyama EK, et al: Management of bronchopleural fistula with differential lung ventilation and positive end-expiratory pressure. Respir Care 25:654–657, 1980
15. Baker WL, Faber LP, Osteermiller WE, et al: Management of bronchopleural fistulas. J Thorac Cardiovasc Surg 62:393–401, 1971
16. Carlon GC, Ray C, Klain M: High-frequency positive-pressure ventilation in management of a patient with bronchopleural fistula. Anesthesiology 52:160–162, 1980
17. Bishop MJ, Benson MS, Sato P, et al: Comparison of high-frequency jet ventilation with conventional ventilation for bronchopleural fistula. Anesth Analg 66:833, 1987
18. Power DJ, Cline CD, Rodman GH: Effect of chest tube suction on gas flow through a bronchopleural fistula. Crit Care Med 13:99–101, 1985
19. Benumof JL: Anesthesia for emergency thoracic surgery. p. 389. In: Anesthesia for Thoracic Surgery. WB Saunders, Philadelphia, 1987
20. Normandale JP: Bullous cystic lung disease. Anaesthesia 40:182–185, 1985
21. Forman S, Weill H, Duker GR, et al: Bullous disease of the lung. Ann Intern Med 69:757–767, 1968
22. Leape LL, Longino LA: Infantile lobar emphysema. Pediatrics 34:246–255, 1964
23. Peters RM: Indications for operative treatment of bullous emphysema. Ann Thorac Surg 35:479, 1983
24. Nakahara K, Nakaola K, Ohno K, et al: Functional indications for bullectomy of giant bulla. Ann Thorac Surg 35:480–487, 1983

25. Ting EY, Klopstocz R, Lyons HA: Mechanical properties of pulmonary cysts and bullae. Am Rev Respir Dis 87:538–544, 1963

26. Eger EI, Saidman LJ: Hazards of nitrous oxide anesthesia in bowel obstruction and pneumothorax. Anesthesiology 26:61–66, 1965

27. McCarthy G, Coppel DL, Gibbons JR, et al: High-frequency jet ventilation for bilateral bullectomy. Anaesthesia 42:411, 1987

28. Benumof JL: Sequential one-lung ventilation for bilateral bullectomy. Anesthesiology 67:268–272, 1987

29. Benumof JL: Anesthesia for special elective therapeutic procedures. p. 357. In: Anesthesia for Thoracic Surgery. WB Saunders, Philadelphia, 1987

30. Laros CD, Gelissen HJ, Bergstein PG, et al: Bullectomy for giant bullae in emphysema. J Thorac Cardiovasc Surg 91:63–70, 1986

31. Pride NB, Barter CE, Hugh-Jones P: The ventilation of bullae and the effect of their removal on thoracic gas volumes and tests of overall pulmonary function. Am Rev Respir Dis 107:83–97, 1973

32. Kirschner PA: Surgical priorities for bullectomy. Case conference. J Cardiothorac Anesth 4:119–126, 1990

33. Cohen E, Kirshner PA, Benumof JL: Case conference. Anesthesia for bullectomy. J Cardiothorac Anesth 4:119–126, 1990

34. Connolly JE, Wilson A: The current status of surgery for bullous emphysema. J Thorac Cardiovasc Surg 97:351–361, 1989

35. Lippman M, Mok MS: Anesthetic management of pulmonary lavage. Anesthesiology 33:401, 1978

36. McClenatian JB, Mussenden R: Pulmonary alveolar proteinosis. Arch Intern Med 133:284–287, 1974

37. Ramirez J, Harlan WJ, Jr: Pulmonary alveolar proteinosis. Nature and origin of alveolar lipid. Am J Med 45:502–512, 1968

38. Smith LJ, Ankin MG, Katzenstein A, et al: Management of pulmonary alveolar proteinosis. Chest 78:765–770, 1980

39. Smith JD, Miller JE, Safar P, Robin ED: Intrathoracic pressure, pulmonary vascular pressures and gas exchange during bronchopulmonary lavage. Anesthesiology 33:401–405, 1970

40. Rogers RM, Szidon JP, Shelburne J, et al: Hemodynamic response of the circulation to bronchopulmonary lavage in mass. N Engl J Med 286:1230–1233, 1972

41. Cohen E, Eisenkraft JB: Bronchopulmonary lavage: effects on oxygenation and hemodynamics. J Cardiothorac Anesth 4:119–130, 1990

42. Alfery DD, Zamost BG, Benumof JL: Unilateral lung lavage: blood flow manipulation by ipsilateral pulmonary artery balloon inflation in dogs. Anesthesiology 55:376–381, 1981

43. Spragg RG, Benumof JL, Alfery DD: New methods for the performance of unilateral lung lavage. Anesthesiology 57:535–542, 1982

44. Hudes ET, Bradley JW, Brebner J: Hydropneumothorax—an unusual complication of lung lavage. Can Anaesth Soc J 33:662, 1986

45. McKenzie B, Wood RE, Bailey A: Airway management for unilateral lung lavage in children. Anesthesiology 70:550, 1989

46. Kubota H, Kubota Y, Toshiro T, et al: Selective blind endobronchial intubation in children and adults. Anesthesiology 67:587–589, 1987

47. Lippman M, Mok MS, Wasserman K: Anesthetic management for children with alveolar proteinosis using extracorporeal circulation. Br J Anaesth 49:173, 1977

48. Wedel M: Massive hemoptysis. pp. 194–200. In Moser K, Spragg RG (eds): Respiratory Emergencies. CV Mosby, St. Louis, 1982

49. Reich DL, Thys DM: Mitral valve replacement complicated by endobronchial hemorrhage: spontaneous, traumatic, or iatrogenic? J Cardiothorac Anesth 2:359–362, 1988

50. Rao TLK, Gorski DW, Laughlin S, El Etr AA: Safety of pulmonary artery catheterization. Anesthesiology 57:A116, 1982

51. McDaniel DD, Stone JG, Faltas AN, et al: Catheter-induced pulmonary artery hemorrhage. J Thorac Cardiovasc Surg 82:1–4, 1981

52. Scuderi PE, Prough DS, Price JD, Comer PB: Cessation of pulmonary artery catheter-induced endobronchial hemorrhage associated with the use of PEEP. Anesth Analg 62:236–238, 1983

53. Barash P, Nardi D, Hammond G, et al: Mechanisms, management, and modifications. J Thorac Cardiovasc Surg 82:5–12, 1981

54. Eisenkraft JB, Eger EI: Nitrous oxide anesthesia may double the balloon gas volume of Swan-Ganz catheters. Mt Sinai J Med (NY) 39:430–432, 1989

55. Benumof JL: Anesthesia for emergency thoracic surgery. pp. 376–381. In: Anesthesia for Thoracic Surgery. WB Saunders, Philadelphia, 1987

56. Pashayan AG: Anesthesia for laser surgery. In: ASA Annual Refresher Course Lectures 1988. No. 124. American Society of Anesthesiologists, Park Ridge, IL, 1988

57. Van der Spek AFL, Spargo PM, Norton ML: The physics of lasers and implications for their use during airway surgery. Br J Anaesth 60:709–729, 1988

58. McLeskey CH: Anesthetic management of patients undergoing endoscopic laser surgery. pp. 135–139. In: 1988 Review Course Lectures. International Anesthesia Research Society, Cleveland, OH, 1988

59. Strong MS, Vaughan CW, Polany J, et al: Bronchoscopic carbon dioxide laser surgery. Ann Otol 83:769, 1974

60. McElvein RB, Zorn GL, Jr: Carbon dioxide laser therapy. Clin Chest Med 6:29, 1985

61. Minton JP, Ketchman AS: The laser, a unique oncolytic entity. Am J Surg 108:845, 1964

62. McDougall JC, Cortest DA: Neodymium-YAG laser therapy of malignant airway obstruction. Mayo Clin Proc 58:35, 1983

63. Boyce JR: Laser therapy for bronchoscopy. Anesth Clin North Am 7:597–609, 1989

64. Strong MS, Vaughan CW, Healy GB, et al: Recurrent respiratory papillomatosis. Ann Otol 85:508, 1976

65. Personne C, Colchen A, Leroy M, et al: Indications and technique for endoscopic laser resections in bronchol-

ogy. A critical analysis based upon 2284 resections. J Thorac Cardiovasc Surg 91:710, 1986

66. Personne C, Colchen A, Toty L, et al: Endoscopic laser resection in bronchology. Our experience based on 1233 sessions using Nd-YAG and rigid bronchoscope. Int Cong Series 609:208, 1983

67. Dedhia HV, Leroy L, Jain PR, et al: Endoscopic laser therapy for respiratory distress due to obstructive airway tumors. Crit Care Med 12:464–467, 1985

68. Parr GVS, Under N, Trout RG, et al: One hundred neodymium-YAG (Nd-YAG) laser resections of major airway obstructing tumors. Anesthesiology 60:230, 1984

69. Gelb AF, Epstein JB: Laser in treatment of lung cancer. Chest 86:662–666, 1984

70. Unger M: Bronchoscopic utilization of the Nd-YAG laser for obstructing lesions of the trachea and bronchi. Surg Clin North Am 64:931–938, 1984

71. Sosis M: Evaluation of a new laser-resistant anesthesia circuit protector, drape, and patient eye shield. Anesth Analg 72:S265, 1991

72. Davis RK, Simpton GT: Safety with the carbon dioxide laser. Otololaryngol Clin North Am 16:801, 1983

73. Tomita Y, Mihashi S, Nagata IC, et al: Mutagenicity of smoke condensates induced by CO_2 laser irradiation and electrocauterization. Mutat Res 89:145–149, 1981

74. McLeskey CH: Anesthetic management of patients undergoing endoscopic laser surgery. Anesth Clin North Am 7:611–629, 1989

75. Paes ML: General anesthesia for carbon dioxide laser surgery within the airway. Br J Anaesth 59:1610–1620, 1987

76. Warner ME, Warner MA, Leonard P: Anesthesia for neodymium-YAG (Nd-YAG) laser resection of major airway obstructing tumors. Anesthesiology 60:230–232, 1984

77. Joyner LR, Moran AG, Sarama R, et al: Neodymium-YAG laser treatment of intrabronchial lesions. A new mapping technique via the flexible fiberoptic bronchoscope. Chest 87:418, 1985

78. Ganfield RA, Chapin JW: Pneumothorax with upper laser surgery. Anesthesiology 56:398, 1982

79. Dumon J, Shapshay S, Bourcereau J, et al: Principles for safety in application of neodymium-YAG laser in bronchoscopy. Chest 86:163–168, 1984

80. Eisenman TS: Ossoff RH: Anesthesia for bronchoscopic laser surgery. Otolaryngol Head Neck Surg 94:45, 1986

81. McElvein RB, Zorn G: Treatment of malignant disease in trachea and mainstem bronchi by carbon dioxide laser. J Thorac Cardiovasc Surg 86:858, 1983

82. Paes ML, Conacher ID, Snellgrove JR: A ventilator for carbon dioxide laser bronchoscopy. Br J Anaesth 58:663,1986

83. Benumof J: Anesthesia for special elective therapeutic procedures. pp. 343–348. In: Anesthesia for Thoracic Surgery. WB Saunders, Philadelphia, 1987

84. Healy G, McGill T, Strong M: Surgical advances in the treatment of lesions of the pediatric airway; the role of the carbon dioxide laser. Pediatrics 61:380, 1978

85. Rontal M, Fuller T, Rontal E, et al: Flexible non-toxic fiberoptic delivery system for the carbon dioxide laser. Ann Otol Rhinol Laryngol 94:357, 1985

86. Sosis M, Braverman B, Ivankovich AD: An evaluation of special tracheal tubes with the KTP laser. Anesth Analg 72:S267, 1991

87. George PJM, Garrett CPO, Nixon C, et al: Treatment for tracheobronchial tumors: local or general anesthesia. Thorax 42:656, 1987

88. Ducket J, McDonnell T, Unger M, et al: General anaesthesia for Nd-YAG laser resection of obstructing endobronchial tumors using the rigid bronchoscope. Can Anaesth Soc J 32:67–72, 1985

89. Fisher J: The power density of surgical laser beam: its meaning and measurement. Lasers Surg Med 2:301–315, 1983

90. Vourc'h G, Fishler M, Michon F, et al: Manual jet ventilation vs high-frequency jet ventilation during laser resection of tracheobronchial stenosis. Br J Anaesth 55:973–975, 1983

91. Conacher ID, Paes ML, Morritt GN: Anaesthesia for carbon dioxide laser bronchoscopy—taking turns in the airway. J Anaesth 57:448, 1985

92. Sosis MB: An evaluation of five metallic tapes for protection of endotracheal tubes during CO_2 laser surgery. Anesth Analg 68:392–393, 1989

93. Sosis M, Heller S: A comparison of five metallic tapes for protection of endotracheal tubes during CO_2 laser surgery. Can J Anesth 40:563, 1988

94. Gupta B, Lingham RP, McDonald JS, Gage F: Hazards of laser surgery. Anesthesiology 61:A146, 1984

95. Williamson R: Why 70 watts to evaluate metal tapes for CO_2 laser surgery? Anesth Analg 72:414–415, 1991

96. Sosis M, Dillon F, Heller S: Hazards of CO_2 laser reflection from laser resistant endotracheal tubes. Anesthesiology 71:A444, 1989

97. Sosis M, Dillon F, Heller S: Saline filled cuffs help prevent laser induced polyvinylchloride endotracheal tube fires. Anesth Analg 72:187–189, 1991

98. Sosis M: Saline-soaked pledgets prevent CO_2 laser-induced tracheal tube cuff ignition. Anesth Analg 72:S266, 1991

99. Hirshman CA, Smith J: Indirect ignition of the endotracheal tube during carbon dioxide laser surgery. Arch Otol 106:639, 1980

100. Sosis M, Dillon F: What is the safest foil tap for endotracheal tube protection during Nd-YAG laser surgery? A comparative study. Anesthesiology 72:553–555, 1990

101. Patel K, Hicks J: Prevention of fire hazards associated with use of carbon dioxide lasers. Anesth Analg 60:885–888, 1981

102. Wolf G, Simpson J: Flammability of endotracheal tubes in oxygen and nitrous oxide enriched atmosphere. Anesthesiology 67:236–239, 1987

103. Meyers A: Complications of CO_2 laser surgery of the larynx. Ann Otol 90:132–134, 1981

104. Treyve E, Yarington CT, Thompson GE: Incendiary characteristics of endotracheal tubes with the CO_2 laser. Ann Otol Rhinol Laryngol 90:328–330, 1981

105. Ossoff R, Duncavage J, Eisenman T, et al: Comparisons of tracheal damage from laser-ignited endotracheal tube fires. Ann Otol Rhinol Laryngol 92:333–336, 1983

106. Sosis M, Dillon F, Heller S: Hazards of a new clear unmarked polyvinylchloride endotracheal tube designed for use with the Nd-YAG laser. Anesthesiology 71:A420, 1989

107. Hunton J, Oswal V: Metal tube anaesthesia for ear, nose and throat carbon dioxide laser surgery. Anaesthesia 40:1210–121, 1985

108. Sosis MB, Heller S: A comparison of special endotracheal tubes for use with the CO_2 laser. Anesthesiology 69:A251, 1988

109. Pashayan AG, Gravenstein JS, Cassis NJ, McLaughlin G: The helium protocol for laryngotracheal operations with CO_2 laser: a retrospective review of 523 cases. Anesthesiology 68:801–804, 1988

110. Casey K, Fairfax W, Smith S: Intratracheal fire ignited by the Nd-YAG laser during treatment of tracheal stenosis. Chest 84:295–296, 1983

111. Snow J, Norton M, Suluja T, et al: Fire hazards during CO_2 laser microsurgery on the larynx and trachea. Anesth Analg 55:146–147, 1976

112. Alfery DD, Benumof JL, Spragg RG: Anesthesia for bronchopulmonary lavage. pp. 403–419. In Kaplan JA (ed): Thoracic Anesthesia. Churchill Livingstone, New York, 1983

17

TRACHEOSTOMY AND TRACHEAL RECONSTRUCTION

Roger S. Wilson, M.D.

TRACHEOSTOMY

General Considerations

Tracheostomy, although a common surgical procedure, lacks uniformity in regard to indications and technique.[1,2] Indications for tracheostomy include (1) upper airway obstruction, (2) access for tracheal toilet, (3) route for administration of positive-pressure ventilation, and (4) airway protection from aspiration of gastric and/or pharyngeal contents. When performed electively, the incidence of complications, including hypoxia, cardiac arrest, injury to structures immediately adjacent to the trachea, pneumothoraxes, and hemorrhage should be minimal. Elective tracheostomy, like any other surgical procedure, should be done in the operating room under "ideal" operating conditions. Such conditions are provided in a well-equipped operating suite with adequate lighting and personnel who understand the procedure to be undertaken. In general, the best operating conditions are provided with prior endotracheal intubation and the patient adequately anesthetized or sedated with use of additional local anesthesia.

Anesthetic requirements are variable and are dictated by the state of patient awareness and the nature and extent of other systemic disease. If necessary, the procedure can be safely done by using local infiltration, supplemented with intravenous sedative and/or narcotic drugs. The advantage of this approach, especially when used for a critically ill patient, is that it allows for the administration of high concentrations of inspired oxygen. In patients in whom cardiovascular stability is not a problem, general anesthesia with any of the inhalational agents may be used with or without supplemental local infiltration. Use of nitrous oxide is dictated by the level of inspired oxygen concentration.

Monitoring, including the use of the electrocardiogram (ECG), intra-arterial pressure, and pulmonary artery pressure is dictated by the complexity of the patient's overall condition. In a patient with normal cardiopulmonary function, the standard ECG and blood pressure cuff monitoring are adequate. The need for additional monitoring is dictated by the presence of concomitant respiratory, cardiovascular, nervous system, or metabolic diseases.

Surgical Procedure

The patient is placed in the supine position with the neck extended, with either a rolled towel or inflatable thyroid bag placed beneath the shoulders. The head can be positioned in a "doughnut" or a head-dish for additional stability. These maneuvers provide for maximal surface exposure, and in most patients bring the trachea from the intrathoracic to the cervical position. After appropriate preparation of the skin and

441

surgical draping, the procedure is accomplished through a short horizontal incision placed at the level of the second tracheal ring (Fig. 17-1). The strap muscles are separated in the midline and the thyroid isthmus is divided and appropriately sutured to obtain hemostasis. Specific identification of the location of the tracheal rings is made by counting down from the easily palpable cricoid cartilage. The second and third rings are opened vertically in the midline for access to

the trachea. The tracheostomy tube should be placed so that it will not erode the first ring and press against the cricoid cartilage. In addition, the opening should not be placed too low, or the tip of the tube and its cuff will be too close to the carina. Low placement of the tracheostomy tube is also hazardous since the innominate artery crosses anteriorly to the trachea low in the neck, and the possibility of erosion into the vessel by either the cuff or tip of the tracheostomy tube is possi-

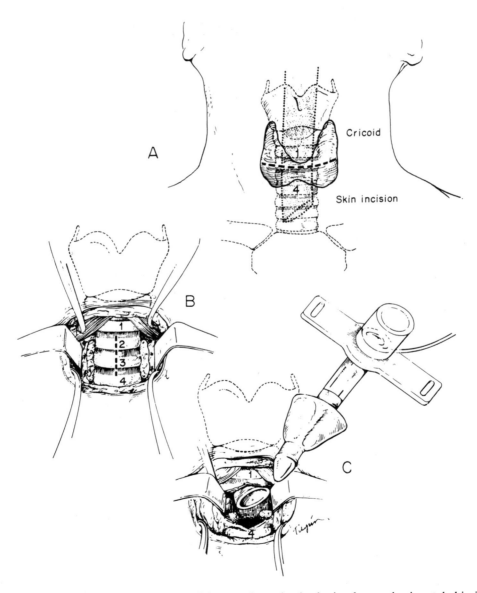

Fig. 17-1. Technique of tracheostomy. **(A)** With an endotracheal tube in place, a horizontal skin incision is made 1 to 2 cm below the cricoid cartilage. **(B)** Strap muscles are spread in the midline and the thyroid isthmus is divided. A vertical incision is made in the second and third cartilaginous rings. **(C)** With thyroid pole retractors holding back the cut edge of the trachea, the endotracheal tube is withdrawn and the tracheostomy tube is inserted. (From Grillo,[42] with permission.)

TABLE 17-1. Tracheostomy Tube Length

Internal Diameter (mm)	Portex Standard (mm)	Portex Extra Length (mm)	Shiley Single Cannula (mm)	Shiley Double Cannula (mm)
5.0	NA	NA	58	NA
6.0	67	NA	67	67
7.0	73	84	80	78
8.0	78	95	89	84
9.0	84	106	89	NA
10.0	84	NA	105	84

Abbreviation: NA, not available.

ble. Segments of the trachea should not be removed, since this might lead to a greater loss of tracheal wall stability and predisposes to stenosis once healing is accomplished following removal of the tube. The lateral tracheal walls are retracted with use of thyroid pole retractors, and the appropriate-size tracheostomy tube is inserted into the airway following slow withdrawal of the previously placed oral or nasal endotracheal tube to a more proximal position in the trachea. As shown in Table 17-1, tracheostomy tube size varies according to type, internal diameter, and length. Once the tracheostomy tube is positioned and an adequate airway demonstrated with use of positive-pressure ventilation and visual inspection of chest wall expansion, the previously placed endotracheal tube is removed from the trachea. The wound is appropriately closed, a skin suture is placed through the flange, and "trach-tape" or a tie is secured around the neck.

Complications

Complications may occur during the intra- and postoperative periods. Intraoperative complications generally occur secondary to either the anesthesia, underlying disease, or surgical procedure. Surgical complications generally fall into three major categories: hemorrhage, injury to structures adjacent to the trachea, and failure to cannulate the airway. Bleeding from the surgical incision is usually easily controlled, but may be complicated by the difficulty of exposure. Vascular structures such as the thyroid isthmus may bleed easily when divided for exposure. Injuries to adjacent structures include damage to recurrent laryngeal nerves, entrance into major vessels, and rare, but possible, laceration of the esophagus. Inability to cannulate the trachea is possible due to inadequate surgical exposure, inability to bring the trachea to a superficial location, or selection of a tracheostomy tube too large to fit into the tracheal stoma. Such complications can be avoided by careful planning and appropriate selection of tubes. In the presence of prior endotracheal intubation, the danger of

loss of the airway is minimized. Long-term complications resulting from the use of endotracheal and tracheostomy tubes will be considered in the discussion of types of tracheostomy tubes and cuffs.

Emergency Tracheostomy

An emergency tracheostomy is occasionally necessary. The need is dictated by the urgency of providing an airway, often due to rapidly progressing airway obstruction. This may occur following head and neck trauma, upper airway compromise due to allergic reactions, angioneurotic edema, epiglottitis, local infection following neck surgery such as thyroidectomy, or an anterior approach for a cervical fusion. Such postoperative problems result from hemorrhage with external compression and potential for total airway obstruction. The ability to accomplish airway control with an endotracheal tube may not be possible. Appropriate emergency procedures include needle tracheostomy, cricothyroidotomy, and standard tracheostomy. Needle tracheostomy is often of limited success since flow through the catheter or needle requires a high-pressure gas source and the immediate availability of appropriate connecting devices between the gas source and the needle or catheter. With this technique, ventilation and, hence, CO_2 elimination are difficult. This maneuver is potentially lifesaving for only a limited time. Formal emergency tracheostomy in general is not technically feasible due to the lack of adequate instruments and lighting and the time required to accomplish it before major circulatory and/or cerebral complications occur.

The technique of cricothyroidotomy has become increasingly popular and has been described in numerous publications.[3,4] One advantage is that it can be done quickly with a minimum amount of equipment. A rolled towel is placed under the shoulders to put the neck in a hyperextended position. A small transverse incision is made through the skin into the cricothyroid membrane using a #11 scalpel blade; the incision is spread with a surgical clamp or a knife handle or with a digital technique. A small (5.0 or 6.0 mm) pediatric endotracheal tube or tracheostomy tube is placed through the cricothyroid membrane into the trachea. This technique has the advantages of simplicity, speed, and minimal bleeding. It also provides an airway sufficient for adequate gas exchange. Potential complications of this technique include injury to the cricoid or thyroid cartilages, with the potential for laryngeal stenosis, injury to the esophagus, hemorrhage from the anterior jugular vein, injury to the carotid artery or internal jugular vein, and infection at the cricothyroid incision. These complications are generally avoidable if the incision is correctly placed, a small tube is used, and the duration of use of the cricothyroidotomy is limited to a short time period, ie, hours or days. Although it may be advisable to convert the cricothyroidotomy to a standard tracheostomy as soon as the patient's overall condition permits, there is no uniform opinion regarding this decision.

Tracheostomy Tube Design

Tracheostomy tubes come in a wide variety of types. They differ in several respects, including (1) rigidity, (2) flange shape, (3) length, (4) internal/external diameter, (5) angle or curvature of the tube body, and (6) cuff shape and characteristics.[5]

Recognition that tracheal intubation with cuffed endotracheal and tracheostomy tubes can produce in-

jury has stimulated improvement in design of both tubes and cuffs. The pathogenesis of tracheal injuries produced by "cuff pressure" has been well documented.[6-9] Complications include tracheal stenosis or disruption of the tracheal wall, with the potential for development of a tracheoesophageal fistula or a fistula into a major vessel. A number of cuff designs and techniques have been developed in the hope of minimizing tracheal injury.[10,11] Approaches have included intermittent cuff inflation and deflation, inflation of cuffs during inspiration only, underinflation with a minimal leak technique, use of double-cuff tubes, and design of high-volume, low-pressure cuffs. The latter has proved to be the most effective way of reducing tracheal injury.[12]

The large-residual-volume, low-pressure cuff has been designed in several configurations by a variety of manufacturers. The general design of this cuff is such that it occludes the lumen of the trachea by conforming to the existing configuration of the cross-sectional area without deforming it (Fig. 17-2). Improved design of the cuff per se does not totally eliminate tracheal injury. Several precautions must be taken regardless of the type of cuff used. The cuff must not be inflated beyond the minimum volume and pressure required to provide a minimal leak.

Excessive pressure within the inflated cuff (generally assumed to be > 25 mmHg) will potentially increase the risk of tracheal injury. Although lateral

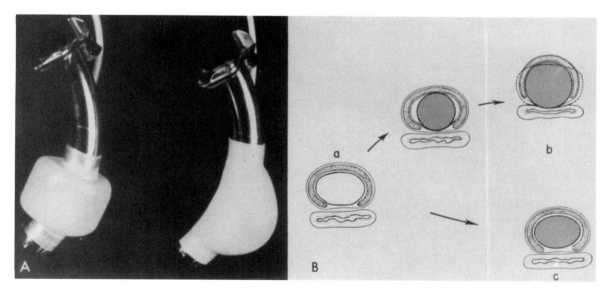

Fig. 17-2. Tracheostomy tube cuffs. **(A)** On the left is a large-volume, high-compliance cuff, adjacent to a partially inflated standard high-pressure cuff. **(B)** When the high-pressure cuff is inflated, the eccentrically shaped trachea *(a)* is not sealed until the airway is deformed with use of high cuff pressures *(b)*. This is in contrast to the low-pressure cuff *(c)*, which fills the eccentrically shaped trachea and provides occlusion without exerting significant pressure. (From Grillo,[42] with permission.)

wall pressure, pressure at the point of contact surface between cuff and tracheal wall, is more important than intracuff pressure, the latter is monitored due to ease of measurement. Excessive cuff pressure is frequently encountered when the tracheostomy tube that has been selected is too small, requiring overinflation of the cuff to completely fill the void between the tube and the trachea. When this occurs, alternative measures, such as an increase in tracheostomy tube size, selection of a tracheostomy tube with a larger cuff, or acceptance of a larger leak, must be undertaken.

Care and Maintenance of the Tracheostomy

Adequate care must be provided to the tracheal stoma to prevent injury. The care should focus on removal of secretions from the region of the stoma and the surrounding skin. Tracheostomy dressings should be changed regularly, eg, every 8 hours. The technique should include use of sterile gloves and cotton-tipped applicators with hydrogen peroxide to cleanse the stoma site. Tracheostomy tapes, which often become soiled, should be changed on a regular basis.

Tracheostomy tubes with inner cannula are beneficial in cases in which secretions are abundant and the risk of tube obstruction exists. The advantage of this type of tube is that it allows removal of the inner cannula for cleaning without removal of the tracheostomy tube from the airway.

It is advisable to change the tracheostomy tube on a regular basis to ensure that the tube may be easily removed. Difficulty in removing tubes occurs as the stoma heals down around the shaft of the tube, the stoma size being reduced so that when the tube is partially withdrawn, the bulk of the cuff does not allow removal from the airway.[13] Elective removal and reinsertion of a new tracheostomy tube on a weekly basis obviates this problem. Elective tube changes should be postponed until 72 to 96 hours following original surgical placement; inadequate development of the stomal tract during the first few days makes such changes dangerous.

Elective tube change should be carefully regulated. The nature of the changing procedure should be explained to the patient. If mechanical ventilation is being used, 100 percent inspired oxygen should be administered for several minutes before the procedure is performed. A laryngoscope, endotracheal tube, and a self-inflating manual resuscitation bag should be readily available. The patient is positioned flat in bed and a rolled towel placed under the shoulders to provide better visualization of the neck area. Following suctioning of the airway, the cuff is deflated and the tube withdrawn. A similar-size tracheostomy tube should be repositioned in the stoma, the cuff inflated, and adequacy of tube placement ascertained by auscultation of breath sounds, with spontaneous or positive-pressure ventilation delivered through the tracheostomy tube. If the patient needs to be returned to mechanical ventilation, the adequacy of breath sounds must again be reconfirmed by use of chest auscultation after the tube is secured in place.

Minitracheostomy

Minitracheostomy, originally described by Matthews and Hopkinson, is a new and novel technique used to provide access for endotracheal suctioning while preserving normal glottic function for cough and speech.[14] This technique uses a commercially available (Mini-Trach II; Portex, Concord, NH) indwelling plastic cannula that is 4.0 mm in internal diameter. This catheter is placed percutaneously through the cricothyroid membrane. Recent clinical experience published by Wain et al described the use of this technique in 56 patients from a variety of surgical and medical services.[15] Indications for catheter placement in this population included (1) excessive postoperative secretions, (2) difficulty with "blind" endotracheal suctioning, (3) preoperative secretions, and (4) acute airway obstruction. Advantages of the technique are its ease of insertion, ability to preserve laryngeal function, and favorable acceptance on the part of the patient. Such catheters can be left in place for periods exceeding 1 month. Minor reported complications include local hematoma, subcutaneous emphysema, and hoarseness. In addition to using the device as a means for tracheal toilet, it has also been described as a method for delivery of high-frequency jet ventilation in patients with respiratory failure.[16]

TRACHEAL RECONSTRUCTION

Etiology of Injuries

Although tracheostomy is one of the most ancient of surgical procedures, techniques of tracheal resection have been advanced only during the past 25 years.[17] Currently, all but the most extensive benign and malignant lesions are potentially surgically resectable. Techniques of tracheal surgery and anesthesia have been developed and refined to a considerable degree. In addition, there has been heightened awareness and understanding of tracheal disease, including neoplastic, inflammatory, and traumatic lesions. The etiologies of tracheal injury are numerous and are outlined in Table 17-2.

**TABLE 17-2. Etiology of
Tracheal Lesions**

Congenital lesions
    Tracheal agenesis/atresia
    Congenital stenosis
    Congenital chondromalacia

Neoplastic lesions
    Primary neoplasms
        Squamous cell carcinoma
        Adenoid cystic carcinoma (cylindroma)
        Carcinoid adenoma
        Carcinosarcoma-chondrosarcoma
    Secondary neoplasms
        Bronchogenic carcinoma
        Esophageal carcinoma
        Tracheal carcinoma
        Breast carcinoma
        Head/neck carcinoma

Postintubation injuries
    Laryngeal stenosis
    Cuff injury
    Ulceration/fistula
    Granuloma formation

Posttracheostomy injury
    Cuff lesions
    Stoma lesions

Trauma
    Penetrating
    Blunt injuries
        Cervical
        Intrathoracic
Infection

Congenital Lesions

As outlined by Grillo, there are a variety of congenital lesions involving the trachea.[18] The extent ranges from those incompatible with life, such as tracheal agenesis or atresia, to regional segmental stenoses. Congenital tracheal stenosis may be associated with a number of other anomalies, such as an aberrant left pulmonary artery or pulmonary artery sling, which produce compression of the posterior tracheal wall. This occurs when the left pulmonary artery originates from the proximal portion of the right pulmonary artery and passes behind the trachea to the left lung. Complete tracheal rings are common in this anomaly, and surgical correction of the vascular anomaly does not necessarily improve airway obstruction. In contrast, vascular ring malformations, when they compress the trachea without associated primary tracheal anomalies, are generally improved by surgical correction. Tracheal compromise of this type occurs with a double aortic arch, a right aortic arch, or a ligamentum arteriosum (see Chapter 19).

In general, surgical repair of pediatric tracheal abnormalities must be approached with caution. The small cross-sectional area of the airway, with its potential for obstruction from edema and secretions, increases the surgical risk in infancy or childhood. In addition, other increased risks of surgery and anesthesia may preclude operation at this time. If possible, it is preferable to use alternative measures, such as tracheostomy, to temporize until some later stage of life.

Neoplastic Lesions

Primary neoplastic lesions, although uncommon, may develop in the trachea (Table 17-3).[19] In several published series, squamous cell carcinoma and adenoid cystic carcinoma are the most common, with a variety of other rare tumors having been cited in all series.[19–21]

Although extensive knowledge concerning the natural history of these lesions is not clear, it is evident that both squamous cell carcinoma and adenoid cystic carcinoma are amenable to early aggressive therapy and are potentially curable. Squamous cell carcinoma may present as a well-localized lesion of the exophytic type or as an ulcerating lesion. Limited experience suggests that spread is first to regional lymph nodes adjacent to the trachea and then direct extension into mediastinal structures. Adenoid cystic

**TABLE 17-3. Primary
Tracheal Tumors**

Benign
    Squamous papillomata
        Multiple
        Solitary
    Pleomorphic adenoma
    Granular cell tumor
    Fibrous histiocytoma
    Leiomyoma
    Chondroma
    Chondroblastoma
    Schwannoma
    Paraganglioma
    Hemangioendothelioma
    Vascular malformation

Intermediate
    Carcinoid
    Mucoepidermoid
    Plexiform neurofibroma
    Pseudosarcoma
    Malignant fibrous histiocytoma

Malignant
    Adenocarcinoma
    Adenosquamous carcinoma
    Small cell carcinoma
    Atypical carcinoid
    Melanoma
    Chondrosarcoma
    Spindle cell sarcoma
    Rhabdomyosarcoma

carcinoma infiltrates the airway in a submucosal fashion, often for longer distances than is evident on gross endoscopic examination. Some lesions of high malignancy have spread by direct invasion into the pleura and lungs by the time the diagnosis is made. The opportunity for complete removal of this type of tumor occurs at the time of the initial surgery with wide resections of the margins. Currently, there is limited experience with the many other types of tumors that may invade the trachea; thus, generalizations concerning their natural history are difficult.

Primary tumors of the trachea present in several ways. Shortness of breath, especially with exertion, is often the primary symptom. As the tumor grows, this begins to worsen, producing limitations with very minimal levels of exercise. Wheezing, which is often confused and misdiagnosed as bronchial asthma, is a common feature. Stridor, with repeated attacks of respiratory obstruction due to a combination of tumor and secretions, may also occur. History of position-dependent airway obstruction, especially in the case of exophytic lesions, is possible. Obstruction may occur in a specific position, such as a lateral position, and be relieved in other positions. This finding is important when a history is taken during the preanesthesia visit, since induction of anesthesia in such patients must occasionally be undertaken in a specific position to ensure initial patency of the airway. Patients can also present with episodes of unilateral and bilateral pneumonia, often unresponsive to antibiotics and physiotherapy. Hemoptysis may accompany several of the aforementioned findings or present as the sole symptom.

Secondary neoplasms may occur throughout the tracheobronchial tree. It is not uncommon for structures adjacent to the airway to involve the trachea by metastases or direct extension. Bronchogenic, laryngeal, and esophageal carcinoma can invade the trachea and main bronchi. In general, metastases of this nature are associated with far advanced disease and obviate tracheal surgery except for palliation.

Secondary neoplasms occurring from thyroid malignancies perhaps are one area in which combined primary resection of the tumor and tracheal reconstruction is warranted. Not uncommonly, late recurrences of carcinoma originating in the thyroid have appeared in the trachea and larynx. Resection of these slow-growing late lesions has produced excellent palliation for several years.

A variety of other tumors can involve the trachea, including metastases from head and neck carcinoma, carcinoma of the breast with mediastinal involvement, and lymphoma. In general, tracheal reconstruction is not indicated in such cases. A recently published review of a 26-year experience with surgical management of primary tracheal tumors at the Massachusetts General Hospital supported an aggressive surgical approach.[19] Of the tumors in 198 patients evaluated, 147 (74 percent) were surgically excised. Overall, 10-year survival was approximately 33 percent for squamous cell carcinoma and 45 percent for adenoid cystic neoplasms. Surgical mortality for resection was 5 percent, 7 deaths in 132 patients, 6 occurring following carinal resection and reconstruction.

Injuries

Direct laryngeal and tracheal trauma can occur from both penetrating and blunt injuries to the cervical portion of the airway.[22] The presentation of penetrating injuries, including knife wounds or gunshot wounds, is dependent on the severity of the injuries and coexisting trauma to other vital structures, such as nerves and vessels.

Blunt injuries may severely damage the cervical trachea and are often complicated in their presentation.[23] Direct blows to the cervical area may be sufficient to lacerate or completely sever the trachea. Supporting tissues may hold the damaged area together, providing an airway that is adequate enough to allow the patient to reach an emergency facility. Total disruption of this airway is often produced at the time of intubation or attempts at emergency tracheostomy. If the airway is adequate, all maneuvers, such as tracheostomy and/or intubation, should be held in abeyance until clinical evaluation and diagnostic tests are performed to delineate the severity of the injury. Adequate facilities, ideally a well-equipped operating room, should be available for optimum management. Laryngeal fracture may occur as a primary or concomitant injury in such cases. The surgical management of such lesions, as described by Montgomery in 1968, is best undertaken after healing of the acute injury.[24]

The intrathoracic trachea and bronchi, like other intrathoracic organs, may also be disrupted during indirect closed-chest trauma.[25,26] One area particularly susceptible to injury is the membranous wall of the trachea, which can be lacerated in a vertical direction with extension at the level of the carina into the right or left mainstem bronchus. Such injuries often present as a pneumothorax, which commonly fails to respond completely to tube thoracostomy and suction. The inability to re-expand a collapsed lung or the persistence of an excessive air leak should always raise the question of tracheal or major disruption. Incomplete separation of the bronchi may occur and only present as a late stenosis following discharge from the hospital.

Infection

Although rare, stricture of the trachea can result from pulmonary tuberculosis or other infectious etiologies, including diphtheria, syphilis, and typhoid, which all have been described in the past. Rarely are chronic inflammatory conditions of the trachea involved with stenosis. Fibrosing mediastinitis and systemic diseases such as Wegener's granulomatosis or amyloidosis can produce benign strictures.

Postintubation and Tracheostomy Injuries

The use of endotracheal or tracheostomy tubes has been shown to produce a variety of tracheal lesions. These have been described in detail in several articles.[6,7] As shown in Figure 17-3, lesions may be produced by the cuff in any of the areas where it contacts the tracheal wall. Laryngeal injury occurs with use of either oral or nasal endotracheal tubes, and at the stoma site with tracheostomy tubes.

Endotracheal intubation can produce a variety of injuries involving the nares, larynx, and trachea, with most injuries resulting from pressure necrosis.[6] At the laryngeal level, the vocal cords are a common site of injury. The extent of injury varies from edema and local irritation to more serious ulceration and erosion, often at the posterior commissure, with subsequent scar formation and/or granulomata. Although the majority of laryngeal lesions are reversible in time, a number require surgical correction.[24] Initial symptoms include hoarseness, sore throat, and stridor. Progression of edema with resulting airway obstruction may require reintubation and, in a limited number of cases, tracheostomy.

Subglottic stenosis may occur as a result of mucosal erosion at the level of the cricoid cartilage. The true incidence of this lesion is unknown. Subglottic stenosis poses a difficult problem due to limitations in surgical repair when the lesion is severe.

Cuff-related lesions with either tracheostomy or endotracheal tubes are similar. The presumed mechanism involves a force applied against the tracheal wall producing necrosis. Although many etiologic factors have been considered, including local infection and toxicity of cuff materials, it is apparent that the single most important factor is the direct pressure exerted by the inflated cuff against the tracheal mu-

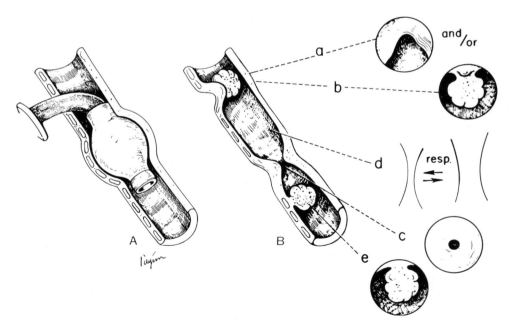

Fig. 17-3. Sites of tracheal injury. **(A)** A cuffed tracheostomy tube is shown in situ with dilation of the trachea at the level of the high-pressure cuff. **(B)** Sites of possible tracheal injuries are shown as follows: (a) erosion of the stoma and subsequent healing produces an anterolateral stricture; (b) granuloma may form also at this level; (c) at the level of pressure exerted by the cuff, circumferential erosion will result in a circumferential stenosis; (d) between the stoma and the level of the cuff, thinning of the tracheal wall with potential loss of cartilage may occur; and (e) the tube tip may produce erosion and/or granulomata. (From Grillo,[42] with permission.)

cosa.[8,9] The degree of injury produced depends on a number of factors, including the length of time the pressure is applied, the healing abilities of the patient, and the total amount of tissue injury produced. The extent of injury may vary from superficial ulceration with minimal sequelae, to extensive erosion involving destruction of cartilage with the potential for fistula formation. The pathophysiology and visual confirmation of such lesions, both in the experimental model and in patients, have been extensively described.[12] The natural evolution of this injury relates to cicatrization during the healing process, which produces a circumferential stenosis (Fig. 17-3).

Tracheomalacia can also be the consequence of a cuff-related injury. This occurs at the level of the cuff, where progressive lateral force weakens a tracheal segment and local inflammation destroys the cartilage. Tracheomalacia also occurs between the level of the tracheostomy stoma and the cuff, where inflammatory changes, perhaps due to pooling of secretions and local bacterial infection, lead to thinning of cartilaginous structures without significant injury to the mucosa itself. Such segmental injuries produce a functional obstruction, particularly when a maximal respiratory effort during inspiration or expiration is produced. The tracheal stoma is a frequent site of stenosis. The mechanism is most likely related to a significant loss of anterolateral tracheal wall and subsequent cicatricial healing, producing an anterolateral stricture. Factors leading to the development of such an injury include extensive surgical resection of anterior tracheal wall, local infection of the tissue in the stomal area, and pressure necrosis created by leverage between ventilator tubing and the tracheostomy tube.

Granulation tissue can develop at several sites in the airway, including the stoma and the tip of the tracheostomy or endotracheal tube, where it impinges on the anterior tracheal wall. Such lesions produce airway obstruction that may be position-related and ball-valve in nature.

Life-threatening complications of tracheal injuries include tracheoesophageal fistula and fistula formation between the airway and major vessels.[27] Tracheoesophageal fistulae are usually manifest by unexplained recurrent episodes of aspiration pneumonia, often associated with an increase or change in the character of tracheal secretions. Presenting features during mechanical ventilation may include the presence of air in the gastrointestinal tract and/or the inability to maintain adequate tidal volume and minute ventilation. Tracheoinnominate artery fistulae manifest themselves by sudden, massive, life-threatening hemorrhage from the tracheobronchial tree or through the stoma. Such lesions are often heralded by

minor episodes of bleeding from the stoma as erosion first begins to develop.

Diagnostic Evaluation

Diagnostic evaluation for patients with obstructive lesions of the airway consists of detailed history and physical examination, pulmonary function studies, roentgenographic studies, and bronchoscopy. The indications for each study and the potential benefit derived from the information vary from patient to patient. In addition, the severity and urgency of airway compromise will often dictate the diagnostic regimen that is followed. In life-threatening situations in which there is a high index of suspicion as to the nature of the tracheal pathology, diagnosis may consist only of bronchoscopy. However, in the patient presenting for elective surgery with symptoms indicative of airway obstruction, a detailed evaluation is generally warranted.[28]

History and Physical Examination

The signs and symptoms produced by airway obstruction will be affected by the anatomic location, degree of airway obstruction, and presence of pre-existing cardiopulmonary disease. The clinical symptoms generally consist of dyspnea, especially with effort, wheezing, which may present as frank stridor, difficulty in clearing secretions, and eventual airway obstruction from inability to clear mucus. Although simple and nonspecific, these symptoms are frequently misdiagnosed. It is not uncommon, especially when dealing with tracheal tumors, to find that patients have been diagnosed as having asthma. In many cases, suspicion as to some other diagnosis is aroused only when the supposed asthma fails to respond to usual treatment modalities, often including use of corticosteroids. It is essential to remember that in any patient with a history of recent intubation and/or tracheostomy, the development of any of the above symptoms should be considered a result of an organic lesion until proven otherwise.

Pre-existing cardiopulmonary disease will often limit exercise. In such cases, tracheal stenosis can progress to a severe stage before symptomatology is present.

Physical examination is essential, but generally of limited value. Audible stridor, either occurring at rest or provoked with a maximal expiratory effort with an open mouth, is a common finding. Chest auscultation frequently reveals diffuse inspiratory and expiratory wheezing, often difficult to differentiate from that typical of asthma. Auscultation of the upper cervical airway may reveal high-pitched inspiratory and expiratory sounds characteristic of obstruction to air flow.

Pulmonary Function Studies

Although standard spirometry is of limited value in diagnosing obstructive lesions, the use of flow-volume loops has been shown to be very reliable.[29] With standard spirometry, measured air flow during inspiration and expiration may be reduced. Maximal expiratory and/or inspiratory flow is affected to a far greater degree than is the 1-second forced expiratory volume (FEV_1). The ratio of peak expiratory flow to FEV_1 has been used as an index of obstruction. When this ratio is 10:1 or greater, it is suggestive of airway obstruction. The flow-volume loop is the most specific test for the diagnosis of upper airway obstruction. During a forced expiration from total lung capacity, the maximal flow achieved during the first 25 percent of the vital capacity is dependent on effort alone. In the case of fixed airway obstruction, the peak expiratory flow is markedly reduced, producing a characteristic plateau. With fixed intra- or extrathoracic lesions, the inspiratory flow has the same characteristic plateau. In the case of a variable obstruction, such as that seen with tracheomalacia, the maximal cutoff of inspiratory or expiratory flow will depend on the location of the lesion. Extrathoracic or cervical lesions produce a plateau during inspiration, with minimal effect on expiratory flow, while intrathoracic lesions that are variable tend to demonstrate alterations in the expiratory flow curve with minimal or no effect on inspiration. In general, stenoses that are circumferential, such as those produced by cuff lesions, are fixed in origin. Tumors and tracheomalacia frequently produce a variety of intermittent obstructions. It is often possible to estimate the functional impairment of the tracheal lesion by using a restricted orifice in the patient's mouthpiece during the flow-volume study. When the limited orifice begins to show additional effect on the flow-volume loop, it can be assumed that the intrinsic lesion has reduced the trachea to that cross-sectional area. In general, airway obstruction must reach 5 to 6 mm in cross-sectional diameter before signs and symptoms become clinically evident. The peak expiratory flow rate decreases to approximately 80 percent of normal when the airway diameter is reduced to 10 mm (see Chapters 1 and 12).

Radiologic Studies

Routine and special radiologic studies will often precisely demonstrate the extent and location of the tracheal pathology (Figs. 17-4 and 17-5).[30,31] In addition to the standard posteroanterior and lateral chest ra-

diographs, the oblique views are of additional benefit. The latter will often show the full extent of the trachea when mediastinal structures are rotated to the side. Lateral cervical views are of value in demonstrating detailed laryngotracheal relationships and deformities impinging on the anterior or posterior tracheal walls. Whenever possible, fluoroscopy is done to determine the functional nature of the lesion and to demonstrate the presence of airway malacia. Once areas of pathology are identified, laminograms or polytome views of the trachea in both anteroposterior and lateral projections and chest computed tomography are used to obtain the definitions and exact positions of the lesions. In general, contrast material should not be used for fear of producing airway obstruction.

Evaluation of patients with endotracheal tubes in place must be undertaken with caution, since optimal examination using radiologic techniques can only be done when the endotracheal or tracheostomy tube has been removed. Although the airway may be adequate immediately following decannulation, it is not uncommon for compromise to occur in a matter of minutes. Hence, any decannulation, especially when done in the x-ray department, must be done under close supervision of someone trained and properly equipped to reinstitute tracheal intubation.

Bronchoscopy

Bronchoscopy is generally the most definitive diagnostic procedure. In general, bronchoscopy is deferred until the time of the proposed corrective operation in order not to precipitate airway obstruction secondary to edema or hemorrhage (see Chapter 12).

Anesthetic Management

Various approaches to the induction and maintenance of anesthesia during surgery for tracheal reconstruction have been described.[32–35] The surgical and anesthetic techniques described in this chapter have been used by Grillo and colleagues and the thoracic anesthesia group for several hundred patients who have undergone tracheal resection and reconstruction at the Massachusetts General Hospital since 1962.[36–41]

Preoperative Assessment

Based on the studies discussed above, preoperative workup should localize the nature, location, and extent of the trachea requiring reconstruction. The preoperative assessment from the anesthesiologist's vantage point should consider, among other things, the degree of airway limitation, the presence of pre-existing disease, especially of the lungs or heart, and the

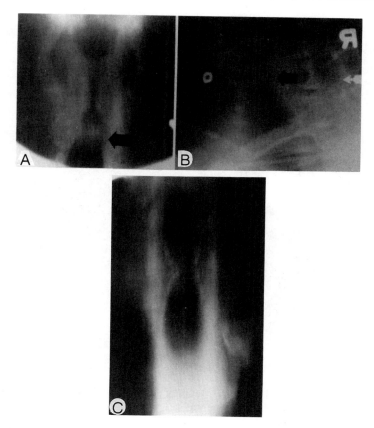

Fig. 17-4. Radiographs of benign tracheal lesions. **(A)** Details of the larynx and upper trachea are shown, with a large granuloma indicated by the arrow. **(B)** The same lesion shown in detail on a soft-tissue lateral view of the neck. The arrow indicates the granuloma within the air column. **(C)** Laminagraph showing stomal stenosis. Above may be seen the normal upper surface of the vocal cords and the bell-shaped subglottic larynx, which terminates at the bottom of the cricoid. (From Grillo,[42] with permission.)

potential problems in the postoperative period. The patient should be evaluated with the understanding that intraoperative difficulties associated with the airway, as well as potential problems during induction, may cause the individual undue stress from hypoxia, hypercarbia, and/or cardiovascular instability. The general approach to the anesthetic technique used and possible alternatives during the procedure must be based on these factors as well as the surgical approach that is anticipated (see Chapter 3).

In most cases, bronchoscopy is done at the time of the contemplated surgical correction. Advantages of this approach are that (1) only one anesthetic is required for total correction, (2) appropriate invasive monitoring need only be undertaken once, and (3) airway compromise following bronchoscopy, in the presence of existing pathology, should not become a life-threatening postoperative problem.

Careful attention to detail must be paid while eval-

uating the anatomic configuration and function of the upper airway. Inspection of jaw motion, adequacy of the oral pharynx, and problems relating to mask fit must be viewed with great concern in the preoperative period, since prolonged induction with inhalation agents will rely heavily on the ability to maintain an adequate natural airway in lieu of the distal airway problems. Arterial blood gases, although possibly affected by pre-existing chronic and acute parenchymal lung disease, are seldom deranged in the presence of pure upper airway stenosis. Occasionally, if obstruction is severe enough, a compensatory hypocarbia may result. Hypercarbia occurs, as with asthma, only as an extremely late event. Occasionally, when severe airway compromise exists in the preoperative period, prophylactic measures may be utilized. These include use of increased inspired oxygen concentrations, increased humidity, and topical steroids or racemic epinephrine. During the course of the workup, a patient

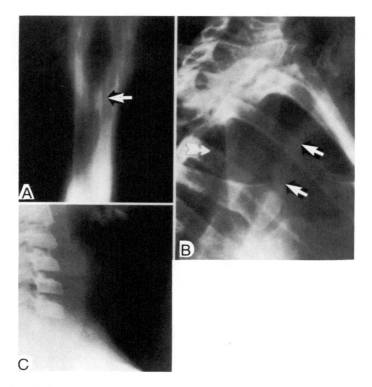

Fig. 17-5. Other tracheal lesions are shown. **(A)** Detail of a cuff stenosis on a tracheal laminagraph is shown. The bell shape of the lower larynx may be seen above with a segment of normal trachea, which tapers abruptly to a narrow stenotic segment. The trachea opens up to a normal diameter below this segment. **(B)** Detail from an oblique view shows the trachea air column reaching a point of maximum narrowing between the two white arrows. **(C)** Ball-like anterior granuloma is shown on a lateral neck view in the lower part of a long cervical trachea. The granuloma formed at the site of anterior erosion where the tip of the tube had pressed against the tracheal wall. (From Grillo,[42] with permission.)

is generally admitted to an intensive care unit if the airway is felt to be extremely marginal. This provides close and continuous observation, available monitors, and required equipment and personnel if emergency intubation should become necessary.

The type of preoperative medication is governed by the extent of airway obstruction. In patients in whom airway obstruction is minimal, the need for tranquilizers, sedatives, and/or drying agents is dictated by the usual criteria. The obvious concern when faced with airway obstruction is the avoidance of oversedation and central respiratory depression. In cases in which anxiety and emotional instability make patient management difficult, appropriate sedation with small doses of tranquilizers and/or barbiturates is relatively safe. In patients in whom airway obstruction is severe, especially when there is obvious stridor and use of accessory respiratory muscles, the administration of atropine and other drying agents should be avoided. Atropine has been reported to produce dry-

ing of secretions, creating a situation in which inspissated plugs form and become impacted in the narrow portion of the airway, creating close to total airway obstruction. When in doubt, all premedication should be withheld until the patient arrives in the operating room and is under the close supervision of the anesthesiologist and surgeon.

In those patients in whom airway obstruction exists but has been bypassed by either an endotracheal tube, tracheostomy tube, or T tube, the use of premedication is governed by the patient's needs and the conditions compatible with safe induction of anesthesia.

Monitoring

The standard approach for monitoring the otherwise uncomplicated patient is the use of an ECG, blood pressure cuff, pulse oximeter, esophageal stethoscope, and radial arterial catheter. The arterial catheter is not only useful for instantaneous monitoring of blood pressure during the intra- and postoperative periods, but is of even greater benefit in facilitating sampling of arterial blood to follow the efficiency of gas exchange. The selection of the site of cannulation is governed not only by the availability of such vessels, but also by the fact that the right radial artery is often lost due to compression or deliberate sacrifice of the innominate artery, which crosses the trachea and, hence, the operative field anteriorly from left to right. Thus, the left radial artery is preferred. In addition, when the approach is via a right thoracotomy and surgical exposure dictates that the right arm be prepared into the surgical field, the left radial, left brachial, dorsalis pedis, or femoral arteries are generally utilized.

A central venous catheter is appropriate when it is anticipated that vasopressor support or other intravenous medications requiring such a route will be used during the intraoperative period. In general, the use of a central venous pressure or pulmonary artery catheter is dictated by a history of existing cardiopulmonary disease. Following intubation, placement of an esophageal stethoscope not only provides useful information pertaining to breath sounds, heart tones, and rhythm, but also provides a foreign body that guides the surgeon in helping to identify the esophagus in the surgical field. Measurement of end-tidal gases should also be performed.

Airway Equipment

In addition to a conventional anesthesia machine and appropriate monitoring, it is necessary to provide several other important pieces of equipment. It is beneficial to have an anesthesia machine with the capabilities of delivering high-flow oxygen, in excess of 20 L/min. This is particularly useful during the induction phase, when air leaks may pose problems, and during rigid bronchoscopy. In addition, appropriate equipment should be provided to facilitate laryngoscopy and topical anesthesia. The choice of a laryngoscope blade is not as important as the individual's ability to use any given one with facility. A long bronchial sprayer, with 4 percent lidocaine, is useful for topicalization of the pharynx and tracheal mucous membranes. The most important equipment to be kept readily available is a variety of tubes, ranging from 20 to 30 French (F) for endotracheal intubation. The optimal size to provide an adequate airway, ability to suction secretions, and enough room for surgical manipulation and suturing of the airway is 28 F. In general, the tube size is selected when visualization of the airway is accomplished during rigid bronchoscopy; the decision is then made as to whether it is feasible to intubate through the stenosis or rely on a

tube placed above it. These decisions are discussed below in detail in connection with the technique for bronchoscopy.

Anesthesia Management

Once the patient is positioned comfortably on the operating room table in the supine position with an appropriate intravenous catheter and monitoring in place, the induction of anesthesia commences. In patients in whom airway obstruction is of minor significance, due to either a good natural airway or the presence of an intratracheal appliance, anesthesia may be induced with thiopental or a similar agent. When airway conditions are consistent with a high degree of obstruction, it is desirable to undertake a gentle, controlled inhalational induction with a volatile anesthetic. First, the patient is denitrogenated with oxygen via a mask for an appropriate period of time. Induction of anesthesia is accomplished with inhalation techniques using enflurane and, on rare occasions, halothane. Relaxants should be avoided, with reliance placed on spontaneous ventilation and assisted breaths when possible, since the ability to intubate the larynx and provide an airway is not always guaranteed. In many cases in which airway obstruction is severe, it is impossible with mask and positive-pressure ventilation to provide adequate gas flow through a limited orifice. However, during spontaneous ventilation, even in the anesthetized state, the patient is able to breathe adequately.

Anesthesia is induced until it is judged that the patient will tolerate direct laryngoscopy. Laryngoscopy is then performed and, at this time, topical anesthesia, generally with 4 percent lidocaine, is applied to the oral pharynx and glottis.

The mask is reapplied, volatile agent-oxygen administered, and a judgment made as to whether the patient has responded unfavorably to this procedure. If conventional signs, including tachycardia, hypertension, tearing, or any other manifestations of light anesthesia are evident, continued induction is carried out for an adequate period of time. When conditions are again favorable, a second laryngoscopy is undertaken and an attempt is made to topicalize the trachea by inserting the tracheal spray immediately below the cords. When an adequate depth of anesthesia is present, bronchoscopy can be undertaken.

During bronchoscopy, it is critical for the anesthesiologist to visually inspect the status of the airway with regard to the nature and extent of the lesion. This is important in terms of appreciating the difficulty of endotracheal tube placement and selection of the appropriate-size tube. There are several potential problems that must be considered at this time. Lesions involving the upper third of the trachea, especially those in the subglottic area, pose special problems with placement because of cuff position. A lesion that is located high in the airway, where the tube cannot be passed through the lesion because of the limited orifice, will not allow the cuff to pass below the cords and results in inability to attain a complete seal of the airway. Selection of a tube that is small enough to pass through the lesion with the cuff below it produces additional problems due to decreased internal diameter, especially when 20 to 24 F tubes are used, and creates problems of potential airway obstruction with secretions and blood during the operative procedure. Lesions located in the mid and lower third of the trachea are less problematic with respect to position. They must be considered in view of the need to pass the tube through the lesion itself to maintain adequacy of ventilation until the trachea is transected and/or the need to dilate the lesion at the time of bronchoscopy in order to provide adequacy of the airway. Dilatation must be considered with great caution due to the risk of significant airway damage, complicated by bleeding or perforation into other structures such as the esophagus or great vessels. Grillo's approach has been to dilate strictures if the airway measures less than 5 mm in diameter.[36] Dilatation is done under direct vision with several rigid pediatric ventilating bronchoscopes. Dilators passed through a large bronchoscope may easily perforate the tracheobronchial wall, especially if the stricture is in the distal trachea. If the airway measures more than 5 mm, an endotracheal tube is generally passed to a point above the stricture in lesions of the mid to lower trachea, and passed through it in lesions of the upper trachea. Caution must be exercised when tumors are present in the airway because of the potential for direct trauma if passage of the endotracheal tube results in obstruction from a dislodged piece of tumor with or without serious hemorrhage in the airway. Strictures of the anterior tracheal wall or stoma strictures are generally easily dealt with, since the mobile posterior membranous tracheal wall usually allows passage of an endotracheal tube or gas flow if the tube is positioned above the lesion.

Once bronchoscopy is completed, endotracheal intubation with the appropriate-size endotracheal tube is performed. This procedure is done in the normal manner using the sniffing position and direct laryngoscopy. As the tube is advanced down the airway, passage of the tube through the area of stricture can often be felt. Once the tube is thought to be in the appropriate position, the chest is auscultated in standard fashion to ensure bilateral lung ventilation. The tube is then secured, the eyes taped, and an esophageal stethoscope passed. Anesthesia is maintained with inhalation agent-oxygen or, in cases in which

normal pulmonary function exists and an adequate airway is present, with a combination of nitrous oxide and oxygen to supplement the anesthetic. Relaxants are avoided, and ventilation is generally accomplished by hand.

Surgical Positioning

As shown in Figure 17-6, several approaches to surgical incisions are used depending on the extent and location of the tracheal lesion. For most lesions located in the upper half of the trachea, an anterior collar incision is used with or without a vertical partial sternal split. For this incision, the patient is positioned supine, with a thyroid bag or bolster placed under the shoulders and the head on a supporting doughnut. The back of the table is elevated approximately 10 to 15 degrees to position the cervical and sternal area parallel to the floor when the head is in the fully extended position. The arms are either left at the side or extended on arm boards at 90-degree angles. Exploration of the lesion is done through the anterior collar incision, and the sternum is divided later if deemed necessary for surgical exposure.

Lesions of the lower half of the trachea are approached through a right posterior lateral thoracotomy incision in the fourth interspace or in the bed of the fourth rib. The position for this incision is a standard left lateral decubitus with the right arm draped and prepared so that it can be moved into the field for easier access to the neck. In this position, it is necessary to have intravenous and monitoring catheters in the left upper or lower extremities. In this position, a thoracotomy can be done and a collar incision added to free the trachea if there is need to perform a laryngeal release. In special cases of extensive or unusual lesions involving a greater area of the trachea, a vertical incision can be extended into the right and left fourth intercostal spaces from the sternal incision, as shown in Figure 17-6.

Reconstruction of the Upper Trachea

The surgical approach for lesions of the upper half of the trachea is shown in Figure 17-7. A low, short collar incision is made across the neck and a T incision is extended vertically over the sternum. Anterior dissection of the trachea is carried from the cricoid cartilage to the carina, with care taken not to injure the innominate artery or other structures adjacent to the trachea. Dissection around the back of the trachea is done at a point inferior to the lesion. If the patient has not been intubated through the stricture, caution must be undertaken during this dissection, since it is possible with release of the external supporting struc-

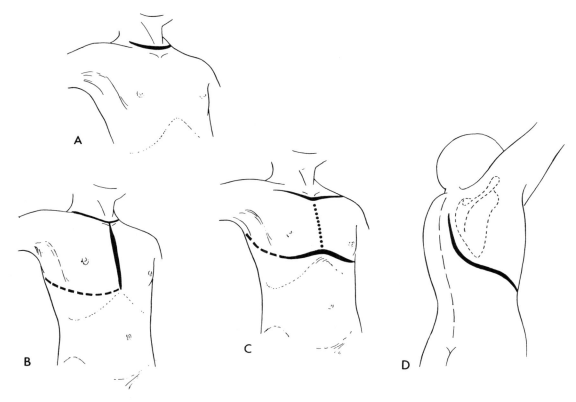

Fig. 17-6. Incisions for tracheal resection. **(A)** Standard collar incision for the majority of benign strictures and neoplastic lesions of the upper trachea. **(B)** Sternotomy extension: the dotted line shows an extension that may be carried through the fourth interspace to provide total exposure of the trachea from cricoid to carina. **(C)** Technique for raising a large bipedicle flap for total exposure and use in cases in which mediastinal tracheostomy is required. **(D)** Posterolateral thoracotomy, carried through the bed of the fourth rib or the fourth interspace for exposure of the lower half of the trachea. (From Grillo,[42] with permission.)

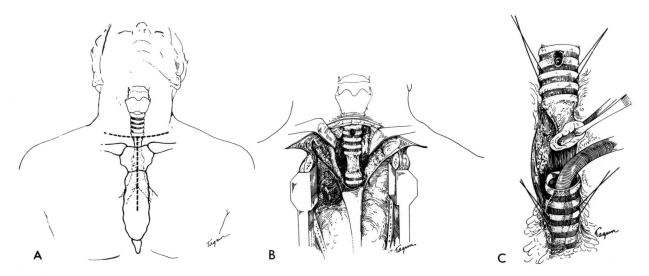

Fig. 17-7. Reconstruction of the upper trachea. **(A)** Collar incision and extension for upper sternotomy. **(B)** Dissection is carried down to isolate the damaged segment. **(C)** Circumferential dissection is carried out immediately beneath the level of pathology. Traction sutures are in place and the distal airway intubated via the operating field. (From Grillo,[42] with permission.)

ture of the trachea to produce progressive, and eventually complete, airway obstruction.

During this portion of the cervical procedure, anesthesia is maintained through a previously placed oral endotracheal tube. At the point at which it is anticipated that the trachea will be divided, nitrous oxide is eliminated from the anesthetic gas mixture and anesthesia is maintained with enflurane, isoflurane, or halothane and oxygen alone. At this point, a tape is placed around the trachea below the lesion, and lateral traction sutures are placed through the full thickness of the tracheal wall in the midline on either side at a point no more than 2 cm below the point of division of the trachea. It is important to anticipate the placement of these sutures so that the cuff on the endotracheal tube may be deflated to prevent it from being injured by the suture needle. The trachea is then transected below the lesion, as demonstrated in Figure 17-7C, and the distal trachea is intubated across the operative field with a flexible armored tube. The necessary sterile connecting equipment, consisting of corrugated tubings and a Y piece, are then passed to the anesthesiologist for connection to the anesthesia machine. The ability to ventilate the lungs is then assessed by use of positive pressure. The surgical dissection continues in order to free and excise the injured portion of the trachea.

Once adequacy of the tracheal lumen and extent of the tracheal resection have been determined, an attempt is made to approximate the two free ends of the trachea. This is accomplished by use of the traction sutures, with the anesthesiologist flexing the neck by grasping the head from above. When it is deemed possible to directly reanastomose the tracheal ends, intermittent sutures are placed into the trachea in a through and through manner, with anesthesia continuing through the tube positioned in the distal airway. In cases in which it is not possible to bring the ends together due to undue tension, a laryngeal release is performed. Once all sutures have been placed, the distal armored tube is removed and the oral endotracheal tube, which has remained in the proximal portion of the trachea, is advanced through the anastomosis into the distal trachea under direct vision (Fig. 17-8). Care must be taken at this point not to pass the tube too far distally into the trachea, since subsequent flexion of the neck for surgical foreshortening of the trachea will potentiate right mainstem bronchial intubation. Prior to this exchange, the airway is suctioned to remove aspirated blood. Anesthesia is then administered through the oral endotracheal tube into the distal trachea as the sutures are tied down to produce an airtight anastomosis. After all sutures have been placed, the patient's neck is flexed and the head supported in the position shown in Figure 17-8.

At the completion of the operation, the patient should be breathing spontaneously; extubation should be anticipated under either "awake" conditions or moderately deep anesthesia. The selection of the "awake" technique, which is designed to afford a good airway, must be balanced against the occasional need to reintubate the patient if laryngeal difficulty and/or other aspects of unresected tracheal disease promote airway obstruction. In most cases, it is prudent to extubate patients at a deeper level of anesthesia and maintain the airway, thus avoiding the potential for struggling, bucking, and excessive motion, which could injure the suture line. In patients in whom intubation was difficult because of upper airway pathology, it is prudent to allow the patient to awaken, supporting the head and neck during the excitement phase to avoid excessive motion. It is generally preferable to attempt extubation in the operating room, where the quality of airway patency may be quickly evaluated. Under such controlled circumstances, reintubation or diagnostic bronchoscopy can be done more easily and safely than in the recovery room or intensive care unit. Once the airway and ventilation are judged to be adequate, the patient can be safely transported, with supplemental oxygen, to the recovery room or intensive care unit.

Reconstruction of the Lower Trachea

The basic incision and surgical approach for the lower trachea have been described above. The general principles concerning intubation and early maintenance of anesthesia are similar to those described for the upper trachea with the exception of tube selection. In dealing with lower tracheal, and especially carinal, lesions it is advantageous to have a tube that is adequate in length to enter either mainstem bronchus. For this purpose, an armored tube with an added extension of some 4 to 5 inches on the proximal portion is used to provide both flexibility at the distal end and adequate length for bronchial intubation (Fig. 17-9). This tube is generally passed with the aid of a stylet and positioned according to the anatomic location and extent of the lesion.

During the thoracotomy and surgical resection of the trachea, positive-pressure ventilation is used while maintaining the ability of the patient to ventilate spontaneously, which is often needed during periods of discontinuity of the airway when positive-pressure ventilation is not possible. Although ventilation is impaired with the open thorax, adequate gas exchange has been maintained with high-flow insufflation of oxygen and anesthetic agent while relying on the dependent lung for the bulk of ventilation.

In general, resection involving the distal trachea

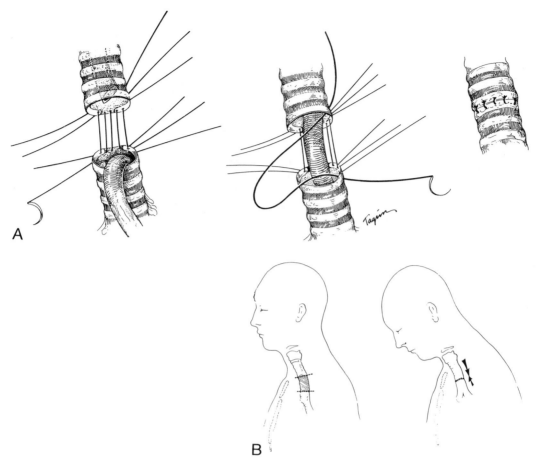

Fig. 17-8. Details of anastomotic technique. **(A)** Original endotracheal tube positioned in the upper trachea with the distal trachea intubated. Once all sutures are in place, the endotracheal tube is advanced and the sutures are tied in serial fashion. **(B)** With cervical flexion, the maximum amount of approximation is obtained. (From Grillo,[42] with permission.)

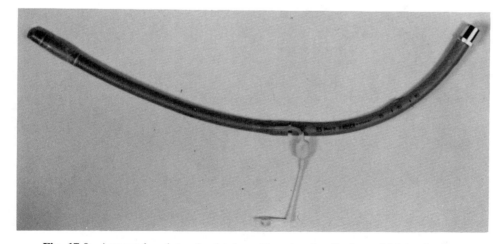

Fig. 17-9. Armored endotracheal tube with extension for bronchial intubation.

and carina is carried out with the endotracheal tube in a position proximal to the lesion. Surgical exposure and resection are much the same as previously described for upper tracheal lesions. Once the trachea is divided, it is common to find that the distal tracheal stump is too short to hold the endotracheal tube and cuff. Under these circumstances, it is often impossible to adequately ventilate both lungs. Generally, the left mainstem bronchus is intubated through the operative field, and ventilation and anesthesia are carried out entirely via the left lung while the diseased segment is excised. Although it is theoretically possible to temporarily eliminate perfusion to the right lung with pulmonary artery clamping, this is technically

very difficult and entails the potential hazard of injury to the right pulmonary artery. In cases in which adequate oxygenation and ventilation are not attainable with one lung, an easy approach is to advance a second tube into the right mainstem bronchus, preferably in the bronchus intermedius. A second anesthesia machine and sterile tubing are used to maintain continuous positive airway pressure (5 cm water) with oxygen to the right lung, while ventilation is carried out in the dependent left lung. With lesions of the distal trachea not involving the carina, anastomosis and tube positioning are carried out in much the same way as for the upper tracheal lesions (Fig. 17-10). Once the anastomosis is complete, it is prudent to

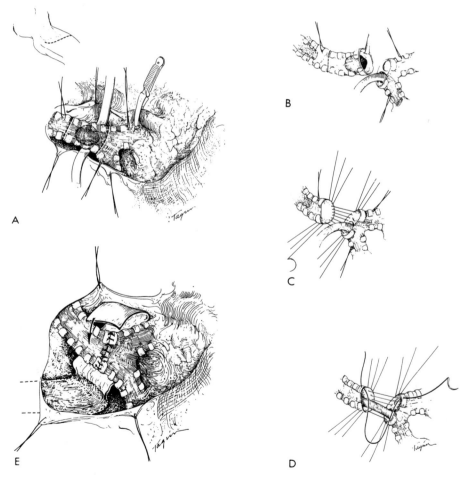

Fig. 17-10. Transthoracic approach. **(A)** The lesion in the distal trachea has been isolated and the right pulmonary artery is shown to be clamped, although this is not done routinely. **(B)** The trachea has been divided above the carina and the left main bronchus intubated. **(C)** Anastomotic sutures are placed by a procedure similar to that used in the upper trachea. **(D)** The endotracheal tube has been advanced through the anastomosis and the remaining sutures appropriately placed. **(E)** Anastomosis completed with a pedicle pleural flap secured for additional support. (From Grillo,[42] with permission.)

withdraw the endotracheal tube back into the proximal trachea so that ventilation goes through the area of anastomosis.

In resections involving the carina in which end-to-end and end-to-side anastomoses between trachea and right and left mainstem bronchi must be carried out, a variety of tube manipulations and combinations of the previously considered maneuvers must be undertaken (Fig. 17-11). Generally, the right mainstem bronchus is anastomosed to the distal trachea and the left bronchus reimplanted in end-to-side fashion into the bronchus intermedius or the distal trachea. It is not uncommon during such procedures to have significant periods of one-lung anesthesia, with the need to insufflate the second lung dictated by the level of arterial oxygenation.

Once all the anastomoses have been completed and adequacy of ventilation is assured by quality of breath sounds and visual inspection of chest wall expansion, closure of the surgical wound is undertaken in standard fashion.

When a right thoracotomy has been used for surgical dissection, the decision as to whether to extubate the airway is of major importance. The potential for inadequacy of ventilation and pulmonary toilet must be balanced against the problems of continued intubation, potential infection, and direct trauma to the suture line. If no significant parenchymal lung disease was present preoperatively, it is generally possible to extubate patients following thoracotomy and major carinal reconstruction without undue consequences. Exceptions are generally those patients in whom bilateral thoracotomy has been undertaken and significant postoperative pain is expected to limit cough and ventilation. These patients require tracheal intubation and some amount of mechanical ventilatory support. Following thoracotomy, the procedures for extubation are similar to those described for the upper airway approach. An exception is that the patient is generally taken out of the lateral position and placed supine prior to extubation. This will facilitate adequate exposure if reintubation is deemed necessary. The patient is transported to the recovery area once stability of circulation and adequacy of ventilation are achieved.

Postoperative Care

Postoperative patients are admitted to the intensive care unit for a minimum of 24 hours. Patients are monitored by using ECG, arterial pressure, and serial arterial blood gases. A radiograph of the chest is obtained shortly following admission to ensure that a pneumothorax is not present. Sufficient oxygen is administered with a high-flow humidified system via a face mask to provide adequate arterial oxygenation and thinning of secretions. The head is maintained in the flexed position by a number of firm pillows placed behind the occiput and sutures located from the chin to the anterior chest. Chest physical therapy and routine nursing procedures are dictated by the nature of other underlying diseases and the ability to effectively maintain gas exchange and pulmonary toilet. Blind nasotracheal suctioning is undertaken with caution in those patients whose cough is inadequate to raise secretions. This is best done by physicians, chest physical therapists, or nurses trained specifically in this procedure. Potential complications include perforation of the anastomotic site and tracheal irritation with subsequent edema and airway obstruction,

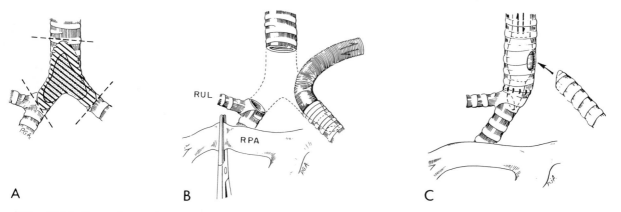

Fig. 17-11. Resection and reconstruction of the carina. **(A)** Tumor position is outlined by the stippled area. **(B)** With the tube positioned in the left main bronchus, the right lung is mobilized and the stump of the right mainstem bronchus sutured into the trachea. **(C)** The left main bronchus is anastomosed in end-to-side fashion into the trachea. (From Grillo,[42] with permission.)

which may induce vomiting and aspiration. In cases in which abundant secretions are a problem, frequent transoral flexible fiberoptic bronchoscopy can be used to provide pulmonary toilet. This is especially true in cases in which the carina has been resected and secretions tend to pool in major bronchi without being propelled by normal mechanisms into the trachea. The need for emergency intubation because of hemorrhage, airway obstruction, or dehiscence of the anastomosis has rarely arisen.

In case of inadequate ventilation, with increasing levels of carbon dioxide and/or deterioration of oxygenation, endotracheal intubation is undertaken. This procedure must be done with caution, generally with the aid of sedation and topical anesthesia; the tube is placed either nasally or orally with direct visualization of the larynx. This can be accomplished with the patient maintained in the flexed position without producing undue stress on the suture line. Following intubation, the need for ventilation is reassessed after pulmonary toilet has been achieved, and therapy is directed at minimizing both positive pressure on the airway and the time for which the intubation is maintained. The latter is especially true in cases in which the endotracheal tube passes through the anastomosis (high tracheal reconstructions) because of the potential for dehiscence in an early stage of recovery. When prolonged intubation, generally considered more than 2 to 3 days, is anticipated, elective tracheostomy should be seriously considered. The hazards of the tracheostomy are dictated by body habitus, the location of the anastomosis, and the ability to safely dissect and position the tracheostomy tube following the reconstructive surgery.

Upper airway obstruction, secondary to laryngeal edema, is an infrequent complication. It has most commonly occurred when there has been a high anastomosis or previous history of laryngeal disease. When there is a history of cord paralysis and/or recurrent episodes of laryngeal edema or when the trachea is anastomosed directly to the larynx at the cricoid cartilage, prophylactic measures are taken to avoid laryngeal edema. This therapy includes use of high humidity and inhalation of topical steroids and racemic epinephrine. Dexamethasone and racemic epinephrine, 0.5 mL of a 1 : 200 dilution in 2.5 mL of water, are administered with a nebulizer every 4 hours. Schedules are arranged so that inhalation of one or the other drug is achieved every 2 hours. This regimen is continued for a minimum of 24 hours or longer if laryngeal edema, as evidenced by stridor and hoarseness, persists.

Patients should be kept in the intensive care unit for 1 or more days until it is deemed safe to return them to a general surgical floor. This is dictated by the ability to discontinue cardiovascular monitoring, the need for repeated measurement of arterial blood gases, and the quality of nursing care. In most cases in which the procedure has been uncomplicated, patients are able to sit out of bed in a chair on the day following surgery and are often able to begin taking clear liquids and/or soft solids by the first postoperative day.

REFERENCES

1. Heffner JE, Miller KS, Sahn SA: Tracheostomy in the intensive care unit. Part 1: indications, technique, management. Chest 90:269–274, 1986
2. Heffner JE, Miller KS, Sahn SA: Tracheostomy in the intensive care unit. Part 2: complications. Chest 90:432–436, 1986
3. Sise MJ, Shackford SR, Cruickshank JO, et al: Cricothyroidotomy for long-term tracheal access. A prospective analysis of morbidity and mortality in 76 patients. Ann Surg 200:13–17, 1984
4. Cole RR, Aguilar EA: Cricothyroidotomy versus tracheotomy: an otolaryngologist's perspective. Laryngoscope 98:131–135, 1988
5. Wilson DJ: Airway appliances and management. pp. 80–89. In Kacmarek R, Stoller J (eds): Current Respiratory Care. BC Decker, Toronto, 1988
6. Lindholm CE: Prolonged endotracheal intubation. Acta Anaesthesiol Scand, suppl. 33:1969
7. Stauffer JL, Olson DE, Petty TL: Complications and consequences of endotracheal intubation and tracheostomy. A prospective study of 150 critically ill adult patients. Am J Med 70:65–76, 1981
8. Ching NPH, Ayres SM, Spina RC, et al: Endotracheal damage during continuous ventilatory support. Ann Surg 179:123–127, 1974
9. Cooper JD, Grillo HC: The evolution of tracheal injury due to ventilatory assistance through cuffed tubes. A pathologic study. Ann Surg 169:334–348, 1969
10. Carroll RG, McGinnis GF, Grenvik A: Performance characteristics of tracheal cuffs. Int Anesthesiol Clin 12:111–135, 1974
11. Crawley BE, Cross DE: Tracheal cuffs. A review in dynamic pressure study. Anaesthesia 30:4–11, 1975
12. Cooper JD, Grillo HC: Experimental production and prevention of injury due to cuffed tracheal tubes. Surg Gynecol Obstet 129:1235–1241, 1969
13. Pavlin EG, Nelson E, Pulliam J: Difficulty in removal of tracheostomy tubes. Anesthesiology 44:69–70, 1976
14. Matthews HR, Hopkinson RB: Treatment of sputum retention by minitracheostomy. Br J Surg 71:147–150, 1984
15. Wain JC, Wilson DJ, Mathisen DJ: Clinical experience with minitracheostomy. Ann Thorac Surg 49:881–886, 1990
16. Matthews HR, Fischer BJ, Smith BE, et al: Minitracheostomy: a new delivery system for jet ventilation. J Thorac Cardiovasc Surg 92:673–675, 1986

17. Grillo HC: Notes on the windpipe. Ann Thorac Surg 47:9–26, 1989
18. Grillo HC: Congenital lesions, neoplasms and injuries of the trachea. In Sabiston DC, Spencer FC (eds): Gibbon's Surgery of the Chest. Vol. 1. WB Saunders, Philadelphia, 1982
19. Grillo HC, Mathisen DJ: Primary tracheal tumors: treatment and results. Ann Thorac Surg 49:69–77, 1990
20. Pearson FG, Todd TRJ, Cooper JD: Experience with primary neoplasms of the trachea. J Thorac Cardiovasc Surg 88:511–516, 1984
21. Grillo HC: Tracheal tumors: surgical management. Ann Thorac Surg 26:112–125, 1978
22. Mathisen DJ, Grillo HC: Laryngotracheal trauma. Ann Thorac Surg 43:254–262, 1987
23. Jones WS, Mavroudis C, Richardson JD, et al: Management of tracheobronchial disruption resulting from blunt trauma. Surgery 95:319–323, 1984
24. Montgomery WW: The surgical management of supraglottic and subglottic stenosis. Ann Otol Rhinol Laryngol 77:534–546, 1968
25. Chesterman JT, Satsangi PN: Rupture of the trachea and bronchi by closed injury. Thorax 21:21–27, 1966
26. Deslauriers J, Beaulieu M, Archambault G, et al: Diagnosis and long-term follow-up of major bronchial disruptions due to nonpenetrating trauma. Ann Thorac Surg 33:33–39, 1982
27. Hood RM, Sloan HE: Injuries of the trachea and major bronchi. J Thorac Cardiovasc Surg 38:458–480, 1959
28. Kryger M, Bode F, Antic R, et al: Diagnosis of obstruction of the upper and central airways. Am J Med 61:85–93, 1976
29. Hyatt RE, Black LF: The flow-volume curve. A current perspective. Am Rev Respir Dis 107:191–199, 1973
30. MacMillan AS, James AE, Jr, Stitik FP, et al: Radiologic evaluation of post-tracheostomy lesions. Thorax 26:696–703, 1971
31. Pearson FG, Andrews MJ: Detection and management of tracheal stenosis following cuffed tube tracheostomy. Ann Thorac Surg 12:359–374, 1971
32. Lee P, English ICW: Management of anesthesia during tracheal resection. Anaesthesia 29:305–306, 1974
33. Clarkson WB, Davies JR: Anesthesia for carinal resection. Anaesthesia 33:815–819, 1978
34. Ellis RH, Hinds CJ, Gadd LT: Management of anesthesia during tracheal resection. Anaesthesia 31:1076–1080, 1976
35. Geffin B, Bland J, Grillo HC: Anesthetic management of tracheal resection and reconstruction. Anesth Analg 48:884–894, 1969
36. Grillo HC: Circumferential resection and reconstruction of mediastinal and cervical trachea. Ann Surg 162:734, 1965
37. Grillo HC: Terminal or mural tracheostomy in the anterior mediastinum. J Thorac Cardiovasc Surg 51:422–427, 1966
38. Grillo HC: The management of tracheal stenosis following assisted respiration. J Thorac Cardiovasc Surg 57:521–571, 1969
39. Grillo HC: Surgical approaches to the trachea. Surg Gynecol Obstet 129:347–352, 1969
40. Grillo HC: Reconstruction of the trachea. Experience in 100 consecutive cases. Thorax 28:667–679, 1973
41. Young-Beyer P, Wilson RS: Anesthetic management for tracheal resection and reconstruction. J Cardiothorac Anesth 2:821–835, 1988
42. Grillo HC: Congenital lesions, neoplasms, and injuries of the chest. In Sabiston DC, Spencer FC (eds): Gibbon's Surgery of the Chest. Vol. 2. WB Saunders, Philadelphia, 1976

18

THORACIC TRAUMA

Brendan T. Finucane, M.D.

When sorrows come, they come not single spies, but in battalions.

Act 4, Scene 5, *Hamlet*

This quotation from Shakespeare perhaps aptly describes thoracic injuries, which are rarely single and are often associated with other serious injuries and, in many cases, death.

In 1896, Paget was quite pessimistic when he wrote, "Surgery of the heart has probably reached the limits set by nature."[1] In that same year, Rehn successfully sutured the myocardium of a patient who had sustained a penetrating wound to the heart.[2] Trauma is a very serious health problem in the United States today. For example, in 1984, 42,200 people died from motor vehicle accidents[3]; 21,114 of these had recordable blood alcohol levels.[4] In that same year, 1.8 million people suffered serious disabling injuries as a result of motor vehicle accidents. The magnitude of this problem is even more sobering in pediatric age groups, in which it accounts for approximately 50 percent of all deaths in children of school age[5] and is the most common cause of death in children under 14 years of age.[6]

In recent years, there has been a tremendous surge in the incidence of drug-related violence in poverty-stricken areas of U.S. cities. This, coupled with the ready availability of handguns, has resulted in a vast increase in the number of murders. Social factors also enter into the equation. For example, males are far more likely to be involved in drug- or alcohol-related motor vehicle accidents than females. There is one other issue that cannot be ignored: the cost of trauma care. It has been estimated that trauma care accounts for approximately 2.3 percent of the gross national product in the United States.[7]

The majority of chest injuries result from blunt trauma secondary to motor vehicle accidents and penetrating injuries secondary to gunshot wounds and stabs. Stab wounds account for the majority of penetrating injuries to the chest in civilian life and high-velocity missile wounds in military populations.[8] Twenty-five percent of all deaths due to motor vehicle accidents are related to chest injury, and chest injuries are a contributing factor in another 25 percent of deaths. Approximately 70 percent of patients who die at the scene of an accident have sustained a major chest injury. Most of these deaths are due to asphyxia and hemorrhage. A significant number of these patients can be sustained by basic cardiopulmonary resuscitation (CPR) until better-equipped emergency medical technicians arrive.

The development of emergency medicine as a specialty has also focused much more attention on trauma, both at the scene of the accident and in emergency rooms. With the aid of sophisticated audiovisual communications and telemetry, decision making by physicians can be brought to the scene of the accident. One of the major corrective actions required to improve the care of the seriously injured patient is regionalization of trauma care. Not every hospital has the equipment or personnel to deal with these patients; therefore, this activity should be confined to those hospitals that do. This simple measure would result in a significant reduction in mortality among trauma victims, not to mention the monetary benefits to the community.

TYPES OF INJURY

Thoracic injuries are classified as penetrating and nonpenetrating (Table 18-1).

Penetrating Injuries

Penetrating injuries to the chest are usually the result of gunshot wounds or stabbings. The amount of destruction occurring secondary to a gunshot wound is related to the kinetic energy (KE) transmitted to the tissues on impact and can be expressed mathematically as follows:

$$KE = \frac{WV^2}{2G}$$

W = weight
V = velocity
G = acceleration of gravity

In simpler language, tissue destruction following gunshot wounds is related to the muzzle velocity of the weapon and the weight of the bullet discharged. Soft bullets, which fragment on impact, cause much more local destruction than hard bullets, which cleanly traverse the tissues. Rifles generally cause more destruction because of the higher velocity and greater mass of the bullet. Close-range shotgun blasts usually cause severe tissue destruction over a wide area.[9] When evaluating patients with gunshot wounds, some of these facts may be helpful in the overall assessment of the injury (Table 18-2). Stabbings, on the other hand, are less complex. The damage inflicted is usually confined to the structures directly underlying the point of contact. These wounds are far less likely to be fatal than gunshot wounds to the chest and are far easier to treat.

TABLE 18-1. Classification of Thoracic Injuries

Penetrating injuries
Gunshot
Stab
Nonpenetrating injuries
Blunt
Deceleration
Blast

TABLE 18-2. Kinetic Energy Calculated for Bullets Commonly Used in the United States

Type Cartridge	Weight Bullet (Grain)	Velocity (ft/s)	Kinetic Energy (ft-lb)
.218 Bee	45	2,860	818
M16 (AR-15)	55	3,250	1,290
.22 Savage	70	2,750	1,175
.243 Winchester	100	3,000	1,998
.257 Roberts	117	2,630	1,797
.270 Winchester	130	3,140	2,846
30/06 Springfield	150	2,750	2,519
.30.30 Winchester	150	2,380	1,887
.300 Savage	180	2,610	2,264
.300 H and H Magnum	220	2,650	3,328
.338 Winchester Magnum	250	2,540	3,899
.375 H and H Magnum	300		4,298

(From Shepard,[9] with permission.)

Nonpenetrating Injuries

The vast majority of chest injuries seen in practice today are a result of blunt trauma to the chest, secondary to motor vehicle accidents. Injuries may range from simple rib fractures to severe destruction of tissues, such as rupture of thoracic viscera. The more serious the injury, the greater the likelihood of rib fractures.[10] Furthermore, fractures of the upper five ribs are usually associated with more serious injuries. Because of the greater flexibility of the thoracic cage in children, it requires greater force to produce fractures. The exact mechanisms producing visceral injury within the thoracic cavity following blunt or decelerating injuries are poorly understood, but, generally, the extent of injury depends on the mass of the offending object, the physical characteristics of the resulting shock wave, and the ability of the target tissue or tissues to dissipate this shock wave. Deceleration injuries can be divided into *impact* and *momentum* injuries. The impact injury usually results in fractures to the sternum and ribs, with minimal damage to underlying structures. Momentum injuries occur to those organs that are suspended within the thoracic cage, such as the heart, lungs, and aorta. When the body is suddenly brought to a grinding halt on impact, these structures continue to move. The amount of destruction is proportional to the shearing forces imparted to the organ involved. Rupture of the descending aorta, at the isthmus, commonly occurs in severe deceleration injuries, such as airline crashes.[11] Other serious injuries that occur following blunt trauma include cardiac contusions and rupture, tracheal and bronchial tears, lung contusions, and diaphragmatic and esophageal injuries.

Injuries to the thoracic cage are among the most

common encountered in practice today. The injury may range from a simple fracture of one or two ribs to the more complex flail chest injury. The one factor common to all rib fractures, simple or complex, is that they cause a disproportionate degree of pain. To the young, healthy adult this is usually of no consequence; however, to the heavy smoker with advanced chronic obstructive pulmonary disease, there may be serious consequences. In the conscious patient, the diagnosis can be made clinically. Patients can usually pinpoint with great accuracy the exact location of the fracture or fractures. A chest radiograph should always be performed, not necessarily to confirm the diagnosis, but to rule out pneumothorax or atelectasis.

The range of treatments used to manage patients with rib fractures includes immobilization, narcotics and analgesics, intercostal nerve blocks,[12] epidural blocks with local anesthetics and narcotics, interpleural injections of local anesthetics,[13] and patient-controlled analgesia (PCA).[14] Immobilization techniques are mentioned only for completeness. This method is obsolete in the modern practice of medicine, and encourages atelectasis and further splinting in predisposed patients. To achieve adequate relief for this condition, large doses of analgesics are required, often resulting in hypoventilation.

BASIC ANESTHESIA REQUIREMENTS FOR MAJOR TRAUMA

Certain basic arrangements must exist in a hospital for optimal care of the seriously injured patient. A trauma team consisting of surgeons at every level of training should be available on a 24-hour basis. This team must have access to a consultant surgeon with expertise in the area of trauma. An anesthesiologist, although usually not an integral member of the team, must be available in the immediate vicinity with similar backup support on a 24-hour basis. Seriously injured patients are best handled in facilities with tertiary care capabilities. Other necessary services for optimal patient care include capable blood bank facilities, a critical care laboratory, and intensive care facilities. Nursing and ancillary personnel familiar with the management of trauma patients are also highly desirable (Table 18-3).

In many major trauma centers in the United States, an anesthesiologist is an active member of the trauma team. MacKenzie[15] has estimated that the Baltimore shock treatment unit has reduced the mortality rate in blunt trauma patients from 25.4 percent in 1972 to

TABLE 18-3. Basic Requirements for Management of Major Trauma Patients

Trauma center
Trauma team
Blood bank (24-hour availability)
Intensive care facilities
Tertiary care facilities

11.6 percent in 1984 by establishing strict protocols and priorities. When confronted with a trauma victim, the treatment unit divides priorities into three components.

First priority

1. Evaluate the airway and ventilation
2. Arrest hemorrhage, establish intravenous access, and administer fluids and blood when necessary.
3. Briefly evaluate central nervous system.
4. Insert central catheter.
5. Draw blood for laboratory evaluation.
6. Establish ECG monitoring and insert a nasogastric tube.

Second priority

1. Cervical spine clearance is obtained if possible. Chest and pelvic bone x-rays are also taken. Additional radiologic investigations are performed depending on the results of the regional x-rays.
2. Peritoneal lavage.
3. Urine catheterization.
4. Splinting of long-bone fractures when indicated.
5. History, if available.
6. Arterial catheter insertion.

Third priority

1. Systematic examination of all major organ systems.
2. Additional x-ray investigations if required.
3. Subspecialty consultation.
4. Consensus opinion about management.

Preoperative Evaluation and Preparation

When an anesthesiologist is a member of the trauma team, valuable time is saved, especially when these patients require surgery. An anesthesiologist should be involved in the resuscitation from the outset, and should be fully familiar with the major problems involved. Then, time permitting, the anesthesiologist should carry out a specific preanesthetic evaluation. In the conscious patient, time permitting, a brief history should be taken that includes the following:

1. Review of systems
2. Past medical history
3. Past surgical history
4. Previous anesthesia difficulties
5. Family history of malignant hyperthermia
6. Current medications
7. Allergies
8. NPO status

Physical examination should include the following:

1. Global assessment
2. Evaluation of the airway
3. Scrutiny of teeth
4. Respiratory and cardiovascular examinations
5. Vital signs

Laboratory investigation should include recent arterial blood gas and hematocrit levels.

As time is such an important element in the survival of a number of patients with thoracic trauma, it is important to be prepared in advance. Ideally, an operating room should be set aside each day for the sole purpose of dealing with trauma victims. Unfortunately, few trauma centers can afford this luxury. In the operating room, monitoring equipment should be calibrated and ready for immediate use; all necessary medications, including emergency cardiac drugs, should be prepared and labeled; blood pumps and blood warming equipment should be immediately available; and a functioning defibrillator must be present.

Monitoring

In addition to basic monitoring for routine cases (ECG, pulse oximeter, automatic blood pressure measuring devices, precordial stethoscope), arterial, central venous pressure (CVP), and urine output monitoring are highly desirable. However, valuable time must not be wasted attempting to place these monitors in unstable, exsanguinating patients.

Induction

Unconscious, moribund patients are intubated immediately without anesthesia, and surgery is performed without anesthesia until vital signs or the patient's state of consciousness indicate a need for anesthesia. Conscious, combative patients with altered mental status can be particularly difficult to handle. Patients who are in a state of shock are particularly susceptible to the adverse effects of thiobarbiturates; therefore, these drugs should be strictly avoided in these situations. Halford, referring to his experiences with thiopental at Pearl Harbor, wrote that it was the "ideal form of euthanasia when used in the presence of shock."[16] Ketamine is the drug of choice for induction of anesthesia in hypovolemic hemorrhaging patients who require anesthesia to allow the surgeon to arrest hemorrhage. Only fractions of the usual doses of medications are necessary in the shock state, owing to a significant reduction in the volume of distribution. For example, 0.5 to 1 mg/kg of ketamine will be adequate for most patients. Shocked patients, who are deprived of adequate hepatic and renal blood flow, may also respond differently compared with normovolemic patients in terms of metabolism and excretion of drugs. Although acute blood loss is not associated with significant hypoproteinemia, replacement of blood loss with large volumes of crystalloid may lead to a relative hypoproteinemia and subsequent pharmacokinetic disturbances.[17] Finally, acid-base and temperature disturbances in these patients may give rise to further pharmacokinetic aberrations.

In the majority of cases, the anesthesiologist will have had sufficient time to replace intravascular fluid deficits; therefore, thiobarbiturates or other induction agents can be safely used. Trauma is frequently associated with a decrease in gastric emptying, which places these patients at greater risk of aspiration pneumonitis, so that a rapid-sequence induction is indicated. Patients should be preoxygenated for 3 to 4 minutes, then d-tubocurarine, 3 mg, should be administered intravenously to prevent excessive muscle fasciculation caused by succinylcholine. During induction with thiopental, etomidate, midazolam, or ketamine and succinylcholine, cricoid pressure is applied and maintained until the trachea has been intubated and the cuff inflated. In stable patients, maintenance of anesthesia is left to the discretion of the anesthesiologist. If major blood loss is anticipated, it is probably advisable to use oxygen, air mixtures, muscle relaxants, and intermittent doses of narcotic with minimal concentrations of inhalation agents. Nitrous oxide is probably best avoided in chest trauma patients who are at risk of pneumothorax.

Maintenance

During surgery for major trauma, the anesthesiologist has the responsibility of providing good operating conditions for the surgeon, and must clinically observe each major organ system for the development of new signs, treating them appropriately. Successful resuscitation of patients with major chest trauma requires teamwork; blood and fluid replacement must be prompt and given in appropriate quantities. If patients do not respond to volume replacement, ongoing hemorrhage, tension pneumothorax, or pericardial tamponade must be suspected. Interruption of the superior vena cava may explain why some patients fail to respond to fluid therapy. In these cases, intravenous access must be established in the lower extremities. After the surgeon has entered the chest cavity, compression of the aorta above the site of bleeding may provide valuable time to restore blood volume. Little, if any, anesthesia is required in patients in shock; however, when the blood volume is restored, consciousness rapidly returns. At this point, anesthesia can be maintained with oxygen, narcotics, neuromuscular blocking drugs, amnestics, and small quantities of inhalation agents if required.

What special precautions are necessary when using neuromuscular blocking drugs in the presence of serious trauma? Succinylcholine, a rapid-acting, depolarizing neuromuscular blocking drug, is usually chosen to provide profound relaxation during rapid-sequence induction of anesthesia. However, caution should be exercised when patients present with extensive muscular damage since potassium levels may rise dangerously following succinylcholine.[18] There are numerous nondepolarizing drugs to choose from during the maintenance of anesthesia. Vecuronium is one of the most useful nondepolarizing neuromuscular blocking drugs used in seriously traumatized patients because it has minimal effects on the circulation. Pancuronium is also a reasonable choice in these patients; however, tachycardia may be undesirable because it may lead to further confusion in distinguishing drug effect from hypovolemia or inadequate levels of anesthesia. d-Tubocurarine and atracurium are best avoided in seriously traumatized patients because of their hypotensive effects. Finally, all neuromuscular blocking agents are subject to aberrant behavior in the presence of changing acid-base status, altered metabolism and excretion, and hypothermia. Also, interactions with certain antibiotics prolong the duration of neuromuscular blockade. For these reasons, intelligent monitoring of neuromuscular function is mandatory.

Hypothermia is a major problem in traumatized patients undergoing exploratory surgery, and every effort should be made to maintain a normal temperature. The anesthesiologist can help reduce this complication by using a heated humidifier and low gas flows. All irrigating and intravenous fluids should be heated. The room should be warmed to an acceptable temperature to allow sufficient functioning of the team. Heating lamps and warming blankets may also play a role. Accessible exposed areas of the body should be covered with a plastic wrap or other heat-preserving material.

Awareness is a major, but unavoidable, hazard of surgery and anesthesia in the unstable, traumatized patient. Bogetz and Katz have shown that the incidence of awareness is as high as 43 percent in unstable patients undergoing trauma surgery.[19] They also demonstrated an 11 percent incidence of awareness in a group of trauma patients who received reduced doses of anesthetic drugs during anesthesia. Reduced minimum alveolar concentration (MAC) values might be expected in a number of traumatized victims because of hypotension, hypothermia, anemia, and acute alcohol intoxication; however, these individuals are often young, unpremedicated, and otherwise healthy with high levels of circulating catecholamines, all of which tend to increase MAC requirements.[20] Scopolamine may be a useful medication in those at risk.

Postoperative Care

The vast majority of patients presenting for surgery secondary to chest trauma require postoperative care in a critical care unit until they achieve an adequate level of physiologic homeostasis. The anesthesiologist can play a significant role in the postoperative care of these patients, especially in the realm of acute pain and ventilatory management (see Chapters 21 and 22).

DIAGNOSIS AND MANAGEMENT OF SPECIFIC INJURIES

Flail Chest

Flail chest may be defined as an abnormal movement of the chest wall occurring as a result of fractures of three or more ribs in two places on the same side. On inspiration, the injured segment tends to encroach on the lung, leading to impairment of ventilation and oxygenation. This injury is most commonly associated with blunt trauma to the chest wall and involves the anterolateral aspect of the chest. The posterior wall is heavily fortified with muscle and, therefore, is rarely involved. Injury to the upper ribs usually signifies serious trauma. The flail chest injury is rarely isolated and is usually an ominous sign, indicating serious underlying injuries to intrathoracic and/or intra-abdominal organs. The thoracic cage in older age groups is more calcified and brittle and, therefore, more susceptible to flail and other serious injuries. In contrast, the thoracic cage in pediatric patients is extremely elastic and resilient, affording much greater protection to underlying structures.[21]

The diagnosis should always be suspected in patients presenting with a history of blunt trauma to the chest or upper abdomen. This condition may go unnoticed for hours and, in some cases, even days, and is sometimes overshadowed by more overt injuries. The diagnosis is particularly difficult when the upper thoracic cage is involved. Chest radiography may not reveal fractures unless films are overpenetrated and oblique views are taken.[22] Radiologic signs of parenchymal damage to the lung may not be evident in the early stages; however, the presence of mediastinal air may signify bronchial or tracheal injury. Serial blood gas measurements can be very helpful in establishing the diagnosis. Repetitive clinical assessment of patients with blunt trauma is the key to early detection of flail chest.

For many years, the major cause of respiratory dysfunction associated with flail chest has been attributed to the *pendelluft phenomenon*, which is a to-and-fro movement of air from the damaged to the normal lung. Recent reports indicate that this theory is no longer tenable.[23,24] In fact, one investigator demonstrated that there was an increase in ventilation and improved gas exchange on the injured side.[25] It is likely that serious damage to the chest wall will lead to disturbances of ventilation. Coupled with parenchymal damage to the underlying lung, this can very readily cause respiratory failure. The primary pathophysiologic defect associated with flail chest injury is inadequate oxygenation.

The management of this condition is controversial. The goals of treatment are directed toward stabilization of the injured segment, maintenance of adequate ventilation, and effective pain relief. All patients with a flail chest should be admitted to a surgical intensive care unit. Temporary stabilization of the flail segment should be carried out as soon as possible by using either sandbags or pillows until a decision about definitive treatment has been made. The treatment varies with the severity of the injury, ranging from simple supportive therapy, such as oxygen enrichment, physical therapy, and pain management, to full ventilatory support. The latter is now considered to be the most effective treatment for patients who develop respiratory failure. Another treatment that has been used is external stabilization of the flail segment by traction on the injured segment.[26] Currently, there are few indications for this mode of treatment. Moore and his colleagues have stabilized the chest wall in selective cases by intramedullary pinning of fractured ribs.[27]

Which patients need endotracheal intubation and ventilatory support? This decision is usually determined by clinical observation, sequential arterial blood gas analysis, and assessment of the vital capacity and inspiratory force over a period of time (Table 18-4). These criteria should only serve as a guide to therapy. Any one alone may not be sufficient grounds for committing a patient to ventilation, but certainly two or more in any one patient would make a strong

TABLE 18-4. Criteria for Intubation

$PaO_2 < 70$ mmHg with O_2 enrichment
$PaCO_2 > 50$ mmHg
pH < 7.25
Tachypnea > 30/min
Vital capacity < 15 mL/kg
Negative inspiratory force < -20 cmH$_2$O

case for doing so. When a decision has been made to institute mechanical support of ventilation, an endotracheal tube is inserted, with use of sedation and topical anesthesia. Nasal intubation is probably more comfortable for the patient; however, some investigators have indicated that nasal intubation causes maxillary sinus infections that may lead to sepsis and, for that reason, opt for the oral route[28,29] (see Chapter 23).

When is a tracheostomy indicated? Historically, patients with a flail chest injury needing ventilation were subjected to tracheostomy at the commencement of therapy. Most clinicians are now convinced that tracheostomy can be a serious source of morbidity and mortality and, therefore, make every effort to avoid it if possible.[30] Unless there is extreme difficulty in clearing secretions, tracheostomy is deferred for up to 2 weeks. There is considerable disagreement among anesthesiologists and surgeons about this issue. All gases delivered to patients should be humidified, as inhalation of dry gases for lengthy periods causes serious disruption of the tracheal mucosa and encourages the formation of mucus plugs and erosions.[31] In the initial stages of treatment, patients are placed on intermittent mandatory ventilation (IMV). The rate per minute is determined by the arterial carbon dioxide tension and the patient's intrinsic rate. An initial IMV rate of approximately 6 per minute is usually adequate. Approximately 5 cmH$_2$O of distending airway pressure is also selected in these patients. The inspired oxygen tension is determined by that concentration of oxygen that maintains the arterial oxygen tension around 80 mmHg. Weaning is attempted when the arterial blood gases are in an acceptable range, the vital capacity approaches 15 mL/kg, and the inspiratory force is approximately -20 cmH$_2$O. Extubation can be carried out when the patient is capable of maintaining normal blood gases on room air, is capable of generating a negative inspiratory force between -30 and -40 cmH$_2$O, and has a vital capacity greater than 20 mL/kg of body weight.

How should these patients be monitored? Because this condition is associated with such a poor prognosis, extensive monitoring, including continuous monitoring of the ECG, is recommended. Chest injuries sufficient to fracture several ribs are often associated with cardiac contusions; therefore, dysrhythmias may be a problem. The need for frequent arterial blood gas and other laboratory data certainly justifies arterial catheterization. The inspired oxygen tension should be monitored with an oxygen analyzer. Pulmonary artery pressure monitoring is extremely useful in this situation, allowing the clinician to calculate the degree of pulmonary shunting, as well as numerous cardiovascular parameters.[32]

Adequate pain relief should be instituted as soon as possible after the injury. In the early stages of treatment, small increments of morphine (3 to 4 mg/70 kg) may be given every 1 to 2 hours. To facilitate the weaning process, other methods of pain relief, such as intercostal nerve blocks, continuous epidural analgesia, and PCA, are preferable. The former method has the serious limitation of requiring repeated injections. Continuous thoracic epidural anesthesia, although not widely practiced, is probably the method of choice in respiratory failure secondary to chest injury. The use of continuous epidural anesthesia, on the other hand, has the serious limitation that much larger volumes of local anesthetic are required to achieve adequate pain relief. The resulting sympathetic block may not be desirable in patients with unstable cardiovascular systems, and urinary retention inevitably develops in noncatheterized patients.

There seems to be no general agreement about the use of prophylactic antibiotics in these patients. However, frequent cultures should be performed and the appropriate antibiotic commenced when indicated. Flail chest injury is associated with significant morbidity and mortality. Shackford and Virgilio performed a prospective study in 36 patients who presented with this injury.[33] Of those patients, 30 percent required mechanical ventilation, 69 percent developed pneumonia, and approximately 30 percent developed adult respiratory distress syndrome. The mean duration of ventilation was 10.5 days. The mortality rate in this group was approximately 10 percent. Depending on the series, the mortality rate may vary anywhere between 6 and 50 percent.[34,35]

Pneumothorax

Pneumothorax occurs secondary to blunt or penetrating trauma to the chest wall. Open pneumothorax is often associated with shotgun wounds to the chest wall at close range. In this situation, intrapleural pressure equalizes with the atmosphere, resulting in a diminished movement of air on the affected side. Venous return is impaired by positive pressure and mediastinal shift. The diagnosis of the "sucking" chest wound is fairly obvious from clinical observation, and the immediate treatment of this condition is to occlude the defect. Definitive treatment involves insertion of a chest tube and repair of the defect. Less obvious pneumothoraxes occur as a result of penetration of the chest wall and lung by sharp objects, such as bullets, knives, ice picks, or rib fragments. The presence of surgical emphysema should signal the possibility of a pneumothorax.

Pneumothoraxes of less than 20 percent are usually not clinically detectable. Patients may complain of chest pain, which is accentuated by deep breathing. Cyanosis may be evident, and the trachea can be deviated with larger pneumothoraxes. Percussion of the chest reveals a tympanitic sound, and breath sounds may be diminished or absent. Conditions that may mimic pneumothorax include hemothorax or atelectasis. Radiologic examination is the best diagnostic aid available, and all films should be taken during expiration.[36] The presence of rib fractures or surgical emphysema should provide a clue to the diagnosis. Pneumothoraxes with a volume greater than 10 percent should be treated by tube thoracostomy in trauma patients.

Tension pneumothorax occurs when air enters the pleural cavity during inspiration, but, owing to a ball-valve action, cannot escape during expiration. In conscious patients, rapid deterioration is noted. Breath sounds are barely perceptible and the trachea is markedly deviated. Cyanosis and cardiovascular collapse are noted (Table 18-5). This condition can be easily confused with pericardial tamponade or shock, secondary to hypovolemia. During general anesthesia, a dramatic decrease in compliance should alert the anesthesiologist to the problem. Nitrous oxide should be discontinued as soon as possible, as it accentuates the size of the pneumothorax.[37]

As soon as a tension pneumothorax is suspected, a large-bore needle should be inserted into the pleural cavity, allowing air to drain freely. If the diagnosis is correct, rapid improvement is noted. This is a surgical emergency and valuable time should not be wasted seeking radiologic confirmation. Figure 18-1A shows a portable radiograph of a 2-month-old infant with a large tension pneumothorax. At the time of the diagnosis, the child was moribund. The arterial blood

TABLE 18-5. Cardinal Signs of Tension Pneumothorax

Cyanosis
Marked decrease in pulmonary compliance
Rapid deterioration of vital signs
Diminished or absent breath sounds
Tracheal deviation

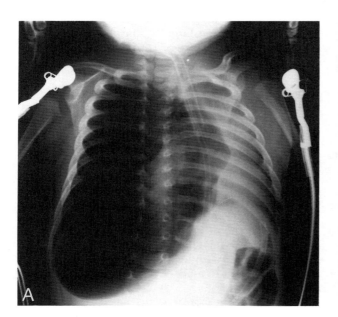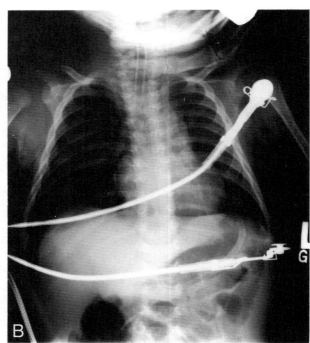

Fig. 18-1. **(A)** Tension pneumothorax in a 2-month-old child. **(B)** Supine chest film 20 minutes later.

gases on 100 percent O_2 were as follows: PaO_2 = 19 mmHg, $PaCO_2$ = 75 mmHg, pH = 6.94, and a base deficit of −18 mEq/L. The repeat radiograph in 20 minutes was much improved, and the blood gases on 100 percent oxygen were PaO_2 = 85 mmHg, $PaCO_2$ = 47 mmHg, pH = 7.21, and base deficit of −9 mEq/L. A radiograph was taken in this instance after initial attempts to decompress the pleural cavity were unsuccessful. This example demonstrates the dramatic reversibility of this potentially lethal condition (Fig. 18-1B).

The incidence of pneumothorax associated with subclavian puncture, even in capable hands, is approximately 2 percent.[38] Despite this fact, in many centers, the subclavian vein is one of the first vessels selected for cannulation in trauma patients. Large antecubital veins are more than adequate for rapid infusion of fluids. If central venous pressure monitoring is warranted, cannulation of the internal jugular vein is an excellent alternative to the subclavian and is associated with fewer serious complications.[39] Hemothorax and hydrothorax are other recognizable complications of subclavian cannulation. The position of the cannula should be verified by intermittently aspirating for blood. The waveform may also be studied with the appropriate electronic equipment. Radiologic confirmation of the catheter tip is not always feasible initially, but should be carried out when time permits.

Acute Traumatic Hemothorax

Hemothorax occurs in approximately 70 percent of all major chest injuries. Gay and McCabe classify penetrating injuries of the chest into three categories based on severity.[40] Those in the first category are patients who are moribund on arrival in the hospital and need immediate treatment. The second category comprises those patients who present in shock, but for whom there is sufficient time to quickly evaluate the injury. The third category comprises those patients who are stable on arrival in the hospital; therefore, a thorough evaluation of the injury can be carried out.

The diagnosis of hemothorax is made on the basis of history and clinical examination of the chest. When a significant quantity of blood has accumulated in the chest cavity, the trachea may be deviated, the chest wall is dull to percussion, and breath sounds are diminished on auscultation. A chest radiograph and an ECG should be obtained for all patients, except those presenting in extremis. Approximately 500 mL of blood must accumulate in the chest cavity before it is radiologically detectable. Upright chest films are preferable, if possible. Hypovolemia from blood loss is the most common presenting problem in patients with significant chest injury. Therefore, the immediate treatment should be directed toward restoring blood volume.

Two large-bore intravenous cannulae should be inserted as soon as possible. Central venous pressure monitoring is invaluable in both the diagnosis and management of patients with a hemothorax. Oxygen therapy is mandatory in those patients who have mechanical interference with ventilation. A chest tube should be inserted as soon as possible in the sixth intercostal space in the midaxillary line on the injured side and connected to suction at a negative pressure of approximately -15 cmH$_2$O. Tube thoracostomy is invaluable in suspected hemothorax because it allows immediate confirmation of the diagnosis. Furthermore, it provides an accurate assessment of the cumulative blood loss and of ongoing losses, facilitates re-expansion of the lung, and simplifies the technique of autotransfusion when major bleeding is encountered. Concurrent pneumothoraxes are frequently present. Thoracostomy tube insertion alone is the only surgical treatment required in more than 80 percent of patients presenting with a hemothorax.[41] In the majority of cases, the source of bleeding is the pulmonary vessels, which normally have low perfusion pressures. On the other hand, bleeding from systemic vessels or the heart is usually more persistent and voluminous and may require thoracotomy (Table 18-6).

In most situations, there is sufficient time to allow the thoracotomy to be performed in the relative comfort of an operating room. Emergency room thoracotomy may be indicated in those patients who present in extremis. Baker et al presented their experience with this mode of therapy in 168 patients over a 5-year period.[42] In this series, optimal results were achieved in patients presenting with penetrating wounds of the chest. The poorest results were obtained in those patients presenting with multiple blunt trauma. The overall survival rate was 19.6 percent. The authors concluded that emergency room thoracotomy was a productive exercise both in terms of patient care and cost effectiveness. Therefore, it appears that this mode of therapy may be lifesaving in selected cases. The rationale behind this treatment is to relieve cardiac tamponade if present and to control arterial bleeding by clamping the aorta above the site of bleeding. The patient is then transported to the operating room for definitive treatment.

The anesthetic requirements for moribund patients undergoing thoracotomy are minimal. An endotracheal tube should be inserted as soon as possible, 100 percent oxygen should be administered, and the thoracotomy should be performed while using controlled ventilation. If and when adequate perfusion pressures are restored, an appropriate level of anesthesia can be provided by using small doses of ketamine or narcotics.

Tracheal and Bronchial Injuries

Tracheal and bronchial injuries are among the most serious encountered in thoracic surgery. Most penetrating wounds to these structures result from gunshot and stab wounds. These injuries also occur following blunt trauma associated with high-speed travel. Bertelsen and Howitz reviewed autopsy findings in approximately 1,220 patients who succumbed to blunt chest trauma, and found a 2.8 percent incidence of tracheobronchial rupture.[43] Approximately 80 percent of tracheobronchial injuries occur within 2.5 cm of the carina. Lloyd et al suggest that when the elastic capability of the lungs has been exceeded as a result of the impact, tears occur, mainly in the vicinity of the carina.[44] A more serious tear results if the impact is delivered during glottic closure. This injury should be suspected in any patient presenting with dyspnea, cough, hemoptysis, subcutaneous emphysema, cyanosis, or atelectasis associated with blunt or penetrating trauma to the neck or upper chest. Auscultation of the heart may reveal a crunching sound associated with pericardial air (Hamman's sign). Tension pneumothorax may occur, especially if the tracheal wound communicates with the pleural cavity. In some cases, a massive air leak may be evident on attempting to ventilate the patient. All patients with suspected tracheal or bronchial injury require diagnostic bronchoscopy as soon as they are stable. Tracheobronchial injuries are often associated with other serious injuries, including cervical spine, esophageal, or diaphragmatic injury, or cardiac and pulmonary contusions. It is most important to deal with the tracheobronchial injury before proceeding with other surgical procedures if possible.

Small tracheal wounds with good apposition may be treated by endotracheal intubation, with the cuff of

TABLE 18-6. Indications for Thoracotomy

Persistent hypotension despite aggressive volume replacement
Bleeding more than 300 mL/h for 4 h
Massive continuing hemorrhage > 2,000 mL
Left hemothorax in the presence of widened mediastinum

the endotracheal tube placed below the wound site. Fiberoptic bronchoscopy is a useful technique for more accurate positioning of endotracheal tubes in tracheobronchial injuries. The tracheal wound should heal within 48 hours.[45] Other clinicians recommend tracheostomy in this situation. Tracheostomy is indicated when there is extensive injury to the larynx and the cervical trachea or when endotracheal intubation cannot be performed. More extensive injuries involving complete separation of the trachea or bronchi require open surgical treatment. The long-term sequelae of these injuries are bronchial and subglottic stenosis. Tracheal and bronchial surgical procedures require close cooperation between the surgeon and anesthesiologist at all times.

Traumatic Rupture of the Diaphragm

Traumatic rupture of the diaphragm usually occurs secondary to blunt trauma to the chest and abdomen. The majority of ruptures occur on the left side in the posterior central area; however, avulsion of the diaphragm from the rib cage has been described.[46,47] In most circumstances, the intra-abdominal pressure exceeds that of the thoracic cavity. This pressure difference is greater during inspiration; therefore, when a deficit occurs in the diaphragm, there is a tendency for abdominal viscera to enter the thoracic cavity. Herniation of abdominal contents does not always take place immediately. Incarceration and strangulation are more likely to occur with small tears.

A patient with this injury may be asymptomatic or may present with respiratory distress. Patients with chronic rupture usually present with symptoms of intestinal obstruction. This injury must be suspected in all patients presenting with blunt trauma. In overt cases, in which viscera have entered the chest, the diagnosis may be obvious on clinical grounds. If the diagnosis is suspected, it can be confirmed by chest radiography and by performing a diagnostic pneumoperitoneum. In Brooks' series of 42 cases, approximately 70 percent were recognized immediately, and 17 percent were diagnosed after a delay varying between 4 and 47 days.[48]

The anesthesiologist should be aware of this condition, which must be suspected when unexplained changes in compliance occur intraoperatively in patients who have sustained serious chest injury. Patients with significant migration of viscera into the chest cavity also appear to be at greater risk from aspiration pneumonitis. Diaphragmatic injuries are quite often associated with fractured ribs and a flail chest and, therefore, frequently require mechanical ventilation for several days. The treatment of this condition, once diagnosed, is operative as soon as the patient's condition permits. The optimal approach to repair this injury is through the thoracic cavity.[49,50]

Penetrating Cardiac Injuries

Penetrating cardiac injuries occur as a result of gunshot or knife wounds to the neck, precordium, or upper abdomen. Gunshot wounds are usually more devastating, causing destruction of one or more chambers. Knife wounds, on the other hand, are usually singular and less destructive. Numerous reports support the fact that approximately 50 percent of all victims of penetrating cardiac wounds die at the scene of the accident.[51]

The right ventricle, which occupies the largest area beneath the precordium, is most commonly penetrated (Table 18-7). Symbas et al's experience with penetrating wounds of the heart revealed on *overall* mortality rate of 18.4 percent in 102 patients.[52] When these data were broken down further, 11.1 percent of the deaths resulted from stab wounds, whereas 27.3 percent occurred as a result of bullet wounds. Several serious effects may result from penetrating cardiac injuries, the most common being cardiac tamponade.

Cardiac Tamponade

The normal heart is surrounded by a fibrous, poorly compliant membrane, which in the adult contains approximately 60 mL of serous fluid. Rapid accumulation of 100 to 200 mL of fluid in this closed space limits the degree of dilation of the heart during diastole. The pericardial sac can accommodate as much as 2 L of fluid if the fluid is allowed to accumulate slowly.

Cardiac tamponade should always be suspected in patients with wounds in the vicinity of the neck, precordium, or upper abdomen. The classic symptoms and signs are not always present (Table 18-8). Patients may appear restless, cyanotic, or clearly in shock. The symptomatology may be misleading in intoxicated patients. Beck's triad, consisting of distention of the neck veins, hypotension, and muffled heart sounds, is

TABLE 18-7. Site of 54 Penetrating Wounds of the Heart

Wound Site	RV	LV	RA	LA
Stab	24	7	4	0
Bullet	3	11	3	2
Percent of total	50	33.3	12.9	3.7

Abbreviations: RV, right ventricle; LV, left ventricle; RA, right atrium; LA, left atrium.

(From Symbas et al,[52] with permission.)

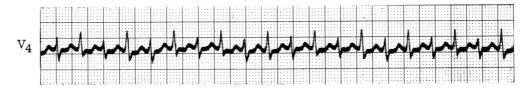

Fig. 18-2. Electrical alternans is demonstrated in a patient with cardiac tamponade. (From Goldman,[135] with permission.)

present in only 41 percent of cases with penetrating cardiac wounds.[53–55] Pulsus paradoxus, which is a decline in systolic blood pressure of 10 mmHg or more on inspiration, is also of limited value in these patients unless continuous arterial pressure monitoring is used.[56] Paradoxic filling of neck veins on inspiration may be too subtle to detect in uncooperative, struggling patients (Kussmaul's sign). Since a number of these patients deteriorate rapidly, there is usually insufficient time to carry out investigations such as echocardiography, which is very accurate diagnostically. The ECG is usually not helpful; however, a patient occasionally will show electrical alternans, which is usually diagnostic of tamponade (Fig. 18-2). Usually, the ECG shows nonspecific ST segment or T wave abnormalities, but it may appear normal. Chest radiographs are also of limited value; occasionally, air may be seen in the pericardial sac. Heavy reliance is placed on clinical impression in patients with cardiac tamponade. Elevation of the central venous pressure in the face of shock or hypotension is clear evidence of the diagnosis and should be acted on immediately.

Experts in the field of thoracic surgery feel that the definitive treatment of this condition is surgery as soon as possible.[57,58] Pericardiocentesis may be used to relieve the tamponade in rapidly deteriorating patients. However, this is of limited value because blood rapidly reaccumulates in the pericardial sac. Aspiration of nonclotting blood from the pericardial sac is diagnostic, but the converse is not true.[59]

Pericardiocentesis should be carried out in a semisitting position. A 16- or 18-gauge metal needle is inserted into the subxiphoid region at an angle of 35 degrees and advanced toward the left shoulder. The hub of the needle can be connected to a V lead of the ECG, and ECG monitoring can be carried out while the needle is advanced toward the pericardial sac. Accidental encroachment of the needle on the ventricular wall will be evident as ST segment elevation. Removal of 30 to 60 mL of blood may result in dramatic improvement. If a plastic catheter is used for aspiration, it should be secured to allow repeated use.

Time will dictate the degree of monitoring carried out on patients with cardiac tamponade. In many situations, basic monitoring techniques are used. Whenever possible, the CVP should be monitored electronically, allowing the anesthesiologist to study the waveform and providing continuous readings. The normal CVP has three waves: the A wave, which coincides with atrial contraction; the C wave, which is due to bulging of the atrioventricular (A-V) valves during isometric contraction; and the V wave, which is due to atrial filling when the A-V valves are closed (Fig. 18-3A). On each side of the V wave there are two pronounced depressions, referred to as X and Y descents, which are used to identify the V wave. In pericardial tamponade or effusion, there is a pronounced systolic X dip with minimal diastolic Y dip (Fig. 18-3B).

Central venous pressure monitoring is not only useful in the diagnosis, but may also be used as a guide to volume replacement. High central venous pressures,

TABLE 18-8. Diagnosis of Cardiac Tamponade
Site of wound
Beck's triad
Kussmaul's sign
Pulsus paradoxus
ECG
Shock and ↑ CVP

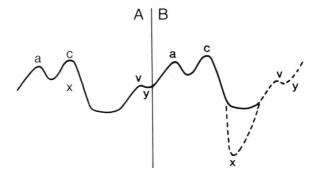

Fig. 18-3. **(A)** Normal A, C, and V waves, with the X and Y descents. **(B)** Pronounced X descent seen with cardiac tamponade.

in the vicinity of 15 to 20 cmH$_2$O, should be maintained until the tamponade is relieved.

Anesthetic Management

The patient should be prepared and draped while conscious, and the incision should be made as rapidly as possible after anesthesia is induced. The classic incision for this lesion is a horizontal cut in the fourth or fifth left intercostal space. The administration of a general anesthetic to a patient with a significant tamponade is potentially lethal.[60,61] Almost any maneuver, other than administration of 100 percent O$_2$ (which is carried out by the anesthestiologist), including positive-pressure ventilation, causes deterioration.[62,63] It is for this reason that experts in the field of anesthesiology recommend local anesthesia for this procedure.[64–66] This may be a satisfactory approach in a moribund, lifeless patient or in patients with large, chronic pericardial effusions, but it is less than optimal in struggling, uncooperative patients with serious penetrating wounds of the heart. The surgeon needs good access in order to find the source of bleeding. It is for this reason that general anesthesia is preferable in most patients with pericardial tamponade secondary to trauma.

What are the choices of general anesthesia under these circumstances? Inhalation agents or thiopental cause further cardiac depression and impairment of diastolic filling. Peripheral vasodilation associated with these agents further impairs filling. The anesthesiologist can effectively manage these patients by maintaining an elevated central venous pressure (> 15 cmH$_2$O) and by avoiding myocardial depressants (Table 18-9). Ketamine, which is a phencyclidine derivative, is ideal for this purpose. It causes cardiac depression in the isolated heart, but, in the intact heart, it has a biphasic action—the initial negative inotropic effect is immediately followed by a positive inotropic effect.[67,68] Tweed studied the effects of ketamine on contractility in four normal subjects and found a consistent increase (Table 18-10).[69] Ketamine has some other features that are beneficial in this situation: (1) it causes dissociative anesthesia; (2) it has excellent analgesic properties so that supplementation with other anesthetic agents is unnecessary; (3)

TABLE 18-9. Ideal Anesthetic Agent in the Presence of Cardiac Tamponade

Positive inotropic and chronotropic action
Peripheral vasoconstriction
Antiarrhythmic action
Anesthetic properties

TABLE 18-10. Myocardial Contractility after Ketamine[a]

Patient No.	Δ dP/dt at CPIP (%)[b]	ΔLVEDP[c]
1	+12	−7
2	+26	−6
3	+45	−2
4	+21	+5
Mean	+26	−2.5
	P < .05	

Abbreviations: CPIP, common peak intraventricular pressure; LVEDP, left ventricular end-diastolic pressure.

[a] Ketamine increased (dP/dt)/CPIP while decreasing LVEDP.

[b] Percent change in the ratio (dP/dt)/CPIP after ketamine.

[c] Change in absolute value of LVEDP after ketamine.

(From Tweed,[69] with permission.)

high inspired oxygen concentrations can be delivered; and (4) cardiac tamponade is frequently associated with ventricular dysrhythmias, and Corssen and others have indicated that ketamine has antiarrhythmic properties.[70–72] These findings further substantiate the use of ketamine for patients with pericardial tamponade. The recommended dose for patients with diminished cardiac output is 0.25 to 0.50 mg/kg. Despite careful anesthetic management, patients may deteriorate before the tamponade is relieved. If deterioration occurs, isoproterenol is the drug of choice.[73] An infusion should be prepared with a concentration of 4 μg/mL. It should be infused at a rate of 0.1 μg/kg/min and titrated to effect. When the pericardium is decompressed, the vital signs usually instantaneously improve. Conservative anesthetic management must prevail even after the tamponade has been relieved to allow the myocardium time to recover from this serious insult.

Coronary Artery Injuries

The incidence of coronary artery laceration following penetrating cardiac wounds is in the region of 4 percent.[74] Division of a coronary artery invariably leads to hemorrhage and tamponade and, depending on the size of the vessel, may cause myocardial infarction. Most injuries involve the left coronary artery or its branches. The right coronary artery is protected by the sternum. These injuries are usually discovered at the time of surgery, and lacerations of larger arteries are reanastomosed if possible. Saphenous vein grafts from the aorta to a coronary artery distal to the injury have been described.[75,76] Blunt injuries may result in occlusion of a coronary artery, eventually leading to myocardial infarction. From an anesthetic stand-

TABLE 18-11. Causes of a Cardiac Contusion

Steering wheel injury	Puck
Fist	Kick
Club	Fall
Ball	Blast

TABLE 18-13. Cardiac Contusion Symptoms

Pain
Dyspnea
Hypotension
Tachycardia
Rhythm disturbances
Conduction abnormalities

point, these patients should be managed similarly to patients with acute myocardial infarctions.

Cardiac Contusions

Blunt trauma to the chest wall resulting in cardiac contusions can occur in a variety of ways (Table 18-11). Rapid deceleration injuries as a result of motor vehicle accidents are the most common cause of cardiac contusions, simply because the heart is suspended by the great vessels in the thoracic cavity. On sudden impact, the heart strikes the inner aspect of the chest wall with great force, often resulting in cardiac contusion and more serious injuries (Table 18-12).

Rhythm disturbances are among the most common presenting signs in patients with cardiac contusion.[77] Conduction disturbances are more commonly associated with injuries to the right atrium and ventricle[78] (Table 18-13).

All patients presenting with blunt or penetrating injuries to the chest should have an ECG as soon as possible after admission. Typical signs of injury may not appear for several hours afterward. There should be a high index of suspicion in patients presenting with rhythm or conduction disturbances. The diagnosis of cardiac contusion is a real dilemma for the clinician. Most routine and sophisticated tests have proved unreliable. Enzyme studies are of little help.[79] However, more recently, two-dimensional echocardiography has proven useful in a number of cases.[80] Patients with these injuries should be handled in the same manner as patients presenting with myocardial infarctions. Many patients with cardiac contusions need immediate surgery for other reasons. Subsequent management may play a major role in the outcome for patients presenting with cardiac trauma.

Injuries to the Great Vessels

The intrathoracic aorta can be injured as a result of penetrating or blunt trauma to the chest. The resulting hemorrhage is usually devastating, allowing only approximately 15 percent of patients to reach a medical facility alive.[81]

The vast majority of aortic ruptures occur as a result of motor vehicle accidents.[82] The most frequent site of aortic rupture is at the isthmus[83] (Table 18-14). The three most common presenting signs are mediastinal widening, hemothorax, and tracheal deviation. Injuries to other major intrathoracic arterial vessels may present with hemorrhagic shock, hemothorax, or tamponade.[84] Caval injuries are among the most difficult to deal with surgically and are associated with an extremely high mortality.[85]

The foremost goal of the anesthesiologist when dealing with major thoracic vessel injuries is simply to maintain an adequate blood volume, allowing the surgeon time to find the source of bleeding and, if possible, to repair the injured vessel. It is only rarely that cardiopulmonary bypass is needed in major thoracic injuries; however, the perfusionist must be ready at a moment's notice to go on bypass if necessary.

Hemorrhagic Shock

Hemorrhagic shock may be defined as inadequate perfusion of the tissues with oxygen and substrate and failure to remove the end products of metabolism. The syndrome may be divided into three distinct stages depending on the overall blood loss and the rate at which blood is lost. Mild shock is present when up to 20 percent of the blood volume is lost, and is usually manifested by anxiety and restlessness. The blood

TABLE 18-12. Cardiac Injuries Resulting from Severe Blunt Trauma

Cardiac contusion
Rupture of a chamber
Tears of valves and connecting structures
Coronary artery injuries
Rupture of pericardium
Left ventricular aneurysm

TABLE 18-14. Site of Aortic Rupture

Site	Early	Chronic	Total
Ascending aorta	3	2	5
Aortic arch	1	2	3
Aortic isthmus	82	114	196
Distal descending aorta	2	2	4
Unspecified	2	—	2

(From Symbas et al,[83] with permission.)

pressure may be normal or even slightly increased, and a slight tachycardia may be evident. Shenkin et al have shown that adults in the supine position may lose up to 1,000 mL of blood with little change in the pulse rate.[86] When patients lose more than 20 percent of their blood volume without treatment, they are in a moderate state of shock, which is characterized by hypotension and tachycardia. The pulse usually feels thready and the extremities feel cool to the touch. At this stage, patients appear apathetic and complain of thirst. Patients who have lost 50 percent or more of their blood volume are in a severe state of shock. They usually appear obtunded and may be comatose. Their systolic blood pressure is usually less than 60 mmHg, there is a marked tachycardia, the extremities appear distinctly cold, the skin appears mottled and cyanotic, and the urine output declines to the point of anuria.

The organism invokes a number of responses to blood loss if given sufficient time. The most important compensatory mechanism is a redistribution of blood from the skin, muscle, and splanchnic vessels to the heart and brain. Normally, approximately 70 percent of the total blood volume is harbored in the venous capacitance vessels. This blood is rapidly redistributed to vital organs. This redistribution of blood is brought about by an elevation in serum catecholamines. Fluid migrates from the interstitial space to the intravascular space as a result of a decline in hydrostatic pressure in the capillaries; serum lactate levels increase in response to the change to anaerobic metabolism. In the final stages of untreated shock, cardiac decompensation occurs. This may be related to the release of a specific myocardial depressant factor or to an increased pulmonary vascular resistance. Animal studies suggest that cardiac decompensation does occur in hemorrhagic shock, but that it is a late event.

Management

Hemorrhagic shock is managed initially by inserting large-bore intravenous cannulae. Antecubital veins are suitable for this purpose. One of the keys to successful resuscitation of seriously traumatized patients is the ability to rapidly infuse fluids. It is possible to infuse as much as 1,400 mL of crystalloid or whole blood in 1 minute by using 5.0 mm internal diameter intravenous tubing in combination with an 8 French introducer or a very large intravenous catheter.[87] In 1984, Iserson and Reeter published a report concerning a simple infusion device that would allow five infusion bags to flow simultaneously through a large intravenous catheter (4.5 mm internal diameter).[88] When pressurized, as much as 1,600 mL of fluid could

be infused in 1 minute. A central venous pressure catheter may be inserted in the internal jugular vein quite safely with minimal risk of pneumothorax. However, the subclavian route may be preferable in the shock state because its patency is maintained by its bony attachments to the first rib and clavicle. A urinary catheter should be inserted as soon as possible after the diagnosis of shock has been made. The optimal treatment of patients in hemorrhagic shock is a combination of blood and Ringer's lactate. Shires et al measured the plasma volume, red blood cell mass, and extracellular fluid volume in dogs using the triple isotope determination.[89] They exsanguinated these animals to the point of severe shock and demonstrated that there was a large deficit in the interstitial space; they concluded that this loss of fluid was shared by both the intravascular and intracellular spaces. Furthermore, they demonstrated that the most effective method of correcting volume deficits secondary to hemorrhagic shock is the use of combinations of whole blood and a balanced salt solution, which in this case was Ringer's lactate. Animals that received combinations of whole blood and plasma had lower survival rates (Fig. 18-4). The findings in this paper have been corroborated by numerous clinicians dealing with patients in hemorrhagic shock.

Infusions of large volumes of balanced salt solutions without protein supplementation interfere with the colloid osmotic pressure. When hydrostatic pressure in the pulmonary capillaries exceeds the colloid osmotic pressure, pulmonary edema occurs. Virgilio et al measured the pulmonary capillary wedge pressure and colloid osmotic pressure in patients receiving both colloid and crystalloid solutions and found that pulmonary edema occurred only when the pulmonary capillary wedge pressure was elevated.[90] If the wedge pressure remained within normal limits, pulmonary edema did not develop, regardless of the colloid osmotic pressure. This is thought to be due to an increased rate of pulmonary lymph removal. There are other studies that support the view that when the colloid osmotic pressure in the pulmonary capillaries is less than the hydrostatic pressure, pulmonary edema occurs, that is, even when the pulmonary capillary wedge pressure is within normal limits.[91,92] It appears that balanced salt solutions should be used in combination with whole blood in the early treatment of hemorrhagic shock and that caution should be exercised when the colloid osmotic pressure is exceeded by the pulmonary capillary wedge pressure.

There is some concern about elevating serum lactate levels in patients with hemorrhagic shock by administering large volumes of Ringer's lactate. Studies performed in both animals and humans do not sup-

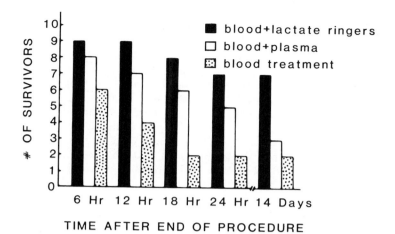

Fig. 18-4. Survival of acutely bled dogs was greatest when they were treated with a combination of blood and crystalloid solution. Colloid treatment alone was not as successful. (From Carrico,[136] with permission.)

port this concern.[93,94] In fact, studies have shown that the combination of blood and Ringer's lactate results in a more rapid return to normal acid-base balance.[95]

A number of blood substitutes can be used in the absence of blood; these include plasma, dextrans, and hetastarch, an artificial starch with a mean molecular weight of 70,000. It is currently being used as a plasma expander in the presence of shock. A 6 percent solution has osmotic properties similar to those of human albumin, approximately 40 percent being excreted in 24 hours. Hetastarch is less likely to cause anaphylaxis or a coagulopathy than dextran 40. Dextran 40 may be used as a plasma expander in the presence of shock, since it remains within the intravascular space for approximately 12 hours. Hypersensitivity reactions to this agent have been reported. It may cause an increased bleeding time by interfering with platelet function when more than 1 L is infused. Dextran causes rouleaux formation and, therefore, may interfere with cross-matching techniques.

There comes a point at which red blood cells are needed to maintain adequate oxygenation to the tissues. It may take as long as 45 minutes to perform satisfactory typing and screening of blood. In massive hemorrhage involving the heart or great vessels, type-specific blood or O negative blood may have to be used.

Cell-Saver Techniques and Rapid-Infusion Devices

Cell-saver techniques involve the collection of blood that, after appropriate preparation and filtration, is returned to the donor.[96] It may be used in elective surgery when massive bleeding is anticipated, and it may also be used in those patients with rare blood groups. Autotransfusion should not be used when the blood is soiled by fecal material. Various devices are used to achieve autotransfusion. Various methods of anticoagulation are used, including citrate-phosphate-dextrose preservative or heparinization. Heparinization should not be used in patients with suspected intracranial bleeding. Symbas et al have shown that it is not necessary to add anticoagulants to defibrinated blood aspirated from the chest.[97] Autotransfusion is frequently associated with damage to the various blood components, which may result in a decreased red blood cell mass, elevated bilirubin level, and hemoglobinuria. When massive quantities of blood are autotransfused (>5,000 mL), coagulopathies frequently develop. Air embolism is a real risk when the equipment is run by untrained personnel. During massive hemorrhage, valuable time is lost preparing blood for retransfusion. In recent years, rapid-infusion devices have been developed that are capable of infusing as much as 2 L of fluid or blood in 1 minute. These devices are invaluable during massive uncontrollable hemorrhage. A heat exchanger is incorporated within the device to prevent hypothermia.

Blood Replacement and Massive Blood Transfusion

Enormous strides have been made in blood transfusion technology and rheology in recent years. Currently, blood is combined with the anticoagulant citrate-phosphate-dextrose and adenine, the addition of which extends the shelf life of the blood to 35 days.

Certain serious hazards are associated with the administration of blood to patients, some of the most serious complications resulting from administration of a mismatched unit. Data from the Food and Drug Administration during a 3-year period in the 1970s revealed that 69 deaths occurred directly as a result of blood transfusion reactions; approximately one-third of these were due to acute hemolytic reactions, all of which resulted from mismatched transfusions secondary to human error.[98] The majority of mistakes were due to incorrect identification of blood or of the patient. It must be re-emphasized that the simple act of administering a unit of blood to a patient carries with it grave responsibility. Therefore, methodic scrutiny of the necessary documentation, including patient identity, is absolutely necessary on each occasion. Hepatitis B now occurs in less than 1 percent of patients who receive transfusions because of improved screening procedures, and the chances of developing non-A and non-B hepatitis are 13 times greater than contracting hepatitis B.[99,100] It has been estimated that approximately 4 percent of all patients receiving blood develop symptoms or signs of infection with this virus. In whole numbers, approximately 120,000 people in the United States are infected as a result of blood transfusions every year. Approximately 1,500 individuals die each year in the United States from non-A non-B hepatitis or induced cirrhosis secondary to blood transfusion (see Chapter 4). The risk of developing the acquired immunodeficiency syndrome (AIDS) from a blood transfusion is approximately 1 in 250,000.[101,102] AIDS testing in trauma victims has revealed an incidence of approximately 11 percent; therefore, health care workers should take all the precautions necessary to prevent contamination. Casual contact with individuals infected with AIDS is unlikely to result in infection. However, the risk of developing non-A non-B hepatitis is much greater. Therefore, gloves, goggles, and protective clothing should be worn when exposure to body fluids is a possibility. Cytomegalovirus has also been implicated as a cause of posttransfusion hepatitis. Investigators have shown that the addition of gamma globulin to stored blood can provide passive immunity to patients receiving blood.[103] Patients receiving pooled plasma are at the greatest risk from serum hepatitis; therefore, this component should be avoided if at all possible. All blood should be warmed during administration. This becomes increasingly important during massive blood replacement, when the temperature may decline to dangerous levels. Certain substances precipitate when mixed with blood; these include bicarbonate, calcium, and lactated Ringer's and dextrose solutions.

There is clear evidence that large quantities of unwanted debris accumulate in stored blood.[104] Therefore, there is general agreement among practitioners that all stored blood should be filtered during transfusion. There is usually considerable debate about the optimal pore size that is most beneficial. Although 20- and 40-μm filters are in general use, there are no objective data to support this practice. In fact, Virgilio compared the incidence of pulmonary dysfunction in patients receiving extensive transfusions using standard (170 μm) and fine filters and found no significant difference between them.[105] In emergency situations, when rapid transfusion is required, fine filters offer considerable impedance to the flow of packed red blood cells. This problem can be easily remedied by the addition of a small quantity of normal saline.

These are some of the problems associated with routine administration of small quantities of blood. Additional complications can be expected when massive blood replacement is required. Massive blood transfusion may be defined as replacement of at least 1.5 times a patient's blood volume in a short period of time. Does massive transfusion predispose patients to pulmonary insufficiency? Simmons et al found a significant correlation between massive transfusion and postoperative hypoxemia.[106] On the other hand, Collins et al found no such relationship.[107] The most definitive information on this topic is also provided by Collins, who demonstrated that patients with peripheral injuries receiving massive blood transfusion did not develop postoperative respiratory failure.[108] Conversely, patients with serious thoracic and abdominal injuries showed a high incidence of respiratory failure in association with massive transfusion. It appears likely that respiratory failure in these cases is related to pulmonary damage rather than to massive transfusion. The other possible causes of postoperative pulmonary insufficiency in these patients are left ventricular failure, microemboli, and denatured proteins. Disseminated intravascular coagulation is often overlooked as a possible etiologic factor.[108]

Dilutional thrombocytopenia is usually the most common cause of a coagulopathy in patients receiving massive blood transfusion.[109,110] When the platelet count declines to less than 65,000/cm^3, spontaneous hemorrhage becomes evident,[111] and 3 U of platelets should be administered for every 10 U of stored blood that has been transfused. It has been estimated that 1 U of platelet concentrate will raise the platelet count by 10,000/cm^3. Although factors V and VIII are markedly reduced in stored blood, these deficiencies rarely lead to coagulopathies by themselves. However, when the levels of these factors fall to less than 20 percent of normal, they add to the primary deficiency. To maintain sufficient levels of these two factors, some researchers previously recommended administering 2 U of fresh frozen plasma for every 10 U of stored blood transfused.[112] Today, it is not recommended to give fresh frozen plasma prophylactically. Disseminated intravascular coagulation (DIC) must be included in the differential diagnosis in any patient presenting with a bleeding diathesis. This is a rather bizarre coagulopathy occurring in patients with trauma and shock and in those receiving large quantities of stored blood.[113] It is characterized by an initial tendency toward coagulation, which is rapidly followed by deficiencies in the clotting mechanism.

The following approach should be used in all patients receiving large quantities of stored blood. When 10 U of blood have been administered to an adult patient, blood should be drawn for a platelet count. A specimen of blood should also be drawn for subsequent evaluation of the clot. Fresh frozen plasma and platelet concentrates should be administered only when needed. Should spontaneous bleeding occur from intravenous sites, an estimation of the platelet count, partial thromboplastin time (PTT), and plasma fibrinogen must be made as soon as possible, and the clot should be examined for evidence of lysis within 2 hours. If the PTT is elevated but the clot remains intact, bleeding is probably due to deficiency of factors V and VIII and can be readily treated with fresh frozen plasma. If, on the other hand, thrombocytopenia, hypofibrinogenemia, and clot lysis occur, DIC is likely[114] (Table 18-15). The definitive diagnosis is made by a determination of the fibrin split products, which distinguishes primary from secondary fibrinolysis. When serious coagulation disturbances occur, the expertise of a hematologist or pathologist well versed in the subject is strongly advised. However, the anesthesiologist is expected to closely monitor the coagulation status of patients receiving large quantities of stored blood and to treat the more common disturbances.

Citrate, when infused intravascularly, binds with calcium. With normal rates of infusion, changes in the ionized calcium level are minimal; however, when infusion rates exceed 1.5 mL/kg/min, symptoms and signs of hypocalcemia may appear. These include hypotension, elevation of the central venous pressure, and tetany. The ECG may show evidence of a prolonged QT interval. Normally, citrate is metabolized in the Kreb's cycle. Therefore, any factor interfering with metabolism, such as hypothermia or hepatic disease, may lead to elevated citrate levels. Hyperventilation causes a decrease in ionized calcium levels and, therefore, should be carefully avoided during rapid infusions of stored blood. Should calcium salts be given prophylactically under these circumstances? Most authorities are opposed to the use of prophylactic calcium because it is extremely difficult to predict the associated changes in ionized calcium levels. Rhythm disturbances associated with hypercalcemia may be more immediately life-threatening than hypocalcemia.[115] Anesthetic depression should be avoided during rapid infusions of stored blood. Measurements of serum ionized calcium levels are readily available in most critical care laboratories and are certainly recommended during massive blood replacement, but calcium therapy should be carried out with caution.

Stored blood contains from 4 to 23 mEq/L of potassium; therefore, hyperkalemia is usually not a problem during normal rates of infusion. Even during rapid infusions, potassium from stored blood enters donor cells or is excreted by the kidneys. Hyperkalemia occurs in adults only when the rates of infusion exceed 120 mL/min; however, infants and children are more prone to this problem than are adults.[116–118]

There appears to be no general agreement about changes in hydrogen ion concentration during massive transfusion. These changes are extremely variable; therefore, bicarbonate should not be given prophylactically.[119] Approximately 14 mmol of hydrogen ions are generated in each unit of stored blood; however, these ions are buffered by the plasma bicarbonate and red blood cells during infusion.

Quantities of 2,3-diphosphoglycerate decline in stored blood in proportion to the duration of storage.[120] This is associated with increased binding of oxygen with hemoglobin and a shift to the left of the oxygen-hemoglobin dissociation curve. The significance of increased oxygen affinity in patients receiving large quantities of stored blood is not clear. Theoretically, at least, this may be important in patients who have lost the ability to regulate regional blood flow to organs, such as the heart, through disease. This problem may be further aggravated by hyperventilation.

Hypothermia is a common occurrence in patients receiving large quantities of stored blood.[121] Every effort should be made to keep the body temperature above 35°C.

TABLE 18-15. Criteria for Differentiating DIC and Dilutional Thrombocytopenia

DIC	Dilutional Thrombocytopenia
Thrombocytopenia	Thrombocytopenia
Hypofibrinogenemia	Normal or slightly reduced fibrinogen
Clot lysis (after 2 hours)	Intact clot (after 2 hours)

In summary, the transfusion of massive quantities of blood induces several biochemical, physiologic, and metabolic changes, which, if not corrected, may cause serious morbidity and mortality.

Inotropes and Vasodilators in Shock

Vasopressors have no logical place in the long-term treatment of shock due to hemorrhage. The primary pathophysiologic defect is inadequate tissue perfusion secondary to blood loss; therefore, the primary treatment should be directed toward replenishing fluid and blood losses. Occasionally, it will be necessary to use vasopressors such as epinephrine in patients presenting in extremis. Vasopressor support is of vital importance in this situation. Those drugs with predominant alpha-stimulating properties appear to be the most beneficial, and drugs with predominant beta-stimulating effects the least. Dopamine, a precursor of norepinephrine, has been used in clinical practice for approximately 12 years and has some interesting properties. In low doses (1 to 6 μg/kg/min), it acts on the beta-adrenergic and dopaminergic receptors. In doses exceeding 10 μg/kg/min, it has a predominant alpha-adrenergic effect in adults. Dopaminergic receptors, when stimulated, dilate the renal and splanchnic blood vessels, redirecting blood to the corresponding organs. Therefore, this vasopressor may be of some definite benefit to patients in shock. However, it is important to replace blood and fluid losses while attempting this therapy. In the terminal stages of shock, dopamine may also provide some inotropic support. Dopamine should always be infused through a central vein. Digitalis is not recommended routinely for patients in hemorrhagic shock. However, it may be of value in older debilitated patients who have been subjected to this insult.

Is there a place for vasodilators in the presence of hemorrhagic shock? A number of animal studies showed increased survival rates when vasodilators were used to treat shock.[122,123] Chlorpromazine, which has alpha-blocking properties, has been used in humans for this purpose.[124] It appears that vasodilator therapy has a firm place in the therapy of cardiogenic shock, but most clinicians are still reluctant to use it in patients with hemorrhagic shock. Again, adequate volume replacement must be achieved before attempting this form of therapy.

Renal Failure

A discussion of thoracic trauma would be incomplete without some reference to renal failure. Although posttraumatic renal failure is uncommon, with an incidence of approximately 3 percent, it is associated with a 60 percent mortality rate.[125] The etiology of renal failure in the trauma setting is predominantly secondary to acute tubular necrosis. Intense renal vasoconstriction accompanying hypovolemic shock accounts for the majority of cases of renal failure in trauma victims. Patients with serious muscle injuries may also develop renal failure secondary to myoglobulinuria. Finally, some patients develop renal failure secondary to drug toxicity in the course of treatment. Aminoglycosides and cephalosporins are known nephrotoxic substances, and radiographic contrast materials are also nephrotoxic.[126,127] It also has been clearly established that enflurane may cause high-output renal failure in association with the production of elevated levels of the fluoride ion.[128,129] Therefore, it would be prudent to avoid this agent in a setting in which renal failure is likely to occur. Interestingly, furosemide has been shown to be a cause of renal failure, despite the fact that it is frequently used to treat the condition.[130,131]

Oliguria, defined as a volume of less than 400 mL of urine in 24 hours, is the most common sign of renal failure following major trauma. The cause of oliguria is uncertain, but may involve renal tubular obstruction, passive backflow of the glomerular filtrate, or intense prerenal vasoconstriction. The predominant effects of filtration failure are the retention of creatinine, urea, and some electrolytes. In complete failure, the serum creatinine will rise by approximately 1.5 mg/dL per day. However, these biochemical changes in blood or urine are of minimal help to the anesthesiologist during surgery. It is mandatory to measure the urine output in all patients presenting with significant blood loss or blunt trauma, and the urine output should be recorded on an hourly basis. The most likely cause of oliguria in the surgical setting is inadequate fluid or blood replacement. Should oliguria occur in the course of a surgical procedure, the most rational approach to the problem is to first rule out any technical problems with the catheter. Patients then should be given a fluid challenge, but this maneuver should be used cautiously in patients with cardiac disease. Measurement of the central venous pressure is an invaluable tool in the assessment of the volume status of traumatized patients. Infusion of 500 mL of a balanced salt solution or free water is recommended and, if there is no response to this approach after approximately 30 minutes, 50 to 100 mL of 25 percent mannitol should be infused over 20 minutes. Mannitol alters the distribution of blood in the renal parenchyma, promoting urine flow.[132] Furosemide has also been recommended in this situation, although a firm basis for its use has not been established.[133,134] The recommended dose of furosemide is 0.5 to 1 mg/kg initially; this dose is doubled every 30 minutes until diuresis is evident or up to 400 mg has been administered. Dopamine is the only vasopressor recommended in renal failure, and the dose should be carefully monitored. Doses in the range of 1 to 5 $\mu g/kg/min$ have a favorable effect on the dopaminergic receptors in the renal vessels causing dilatation. Acute renal failure is an important entity occurring in patients with serious trauma, and the anesthesiologist, who is usually first to detect the onset of this condition, must aggressively treat oliguria in these patients.

SUMMARY

Trauma is the penalty modern society pays for high-speed travel, illicit drug and alcohol use, and the ready availability of handguns. The anesthesiologist plays a very important role in the management of patients with serious thoracic trauma. In the majority of cases, the anesthesiologist is confronted with patients who are seriously hypovolemic. Whenever possible, the blood volume must be replaced before the patients are subjected to anesthesia. Occasionally, time will not permit adequate restoration of blood volume, especially when major arterial bleeding occurs. In this situation, the anesthesiologist is expected to proceed with minimal information about the patient. With reasonable care, attention, and aggresive therapy, a number of these patients survive and return to normal lives.

REFERENCES

1. Paget S: Surgery of the Chest. p. 121. Wright, London, 1896
2. Rehn L: Ueber penetrirende herzuden and herznaht. Arch Klin Chir 55:315, 1897
3. Maull KI, Kinning LS, Hickman JK: Culpability and accountability of hospitalized injured alcohol-impaired drivers: a prospective study. JAMA 252:1880–1883, 1984
4. Accidents Facts. National Safety Council, Chicago, 1987
5. Mayer T, Walker ML, Johnson DG, et al: Causes of morbidity and mortality in severe pediatric trauma. JAMA 245:719–721, 1981
6. Cowley RA, Trump B: Today's neglected disease—trauma. Bull Univ Md Sch 56:19–23, 1971
7. Munoz E: Economic cost of trauma, United States 1982. J Trauma 24:237–244, 1984
8. Symbas PN: Cardiothoracic Trauma. WB Saunders, Philadelphia, 1989
9. Shepard GH: High-energy, low-velocity close-range shotgun wounds. J Trauma 20:1065–1067, 1980
10. Attar S, Kirby WH: The forces producing certain types of thoracic trauma. p. 4. In Daughtry DC (ed): Thoracic Trauma. Little, Brown, Boston, 1980
11. Attar S, Kirby WH: The forces producing certain types of thoracic trauma. p. 7. In Daughtry DC (ed): Thoracic Trauma. Little, Brown, Boston, 1980
12. Faust RJ, Nauss LA: Post-thoracotomy intercostal block: comparison of its effects on pulmonary function with those of intramuscular meperidine. Anesth Analg 55:542–546, 1976
13. Reiestad F, Stromskag KE: Interpleural catheter in the management of postoperative pain: a preliminary report. Reg Anaesth 11:89–91, 1986
14. Ferrante FM, Ostheimer GW, Covino BG: Patient-Controlled Analgesia. Year Book Medical Publishers, Chicago, 1989
15. Mackenzie C: Advances in Trauma Emergency Care. Anesthesia Review 4. Churchill Livingstone, New York, 1986
16. Dundee JW, Wyant GM: Intravenous Anesthesia. pp. 3–4. Churchill Livingstone, London, 1974
17. Cloutier CT, Lowery BD, Carey LC: The effect of hemodilutional resuscitation on serum protein levels in humans in hemorrhagic shock. J Trauma 9:514–521, 1969
18. Mazze RI, Escue HM, Houston JB: Hyperkalemia and cardiovascular collapse following administration of succinylcholine to the traumatized patient. Anesthesiology 31:540–547, 1969
19. Bogetz MS, Katz JA: Recall of surgery for major trauma. Anesthesiology 61:6–9, 1984
20. Wolfson B, Freed B: Influence of alcohol on anesthetic requirements and acute toxicity. Anesth Analg 59:826–830, 1980
21. Bloomer WE: Chest trauma as effected by age and pre-existing disease. p. 201. In Daughtry DC (ed): Thoracic Trauma. Little, Brown, Boston, 1980
22. Gay WA, McCabe JC: Trauma to the chest. p. 263. In Shires CT (ed): Care of the Trauma Patient. McGraw-Hill, New York, 1979
23. Maloney JV, Jr, Shmutzer KJ, Raschke E: Paradoxical respiration and "pendelluft." J Thorac Cardiovasc Surg 41:291–298, 1961
24. Sarnoff SJ, Gaensler EA, Maloney JV: Electrophrenic respiration. The effectiveness of contralateral ventilation during activity of one phrenic nerve. J Thorac Cardiovasc Surg 19:929–937, 1950
25. Duff JH, Goldstein M, McLean APH, et al: Flail chest: a clinical review and physiological study. J Trauma 8:63–74, 1968
26. Jones TB, Richardson EP: Traction on the sternum in the treatment of multiple fractured ribs. Surg Gynecol Obstet 42:283, 1926
27. Moore BP: Operative stabilization of nonpenetrating chest injuries. J Thorac Cardiovasc Surg 70:619–630, 1975
28. Arens JF, LeJume FE, Webre DR: Maxillary sinusitis: a complication of nasal tracheal intubation. Anesthesiology 40:415, 1974
29. Deutschman CS: Paranasal sinusitis associated with nasotracheal intubation: a frequently unrecognised and treatable source of sepsis. Crit Care Med 14:111, 1986
30. Dane TEB, King EG: A prospective study of complications after tracheostomy for assisted ventilation. Chest 67:398–404, 1975

31. Chalon J, Loew DAY, Malebranche J: Effects of dry anesthetic gases on tracheobronchial ciliated epithelium. Anesthesiology 37:338–343, 1972

32. Swan HJC, Ganz W, Forrester J, et al: Catheterization of the heart in man with use of a flow-directed balloon tipped catheter. N Engl J Med 283:447–451, 1970

33. Shackford SR, Virgilio RW: Selective use of ventilator therapy in flail chest injury. J Thorac Cardiovasc Surg 81:194–201, 1981

34. Sankaran S, Wilson RF: Factors affecting prognosis in patients with flail chest. J Thorac Cardiovasc Surg 60:402–410, 1970

35. Thomas AN, Baisdell FW, Lewis FR, et al: Operative stabilization for flail chest after blunt trauma. J Thorac Cardiovasc Surg 75:793–801, 1978

36. Murphy CH, Murphy MR: p. 67. Radiology for Anesthesia and Critical Care. Churchill Livingstone, New York, 1987

37. Eger EI II, Saidman LJ: Hazards of nitrous oxide anesthesia in bowel obstruction and pneumothorax. Anesthesiology 26:61–66, 1965

38. Defalque RJ: Subclavian venipuncture: a review. Anesth Analog 47:677–682, 1968

39. Defalque RJ: Percutaneous catheterization of the internal jugular vein. Anesth Analg 53:116–121, 1974

40. Gay WA, McCabe JC: Trauma to the chest. pp. 275–276. In Shires GT (ed): Care of the Trauma Patient. McGraw-Hill, New York, 1979

41. Symbas PN: Acute traumatic hemothorax. Ann Thorac Surg 26:195–196, 1978

42. Baker CC, Thomas AN, Trunkey DD: The role of emergency room thoracotomy in trauma. J Trauma 20:848–855, 1980

43. Bertelsen S, Howitz P: Injuries of the trachea and bronchi. Thorax 27:188–194, 1972

44. Lloyd JR, Heydinger DK, Klassen KP, et al: Rupture of the main bronchi in closed chest injury. Arch Surg 77:597, 1958

45. Symbas PN, Hatcher CR, Boehm GA: Acute penetrating tracheal trauma. Ann Thorac Surg 22:473–477, 1976

46. Brooks JW: Blunt traumatic rupture of the diaphragm. Ann Thorac Surg 26:199–203, 1978

47. Hood RM: Traumatic diaphragmatic hernia. Ann Thorac Surg 12:311–324, 1971

48. Brooks JW: Blunt traumatic rupture of the diaphragm. Ann Thorac Surg 26:199–203, 1978

49. Brooks JW, Seiler HH: Traumatic hernia of the diaphragm. pp. 175–193. In Daughtry DC (ed): Thoracic Trauma. Little, Brown, Boston, 1980

50. Ebert PA: Physiologic principles in the management of the crushed-chest syndrome. Monogr Surg Sci 4:69–94, 1967

51. Parmley LF, Mattingly TW, Manion WC: Penetrating wounds of the heart and aorta. Circulation 17:953–973, 1958

52. Symbas PN, Harlaftis N, Waldo WJ: Penetrating cardiac wounds: a comparison of different therapeutic methods. Ann Surg 183:377–381, 1976

53. Beck CS: Two cardiac compression triads. JAMA 104:714–716, 1935

54. Asfaw I, Arbulu A: Penetrating wounds of the pericardium and heart. Surg Clin North Am 37–48, 1977

55. Yao ST, Vanecko RM, Printen K, et al: Penetrating wounds of the heart: a review of 80 cases. Ann Surg 168:67–78, 1968

56. Trinkle JK, Marcos J, Grover FL, et al: Management of the wounded heart. Ann Thorac Surg 17:230–236, 1973

57. Beach PM, Jr, Bognolo D, Hutchinson JE: Penetrating cardiac trauma. Am J Surg 131:411–414, 1976

58. Lemos PCP, Okumura M, Acevedo AC, et al: Cardiac wounds: experience based on a series of 121 operated cases. J Cardiovasc Surg 17:1–8, 1976

59. Warburg E: Myocardial and pericardial lesions due to nonpenetrating injury. Br Heart J 2:271–280, 1940

60. Cassell P, Cullum P: The management of cardiac tamponade: drainage of pericardial effusions. Br J Surg 54:620–626, 1967

61. Proudfit WL, Effler DB: Diagnosis and treatment of cardiac pericarditis by pericardial biopsy. JAMA 161:188–192, 1956

62. Guntheroth WG, Morgan BC, Mullins GL: Effect of respiration on venous return and stroke volume in cardiac tamponade: mechanism of pulsus paradoxus. Circ Res 20:381–390, 1967

63. Morgan BC, Guntheroth WG, Dillard DH: Relationship of pericardial to pleural pressure during quiet respiration and cardiac tamponade. Circ Res 16:493–498, 1965

64. Stanley TH, Weidauer HE: Anesthesia for the patient with cardiac tamponade. Anesth Analg 52:110–114, 1973

65. Kaplan JA: Pericardial diseases. p. 495. In Kaplan JA (ed): Cardiac Anesthesia. Grune & Stratton, Orlando, FL, 1979

66. Kaplan JA, Bland JW, Jr, Dunbar RW: The perioperative management of pericardial tamponade. South Med J 69:417–419, 1976

67. Dowdy EG, Kaya K: Studies of the mechanism of cardiovascular responses to CI-581. Anesthesiology 29:931, 1968

68. Traber DL, Wilson RD, Priano LL: Differentiation of the cardiovascular effects of CI-581. Anesth Analg 47:769–778, 1968

69. Tweed WA: Ketamine and the cardiovascular system. pp. 37–43. In: Ketalar. Parke, Davis and Company, Ltd., Montreal, 1971

70. Williams C, Soutter L: Pericardial tamponade. Arch Intern Med 94:571–584, 1954

71. Corssen G, Allarde R, Brosch F, et al: Ketamine as the sole anesthetic in open-heart surgery—a preliminary report. Anesth Analg 49:1025–1031, 1970

72. Dowdy EG, Kaya K: Studies of the mechanism of cardiovascular responses to CI-581. Anesthesiology 29:931, 1968

73. Fowler NO, Holmes JC: Hemodynamic effects of isoproterenol and norepinephrine in acute cardiac tamponade. J Clin Invest 48:502, 1969

74. Rea WJ, Sugg WL, Wilson LC, et al: Coronary artery lacerations—an analysis of 22 patients. Ann Thorac Surg 7:518–528, 1969

75. Tector AJ, Reuben CF, Hoffman JF, et al: Coronary artery wounds treated with saphenous vein bypass grafts. JAMA 225:282–284, 1973

76. Levitsky S: New insights in cardiac trauma. Surg Clin North Am 43–55, 1975

77. Kissane RW: Traumatic heart diseases, especially myocardial contusion. Postgrad Med 15:114–119, 1954

78. Moseley RE, Vernick JJ, Doty DB: Response to blunt chest injury: a new experimental model. J Trauma 10:673–683, 1970

79. Watson JH, Bartholomae WM: Cardiac injury due to nonpenetrating chest trauma. Ann Intern Med 52:871–880, 1960

80. Rothstein RJ: Concepts in emergency and critical care. JAMA 250:2189–2191, 1983

81. Parmley LF, Mattingly TW, Marion WC: Nonpenetrating traumatic injury of the aorta. Circulation 17:1086–1101, 1958

82. Greendyke RM: Traumatic rupture of aorta: special reference to automobile accidents. JAMA 195:527–530, 1966

83. Symbas PN, Tyras DW, Ware RE, et al: Traumatic rupture of the aorta. Ann Surg 178:6–12, 1973

84. Symbas PN, Kourias E, Tyras DH, et al: Penetrating wounds of great vessels. Ann Surg 179:757–762, 1974

85. Bricker DL, Morton JR, Okies JE, et al: Surgical management of injuries to the vena cava: changing patterns of injury and newer techniques of repair. J Trauma 11:725–735, 1971

86. Shenkin HA, Cheney RH, Govons SR, et al: On the diagnosis of hemorrhage in man—a study of volunteers bled large amounts. Am J Med Sci 208:421–436, 1944

87. Milliken JS, Cam TL, Hansborough J: Rapid volume replacement for hypovolemic shock: a comparison of techniques and equipment. J Trauma 24:237–244, 1984

88. Iserson KV, Reeter AK: Rapid fluid replacement: a new methodology. Ann Emerg Med 12:97–100, 1984

89. Shires T, Coln D, Carrico J, et al: Fluid therapy in hemorrhagic shock. Arch Surg 88:688–693, 1964

90. Virgilio RW, Smith DE, Rice CL, et al: Effect of colloid osmotic pressure and pulmonary capillary wedge pressure on intrapulmonary shunt. Surg Forum 27:168–173, 1976

91. Stein L, Berand J, Morissette M, et al: Pulmonary edema during volume infusion. Circulation 52:483–489, 1975

92. Stein L, Berand J, Cavanilles J, et al: Pulmonary edema during fluid infusion in the absence of heart failure. JAMA 229:65–68, 1974

93. Baue AE, Tragus ET, Wolfson SK, et al: Hemodynamic and metabolic effect of Ringer's lactate solution in hemorrhagic shock. Ann Surg 166:29–38, 1967

94. Trinkle JK, Rush BF, Eiseman G: Metabolism of lactate following major blood loss. Surgery 63:782–787, 1968

95. McClelland RN, Shires GT, Baxter CR: Balanced salt solution in the treatment of hemorrhagic shock. JAMA 199:830–834, 1967

96. Stehling LC, Zauder HL, Rogers W: Intraoperative autotransfusion. Anesthesiology 43:337–345, 1975

97. Symbas PN, Levin JM, Ferrier FL, et al: A study on autotransfusion from hemothorax. South Med J 62:671–674, 1969

98. Schmidt PJ: Transfusion mortality; with special reference to surgical and intensive care facilities. J Fla Med Assoc 67:151–153, 1980

99. Dienstag JL, Alter HJ: Non-A, non-B hepatitis: evolving epidemiologic and clinical perspective. Seminars in Liver Disease 6:67–81, 1986

100. Lever AM: Non A/non B hepatitis. J Hosp Infect, suppl. A. 11:150–160, 1988

101. Zuck TF, Sherwood WC, Bove JR: A review of recent events related to surrogate testing of blood to prevent non-A, non-B posttransfusion hepatitis. Transfusion 27:203–206, 1987

102. Berry AJ: Transmission of infection in the operating room. p. 145. ASA Refresher Course Lectures, 1989

103. Katz R, Rodriguez J, Ward R: Post-transfusion hepatitis—effect of modified gammaglobulin added to blood in vitro. N Engl J Med 285:925–932, 1971

104. Solis RT, Goldfinger D, Gibbs MB, et al: Physical characteristics of microaggregates in stored blood. Transfusion 14:538–550, 1974

105. Virgilio RW: Blood filters and postoperative pulmonary dysfunction. Weekly Anaesthesiol Update 2:2–8, 1979

106. Simmons RL, Heisterkamp CA, Collins JA, et al: Respiratory insufficiency in combat casualties. Ann Surg 170:53–62, 1969

107. Collins JA, Gordon WC, Hudson TL, et al: Inapparent hypoxemia in casualties with wounded limbs: pulmonary fat embolism? Ann Surg 167:511–520, 1968

108. Collins JA: Massive transfusion: What is current and important? pp. 1–16. In Nusbacher J (ed): Massive Transfusion 1978. American Association of Blood Banks, Washington, DC, 1978

109. Miller RD, Robbins TO, Tong MJ, et al: Coagulation defects associated with massive blood transfusions. Ann Surg 174:794–801, 1971

110. Krevans JR, Jackson DP: Hemorrhagic disorder following massive whole blood transfusions. JAMA 159:171–177, 1955

111. Miller RD: Complications of massive blood transfusions. Anesthesiology 39:82–93, 1973

112. Gill W, Champion HR: Volume resuscitation in critical major trauma. pp. 77–105. In Dawson RD (ed): American Association of Blood Banks, Technical Workshop, Transfusion Therapy. Gunthrop-Warren Printing, Chicago, 1974

113. Rodriguez-Erdmann F: Bleeding due to increased intravascular blood coagulation. N Engl J Med 273:1370–1378, 1965

114. Deykin D: The clinical challenge of disseminated intravascular coagulation. N Engl J Med 283:636–644, 1970

115. Bunker JP: Metabolic effects of blood transfusion. Anesthesiology 27:446–455, 1966

116. Taylor WC, Grisdole LC, Steward AG: Unexplained death from exchange transfusion. J Pediatr 52:694–700, 1958

117. Bolande RP, Traisman HS, Philipsborn HF: Electrolyte consideration in exchange transfusions for erythroblastosis fetalis. J Pediatr 49:401–406, 1956

118. Kates RA, Finucane BT: Massive transfusion in neonates. South Med J 77:516–517, 1984

119. Miller RD, Tong MJ, Robbins TO: Effects of massive transfusion of blood on acid-base balance. JAMA 216:1762–1765, 1971

120. Bunn HF, May MH, Kocholaty WF, et al: Hemoglobin function in stored blood. J Clin Invest 48:311–321, 1969

121. Boyan CP, Howland WS: Blood temperature: a critical factor in massive transfusion. Anesthesiology 22:559–563, 1961

122. Wiggers HC, Ingraham RC, Roehild F, et al: Vasoconstriction and the development of irreversible hemorrhagic shock. Am J Physiol 153:511–520, 1948

123. Baez S, Zweifach BW, Shorr E: Protective action of Dibenamine against the fatal outcome of hemorrhagic and traumatic shock in rats. Fed Proc 11:7, 1952

124. Collins VJ, Jaffee R, Zahony I: Anesthesia conference; shock—a different approach to therapy. IMJ 121, 122:350–353, 1962

125. Baek S, Makabali GG, Shoemaker WC: Clinical determinants of survival from postoperative renal failure. Surg Gynecol Obstet 140:685–689, 1975

126. Silverblatt FJ: Antibiotic nephrotoxicity—a review of pathogenesis and prevention. Urol Clin North Am 557–567, 1975

127. Ansari Z, Baldwin DS: Acute renal failure due to radiocontrast agents. Nephron 17:28–40, 1976

128. Cousins MJ, Mazze RI, Barr GA, et al: A comparison of the renal effects of isoflurane and methoxyflurane in Fischer 344 rats. Anesthesiology 38:557–563, 1973

129. Cousins MJ, Greenstein LR, Hitt BA, et al: metabolism and renal effects of enflurane in man. Anesthesiology 44:44–53, 1976

130. Loughridge L: Anesthesia and the kidneys. p. 321. In Scurr C, Feldman S (eds): Scientific Foundations of Anaesthesia. William Heinemann Medical Books, London, 1974

131. Baek SM, Brown RS, Shoemaker WC: Early prediction of acute renal failure and recovery: renal function response to furosemide. Ann Surg 178:605–608, 1973

132. Epstein M, Schneider NS, Befeler B: Effect of intrarenal furosemide on renal function and intrarenal hemodynamics in acute renal failure. Am J Med 58:510–516, 1975

133. Baek SM, Brown RS, Shoemaker WC: Early prediction of acute renal failure and recovery: renal function response to furosemide. Ann Surg 178:605–608, 1973

134. Epstein M, Schneider NS, Befeler B: Effect of intrarenal furosemide on renal function and intrarenal hemodynamics in acute renal failure. Am J Med 58:510–516, 1975

135. Goldman MJ: Principles of Clinical Electrocardiography. 10th Ed. Lange Medical Publications, Los Altos, CA, 1979

136. Carrico CJ: Fluid resuscitation following injury: rationale for the use of balanced salt solutions. Crit Care Med 4:48, 1976

19

ANESTHESIA FOR PEDIATRIC AND NEONATAL THORACIC SURGERY

James W. Bland, Jr., M.D.
Keith K. Brosius, M.D.

Thomas J. Mancuso, M.D.
Stephen R. Tosone, M.D.

The great increase in medical knowledge, intelligence, and technology that has occurred during the last half of this century has significantly influenced the ability to deal effectively with congenital anomalies, disease states, and trauma seen in the pediatric, neonatal, and adolescent populations. Progress in the surgical management of pathophysiologic states in young patients has been accompanied by equally important improvements in pediatric anesthesiology and intensive care, neonatology, cardiology, and pulmonology. Further advances in nutritional support methods, antimicrobial therapy, understanding of the effects of the stress response in the neonate, aspects of organ transplantation and its immunologic implications, and information storage, retrieval, and exchange have all been extremely useful to the entire pediatric health care team. Specific examples of pharmacologic and technologic growth in pediatric anesthesiology and intensive care include greater understanding of the physiology of the fetus and the neonate; development of nonflammable anesthetic agents with fewer detrimental effects on the cardiovascular system; introduction of safer narcotics and muscle relaxants, and further understanding of their pharmacodynamics in the pediatric population; better physiologic monitoring systems for the cardiovascular and pulmonary systems applicable to a wide variety of patients; improved systems for providing respiratory support in the intensive care unit and at home for patients requiring long-term ventilation; and ultramicroanalysis for blood pH, blood gas values, and biochemical measurements.

Anesthesia for thoracic operations in infants and children is extremely demanding and requires the most meticulous cooperation and communication among the anesthesiology staff, surgeon and surgical assistants, intensivists, and nursing personnel. Each member of the care team must understand and appreciate the problems encountered by the others if the best results are to be obtained. Betts and Downes' assertion that good pediatric anesthesia demands adequate analgesia, life support, intensive surveillance,

485

and appropriate operating conditions for the surgical team should continue to be the goal of every anesthesiologist.[1]

UNIQUENESS OF THE PEDIATRIC PATIENT

Not only are children as a group different from adults, they are very different within that group. Although both an 80 kg, 17-year-old boy presenting for pectus excavatum repair and a 1.0 kg premature infant presenting for repair of tetralogy of Fallot have some anesthetic considerations that adults do not, they are not members of a homogenous group called *children*. Since conduct of anesthesia in a careful and safe manner is paramount, knowledge of the anatomic and physiologic differences between children and adults is essential. However, once safety is assured, consideration of the important psychological differences of children of various ages is essential if the child is to have as pleasant an experience as possible during the perioperative period. Some of these important differences are summarized in Table 19-1. To assure the efficient conduct of a safe surgical procedure, the pediatric anesthesiologist must carefully consider these age- and size-related variables, as well as factors related to the specific disease process being treated, the operation being performed, the level of postoperative care available, and the preferences of the individual surgeon. Indeed, the anesthetic management of the premature infant is virtually a specialty in itself, requiring a high degree of coordination among the anesthesiologist and the many other members of the team caring for the high-risk newborn.[2] As the child grows, matures, and passes into an "age of awareness," psychological factors play an increasingly important role in anesthetic management if the trauma associated with hospitalization, fear, pain, and separation of child and parents is to be minimized.

Changes Related to Birth

The fetus has intrauterine renal, hepatic, endocrine, hematopoietic, and neural function. Maternal organ systems may assist fetal function to some extent by placental exchange, but, for the most part, these systems are functional at birth, requiring no great transition. The gastrointestinal and neuromuscular systems certainly continue to develop after birth, but they are usually capable of immediately meeting the infant's needs. The greatest changes required in adapting to extrauterine life involve the cardiovascular and respiratory systems.

Fetal Respiration

Fetal respiration takes place at the capillary interfaces of the placenta. Maternal oxygen diffuses across the placenta to the fetal blood because of the gradient that exists between the mother's arterial blood (PO_2, 90 to 100 mmHg) and that of the fetus (PO_2, 30 to 35 mmHg). Fetal carbon dioxide diffuses similarly by the Haldane and Bohr effects, respectively.[3] Obviously, fetal lungs contain no air; circulation of blood to the lungs is thus much less than normal prior to birth, since the lungs are performing no ventilatory function.

Fetal Circulation

During intrauterine life, the fetus depends on three forms of communication, or "shunts," not normally present after birth—the ductus arteriosus, foramen ovale, and ductus venosus. Each of these types of communication plays a vital role in maintaining efficient fetal circulation in utero, allowing the fetal blood to

TABLE 19-1. Normal Values

Age		Heart Rate (beats/min)	Blood Pressure (mmHg)	Respiratory Rate (breaths/min)	Hematocrit (%)	Blood Volume (mL/kg)	Maintenance Fluids (mL/kg/24 h)	Caloric Requirements (cal/kg/24 h)
Premature (<2,000 g)	Preterm	140–160	50/30	40–60	40–50	100	100–120	120
Neonate	0–28 d	120–140	60/40	40–60	40–60	100	80–100	100
Infant	28 d–1 yr	80–120	60–90 40–60	30–50	30–40	80	80	80–100
Child	1–10 yr	80–100	80–120 40–70	20–30	30–40	70	60–80	40–80
Young adult	11–16 yr	60–90	90–140 50–80	10–20	35–45	60–70	60	40–60

bypass the nonaerated lungs, and in making the transition to the normal adult-like extrauterine circulation as the lungs inflate and the pulmonary vascular resistance (PVR) falls after birth.

Relatively oxygenated placental blood having a PO_2 of 60 mmHg flows from the low-pressure side of the placenta via the fetal umbilical vein to the fetal liver, through which it enters the inferior vena cava via the ductus venosus. This oxygenated blood mixes with fetal inferior vena caval blood and, to a lesser degree, superior vena caval blood, resulting in blood with a PO_2 of approximately 35 to 40 mmHg that flows into the right atrium. The anatomic characteristics of the atrial septum with the "trap-door" flap of the foramen ovale direct most of this oxygen-rich blood across to the left atrium. The higher pressure in the right atrium keeps the foramen ovale open prior to birth; reversal of this pressure gradient at birth allows functional closure of the foramen ovale even though it may not anatomically close for many years. Left atrial blood then mixes with the small amount of pulmonary venous blood, crosses the mitral valve into the left ventricle, and is pumped into the aorta and systemic circulation. The brachiocephalic and coronary vessels receive the relatively well-saturated arterial blood.

Venous blood from the superior vena cava enters the right atrium, mixing minimally with blood from the inferior vena cava and placenta before crossing the tricuspid valve into the right ventricle. A small percentage of the blood ejected by the right ventricle goes to the lungs. The lower PO_2 of this blood results in pulmonary vasoconstriction and elevation of the PVR. This small fraction of right ventricular output that goes to the lungs mixes with blood from the bronchial arteries and drains into the left atrium. The remaining blood pumped from the right ventricle follows the path of least resistance, passing from the pulmonary artery into the aorta via the ductus arteriosus to perfuse the lower portion of the systemic vascular bed and the fetal portion of the placenta via the two umbilical arteries. Because of the streaming of caval blood in the right atrium, the blood in the lower body is not as well oxygenated as that of the aortic arch and brachiocephalic vessels.

In contrast to the extrauterine circulation, the arterial side of the fetal circulation is the low pressure-low resistance circuit due to the runoff into the low-resistance placenta. Pulmonary vascular resistance greatly exceeds systemic vascular resistance until the first breath is taken and the umbilical cord is clamped. These two actions cause a simultaneous decrease in PVR and an increase in systemic vascular resistance. As the arterial PO_2 rises, PVR falls further, and left-to-right (aortic-to-pulmonary arterial) shunting may oc-

cur across the still-patent ductus arteriosus. With further increases in PO_2, the ductus begins to close and systemic vascular resistance rises, effectively closing the foramen ovale by increasing the left atrial pressure. Pulmonary vascular resistance continues to fall over a period of approximately 7 days, but normal values for PVR may not be achieved for several weeks after birth, as the pulmonary vessels thin out and become more compliant.[4,5]

The Transitional Circulation

A healthy full-term newborn has successfully made the transition from intrauterine life, when the placenta is the organ of gas exchange and the lungs are filled with amniotic fluid, to extrauterine life, when the lungs receive the entire output from the right ventricle and perform gas exchange. This change, although necessarily sudden at birth, is neither functionally nor anatomically permanent until at least several days after birth. The pulmonary vasculature is very reactive to many stimuli, and PVR may increase dramatically in response to hypoxemia, acidemia, hypercarbia, hypoglycemia, anemia, polycythemia, sepsis, and hypothermia.[6] Even in a healthy newborn, PVR is higher than it is in adults and only gradually decreases during the first few months of life, but may not reach adult levels for several years.[7]

The transitional nature of the circulation in neonates is important to the anesthesiologist. If, during anesthesia, a baby develops hypoxemia, hypercarbia, or acidemia, and PVR increases with a resultant decrease in pulmonary blood flow, gas exchange will worsen and a downward spiral may occur, with blood flow returning to a pattern similar to that seen during fetal life. The foramen ovale will open, as will the patent ductus arteriosus (PDA), and pulmonary blood flow will markedly diminish; however, now there is no placenta. This condition, variously called *persistent fetal circulation* (PFC) or *persistent pulmonary hypertension of the newborn*,[8,9] is very difficult to treat, often requiring systemic catecholamine infusions as well as infusions of pulmonary vasodilators, along with vigorous efforts to correct the precipitating factor(s) (ie, hypoxemia, hypercarbia, acidemia). It is much better to prevent this syndrome with careful attention to arterial blood gases, pH, and patient temperature, as well as careful administration of adequate anesthesia to blunt the increased sympathetic tone associated with surgical stress. Persistent fetal circulation may be associated with infection, polycythemia, diaphragmatic hernia, hypoglycemia, hypocalcemia, meconium aspiration, fetal asphyxia, or central nervous system (CNS) abnormalities. There is, however, an idiopathic form with no apparent cause. Differentiation of PFC from congenital heart disease may be quite difficult without the use of echocardiography and, in some cases, cardiac catheterization and cineangiography.

Neonatal Hepatic Function

Neonatal hepatic function is, for all practical purposes, intact at birth. The capacity of the neonate's liver to metabolize bilirubin, however, is almost equal to the normal load of hemoglobin presented. The result is that any stress that may impede metabolism or increase hemolysis may exceed the liver's capacity to conjugate bilirubin, with resultant hyperbilirubinemia. The glucuronyl transferase system requires a period of 6 to 7 days to reach full functional capacity. Elevated levels of unconjugated bilirubin may result in bilirubin encephalopathy (kernicterus). When bound to albumin, unconjugated bilirubin tends not to enter the CNS; therefore, any condition that increases the presence of unbound bilirubin increases the possibility of permanent brain damage from kernicterus. Those conditions most commonly seen and most preventable are hypoalbuminemia, acidosis, hypoglycemia, hypoxia, hypothermia, and competition for or displacement from albumin binding sites by drugs such as sulfisoxazole and salicylates. Less preventable are sepsis and hemolysis.

Vitamin K_1 is usually given to newborn infants in the United States to prevent hemorrhagic disease. The synthesis of coagulation factors II, VI, IX, and XI is dependent on the presence of vitamin K_1, of which the newborn may be deficient. Therefore, vitamin K_1 (0.5 to 1.0 mg IM or SC) should be given prior to surgery during the newborn period, especially if the child has never been fed. Carbohydrate, fat, protein, and drug metabolism are less influenced by hepatic immaturity, but may become important during periods of stress[10] (see the section *Hypoglycemia*).

Neonatal Renal Function

The neonatal kidney is functionally suited for antenatal life and shares responsibility with the placenta and the mother's kidneys for removal of metabolites. After birth there is a period of maturation when the kidney assumes greater functional capacity and growth by the increased workload. Glomerular filtration rate doubles soon after birth, continues to rise, and quadruples when fully mature. Unlike the liver, the period of renal maturation is much longer. However, by the age of 1 year, it is nearly complete; it reaches its peak capacity at 2 to 3 years, then begins to decline.[11] Traditionally, the neonatal kidney has been

thought to be unable to excrete sodium loads or to concentrate urine to a significant degree. More recently, this theory has been modified to state that because of the higher extracellular fluid volume in the neonatal period and reduced solute loads, eg, urea and sodium, the neonatal kidney *appears* not to concentrate.[12,13] For the normal neonate, unstressed and not undergoing surgery, the large extracellular fluid volume provides the necessary electrolytes to maintain normal serum sodium concentrations in the first week of life, while the excess extracellular fluid is passed as dilute urine. It is for this reason that salt-free fluids are frequently given to the newborn. However, the neonatal surgical candidate may translocate fluids the same as any other patient and needs electrolyte replacement. Therefore, salt-containing fluids should be given and electrolytes regularly measured.

Fluid, Electrolyte, and Caloric Requirements

Maintenance requirements for fluids and calories are summarized in Table 19-1. Sodium, potassium and chloride requirements are all similar to adults at 1 to 3 mEq/kg/24 h. It must be stressed that these are accepted maintenance requirements and should be used only as a guideline. Adjustments should be made for third space losses, the presence of congestive heart failure, existing deficits, changes in insensible losses, and drainage losses during surgery. Babies under phototherapy for hyperbilirubinemia or under infrared warmers for temperature maintenance may have as much as a 20 percent increase in fluid requirements because of increased evaporative losses.[14]

Glucose requirements are 2 to 6 mg/kg/min under normal circumstances, and may be reduced under anesthesia. The basic glucose requirement is fulfilled by using 5 percent dextrose in H_2O, but higher concentrations of glucose may be needed. Caution must be exercised in conditions in which large volumes of fluid are administered (eg, replacement of intraoperative volume loss) not to administer an excess of glucose, since hyperosmolarity will result. Hyperosmolarity secondary to hyperglycemia or hypernatremia may play a part in the pathogenesis of intraventricular hemorrhage in neonates.[15,16] It cannot be overemphasized that premature infants, term newborns, and infants undergoing major thoracic procedures need careful monitoring of glucose, sodium, potassium, and calcium, as well as monitoring of their blood pressure, heart rate, and blood gases. The administration of hypotonic fluids in excess of maintenance volumes (eg, 5 percent dextrose in 0.225 percent saline) may result in significant hyponatremia and should be avoided.[17]

Airway Anatomy

Anatomically, the child, and especially the infant, is different enough from the adult to make intubation more difficult (Table 19-2 and Fig. 19-1). The head is larger in proportion to the rest of the body, sometimes making it less stable; however, this disparity, particularly of the occiput, can be used to advantage during intubation by affording a natural "sniffing" position. In a normal newborn infant, the neck is short in comparison to the adult. The tongue, like the head, is relatively larger in children than in adults, and may cause obstruction during induction and ventilation by mask. The larynx is more cephalad in the child, lying approximately at the level of C_{2-3} as compared with C_5 in adults. It is not, however, more anterior, although it may seem so due to its cephalad placement and the large tongue. Beyond the larynx, the trachea to carina distance is only 4 cm in the infant. Extreme caution must be taken in passing the endotracheal tube past the cords by only 1.5 to 2.0 cm to avoid bronchial intubation. The epiglottis projects cephalad at approximately 45 degrees from the anterior wall of the larynx. This often makes the epiglottis easier to visualize, but more difficult to displace to allow intubation. Finally, the air passages themselves, the nose, nasopharynx, and trachea, must be considered. Being small, but not out of proportion to the infant, they may be easily obstructed, due to, for example, mucus, edema, nasogastric tubes, tape, or endotracheal tubes. Care to prevent inadvertent obstruction must be exercised at all times.

When placement of a nasotracheal tube is planned, it may be advantageous to initially secure the airway with an oral endotracheal tube. It is better to discover that the endotracheal tube size is incorrect after oral placement than to be faced with replacing a nasotracheal tube. Additionally, since nasotracheal intubation is technically more difficult in infants and children than in adults due to anatomic considerations, having an oral endotracheal tube for ventilation and oxygenation allows for careful passage of the nasotracheal tube. The nasal tube is positioned near the glottis with McGill forceps; an assistant can then remove the oral endotracheal tube, and the trachea can be intubated with the nasal tube.

The Premature Infant

Infants of 37 weeks' gestation or less are classified as premature. These infants have not had the time to fully develop and all organ systems are immature and, therefore, not as ready for extrauterine life. Additionally, since premature infants are even smaller (sometimes much smaller) than full-term infants, access to them is very limited once draping and positioning have occurred. For this reason, the endotracheal tube, vascular catheters, and all monitors must be carefully secured before surgery begins. In addition to gestational age, newborns may be classified according to birth weight for a given gestational age (ie, appropriate, large, or small for gestational age). This is especially important for small for gestational age (SGA) premature infants. Since SGA infants are usually subject to extraordinary stress during gestation, liver glycogen stores, iron stores, and muscle mass will be less than for other premature infants of the same gestational age. Often, pulmonary development is accelerated in SGA infants, so that the degree of respiratory distress they exhibit is less than expected. Morbidity and mortality figures increase dramatically in neonates weighing less than 2,000 g and of less than 37 weeks' gestation.[18] Reducing these figures and providing a better quality of life for those who survive are the aims of the neonatal intensivists and others, including anesthesiologists caring for these infants. Consequently, the appearance of "prematures" in the

---

TABLE 19-2.   Unique Features of Infant Airway Anatomy

1. Relatively large head (occiput more prominent).
2. Short neck.
3. Relatively large tongue.
4. Small nares easily obstructed by secretions. Infants are obligate nose breathers until approximately 2 months of age and will not open mouth to breathe even if nares are totally obstructed for any reason (eg, secretions, edema, choanal atresia).
5. The infant's larynx is located more cephalad than that of the older child or adult. At term, the larynx has descended somewhat so that the lower border of the cricoid cartilage is located opposite the middle of C_6. In the adult, the lower border of the cricoid cartilage lies opposite the lower border of C_6.
6. Narrowest portion of the infant's airway is the subglottic area at the level of the cricoid cartilage. Edema at that level greatly diminishes the cross-sectional diameter of the airway and can result in stridor or varying degrees of airway obstruction.
7. Epiglottis is relatively long and usually rather stiff. It is omega-shaped and extends from the base of the tongue at 45 degrees posterior and cephalad.
8. Trachea is short (approximately 4 cm); thus, carina is more cephalad, making endobronchial intubation more likely if careful placement of endotracheal tube is not carried out. In adults, carina is at level of T_5; in infants, carina is at level of T_3.
9. The angles formed by the main bronchi with the trachea vary considerably in infants: 10–35 degrees on the right and 30–50 degrees on the left.
10. Thorax is relatively small; sternum soft, ribs are horizontally placed; diaphragms relatively high; accessory muscles of respiration weak.

ANATOMY

HEAD SIZE

SHORT NECK

LARGE TONGUE

LARYNX — C2-4 (ADULT C5)

        — NOT MORE ANTERIOR

LARYNX TO CARINA DISTANCE 4 cm VS. "12 – 15"

EPIGLOTTIS—45°∠   FROM ANTERIOR WALL — MORE VERTICAL

SMALL AIRWAYS

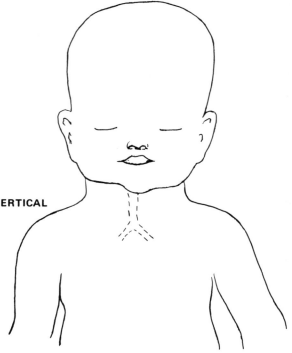

Fig. 19-1. Infant airway anatomy.

operating rooms has become more commonplace and requires anesthetic expertise that gives consideration to their unique problems.

Respiratory Distress Syndrome

Until the advent of continuous positive airway pressure (CPAP), premature infants most frequently succumbed to hyaline membrane disease or respiratory distress syndrome (RDS) of the newborn. Advances in neonatal respiratory care and equipment have reduced the deaths from RDS; however, other causes of death, such as intraventricular hemorrhage, necrotizing enterocolitis, and sepsis, have increased due to the longer survival of premature infants. Respiratory distress syndrome is a disease of atelectasis based on the deficiency of surfactant normally secreted by the type II alveolar cells. Surfactant acts to reduce surface tension in the alveolus, allowing for expansion during respiration.

Infants born prematurely have pulmonary disease resulting from both a decreased amount of and immature form of surfactant. As a result of this lack of surfactant, surface tension in the alveoli is increased, which leads to widespread atelectasis. This decrease or loss of functional residual capacity (FRC) is the important pathophysiologic problem in RDS. The FRC can be partially re-established with the applica-

tion of end-expiratory pressure (the end-expiratory grunting done by infants with mild RDS is a form of self-administered positive end-expiratory pressure [PEEP]). For cases of more severe RDS, CPAP and mechanical ventilation with PEEP and increased F_1O_2 are used as treatments. It is important to continue mechanical ventilation in the operating room in the same manner as was being done in the intensive care nursery. Ventilators on anesthesia machines may not be flexible enough to accomplish this, so that it may be necessary for the infant's own ventilator to be brought into the operating room. Of course, if these infants are to undergo a thoracic procedure, the inspired oxygen concentration, as well as some ventilator parameters, may require adjustment to maintain optimal gas exchange (Fig. 19-2).

Retrolental Fibroplasia or Retinopathy of Prematurity

Oxygen sensitivity is another unique feature of the premature newborn and is a consideration until they reach 40 to 44 weeks' gestational age. Unlike adult RDS patients, the usual neonate with RDS is premature and subject to retrolental fibroplasia if the retinal arteries are exposed to high partial pressures of oxygen. The degree of damage is mostly influenced by the maturity and vascularization of the retina itself when

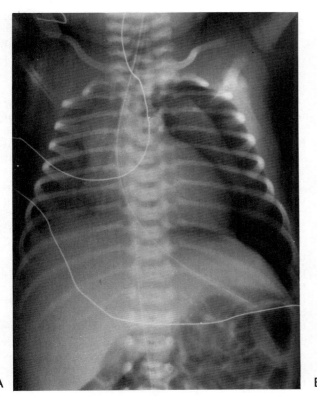 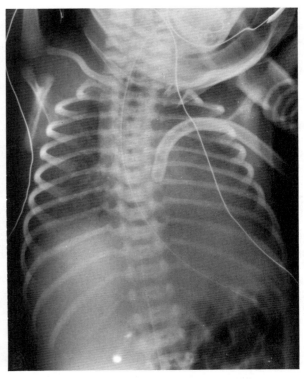

Fig. 19-2. Newborn premature infant with RDS and tension pneumothorax. **(A)** Pretreatment chest radiograph shows collapse of left lung with shift of heart and mediastinum to right. Note also widening of intercostal spaces on the left and depression of left hemidiaphragm. **(B)** Repeat film following insertion of thoracotomy tube shows re-expansion of left lung and return of mediastinal structures to normal position.

the hyperoxygenation takes place.[19-21] The anesthesiologist's responsibility is to maintain the PO_2 of the arterial blood between 60 to 80 mmHg, if possible. Use of nitrous oxide as a diluting gas or an air/oxygen blender is recommended. Arterial blood gases and pulse oximetry are necessary, and oxygen tension should be measured frequently during surgery, especially during thoracic procedures, to ensure adequate oxygenation, but not hyperoxia. There appear to be multiple risk factors in the development of retrolental fibroplasia, of which oxygen is only one.[21] While every attempt should be made to avoid administering more oxygen than is needed to maintain adequate PO_2 levels, it must be remembered that hypoxia which may lead to encephalopathy or even death is far more dangerous than hyperoxia that may contribute to retinopathy of prematurity.[22]

Postanesthetic Apnea

Premature and ex-premature infants who undergo surgery and anesthesia are at risk for postanesthetic apnea. This problem was noted initially in premature infants[23-25]; however, as it was studied further, older and older ex-premature infants were found to exhibit postanesthetic apnea as well.[26,27] *Postconceptual age,* which is the sum of gestastional age and postnatal age, is the term used by most investigators when grouping infants chronologically in studies involving postanesthetic apnea. Although it is not entirely consistent, most investigators define apnea in these babies as cessation of respiratory effort (not obstruction) at end-exhalation for 15 seconds or longer. Although 15 seconds of apnea in an infant may be associated with changes in color or vital signs, these are not included in the definition.

At this institution, all ex-premature infants considered at risk for postanesthetic apnea are monitored for at least 12 hours postoperatively. If postanesthetic apnea occurs, monitoring is continued until there have been 12 continuous hours without apnea. Kurth et al, in a prospective study of 47 preterm infants (preterm defined as a gestational age of 37 weeks or less), found that the incidence of postanesthetic apnea was inversely correlated with postconceptual age and even occurred in infants between 55 to 60 weeks of postconceptual age.[28] Of note is that there were infants who developed postanesthetic apnea who had neither a history of preoperative apnea nor a preoperative pneumogram that showed apnea. In addition, some infants with postanesthetic apnea had normal breathing in the recovery room but became apneic several hours later.

Since most neonates or ex-premature infants who are younger than 60 weeks' postconceptual age and undergo thoracic surgical procedures will be monitored in an intensive care unit after operation, this problem is unlikely to go unnoticed or untreated. Nevertheless, when postoperative apnea occurs, it is important to recognize it and not to overreact with reintubation and excessive increases in F_iO_2. Therefore, an awareness of this problem and familiarity with its epidemiology is very helpful in the postoperative care of all neonates and ex-premature infants.

There are many possible causes for this potentially fatal postoperative event. Halogenated inhalational agents depress the respiratory response to hypoxia, and hypercarbia and narcotics alter the CO_2 response curve. Endorphins have been found to cause apnea in infants, and these may be elevated postoperatively.[29] The cause of apnea of prematurity (independent of any exposure to anesthetic agents or narcotics) is still far from clear. Although there is substantial evidence for "central immaturity," it seems likely that general anesthetic agents and narcotics could easily augment this "central immaturity" with apnea as the result.

Although there have been reports suggesting the use of various mechanical devices or respiratory stimulants (caffeine, theophylline, doxapram) to treat the apnea of prematurity as well as postanesthetic apnea, and there appears to be some promise that at-risk infants given only regional anesthesia do not develop apnea, the most prudent course currently is careful postoperative monitoring of infants at risk until 12 hours without apnea have elapsed.[30–34] The catastrophic result if an unmonitored infant fails to be roused from an apneic spell should always be borne in mind.

Hypoglycemia

The occurrence of hypoglycemia in the newborn period is quite common. In SGA infants, it is the most common form of morbidity, approaching 67 percent.[35,36] Lower values of blood sugar are accepted as normal in infants, and hypoglycemia is defined as a blood sugar of less than 30 mg/dL during the first 72 hours of life, and less than 40 mg/dL after 72 hours. In low-birth-weight infants, ie, term infants less than 2,500 g, hypoglycemia is defined as a blood sugar of less than 20 mg/dL.

Prior to delivery, both the fetal and the maternal pancreas regulate the blood sugar with some degree of placental crossover. At birth, the interruption of this interdependence may manifest itself as a delayed assumption of normal glucose metabolism in the newborn. The most common example is that of the infant of a diabetic mother. Fetal insulin production is quite high, in an attempt to make up for maternal hypoinsulinism and hyperglycemia. At birth, insulin output is still quite high, or at least the response to increases in blood sugar is greater than normal, resulting in severe hypoglycemia.

Other conditions that contribute to the incidence of hypoglycemia in the newborn period are perinatal distress of any kind, toxemia, twinning, erythroblastosis fetalis, sepsis, asphyxia, CNS defects, hypothermia, hypocalcemia, congenital heart disease, maternal medications, endocrine deficiency (hypothyroidism), adrenal hemorrhage, polycythemia, hyperbilirubinemia, and abrupt withdrawal of glucose. The history of any of these conditions should make the anesthesiologist aware of the possibility of hypoglycemia and the need to determine blood glucose levels in the perioperative period. Normal sugar requirements for prematures and other newborns are 2 to 6 mg/kg/min, and may need to be considerably higher under stressful conditions to prevent hypoglycemia. If hypoglycemia is present prior to anesthesia, the occurrence of hyperglycemia and the dangers of hyperosmolarity must be prevented once the child is anesthetized, since anesthesia may reduce glucose requirements. It may become necessary to stop glucose therapy during anesthesia or change to solutions of lower glucose concentration.

Hypocalcemia

While hypocalcemia may be seen in all newborns, it is most prevalent in stressed infants and prematures. Usually hypocalcemia, defined as less than 7 mg/dL, presents as the jitters or a high-pitched cry, but may present with frank tetany. Since it is frequently seen with hypoglycemia, the first sign may be a convulsion. Hypocalcemia occurs most commonly in prematurity, infants of diabetic mothers, sepsis, asphyxiated infants, and infants with RDS. As with hypoglycemia, awareness on the part of the anesthesiologist should be the rule, and treatment should be available. An appropriately rapid infusion of 10 mg/kg of calcium chloride or 30 mg/kg of calcium gluconate is usually effective in reversing tetany. Maintenance therapy should start at 250 mg/kg/24 h of calcium chloride or 750 mg/kg/24 h of calcium gluconate. Signs of hypoglycemia and hypocalcemia may be masked during anesthesia when muscle relaxants are used with artificial ventilation.

Neonatal hypocalcemia is related to low parathyroid hormone activity and decreased stores of available calcium.[37] Parathyroid hormone activity is normal after approximately 3 days in the term infant, but may not be normal for up to several weeks in the premature.[38,39]

Thermoregulation

Hypothermia in the newborn and small child undergoing surgery continues to be a problem, particularly in major surgery of the chest in which a large surface area is exposed to the air, allowing high evaporative and convective heat loss. Both anesthesiologist and surgeon should attempt to *prevent* the heat loss rather than try to correct it after it occurs. The consequences of unintentional hypothermia in the newborn have been reported since 1900, when Budin reported 90 percent mortality in newborns whose temperatures were allowed to fall to 32°C.[40] It has been shown that not only the degree of hypothermia, but the frequency of deviation from normothermia, even without extreme temperature changes, contribute significantly to morbidity and mortality in the newborn period.[41] It is, therefore, the responsibility of those caring for the premature infant and newborn undergoing surgery to prevent unintentional hypothermia, which results in acidosis and cardiovascular depression, and to minimize fluctuations of temperature. Thermoneutrality is a delicate balance between heat production and heat conservation. The newborn and small child have a limited ability to produce heat, mostly through the metabolism of brown fat. Premature infants have reduced stores of brown fat. To maintain thermoneutrality, the premature infant, newborn, and small child must depend heavily on heat conservation. Because of a higher alveolar ventilation, the rate of heat lost to unheated, dry anesthetic gases by an infant is greater than that of an adult, and the development of hypothermia may be quite rapid. Anesthesia ablates the body's response to cold stress, making heat conservation in the operating room essential if the morbidity of hypothermia is to be avoided. Accepted techniques include raising the ambient temperature of the operating room, warming and humidifying anesthetic gases, using only warm scrub and irrigating solutions, using swaddling and other insulation and protection from wetting, non-ionizing heat lamps, thermal mattresses, and warming of all intravenous fluids. The importance of using as many of these heat conservation methods as possible cannot be overemphasized if thermoneutrality is to be preserved. In children, oxy-

gen consumption has been shown to double in the immediate postoperative period if the child is allowed to emerge from anesthesia in a hypothermic state.[42] If respiratory function is even mildly depressed by narcotics, relaxants, or intrinsic disease, the child may not be able to meet oxygen demands and can deteriorate rapidly. If unintentional hypothermia does occur during surgery, it must be corrected prior to removal of respiratory support. Equally important is maintenance of temperature during transport to and from the operating room. Portable heated isolettes and open beds equipped with warming lights or radiant heaters are available for this purpose.

Stress Response of Neonates to Surgery

Until recently, it was believed that neonates neither perceived pain nor experienced suffering when subjected to noxious stimuli. Even today, the emotional aspects of pain perception (ie, suffering) cannot be understood in neonates, since their experiences cannot be comprehended. However, the neural structures necessary for processing proprioceptive information are present, and various measures of cortical function suggest that the sensory cortex is very active in neonates.[43,44] Whether or not the concept that neonates experience pain and, therefore, suffering is accepted, it is clear that noxious stimuli evoke a whole spectrum of responses in the newborn infant characterized as the stress response to surgery.

There are marked changes in cardiorespiratory variables.[45,46] Heart rate and blood pressure both increase during noxious procedures, such as circumcision or blood drawing, and can be blunted by the prior administration of local anesthesia.[47–49] During circumcisions, infants given local anesthesia do not show the decreased transcutaneous partial pressure of oxygen exhibited by neonates not given anesthesia or analgesia. Palmar sweating has been measured in neonates and has been correlated with the state of arousal; marked changes are noted during heelstick blood drawing.[50]

There is a growing body of knowledge regarding hormonal and metabolic responses of neonates to surgical stimulation.[51] In infants undergoing circumcision without anesthesia, as well as more stressful procedures with minimal anesthesia, marked increases in serum cortisol have been documented.[52] Both pre- and full-term infants have been studied by Anand et al, considering the hormonal and metabolic responses of neonates to surgical stress.[53] These investigators found marked alteration in levels of many hormones, as well as significant effects on metabolism that sometimes persisted for significant periods beyond the surgical procedure.[53–55] In neonates who had minimal anesthesia, there appeared to be increased protein breakdown. Clinically, a group of neonates who underwent surgery with fentanyl/O_2/N_2O anesthesia had significantly fewer postoperative complications than a similar group who underwent surgery with O_2/N_2O anesthesia.

These hormonal and metabolic derangements lasting for as long as several days after surgery in patients given only minimal anesthesia support the findings in some behavioral studies. Neonates who were given anesthesia for circumcision were more attentive to a variety of stimuli, were less irritable, and quieted themselves better when disturbed.

The CNS and structures required for long-term memory are well developed during the neonatal period; however, there is not yet firm evidence that neonates remember early painful experiences. However, given the strong evidence regarding the profound influence noxious stimuli have on the neonates' behavior, changes in cardiorespiratory function, and metabolic alterations, it seems incorrect to assume that neonates neither experience nor record painful events, since many of the responses to noxious stimuli

may be harmful and the responses can be blunted by carefully administered anesthesia. There are few, if any, indications to warrant a surgical procedure being performed on a neonate without adequate anesthesia.

PREOPERATIVE ASSESSMENT

All too often, the amount of preoperative information available to the anesthesiologist is inversely related to the severity of the disease being treated. The critically ill, cyanotic newborn may be transferred from another facility and must be evaluated quickly by the receiving physicians to establish a diagnosis. Investigative procedures such as radiographs, echocardiography, cardiac catheterization, and laboratory evaluation must be accomplished quickly so that lifesaving measures may be taken.

Evaluation of the cyanotic newborn infant poses special problems, since there are multiple causes resulting in arterial desaturation. Congenital heart defects must be considered, but other causes of hypox-

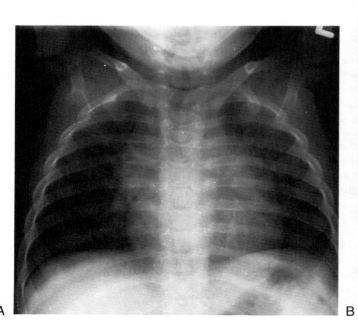
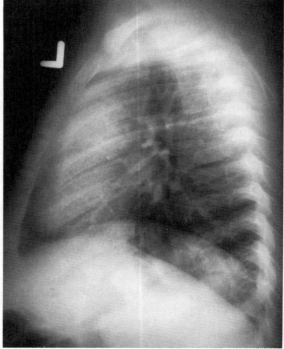

A   B

Fig. 19-3. (A) Normal infant's chest radiograph showing widening of mediastinum due to normal thymic shadow, horizontal ribs, and relatively high diaphragm. The buckling of the trachea toward the right is normal with expiration. **(B)** The lateral radiograph shows retrosternal fullness also due to normal thymic shadow.

emia include congenital diaphragmatic hernia, tracheoesophageal fistula with aspiration pneumonia, other forms of pneumonia, sepsis, pneumothorax, congenital pulmonary space-occupying defects, and upper airway obstruction[56] (Figs. 19-3 to 19-5).

Older children scheduled for elective thoracic operations are now rarely admitted more than 1 day in advance of surgery. Thus, consultations with pulmonologists, cardiologists, or other specialists may not be available until just before the operation (unless performed as an outpatient). It is of particular importance for the anesthesiologist to obtain a careful and thorough history and physical examination. Prior to elective thoracic procedures, the presence of upper respiratory infections, contagious childhood diseases, febrile episodes, or gastrointestinal symptoms are of special concern.

When dealing with congenital anomalies such as tracheoesophageal fistula or certain forms of congenital heart disease, the anesthesiologist should always be aware that other associated anomalies may be present.[57–59] Such defects should be discussed with the parents, and their expected influence on the immediate and late outcome of the proposed operation considered. Nutritional status should be evaluated by the history and the anesthesiologist's physical examination. The upper airway and mobility of the mandible and the cervical spine are examined. Pulmonary function may be evaluated by careful auscultation of the lungs, observation of the child's breathing pattern, and the results of arterial or capillary blood gases, the chest radiograph, and any indicated pulmonary function tests. The need for ventilatory support following thoracic operations can often be determined during the preoperative visit.

Cardiac function can be estimated from details in the history and physical examination recorded by the referring physician. The degree of compensation for congestive heart failure can be judged by the ability of the child to eat, presence of excessive sweating, and overall growth, especially in response to medical therapy. The extent and duration of cyanosis are usually proportional to the hematocrit, except when nutritional problems intervene to prevent compensatory

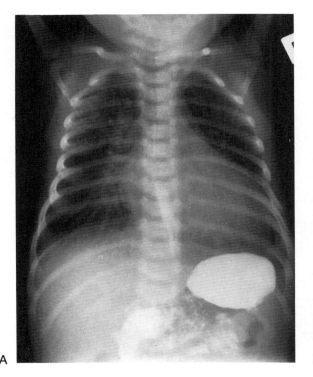
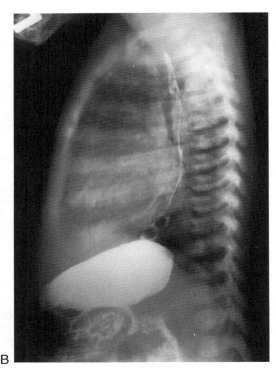

A B

Fig. 19-4. Six-week-old female infant with transposition of the great arteries and ventricular septal defect. **(A)** Chest radiograph showing large transverse cardiac silhouette with narrow base ("egg-on-a-string" configuration) related to superimposition of aorta and pulmonary artery shadows in the anteroposterior view, absence of thymic shadow, increased pulmonary blood flow, and mild interstitial pulmonary edema. **(B)** In lateral view, note increase in heart size.

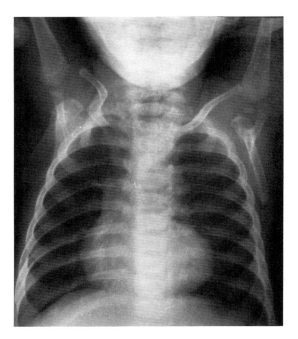

Fig. 19-5. Four-month-old male with tetralogy of Fallot. Anteroposterior chest radiograph shows ''boot-shaped heart'' (coeur en sabot) with upturned apex; concave pulmonary artery segment; decreased pulmonary vascular markings; and right aortic arch proven at catheterization.

polycythemia. The anesthesiologist's own examination of the precordium, peripheral pulses, perfusion, color, and general habitus of the patient will also be helpful. Hepatic and renal function may be affected by the presence or absence of cardiac dysfunction. Palpation of the liver edge and a careful review of significant laboratory data, including blood urea nitrogen, creatinine, and liver enzymes, may help elucidate the status of these organs.

Whenever possible, a patient's previous anesthetic history should be evaluated by noting the response during previous hospitalizations if surgery was performed, and by discussing the patient's past history with the parents. Important also is the determination of any family history suggesting problems associated with anesthesia, including such entities as malignant hyperthermia or pseudocholinesterase deficiency.

An understanding of the details of the planned surgical procedure is essential for the anesthesiologist caring for any patient. In thoracic operations, which are frequently complex, the information is best obtained by direct communication with the attending surgeon. It is also helpful to ascertain the status of the opposite lung in cases involving a thoracotomy. This information can frequently be obtained in discussions with the surgeons and other physicians involved in the care of the patient.

The preoperative visit by the anesthesiologist with the patient and the family is extremely important in the overall management of any operation, but especially for thoracic surgery. Besides obtaining the needed information concerning the patient, the anesthesiologist's preoperative visit is helpful in allowing the parents and patient to ask questions, to express fears and anxieties, and to understand more clearly what is planned. An explanation is given to the parents as to the plan for premedication drugs, induction techniques, expected time for surgery, and the need for intensive care unit or respiratory support postoperatively. A discussion of anticipated anesthetic risk with the parents (and patient, if appropriate) is necessary for informed consent. This should serve to reassure rather than frighten, as anesthetic risk is generally quite low, even for extensive procedures.

PREOPERATIVE ORDERS AND PREMEDICATION

It is unnecessary, and may indeed be harmful, to withhold oral feedings for long periods before operation. This is especially true in the young infant or the cyanotic, polycythemic child. Except in the very ill patient, gastric emptying time is sufficiently rapid to allow oral intake of glucose-containing clear liquids up to 2 hours prior to induction of anesthesia.[60–63] Breast-fed babies may be breast-fed, with the last feeding being completed 2 to 4 hours prior to induction, since the curd of breast milk is more quickly digested in the infant's stomach.[64] Newborn infants requiring surgery usually are not being fed due to the condition prompting the operation (eg, tracheoesophageal fistula, diaphragmatic hernia, cyanotic congenital heart defects), but will usually be nourished with parenteral glucose-containing fluids.

Steward states that premedication for children should be effective for the purpose (an adequate dose of appropriate drug(s), not a routine regimen, and as painless as possible)[65]; and that premedicants should be given to block unwanted autonomic reflex (vagal) responses, result in preoperative sedation and tranquility, and reduce general anesthetic requirements.[66] Certainly, all children do not require premedication. Traditionally, however, children above the age of 1 year presenting for thoracic surgery have commonly been given substantial sedation preoperatively, usually an orally administered sedative or tranquilizer and an injection of a narcotic-anticholinergic combination.[67–72] It is now common practice in many centers to use only oral premedication.[73–77] This method

TABLE 19-3.   Anesthetic Premedication

Medication	Dosage (mg/kg)	Route
Anticholinergics		
Atropine	0.01	IV, PO, IM
Scopolamine	0.005	IV, IM
Glycopyrrolate (Robinul)	0.005	IV, IM
Narcotics		
Morphine	0.1	IV, IM
Meperidine (Demerol)	2.0	PO
Hypnotics		
Pentobarbital (Nembutal)	1–2	PO, IV, IM
Thiopental (Pentothal)	10–15	PR
Methohexital (Brevital)	15–30	PR
Chloral hydrate	20–50	PO, PR
Tranquilizers		
Promethazine (Phenergan)	0.3	PO, IV, IM, PR
Hydroxyzine (Vistaril)	2.0	PO, IM
Diazepam (Valium)	0.1–0.3	PO, IV
Midazolam (Versed)	0.05–0.2	PO, IV, IM, PR
Droperidol (Inapsine)	0.05–0.1	IV, IM

has proven quite satisfactory (Tables 19-3 and 19-4). The anticholinergic agents are often omitted in patients with asthma or cystic fibrosis, or in those with a relatively fixed cardiac output (eg, aortic stenosis, pulmonary stenosis, or mitral stenosis) in whom a significant increase in heart rate is undesirable. The efficacy of newer agents and innovative routes of administration, such as rectal midazolam, intranasal sufentanil, and transmucosal fentanyl, remains to be determined.

Patients with certain forms of congenital heart disease may present unique premedication problems. Children with tetralogy of Fallot may experience intermittent hypercyanotic episodes ("spells") due to an increase in right ventricular outflow tract obstruction and an increase in the right to left shunt. These spells may be precipitated by agitation, anger, and trauma, or they may occur without any apparent cause. They are usually treated with morphine and oxygen, and by placing the infant or child in the knee-chest position, thus increasing venous return and arterial resistance, with resulting improvement in pulmonary blood flow. Morphine is theoretically a desirable premedicant drug for patients demonstrating these spells. Some patients with tetralogy of Fallot who experience hypercyanotic spells are given propranolol to ameliorate the severity and frequency of these dangerous episodes.[78–81] Propranolol has been effective in terminating the acute increase in outflow obstruction that may precipitate these attacks, and such patients may receive propranolol on a chronic basis. If these patients present as candidates for palliation or for thoracic

TABLE 19-4.   Oral Premedication Guidelines

I. The pharmacy prepares a mixture of meperidine and atropine in a palatable syrup:
  A. For patients older than 12 months:
      0.4 mL contains 3 mg meperidine and 0.02 mg atropine (1 mL contains 7.5 mg meperidine and 0.05 mg atropine)
      Dosage: 0.4 mL/kg (maximum volume, 14 mL)
  B. For patients younger than 12 months:
      Atropine alone may be used and is taken from the multiple-dose vial and given orally:
        0.02 mg/kg (0.04 mg/mL)

II. Pentobarbital may be useful as an added oral medication and administered in a dosage range of
    0–4 mg/kg pentobarbital (Nembutal)

III. Example of premedication regimen:
    20-kg 4-year-old presenting for pectus excavatum repair at 8:00 AM:
      1. May have clear liquids up until 4:00 AM.
      2. No oral food or liquids after 4:00 AM except for medications.
      3. Preoperative oral medication to be given at 7:00 AM: D-A (Demerol-atropine) mixture, 8 mL, and pentobarbital 40 mg

surgical procedures other than correction, it is preferable not to discontinue this drug prior to anesthesia if signs of excessive beta-blockade are absent. In addition, propranolol diluted to 0.1 mg/mL should be available. If a spell occurs, as evidenced by increasing cyanosis, developing acidosis, or the disappearance of the systolic ejection murmur indicating infundibular spasm, propranolol should be given intravenously (0.01 mg/kg up to a total dose of 1 mg). Alternatively, a bolus of the ultrashort-acting beta-blocker, esmolol, can be given (500 μg/kg/min over 1 minute, followed by an infusion, 100 μg/kg/min)[82,83] if the spell persists. Other methods of managing hypercyanotic episodes include the administration of morphine, an increase in F_IO_2 to 100 percent, volume expansion, and/or the administration of a pure alpha-adrenergic agonist to increase peripheral resistance.[84]

Atropine effectively blocks the action of the cardiac vagus nerve and may obviate the fall in cardiac output seen with induction doses of the potent anesthetic agents halothane and isoflurane.[66,85,86] Atropine probably should always be administered prior to the administration of succinylcholine, even in patients with asthma or cystic fibrosis, and to patients who receive ketamine for induction of anesthesia. It probably should not be given to children who have a history of a recent significant elevation of body temperature. In patients undergoing insertion of permanent pacemakers, atropine may theoretically cloud the issue of pacemaker capture if the heart rate is faster than the desired rate of the pacemaker being inserted. However, this is not usually a problem, since most pacemakers used in children are placed to treat congenital complete heart block, which does not respond to atropine.

ANESTHETIC MANAGEMENT

In general, the pathologic condition prompting the need for surgery, as well as the physical status of the patient, determine the choice of the anesthetic technique to be used. Infants and children requiring thoracic operations may be American Society of Anesthesiologists (ASA) physical status I or II (eg, an asymptomatic patent ductus arteriosus), but more often than not, young patients for thoracic operations will be ASA physical status III or IV. Sicker patients will usually come to the operating room with intravenous catheters and monitoring devices in place. This often facilitates the induction of anesthesia, since the administration of narcotics and muscle relaxants can be titrated to the desired effect.

If no direct monitoring devices are in place, the es-

sential monitoring instruments are applied before induction is begun. These include the following:

1. The precordial stethoscope applied so that both heart sounds and breath sounds are audible
2. A blood pressure cuff (usually either a Doppler-principle device [Arteriosonde or Infrasonde] or oscillometric type [Dinemapp]
3. The oscillographic display of the ECG
4. A pulse oximeter

Induction of anesthesia is then begun by one of several methods, depending on the overall anesthetic plan and the condition being treated.

Induction Techniques

In the very sick patient, preoxygenation is desirable before any drugs are administered. If the presence of the mask is disturbing to the child, holding the mask a few inches above the face between cupped hands and giving a high flow of oxygen from the anesthesia machine will suffice. If no intravenous catheter is established, a large-bore cannula can be inserted during preoxygenation after appropriate local anesthesia of the skin. An alternative method of intravenous induction, especially useful in older healthier children, is to give induction medications (usually thiopental and atropine) via a very small-bore needle (27 gauge) followed by succinylcholine (from a separate non-Leur-Lok syringe). This needle is removed after induction is complete and the trachea intubated; a large-bore intravenous catheter is then inserted when the patient is asleep.

Thiopental, in standard induction doses, is rarely used in patients classified ASA IV because of its direct depressant effect on the heart. Rather, small doses (1 mg/kg) may be added to a narcotic, such as fentanyl, and/or a benzodiazepine, and titrated to loss of the lid reflex.

For either cyanotic or acyanotic patients who are stable hemodynamically, an inhalation induction with halothane is often used. The gradual addition of increasing concentrations of volatile agent to a mixture of nitrous oxide and oxygen provides a smooth, safe induction, even in patients with cyanotic congenital cardiac malformations. It is apparent that the depression of cardiac output induced by the volatile anesthetic must be coupled with a reduction in oxygen consumption, since further arterial desaturation is rare.[87] Furthermore, this mild myocardial depression may be especially beneficial in patients with the physiology of tetralogy of Fallot by preventing catecholamine-induced outflow tract obstruction and a subsequent hypercyanotic spell. Duration of the induction period is not obviously prolonged in cyanotic patients despite the reduced pulmonary blood flow. These patients must have careful blood pressure monitoring during induction because an overdose of volatile anesthetic with severe myocardial depression, reduced cardiac output, and worsening cyanosis is difficult to reverse due to the impaired pulmonary perfusion and limited elimination of the anesthetic. After the patient is asleep, intravenous catheters are inserted, muscle relaxants administered, and the volatile agent reduced to a maintenance level. Other adjuvant drugs are also given and further monitoring established.

For the unstable or severely cyanotic patient, ketamine, given either intramuscularly (up to 5 mg/kg) or intravenously (1 to 2 mg/kg) may be selected for induction of anesthesia. The theoretic disadvantage of ketamine is its sympathomimetic action, which produces increases in heart rate, systemic blood pressure, and oxygen consumption. In patients with tetralogy of Fallot, ketamine might also increase the right-to-left shunt by precipitating infundibular spasm. In addition, ketamine produces dose-related myocardial depression in isolated heart preparations.[88,89] However, if the sympathetic nervous system is intact or only slightly depressed, the hemodynamic effects of a ketamine induction result in no deterioration in arterial oxygen saturation even with a severe tetralogy.[90,91] There should be a beta-adrenergic blocking drug available to treat a hypercyanotic spell should it occur during induction of ketamine anesthesia. These spells happen much more frequently during manipulation of the heart than during any anesthetic induction technique, and probably result from changes in venous return, resulting in relative or actual hypovolemia.

Monitoring During Thoracic Operations

The monitoring selected by the anesthesiologist depends on several factors: (1) the physical status of the patient, (2) the operation anticipated, and (3) the expected postoperative course. Even the simplest operation in the very sick infant or child may warrant extensive monitoring. Many children undergoing thoracic surgery require accurate and reliable monitoring in the operating room and intensive care unit.

No matter how many physiologic parameters are measured, no monitoring scheme is infallible. Correct interpretation by the anesthesiologist of the data provided is essential. Each additional monitoring technique must be evaluated from the standpoint of (1) its ease of application, (2) the risk/benefit ratio, and (3) the cost/benefit ratio.[92]

Even the most sophisticated monitoring systems available today fail to tell what is really necessary to know: the presence of pain, the accurate assessment of regional perfusion, and the metabolic changes occurring within the cell.[93] The anesthesiologist is the "ultimate" monitor; the instruments used, either simple or complex, are only data-collecting devices that enable the anesthesiologist to receive, process, and assimilate data, and to respond appropriately.

Table 19-5 lists the monitoring devices that should be considered for use in patients undergoing thoracic operations. Such an outline is useful for monitoring most patients, but additional measurements may be indicated in specific patients.

TABLE 19-5. Monitoring of the Pediatric Thoracic Surgical Patient

1. Preinduction
   a. Precordial stethoscope
   b. Blood pressure cuff (usually Dinemapp)
   c. ECG
   d. Nerve stimulator
   e. Temperature (usually axillary probe or cutaneous strip)
   f. Pulse oximeter

2. Postinduction, prior to start of operation
   a. Intra-arterial catheter[a]
   b. Central venous pressure catheter[b]
   c. Urinary bladder catheter
   d. Rectal temperature thermistor probe (or esophageal or nasopharyngeal)[c]
   e. Esophageal stethoscope (often with temperature thermistor incorporated)
   f. Nerve stimulator (determine twitch, tetanus, and train-of-four responses before administering neuromuscular blocking agents)

3. Before closure of surgical incisions
   a. Pacing wires (atrial and/or ventricular)[d]
   b. Atrial pressure catheters (left and/or right)[d]
   c. Pulmonary artery catheters (for pressure measurement and administration of medications directly into the pulmonary circulation)[d]
   d. Pulmonary artery thermistor catheter (for cardiac output determination)[d]
   e. Pulmonary artery oximetric catheter (for mixed venous oxygen saturation determination)[d]

[a] Blood pressure cuffs and intra-arterial lines are placed on the contralateral side of a previous or proposed Blalock-Taussig shunt procedure or on the right side during repair of coarctation of the aorta.

[b] Usually the right internal jugular vein placed percutaneously or, rarely, via the external jugular vein using a J wire; occasionally via either antebrachial vein. The subclavian vein approached from the infraclavicular route may also be used.

[c] Esophageal stethoscopes and temperature probes should be avoided when possible during operations involving the esophagus. If used, the surgeon should always be informed of the presence of such devices.

[d] Used in selected patients.

Electrocardiography

The use of the ECG as a monitoring device in the operating room has been a relatively late development, coming during the early 1960s.[94,95] Leads should be placed to clearly demonstrate atrial depolarization (P wave), ventricular depolarization (QRS), and the repolarization complex (T wave), so that dysrhythmias arising from atrium or ventricle and changes in repolarization due to drug effect or electrolytes (K^+ or Ca^{++}) can be appreciated. Lead placement should also take into account the planned surgical field and patient position to avoid contamination or injury. While the ECG is a valuable source of information concerning the cardiovascular system, it must be remembered that it is only an electrical signal and gives no information as to the actual function of the heart.

The resting heart rate of the infant or child is normally more rapid than that of the adult. Therefore, the definitions of significant tachycardia and bradycardia are different.[96] In infants, a heart rate greater than 180 beats/min or less than 100 beats/min should be carefully evaluated.

Pulse Oximetry

In no field of surgical endeavor has pulse oximetry proven of greater value than in pediatric thoracic procedures. When an infant or child has a disease already compromising cardiac and/or pulmonary function and these structures are manipulated or retracted during the course of an operation, life-threatening arterial hypoxemia is a common occurrence. Previously, hypoxia-induced bradycardia was the earliest "on-line" monitor during procedures such as bronchoscopy, repair of diaphragmatic hernia, and aortopulmonary shunt creation. Now, a functioning pulse oximeter allows the surgeon, as well as the anesthesiologist, to appreciate any degree of hypoxemia.

Probe placement is critical. If severe coarctation or interruption of the arch is present, venous blood will perfuse the lower body (and perhaps the left arm) via the patent ductus arteriosus. In severely ill children, distal extremity perfusion may be inadequate to provide reliable oximeter data.[97,98] Loss or deterioration of a previously strong signal could be due to probe placement, but may also indicate diminished perfusion.

Capnometry

Monitoring of expired levels of carbon dioxide has also proven extremely valuable for the same reasons found for pulse oximetry.[99] Manipulation of intra-thoracic structures alters pulmonary compliance and ventilation-perfusion relationships, and can result in change in endotracheal tube position. Capnometry allows continuous adjustments in ventilation to be made in compensation. Neonates with pulmonary hypertension may require moderate hyperventilation to control the pulmonary vascular resistance and minimize right-to-left shunting via a persistent fetal-type circulation (see the section Congenital Diaphragmatic Hernia). Intermittent sampling of arterial blood gases may provide an acceptable level of monitoring for such patients in a relatively static setting, such as the intensive care unit, but, during thoracic surgery, a continuous monitor of ventilation is preferred.

Capnometry also provides information regarding quantity of pulmonary blood flow in children with right-to-left shunts. If right-to-left shunting is extreme (or a newly created aortopulmonary shunt inadequate), a large discrepancy exists between the normal or elevated arterial carbon dioxide and a low end-expiratory value. Appropriate interventions to reduce the extent of shunting will narrow this gap.

Arterial Blood Pressure

The systemic arterial pressure is determined by blood volume, cardiac output, peripheral resistance, elasticity of the arterial wall, proximal patency of the artery, and the characteristics of the recording system. Systemic arterial pressure and organ perfusion are related through vascular resistance. Blood flow to any given organ may be adequate even when there is relative hypotension; conversely, organ flow may be inadequate when the blood pressure is normal or even elevated. Nevertheless, the accurate measurement and recording of systemic blood pressure, either directly or indirectly using oscillometric or Doppler devices, are important in assessing adequacy of cardiac function.

Most, but not all, thoracic operations require the insertion of intra-arterial catheters for direct pressure measurement. If intra-arterial pressure measurement is not considered necessary, an oscillometric system (eg, Dinamapp) can be used in cases in which blood pressure measurement is needed frequently throughout the surgery. The cuff should be placed on an extremity opposite that in which intravenous infusions are being given, since the time for inflations and deflations of the cuff interfere with fluid and drug administration. If intra-arterial monitoring is used, the cannula is placed in a location convenient to the anesthesiologist to allow frequent arterial blood sampling for measurements of blood gases, hematocrit, serum electrolytes, blood glucose, and other necessary parameters. The radial artery is usually selected for percutaneous catheterization just proximal to the volar carpal ligament. Stopcocks should not be used at the hub of the 22-gauge 1-in. plastic cannula. A T connector with a rubber diaphragm may be used instead of a stopcock to reduce the risk of inadvertent injection of air, frequent motion and arterial trauma produced by turning the stopcock handle, and bacterial contamination from the open end of the stopcock. The rubber diaphragm of the T connector can be used for sampling by puncturing it with a small-bore needle and allowing a few drops of blood to drip out to clear the cannula of flush solution. Little or no negative pressure need be applied to the syringe during sampling, since it will fill from the force of the intra-arterial pressure. Negative pressure tends to collapse the very small vessel and leads to thrombogenic trauma, spasm, and early loss of the monitoring catheter.

The indwelling arterial cannula is connected to a pressure transducer and the waveform displayed on an oscilloscope. The cannula should be continuously flushed with a solution of normal saline containing 1,000 U of heparin/100 mL of fluid at a rate of 2 mL/h. The arterial cannula, cannulation site, and T connector should be conspicuously labeled to avoid inadvertent injection of medications or air into the artery.

When the radial artery on either side is not patent or otherwise not available, alternative sites of cannulation must be considered. The left radial artery should not be used for monitoring during operations for repair of coarctation of the aorta or vascular rings, since the left subclavian artery will be clamped during the repair and the radial artery trace lost. When a Blalock-Taussig shunt operation has been or is being done, the radial artery on the ipsilateral side cannot be used, since the subclavian artery is used to construct the shunt. An alternative site is the axillary artery, cannulated either directly or using a modified Seldinger technique. This site is accessible to the anesthesiologist, comfortable for the patient, and provides excellent sampling and waveforms due to the large size of the artery. Excellent collateral circulation around the shoulder provides safety from vascular compromise. No neurologic damage to the brachial plexus has been found.[100] Careful flushing to avoid central arterial embolization, as with all arterial catheters, is advised. Superficial temporal artery cannulation is another alternative. Direct femoral arterial cannulation[101] may be necessary in cases in which radial and temporal arteries have already been used, but this is quite inconvenient since blood sampling must be done from the leg. Axillary arterial catheters are often utilized when radial or femoral catheters are not useable and their safety and practi-

cality have been demonstrated.[100,102] Umbilical arterial catheters are useful if present in the neonate undergoing an intrathoracic operation. However, in repair of a coarctation in the newborn infant with an umbilical arterial catheter in place, a second arterial catheter should probably be placed to measure pressures and oxygenation proximal to the narrowed aorta. Blood sampling for blood gases from an umbilical arterial catheter, in the presence of increased PVR and a patent ductus arteriosus, may be misleading. In this case, blood shunted right-to-left through the ductus will cause the PaO_2 below the ductus to be falsely low. Blood leaving the heart and perfusing the retinal arteries may have a dangerously high PaO_2, placing the susceptible patient at risk for retrolental fibroplasia.[103–106]

Central Venous Pressure

Central venous pressure (CVP) measurement is indicated when the volume status of the child is unstable or likely to change rapidly, as would be expected when massive blood or third space loss is anticipated. Catheters for monitoring CVP can be inserted percutaneously through the brachial vein in older children, and sometimes in younger ones undergoing thoracic operations. This relatively large-bore catheter also provides a useful route for the injection of irritating medications such as calcium, vasopressors, or blood products.

Central venous catheters can also be inserted via the external jugular veins in children. An 18-gauge, 1.25-in. intravenous catheter is introduced into an external jugular vein through which a J wire is passed and manipulated into the chest. The CVP catheter is then placed over the J wire and advanced into the central circulation. Percutaneous internal jugular vein catheterization can also be easily accomplished in pediatric patients having thoracic operations. A low incidence of complications is reported by advocates of this technique.[107–110] A high approach to the internal jugular vein is advisable in children to avoid the lung.[111] The subclavian vein may also be used via an infraclavicular approach for CVP catheter insertion.[112]

Extreme caution should be exercised in the care of centrally placed catheters and, indeed, all venous catheters in children with cyanotic congenital heart disease. Even very small air bubbles in any intravenous catheter, tubing, or connectors pose potentially lethal hazards due to the possibility of an air embolus to the brain, coronary arteries, or other vital organs. In the acyanotic child, air in the venous system may also reach the systemic circulation through either a patent foramen ovale, atrial or ventricular septal defect, or patent ductus arteriosus during coughing, a Valsalva maneuver, or positive-pressure ventilation.

Transthoracic right and left atrial catheters are used in lieu of CVP catheters in some cardiac surgical procedures not requiring cardiopulmonary bypass, and in most cases in which cardiopulmonary bypass is used. The catheters are passed through the chest wall, secured to the skin, and kept patent using a constant infusion of saline and heparin. When no longer needed, these catheters are withdrawn through the chest wall; surprisingly, the incidence of complications (bleeding, catheter entrapment, sepsis, thrombosis) is very low.

Temperature

The importance of monitoring and maintaining body temperature near normal in children during surgery and anesthesia is well documented.[113–122] Changes in body temperature during anesthesia may result from exposure to a cold environment, reaction to anesthetic drugs, infusion of cold intravenous fluids or blood, and vasoconstriction or vasodilation. Uncontrolled hypothermia in any patient is undesirable, but in the neonate and premature infant produces metabolic acidosis and myocardial and respiratory depression. Hyperthermia is also dangerous, since oxygen consumption significantly increases.[113,122] For this reason, significant hyperthermia is especially detrimental in patients with cyanotic forms of congenital heart disease.

Temperature should be monitored in every pediatric patient by use of a thermistor probe placed in the nasopharynx, or orally into the upper esophagus. During bronchoscopy or esophagoscopy, axillary or rectal temperature should be measured.

Urinary Output

Continuous monitoring of urine output during surgery is one of the most reliable signs of adequate hydration, blood volume, and cardiac output. Almost all patients undergoing cardiovascular surgery or other complex intrathoracic procedures should have a urinary bladder catheter placed for accurate timed measurements of urine volume and, at times, specific gravity and osmolarity. In short procedures, such as ligation of a patent ductus, urinary catheters are often safely omitted. The urethral meatus of the newborn or premature infant may be too small to accept even the smallest Foley catheter. If this is the case, a small infant feeding tube (8 Fr) can be inserted just beyond the point of first urine drainage, and fixed in place to the skin either with a suture or using benzoin and adhesive tape. Adequate urine production is considered to be 1 mL/kg body weight/h.[68,69,123–125]

Neuromuscular Blockade

Muscle relaxants are used as anesthetic adjuncts in many thoracic operations. Like other drugs, they should be administered in a safe and controlled manner. For neuromuscular blockade monitoring, two ECG electrodes are attached over the ulnar aspect of the wrist. Muscle twitch, tetanus, and train-of-four responses are determined prior to the administration of any muscle relaxants and checked periodically throughout the operation; additional muscle relaxants are given as needed based on frequently observed responses. If postoperative mechanical ventilation is not needed, nondepolarizing muscle relaxants are reversed at the end of operation and the blockade monitor used as one indicator of adequacy of reversal.

Arterial Blood Gases, Electrolytes, Hemoglobin, and Glucose

Blood obtained from the arterial cannula is periodically analyzed for blood gases, sodium, potassium, hemoglobin/hematocrit, glucose, and ionized calcium. No particular interval between these samples is recommended, the frequency being determined by the hemodynamic stability of the patient and, to some extent, by the experience of the anesthesiologist. It is important to make some or all of these determinations shortly after induction of anesthesia to determine acid-base status, adequacy of ventilation, and baseline serum electrolytes and glucose.

Assessment of Blood Loss

Accurate estimation of blood loss is difficult, at best; however, careful attention must be paid to this aspect of thoracic operations in patients of all ages, especially in the very young infant. This is best accomplished by the following:

1. Close observation of the operative field.
2. Careful monitoring of pulse rate, estimation of pulse volume, and frequent measurement of blood pressure. The systolic blood pressure is probably the most reliable indicator of blood volume in the infant.[126]
3. Weighing of all sponges and laps before they begin to dry out, and subtracting known dry weight from weight of bloody sponges or laps.
4. Measuring blood suctioned from the surgical field in low-volume graduated suction bottles easily visible or accessible to the anesthesiologist.

5. Keeping an accurate record of irrigation used in the surgical field to avoid confusion with actual blood loss on sponges or in suction containers.
6. Estimation of blood on drapes.

A running total of estimated blood loss should be recorded on the anesthesia record at appropriate intervals, and the final total as well as the amount replaced reported to the surgeon and to the nurse caring for the patient postoperatively.

Intubation of the Trachea

For children undergoing intrathoracic surgical procedures, the choice of nasal versus oral intubation is relatively easy. Any child who is expected to need postoperative ventilatory support may benefit from nasotracheal intubation. A nasotracheal tube may be placed initially in some patients, or an orotracheal tube may be replaced by a nasal tube after the surgical procedure is completed. Nasal tubes are easier to secure, tolerated better with less chewing and gagging, and the need for an uncomfortable oral airway is eliminated. If heparin is used during surgery, caution must be exercised during insertion of the nasotracheal tube to avoid bleeding from the nasal mucosa. Nasotracheal intubation should probably be deferred until heparin reversal has been given.

In preparation for intubation, all needed equipment should be tested and at hand. The low oxygen reserves of the premature newborn allow little time for intubation, and not enough for stopping to obtain equipment. The choice of laryngoscope blades depends on personal preference. Anatomic considerations, ie, the short neck and bulky tongue, make the use of straight blades generally more desirable in the newborn and small child. Most premature and SGA infants require a Miller 0 or Guedel 1 blade; the Miller 1 is more suitable for full-term infants. Beyond the age of 2 years, curved blades become an equally acceptable choice. In all cases, more than one size of blade should be on hand should the primary choice be unsuitable.

Choice of appropriate tube size and type should be based on the patient's age and size (Table 19-6). Other considerations, such as a previous recent intubation, history of prolonged intubation, or previous surgery, may modify the selection of the expected tube size. Cuffed tubes less than 5.0 mm internal diameter are not recommended, even though they are available. The presence of the cuff occupies vital space, increasing resistance and possibly hampering adequate ventilation. If prolonged intubation in older children is anticipated, the high-volume, low-pressure (Lanz-type) cuffs are recommended. The Cole type, or tapered tubes, are not recommended for long-term use in neonates. Double-lumen tubes are not available in pediatric sizes, but selective mainstem intubation and bronchial blockade using a Fogarty catheter have been used to achieve one-lung ventilation.[127]

Tradition has held that newborns should be intubated awake. This attitude is a carryover from the days of ether anesthesia and should be modified to accommodate today's anesthetic techniques. There are surgical indications for awake intubation without relaxation or assisted ventilation, eg, tracheoesophageal fistula, where gas introduced under pressure may pass from the trachea into the distal esophagus and distend the stomach; in addition, there are airway indications in which muscle relaxants are relatively contraindicated, eg, severe Pierre-Robin syndrome,

---

TABLE 19-6. Selection of Endotracheal Tubes

A. Guidelines for selection of endotracheal tube, measured in millimeters of internal diameter:

Premature or small for gestation age	2.5–3.0 mm
Normal term newborn	3.5 mm
6 mo to 2 yr	4.0–4.5 mm
Greater than 2 yr	$\dfrac{\text{age (yr)} + 18}{4}$

B. Guidelines for proper depth of insertion of endotracheal tubes (approximate)

$$\frac{\text{age (yr)}}{2} + 12 = \text{cm depth of insertion at teeth}$$

or

	Oral	Nasal
Newborn	9.5 cm	Crown-heel length × 0.21 cm
6 mo	10.5–11 cm	Crown-heel length × 0.16 + 2.5 cm
>1 yr	age + 12 cm	Crown-heel length × 0.16 + 2.5 cm

when management of the airway may become difficult or impossible if muscle relaxants are used. Just as an awake intubation in an older child or adult would not be considered without some form of sedation (except in the "full stomach" situation), the use of small amounts of sedation is probably indicated before intubation in most children.

Preoxygenation plays a critical role in the safety of intubation in the infant and small child. These patients are already at a disadvantage by having increased oxygen demands (4 to 6 mL/kg/min) and proportionately less alveolar surface through which to absorb oxygen. Their alveolar ventilation is normally twice that of an adult. Thus, it is understandable why the time elapsed between loss of oxygen supply or alveolar ventilation and the onset of hypoxemia is very short. When other pathology exists, such as congestive heart failure, pneumonia, or respiratory distress of the newborn, borderline hypoxemia may already exist and can be dangerously exaggerated during intubation if preoxygenation is not used. Preoxygenation prior to intubation should be done in most children using 100 percent oxygen. An exception to this is in the premature infant who is at risk for developing retrolental fibroplasia in whom an oxygen concentration no more than 10 percent greater than that which is the therapeutic level prior to surgery should be used for preoxygenation.

Intubation technique should include the following points:

1. *Stabilize the head.* The prominent occiput and relatively large head size make the infant's head roll easily on the table. The use of a foam rubber "doughnut" or similar device is useful in stabilizing the head and placing the head in the sniffing position.
2. *Identify both esophagus and trachea.* The vocal apparatus of the newborn and small child does not resemble that of the adult. Care is required to avoid inadvertent esophageal intubation. The placement of a suction catheter or nasogastric tube into the esophagus may aid in identifying airway structures.
3. *Visually assess endotracheal tube passage beyond the cords.* The short distance (4 to 6 cm) between the vocal apparatus and carina makes accidental passage into the right or left mainstem bronchus relatively easy, but can be prevented by careful observation of the endotracheal tube as it is inserted. The formulas for depth of insertion shown in Table 19-6 are only guidelines. Immediate auscultation after intubation should be done to determine that breath sounds are equal bilaterally. Radiographic confirmation should be used when needed.

4. *Avoid excessive manipulation of the vocal cord structures.* Multiple attempts at intubation result in tissue edema and bleeding, both of which can complicate extubation. Of all the causes of postintubation croup, multiple attempts at intubation have been cited as some of the most important.[128] The small airways of the infant and small child are extremely susceptible to obstruction secondary to edema.
5. *Do not prolong attempts to intubate.* Infants and small children do not have the oxygen reserves present in older children and adults. Although the use of the pulse oximeter is very helpful during intubation, it should be kept in mind that an early sign of hypoxemia may be bradycardia. If oxygenation decreases significantly during intubation, or bradycardia occurs during attempts to intubate, the anesthesiologist should stop immediately, reoxygenate, and then proceed. Vagal stimulation may also decrease the heart rate and should be blocked with atropine (0.01 mg/kg IV). However, atropine should not be used to treat bradycardia under anesthesia unless hypoxemia has been ruled out as the cause.

Proper anchoring of the endotracheal tube is essential, since the patient may be virtually inaccessible during thoracic surgery. Nasal intubation requires anchoring that will prevent the in-and-out motion of the tube and avoid compression of the nares. Oral intubation requires both lateral stabilization and prevention of the in-and-out motion. Tincture of benzoin can be applied to the face and to the tube prior to taping, since saliva will dissolve most adhesives. If the patient will be positioned so that secretions will drain out of the mouth onto the endotracheal tube, a bite block made of an absorbent material may be placed in the mouth to prevent secretions from reaching the tape. Newborn infants have a waxy layer of material on the skin known as vernix caseosa. This material may interfere with adhesives (eg, tape, ECG, and grounding pads), and should be removed with mild soap or alcohol prior to surgery. After the endotracheal tube is well anchored, the stomach should be aspirated to remove any air or other material contents.

The complications of intubation in infants and children are the same as in adults. Hypoxia is the most common, followed by soft tissue damage and tooth dislocation. Perforation of the trachea or esophagus is, fortunately, a rare complication, but does occur. The use of stylets on a routine basis is discouraged for this reason.

The minimum criteria for extubation are listed in Table 19-7. A postextubation chest radiograph is usually indicated after any thoracic surgical procedure,

TABLE 19-7. Minimum Criteria for Extubation

1. Inspired oxygen ≤40%
2. IMV ≤2
3. CPAP or PEEP ≤4 cmH₂O
4. Stable blood gases
   PaO₂ 80–100 mmHg
   PaCO₂ 35–45 mmHg
   pH 7.30–7.40
5. Cardiovascular stability—no vasopressors
6. Metabolism or reversal of muscle relaxants and respiratory depressants
7. CNS stability—no active seizure disorder or progressive coma
8. Electrolyte balance—including glucose and calcium

since right upper lobe atelectasis is quite common after prolonged intubation in children. Competency of the glottic structures to prevent aspiration may not be regained for as long as 8 hours after extubation; therefore, cautious feedings of clear liquids should be given initially and progressed only as tolerated (see Appendix 19-1).[129]

Maintenance of Anesthesia

After induction of anesthesia has been accomplished, intravenous and monitoring catheters established, the trachea intubated, and the endotracheal tube secured, the appropriate level of anesthesia is usually maintained with a combination of nitrous oxide/oxygen and halothane or isoflurane in low concentrations, along with a nondepolarizing muscle relaxant. In higher risk patients, the potent anesthetics are omitted and a narcotic substituted.

In most pediatric thoracic operations, a sump-type nasogastric tube is inserted into the stomach to avoid gastric distention intraoperatively from swallowed air or from anesthetic gases that may leak around the endotracheal tube. Gastric distention may interfere with the surgical exposure, especially during operations in the left hemithorax, and can cause reflex bradycardia and hypotension. An esophageal stethoscope is placed with its tip in the midesophagus to monitor heart sounds and breath sounds during surgery. In thoracic procedures, the surgeon should always be informed of the presence of an esophageal stethoscope, since palpation of the instrument in the esophagus may cause the surgeon to believe the esophagus is the trachea (see discussion of tracheoesophageal fistula below).

It is important that the anesthesiologist have a clear view of the operative field to keep up with the progress of the operation and to be able to correlate hemodynamic changes with surgical manipulations. He can assist the surgeon with the intrathoracic exposure by hypoventilating during crucial maneuvers and

ventilating adequately when these measures are accomplished. Ventilation should be decreased or stopped during placement of pericostal sutures to prevent puncture or laceration of the lung parenchyma. In perhaps no other type of surgery is such close cooperation between the surgeon and anesthesiologist as vital as operations within the chest, since what each does profoundly affects the other. Close observation of the surgical field by the anesthesiologist, as well as an appreciation of anesthesia problems by the surgeon, are imperative for a successful outcome.

The maintenance of a patent airway (endotracheal tube) during thoracic operations is the primary responsibility of the anesthesiologist. The use of humidified anesthetic gases decreases the likelihood of obstruction due to secretions or small amounts of blood that can enter the tracheobronchial tree during surgery. The judicious use of small amounts of normal saline as irrigation (0.5 to 2.0 mL) followed by gentle suctioning at an appropriate point in the operation may prevent catastrophic obstruction of the airway. Mechanical ventilation is used in some patients during thoracic operations (rarely, if ever, in the newborn or very small patient), but manual ventilation is necessary for the detection of subtle or gross changes in compliance.

Termination of Operation, Immediate Postoperative Measures, and Transport to Intensive Care Unit

Once the planned operation is complete, and before chest closure, an attempt should be made to correct any atelectasis that may have occurred due to lung compression. This should be done gently, gradually, and under direct vision, so that excessive pressures are not applied to the airways, which could result in a pneumothorax on the contralateral side. During the placement of chest tubes, and especially during the puncture of the pleura, ventilation should be temporarily interrupted. If the chest tube is to be removed in the operating room and not left in place during the immediate postoperative period (as with an uncomplicated patent ductus arteriosus ligation), it is usually placed directly through the incision and the pericostal sutures pulled together tightly around it. It can safely be removed after several positive-pressure breaths are given. A chest radiograph in the operating room is taken to confirm re-expansion of the lung on the affected side.

Intercostal or interpleural nerve blocks may be used to alleviate some of the immediate postoperative pain in patients older than 5 or 6 months.[130–132] The surgeon may inject the local anesthetic as far posteriorly as possible at the level of the incision, as well as one or two segments above and below, or the block may be placed transcutaneously by the anesthesiologist at the conclusion of the operation. Bupivacaine, 0.25 percent, maximum total dose of 2 mg/kg body weight, is usually selected due to its long duration of action. This is especially helpful in patients who undergo early extubation, since it minimizes the splinting often encountered in the immediate postextubation period (see the section *Postoperative Pain*).

The need for postoperative ventilatory support should be anticipated preoperatively, discussed with the parents, and explained to the patient if of an appropriate age. It is based on the preoperative condition of the patient, the specific operation planned, the anesthetic technique used, and the expected postoperative course. In very small infants and in almost all newborn babies undergoing thoracic operations, the endotracheal tube is left in place and mechanical ventilation used for several hours to days, depending on the general condition of the patient. Weaning is begun as soon as hemodynamic and respiratory parameters appear stable.

It is important that a well-defined system for transfer of the patient to the care of the intensive care unit nurses from that of the anesthesia personnel be clearly understood by both to ensure a safe and effective transition. In critically ill children, a battery-powered monitor should be used to display the arterial pressure and ECG during transport. On arrival, the arterial pressure monitoring system is transferred to the intensive care unit equipment from the transport monitor. The venous or atrial monitoring catheters are then connected to the appropriate transducers. While this is being done, the anesthesiologist or respiratory therapist should continue to ventilate the patient by hand, and not until after the pressure monitors are connected and displayed should hand ventilation be discontinued and the patient placed on mechanical ventilation. The ventilator settings can be preset by the respiratory therapist before the patient arrives in the intensive care unit, after communication with the anesthesia personnel in the operating room. Examination by the anesthesiologist and respiratory therapist after institution of mechanical ventilation should be done to ensure adequate chest expansion, presence of bilateral breath sounds, the need for suctioning of the endotracheal tube, and the rate of actual ventilation. Blood gas values should be obtained to determine the adequacy of ventilation shortly after arrival in the intensive care unit.

A detailed report by the anesthesiologist to the intensive care unit nurse responsible for the patient should be given as soon as both feel the patient is stable. This report should include the procedure performed, anesthetic technique used, total amount of drugs, fluids, and blood administered, drugs reversed at the end of surgery (eg, muscle relaxants, heparin), problems encountered during the case, urine output, and any anticipated postoperative difficulties.

MANAGEMENT OF POSTOPERATIVE COMPLICATIONS

Infants and children undergoing thoracic surgical procedures are subject to several postoperative complications involving the lungs, airway, heart, great vessels, upper gastrointestinal tract, and lymphatic system (see Chapter 26). Most of these complications can be prevented by meticulous attention to intraoperative detail by both the surgeon and anesthesiologist. Morbidity and mortality from intrathoracic operations can be further reduced by systematic postoperative assessment and the application of a few simple principles of general postoperative support.

Postoperative Pain

The consideration and treatment of postoperative pain is an important part of any well-conducted anesthetic procedure. The myths regarding children and pain perception are fading, but even though there is agreement that even the youngest infants perceive pain, treatment of pain in children is often inadequate.[133,134]

The same reasons for providing adequate postoperative analgesia for adults also apply to children; namely, the humanitarian responsibility of physicians (especially anesthesiologists), and because postoperative complications are probably more likely to occur if pain is treated inadequately, especially after thoracic procedures.[135] Effective pain relief has been shown to influence recovery from major surgery in adults,[136,137] and there is no reason to believe that the same benefits should not be achieved in children.

Parenteral narcotic analgesics are used frequently after thoracic operations, and usually provide effective pain relief. When administering narcotics, it is important to maintain an adequate plasma level at all times. While such a goal may be possible in adults using an "as required" schedule, recent work suggests that an adequate analgesic level of morphine may not be achieved in children using a conventional "as required" method. It is probably unrealistic to expect a child to ask for an intramuscular injection for pain relief or to understand that an intravenously administered narcotic will not be a painful "shot." For these reasons, narcotics should usually be administered intravenously, either as a continuous infusion or on a schedule. Intermittent intravenous injections do not require a special infusion pump, and may maintain a near-constant analgesic plasma level. There is also the added advantage that intermittent, but regularly administered, narcotic allows the patient to be more carefully monitored during the time of drug administration. Common side effects, including nausea, somnolence, urinary retention, and pruritus, can usually be managed and the pediatric patient provided adequate pain relief. Most children who undergo thoracic procedures are monitored in an intensive care unit during the immediate postoperative period. Therefore, parenteral narcotics may be given safely, the individual patient's response noted, and the narcotic dose appropriately modified. Meperidine is generally avoided because of its CNS side effects,[138] and morphine or methadone, using an interim intravenous dosing schedule, or fentanyl or sufentanil, as continuous infusions, are preferred.

Newborns and infants may be more sensitive to the respiratory depressant effects of narcotics,[139,140] and therefore require special monitoring when these drugs are given. Nonintubated infants younger than 3 months who are given narcotics should be monitored in an intensive care unit setting. Infants and children who are intubated may be safely given larger doses of narcotic analgesics; however, prolonged use of excessive doses will depress the ventilatory response to $PaCO_2$, and weaning from mechanical ventilation may be prolonged. When patients are difficult to manage postoperatively on mechanical ventilation, other sedative medications may be added to the narcotic regimen. One of the intravenous benzodiazepines, such as midazolam or diazepam, is often used. Artificially ventilated children are usually already on parenteral narcotics, so the initial dose of midazolam is on the low side, ie, 0.03 to 0.05 mg/kg.

Patient-controlled analgesia (PCA) is very well-suited for management of postoperative pain in older children[141] (see Chapter 21). As more experience is gained with this technique in children, its safety and wide applicability are becoming more and more apparent.[142] Age is probably not as important a factor in deciding which children to treat with a PCA pump as is the patient's ability to understand how to use the device. An intelligent 5- or 6-year-old can be successfully instructed to use the PCA device. Morphine is usually the narcotic of choice. However, meperidine or methadone may also be used via PCA infusion pumps. A loading dose of narcotic is needed to reach adequate plasma levels and is usually given in the operating room before termination of the case using 0.05 to 0.1 mg/kg of morphine or the equivalent. The PCA dose is 0.01 to 0.02 mg/kg, depending on the surgical procedure, and the lockout time 6 to 10 minutes. Currently available PCA pumps are equipped with 4-hour limits that are set (in a multiple of 5 mg) at 0.25 mg/kg. It has been seen that the children are very comfortable with these doses and settings, and many of them use only 0.7 to 1.0 mg/kg/d of morphine (Table 19-8).

Many regional techniques are applicable to the management of postoperative pain in children who have undergone thoracic procedures. Caudal blocks are probably the easiest and safest of all regional tech-

TABLE 19-8. Analgesics

Drug	Route of Administration	Dose Range
Acetaminophen	PO, P	10–15 mg/kg q4h
Ibuprofen	PO	3–30 mg/kg q6h
Codeine	PO, IM[a]	0.5–1.0 mg/kg q4–6h
Morphine[b]	PO	0.2–0.6 mg/kg q4h
	IV, IM[a]	0.05–0.1 mg/kg q3–4h
Meperidine[b]	PO	1–1.5 mg/kg/4h
	IV, IM[a]	1 mg/kg q4h
Methadone	PO	0.1–0.2 mg/kg q8–12 h
	IV	0.05–0.1 mg/kg q4–6h
Fentanyl[c]	IV	1–3 μg/kg/h
Sufentanil[c]	IV	0.1–0.3 μg/kg/h

[a] Intramuscular injection can be quite painful and should be avoided in children when possible.
[b] The dosages of morphine or meperidine for use in PCA are given in the text.
[c] The short duration of action of the synthetic narcotics fentanyl and sufentanil makes administration by constant infusion practical.

niques[143] and their success rate is very high. Although more experience has been gained with the use of local anesthetic administration, particularly bupivacaine,[144] several researchers have recently reported the use of caudal morphine for relief of postoperative pain in children.[145,146] These studies indicate that good postoperative analgesia may be achieved when caudal, preservative-free morphine is given in doses from 0.05 to 0.1 mg/kg diluted with preservative-free saline. Side effects similar to those reported with adults were seen, and included nausea, pruritus, and urinary retention. Respiratory depression may also occur. Rosen and Rosen administered 0.075 mg of morphine in preservative-free saline (5 to 10 mL) into the caudal space of children who had undergone cardiac surgery.[145] These investigators noted that the patients had decreased analgesic requirements for 24 hours, as well as an average pain-free interval of 6 hours. Children below the age of 2 years were not included in this study. Children in whom caudal morphine is used should be monitored for respiratory depression for at least 24 hours after the morphine is given.[147] Krane reported a case of respiratory depression in a 2 1/2-year-old child who was given 0.1 mg/kg of morphine via the caudal route.[148] The episode of respiratory depression initially occurred 3.5 hours after administration of the morphine, but the patient required a naloxone infusion (10 to 14 μg/kg/h) for 14 hours. In a study of CO_2 sensitivity in children receiving caudal morphine, the slopes $V_E/P_{ET}CO_2$ and V_E55 were found to still be significantly depressed 22 hours following the caudal morphine administration.[147] Caudal morphine seems to be a useful technique for relief of postoperative pain in certain children if appropriate monitoring is provided. Children with natural airways should be monitored in an intensive care unit for 24 hours following caudal narcotics.

Lumbar and thoracic administration of local anesthetics have been used for postoperative analgesia in children, although most reports indicate the usefulness is usually after abdominal and lower extremity surgery.[149–152] Several factors should be kept in mind when considering the use of epidural local anesthetics for postoperative analgesia in children. If the technically less difficult lumbar approach is used, a large volume of local anesthetic must be given, and there is the potential for toxicity.[153–155] However, placement of a thoracic epidural catheter is technically more difficult. There is one report that describes placement of a catheter in the thoracic epidural space in neonates via the caudal canal. These researchers used x-ray films to confirm catheter position in these small (2.7 to 6.5 kg) infants. They reported successful analgesia in all patients. No hypotension or dysrhythmias were reported. The dose of bupivacaine in this report was 0.5 mL/kg of a 0.5 percent solution (2.5 mg/kg total dose).[156]

Intrapleural administration of local anesthetics has been shown to be an effective and safe way to achieve post-thoracotomy analgesia in adults.[157,158] Bupivacaine, 0.5 percent, was administered and the measured serum levels were below the toxic range. McIlvaine and Knox reported a series of 14 children in whom intrapleural 0.25 percent bupivacaine was used to provide postoperative analgesia.[159] In all of their patients, the catheter was placed intraoperatively before chest closure. No patient required supplemental narcotics during the 24-hour period while receiving the infusion of 0.25 percent bupivacaine given at 0.5 to 1.0 mL/h. Plasma levels were high, however, exceeding 2 μg/mL in 11 of 14 children and 4 μg/mL in five of 14 children. No patient exhibited CNS or cardiovascular signs of toxicity. These investigators recommend that the infusion rate of 0.25 percent bupivacaine with 1:200,000 epinephrine not exceed 0.5 mL/kg/h.

Pneumothorax

Pneumothorax is an accumulation of air outside the lung, but within the pleural cavity and/or mediastinum, which occupies space needed for full lung inflation and cardiac filling. Air may remain in the chest following any intrathoracic operation, or it may accumulate postoperatively from an air leak in the lung or tracheobronchial tree. A rubber or plastic tube is usually left in the pleural cavity following thoracotomy, or in the mediastinum when a median sternotomy incision is used. This tube is connected to a collection and drainage system that allows air, blood, and fluid to escape while preventing air from entering the chest. Most drainage systems use the water-seal principle. However, some surgeons prefer not to leave a chest tube in place following relatively simple intrathoracic procedures in which the lung itself has not been incised and bleeding is negligible. In that case, air is evacuated from the chest as the ribs and muscle are approximated, and positive pressure is maintained on the airways by the anesthesiologist until the chest is completely closed. A radiograph is obtained immediately following completion of the operation to be sure that no more air remains. A small residual pneumothorax will usually resolve spontaneously in a few hours without causing difficulty, but careful follow-up is required.

Two specific problems related to pneumothorax deserve special consideration. First, the development of a tension pneumothorax in which air continues to leak from the lung or tracheobronchial tree into the undrained pleural space or mediastinum requires the immediate insertion of a chest tube to prevent compression of the lung, shift of the mediastinum, and life-threatening hypoxia, hypercarbia, and low cardiac output. A tension pneumothorax can occur from the rupture of the lung surface or rupture of a small bleb due to excessive positive pressure, coughing, intraoperative trauma, or agitation in a patient receiving mechanical ventilation. It is diagnosed by clinical deterioration in the patient's vital signs (hypertension followed by hypotension, tachycardia followed by bradycardia, and respiratory distress), acute reduction in breath sounds, decreased pulmonary compliance, displacement of the cardiac point of maximal impulse, and by hypoxemia, hypercarbia, and acidosis as reflected in the arterial blood gases. A chest radiograph can be used to confirm the diagnosis.

The second important problem relates to the development of a pneumothorax in the unoperated pleural cavity, where a chest tube is not likely to be in place. This problem is dangerous and so likely to be overlooked that some surgeons open and drain both pleural cavities in addition to the mediastinum in critically ill patients undergoing certain intrathoracic operations, particularly when a median sternotomy is done. Chest tubes are left in place for 24 to 48 hours postoperatively, or until drainage of blood and fluid ceases. They are "stripped" frequently to avoid the accumulation of a blood clot that might prevent adequate drainage of air and blood. The tubes are not removed if there is evidence of a continued air leak within the chest. At the time of removal, precautions need to be taken to avoid entry of air into the chest through the opening in the chest wall or through the holes in the tubes themselves. A chest radiograph is obtained shortly after removal of the tubes to confirm that no pneumothorax remains, and the patient is observed carefully for the next few hours for signs of respiratory distress or deterioration in vital signs suggestive of a recurrent pneumothorax. Occlusive dressings are placed over the chest tube tracts; in addition, in small infants with thin chest walls, a suture can be placed around the chest tube, and is tied down to occlude the wound as the tube is withdrawn. Even a small residual pneumothorax increases the chances for blood and fluid accumulation within the pleural cavity and may lead to postoperative empyema.

Hemothorax and Hemomediastinum

Blood loss and postoperative bleeding are quite variable during and following intrathoracic operations. In cases of lung biopsy, lobectomy, or patent ductus arteriosus ligation, for example, virtually no blood loss is expected. In contrast, massive bleeding and prolonged postoperative drainage may be encountered during and after reoperation for a complex congenital heart defect. Chest drainage tubes are inserted following an operation within the chest or mediastinum in which even minimal postoperative bleeding is expected. Excessive bleeding requires re-exploration of the chest for control. A table of acceptable rates for postoperative bleeding as a function of the size of the patient has been proposed by Kirklin et al.[160] Rates of bleeding in excess of these limits require re-exploration. Serious complications may occur as a result of waiting too long in the hope that conservative measures and time will take care of the bleeding. Chest tubes are of only limited effectiveness in draining blood from the pleural cavities and mediastinum. Proper position, suction, and "stripping" are important; however, once clots begin to collect within the chest, tube function deteriorates and the likelihood of re-exploration for evacuation of the clot and control of bleeding increases. Accumulation of blood within the chest seriously compromises pulmonary function and cardiac output. Cardiac dysrhythmias and tamponade occur quickly in children and may even require urgent reopening of the incision in the intensive care unit to prevent death. Prior to re-exploration of the chest, all possible measures should be taken to restore normal blood coagulation, including the administration of fresh frozen plasma, platelets, and protamine. In selected patients, antifibrinolytic agents, fresh whole blood, factor-specific cryoprecipitates, and vitamin K may be indicated. Normal body temperature should be restored as quickly as possible; 5 to 10 cm of PEEP can be tried to reduce postoperative intrathoracic bleeding.[161] Agitation and hypertension should be pharmacologically controlled. In spite of all these potentially useful measures, a very low threshold for re-exploration to control postoperative bleeding and to evaluate a hemothorax or hemomediastinum is the best insurance of a subsequent complication-free recovery.

Chylothorax

The accumulation of lymph within the pleural cavity is a relatively late complication of intrathoracic operations. The thoracic duct may be injured in either pleural cavity, but it most often occurs during dissection around the descending thoracic aorta in the left hemithorax. It is particularly at risk during operations for patent ductus arteriosus and coarctation of the aorta. In some cases, an unusually large amount of straw-colored or milky-white fluid may be noted in the chest tube drainage before the tube is removed. In such situations, the tube should be left in place and the patient not allowed to receive oral food or liquids or at least kept on a low-fat diet for several more days.

It is more common for a chylothorax to be discovered several days after the chest tube has been removed when the patient has resumed a normal diet. Acute respiratory distress may develop, with respirations becoming increasingly labored and breath sounds diminished over the hemithorax involved. Chest radiographs will reveal an opaque hemithorax or a large accumulation of fluid. A chest tube should be inserted to drain the fluid and fully re-expand the lung. The tube should be left in place for several days, since most leaks in the thoracic duct will seal during this time and no further treatment will be required. Dietary restriction of fat and the use of short-chain triglycerides may facilitate spontaneous closure of the lymph fistula. Exploration and surgical control of the leak may be required if significant drainage continues or if nutritional depletion becomes a problem. The use of total parenteral nutrition during the early management of chylothorax has been useful in prolonging the time before surgical intervention is required and allowing a greater chance for spontaneous sealing of the leak to occur. Even at the time of re-exploration, the surgeon may find it quite difficult to locate and eliminate the source of lymphatic drainage, especially in the small infant.

Atelectasis

Postoperative atelectasis is, to a greater or lesser degree, an almost universal occurrence following intrathoracic operations in infants and small children. Surgical manipulation of the small, fragile, and often congested lung, associated with postoperative incisional pain and the child's instinctive reluctance to cooperate with even the most skillfully designed program for pulmonary toilet, often complicate recovery. Children with congenital cardiac defects are frequently weak and debilitated, and increased pulmonary blood flow or pulmonary venous congestion from left ventricular failure further complicate the problem.

Management of atelectasis in the older child should begin during the preoperative orientation, when the child is taught to cooperate with nurses and respiratory therapists during the conduct of chest percussion, deep breathing, coughing, and suctioning. Incentive spirometry is particularly effective in the older child, especially when one of the clown-like or ball-containing "game" devices is used during preoperative training.

When postoperative fever, tachycardia, tachypnea, and diminished breath sounds suggest atelectasis, a chest radiograph usually confirms the presence of areas of uninflated lung. If vigorous chest physical therapy and incentive spirometry fail to eliminate the atelectasis, nasotracheal aspiration is used. In patients who are still intubated, suctioning, irrigation, and positive-pressure ventilation usually re-expand the atelectatic segments, unless the tube itself is obstructing one or more bronchi; the right upper lobe is particularly susceptible to obstruction by an improperly placed endotracheal tube. Reintubation with endotracheal suctioning and positive-pressure ventilation can be used for a few hours in infants with persistent atelectasis. Bronchoscopy may be required to examine each bronchial orifice and directly extract obstructing mucus plugs or blood clots. It is particularly useful following an episode of vomiting and suspected aspiration, and can be done at the bedside in the intensive care unit, even using rigid bronchoscopes.

Children with neuromuscular disorders, scoliosis, small airways, cardiac disease, chronic debilitation, and cystic fibrosis pose particularly troublesome problems and may even require a tracheostomy to manage persistent or recurrent postoperative atelectasis. If atelectasis is not prevented or promptly corrected, pneumonitis and life-threatening sepsis may develop within a few days (Fig. 19-6).

Gastric Distention

The use of an uncuffed endotracheal tube with positive-pressure ventilatory assistance may lead to the accumulation of a significant quantity of air in the

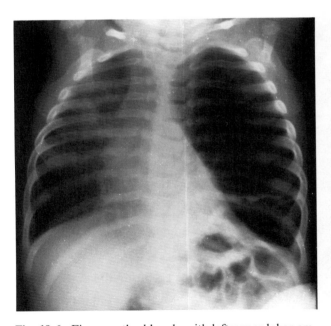

Fig. 19-6. Five-month-old male with left upper lobar emphysema. Preoperative chest radiograph showing hyperlucency and decreased vascular markings of left upper lung field, compression atelectasis of left lower lobe, and shift of heart and mediastinal structures toward right.

stomach and upper gastrointestinal tract of the infant or child, both during anesthesia and in the postoperative period. This problem is compounded by the swallowing reflex of the infant. Gastric distention may lead to acute severe bradycardia and respiratory distress, and to subsequent diffuse abdominal distention, pain, ileus, and respiratory insufficiency. Gastric perforation may even occur as a result of gaseous distention of the stomach. These complications are avoided by the presence of a functional nasogastric tube inserted after the induction of anesthesia, and kept in place until after the child is extubated and no longer requires positive-pressure ventilation. A sump-type catheter, which is irrigated periodically and connected to intermittent suction, can be used. Tube position is confirmed in the stomach by auscultation of an injected bolus of air, palpation, aspiration, and x-ray examination.

Upper Airway Obstruction

Upper airway obstruction following extubation of the infant or child is far more common than in the adult. The likelihood of such obstruction occurring is increased by a difficult intubation, multiple attempts at intubation, overhydration, congestive heart failure, and prolonged intubation. If the child has been agitated or overly active during awakening from anesthesia, trauma to the cords and trachea can produce edema that may result in some degree of upper airway obstruction following extubation. Small infants with large tongues and short necks are particularly at risk, especially those with craniofacial anomalies involving the upper airway or myxedema.

To minimize the likelihood of postextubation upper airway obstruction, the intubated child can be heavily sedated and all gases humidified. In those children particularly at risk of obstruction, dexamethasone, 0.1 mg/kg, should be given 30 minutes prior to extubation, and all equipment necessary for prompt reintubation should be kept at the bedside until a satisfactory upper airway is assured. When prolonged ventilatory support is required, a tracheostomy should be considered to minimize trauma to the vocal cords and to eliminate the pressure and potential necrosis with subsequent stenosis at the level of the narrow subglottic cricoid ring. With meticulous care, however, infants are now ventilated for many weeks with endotracheal intubation alone.

Low Cardiac Output

Infants and children with cardiothoracic conditions requiring operation are obviously more at risk of having an inadequate cardiac output during the postoperative period than patients with less critical illnesses.

The low cardiac output syndrome is characterized by oliguria, obtundation of otherwise abnormal mental status, and progressive respiratory and hepatic deterioration. When it can be determined, the mixed venous oxygen saturation or tension will be low due to the wide arteriovenous oxygen difference, indicative of a large extraction of oxygen.

Five factors determine the adequacy of cardiac output: heart rate, cardiac rhythm, vascular volume, vascular resistance, and myocardial contractility. Proper management of cardiac output in the pediatric thoracic surgical patient requires that bodily demands for cardiac output be kept to a minimum. Fever must be prevented or promptly controlled, and agitation and pain reduced with analgesics and sedatives. The work of breathing is reduced by the use of mechanical ventilatory assistance when necessary.

ANESTHESIA FOR SPECIFIC PEDIATRIC THORACIC PROCEDURES (Tables 19-9 and 19-10)

Bronchoscopy and Bronchography

Therapeutic and diagnostic bronchoscopy in the pediatric patient is not an uncommon procedure and requires skill and cooperation between the endoscopist and anesthesiologist since the airway must be "shared" and each must understand and appreciate the problems of the other.

The development of the pediatric magnifying bronchoscope (Storz Endoscopy Co., Tuttlingen, West Germany; K. Storz Endoscopy American, Los Angeles, CA) has greatly enhanced the safety and effectiveness of bronchoscopy in infants and children. This system provides sheaths of varying sizes and lengths to be used on even the smallest infants, although ventilation is more difficult with the 3.0 mm instrument due to the resistance of the system itself when the light source and magnifying lens are in place. The larger instruments furnish adequate ventilating capabilities and allow the surgeon to continue the visual examination while the patient is being ventilated via the 15 mm side arm attached to the anesthesia system. With these larger instruments, small biopsy forceps or grasping forceps can be passed through the instrument channel while ventilation is maintained with the telescope in place. If larger forceps are needed, the telescope must be removed and biopsy or foreign body extraction accomplished without optical magnification via the main channel of the bronchoscope.[162]

Indications for diagnostic bronchoscopy in children include determination of the cause of stridor such as laryngotracheomalacia, laryngeal webs, postintubation or post-tracheotomy stenosis; determination of

TABLE 19-9.   Selected Thoracic Abnormalities and Anesthetic Considerations Requiring Operation in Infants and Children

Condition	Description	Anesthetic and Perioperative Considerations
Achalasia	Motor disturbance of the esophagus in which cardia does not relax during swallowing, resulting in esophageal dilation, esophagitis, regurgitation, failure to thrive, and, often, aspiration pneumonitis.	Pre-existing chronic aspiration pneumonitis and poor nutritional status often necessitate postoperative mechanical ventilation and vigorous chest physiotherapy, and sometimes a regimen of total parenteral nutrition.
Agenesis, aplasia, or hypoplasia of lung or lobe(s)	Embryologic defects; symptoms vary from none to severe respiratory insufficiency.	Mediastinum may be markedly shifted toward affected side; trachea may be kinked; associated vascular hypoplasia and pulmonary arterial hypertension; therapeutic or diagnostic bronchoscopy often necessary for severe respiratory infections.
Bronchiectasis	Dilatation of bronchi from inflammatory destruction of bronchial and peribronchial tissues; exudate often accumulates in dependent areas or affected lung.	Bronchoscopy and bronchography are often helpful in defining extent of process and in obtaining cultures directly from affected areas. If medical therapy fails, lobectomy is indicated.
Bronchobiliary fistula	A fistula connecting right middle lobe bronchus and the left hepatic duct.	Bronchoscopy and bronchography for diagnosis and surgical excision of the intrathoracic portion of the fistula. Severe recurrent respiratory infections and atelectasis dictate vigorous pre- and postoperative chest physiotherapy and often repeated therapeutic bronchoscopy.
Bronchopulmonary dysplasia	Chronic lung disease resulting in preterm infants with hyaline membrane disease who require long-term artificial ventilation. Thought due to a combination of factors, including barotrauma, oxygen, infection, scarring. Patients usually manifest hypoxemia, hypercarbia, and increased pulmonary vascular resistance. Cor pulmonale and congestive heart failure may also be present.	Effects of bronchopulmonary dysplasia may persist well beyond first year of life. Infants are frequently on chronic bronchodilator and diuretic therapy, which may need adjustment in the perioperative period. Careful attention to electrolytes and fluid administration is necessary. Nitrous oxide, as a part of the anesthetic regimen, may be contraindicated due to emphysematous airtrapping. Ventilatory patterns during anesthesia should be designed to allow for adequate expiratory time and to avoid excessive airway pressure to minimize the possibility of pneumothorax. Postoperative apnea monitoring and pulse oximetry are usually indicated for up to 24 hours and longer under some circumstances.
Chylothorax	Chylous pleural effusion; may be congenital due to birth injury to thoracic duct or due to trauma, especially after palliative cardiovascular procedures involving a left thoracotomy.	Conservative management usually suffices (repeated aspiration and insertion of thoracostomy tube connected to underwater seal). Persistent drainage (longer than 3 or 4 weeks) after appropriate conservative measures may be treated surgically by ligation of the thoracic duct just above the diaphragm. Loss of protein and fats often results in severe nutritional problems, and hyperalimentation is usually required.
Coarctation of the aorta	Narrowing of aorta usually just distal to left subclavian artery. Preductal coarctation usually longer segment of narrowing; postductal coarctation usually discrete narrow segment.	Symptomatic infants usually have associated cardiovascular defects, eg, ventricular septal defects, patent ductus. Beyond infancy, children are usually asymptomatic but often hypertensive. In older children, extensive collateral vessels may result in massive blood loss during thoracotomy. Cross-clamping of the aorta during repair usually results in significant hypertension in vessels proximal to the cross-clamp and requires pretreatment with vasodilators.

(continued)

TABLE 19-9 (*continued*). **Selected Thoracic Abnormalities and Anesthetic Considerations Requiring Operation in Infants and Children**

Condition	Description	Anesthetic and Perioperative Considerations
Corrosive or caustic burns of the esophagus	Chemical burns of mucosa	Initially, esophagoscopy usually done to determine extent of damage. Burns of epiglottic and laryngeal mucosa may compromise airway and make intubation difficult.
Croup (infectious)	Acute laryngotracheal bronchitis. Nondiphtheritic infections usually caused by viral agents.	Must differentiate from acute epiglottitis (see below). Usually does not progress beyond stridor or slight dyspnea. In severe cases, may require artificial airway.
Cystic adenomatoid malformation	Malformed bronchi lead to irregular aeration. Air accumulates in the potential cystic structures.	Sudden massive blood loss may result during removal from avulsion of vessels arising from the aorta and entering cystic areas. Preoperative arteriography should define extent and location of blood supply. May mimic congenital diaphragmatic hernia on chest x-ray.
Cystic fibrosis	Multisystem disease of exocrine glands especially affecting lungs and pancreas.	Chronic lung disease leading to pulmonary insufficiency in many patients. Pulmonary complications include pneumothorax and massive hemoptysis from erosion of enlarged thin-walled bronchial vessels. Bronchoscopy for therapeutic bronchial lavage or for localization of bleeding site with subsequent resection or embolization of bleeding bronchial vessels may be necessary. For selected patients with more localized lung disease, pulmonary resection may be done. Respiratory support with tracheal intubation and mechanical ventilation during infectious exacerbations is not uncommon (see text, bronchoscopy).
Cystic hygroma	A cystic tumor arising along the course of the primitive lymphatic sacs.	Most commonly seen in the neck region. They may be very large and impinge on normal airway structures and result in obstruction of the upper airway, making intubation difficult; occasionally may extend into the mediastinum.
Diaphragmatic hernia Foramen of Bochdalek hernia	Posterolateral (usually left) diaphragmatic defect allowing herniation of abdominal contents into thoracic cavity with compression of ipsilateral lung and shift of mediastinum toward contralateral side.	Often, the most serious of all neonatal surgical problems because of rapidly progressive respiratory failure and early death if not corrected quickly. Resuscitative measures (intubation, ventilation, and treatment of metabolic and respiratory acidosis) must be instituted immediately. Extracorporeal membrane oxygenation may be beneficial.
Foramen of Morgagni hernia	Retrosternal herniation of portion of bowel. Usually presents later and less dramatically than Bochdalek hernia.	May be asymptomatic. Surgical repair indicated when diagnosed due to risk of incarceration. May occur in pericardium, resulting in compromise of cardiac output.
Ectopic bronchus (eparterial bronchus, "pig bronchus")	Origin of right upper lobe bronchus from trachea.	Endotracheal intubation may block right upper lobe bronchus, resulting in atelectasis; may be associated with chronic right upper lobe infection and bronchiectasis.

(*continued*)

TABLE 19-9 (*continued*).   Selected Thoracic Abnormalities and Anesthetic Considerations Requiring Operation in Infants and Children

Condition	Description	Anesthetic and Perioperative Considerations
Empyema	Accumulation of pus within the pleural space, often associated with staphylococcal pneumonia.	Large empyemas may compress lung and compromise respiratory function; usually managed with thoracostomy tube placed under local anesthesia. Chronic empyema may require decortication of fibrinous covering on parenchymal and pleural surfaces to re-expand affected lung.
Erb-Duchenne palsy	Injury (usually birth trauma) to upper brachial plexus (fifth and sixth cervical nerves) resulting in loss of ability to abduct the arm from shoulder, externally rotate arm, supinate forearm. Muscle function of hand is retained.	This and other forms of brachial plexus injuries may be associated with phrenic nerve injuries, with paralysis of the diaphragm on the involved side.
Epiglottitis	Usually bacterial infection (most commonly *Haemophilus influenza*) of epiglottis and surrounding structures, including larynx.	Severe, life-threatening, rapidly progressive disease that may result in total obstruction of upper airway. Should be managed by endotracheal intubation (orotracheal initially to establish the airway, followed by nasotracheal, if possible, to accomplish safely) under anesthesia in operating room with surgeon standing by to do tracheotomy if endotracheal tube cannot be passed. Infectious process rapidly responds to intravenous antibiotics and endotracheal tube can be removed usually in 48 to 72 hours as swelling subsides, as proven by direct laryngoscopy.
Esophageal duplication (enteric cyst)	Spherical or tubular posterior mediastinal structures with muscular walls and lining of any type of gastrointestinal epithelium or ciliated epithelium. Associated anomalies include hemivertebrae of upper thoracic spine and intra-abdominal enteric cysts. Usually do not communicate with the lumen of the esophagus, but may be connected to the small bowel.	Large cysts may compress the lung. Because they frequently contain acid-secreting gastric mucosa, peptic ulceration may occur and erode into lung, bronchus, or esophagus with resulting hemorrhage.
Esophageal perforation	Usually traumatic, caused by instrumentation for pre-existing disease. May occur in newborn, usually on right side, from birth trauma, and presents a sudden respiratory collapse accompanied by hydropneumothorax.	Esophagoscopy for pre-existing disease (stricture of esophagus from corrosive burns or tracheoesophageal fistula) is common procedure in pediatric patients. Anesthesia must be appropriately deep to prevent coughing while esophagoscope is in place. In newborn presenting with hydropneumothorax from esophageal perforation, immediate aspiration is necessary followed by thoracotomy and repair of perforation.
Esophageal stenosis	Rarely, congenital defect associated with tracheoesophageal fistula without esophageal atresia or as isolated congenital stenosis in which esophageal wall contains tissues of respiratory tract origin, including ciliated epithelium and cartilage. More often acquired and associated with esophageal reflux.	Excision is required if ectopic tissue is present. Repeated esophageal dilations either with esophagoscope or by bougienage to alleviate restenosis due to scar tissue formation. Esophageal perforation is always a possible complication. Infants are often malnourished and require total parenteral nutrition.
Esophageal stricture	The result of trauma to the esophagus from several causes: tracheoesophageal fistula repair; corrosive burns of esophagus, congenital esophageal stenosis.	Require repeated dilations with perforation always a possible complication. Colon interposition (or other visceral esophageal bypass) may be necessary.

(continued)

TABLE 19-9 (*continued*). Selected Thoracic Abnormalities and Anesthetic Considerations Requiring Operation in Infants and Children

Condition	Description	Anesthetic and Perioperative Considerations
Esophagitis	In infants, may be the result of gastroesophageal reflux with or without hiatal hernia; may subside spontaneously by 12–15 months of age if not associated with a large hiatus hernia.	May present as recurrent apnea or failure to thrive from recurrent vomiting during early infancy, and respiratory infections from repeated aspirations may be quite severe. If symptoms cannot be controlled by propping baby in infant seat to prevent reflux, some form of antireflux procedure may be indicated. Anemia may result from chronic blood loss. (See gastroesophageal reflux below.)
Eventration of the diaphragm	Congenital defect of muscular layer of diaphragm allowing usually minor herniation of part of abdominal organs into chest. Usually on right. May be asymptomatic or, rarely, may present like Bochdalek hernia. Respiratory symptoms depend on extent of herniation of abdominal contents and range from minimal to severe; gastric volvulus may result when there is significant eventration of the left hemidiaphragm.	On chest x-ray there is usually a smooth dome-shaped elevation of the diaphragmatic shadow on the affected side with loss of lung volume. Small asymptomatic eventration should be corrected whether or not they are symptomatic. If respiratory infection is present, appropriate medical therapy with antibiotics, chest physiotherapy, and even therapeutic bronchoscopy is usually indicated prior to correction.
Gastroesophageal reflux (chalasia)	Results from failure of proper valvular function of esophagogastric junction; may or may not be associated with hiatus hernia.	Vomiting, malnutrition, failure to thrive, recurrent respiratory infections, and chronic anemia characterize these infants. Condition may clear spontaneously by 12–18 months of age with conservative treatment (frequent feedings and propping baby in infant seat). Hyperalimentation often necessary. Indications for antireflux procedure include esophagitis, esophageal stricture, significant hiatus hernia, and recurrent and unresponsive pulmonary problems resulting from aspiration. Ventilatory support after repair is often required due to poor general condition of patient as well as preexisting pulmonary infection.
Hemothorax and hemopneumothorax	Usually the result of trauma either accidental or surgically induced. Usually there is coexisting pneumothorax.	Must be drained with thoracostomy tube(s) usually employing local anesthesia. Blood loss into chest cavity may be massive; portions of the lung may become trapped by clotted blood that will not drain via thoracostomy tube, and open thoracotomy may be required to remove clot and re-expand lung. Traumatic left-sided hemothoraxes are more commonly associated with injuries to the great vessels, while those on the right are usually due to injury to the pulmonary hilum. Respiratory support may be necessary during recovery.
Hiatal hernia	Herniation of upper part of the stomach into the left hemithorax; sliding type more common than paraesophageal type.	See gastroesophageal reflux and esophagitis above. Treatment is usually directed at associated gastroesophageal reflux. Chronic aspiration and pulmonary pathology may be significant.
Hyaline membrane disease	Idiopathic respiratory distress syndrome primarily seen in premature newborn as a result of surfactant deficiency. Primarily seen in the premature newborn, but may occur in infants of diabetic mothers at a greater gestational age or those born by cesarean section and under other stressful conditions during labor and delivery.	Hypoaerated and poorly compliant lungs. Long-term ventilatory support may be required. Damage to upper airway may result in subglottic stenosis. Ligation of patent ductus arteriosus may be required during the course of treatment (see text). Bronchopulmonary dysplasia (chronic lung disease) is not an uncommon sequela (see above).

(continued)

TABLE 19-9 (continued). Selected Thoracic Abnormalities and Anesthetic Considerations Requiring Operation in Infants and Children

Condition	Description	Anesthetic and Perioperative Considerations
Kartagener's syndrome	Situs inversus totalis, paranasal sinusitis, bronchiectasis	May require excision of bronchiectatic segments of lung.
Lobar emphysema, congenital	Obstructive emphysema usually of one of upper lobes (left upper lobe, most commonly). May be the result of defective bronchial cartilage to affected lobe.	May cause severe respiratory symptoms in newborn period requiring immediate surgical intervention, or may not become symptomatic for as long as 5 to 6 months. Lobectomy is treatment of choice. Intubation and positive-pressure ventilation may further overinflate the lobe and compromise respiratory exchange in other parts of the lung. During induction of anesthesia, spontaneous ventilation should be preserved until chest is opened and emphysematous lobe is brought out of the operative site. Nitrous oxide should not be used until after lobectomy is accomplished. After the lobectomy is accomplished, the remaining lung tissue should be gently re-expanded under direct vision before closure of the thoracotomy is begun.
Lobar emphysema, acquired	Usually the result of localized obstruction from foreign bodies, inflammatory reaction, extrinsic compression of bronchus or bronchiole by lymph nodes, or tumor in mediastinum. (Extrinsic bronchial compression usually results in atelectasis, but emphysema may rarely result.)	Bronchoscopy is usually required for diagnosis and is therapeutic in the instance of a suspected or known foreign body. (See text—bronchoscopy). Anesthetic considerations similar to those stated above (congenital lobar emphysema).
Lung abscess	In infants and children, usually results from aspiration of infected material when pulmonary defense mechanisms are overwhelmed or when there is serious systemic disease or immunosuppression.	Bronchoscopy may be diagnostic as well as therapeutic. Long-term medical therapy with large doses of intravenous antibiotics plus intermittent bronchoscopy to promote drainage usually suffices. Although resection is difficult in children, it may be accomplished using a balloon-tipped Fogarty catheter placed in the bronchus during bronchoscopy (see text—bronchoscopy).
Lung cysts—bronchogenic	Usually unilobar and thick-walled structures lined with respiratory epithelium; may be located within the lung, mediastinum, or pericardial sac adjacent to main bronchi. Only occasionally communicates with bronchus.	May not be seen on x-ray, but may produce compression of trachea or bronchus. May be difficult to find and to dissect, especially if within the mediastinum. Injury to phrenic nerve or other mediastinal structures may complicate postoperative course.
True congenital lung cysts	May be unilobar or multilobar, with extensive compromise of adjacent lung tissue and other intrathoracic structures.	Communications with bronchial air passages make infection almost inevitable. Appropriate antibiotics and therapeutic bronchoscopy may be indicated prior to excision of cystic lobe, but significant compromise of lung function either from compression or infection may make excision urgent. Postoperative ventilator support, especially in the chronically ill and malnourished infant or child, may be necessary.

(continued)

TABLE 19-9 (*continued*). **Selected Thoracic Abnormalities and Anesthetic Considerations Requiring Operation in Infants and Children**

Condition	Description	Anesthetic and Perioperative Considerations
Mediastinal emphysema (pneumomediastinum)	Air in mediastinum	Often associated with RDS of prematures and in children with respiratory distress from any cause. Usually associated with pneumothorax, which may necessitate drainage via catheter or thoracotomy tube. May be seen after tracheotomy or esophageal or tracheal perforation. Tension pneumothorax or large pneumopericardium resulting in tamponade requires immediate treatment to remove air. Nitrous oxide should not be used as part of anesthetic management in patients with pneumomediastinum or pneumothorax.
Mediastinal masses, cysts, and tumors	Epithelium-lined cystic masses of enteric, neurogenic, bronchogenic or coelomic origin; or solid vascular or granulomatous tumors, malignant or benign, primary or metastatic.	May be asymptomatic, even occasionally, when quite large. Clinical manifestations appear from expanding, space-occupying structure and depend on location. Tracheal or bronchial compression may result in respiratory distress, making thoracotomy urgent. Intubation may be difficult if tracheal deviation is present, and appropriate measures to cope with difficult intubation should be taken before anesthesia is begun, including preparation for bronchoscopy and tracheotomy. May present with respiratory (shortness of breath, positional dyspnea, etc) or cardiovascular (caval compression, positional intolerance, etc) symptoms. *Induction of anesthesia may result in acute airway obstruction and inability to ventilate or cardiovascular collapse.* Ventilatory support may be necessary postoperatively.
Mediastinitis	Severe systemic infection of mediastinal structures. May follow pharyngeal, esophageal, or tracheal perforation from any cause; thoracic or cervical operations complicated by wound infection; or rupture of infected mediastinal lymph nodes.	Incision and drainage and massive antibiotic therapy required. May also require intermittent instillation of bacteriocidal solutions (such as Betadine) via mediastinal drainage tubes. A plastic surgical procedure involving a rectus flap transfer graft is effective in many cases of severe mediastinitis following sternotomy. Ventilatory support usually necessary postoperatively.
Myasthenia gravis	Autoimmune disorder in which acetylcholine receptors in muscle are affected, resulting in weakness. May be seen in pediatric patients even in neonatal period and should always be suspected in infants of mothers with myasthenia. May be on cholinesterase inhibitors.	In infant of myasthenia gravis mother, may be transient or persistent and may require ventilatory support in newborn period. Muscle relaxants as adjunctive anesthetic agents are rarely, if ever, needed in myasthenic patients. Thymectomy may be indicated in patients unresponsive to medical management, and postoperative ventilatory support after thymectomy may be necessary. Cholinesterase inhibitor therapy should be part of the anesthetic considerations.

(*continued*)

TABLE 19-9 (*continued*). **Selected Thoracic Abnormalities and Anesthetic Considerations Requiring Operation in Infants and Children**

Condition	Description	Anesthetic and Perioperative Considerations
Pectus deformities Pectus excavatum	Funnel chest; severity varies from very mild (usually not requiring surgical correction) to severe, requiring early surgical intervention. Usually sporadic incidence, but familial occurrence not rare; may often be seen in patients with Marfan syndrome. Frequently progressive.	Usually thought to be "asymptomatic" in infancy and childhood, but subtle cardiac and pulmonary abnormalities have been shown to be present in many patients and are related to displacement and compression of the heart and to a decrease in intrathoracic volume. Besides the psychologic, cosmetic, and orthopedic reasons for correction, these pathophysiologic changes may become severe with progression over time. Anesthetic considerations during and after repair include the possibility of pneumothorax, and the production of a "flail chest" if surgical dissection is extensive, and postoperative atelectasis from splinting due to pain.
Pectus carinatum	Pigeon breast; usually not apparent at birth, but becomes evident at 3 or 4 years of age. May be seen in patients with Marfan syndrome or congenital heart disease.	The more severe forms may cause compression and displacement of the heart and reduction of intrathoracic volume, as may be seen in pectus excavatum deformities. The same perioperative considerations apply (see above).
Pericardial problems Absence of the pericardium	May be total or partial; left (most common), right, or diaphragmatic. May be associated with congenital diaphragmatic hernia or heart disease. Arises from defective formation of pleuropericardial membrane or of the septum transversum.	Total absence of the pericardium usually does not require surgical correction. Partial defects on the left may result in herniation of ventricles or left atrial appendage with strangulation. Right-sided defects may result in obstruction of the superior vena cava. Surgical treatment includes enlargement of defect to prevent strangulation or closure using a portion of the mediastinal pleura. When associated with diaphragmatic hernia or congenital heart disease, clinical findings usually are primarily due to the associated defect.
Pericardial cysts	Coelomic cyst—rare in childhood	Usually asymptomatic. Surgical removal usually done to establish diagnosis.
Pericarditis (acute)	May be primary (eg, viral, rheumatic, bacterial, postpericardotomy) or a secondary manifestation of systemic disease.	Except for bacterial (purulent) pericarditis, usually self-limited and rarely requires surgical intervention except for removal of fluid if signs of cardiac tamponade are present. Purulent pericarditis is usually secondary to a severe infectious process such as pneumonitis, osteomyelitis, or meningitis—*Staphylococcus aureus* and *H influenzae* most common. Purulent pericarditis requires surgical drainage, vigorous antibiotic therapy, and general postoperatative support measures with close monitoring.
Chronic constrictive pericarditis	Rare in childhood; etiology usually unknown, but may follow purulent or viral pericarditis	Radical pericardectomy via median sternotomy with extensive resection of visceral and parietal pericardium from atria, cavae, and ventricles. Intra- and postoperative monitoring should include arterial and pulmonary artery catheters and urinary output. Postoperative ventilatory support is usually required.

(continued)

TABLE 19-9 (*continued*). Selected Thoracic Abnormalities and Anesthetic Considerations Requiring Operation in Infants and Children

Condition	Description	Anesthetic and Perioperative Considerations
Pericardial effusion with cardiac tamponade	Unusual in childhood, except after cardiovascular surgical procedures, including non-open heart operations.	Cardiac tamponade occurs when blood, fluid, or air within the pericardium interferes with ventricular filling during diastole and reduces stroke volume and cardiac output. Most commonly seen after cardiac surgery and must be considered first in differential diagnosis, if a low cardiac output state exists in such patients. Treatment of acute tamponade in postoperative patient is immediate opening of chest incision to relieve compression and to control bleeding; tamponade in other situations (rheumatic, viral, or bacterial infections) may be treated initially with needle drainage in emergent situations, but almost always requires surgical drainage (see above). Cardiac depressant drugs such as thiopental and the potent inhalational anesthetics should be avoided during anesthesia, as in any patient who has a significantly depressed cardiac output.
Pneumomediastinum	Air in mediastinum	(See mediastinal emphysema above)
Pneumopericardium	Air in the pericardium	May be associated with pneumothorax and pneumomediastinum in premature newborns with RDS. Sufficient quantities of air, like blood or other fluids, may result in cardiac tamponade and require removal by pericardiocentesis.
Pneumothorax	Air in the pleural space	May occur during anesthesia, especially in patients requiring high inflation pressure to expand lungs due to any cause (eg, infants with idiopathic respiratory distress or congenital diaphragmatic hernia). Treatment of significant pneumothorax (probably >30%) is needle aspiration or thoracostomy tube so that the lung can be expanded. The presence of a pneumothorax precludes the use of nitrous oxide during anesthesia, at least until the chest is opened or a thoracotomy tube is inserted. Tension pneumothorax (see below).
Pneumatocele	Emphysematous blebs or cysts resulting from rupture of alveoli so that single or multilocular cavities occur; usually the result of *S aureus* pneumonia, but may be congenital (bullous emphysema).	Pneumatoceles in patients with *S aureus* pneumonia may require thoracostomy drainage to treat respiratory distress or tension pneumothorax. These complications may occur suddenly and without warning.
Phrenic nerve palsy	Traumatic origin	Trauma to either phrenic nerve from birth injury (eg, breech delivery) or surgical trauma (eg, Blalock-Taussig or Blalock-Hanlon operation) results in upward displacement and decreased movement of the ipsilateral diaphragm. Lung volume is decreased and ventilatory exchange impaired. Must be differentiated from eventration of diaphragm or diaphragmatic hernia. Spontaneous recovery may occur, but, occasionally, plication of the diaphragm on the affected side is necessary to improve respiratory function.

(continued)

TABLE 19-9 (*continued*). **Selected Thoracic Abnormalities and Anesthetic Considerations Requiring Operation in Infants and Children**

Condition	Description	Anesthetic and Perioperative Considerations
Poland's syndrome	A spectrum of defects, usually unilateral, in which there is absence of the pectoralis minor and part of pectoralis major muscles, along with defects of costal cartilages and ribs at the sternal insertions, hypoplasia of subcutaneous tissue, and upward displacement and hypoplasia of the nipple and breast on the affected side. Hand deformities may also be associated.	Paradoxic movement with respirations is seen in larger defects. Usually asymptomatic, but may be surgically corrected to prevent progressive deformity of chest wall, as well as for psychological and cosmetic reasons. After correction of larger defects, ventilatory support may be required as with more extensive pectus repairs (see above).
Pulmonary artery sling	Anomalous left pulmonary artery arising from right pulmonary artery and coursing toward the left side over the right mainstem bronchus and behind the lower trachea between the trachea and esophagus.	One of the most severe types of vascular malformations that compress the trachea and esophagus. Compression of right mainstem bronchus may result in obstructive emphysema and/or atelectasis of right lung. Hypoplasia of distal trachea and right bronchus along with defective tracheal and bronchial cartilages make ventilatory management difficult. High incidence of associated congenital cardiac defects (see text—vascular rings).
Pulmonary arteriovenous fistula	Fistulous and often aneurysmal connection between pulmonary artery and vein; may be single, but often multiple. High incidence in patients with Osler-Weber-Rendu hereditary hemorrhagic telangiectasia.	Signs and symptoms depend on the size and extent of shunt of unsaturated blood into the systemic circulation. Cyanosis and polycythemia may be severe. Brain abscess, hemoptysis, or hemorrhage into the pleural space may occur. Congestive heart failure is rare. Surgery is indicated in most cases unless there are multiple fistulae involving both lungs. Anesthetic considerations are the same as with any patient with a right-to-left shunt. Postoperative ventilatory support may be necessary if the dissection is extensive.
Pulmonary sequestration	Accessory lower lobe almost always located in the left hemithorax. Nonfunctioning pulmonary tissue usually with no connection to airway system or pulmonary arterial tree; blood supply from systemic circulation.	May be asymptomatic or may present as recurrent pneumonia in region of left lower lobe. Surgery indicated because of high incidence of infection in sequestered lobes. Aortography to determine origin of blood supply is helpful in avoiding significant blood loss during surgical removal.
Right middle lobe syndrome	Extrinsic compression and obstruction of right middle lobe bronchus resulting in pneumonitis, atelectasis, and eventually bronchiectasis. Compression usually due to mediastinal lymph nodes.	Diagnostic and therapeutic bronchoscopy often required. Persistent or recurrent right middle lobe collapse often makes lobectomy necessary.
Scimitar syndrome	Anomalous venous return from right lung to inferior vena cava with an intact atrial septum.	Correction requires cardiopulmonary bypass. Physiology and hemodynamics similar to that found in secundum atrial septal defects. There may be abnormalities of the lung parenchyma, as well as the pulmonary arterial tree on the right.
Sternal clefts	May vary from small V-shaped defects in upper sternum to complete separation of the sternum with the heart outside the pericardium and the chest wall (ectopia cordis).	With larger clefts, the heart and great vessels are covered only by skin and subcutaneous tissue. Direct closure may compress the heart and lungs. May be associated with diaphragmatic and abdominal wall defects. True ectopia cordis is very rare and carries a grave prognosis, since severe anomalies of the inside of the heart and of the great vessels are invariably present.

(*continued*)

TABLE 19-9 (*continued*). Selected Thoracic Abnormalities and Anesthetic Considerations Requiring Operation in Infants and Children

Condition	Description	Anesthetic and Perioperative Considerations
Subcutaneous emphysema	Air in the subcutaneous tissues.	Usually due to rupture of alveoli into mediastinal structures with subsequent dissection of air into mediastinum and into subcutaneous tissues of chest, neck, and face. May occur after tracheostomy or be associated with pneumothorax and pneumomediastinum in RDS. Treatment directed at underlying cause.
Subglottic stenosis	Narrowing of the cricoid area of the upper airway.	May be congenital, but usually results from trauma due to instrumentation or endotracheal intubation for prolonged periods; usually granulomatous or due to cartilaginous defects. Bronchoscopy often required to determine extent of stenosis, and tracheostomy may be required. Endoscopic resection with laser ablation of granulomatous lesions may result in relief of obstruction, but they may recur.
Tension pneumothorax	Air under pressure in pleural space.	When the amount of air in the pleural space is large enough to cause the intrapleural pressure to exceed atmospheric pressure, the collapsed lung, the heart and other mediastinal structures shift to the opposite side, compressing the other lung. In addition, venous return is impaired and torsion on the great vessels may markedly impair cardiac function; circulatory collapse may occur. Immediate aspiration followed by insertion of a chest tube is mandatory. This may occur during anesthesia or mechanical ventilation.
Thymus conditions	The thymus normally occupies the anterior-superior mediastinum and may give the impression of cardiac enlargement of mediastinal widening on chest x-ray films of young children.	Thymic tissue may extend into the neck, and thymic cysts may occur in these areas, as well as in the mediastinum. Thymic cysts may enlarge rapidly and produce symptoms. Thymic tumors are rare, but may be seen in infancy and childhood.
Tracheal stricture (acquired)		Abnormal mediastinal structures of many varieties may produce significant tracheal (or bronchial) compression and result in severe respiratory distress. Endotracheal intubation or tracheostomy may not relieve the obstruction and selective right or left mainstem bronchial intubation or instrumentation with a rigid bronchoscope may be necessary.
Tracheomalacia	Partial or nearly complete collapse of trachea during inspiration.	Common cause of stridor and partial upper airway obstruction in infants and small children. Due to incomplete formation or weakness of tracheal wall, especially cartilaginous rings. Laryngomalacia produces similar symptoms and is due to weakness or incomplete formation of rigid laryngeal structures. Bronchoscopy and laryngoscopy are often necessary to make the diagnosis and to rule out other causes of upper airway obstructive symptoms (eg, foreign body, subglottic stenosis, vocal cord paralysis, etc).

(*continued*)

TABLE 19-9 (*continued*). Selected Thoracic Abnormalities and Anesthetic Considerations Requiring Operation in Infants and Children

Condition	Description	Anesthetic and Perioperative Considerations
Vascular rings	See text.	See text.
Vocal cord paralysis	May result from birth trauma, damage to recurrent laryngeal nerve during surgical procedures involving chest or neck, or as part of the Arnold-Chiari malformation.	Laryngoscopy with patient breathing spontaneously is necessary to diagnose vocal cord paralysis. Common cause of stridor following transcervical approach for division of tracheoesophageal fistula or cervical esophagostomy for esophageal atresia. May also follow ligation of a patent ductus or a Blalock-Taussig shunt.

the origin of hemoptysis; the investigation of persistent pneumonia or atelectasis; and the workup of a suspected tracheoesophageal fistula (in combination with esophagoscopy).

Therapeutic bronchoscopy in children is usually done to remove aspirated foreign bodies or for the treatment of cystic fibrosis (see below). Removal of foreign bodies may be especially treacherous, depending on the size and nature of the aspirated material, since fragmentation may occur, producing glottic, tracheal, or bilateral mainstem bronchus obstruction. In some cases, the endoscopist may be forced to push the foreign material down into the right or left mainstem bronchus to allow ventilation of the unobstructed air passages. If the foreign body is impacted in a bronchus, a Fogarty catheter may be slipped past the object with the balloon deflated and, once beyond the foreign body, the balloon inflated and pulled toward, or even into, the bronchoscope.[162] If the foreign body material is vegetal (peanut or bean), vegetal or arachidic bronchitis will result, particularly if the object has been present for some time. This condition is characterized by cough, a septic fever pattern, and dyspnea.[163] Treatment includes removal of the foreign body and appropriate antibiotic coverage, as well as chest physiotherapy and postural drainage.[164]

The anesthetic technique for bronchoscopy is tailored to the condition of the patient and the indication for the procedure. Many patients requiring bronchoscopy, either diagnostic or therapeutic, will arrive in the operating room with an intravenous infusion in place so that thiopental in appropriate doses may be used for induction. Atropine is usually given prior to bronchoscopy to avoid untoward vagal reflexes during the procedure. Halothane/nitrous oxide/oxygen or halothane/oxygen can be used as an alternative to an intravenous induction if an intravenous catheter has not been placed. If nitrous oxide is used with halothane and oxygen for induction, it should be discontinued several minutes prior to the insertion of the

bronchoscope to ensure optimal oxygenation during the procedure. Succinylcholine may be needed to facilitate insertion of the appropriate-sized bronchoscope. Once the bronchoscope has passed the cords, the breathing circuit is attached to the side arm of the instrument and ventilation assured. Significant leaks and inadequate ventilation may occur until all the openings at the tip of the bronchoscope have passed beyond the vocal cords. In patients with various forms of chronic lung disease in which the upper airways are deflated (eg, cystic fibrosis), even the largest available bronchoscope may not fill the trachea enough to prevent significant leaks that impair adequate ventilation, particularly in the presence of increased airway resistance. In such cases, the leak can be minimized or eliminated by gently compressing the glottic structures around the bronchoscope with the thumb and index fingers applied to the cricoid cartilage.

Bronchoscopic or laryngoscopic instrumentation of the upper airway always carries with it the possibility of significant laryngeal or subglottic edema, especially in smaller infants and children. Management of this complication includes postoperative humidification of inspired gases, adequate hydration, intermittent positive-pressure breathing or racemic epinephrine (0.5 mL of racemic epinephrine diluted with 3.5 mL of normal saline) every 2 to 3 hours, and dexamethasone.[165] Endotracheal intubation may be required if these measures do not suffice.

Bronchography may be necessary to define the extent of certain parenchymal diseases of the lung, such as segmental bronchiectasis. Contrast material is introduced with a catheter passed via the bronchoscope or an endotracheal tube, depending on the ease with which the catheter can be placed into the desired area of the bronchial tree. This procedure is usually done in the radiology department in order to use fluoroscopy, and the patient may need to be turned into several positions to obtain adequate diagnostic films. After the necessary radiographs are obtained, as much

TABLE 19-10.   Cardiovascular Procedures in Infants and Children Not Requiring Cardiopulmonary Bypass

Procedure	Description	Anesthetic and Perioperative Considerations
Blalock-Hanlon atrial septectomy	Surgical excision of atrial septum to increase mixing of systemic and pulmonary venous blood in patients with transposition of the great arteries.	Rashkind balloon septostomy at cardiac catheterization may prove inadequate, and surgical intervention will be needed to provide adequate mixing. Patients are cyanotic and usually manifest the signs and symptoms of congestive heart failure. Surgical septostomy is done through a right thoracotomy and may involve inflow occlusion and cardiac standstill. Resuscitative drugs and the ability to replace blood rapidly are important considerations for the anesthesiologist. Nitrous oxide/narcotic/relaxant anesthetic techniques are usually employed. Postoperative ventilatory support is usually required.
Blalock-Taussig shunt	Anastomosis of the right or left subclavian artery (depending on the presence of a right or left aortic arch) to the pulmonary artery to increase inadequate pulmonary blood flow for patients with tetralogy of Fallot physiology (pulmonary stenosis and right to left shunt through a ventricular septal defect, atrial septal defect, patent ductus, or patent foramen ovale). May be "modified" to use an interposed synthetic tube graft between subclavian and pulmonary arteries.	Hypoxemia usually severe. Anatomy of intracardiac defects usually precludes total correction, although age and size may influence selection of surgical procedure for a given defect. Anastomosis may be surgically difficult due to small size of subclavian artery, and heparinization is necessary to ensure patency. This requires the expectation of postoperative bleeding and blood replacement, as well as maintenance of at least partial heparinization to keep shunt from clotting. Postoperative ventilatory support may be necessary, but excessive inspiratory pressures must be avoided to minimize the ventilatory effects on intrathoracic blood flow.
Waterston	Anastomosis of the ascending aorta to the right pulmonary artery to increase pulmonary blood flow for patients with tetralogy of Fallot physiology (see above).	Same anesthetic considerations as with Blalock-Taussig shunts; Waterston shunts may kink pulmonary artery and result in differential pulmonary blood flow and make total correction of associated defect more difficult. Technically easier to perform than Blalock-Taussig shunt, but more difficult to correct when total correction of defect is anticipated. "Overshunting" may occur, resulting in congestive heart failure.
Pulmonary artery banding	Used to decrease torrential flow to lungs in large left to right shunts in which increased pulmonary blood volume results in congestive heart failure and pulmonary edema. May be used in conjunction with Blalock-Hanlon atrial septostomy to decrease pulmonary flow while increasing intracardiac mixing in patients with transposition of the great arteries or in patients with associated ventricular septal defects.	Congestive heart failure usually predominates the clinical picture. Preoperative ventilatory support with PEEP or CPAP is often required prior to surgery as well as in the immediate postoperative period. Nitrous/narcotic/relaxant anesthetic techniques are usually employed for these patients.
Coarctation of the aorta	Symptomatic coarctation of the aorta in infancy is usually associated with other congenital cardiac anomalies including ventricular septal defects, patent ductus, aortic stenosis, and transposition of the great arteries. In childhood, but beyond infancy, coarctation of the aorta is usually asymptomatic and is less often associated with other congenital heart defects except for a bicuspid aortic valve with or without stenosis or insufficiency. Systemic arterial hypertension usually accompanies isolated coarctation and may represent the presenting abnormality.	Congestive heart failure from obstructive circulatory disease usually predominates clinically, and preoperative ventilatory support along with medical anticongestive measures are often necessary. After subclavian flap angioplasty or primary repair of infantile coarctation by end-to-end repair, postoperative ventilation is useful in treating residual pulmonary edema. Mild hypothermia (34°C) is used for spinal cord protection. Postcoarctectomy hypertension readily responds to esmolol.

(continued)

TABLE 19-10 (*continued*). Cardiovascular Procedures in Infants and Children Not Requiring Cardiopulmonary Bypass

Procedure	Description	Anesthetic and Perioperative Considerations
Division of vascular rings	Pathophysiology results from vascular malformations that compress the trachea, bronchi, or esophagus.	See text.
Ligation and/or division of patent ductus arteriosus	Persistent patent ductus arteriosus occurs as an isolated anomaly, associated with complex congenital heart disease or with respiratory disorders of the newborn, such as idiopathic RDS of premature infants or in association with persistent fetal circulation of the stressed newborn.	Asymptomatic persistent patency of the ductus arteriosus requires surgical correction as an elective procedure and should be treated as such by the anesthesiologist. The anesthetic and immediate postoperative considerations are relatively simple and encompass the usual precautions undertaken during any type of elective thoracotomy. Sophisticated monitoring techniques in uncomplicated patent ductus are not usually necessary. An intercostal bupivacaine block from within the thorax prior to closure is often useful in preventing respiratory complications in the immediate postoperative period. Ligation of the ductus arteriosus in the premature newborn with respiratory distress is discussed in the text.
Pacemaker implantation	Implantation of permanent epicardial pacing electrode and abdominal wall or intrathoracic power source is required in symptomatic infants with congenital complete heart block and in young patients who develop complete heart block after intracardiac repair of congenital or acquired defects.	Transvenous or temporary epicardial pacing may be warranted prior to induction of anesthesia regardless of the anesthetic technique used. Since children may require a much higher stimulating threshold than adults, care should be taken at the time of surgery that the diaphragm is not stimulated to contract by the pacing signal. The use of nondepolarizing muscle relaxants may mask diaphragmatic pacing. A carefully controlled, constant infusion of succinylcholine can be used at the time of determination of required pacemaker threshold.
Central Gortex shunts	Prosthetic material used to connect pulmonary artery to aorta to increase pulmonary blood flow.	Same anesthetic considerations as with Blalock-Taussig shunts. Blood loss through wall of prosthesis may be massive, especially if heparinization is required to prevent thrombosis.
Glenn shunt	Anastomosis of superior vena cava to main pulmonary artery to increase pulmonary blood flow in patients with tricuspid atresia and decreased pulmonary flow.	Has become popular in a "modified" form (superior vena cava end-to-side to pulmonary artery) as either first stage or part of definitive Fontan-type repair. CVP catheters in SVC should be positioned distally. Will reveal pulmonary artery pressure after repair.
Aortopulmonary artery anastomosis (creation of aorticopulmonary window)	Done to increase pulmonary blood flow.	Can sometimes be done without cardiopulmonary bypass if anatomy of great vessels allows partial occlusion side-biting clamps to be used during the anastomosis.

of the contrast material as possible is suctioned from the bronchial tree. Anesthesia should be sufficiently deep to prevent coughing when the contrast is introduced, since coughing may spread the material and result in poor-quality radiographs.

Anesthesia for bronchography is similar to that for bronchoscopy using either an intravenous induction and halothane/oxygen maintenance or an inhalation induction as described above. If an endotracheal tube is used instead of a bronchoscope to pass the contrast catheter, a curved 15 mm connector with a removable cap "chimney" side arm is used so that ventilation can be maintained while manipulation of the catheter is under way.

Flexible fiberoptic bronchoscopy is a technique that has several important uses in pediatrics,[166,167] including bronchial lavage (see below). This technique is well suited for evaluation of the upper airway and for evaluation of tracheostomies. The fiberoptic bronchoscope may be used to intubate infants and children who have difficult airways, such as those with Pierre-Robin syndrome.

Although this procedure can be done with topical anesthesia and intravenous sedation, especially in older children, another technique is often used. General anesthesia is induced using an inhalation induction with O_2 and halothane by mask. It is important to remember that in children who have partial airway obstruction, the time needed to accomplish an inhalation induction may be quite prolonged. Once an adequate level of general anesthesia and a secure intravenous catheter have been established, and with the patient breathing spontaneously, a face mask with a hole cut into it above the connection to the breathing circuit is used. The flexible bronchoscope is passed through the hole into the nose. The airway can then be evaluated. Using this technique, the patient is kept well anesthetized and well oxygenated since oxygen and halothane are being breathed during airway visualization. Since the child is breathing spontaneously, vocal cord motion can also be evaluated. If the procedure is being done to secure the airway, an endotracheal tube can be passed over the bronchoscope through the mask and into the trachea. This should be done expeditiously since in infants, nearly complete airway obstruction will exist as long as both the bronchoscope and the endotracheal tube are in the trachea. Currently, ultrathin flexible fiberoptic bronchoscopes are available in sizes small enough to allow passage of a 3.0 mm endotracheal tube.

Bronchoscopy and bronchial lavage in patients with cystic fibrosis (and other chronic lung diseases) are done to attempt to open airways obstructed by thick inspissated secretions characteristic of these conditions. Lavage is done using generous amounts of half-normal saline and dilute sodium bicarbonate as well as diluted acetylcystine.

These patients are often quite ill, with borderline or overt respiratory failure, superimposed pneumonia, and cor pulmonale. The anesthetic management must take into account all of these factors. The uptake of the inhalation agents is slow due to the lung disease, and the cardiovascular depressant effects of induction doses of barbiturates may preclude their use. Narcotics are also relatively contraindicated in these patients due to their suppression of the cough reflex. Intravenous ketamine, 1 to 2 mg/kg, along with diazepam, 0.1 to 0.2 mg/kg, have been used for induction.[168] Additional doses of each of these drugs may be necessary, but are usually not required if the procedure is not prolonged. Very small incremental doses of thiopental, 0.5 to 1.0 mg/kg, have also been added to this regimen in some patients. Atropine is not contraindicated in patients with cystic fibrosis undergoing bronchoscopy, since its drying properties are minimal if given intravenously prior to the administration of ketamine and succinylcholine. It should be used during bronchoscopy in such patients to avoid undesired vagal responses from succinylcholine and manipulation of the airway.

Esophagoscopy

Indications for upper gastrointestinal tract endoscopy include management of acquired or congenital esophageal stricture, evaluation of the extent and degree of caustic or acid burns of the esophagus, removal of foreign bodies, determination of the extent of reflux esophagitis in patients with dysfunction of the gastroesophageal sphincter, identification and treatment of esophageal varices, and evaluation of a tracheoesophageal fistula in conjunction with bronchoscopy. The flexible fiberoptic esophagogastroscope is sometimes used in children; however, the rigid instruments are usually employed, especially in the removal of foreign bodies and in the management of esophageal strictures, the most common reasons for esophagoscopy in the pediatric patient.[169]

In adult patients, sedation may suffice along with topical anesthesia for upper gastrointestinal endoscopy. However, patient cooperation is necessary; for this reason, general anesthesia is almost always required in the pediatric age group. The exception to this may be for the removal of coins in the esophagus, which can sometimes be accomplished using light sedation and insertion of a Foley catheter into the esophagus through the nose. Under fluoroscopic visualization, the coin is pulled from the esophagus by inflating the balloon tip as it lies beyond the coin.[170]

For many patients undergoing esophagoscopy, a rapid-sequence induction using preoxygenation, thiopental, succinylcholine, and cricoid pressure is probably the safest method, especially if there is known to be esophageal dilation above a stricture with the possibility of retained material. A few small infants may require awake intubation (see discussion on tracheoesophageal fistula). Elective esophagoscopy for other conditions can be safely done using an inhalation induction. Maintenance of anesthesia after intubation of the trachea is accomplished with deep levels of inhalational agents, since light levels of anesthesia that allow coughing or movement may result in esophageal or pharyngeal perforation and must be avoided.

In very small infants, the esophagoscope may impinge on the endotracheal tube and cause obstruction. This complication, as well as the possibility of accidental extubation during the procedure, must be watched for at all times. Stridor may also result after esophagoscopy and should be managed as outlined in the section on bronchoscopy. Sharp foreign bodies may perforate small or major blood vessels, and significant bleeding may require blood replacement.

Congenital Diaphragmatic Hernia

Congenital diaphragmatic hernia (CDH) presenting in the immediate newborn period is one of the most life-threatening, yet surgically correctable conditions encountered by the anesthesiologist. The incidence of CDH is approximately 1 in 5,000 live births.[171–173] Despite advances in surgical, anesthetic, and neonatal intensive care in the last 25 years, the overall mortality for infants with CDH presenting in the first 6 hours of life remains between 40 and 60 percent.[173–179]

Congenital diaphragmatic hernia is classified according to the anatomic location of the diaphragmatic defect. Herniation of abdominal viscera may occur at any of three diaphragmatic locations: the posterolateral foramen of Bochdalek, the anterior foramen of Morgagni, or the esophageal hiatus (Figs. 19-7 and 19-8). Unilateral Bochdalek hernias account for more than 80 percent of all defects and are the most likely to present with severe symptoms in the neonatal period. Left-sided defects are four to five times more frequent than right-sided defects, and bilateral defects are rare. Two to four percent of hernias are of the Morgagni type. These are anteriorly located, tend to be small, and typically present well beyond the neonatal period. Symptoms are usually mild and diagno-

sis is occasionally made as an incidental finding on chest radiograph. Hiatal hernias account for the remainder and also typically present beyond the newborn period, with gastrointestinal rather than pulmonary findings.[171,173]

Embryologically, the earliest precursor of the diaphragm is the septum transversum, formed at approximately 4 weeks' gestation from mesenchyme located between the heart and coelomic cavity. It is joined by the dorsal mesentery of the foregut to form the central tendon of the developing diaphragm. At this time, the pleuroperitoneal cavity exists as a single, undivided space. From the developing central tendon and from the posterolateral coelomic wall, pleuroperitoneal folds develop and gradually extend medially to divide the cavity into distinct pleural and peritoneal compartments. An ingrowth of mesenchyme between the layers of the pleuroperitoneal membrane provides the muscular component. Closure is usually complete by the ninth week of gestation, the posterolateral portions being the last to close and the right side closing earlier than the left. Coincident with development and closure of the diaphragm, the developing midgut undergoes rapid elongation in the umbilical stalk and returns to the peritoneal cavity. If either the gut returns prematurely or diaphragmatic closure is delayed, herniation of abdominal viscera into the pleural cavity may occur.[171,173,180,181]

The presence of abdominal viscera within the fetal pleural space results in a maturational disturbance of the developing lung. Necropsy specimens of lungs of infants dying of CDH are remarkable for a decrease in total lung mass, a severe reduction in the number of airway generations, and a parallel reduction in alveolar number. The ipsilateral lung, especially the ipsilateral lower lobe, is more severely affected than the contralateral. Associated abnormalities are present within the pulmonary vascular tree. The main pulmonary arteries are small in proportion to the reduced lung mass, and there is a reduction in vascular tree branching generations. Also, there is muscular hypertrophy of the media with the presence of smooth muscle within the walls of small-diameter vessels normally devoid of a muscular component.[175,182–184]

Infants born with the common left-sided Bochdalek hernia frequently present with the classic triad of cyanosis, dyspnea (respiratory distress), and cardiac dextroposition. Physical findings may include tachypnea, nasal flaring, suprasternal and subcostal retractions, an abnormally scaphoid abdomen, and unilateral or bilateral diminished breath sounds. Audible peristaltic sounds over the affected hemithorax may be present, but this is an inconsistent finding. Anteroposterior chest radiographs demonstrate a shift of mediastinal structures to the side opposite the hernia, as

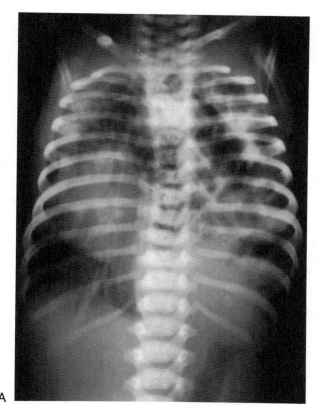

Fig. 19-7. (A & B) Two different newborn patients with congenital diaphragmatic hernias through the foramen of Bochdalek. Preoperative chest radiographs show intestinal organs mostly within the left hemithorax and herniation of the mediastinal structures into the right side; there is absence of most gas shadows from the abdomen, except for a small amount in the stomach and descending colon.

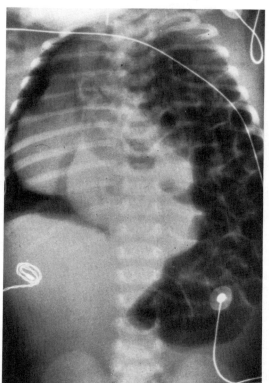

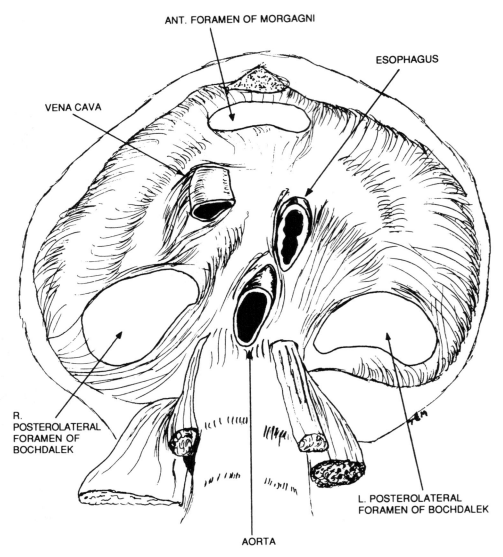

ANT. FORAMEN OF MORGAGNI

ESOPHAGUS

VENA CAVA

R.
POSTEROLATERAL
FORAMEN OF
BOCHDALEK

L. POSTEROLATERAL
FORAMEN OF BOCHDALEK

AORTA

Fig. 19-8. Sites of potential herniation in congenital diaphragmatic hernia.

well as air-filled bowel loops within the thoracic cavity. The abdomen generally shows a paucity of gas, and a nasogastric tube placed for gastrointestinal decompression may be found to have the tip located within the thorax. If the diagnosis remains unclear, air or radiopaque contrast material may be instilled through the nasogastric tube to better delineate the location of the gastrointestinal tract.[171,173] Both age at presentation and the severity of symptoms have prognostic significance. Those infants with the greatest degree of pulmonary hypoplasia and associated pulmonary vascular disease present early on the first day of life. Mortality is correspondingly greater for those infants diagnosed at less than 6 hours of age and remains at approximately 50 percent despite treatment.

Infants presenting beyond 18 to 24 hours of age have less severe anatomic and physiologic derangements and can be expected to have near 100 percent survival.[174,185]

Associated congenital anomalies occur in approximately 10 to 30 percent of infants with CDH.[174,176] The incidence of other anomalies is approximately two times as frequent in right-sided as opposed to left-sided defects.[5] A wide range of associated malformations has been reported affecting virtually every organ system, and may occur in isolation or as a part of multiple anomalies within a single patient. As expected, mortality is increased in the presence of major associated anomalies.[176,186] This is particularly true when the cardiovascular system is involved. In Green-

TABLE 19-11.   Associated Anomalies Found in Infants With Congenital Diaphragmatic Hernias

Organ System	Malformation
Cardiovascular	Any form of cyanotic or acyanotic defect
Gastrointestinal	Tracheoesophageal fistula, malrotation, various atresias, omphalocoele
Genitourinary	Hypospadius, hydronephrosis, renal dysplasia
Central nervous system	Spina bifida defects, hydrocephalus, cerebral dysgenesis
Musculoskeletal	Syndactyly, amelias
Chromosomal	Trisomy 18, trisomy 21

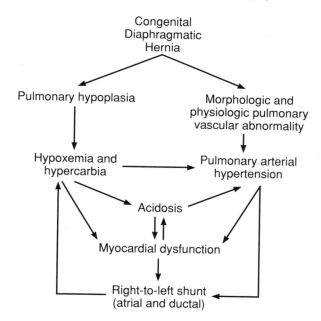

Fig. 19-9. Cycle of pathophysiologic events that occur in infants with severe congenital diaphragmatic hernias.

wood et al's series of 48 infants, 23 percent had associated cardiovascular abnormalities. Mortality in this group was 73 percent in contrast to a 27 percent mortality in those without cardiac abnormalities.[186] Table 19-11 provides a representative inventory of reported anomalies categorized by organ system.[174,176]

The pathophysiologic derangements produced by CDH are a consequence both of pulmonary parenchymal hypoplasia and abnormalities in structure and function of the pulmonary vasculature. Affected infants can be broadly classified into three physiologic categories. The first group comprises those infants who experience severe compression of fetal lung buds producing profound bilateral pulmonary hypoplasia, prohibiting extrauterine survival regardless of therapeutic interventions. On the other extreme are those infants who have only mild ipsilateral pulmonary hypoplasia and near-normal pulmonary vascular hemodynamics and in whom near 100 percent survival is anticipated. Comprising the third group are those infants with more severe pulmonary maldevelopment accompanied by a *persistent fetal circulation*.[187] Survival of infants in this group is in large degree influenced by proper therapeutic management, although overall mortality remains at approximately 50 percent. It is toward this group that current research is directed in an effort to diminish the high mortality.

Figure 19-9 summarizes the pathophysiologic alterations accompanying large Bochdalek hernias. Functionally, the lungs of affected infants are noncompliant because of the severe reduction in lung mass and a relative deficiency of surfactant.[177,178,188] This results in altered gas exchange leading to hypercarbia and hypoxemia. Supranormal inflating pressures and respiratory rates to provide adequate tidal volume and minute ventilation often result in significant barotrauma, and contralateral pneumothorax is not uncommon.[176]

Pulmonary vascular hypertension occurs as a consequence of reduced total cross-sectional area of the pulmonary vascular bed, abnormal muscularity of pulmonary vessels, and abnormal hypersensitivity of the vessels to vasoconstrictor stimuli, principally hypercarbia and hypoxia. Acidosis, hypothermia, and elevated airway pressures also may contribute to sustained elevations in PVR.[175,182,189,190] With patency of the ductus arteriosus the parallel arrangement of the pulmonary and systemic circulation characteristic of the fetal circulatory pattern persists. The magnitude and direction of flow of right ventricular output will depend on the relative resistance to flow within the two vascular beds: pulmonary via the pulmonary artery and systemic via the ductus arteriosus. In the face of significantly increased PVR, flow will be preferentially directed right-to-left across the ductus arteriosus, further contributing to systemic hypoxemia. A right-to-left shunt also may occur at the atrial level as right ventricular and right atrial pressures increase due to elevated right ventricular afterload. Left atrial pressure may coincidentally decrease due to a falling pulmonary venous return, further contributing to an atrial pressure gradient that favors right-to-left shunting of blood. Primary myocardial dysfunction occurs as a consequence of elevated afterload, persistent hypoxemia, and acidosis. Left ventricular hypoplasia, perhaps due to in utero mediastinal compression, may also be present in infants with CDH.[191]

The combined effect of these pathophysiologic alterations is the establishment of a vicious cycle of hypoxemia, hypercarbia, pulmonary hypertension, myocardial dysfunction, and right-to-left shunting of blood through persistent fetal channels. If uninterrupted, this sequence of events ultimately proves fatal. The goal of preoperative stabilization and subsequent intraoperative anesthetic management is to interrupt this cycle. The focus of management is the reduction of PVR and associated right-to-left shunts. This is accomplished through a combination of optimizing ventilation, supporting myocardial function, and correcting metabolic derangements (acidosis, electrolytes, glucose, temperature).

Once the diagnosis of CDH is made, all patients should be placed in an oxygen-enriched atmosphere. A large-gauge nasogastric tube (10 to 14 Fr) should be inserted to decompress the stomach and prevent further accumulation of air, which will adversely affect ventilatory mechanics. If respiratory distress and cyanosis persist, endotracheal intubation should be accomplished after preoxygenation with 100 percent oxygen. Muscle relaxants and intravenous narcotics may be used to facilitate intubation, but positive-pressure ventilation by mask should be minimized so that further gastrointestinal distention does not occur. For this reason, awake intubation by skilled personnel may be preferable. Neuromuscular blockade is usually advisable to facilitate ventilation and to avoid wide swings in airway pressure that may adversely affect pulmonary hemodynamics. An attempt should be made to produce a respiratory alkalosis while maintaining the lowest possible mean airway pressure and peak inspiratory pressure. In the face of significant primary pulmonary hypertension, elevation of pH above 7.5 is often required to induce pulmonary vasodilation of a degree sufficient to reduce right-to-left shunting.[192] Ventilatory parameters necessary to achieve this goal will obviously vary according to the degree of pulmonary hypoplasia. Indeed, hypocarbia may not be attainable despite high airway pressures and respiratory rates in the most severely affected infants. Prognostically, this is a very ominous sign. An additional risk directly related to the severity of pulmonary hypoplasia and the magnitude of ventilatory support efforts is the development of a contralateral pneumothorax, which should be suspected whenever an acute deterioration in oxygenation or hemodynamics occurs.[176] Prompt therapy is mandatory as the attendant hypoxemia, acidosis, and hemodynamic compromise can result in abrupt increases in PVR and a return to a fetal circulatory pattern that may have previously been corrected. The development of a pneumothorax in the perioperative period is associated with a high mortality (75 to 80 percent), and early use of neuromuscular blockade appears to reduce its incidence.[176] Some centers advocate placement of a prophylactic chest tube in the contralateral hemithorax at or before repair to prevent this potentially catastrophic complication.

While ventilatory management will be the primary focus of preoperative stabilization, several other points should be addressed. A warm environment is essential and the temperature of the environment and infant should be monitored throughout the perioperative period because of the adverse effects of hypothermia on oxygen consumption and acid-base balance. Metabolic acidosis should be judiciously treated with intravenous $NaHCO_3$ as an adjunct to elevating pH to a level beneficial to the pulmonary vasculature and myocardial performance. The dosage is calculated according to the following formula:

$$NaHCO_3 \text{ (mEq)} = \text{body wt (kg)} \times \text{base deficit} \times 0.3\text{–}0.5*$$

Intravenous fluids should be provided at a basal level of 50 to 60 mg/kg/d of 10 percent dextrose in water. Additional fluids may be required and should be administered based on assessment of hemodynamics, electrolytes, and urine output. If volume supplementation fails to correct hemodynamics and urine flow, addition of an inotrope should be considered. Isoproterenol, 0.1 to 1.0 μg/kg/min, has the theoretic advantage of pulmonary vasodilation, but dopamine, 1 to 10 μg/kg/min, has been used successfully in this clinical situation.[192–195]

Theoretically, selective dilatation of the pulmonary vasculature would result in a reduction of pulmonary artery pressure, increase of pulmonary blood flow, and correction of right-to-left shunting at the ductal and atrial levels. Unfortunately, no specific pulmonary vasodilator exists. A variety of vasodilating agents have been used in the setting of primary pulmonary hypertension.[187] Tolazoline is probably the most widely used and studied agent for this purpose. The pharmacologic mechanism of action of tolazoline is complex. Its vasodilating properties have been ascribed to alpha-adrenergic antagonism, a direct effect on vascular smooth muscle, histaminergic agonist effects, and cholinergic agonist effects.[196] It possesses both systemic as well as pulmonary vasodilating effects, although the relative effect on the two beds is variable. In one study of infants monitored with pulmonary artery catheters, the combination of dop-

---

* The volume of distribution of bicarbonate is increased in the newborn period due to an increased amount of extracellular water.

amine with tolazoline resulted in a decrease in the pulmonary artery pressure to systemic arterial pressure (SAP) ratio.[192] Tolazoline may be administered to neonates with refractory hypoxemia (postductal PaO_2 <60 mmHg) at an initial dose of 1 to 2 mg/kg as a bolus, followed by continuous intravenous infusion of 1 to 4 mg/kg/h. There is a theoretic advantage to delivering the infusion directly into the pulmonary artery and monitoring pulmonary artery pressures, although this is technically difficult and time-consuming to achieve. Those who respond to tolazoline will almost invariably do so within the first 2 hours of therapy. Response is quite variable, and, if a beneficial response occurs, it may not be sustained.[173] Adverse effects of tolazoline therapy include severe systemic hypotension, cutaneous flushing, gastrointestinal and pulmonary hemorrhage, thrombocytopenia, renal insufficiency, and seizures. Its reported half-life in neonates ranges from 3.3 to 33 hours, and persistence of pharmacologic effect must be anticipated for several hours after discontinuation of infusion.[196] Because of tolazoline's unpredictable hemodynamic effects, the frequency of other adverse effects, and its duration of action, its use should probably be restricted to those infants who are unlikely to survive with more conventional therapy.

Traditional wisdom has dictated that severely symptomatic infants with CDH undergo surgical repair as early as possible. This approach is based on the assumption that surgical decompression of the herniated viscera will result in prompt improvement in pulmonary mechanics and gas exchange. The premise is that mechanical compression of the lung is the major factor in pulmonary dysfunction of CDH. This traditional approach is currently undergoing re-evaluation. Several investigators have demonstrated that the condition of many infants may be substantially improved prior to operative repair if a longer period of preoperative stabilization is allowed.[194,195,197] This may be associated with a significant decrease in early mortality. Preoperative stabilization is continued until no further improvements in metabolic, pulmonary, or hemodynamic condition can be achieved. This end point is generally attainable within 4 to 18 hours of arrival in a tertiary care facility. This approach is particularly advocated for those infants with the most severe derangements of cardiorespiratory function in order to optimize their condition prior to operative intervention. None of the studies have shown a detrimental effect on mortality by using this strategy.[194,195,197] In support of this view is the work of Bohn, who studied pulmonary compliance pre- and postoperatively in infants with CDH. Not only did operative reduction of the hernia fail to im-

prove this measure of pulmonary function, it actually had a detrimental effect on compliance in seven of nine infants studied, improved compliance in one infant, and had no significant effect on measured compliance in the remaining patient.[195]

Routine intraoperative monitors should be used for all neonates undergoing operative repair of CDH. However, additional monitoring is nearly always required for these infants due to the severity of their illness and the peculiar pathophysiologic derangements characteristic of their disease. Breath sounds should be continuously monitored with a precordial stethoscope placed over the contralateral hemithorax to facilitate early detection of a pneumothorax. An arterial catheter is indicated for frequent sampling of arterial blood gases as well as continuous blood pressure monitoring. Right radial artery cannulation is preferred, as this supplies a measure of preductal blood perfusing the cerebral circulation. Umbilical artery catheters with their tip in the postductal aorta provide a better assessment of the total magnitude of the right-to-left shunt (atrial and ductal). While two arterial catheters may be ideal (pre- and postductal), a reasonable alternative is to place a pulse oximeter probe on an extremity with a ductal location opposite that of the arterial catheter (ie, preductal if the arterial catheter is postductal, or vice versa). Reliable venous access is essential for the administration of blood products, fluids, and medications. Peripheral intravenous catheters should be preferentially placed in upper extremities, as abdominal closure following reduction of the hernia carries the potential for compromise of lower extremity venous return. Central venous catheter insertion via an internal jugular vein will provide reliable venous access. Additionally, it can provide useful information regarding right-sided filling pressures and venous oxygen saturation. A urinary catheter should also be used for continuous monitoring of urine volume and intermittent assessment of urinary chemistries and concentration. The latter measurements may have greater importance postoperatively, as it has recently been demonstrated that CDH infants may develop a syndrome consistent with SIADH (syndrome of inappropriate secretion of antidiuretic hormone) in the postoperative period.[198]

Surgical repair of a diaphragmatic hernia is usually carried out through an abdominal approach with the patient in the supine position. The hernia is reduced by gentle traction on the intestine and the diaphragmatic defect closed by direct suture. Prior to diaphragmatic closure, a chest tube is placed in the ipsilateral pleural space and connected to waterseal. Large defects may require the use of a prosthetic graft to achieve closure. If the patient's condition permits,

Ladd's procedure is performed for correction of associated malrotation. Abdominal closure follows, which also may require incorporation of prosthetic material depending on the severity of cardiorespiratory compromise associated with this part of the procedure.

Anesthetic management of the infant undergoing repair of CDH primarily consists of intraoperatively continuing those therapeutic maneuvers used during preoperative stabilization. Sufficient depth of anesthesia is required to minimize sympathetic responses to surgical stimulation that could adversely affect pulmonary vascular resistance. A stable systemic and pulmonary hemodynamic state needs to be maintained. This can usually be provided with a basic narcotic-oxygen-relaxant anesthetic technique. Nitrous oxide should be avoided for several reasons. First, it increases the potential for overdistention of the bowel, leading to further respiratory embarrassment. Second, use of nitrous oxide in significant concentrations will, by necessity, limit the concentration of delivered oxygen. In the most severely affected neonates, 100 percent oxygen is almost always required because of its beneficial effect of lowering PVR. Third, there is the theoretic concern that nitrous oxide, independent of its effect on lowering F_IO_2, may have pulmonary vasoconstrictive properties. In premature neonates at risk for retinopathy of prematurity who are maintaining PaO_2 in excess of 100 mmHg, air may be added to the inspired gas to achieve a safe reduction in F_IO_2.

Fentanyl in a total dose of 10 to 50 μg/kg will usually provide adequate depth of anesthesia while maintaining stable hemodynamics. Fentanyl is administered in 2 to 5 μg/kg boluses, assessing hemodynamic response between doses. A minimum of 10 μg/kg administered prior to initial surgical incision is usual. If surgical stimulation results in excessive elevations of pulse or blood pressure, or if there is evidence of increasing right-to-left shunt, further incremental doses of narcotic are administered until stability is restored. Small concentrations of one of the volatile agents may be used as an adjunct to narcotics in the more stable patients undergoing repair.

Neuromuscular blockade is a necessary adjunct to the chosen anesthetic. Paralysis facilitates surgical repair of the defect, especially diaphragmatic and abdominal closure. Additionally, it minimizes fluctuations in airway pressure that may adversely affect PVR and increase the likelihood of a contralateral pneumothorax. Pancuronium is usually given for this purpose, since it provides prolonged neuromuscular blockade and does not result in significant histamine release.

Intraoperatively, ventilation is probably better controlled by hand than by machine. Most researchers recommend maintaining peak inspiratory pressures below 30 cmH_2O to avoid adverse effects on pulmonary blood flow and to reduce the potential for pneumothorax. Rapid rates of 60 to 120 breaths/min may be required. The goal is to produce hypocarbia at the lowest feasible peak and mean airway pressures. Any sudden change in compliance or oxygen saturation may indicate a contralateral pneumothorax, which should be immediately investigated and treated. Following reduction of the herniated viscera, vigorous attempts to inflate the hypoplastic ipsilateral lung should be avoided since it is usually futile and increases the potential for contralateral pneumothorax. During abdominal closure, it is important to pay close attention to changes in compliance and hemodynamics. Excessive elevations of intra-abdominal pressure associated with closure of the abdominal wall may impede both ventilation and venous return from the lower half of the body. Creation of a ventral hernia by closing only skin without fascial closure is one option. Silastic prostheses, such as those used for repair of abdominal wall defects, may be required in extreme cases.

Throughout the intraoperative course, frequent sampling of arterial blood for measurement of blood gases, glucose, electrolytes, and hematocrit is necessary. Maintenance fluid consisting of 10 percent dextrose in water is supplemented with sodium chloride. Third space losses may be high (5 to 10 mL/kg/h) and are replaced with isotonic fluid as indicated by pulse, blood pressure, CVP, and urine volume. Serum glucose requires frequent monitoring since infants may become hyperglycemic while receiving 10 percent dextrose. Substitution of lesser concentrations of dextrose may be necessary to avoid hyperglycemia and osmotic diuresis. Blood loss is usually small, but blood should be available and administered to maintain a hematocrit of 40 percent or greater.

At the termination of surgery, infants are transported to the neonatal intensive care unit with the endotracheal tube in place. Ventilation with 100 percent oxygen is continued; neuromuscular blockers are not reversed and narcotic administration at a dosage of 2 to 5 μg/kg/h of fentanyl is maintained. Provisions for proper temperature maintenance and monitoring should be made for transport. Therapy directed at alleviating PFC is continued in the intensive care unit. The duration of ventilatory assistance and choice of other therapeutic modalities will depend on the infant's response in the early postoperative period.

As stated earlier, CDH infants fall into one of three general categories based on the severity of their disease. One group is characterized by mild pathophysiologic derangements, has minimal pulmonary hypoplasia, does not revert to a fetal circulatory pattern, and requires little special postoperative management.

Occasionally, these patients may even be candidates for tracheal extubation at the end of the operative procedure. A second group of patients is characterized by such severe bilateral pulmonary hypoplasia that survival is impossible, despite the use of all currently available means of support. The CDH in the remaining group of infants is intermediate in severity, and survival is in large degree dependent on proper therapeutic management. Most of these infants will experience a postoperative period of adequate oxygenation (the "honeymoon" period). Ventilatory and pharmacologic therapy aimed at reducing PVR may sustain oxygenation, allowing for gradual weaning of support and ultimate survival. In others, the honeymoon period is transient, followed by a reversion to a fetal circulatory pattern and attendant severe hypoxemia. Finally, some infants who are potentially salvageable may never experience a honeymoon period. Severe pulmonary vascular hypertension, right-to-left shunting, and persistent hypoxemia are manifest in the immediate postoperative period and are not amenable to conventional therapy.

Currently, there is no consistently reliable method to identify those infants who are unable to survive due to severe bilateral pulmonary hypoplasia.[193] If these infants could be conclusively identified, then further supportive care could be justifiably withheld, as no form of therapy will affect outcome. Although absolute identification of this subgroup remains problematic, a variety of clinical measurements are available that aid in quantifying the degree of pulmonary hypoplasia. These measurements are useful in directing therapeutic strategy and estimating overall mortality. Because standard practice has been early operative intervention for severely affected infants, studies aimed at predicting outcome have relied primarily on assessments made postoperatively during conventional therapy. The components of conventional therapy differ somewhat from institution to institution, but generally include (1) conventional mechanical ventilatory support to produce respiratory alkalosis, (2) support of intravascular volume and correction of metabolic derangements (acidosis, electrolytes), (3) inotropic support as indicated, (4) various combinations of sedatives, narcotics, and neuromuscular blocking agents, (5) appropriate interventions for barotrauma, and (6) possibly a trial of vasodilators. Identification of patients unlikely to survive with conventional support becomes important as extracorporeal membrane oxygenation (ECMO) has been successfully used in this subgroup and has reduced overall mortality. Conversely, because ECMO is associated with significant risks, it should possibly be reserved for this group of high-risk patients.[199,200]

Generally, ECMO selection criteria are based on the outcome studies alluded to above. Several studies predicting survival with conventional therapy will be briefly highlighted. In Harrington et al's series of 39 patients, a postreduction A-aDO$_2$ of less than 400 mmHg was predictive of survival; an A-aDO$_2$ of more than 500 mmHg predicted nonsurvival, and between 400 and 500 mmHg indicated that prognosis was uncertain.[201] Krummel et al noted that an A-aDO$_2$ of more than 620 mmHg persisting for longer than 12 hours was predictive of 100 percent mortality in their institution.[199] O'Rourke et al have demonstrated a correlation between postductal PaO$_2$, pulmonary vascular hypoplasia, and mortality.[179] Infants achieving at least one PaO$_2$ above 100 mmHg in the first 24 hours had 23 percent mortality on conventional therapy. A 100 percent mortality was associated with the inability to achieve a postductal PaO$_2$ of 100 mmHg and correlated with a high degree of pulmonary vascular hypoplasia measured angiographically. In a small series of patients, Bloss et al correlated the response to vasodilator therapy with mortality.[202] Infants experiencing an increase in PaO$_2$ of more than 100 mmHg in response to tolazoline survived. The group with a 20 to 100 mmHg increase had 67 percent mortality, and the group with a less than 20 mmHg increase had 100 percent mortality.

All the aforementioned analyses correlate measures of postreduction oxygenation with mortality. Bohn et al have been able to correlate the level of delivered ventilatory support with outcome.[177,178] Plotting the ventilatory index defined as the product of mean airway pressure and respiratory rate, against arterial PCO$_2$, yields a grid of expected mortality. Figure 19-10 summarizes mortality data derived from 54 infants with measurements obtained 2 hours following surgical repair of CDH. Data derived from 58 infants measured preoperatively yielded similar results.

High-frequency oscillatory ventilation was used postoperatively in 16 patients with persistent hypercarbia. While this technique resulted in a significant reduction in PaCO$_2$ and an increase in PaO$_2$, it was sustained in only two patients, with the remaining 14 ultimately succumbing to their disease.[177,178]

Selection criteria for ECMO typically include one or more of the following: (1) demonstrating inadequate oxygenation on conventional therapy (PaO$_2$ <40 to 60, A-aDO$_2$ >500 to 600 mmHg), (2) an acute deterioration in cardiorespiratory status (abrupt decrease in PaO$_2$, unresponsive acidosis, hemodynamic instability), or (3) unrelenting barotrauma. Exclusionary criteria typically include (1) serious coexisting anomaly (chromosomal, cardiac, or neurologic), (2) more than 7 to 10 days of ventilatory support, (3) birth weight less than 2 kg or gestastional age less than 35 weeks, or (4) pre-existing intracranial hemorrhage.[193,200,203]

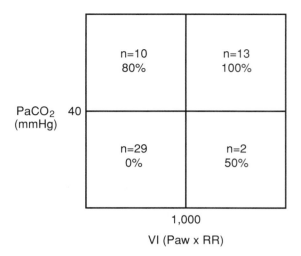

Fig. 19-10. Relationship between ventilatory index (VI), $PaCO_2$, and expected mortality in infants with congenital diaphragmatic hernia receiving conventional therapy. % = expected mortality. (Modified from Bohn et al,[177] with permission.)

Complications are significant and mainly relate to the need for systemic anticoagulation. Significant bleeding problems occur in approximately 25 to 40 percent of CDH patients treated with ECMO, approximately half of which are fatal. In spite of its drawbacks, ECMO has been used successfully in infants who would likely have died if treated with conventional therapy.[193,200,203] Redmond et al reported a 50 percent long-term survival in ECMO-treated infants with a predicted 100 percent mortality according to Bohn et al's original criteria.[193] Similarly, Heiss et al found an 83 percent survival rate in a group of ECMO-treated infants who were predicted by Bohn et al to have 50 percent mortality, and one of two infants who fell within the 100 percent mortality range survived.[200] The overall survival rate in ECMO-treated patients is conservatively 50 percent for a population whose expected survival is less than 25 percent with conventional therapy.[185,193,200,203] Truog et al[204] recently reported surgical repair of congenital diaphragmatic hernia during ECMO, with only one survivor in their five patients. However, this approach to the treatment of CDH may well deserve further scrutiny (see Chapter 24).

Repair of CDH before birth is an exciting and revolutionary concept with far-reaching possibilities for lower mortality and morbidity as well as more normal lung development. The report of Harrison et al of intrauterine repair of a congenital diaphragmatic hernia is particularly noteworthy and may well be the first step in a new mode of management of this often fatal anomaly.[205]

Follow-up studies of patients with repaired diaphragmatic hernias are generally encouraging, although most series do detect a variety of subtle abnormalities. It appears that there is persistence in the reduction of the number of branches of both bronchi and pulmonary arteries on the affected side, resulting in a decrease in ventilation and perfusion.[183,206,207] Plain chest radiographs are frequently normal, but may reveal a decrease in vascularity on the affected side.[208] Lung scans may confirm the hypoperfusion suggested on plain film.[209] Measurements of lung volumes are usually normal, although some investigators suggest that this may be due to overexpansion of existing alveoli rather than growth in alveolar number, as normally occurs.[207–209] An asymptomatic pre-emphysematous state may exist in older individuals.[208] Despite these abnormalities, it appears that patients surviving repair of CDH develop sufficient lung function to allow normal activity without symptoms, at least into adolescence and early adulthood.

Follow-up of patients with neonatal respiratory failure treated with ECMO has also been encouraging. The overall incidence of significant neurologic or pulmonary sequelae appears to be similar in ECMO- and conventionally treated patients. Approximately 30 percent of patients at follow-up will have readily detectable neurologic sequelae in each treatment group, although asymptomatic electroencephalographic abnormalities may be somewhat higher in ECMO-treated patients. Congenital diaphragmatic hernia infants represent a small percentage of patients in these series, and specific follow-up information on ECMO-treated CDH infants has not yet been reported.[210–212]

Esophageal Atresia and Tracheoesophageal Fistula

Esophageal atresia (EA) with or without a tracheoesophageal fistula (TEF) is not an uncommon congenital anomaly, and requires early surgical intervention. The incidence of these related defects occurs in approximately one in 3,000 live births.[213]

The presence of polyhydramnios during pregnancy may indicate some form of intestinal obstruction in the fetus; if it is present, the diagnosis of esophageal atresia can be made at the time of delivery or shortly afterward by carefully attempting to insert a soft radiopaque catheter into the stomach either nasally (which may also rule out the presence of choanal atresia) or through the mouth. If atresia is present, the catheter will be seen to coil in the upper blind pouch of the atretic esophagus. If further anatomic definition is needed and contrast medium required, the use of a small amount of dilute barium (2 mL or less) is considered to be the lesser of several evils (Ball TI, personal communication). The use of oil-based or water-soluble contrast materials may often result in a chemical pneumonitis if an associated TEF exists. Newborn infants do not clear these substances from the lungs and airways, due to an ineffective cough and impaired ciliary function. Any infant showing early signs of gagging and coughing on secretions with feedings, and subsequent respiratory distress and cyanosis, should be suspected of having some form of esophageal defect, and appropriate steps should be taken to make a diagnosis so that early intervention can prevent the development of pneumonia and even death. If an H-type fistula exists (see below) without EA, early signs of respiratory distress are not usually present (gagging, coughing, cyanosis, rapid respirations), and the diagnosis may not be suspected until the child is several months old, when recurrent pneumonia suggests the presence of this type of defect.

Several anatomic combinations of EA and TEF include the following (Fig. 19-11):

A. EA without TEF (8 percent)
B. EA with the fistula between the proximal esophageal segment and the trachea (less than 1 percent)
C. EA with the fistula between the distal esophagus segment and the distal trachea (87 percent)
D. EA with the fistula between both proximal and distal esophageal segments and the trachea (less than 1 percent)
E. TEF without esophageal atresia (H-type) (4 percent)

There is a very high incidence (perhaps as high as 50 percent) of associated congenital anomalies in patients with EA, with or without TEF.[214] Calverly and Johnston reported that factors influencing survival in patients with TEFs were associated congenital anomalies, prematurity, and pulmonary complications.[215]

The overall mortality among infants with TEF/EA is approximately 10 percent. Gestational age, birth weight, the presence of cardiorespiratory compromise (congenital anomalies, pneumonia) all have been

shown to decrease survival.[216,217] The sickest infants will often undergo a staged repair with ligation of the fistula and placement of a gastrostomy with anastomosis of the esophagus delayed. However, many centers are performing primary repair on smaller and more compromised infants.[218] This discussion concerns itself with the anesthetic management of type 1 EA with TEF.

Anomalies in other parts of the gastrointestinal tract occur in approximately 20 percent of patients with EA/TEF; the genitourinary system in approximately 10 percent (usually absent kidney), the musculoskeletal system in 10 to 30 percent, and craniofacial defects in 5 percent.[219] Further evidence of the importance of associated anomalies with EA/TEF affecting mortality figures has been reported by Barry and Auldist,[220] who conclude that the mortality rate for patients with isolated TEF is 6 percent, but 50 percent for those with TEF and multiple defects. Quan and Smith described the VATER association of defects.[221] VATER is a mnemonic suggesting the association of *v*ertebral *a*nomalies, *a*nal atresia, *t*racheoesophageal fistula with esophageal atresia, *r*enal anomalies, and *r*adial limb dysplasias.

Low birth weight is not necessarily an indication of prematurity, but most investigators reporting series of patients with EA/TEF accept a birth weight of less than 2,500 g as indicating a state of immaturity with its concomitant ramifications for management and survival. Smith reported that the incidence of prematurity or a birth weight of less than 2,500 g is 50 percent in patients with EA/TEF, which is significantly higher than with any other defect.[222] In his series, the premature infant with EA/TEF, unless extremely small (<1,500 g), posed no particular problem with management because of size or maturity.

Pulmonary complications (atelectasis, pneumonitis, consolidation, and varying degrees of respiratory insufficiency) are related to the age at which the diagnosis is made and surgical intervention under-

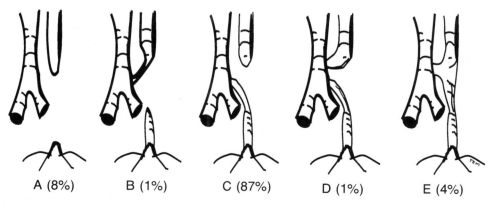

A (8%) B (1%) C (87%) D (1%) E (4%)

Fig. 19-11. (A–E) Drawing showing the most common types of tracheoesophageal fistulas.

taken.[215,223] Aspiration of secretions or feedings from the proximal esophageal segment almost always results in atelectasis or pneumonitis of the right upper lobe. Regurgitation of gastric contents via the fistula results in a chemical pneumonitis that is resistant to treatment. The advantages of diagnosis before the infant is fed for the first time are obvious, since the morbidity and mortality observed in infants with this condition is significantly higher if diagnosis and appropriate treatment are delayed.

Pulmonary complications may be avoided or minimized by withholding feedings, inserting a suction system into the upper pouch of the atretic esophagus to remove secretions, and nursing the infant in a 45-degree head-up position. Gastrostomy should be performed as soon as possible to prevent the increased risk of regurgitation of gastric contents, as well as upward displacement of the left hemidiaphragm and a decrease in lung volume associated with gastric distention. Early intubation to protect the lungs and airways may be useful in esophageal atresia without TEF, but is of no use when there is a communication between the trachea and the stomach, since most of the gas will travel into the stomach rather than the lungs.

The intraoperative management of patients with EA/TEF requires great skill and patience from both surgeon and anesthesiologist. Successful outcome depends on recognition that the condition exists, appropriate preoperative therapeutic measures, and meticulous cooperation between surgeon and anesthesiologist, since both are required to work in virtually the same small area.

Gastrostomy is usually carried out in the operating room with local anesthesia using 1 percent lidocaine (2 to 4 mg/kg). The infant is maintained in the 45-degree head-up position to minimize the possibility of aspiration, and atropine, 0.01 mg/kg, is administered intravenously on arrival in the operating room. The infant should be monitored during the procedure with a precordial stethoscope, blood pressure cuff, temperature probe, and pulse oximeter. Esophageal stethoscopes and temperature probes are avoided for obvious reasons during gastrostomy, as well as during subsequent procedures for EA/TEF. Appropriate oxygen is given as necessary and careful attention paid to maintenance of body temperature, as well as proper fluid, electrolyte, and glucose administration.

For more definitive repairs of EA/TEF, general anesthesia with endotracheal intubation is required. The monitoring technique is usually dictated by the general condition of the infant: the sicker the infant, the more complex the monitoring regimen. Newborn infants requiring surgery often arrive in the operating room with umbilical arterial and venous catheters in place that are used for pressure measurements and administration of fluids and blood. Even if an umbilical arterial catheter is used for direct pressure measurement and blood sampling, a back-up indirect pressure measurement system should be applied in case the umbilical arterial catheter becomes inoperative during surgery. Heart and breath sounds are monitored with a stethoscope placed against the left hemithorax after the infant is positioned for a right thoracotomy. This may be the most important monitor because during much of the operation, the right lung receives little ventilation, since it is retracted out of the surgeon's way. If breath sounds are lost from the left axillary stethoscope, even for a few breaths, hypoxemia will surely follow.[224]

A secure intravenous catheter should be established first; the airway is then secured after preoxygenation using an awake intubation or, alternatively, after induction of general anesthesia and muscle relaxant administration through the catheter. An awake laryngoscopy has the advantage that in the event intubation is unsuccessful, the infant still has the ability to breathe. If intravenous agents are used, the dose of the induction agent must be tailored to the patient's clinical condition.

An inhalational technique with spontaneous respiration should be used for maintenance, but some infants are very difficult to maintain this way, either being anesthetized inadequately (and moving and coughing) or too deeply (and developing apnea and hypotension). Infants with decreased pulmonary compliance, usually caused by hyaline membrane disease or pneumonia, present a substantial challenge to the anesthesiologist when controlled ventilation is used. If a gastrostomy is not placed beforehand, severe gastric distention may occur when positive-pressure ventilation is begun, and both cardiac arrest and gastric rupture have been reported to occur in this situation.[225,226] When a gastrostomy has been performed, before positive-pressure ventilation is begun, ventilation may be ineffective because of the pop-off effect of the open gastrostomy. There are reports of various maneuvers, including placement of the open end of the gastrostomy tube under water[227] and occlusion of the esophageal end of the fistula by retrograde placement of a Fogarty balloon-tipped catheter.[228] A Fogarty catheter has also been placed through a bronchoscope into the fistula to prevent escape of gas into the stomach during positive-pressure ventilation.[229]

Secretions may be a problem, and obstruction of the endotracheal tube can occur. Suctioning of the endotracheal tube should be done carefully and with the knowledge and cooperation of the surgeon. The use of a humidification system in the anesthetic circuit is useful in preventing inspissation of secretions in the endotracheal tube, and has an added advantage in reducing heat loss via the lungs.

As mentioned above, after intubation and proper securing of the endotracheal tube, anesthesia can be induced and maintained with low concentrations of halothane or isoflurane along with nitrous oxide and oxygen. If significant pneumonia exists, a high inspired oxygen concentration may be necessary to maintain the PaO_2 between 80 to 100 mmHg. If the potent anesthetic agents are not tolerated, a nitrous oxide/narcotic/relaxant technique can be used, but requires controlled ventilation.

The integrity of the fistula repair can be assured in the following manner: the surgeon places a small amount of saline into the wound and the anesthesiologist applies 20 cmH_2O constant positive pressure to the airway while looking for any leak in the tracheal suture line. If, after ligation of the fistula, primary repair of the esophageal atresia is undertaken with anastomosis of the proximal and distal segments, the surgeon may ask the anesthesiologist to pass a small suction catheter into the proximal segment until it can be felt near the end of the atretic esophageal pouch. When the catheter is palpable and placed properly, the anesthesiologist can mark it at the level of the infant's upper alveolar ridge with a suture or umbilical tape with the head in a neutral or slightly flexed position. It is then withdrawn and carefully measured to determine the maximum safe distance that catheters should be inserted for postoperative oropharyngeal suctioning to avoid disruption of the anastomosis. Extension of the neck after repair is avoided for the same reason.

Most infants undergoing repairs for EA/TEF are kept intubated for several hours to several days after surgery. Weaning from the ventilator begins as soon as possible after blood gas values and radiologic findings indicate improvement in atelectasis or pneumonia.

Complications after the repair include persistent pneumonia or atelectasis, pneumothorax, leakage or breakdown of the anastomosis, or reopening of the fistula into the trachea. Other tracheal complications (tracheal stenosis or granulomas) are rare.[230]

Mediastinal Masses

Children with masses of the anterior and middle mediastinum often require surgery for biopsy or removal of these masses, and general anesthesia is usually necessary. Abnormal masses contained within the anterior and middle mediastinum in children include teratomas, thymic masses, lymphomas, foregut duplication cysts, angiomatous tumors, and hilar adenopathy.[231–233] Unfortunately, the usual laboratory studies,

such as blood counts, bone marrow aspiration, and serum chemistries, fail to provide an adequate pathologic diagnosis, and biopsy is often necessary.[234] Surgical excision may be the treatment of choice, either alone or in combination with radiation therapy or chemotherapy, and such children usually require general anesthesia.

There are numerous reports of catastrophies involving these patients with mediastinal masses during all stages of general anesthesia (induction, maintenance, and emergence),[231,235–237] including cardiovascular collapse and/or partial or complete airway obstruction. When the vital structures contained within the anterior and middle mediastinum (the heart, pericardium, great vessels, trachea, and the recurrent laryngeal nerve) are considered, it is surprising that so many children with mediastinal masses undergo general anesthesia without difficulty and that many of them have little or no cardiorespiratory signs or symptoms preoperatively.[238]

In addition to the usual history, it is important to ask the child and the parents specifically about the presence of syncope and dyspnea, as well as intolerance of, or preference for, any certain anatomic position, since these may indicate airway compromise or impairment of venous return or stroke volume. In the physical examination of the cardiorespiratory system, evidence of the superior vena cava syndrome (ie, stridor, facial cyanosis, distention of neck veins, head and neck edema) should be sought. Mediastinal masses may first be noted on a chest x-ray taken for various reasons, and these should be reviewed. Since these masses may grow rapidly, all x-ray studies should be recent. However, since a plain chest x-ray may be very misleading with regard to airway obstruction and is of very limited value in the assessment of cardiovascular compromise, other laboratory studies are indicated before beginning anesthesia. These studies include echocardiography, a respiratory flow/volume loop if the patient will cooperate, chest and upper airway computer tomography (CT) scan,[239] and, occasionally, awake fiberoptic bronchoscopy (Fig. 19-12). If there are signs of airway obstruction or involvement of the heart and great vessels (ie, superior vena cava syndrome, tamponade, new cardiac murmurs), upright and supine echocardiograms as well as a chest CT scan should be done. Interestingly, the anesthesiologist may first encounter the patient with a mediastinal mass when consulted to provide anesthesia for the CT scan, which is requested by the oncologist as part of a preoperative workup. A flow/volume loop may demonstrate intrathoracic airway obstruction, but not all children will cooperate for this test.[235] Awake fiberoptic bronchoscopy may be used both for airway evaluation and for intubation, but should be

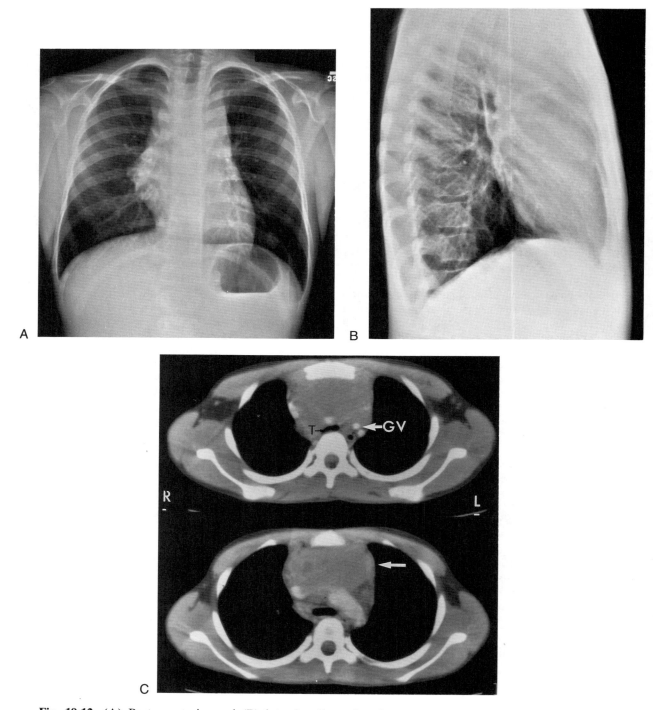

Fig. 19-12. (A) Posteroanterior and **(B)** lateral radiographs of a 15-year-old patient with large anterior mediastinal mass showing posterior displacement and some narrowing of tracheal lumen. **(C)** CT scan demonstrates the mass (*lower arrow*) displacing and compressing the great vessels (*GV*) and the trachea (*T*).

TABLE 19-12. Mediastinal Mass on Chest X-ray

I. High risk for general anesthesia
    A. Positive history and physical examination.
    B. Computed tomography scan with tracheal lumen narrowed by ≥35 percent.
    C. Abnormal flow/volume loop.
    D. Abnormal airway seen during awake fiberoptic bronchoscopy.
  Management plan
    A. Biopsy peripheral lymph node with local anesthesia.
    B. Needle biopsy (? CT-directed) lymph node if possible.
    C. Presumptive treatment with radiation and/or steroids to decrease tumor size; when patient meets criteria for the lower risk group, perform indicated procedure (biopsy or excision) with general anesthesia.
                        or
      if general anesthesia is absolutely necessary to establish the diagnosis; place all monitors preinduction, have femoral-femoral bypass immediately available, inhalation induction (O_2-halothane), avoid neuromuscular blockade, begin with the child in the most comfortable position, be able to change the position easily and quickly, and have rigid and flexible bronchoscopes available.
II. Low-risk group
  Children without signs and symptoms of cardiorespiratory compromise and whose diagnostic studies are within normal limits.
  Management plan
    A. If possible, biopsy a peripheral lymph node using local anesthesia.
    B. If administering general anesthesia, inhalation induction, maintain spontaneous ventilation.
    C. Avoid neuromuscular blocking agents.
    D. Be able to change the patient's position quickly.
    E. Have rigid bronchoscopy available.

done only by a skilled pediatric bronchoscopist. Some investigators report that fiberoptic bronchoscopy is not useful and is possibly hazardous.[238]

There is no clear consensus regarding the preoperative diagnostic laboratory studies necessary for a child with a mediastinal mass found on chest x-ray film who has no signs or symptoms of cardiorespiratory compromise before inducing general anesthesia[239] (see Chapter 16).

These children may be divided into two categories based on the risk of airway obstruction or cardiovascular collapse during general anesthesia: high risk and moderate risk (Table 19-12).

High Risk

High-risk children are those with signs and symptoms of moderate to severe cardiorespiratory compromise, abnormal flow/volume loops, or CT scan showing tracheal narrowing to less than 70 percent of normal or tumor involvement of the heart or great vessels.

Moderate Risk

Moderate risk children are those without signs and symptoms of cardiorespiratory compromise, who do not show tracheal, bronchial, or cardiac abnormalities on chest CT scan, echocardiogram, or flow/volume loop.

Although much of the information regarding the anesthetic management of children with mediastinal masses is in the form of brief reports or reviews of experience with small groups, several points emerge with some consistency. Children with signs and symptoms of respiratory or cardiovascular compromise are much more likely to experience difficulty during general anesthesia. Although attention is often focused on the airway, involvement of other mediastinal structures (ie, heart, pericardium, great vessels) is not uncommon and may cause problems equally as devastating as those caused by tracheal obstruction. If the patient's condition deteriorates with adequate ventilation and oxygenation, it must be assumed that there is cardiovascular involvement (tamponade, decreased ventricular filling, outflow obstruction), and therapeutic efforts must be directed toward these possibilities. Mediastinal tumors may grow quite rapidly, and recent diagnostic studies are essential. As always, effective communication between the surgeon and anesthesiologist may prevent problems, especially if such communication occurs before the child appears in the operating room. It may be helpful to arrange a multidisciplinary conference involving pediatric medicine, surgery, radiology, hematology/oncology, anesthesiology, and pulmonology to be sure that all aspects of the procedure have been considered and that no catastrophe occurs.

Patent Ductus Arteriosus in the Premature Infant

Persistent patency of the ductus arteriosus in infants born prematurely is well documented.[240–245] During the last two decades, improvements in the techniques for ventilatory support in the treatment of

RDS and for metabolic and nutritional requirements of preterm babies have significantly improved survival and quality of life.

The vasoconstrictor response of the ductus to an increase in the partial pressure of oxygen during early neonatal life is proportional to gestational age: the lower the gestational age, the greater the likelihood of patency of the ductus.[246] Forty-two percent of babies who weigh less than 1,000 g and 20.2 percent of those weighing less than 1,750 g will have clinical evidence of patency of the ductus.[240,247]

As is seen in other varieties of left-to-right shunts, the clinical findings depend on the size of the ductus and the relationship between pulmonary and systemic resistances. Because many infants born prematurely have RDS,[248] the severity of the disease determines the degree of left-to-right shunting. In more severe RDS, pulmonary resistance remains higher in relation to systemic resistance and results in less shunting. In the most severe forms of RDS, pulmonary resistance exceeds systemic resistance, and right-to-left shunting through the ductus results in a decrease in PaO_2 distal to the ductal connection to the aorta. As RDS improves and pulmonary resistance falls below systemic resistance, more and more left-to-right shunting may take place and congestive heart failure may ensue, requiring pharmacologic maneuvers to attempt to cause the ductus to close or, if these fail, surgical closure.

There appears to be some relationship between the presence of a patent ductus and the development of necrotizing enterocolitis in the preterm infant. Because of the vascular effects of a large run-off from the aorta to the pulmonary circulation, a steal phenomenon from the splanchnic circulation takes place causing bowel ischemia. The clinical picture of abdominal distention and bloody stools, together with dilated loops of intestine seen on the x-ray film, suggest the presence of necrotizing enterocolitis with resulting intestinal perforation and/or bowel necrosis.[249,250]

Medical therapeutic measures in managing congestive heart failure in the preterm infant with RDS and a patent ductus initially include fluid restriction and diuretics. These may suffice and buy time while the infant matures, and the ductus may close spontaneously. Fluid restriction and diuretic therapy necessarily result in varying degrees of dehydration; this should be kept in mind by the anesthesiologist when evaluating such patients for any surgical procedure including ligation of the ductus.[251]

The prostaglandin inhibitor, indomethacin, is often useful for pharmacologic closure of the patent ductus and may be given intravenously or enterally via a gastric tube. The usual dose range is 0.1 to 0.3 mg/kg and ductal closure may be expected to occur within 24 hours.[252–254]

As with any pharmacologic intervention, indomethacin is not entirely without risk and may result in decreased renal function and clotting abnormalities, but these effects may be expected to clear if prostaglandin inhibitor therapy is stopped. Indomethacin treatment is not used if there is the suspicion that necrotizing enterocolitis is present, if renal function is already compromised, or in the presence of hyperbilirubinemia or clotting abnormalities.[255,256]

If medical therapy is not successful in causing closure of the ductus, surgical intervention is indicated. Once the decision is made by the neonatologist, cardiologist, and surgeon, the anesthetic management is usually simply an extension of the preoperative management except, perhaps, for the volume status of the infant.[251,257] Infants are transported to the operating room in a thermoneutral environment (the operating room should be warmed to help maintain the baby's temperature at normal level), often with monitoring and intravenous catheters already in place. Nondepolarizing muscle relaxants are often used by the neonatologists to improve artificial ventilatory efficiency.[258] If an umbilical or other arterial catheter is already established, it is useful for monitoring and blood sampling. If one is not present at the time of surgery, placement is not usually attempted, since oximetric and noninvasive blood pressure measurements are usually adequate for monitoring during the usually very short operative procedure in which time is of the essence in overall patient care. During the operation, ventilatory parameters are maintained as close to preoperative settings as possible (taking into account the left lateral decubitus position required for surgical exposure). Either hand ventilation or anesthesia machine ventilation is used, based on measurements of oxygenation by oximetry and carbon dioxide elimination by capnography or mass spectrometry.

Measures to prevent hyperoxia should be taken to avoid the inherent risks of retinopathy of prematurity or retrolental fibroplasia.[259–265] This condition undoubtedly has a multifactorial etiology, with hyperoxia probably being only one in a number of contributing causes, but it seems best based on current data to maintain the PaO_2 at normal levels during anesthesia and surgery for the premature infant. Gregory states that if an infant is less than 44 weeks' gestational age, it may be appropriate to maintain the SaO_2 between 86 and 92 percent.[266]

In older infants, children, and adults, division and suture of the ductal tissue at surgery is the preferred operation, since this eliminates the possibility of recanalization, the formation of a false aneurysm, or the need for reoperation. However, ligation and division are associated with greater surgical difficulty and risk. Therefore, simple ligation of the ductus is usually performed on the premature infant to minimize operative time and to decrease the possibility of hypothermia or hemorrhage.[267]

Anesthesia for ligation of the ductus in the premature infant is usually tolerated quite well. Nitrous oxide/air/oxygen, a nondepolarizing muscle relaxant, and a narcotic (usually fentanyl, 10 to 50 μg/kg) are usually employed. Continuation of supportive measures to maintain body temperature and to provide proper fluids, electrolytes, glucose, and calcium are part of the intraoperative care. Correction of metabolic acidosis beyond a base deficit of -5 mEq/L is probably prudent.* Although blood loss is usually minimal, the possibility of ductal tear during dissection with resultant massive hemorrhage must be kept in mind, and preparation for needed transfusion of blood includes adequate vascular access and blood or blood substitutes immediately available. Resuscitation drugs including diluted epinephrine, calcium, and bicarbonate should always be prepared and ready for use.

One important consideration in the management of the preterm infant with a patent ductus is the maintenance of adequate levels of hemoglobin. When the hemoglobin falls significantly, the cardiac output must rise to maintain adequate systemic oxygenation. In the premature infant with a ductus and a sizeable left-to-right shunt, the myocardium may already be compromised and anemia will make the situation worse. Even the small amounts of blood taken for laboratory analyses may become significant over several days because of a small blood volume. The hematocrit should be maintained above 45 percent if possible in the face of a normal blood volume. The administration of stored blood to the anemic preterm infant results in

---

* An arterial pH of less than 7.30 due to a metabolic component or base deficit of 5 or greater should be corrected using sodium bicarbonate, calculating the dose to be administered using the following formula:

$$mEq\ NaHCO_3 = weight\ (kg) \times base\ deficit\ correction\ desired \times 0.5$$

The mEq of $NaHCO_3$ should be diluted with an equal amount of sterile distilled water to lower the very high osmolarity of bicarbonate. Hyperosmolarity has been suggested as a cause of spontaneous intracranial hemorrhage in the premature newborn. Full correction of the total base deficit is not usually recommended. Rather, correction of approximately one-half of the measure deficit is carried out and blood gases remeasured before further correction is attempted.

more efficient peripheral oxygen delivery, since fetal hemoglobin is less effective at the tissue level in unloading oxygen than is adult hemoglobin. However, for several reasons, including the transmission of blood-borne infections and the possibility that adult hemoglobin may increase the risk of retinopathy of prematurity,[266] transfusion must be used with great care.

Tracheostomy

Fortunately, the need for urgent tracheostomy in infants and children is rare. Endotracheal intubation is usually possible even in cases of relatively severe acute epiglottitis.[268–270] Tracheostomy can be a difficult and dangerous procedure in the small infant with a short, fat neck, especially when the child is agitated and struggling. Every effort should be made to gain satisfactory control of the airway by endotracheal intubation and/or bronchoscopy, and to perform the tracheostomy under the ideal circumstances of the operating room and general anesthesia with controlled ventilation.

Tracheostomy is considerably simplified by the presence of a ventilating bronchoscope in the trachea. The rigid instrument can be manipulated by the anesthesiologist to displace the trachea directly anteriorly beneath the skin. Major arteries and veins thus fall to either side, while good ventilation is assured. Supplemental local infiltration anesthesia can be used to allow a "light" level of general anesthesia. The electrocautery is used to dissect and control bleeding, since even minimal postoperative bleeding can be dangerous and difficult to control.

Tracheostomy tubes of several appropriate sizes should be available in the operating room, and proper adaptors for the ventilation system tested for compatibility. Cuffed tracheostomy tubes are usually not necessary in children, and their use is discouraged since mucosal erosion, necrosis, and subsequent tracheal stenosis are more likely when cuffed tubes are used. The carina is very high in the infant and small child, and it is not unusual to have to shorten the tracheostomy tube in order to assure good ventilation of both lungs. A tracheostomy tube resting on or very near the carina will also be difficult to suction and will provoke paroxysms of coughing.

Postoperatively, a chest radiograph is obtained and the child is observed carefully in the intensive care unit. Many children having tracheostomies will require controlled positive-pressure ventilation postoperatively due to the underlying pathology that necessitated the procedure. Even those seemingly healthy children who required tracheostomy for acute upper airway obstruction (epiglottitis) must be observed very carefully. Accidental removal or obstruction of the tube must be detected immediately if life-threatening hypoxemia is to be prevented. Humidified air with the desired F_1O_2 should be delivered to the tracheostomy. Removal of a tracheostomy tube that has been in place for several weeks or more should be preceded by a diagnostic bronchoscopy to ensure that the upper airway is patent and that there is no obstructing granuloma at the site of the tracheostomy (see Appendix 19-1).

Vascular Rings

The most common vascular abnormalities requiring operation to relieve airway obstruction include the double aortic arch, a right aortic arch with a left-sided ligamentum arteriosum, and an anomalous origin of the innominate artery (the "innominate arterial compression syndrome").[271,272] The first two of the anomalies are true "vascular rings," the trachea and esophagus being squeezed in a circle formed by these continuous vessels.

Vascular rings usually present in early childhood. Symptoms include wheezing, stridor, coughing, noisy breathing, difficulty in feeding, and even frank cardiorespiratory arrest. The diagnosis can usually be established by a chest radiograph with barium swallow, the barium-filled esophagus being indented posteriorly by the vascular structure. Angiography may be used to further delineate the anomaly, although it is probably not necessary in most cases. Bronchoscopy with or without bronchography will clearly demonstrate the flattened and obstructed trachea just above the carina. Simple "air tracheograms" visible on properly performed plain chest radiographs usually demonstrate the abnormality quite satisfactorily.

The tracheal compression caused by the vascular ring can be relieved by division of the ring at an appropriate point, care being required to maintain the proper relationship of vessels needed for circulation to the head and lower body. Operation is usually performed through a left thoracotomy. Anesthetic management must take into consideration the child's airway obstruction, but, fortunately, ventilation usually improves once an endotracheal tube is in proper position. The trachea is usually compressed just above the carina, so the tube must often be pushed down lower than would ordinarily be the case. Occasionally, direct left mainstem intubation is required, with a sidehole in the endotracheal tube facilitating ventilation of the right lung. The surgeon will need to partially collapse the left lung to gain exposure to the vascular structures. Comparison of palpable pulses in the head

and arms may assist the surgeon in identifying the proper location for division of the ring.

Correction of the innominate artery syndrome requires only that the innominate artery be pulled forward, away from the trachea that it is compressing. The artery is usually sutured to the posterior periosteum of the sternum to hold it away from the trachea. The results of the operation are excellent in most cases.

Postoperatively, relief of the tracheal obstruction is usually clearly evident and dramatic. Occasionally, however, there will have been substantial tracheomalacia produced by the chronic presence of the offending vessel. Symptoms of airway obstruction may persist for some time, particularly if the child is over-hydrated, suffering from congestive heart failure, or quite small. A traumatic intubation or the need for prolonged postoperative intubation will increase mucosal edema, producing more symptoms of airway obstruction at an already compromised site in the trachea. Symptoms are more severe when the child is agitated, since the trachea is more likely to collapse during forceful inspiration. Obviously, this is a "vicious circle," which is best interrupted by the judicious use of sedation, fluid restriction, diuretics, steroids, humidified oxygen, and racemic epinephrine.

One form of partial vascular ring, the pulmonary arterial sling, may require the use of cardiopulmonary bypass for correction. In this anomaly, the left pulmonary artery passes to the right of the trachea before crossing back posteriorly to the left lung. This "sling" thus pulls on and compresses the trachea and right mainstem bronchus at the carina. Correction requires division of the left pulmonary artery, removal of the left pulmonary artery from behind the trachea, and reanastomosis of the vessel to the main pulmonary artery just distal to the pulmonary valve.

PREVENTION OF BACTERIAL ENDOCARDITIS DURING DIAGNOSTIC OR THERAPEUTIC SURGICAL PROCEDURES

Certain patients with rheumatic or congenital heart defects may require diagnostic or therapeutic procedures that necessitate the administration of appropriate antibiotics to prevent endocarditis. During the preoperative evaluation, the anesthesiologist should be aware of the incumbent risks of endocarditis if prophylaxis is omitted, the types of procedures and the defects for which antibiotic coverage is recommended, and the dosage and time of administration of

TABLE 19-13. Recommended Antibiotic Protocol for Dental/Respiratory System Procedures in Adults and Adult-Sized Children

Procedure	Conditions	Recommendation
Standard	For dental surgery, which may cause gingival bleeding and oral/respiratory tract surgical procedures.	Penicillin V (2.0 g orally 1 h before then 1.0 g later); patients unable to take oral medications: 2 million units aqueous penicillin G IV or IM 30 to 60 min before procedure and 1 million units; 6 hours later.
Special	Parenteral regimen for maximal protection is necessary: eg, systemic-pulmonary shunts or prosthetic valves are present.	Ampicillin (1.0–2.0 g IM or IV) plus gentamicin (1.5 mg/kg IV or IM) one-half hour before proposed procedure. Follow with 1 g oral penicillin V 6 hours later. Alternatively, parenteral regimen can be repeated once 8 hours later.
	Oral regimen for penicillin-sensitive patients.	Erythromycin (1 g orally, 1 h before and 500 mg 6 h later)
	Parenteral regimen for penicillin-sensitive patients.	Vancomycin (1 g slowly over 1 h before; no repeat dosage necessary)

the appropriate antimicrobial medications. It should be remembered that even hemodynamically insignificant defects (eg, mild rheumatic mitral valve insufficiency, small ventricular septal defects, mild pulmonic or aortic valve stenosis including a congenital bicuspid valve) require antibiotic administration during certain procedures to prevent this very serious complication of heart disease.

The Committee on Rheumatic Fever and Bacterial Endocarditis of the Council on Cardiovascular Disease in the Young of the American Heart Association recommends that procedures requiring antibiotic prophylaxis include the following[273]:

1. All dental procedures that are likely to induce gingival bleeding. (Simple adjustment of orthodontic devices or shedding of deciduous teeth are not included.)
2. Diagnostic or therapeutic procedures of the upper or lower respiratory tract including tonsillectomy, adenoidectomy, rigid bronchoscopy,[274]* esophagoscopy, or other operation that may cause disruption of the respiratory mucosa. (Laryngoscopy and endotracheal intubation for anesthesia via the oral route are excluded if trauma to the oral, pharyngeal, or glottic structures does not occur. Nasotracheal intubation is an indication for prophylaxis.)
3. Genitourinary tract surgery or instrumentation, including cystoscopy, urethral catheterization, prostatic and bladder surgery.
4. Gastrointestinal and gallbladder surgery or instrumentation, including esophagoscopy, esophageal dilation, sclerotherapy for varices, rectal and colon procedures including colonoscopy and proctosigmoidoscopic biopsy, and upper gastrointestinal endoscopy.
5. Surgery of the heart and great vessels, including patent ductus arteriosus ligation, systemic to pulmonary artery shunting procedures, pulmonary artery banding, and all "open heart" operations.†
6. Surgical procedures involving any infected or contaminated tissues, eg, incision and drainage of abscesses and circumcision.

---

* The risk with flexible bronchoscopy is low, but the necessity for prophylaxis is not yet defined.

† Endocarditis associated with most cardiac operations is usually due to *Staphylococcus aureus*, coagulase-negative staphylococci, or diphtheroids. Streptococci, gram-negative bacteria, and fungi are less common. Prophylaxis, therefore, should be directed primarily against staphylococci and is best of short duration. Penicillinase-resistant penicillins, such as the first-generation cephalosporins, are usually given, although the choice of drug should be based on each hospital's antibiotic susceptibility profile.

TABLE 19-14. Pediatric Doses for Endocarditis Prophylaxis

Ampicillin: 50 mg/kg per dose.
Erythromycin: 20 mg/kg for first dose and 10 mg/kg second dose.
Gentamicin sulfate: 2 mg/kg/dose.
Penicillin V: full adult dose if weight is greater than 27 kg (60 lb); one-half adult dose if weight less than 27 kg (60 lb); aqueous penicillin G sodium (50,000 U/kg; 25,000 U/kg follow-up); Vancomycin 20 mg/kg per dose). Intervals between doses are same as for adults. Total doses should not exceed adult doses.

7. Patients with long-term indwelling vascular catheters, eg, hyperalimentation.
8. Following cardiac surgery for any of the above listed types of surgery. Exceptions include patients with uncomplicated atrial septal defects of the secundum variety closed with direct suturing without a prosthetic patch, patients who have had ligation or division of a patent ductus arteriosus more than 6 months prior to present procedure, and patients who have had coronary artery bypass grafts.*
9. Any patient with a documented previous episode of endocarditis, even if there is no clinically detectable heart defect.

The patient taking ordinary rheumatic fever prophylactic antibiotics cannot be considered to be covered adequately for prevention of endocarditis for the surgical and diagnostic procedures listed above.

The planned operation determines the antibiotic regimen to be followed for the prevention of endocarditis. Thoracic operations including bronchoscopy and esophagoscopy require the administration of appropriate doses of penicillin, ampicillin, or amoxicillin given orally or parenterally (Tables 19-13 and 19-14), and sometimes gentamicin as well. Penicillin-sensitive patients may be given oral erythromycin or parenteral vancomycin. The parenteral administration of vancomycin should be done with extreme caution, since rapid injection intravenously can result in significant untoward reactions.[275]

ACKNOWLEDGMENT

Radiographs are courtesy of Turner Ball, Jr., M.D., Brit Gay, M.D., and Ellen Patrick, M.D., Department of Radiology, Henrietta Egleston Hospital for Children, Emory University School of Medicine, Atlanta, GA. Diagrams are by Mr. Terry E. Morris, M.M.Sc.

* The risk of endocarditis appears to continue indefinitely and is particularly significant in those patients with prosthetic heart valves in whom the mortality is considerable and in those patients with systemic-pulmonary artery shunts.

REFERENCES

1. Betts EK, Downes JJ: Anesthesia. p. 50. In Welch KJ, Randolph JG, Ravitch MM, et al (eds): Pediatric Surgery. 4th Ed. Year Book Medical Publishers, Chicago, 1986
2. Cook DR, Marcy JH (eds): Neonatal Anesthesia. Appleton-Davis, Pasadena, CA, 1989
3. Smith CA, Nelson NM (eds): The Physiology of the Newborn Infant. Charles C Thomas, Springfield, 1976
4. Rudolph AM: Fetal circulation and cardiovascular adjustments after birth. pp. 1219–1223. In Rudolph AM (ed): Pediatrics. 18th Ed. Appleton & Lange, East Norwalk, CT, 1987
5. Rudolf AM: The changes in the circulation after birth: their importance on congenital heart disease. Circulation 41:343, 1970
6. Hickey PR, Hansen DD: Anesthesia and cardiac shunting in the neonate: ductus arteriosus, transitional circulation and congenital heart disease. Semin Anesth 3:106–116, 1984
7. Bohn D: Anomalies of the pulmonary valve and pulmonary circulation. pp. 269–297. In Lake CL (ed): Pediatric Cardiac Anesthesia. Appleton & Lange, East Norwalk, CT, 1988
8. Hickey PR, Crone RK: Cardiovascular physiology and pharmacology in children: normal and diseased pediatric cardiovascular systems. pp. 175–193. In Ryan JF, Todres ID, Cote CJ, Goudsouzian NG (eds): A Practice of Anesthesia for Infants and Children. WB Saunders, Philadelphia, 1986
9. Reid LM: Structure and function in pulmonary hypertension. Chest 89:279–288, 1986
10. Phibbs RH: Supportive care of the premature and sick newborn. pp. 130–138. In Rudolph AM (ed): Pediatrics. 18th ed. Appleton & Lange, East Norwalk, CT, 1987
11. Martyn JAJ: Pediatric clinical pharmacokinetics—principles and concepts. p. 65. In Ryan JF, Todres ID, Cote CJ, Goudsouzian NG (eds): A Practice of Anesthesia for Infants and Children. WB Saunders, Philadelphia, 1986
12. Arant BS: The newborn-kidney. pp. 1143–1146. In Rudolph AM (ed): Pediatrics. 18th Ed. Appleton & Lange, East Norwalk, CT, 1987
13. Bennett EJ: Fluids for anesthesia and surgery in the newborn and the infant. Charles C Thomas, Springfield, 1975
14. Williams PR, Oh W: Effect of radiant heaters on insensible water loss in newborn infants. Am J Dis Child 128:511–514, 1974
15. Volpe JJ: Neonatal periventricular hemorrhage: Past, present, and future. J Pediatr 92:693–696, 1978
16. Simmons MA, Adcock EW, Bard H, et al: Hypernatremia and intracranial hemorrhage in neonates. N Engl J Med 291:6–10, 1974
17. Dabbagh S, Ellis D: Regulation of fluids and electro-

lytes in infants and children. p. 118. In Motoyama EK, Davis PJ (eds): Smith's Anesthesia for Infants and Children. 5th Ed. CV Mosby, St. Louis, 1990

18. Lubchenco LO: The high-risk infant. In: Major Problems in Clinical Pediatrics. Vol. 14. WB Saunders, Philadelphia, 1976

19. Avery GB: Neonatology: Pathophysiology and Management of the Newborn. 3rd Ed. JB Lippincott, Philadelphia, 1987

20. Lucey JF, Dangman B: A reexamination of the role of oxygen in retrolental fibroplasia. Pediatrics 73:82–96, 1984

21. Hoon AH, Jan JE, Whitfield MF, et al: Changing pattern of retinopathy of prematurity: a 37-year clinic experience. Pediatrics 82:344–349, 1988

22. Gibson DL, Sheps SB, Schechter MT, et al: Retinopathy of prematurity: a new epidemic? Pediatrics 83:486–492, 1989

23. Cote CJ: Practical pharmacology of anesthetic agents, narcotics, and sedatives. pp. 84–85. In Ryan JF, Todres ID, Cote CJ, Goudsouzian NG (eds): A Practice of Anesthesia for Infants and Children. WB Saunders, Philadelphia, 1986

24. Gregory GA: Anesthesia for premature infants. p. 813. In Gregory GA (ed): Pediatric Anesthesia. 2nd Ed. Churchill Livingstone, New York, 1989

25. Steward DJ: Preterm infants are more prone to complications following minor surgery than are term infants. Anesthesiology 56:304–306, 1982

26. Liu LMP, Cote CJ, Goudsouzian NG, et al: Life-threatening apnea in infants recovering from anesthesia. Anesthesiology 59:506–510, 1983

27. Welborn LG, Ramirez N, Oh TH, et al: Post-anesthetic apnea and periodic breathing in infants. Anesthesiology 65:658–661, 1986

28. Kurth DC, Spitzer AR, Broennle AM, Downes JJ: Postoperative apnea in preterm infants. Anesthesiology 66:483–488, 1987

29. Martin RJ, Miller MJ, Waldeman AC: Pathogenesis of apnea in preterm infants. J Pediatr 109:733–741, 1986

30. Welborn LG, DeSoto H, Hannallah RS, et al: The use of caffeine in the control of post-anesthetic apnea in former premature infants. Anesthesiology 68:796–798, 1988

31. Belin B, Vatashsky E, Aronson NB, et al: Naloxone reversal of postoperative apnea in a premature infant. Anesthesiology 63:317–318, 1985

32. Barrington KJ, Finer NN, Peters KL: Physiology effects of doxapram in idiopathic apnea of prematurity. J Pediatr 108:124–129, 1986 (Letter 109:563, 1986)

33. Welborn LG, Rice LJ, Hannallah RS: Postoperative apnea in former preterm infants: prospective comparison of spinal and general anesthesia. Anesthesiology 72:838–842, 1990

34. Muttitt SC, Tierney AJ, Finer NN: The dose response of theophylline in the treatment of apnea of prematurity. J Pediatr 112:115–121, 1988

35. Lubchenco LO, Bard H: Incidence of hypoglycemia in newborn infants classified by birth weights and gestational age. Pediatrics 47:831–838, 1971

36. Cowett RM, Andersen GE, Maguire CA, Oh W: Ontog-

eny of glucose homeostasis in low birth weight infants. J Pediatr 112:462–465, 1988

37. Bakwin H: Tetany in newborn infants: relation to physiologic hypoparathyroidism. J Pediatr 14:1–10, 1939

38. Tsang RC, Chen I, Friedman MA, et al: Neonatal parathyroid function: role of gestational age and postnatal age. J Pediatr 83:728–738, 1973

39. Schediwie HE, Odell WD, Risher DA, et al: Parathormone and perinatal calcium homeostasis. Pediatr Res 13:1–6, 1979

40. Oliver TK, Jr: Temperature regulation and heat production in the newborn. Pediatr Clin North Am 12:765–779, 1966

41. Pearlstein PH, Edwards NK, Atherton MD, et al: Computer assisted newborn intensive care. Pediatrics 57:494–501, 1976

42. Roe CF, Santulli TV, Blair CS: Heat loss in infants during general anesthesia and operations. J Pediatr Surg 1:266–274, 1966

43. Rizvi T, Wadhwa S, Bijlan V: Development of spinal substrate for nociception. Pain, suppl. 4:195, 1987

44. Humphrey T: Some correlations between the appearance of human fetal reflexes and the development of the nervous system. Prog Brain Res 4:43–135, 1964

45. Williamson PS, Williamson ML: Physiologic stress reduction by a local anesthetic during newborn circumcision. Pediatrics 71:36–40, 1983

46. Holve RL, Bromberger PJ, et al: Regional anesthesia during newborn circumcision. Clin Pediatr 22:813–818, 1983

47. Maxwell LG, Yaster M, Wetzell RC: Penile nerve block reduces the physiologic stress of newborn circumcision. Anesthesiology 65:A432, 1986

48. Rawlings DJ, Miller PA, Engle R: The effect of circumcision in transcutaneous PO_2 monitoring in infants. Am J Dis Child 134:676–678, 1980

49. Messner JT, Loux PC, Grossman LB: Intraoperative transcutaneous PO_2 monitoring in infants. Anesthesiology 51:S319, 1979

50. Harrin VA, Rutter H: Development of emotional sweating in the newborn infant. Arch Dis Child 57:691–695, 1982

51. Srinivasan G, Jarn R, Pildes R, et al: Glucose homeostasis during anesthesia and surgery in infants. J Pediatr Surg 21:718–721, 1986

52. Obara H, Sugiyama D, Tanaka O, et al: Plasma cortisol levels in paediatric anesthesia. Can Anaesth Soc J 31:24–27, 1984

53. Anand KJS, Brown MJ, Causon R, et al: Can the human neonate mount an endocrine and metabolic response to surgery? J Pediatr Surg 20:41–48, 1985

54. Anand KJS, Brown MJ, Bloom S, et al: Studies on the hormonal regulation of fuel metabolism in the human neonate undergoing anesthesia and surgery. Hormone Res 22:115–128, 1985

55. Anand KJS, Hickey PR: Pain and its effects in the human neonate and fetus. N Engl J Med 317:1321–1329, 1987

56. Bland JW, Williams WH: Anesthesia for treatment of congenital heart defects. p. 287. In Kaplan JA (ed): Cardiac Anesthesia. Grune & Stratton, Orlando, FL, 1979

57. Thein RMH, Epstein BS; General surgical procedures in the child with a congenital anomaly. p. 88. In Stehling LC, Zauder HL (eds): Anesthesia Implications of Congenital Anomalies in Children. Appleton-Century-Crofts, East Norwalk, CT, 1980

58. Noonan JA: Association of congenital heart disease with other defects. Pediatr Clin North Am 25:797–816, 1978

59. Greenwood RD, Rosenthal A, Nadas AS: Cardiovascular abnormalities associated with diaphragmatic hernia. Pediatrics 57:92–97, 1976

60. Schreiner MS, Triebwasser A, Keon TP: Ingestion of liquids compared with preoperative fasting in pediatric outpatients. Anesthesiology 72:593–597, 1990

61. Splinter WM, Stewart JA, Muir JG: The effect of preoperative apple juice on gastric contents, thirst and hunger in children. Can J Anaesth 36:55–58, 1989

62. Maltby JR, Koehli N, Ewen A, Shaffer EA: Gastric fluid volume pH and emptying in elective inpatients: influences of narcotic-atropine premedication, oral fluid, and ranitidine. Can J Anaesth 35:562–566, 1988

63. Meakin G, Dingwal AE, Addison GM: Effects of preoperative feedings on gastric pH and volume in children. Br J Anaesth 59:678–682, 1987

64. Barnes LA: Nutrition and nutritional disorders. pp. 113–122. In Vaughn VC, McKay RJ, Behrman RE (eds): Nelson's Textbook of Pediatrics. 13th ed. WB Saunders, Philadelphia, 1987

65. Steward DJ: Pediatric anesthetic techniques & procedures, including pharmacology. pp. 19–56. In: Manual of Pediatric Anesthesia. Churchill Livingstone, New York, 1979

66. Steward DJ: Pediatric anesthetic techniques and procedures, including pharmacology. pp. 39–110. In: Manual of Pediatric Anesthesia. 3rd Ed. Churchill Livingstone, New York, 1990

67. Moffitt EA, McGoon DC, Ritter DG: The diagnosis and correction of congenital cardiac defects. Anesthesiology 33:144–160, 1970

68. Laver MB, Bland JHL: Anesthesia management of the pediatric patient during open heart surgery. Int Anesthesiol Clin 13:149–182, 1975

69. Santoli FM, Pensa PM, Azzolina G: Anesthesia in open-heart surgery for correction of congenital heart diseases in children over one year of age. Int Anesthesiol Clin 14:165–204, 1976

70. Hansen DD: Anesthesia. In Sade RM, Cosgrove DM, Castaneda AR (eds): Infant and Child Care in Heart Surgery. Year Book Medical Publishers, Chicago, 1977

71. Bland JW, Williams WH: Anesthesia for treatment of congenital heart defects. p. 291. In Kaplan JA (ed): Cardiac Anesthesia. Grune & Stratton, Orlando, FL, 1979

72. Koch F: Perioperative management of the pediatric cardiac patient. p. 75. In Lake CL: Pediatric Cardiac Anesthesia. Appleton & Lange, East Norwalk, CT, 1988

73. Roxas R, Jewell M: Pediatric cardiac anesthesia. p. 38. In Arciniegas E: Pediatric Cardiac Surgery. Year Book Medical Publishers, Chicago, 1985

74. Nicholson SC, Jobes DR: Hypoplastic heart syndrome. p. 248. In Lake CL: Pediatric Cardiac Anesthesia. Appleton & Lange, East Norwalk, CT, 1988

75. Walters J, Christianson L, Betts EK, et al: Oral vs intramuscular premedication for pediatric inpatients. Anesthesiology 59:SA454, 1983

76. Brzustowicz RM, Denkin AN, Betts EK, et al: Efficacy of oral premedication for pediatric outpatient surgery. Anesthesiology 60:475–477, 1984

77. Nicolson SC, Betts EK, Jobes DR, et al: Comparison of oral and intramuscular preanesthetic medication for pediatric inpatient surgery. Anesthesiology 71:8–10, 1989

78. Ponce FE: Propranolol palliation of tetralogy of Fallot: experience with long-term drug treatment in pediatric patients. Pediatrics 52:100–108, 1973

79. Honey M, Chamberlin DA, Howard J: The effect of beta-sympathetic blockade on arterial oxygen saturation in Fallot's tetralogy. Circulation 30:501–510, 1964

80. Cummings GR: Propranolol in tetralogy of Fallot. Circulation 41:13–15, 1970

81. Garson A, Gillette PC, McNamara DG: Propranolol: the preferred palliation for tetralogy of Fallot. Am J Cardiol 47:1098–1104, 1981

82. Frishman WH, Murthy S, Strom JA: Ultra-short acting adrenergic blockers. Med Clin North Am 72:359–372, 1988

83. Sacks EJ, Laddu AR: Esmolol (Brevibloc) to assess dynamic subpulmonary stenosis in a child after repair of complete transposition: a case report. Int J Clin Pharmacol Ther Toxicol 27:117–119, 1989

84. Zuberbuhler JR: Tetralogy of Fallot. p. 285. In Adams FH, Emmanouilides GC, Fiemenschneider TA (eds): Moss' Heart Disease in Infants, Children and Adolescents. 4th Ed. Williams & Wilkins, Baltimore, 1989

85. Eger EI, Kraft ID, Keasling HH: A comparison of atropine, or scopolamine, plus pentobarbital, meperidine, or morphine as pediatric preanesthetic medication. Anesthesiology 22:962–969, 1961

86. Merin RG: Effects of anesthetics on the heart. Surg Clin North Am 55:759–774, 1975

87. Greeley WJ, Bushman GA, Davis DP, et al: Comparative effects of halothane and ketamine on systemic arterial oxygen saturation in children with cyanotic heart disease. Anesthesiology 65:666–668, 1986

88. Schwartz DA, Horwitz LD: Effects of ketamine on left ventricular performance. J Pharmacol Exp Ther 194:410–414, 1975

89. Traber DL, Wilson RD, Priano LL: The effect of beta-adrenergic blockade on the cardiopulmonary response to ketamine. Anesth Analg 49:601–613, 1970

90. Morray JP, Lynn AM, Stamm SJ: Hemodynamic effects of ketamine in children with congenital heart disease. Anesth Analg 63:895–899, 1984

91. Hickey PR, Hansen DD, Cramolina GM: Pulmonary and systemic hemodynamic responses to ketamine in infants with normal and elevated pulmonary vascular resistance. Anesthesiology 61:A438, 1984

92. Gibbs RM: Monitor liability. Anesthesiol News 3:1, 1978

93. Smith RM: The pediatric anesthetist. 1950–1975. Anesthesiology 43:144–155, 1975

94. Cannard TH, Dripps RD, Helwig J, et al: The ECG during anesthesia and surgery. Anesthesiology 21:194–202, 1960

95. Mazzia VDB, Ellis CH, Siegal H, et al: The electrocardiogram as a monitor of cardiac function in the operating room. JAMA 198:103–107, 1966

96. Nadas AS, Fyler D: p. 191. Pediatric Cardiology. 3rd Ed. WB Saunders, Philadelphia, 1972

97. Yelderman M, New W: Evaluation of pulse oximetry. Anesthesiology 59:349–352, 1983

98. Barker SJ, Tremper K, Gamel DM: Clinical comparison of transcutaneous PO_2 and pulse oximetry in the operating room. Anesth Analg 65:805–808, 1986

99. Severinghaus JW. Monitoring anesthetic and respiratory gases. pp. 265–290. In Blitt CD (ed): Monitoring in Anesthesia and Critical Care Medicine. Churchill Livingstone, New York 1985

100. Lawless S, Orr R: Axillary arterial monitoring of pediatric patients. Pediatrics 84:273–275, 1989

101. Glenski JA, Beynum FM, Brady J: A prospective evaluation of femoral artery monitoring in pediatric patients. Anesthesiology 66:227–229, 1987

102. Gordon LH, Brown M, Brown OW, Brown EM: Alternative sites for continuous arterial monitoring. South Med J 77:1498–1500, 1984

103. Kinsey VE, Arnold HJ, Kalina RD, et al: PaO_2 levels and retrolental fibroplasia: A report of the cooperative study. Pediatrics 60:655–668, 1977

104. Motoyama EK, Cook DR, Oh TH: Respiratory insufficiency and pediatric intensive care. p. 632. In Smith RM (ed): Anesthesia for Infants and Children. 4th Ed. CV Mosby, St. Louis, 1980

105. James LS, Lanman JT: History of oxygen therapy and retrolental fibroplasia. Pediatrics 57:591–642, 1976

106. McGoldrick KE: Anesthesia for ophthalmic surgery. pp. 640–643. In Motoyama EK, Davis PJ (eds): Smith's Anesthesia for Infants and Children. 5th Ed. CV Mosby, St. Louis, 1990

107. Prince SR, Sullivan RL, Hackel A: Percutaneous catheterization of the internal jugular vein in infants and children. Anesthesiology 44:170–174, 1976

108. Cote CJ, Jobes DR, Schwartz AJ, et al: Two approaches to cannulation of a child's internal jugular vein. Anesthesiology 50:371–373, 1979

109. Nicholson SC, Steven JM, Betts EK: Monitoring the pediatric patient. In Blitt CD (ed): Monitoring in Anesthesia and Critical Care Medicine. 2nd Ed. Churchill Livingstone, New York, 1990

110. Swedlow DB, Cohen DE: Invasive assessment of the failing circulation. In Swedlow DB, Raphaely RC (eds): Cardiovascular Problems in Pediatric Critical Care, Clinics in Critical Care Medicine. Churchill Livingstone, New York, 1986

111. Kaplan JA: Hemodynamic monitoring. In Kaplan JA (ed): Cardiac Anesthesia. Grune & Stratton, Orlando, FL, 1979

112. Pybus DA, Poole JL, Crawford MC: Subclavian venous catheterization in small children using a Seldinger technique. Anaesthesia 37:451–453, 1982

113. Adamsons K, Towell MR: Thermal homeostasis in the fetus and newborn. Anesthesiology 26:531–548, 1965

114. Stern L, Lees MA, Ledac J: Environmental temperature, oxygen consumption, and catecholamine excretion in newborn infants. Pediatrics 36:367–373, 1965

115. Buetow KC, Kline SE: Effect of maintenance of "normal" skin temperature on survival of infants of low birth weight. Pediatrics 34:163–170, 1964

116. Gandy GM, Adamsons K, Cunningham N, et al: Thermal environment and acid-base homeostasis in human infants during the first few hours of life. J Clin Invest 43:751–758, 1964

117. Goudsouzian NG, Morris RH, Ryan JF: The effects of a warming blanket on the maintenance of body temperatures in anesthetized infants and children. Anesthesiology 39:351–353, 1977

118. Bennett EJ, Patel KP, Grundy EM: Neonatal temperature and surgery. Anesthesiology 46:303–304, 1977

119. Davis PJ: Temperature regulation in infants and children. pp. 143–156. In Motoyama DK, Davis PJ (eds): Smith's Anesthesia for Infants and Children. 5th Ed. CV Mosby, St. Louis, 1990

120. Vicanti FX, Ryan JF: Temperature regulation. pp. 19–23. In Ryan JF, Todres ID, Cote CJ, Goudsouzian NG (eds): A Practice of Anesthesia for Infants and Children. WB Saunders, Philadelphia, 1986

121. Lake CL: Monitoring of the pediatric cardiac patient. pp. 87–120. In Lake CL (ed): Pediatric Cardiac Anesthesia. Appleton & Lange, East Norwalk, CT, 1988

122. LaFarge CG, Miettinen OS: The estimation of oxygen consumption. Cardiovasc Res 4:23–30, 1970

123. Sade RM, Cosgrove DM, Castaneda AT: Infant and Child Care in Heart Surgery. Year Book Medical Publishers, Chicago, 1977

124. Janssen PJ: Anesthesia for corrective open heart surgery of congenital defects beyond infancy. Int Anesthesiol Clin 14:205–238, 1976

125. Roxas R, Jewell M: Pediatric cardiac anesthesia. p. 40. In Arciniegas E (ed): Pediatric Cardiac Surgery. Year Book Medical Publishers, Chicago, 1985

126. Steward DJ: p. 92. Manual of Pediatric Anesthesia. Churchill Livingstone, New York, 1990

127. Rao CC, Krishna G, Grosfeld JL, et al: One-lung pediatric anesthesia. Anesth Analg 60:450–452, 1981

128. Koka BV, Jeon IS, Andre JM, et al: Postintubation croup in children. Anesth Analg 56:501–505, 1977

129. Burgess GE, Cooper JR, Marino RJ, et al: Laryngeal competence after tracheal extubation. Anesthesiology 51:73–77, 1979

130. Rothstein P, Arthur CR, Feldman HS, et al: Bupivacaine for intercostal nerve blocks in children: blood concentrations and pharmacokinetics. Anesth Analg 65:625–632, 1986

131. Rice LJ, Hannallah RS: Local and regional anesthesia. pp. 419–421. In Motoyama EK, Davis PJ (eds): Smith's Anesthesia for Infants and Children. 5th Ed. CV Mosby, St. Louis, 1990

132. Arthur DS, McNichol LR: Local anaesthetic techniques in paediatric surgery. Br J Anaesth 58:760–778, 1986

133. Schecter NL, Allen DA, Hanson K: Status of pediatric pain control: a comparison of hospital analgesic usage in children and adults. Pediatrics 77:11–15, 1986

134. Beyer JE, DeGood DE, Ashley L, et al: Patterns of postoperative analgesic use with adults and children following cardiac surgery. Pain 17:71–81, 1983

135. Tyler DC: Respiratory effects of pain in a child after thoracotomy. Anesthesiology 70:873–874, 1989

136. Fleming WH, Sarafian LB: Kindness pays dividends: the medical benefits of intercostal nerve block following thoracotomy. J Thorac Cardiovasc Surg 74:273–274, 1977

137. Kaplan JA, Miller ED, Gallagher FG: Postoperative analgesia for thoracotomy patients. Anesth Analg 54:773–777, 1975

138. Shochet RB, Murray GB: Neuropsychiatric toxicity of meperidine. J Intensive Care 3:246–252, 1988

139. Koren G, Butt W, Pape K, et al: Postoperative morphine infusion in newborn infants: assessment of disposition characteristics and safety. J Pediatr 107:963–967, 1985

140. Way WL, Costly EC, Way EL: Respiratory sensitivity of the newborn infant to meperidine and morphine. Clin Pharmacol Ther 6:454–461, 1965

141. Rodgers BM, Webb CJ, Stergios D, et al: Patient-controlled analgesia in pediatric surgery. Pediatr Surg 23:259–262, 1988

142. Brown RE, Broadman LM: Patient-controlled analgesia (PCA) for postoperative pain control in adolescents. Anesth Analg 66:S22, 1987

143. Broadman LM, Hannallah RS, McGill W, et al: "Kiddie caudals": experience with 1154 consecutive cases without complications. Anesth Analg 66:S18, 1987

144. Broadman LM, Hannallah RS, Norrie W, et al: Caudal analgesia in pediatric outpatient surgery: a comparison of three different bupivacaine concentrations. Anesth Analg 66:S19, 1987

145. Rosen KR, Rosen DR: Caudal epidural morphine for control of pain following open heart surgery in children. Anesthesiology 70:418–421, 1989

146. Krane EJ, Jacobson LE, Lynn A, et al: Caudal morphine for postoperative analgesia in children: a comparison with caudal bupivacaine and intravenous morphine. Anesth Analg 66:647–653, 1987

147. Attia J, Ecoffey C, Gross J, et al: Epidural morphine in children: pharmacokinetics and CO_2 sensitivity. Anesthesiology 65:590–594, 1986

148. Krane EJ: Delayed respiratory depression in a child after caudal morphine. Anesth Analg 67:79–82, 1988

149. Ecoffey C, Dubousset A, Sanii K: Lumbar and thoracic epidural anesthesia for urologic and upper abdominal surgery in infants and children. Anesthesiology 65:87–90, 1986

150. Dalens B, Tanguy A, Haberer J: Lumbar epidural anesthesia for operative and postoperative pain relief in infants and young children. Anesth Analg 65:1069–1073, 1986

151. Shulman M, Sandler AN, Bradley J, et al: Post-thoracotomy pain and pulmonary function following epi-dural and systemic morphine. Anesthesiology 61:569–575, 1984

152. Jones SF, Beasley JM, Davis J, et al: Intrathecal morphine for postoperative pain relief in children. Br J Anaesth 56:137–140, 1984

153. McGown RG: Caudal analgesia in children. Anaesthesia 37:806–818, 1982

154. Schulte-Steinberg O, Rahlfs VW: Spread of extradural analgesia following caudal injection in children. Br J Anaesth 49:1027–1034, 1977

155. Satoyoshi M, Kamiyama Y: Caudal anaesthesia for upper abdominal surgery in infants and children: A simple calculation of the volume of local anesthetic. Acta Anaesthesiol Scand 28:57–60, 1984

156. Armitage EN: Caudal block in children. Anaesthesia 34:396–398, 1979

157. Reistad F, Stromskag KE, Holmquist E: Intrapleural administration of bupivacaine in postoperative management of pain. Anesthesiology 65:S204, 1986

158. Reistad F, Stromskag KE: Interpleural catheter in the management of postoperative pain: a preliminary report. Regional Anesth 2:8991, 1986

159. McIlvaine WB, Knox RF: Continuous infusion of bupivacaine via intrapleural catheter for analgesia after thoracotomy in children. Anesthesiology 69:261–0264, 1988

160. Kirklin JW, Karp RB, Bargeron LA: Surgical treatment of ventricular septal defect. p. 1044. In Sabiston DC, Spencer FC (eds): Surgery of the Chest. 3rd Ed. WB Saunders, Philadelphia, 1976

161. Ilabaca PA, Ochsner JL, Mills NL: Positive end-expiratory pressure in the management of the patient with a postoperative bleeding heart. Ann Thorac Surg 30:281–284, 1980

162. Johnson DG: Bronchoscopy. pp. 619–621. In Welch KJ, Randolph JG, Ravitch MM, et al (eds): Pediatric Surgery. 4th Ed. Year Book Medical Publishers, Chicago, 1986

163. Stern RC: Foreign bodies in the larynx, trachea, and bronchi. p. 891. In Berhman RE, Vaughn VC (eds): Nelson's Textbook of Pediatrics. 13th Ed. WB Saunders, Philadelphia, 1988

164. Law D, Kosloske AM: Management of tracheobronchial foreign bodies in children: a reevaluation of postural drainage and bronchoscopy. Pediatrics 58:362–367, 1976

165. Jordan WS, Graves CL, Elwyn RA: New therapy for postintubation laryngeal edema and tracheitis in children. JAMA 212:585–588, 1970

166. Nussbaum E: Flexible fiberoptic bronchoscopy and laryngoscopy in children under 2 years of age. Crit Care Med 10:770–772, 1982

167. Fitzpatrick SB, Marsh B, Stokes D: Indications for flexible fiberoptic bronchoscopy in pediatric patients. Am J Dis Child 137:595–597, 1983

168. Meyer BW: p. 158. Pediatric Anesthesia. JB Lippincott, Philadelphia, 1981

169. Johnson DG: Esophagoscopy. pp. 677–681. In Welch KJ, Randolph JG, Ravitch MM, et al (eds): Pediatric Surgery. 4th Ed. Year Book Medical Publishers, Chicago, 1986

170. Campbell JB, Quattromani FL, Foley LC: Catheter technique for removal of foreign bodies: experience with 100 cases. Pediatr Radiol 11:174–175, 1981

171. Holder TM, Ashcraft KW: Congenital diaphragmatic hernia. pp. 432–445. In Ravitch MM (ed): Pediatric Surgery. 3rd Ed. Year Book Medical Publishers, Chicago, 1979

172. Harrison MR, Bjorda RI, Langmark F, et al: Congenital diaphragmatic hernia: the hidden mortality. J Pediatr Surg 13:227–230, 1978

173. Cullen ML, Klein MD, Philippart AI: Congenital diaphragmatic hernia. Surg Clin North Am 61:1115–1138, 1985

174. Reynolds M, Luck SR, Lappen R: The "critical" neonate with diaphragmatic hernia: a 21-year perspective. J Pediatr Surg 19:364–369, 1984

175. Dibbins AW: Congenital diaphragmatic hernia—hypoplastic lung and pulmonary vasoconstriction. Clin Perinatol 5:93–104, 1978

176. Hansen J, James S, Burrington J, et al: The decreasing incidence of pneumothorax and improving survival of infants with congenital diaphragmatic hernia. J Pediatr Surg 19:385–388, 1984

177. Bohn D, Tamura M, Perrin D, et al: Ventilatory predictors of pulmonary hypoplasia in congenital diaphragmatic hernia, confirmed by morphologic assessment. J Pediatr 111:423–431, 1987

178. Bohn D, Jame I, Filler R, et al: The relationship between $PaCO_2$ and ventilation parameters in predicting survival in congenital diaphragmatic hernia. J Pediatr Surg 19:666–671, 1984

179. O'Rourke PP, Vacanti JP, Crone RK, et al: Use of the postductal PaO_2 as a predictor of pulmonary vascular hypoplasia in infants with congenital diaphragmatic hernia. J Pediatr Surg 23:904–907, 1988

180. Wells LJ: Development of the human diaphragm and pleural sacs. Contrib Embryol 35:109–133, 1954

181. Wesselhoeft CW, DeLuca FG: Neonatal septum transversum defects. Am J Surg 147:481–485, 1984

182. Geggel RL, Reid LM: The structural basis of PPHN. Clin Perinatol 3:525–551, 1984

183. Kitagawa M, Hislop A, Boyden EA, et al: Lung hypoplasia in congenital diaphragmatic hernia. Br J Surg 58:342–346, 1971

184. Reale FR, Esterly JR: Pulmonary hypoplasia: a morphometric study of the lungs of infants with diaphragmatic hernia, anencephaly and renal malformations. Pediatrics 51:91–96, 1973

185. Wiener ES: Congenital posterolateral diaphragmatic hernia: new dimensions in management. Surgery 92:670–681, 1982

186. Greenwood RD, Rosenthal A, Nadas AS: Cardiovascular abnormalities associated with congenital diaphragmatic hernia. Pediatrics 57:92–97, 1976

187. Ein SH, Barker G, Olley P, et al: The pharmacologic treatment of newborn diaphragmatic hernia—a 2-year evaluation. J Pediatr Surg 15:384–394, 1980

188. Sakai, H, Tamura M, Hosokawa Y, et al: Effect of surgical repair on respiratory mechanics in congenital diaphragmatic hernia. J Pediatr 111:432–438, 1987

189. Peckham GJ, Fox WW: Physiologic factors affecting pulmonary artery pressure in infants with persistent pulmonary hypertension. J Pediatr 93:1005–1010, 1978

190. Ehrlich FE, Salzberg AM: Pathophysiology and management of congenital posterolateral diaphragmatic hernias. Amer Surg 44:26–30, 1978

191. Siebert JR, Haas JE, Beckwith JB: Left ventricular hypoplasia in congenital diaphragmatic hernia. J Pediatr Surg 19:567–571, 1984

192. Drummond WH, Gregory GA, Heymann MA, et al: The independent effects of hyperventilation, tolazoline, and dopamine on infants with persistent pulmonary hypertension. J Pediatr 98:603–611, 1981

193. Redmond C, Heaton J, Calix J, et al: A correlation of pulmonary hypoplasia, mean airway pressure, and survival in congenital diaphragmatic hernia treated with extracorporeal membrane oxygenation. J Pediatr Surg 22:1143–1149, 1987

194. Hazebroek F, Tibboel D, Bos A, et al: Congenital diaphragmatic hernia: impact of preoperative stabilization. A prospective pilot study in 13 patients. J Pediatr Surg 23:1139–1146, 1988

195. Langer JC, Filler RM, Bohn DJ, et al: Timing of surgery for congenital diaphragmatic hernia: is emergency operation necessary? J Pediatr Surg 23:731–734, 1988

196. Ward RM: Pharmacology of tolazoline. Clin Perinatol 11:703–711, 1984

197. Cartlidge P, Mann N, Kapila L: Preoperative stabilization in congenital diaphragmatic hernia. Arch Dis Child 61:1226–1228, 1986

198. Rose MI, Smith SD, Chen H: Inappropriate fluid response in congenital diaphragmatic hernia: first report of a frequent occurrence. J Pediatr Surg 23:1147–1153, 1988

199. Krummel TM, Greenfield LJ, Kirkpatrick BV, et al: Clinical use of an extracorporeal membrane oxygenator in neonatal pulmonary failure. J Pediatr Surg 17:525–531, 1982

200. Heiss K, Manning P, Oldham KT, et al: Reversal of mortality for congenital diaphragmatic hernia with ECMO. Ann Surg 209:225–230, 1989

201. Harrington J, Raphaely RC, Downes JJ: Relationship of alveolar-arterial oxygen tension difference in diaphragmatic hernia of the newborn. Anesthesiology 56:473–476, 1982

202. Bloss RS, Aranda JV, Beardmore HE: Vasodilator response and prediction of survival in congenital diaphragmatic hernia. J Pediatr Surg 16:118–121, 1981

203. Johnston PW, Bashner B, Liberman R, et al: Clinical use of extracorporeal membrane oxygenation in the treatment of persistent pulmonary hypertension following surgical repair of congenital diaphragmatic hernia. J Pediatr Surg 23:908–912, 1988

204. Truog RD, Schena JA, Hershenson MB, et al: Repair of congenital diaphragmatic hernia during extracorporeal membrane oxygenation. Anesthesiology 72:750–753, 1990

205. Harrison MR, Adzick NS, Longaker MT, et al: Successful repair in utero of a fetal diaphragmatic hernia after removal of herniated viscera from the left thorax. N Engl J Med 322:1582–1584, 1990

206. Thurlbeck WM, Kida K, Langston C, et al: Postnatal

lung growth after repair of diaphragmatic hernia. Thorax 34:338–343, 1979

207. Wohl M, et al: The lung following repair of congenital diaphragmatic hernia. J Pediatr 90:405–414, 1977

208. Reid IS, Hutcherson RJ: Long-term follow-up of patients with congenital diaphragmatic hernia. J Pediatr Surg 11:939–942, 1976

209. Chatrath RR, et al: Fate of hypoplastic lungs after repair of congenital diaphragmatic hernia. Arch Dis Child 46:633–635, 1971

210. Andrews AF, Nixon CA, Cilley RE, et al: One to three year outcome for 14 neonatal survivors of extracorporeal membrane oxygenation. Pediatrics 78:692–698, 1986

211. Krummel TM, Greenfield LJ, Kirkpatrick BV, et al: The early evaluation of survivors after extracorporeal membrane oxygenation for neonatal pulmonary failure. J Pediatr Surg 19:585–590, 1984

212. Towne BH, Lott IT, Hicks DA, et al: Long-term follow-up of infants and children treated with extracorporeal membrane oxygenation (ECMO). J Pediatr Surg 20:410–414, 1985

213. Waterston DJ, Bonhan-Carter RE, Aberdeen E: Congenital tracheoesophageal fistula in association with esophageal atresia. Lancet 2:55–57,1963

214. Greenwood RD, Rosenthal A, Nadas AS: Cardiovascular abnormalitites associated with diaphragmatic hernia. Pediatrics 57:92–97, 1976

215. Calverly RK, Johnston T: The anesthetic management of tracheoesophageal fistula: a review of ten years' experience. Can Anaesth Soc J 19:270–282, 1972

216. Randolph JG, Newman KD, Anderson KD: Current results in repair of esophageal atresia with tracheoesophageal fistula using physiologic status as a guide to therapy. Ann Surg 209:526–531, 1989

217. Sillen V, Hagberg S, Rubenson A, Werkmaster K: Management of esophageal atresia: review of 16 years' experience. J Pediatr Surg 23:805–809, 1988

218. Pohlson EC, Schaller RT, Tapper D: Improved survival with primary anastomosis in the low birth weight neonate with esophageal atresia and tracheoesophageal fistula. J Pediatr Surg 23:418–421, 1988

219. Thein RMH, Epstein BS: General surgical procedures in the child with a congenital anomaly. p. 91. In Stehling LC, Zauder HL (eds): Anesthetic Implications of Congenital Anomalies in Children. Appleton-Century-Crofts, East Newalk, CT, 1980

220. Barry JE, Auldist AW: The VATER association: one end of a spectrum of anomalies. Am J Dis Child 128:769–771, 1974

221. Quan L, Smith DW: The VATER association, vertebral defects, anal atresia, T-E fistula with esophageal atresia, radial and renal dysplasia: A spectrum of associated defects. J Pediatr 82:104–107, 1973

222. Smith RM: Anesthesia for Infants and Children. 4th Ed. CV Mosby, St. Louis, 1980

223. Bedard P, Givran DP, Shandling B: Congenital H-type tracheoesophageal fistula. J Pediatr Surg 9:663–668, 1974

224. Buchino JJ, Keenan WJ, Pretsch JB, et al: Malposition-ing of the endotracheal tube in infants with tracheoesophageal fistula. J Pediatr 109:524–525, 1986

225. Jones TB, Kirchner SG, Lee F, et al: Stomach rupture associated with esophageal atresia, tracheoesophageal fistula and ventilatory assistance. AJR 134:675–677, 1980

226. Baraka A, Slim M: Cardiac arrest during IPPV in a newborn with tracheoesophageal fistula. Anesthesiology 32:564–565, 1970

227. Fann JI, Hartman GE, Shochat SJ: Waterseal gastrostomy in the management of premature infants with tracheoesophageal fistula and pulmonary insufficiency. J Pediatr Surg 23:29–31, 1988

228. Karl HW: Control of life-threatening air leak after gastrostomy in an infant with respiratory distress syndrome and tracheoesophageal fistula. Anesthesiology 62:670–672, 1985

229. Filston HC, Chitwood WR, Schkolne B: The Fogarty balloon catheter as an aid to management of the infant with esophageal atresia and tracheoesophageal fistula complicated by severe RDS or pneumonia. J Pediatr Surg 17:149–151, 1982.

230. Myers NA, Aberdeen E: Congenital esophageal atresia and tracheoesophageal fistula. p. 459. In Ravitch MM, Welch KJ, Benson CD, et al (eds): Pediatric Surgery. 3rd Ed. Year Book Medical Publishers, Chicago, 1979

231. Northrip DR, Bohman BK, Tsueda K: Total airway occlusion and superior vena cava syndrome with an anterior mediastinal tumor. Anesth Analg 65:1079–1082, 1986

232. Mackie AM, Watson CB: Anaesthesia and mediastinal masses. Anaesthesia 34:899–903, 1984

233. Ravitch MM: Mediastinal cysts and tumors. In Welch KJ, Randolph JG, Ravitch MM, et al (eds): Pediatric Surgery. 4th Ed. Year Book Medical Publishers, Chicago, 1986

234. Miller RM, Simpson JS, Ein SH: Mediastinal masses in infants and children. Pediatr Clin North Am 26:677–690, 1979

235. Prakash VBS, Abel MD, Hubmayr RD: Mediastinal mass and tracheal obstruction during general anesthesia. Mayo Clin Proc 63:1004–1011, 1988

236. John RE, Narang VPS: A boy with an anterior mediastinal mass. Anaesthesia 43:864–866, 1988

237. Fletcher R, Nordstrom L: The effects on gas exchange of a large mediastinal tumor. Anaesthesia 41:1135–1138, 1986

238. Azizkham RG, Dudgeon DL, Buck JR, et al: Life-threatening airway obstruction as a complication of the management of mediastinal masses in children. J Pediatr Surg 20:816–822, 1985

239. Kirks DR, Fram EK, Vock P, et al: Tracheal compression by mediastinal masses in children: CT evaluation. AJR 141:647–651, 1983

240. Ellison RC, Peckham GJ, Lang P, et al: Evaluation of preterm infant for patent ductus arteriosus. Pediatrics 71:364–372, 1983

241. Heymann MA: Patent ductus arteriosus. pp. 209–224. In Adams FH, Emmanouilides GC, Riemenschneider TA (eds): Moss' Heart Disease in Infants, Children, and

Adolescents. 3rd Ed. Williams & Wilkins, Baltimore, 1989

242. Clarkson PM, Orgill AA: Continuous murmurs in infants of low birth weight. J Pediatr 84:208–211, 1974

243. Rudolph AM: p. 176. Congenital Diseases of the Heart. Year Book Medical Publishers, Chicago, 1974

244. Neal WA: Patent ductus arteriosus complicating respiratory distress syndrome. J Pediatr 86:127–132, 1975

245. Thibeault DW: Patent ductus arteriosus complicating the respiratory distress syndrome in preterm infants. J Pediatr 86:120–126, 1975

246. McMurphy DM, Heyman MA, Rudolph AM, Mclmon KL:. Developmental change in constriction of the ductus arteriosus: response to oxygen and vasoactive substances in the isolated ductus arteriosus of the fetal lamb. Pediatr Res 6:231–238,1972

247. Taylor SP: Aortic valve and aortic arch anomalies. p. 339. In Lake CL: Pediatric Cardiac Anesthesia. Appleton & Lange, East Norwalk, CT, 1988

248. Tooley WH: Hyaline membrane disease (neonatal respiratory distress syndrome). pp. 1381–1390. In Rudolph AM (ed): Pediatrics. Appleton & Lange, East Norwalk, CT, 1987

249. Gregory GA: Anesthesia for premature infants. p. 809. In Gregory GA (ed): Pediatric Anesthesia. 2nd Ed. Churchill Livingstone, New York, 1989

250. Hudak ML: Necrotizing enterocolitis. pp. 930–933. In Rudolph AM (ed): Pediatrics. Appleton & Lange, East Norwalk, CT, 1987

251. Robinson S, Gregory FA: Fentanyl-air-oxygen anesthesia for ligation of patent ductus arteriosus in preterm infants. Anesth Analg 60:331–334, 1981

252. Heymann MA, Rudolph AM, Silverman NH: Closure of the ductus arteriosus in premature infants by inhibition of prostaglandin synthesis. N Engl J Med 295:530–533, 1976

253. Friedman WF: Pharmacologic closure of patent ductus arteriosus in the premature infant. N Engl J Med 295:526–529, 1976

254. Nadas AS: Patent ductus revisited (editorial). N Engl J Med 295:563, 1976

255. Wagner HR, Ellison RC, Zierler S, et al: Surgical closure of patent ductus arteriosus in 268 preterm infants. J Thorac Cardiovasc Surg 87:870–875, 1984

256. Taylor SP: Aortic valve and aortic arch anomalies. p. 340. In Lake CL (ed): Pediatric Cardiac Anesthesia. Appleton & Lange, East Norwalk, CT, 1988

257. Neuman GG, Hansen DD: The anesthetic management of preterm infants undergoing ligation of patent ductus arteriosus. Can Anesth Soc J 27:248–253, 1980

258. Stark AR, Bascom FA, Frantz ID: Muscle relaxation in mechanically ventilated infants. J Pediatr 94:439–443, 1979

259. Betts EK, Downes JJ, Schaffer DB, et al: Retrolental fibroplasia and oxygen administration during general anesthesia. Anesthesiology 47:518–520, 1977

260. Phibbs RH: Oxygen therapy: a continuing hazard to the premature infant. Anesthesiology 47:486–487, 1977

261. Merritt JC, Sprague DH, Merritt WE, et al: Retrolental fibroplasia: a multifactorial disease. Anesth Analg 60:109–111,1981

262. Adamkin DH, Shott RJ, Cook LN, et al: Nonhyperoxic retrolental fibroplasia. Pediatrics 60:828–830, 1977

263. Purohit DM, Ellison RC, Zierle S, et al: Risks of retrolental fibroplasia: experience with 3,025 premature infants. Pediatrics 76:339–344, 1985

264. Lucey JF, Dongman B: A reexamination of the role of oxygen in retrolental fibroplasia. Pediatrics 73:82–96, 1984

265. Wasunna A, Whitelaw AGL: Pulse oximetry in preterm infants. Arch Dis Child 62:957–958, 1987

266. Gregory GA: Anesthesia for premature infants. p. 813. In Gregory GA (ed): Pediatric Anesthesia. 2nd Ed. Churchill Livingstone, New York, 1989

267. Ashmore PG: Patent ductus arteriosus. p. 114. In Arciniegas E (ed): Pediatric Cardiac Surgery. Year Book Medical Publishers, Chicago, 1985

268. Sweeney DB, Allen TH, Steven IM: Acute epiglottitis: management by intubation. Anesth Intensive Care 1:526–528, 1973

269. Oh TH, Motoyama EK: Comparison of nasotracheal intubation and tracheostomy in management of epiglottitis. Anesthesiology 46:214–216, 1977

270. Diaz JH: Croup and epiglottitis in children: the anesthesiologist as diagnostician. Anesth Analg 64:621–633, 1985

271. Arciniegas E: Vascular rings. pp. 119–127. In Arciniegas E (ed): Pediatric Cardiac Surgery. Year Book Medical Publishers, Chicago, 1985

272. Taylor SP: Aortic valve and aortic arch anomalies. pp. 343–346. In Lake CL (ed): Pediatric Cardiac Anesthesia, Appleton & Lange, East Norwalk, Ct, 1988

273. Shulman ST, Amren DP, Bisno AL, et al: Prevention of bacterial endocarditis. Circulation 70:1123A–1127A, 1984

274. Shulman ST, Amren DP, Bisno AL, et al: Prevention of bacterial endocarditis. Am J Dis Child 139:232–235, 1985

275. Wilkinson PL, Ham J, Miller RD: p. 165. Clinical Anesthesia. CV Mosby, St. Louis, 1980

Appendix 19-1.
RESPIRATORY CARE OF PEDIATRIC PATIENTS

A. Tracheal airway care (applies to endotracheal tubes and tracheostomies)
   1. Use sterile tracheal apparatus.
   2. Humidify and warm inspired air.
   3. Instill sterile saline (0.5 mL to 2 mL) every 1 to 3 hours to prevent drying of secretions.
   4. Induce coughing or positive pressure to inflate lungs and use chest physiotherapy.
B. Suctioning of endotracheal tubes and tracheotomies
   1. Use sterile equipment (suction catheter, sterile saline, sterile gloved hand) for suctioning.
   2. Have second person ventilate patient with 100 percent oxygen before and after each suctioning maneuver and to instill sterile saline for wash.
   3. Suction only 5 to 15 seconds at a time followed by five to 10 positive-pressure breaths of 100 percent oxygen.
   4. After suctioning of endotracheal tube is complete, suction mouth; also suction nose if necessary.
   5. Reconnect patient's endotracheal tube to the ventilator.
   6. Check ventilator or supportive apparatus (CPAP of PEEP) and observe patient closely to ensure proper chest expansion.
C. Removal of endotracheal tubes
   1. Have patient breathe 100 percent oxygen. In some patients, mild sedation (10 to 20 mg/kg chloral hydrate may be helpful in very active child).
   2. Suction nose and mouth thoroughly. (Keep in mind that newborn infants are obligate nose breathers up until approximately 6 weeks of age).
   3. Empty stomach of any contents by suctioning.
   4. Change to sterile catheter and put on sterile glove for suctioning endotracheal tube if necessary.
   5. Ventilate patient with 100 percent oxygen for 2 to 3 minutes. Do not hyperventilate to the point of apnea. Allow PCO_2 to remain at breathing threshold.
   6. Remove endotracheal tube at the end of a full positive-pressure inspiration.
   7. Place patient in an atmosphere with oxygen concentration 20 percent higher than that prior to extubation.
   8. Suction mouth and throat every 30 to 60 minutes after extubation if necessary to remove secretions for 4 to 6 hours. Give bag and mask ventilation with 100 percent oxygen after each suctioning and after chest physiotherapy.
   9. Preferably feed patient via nasogastric tube (infants propped at 45-degree angle) for at least 8 hours following extubation. Administer intravenous fluids to account for deficits.
   10. Steroid administration continues to be controversial, but, if the decision to use them is made, they should probably be given intravenously at least an hour prior to extubation (0.2 mg/kg dexamethasone) as a one-shot dose.

11. If stridor is present after extubation, racemic epinephrine in 1 : 8 dilution administered as an aerosol via intermittent positive-pressure breathing may be helpful. Frequency and duration of treatment should not be more often than 5 minutes every 20 minutes for three to four treatments.

D. Endotracheal tube sizes

Endotracheal (Clear) Tubes ThinWall—Uncuffed

Internal Diameter	Age of Patient	Length (cm) to Midtrachea	
		Oral	Nasal
2.5–3.0	Premature	11	13.5
3.5	Newborn	12	14
4.0	6 mo	13	15
4.5	1 yr	14	16
5.0	2 yr	15	17
5.5	4 yr	17	19
6.0	6 yr	19	21
6.5	8 yr	20	22
7.0	10 yr	21	22
7.5	12 yr	22	23
8.0	14 yr	23	24
8.5	16 yr	24	25
9.0	18 yr	25	26
9.5	Adult	26	27

Formula: Size of tube (internal diameter) = age of patient/4 + 4.5
or
Size of tube (internal diameter) = 18 + age of patient/4
Length to midtrachea from alveolar ridge: age of patient (yr)/2 + 12

E. Parameters useful in determining need for respiratory support

Parameter	Normal	Wean or Extubate
PaO_2 ($F_IO_2 = 1.0$)	>600 mmHg	>300 mmHg
PaO_2 ($F_IO_2 = 0.21$)	75–100 mmHg	50 mmHg
$PaCO_2$	35–45 mmHg	45–50 mmHg
VC	70 mL/kg	15 mL/kg
Negative inspiratory force	< −100 mmHg	< −25 mmHg

F. Oral versus nasotracheal intubation
   Oral
      Advantages
         Easier to place
         Larger size possible
         Easier to suction

      Disadvantages
         More difficult to maintain in place
         More vocal cord damage possible

   Nasal
      Advantages
         Better tolerated by patient
         Harder to dislodge in either direction

      Disadvantages
         Smaller size
         Nasal bleeding

Less movement at cords	More difficult to suction
Better oral hygiene possible	Bacteremia
Oral feedings possible	Sinus infection
	Necrosis of naris possible

Some complications arising from orotracheal or nasotracheal intubation:
1. Tracheal stenosis
2. Tracheal and or vocal cord erosion
3. Pharyngoesophageal perforation
4. Granulomas of cords
5. Right mainstem bronchus intubation
6. Obstruction of tube by secretions or blood

G. Tracheostomy

Rare done in infants and children except as a last resort because of common use of nasal or oral tracheal intubation. Tracheostomy should be done in controlled conditions of the operating room with the airway secured with an endotracheal tube or bronchoscopy.

Indications (relative)
1. Inability to maintain adequate airway with an endotracheal tube.
2. Profuse secretions requiring almost constant suctioning and potentially causing obstruction of the endotracheal tube.
3. Upper airway obstruction not safely managed with an endotracheal tube.
4. Ultra–long-term need for ventilatory support.
5. Subglottic stenosis.

Complications of tracheostomy
1. Tracheal stenosis
2. Tracheal erosion
3. Mediastinitis
4. Pneumothorax, pneumopericardium, pneumomediastinum
5. Hemorrhage or hemothorax
6. Infection and pneumonitis
7. Surgical error (high tracheostomy, damage to vocal cords)
8. Erosion into esophagus or into the innominate artery
9. Mechanical obstruction
10. Accidental decannulation
11. Difficulties in closing stoma after removal of tracheostomy

20

PULMONARY TRANSPLANTATION

Wilfred A.P. Demajo, M.D.

Lung transplantation was first attempted in humans in 1963[1] and, until 1983, approximately 43 lung transplants were performed, with only 1 long-term success.[2] The reasons for this failure have been attributed to various factors, among which are bronchial dehiscence, pneumonias, and infection. In 1983, the Toronto Lung Transplant group, after research to address some of these problems[3,4] and as a consequence of better immunosuppression, especially the introduction of cyclosporine,[5] embarked on a lung transplantation program. Since then, more than 31 single-lung, 18 double-lung, and 20 sequential single-lung transplants have been done. The longest surviving single-lung transplant patient is 6 years from his operation, while the longest surviving double-lung transplant patient is 4 years posttransplant. Ten of the single-lung patients and 5 of the double-lung patients died of various causes.

HISTORY

Review of the literature up to 1983 reveals a paucity of data relating to the pre- and intraoperative condition and management of patients undergoing lung transplantation. There were 21 lung transplants and two heart-lung transplants performed; of the lung transplants, 4 involved transplantation of only the left lower lobe and, in one case, double lungs were transplanted. Useful clinical data are available in 11 cases; of these, 5 were suffering from chronic obstructive lung disease (ie, emphysema) and 6 had restrictive lung disease (2 paraquat, 1 smoke inhalation, 1 silicosis, 1 fibrosis, and 1 cavitary tuberculosis).[6,7]

Pulmonary function tests revealed severe abnormalities in both groups. The diffusion capacity was 25 percent and 31 percent of predicted in the chronic obstructive and the restrictive disease groups, respectively. The data on arterial oxygenation were not interpretable, as the oxygen concentration was not indicated in a number of cases; however, the range was 40 to 63 mmHg in the obstructive group and 37 to 60 mmHg in the restrictive group. The arterial carbon dioxide was elevated in both groups, with the obstructive group showing a mean of 66 mmHg (range, 49 to 100 mmHg) and the restrictive group showing a mean of 72 mmHg (range, 34 to 100 mmHg); 5 patients were ventilated preoperatively.

Hemodynamic data are available for 7 patients (4 obstructive, 3 restrictive). All had pulmonary hypertension. Extracorporeal bypass was used in 15 of the 43 patients. In 4 patients, it was used because either heart-lung or double-lung transplantation was performed. In the other 11 patients, 8 were placed on bypass electively as it was felt to be the optimal way to perform single-lung transplantation, 1 required bypass because of intraoperative hypoxemia, and the other 2 had pre- and intraoperative venovenous femoral partial bypass to ameliorate hypercarbia and/or hypoxemia. Of those in whom bypass was not used, 3 cardiac arrests were reported, 1 due to right ventricular failure[8]; the cause of cardiac arrest in the other 2 patients was not reported.

The anesthetic technique and intraoperative course used were reported in detail for only 2 cases. In the case reported by White et al, the patient had arterial and central venous pressure (CVP) catheters inserted.[8]

Induction was done with thiopental; the patient was paralyzed with succinylcholine and intubated with a Carlen's double-lumen tube. Ventilation was performed with an Air Shields Ventimetre respirator and oxygen, ± nitrous oxide, and halothane were used. On one-lung ventilation and an F_iO_2 of 1.0, arterial blood gases were PaO_2 130 mmHg and $PaCO_2$ 82 mmHg, and pH 7.15. Severe hypotension (systolic, 50 mmHg) occurred at the time of one-lung ventilation and progressed to a cardiac arrest with a CVP of 40 cmH$_2$O. The patient was responsive to isoproterenol and the systolic blood pressure improved to 60 mmHg. Following the opening of the transplanted lung, the CVP fell to 3 cmH$_2$O and blood pressure returned to normal. Arterial blood gas values at this point on F_iO_2 of 1.0 were PaO_2 211 mmHg, PCO_2 60 mmHg, and pH 7.25. The patient reported by Rolly et al was anesthetized in the same manner, except that a CVP catheter was not used.[9] On one-lung ventilation (F_iO_2 = 1.0), arterial blood gases were PaO_2 160 mmHg, PCO_2 110 mmHg, and pH 7.21; there were no episodes of hypotension, and the operation was completed uneventfully.

These cases pointed out that the major potential intraoperative problems in the performance of lung transplantation are hypoxemia, hypercarbia, and right ventricular failure. In addition, it was speculated that the use of heparin for bypass in these types of patients, who are likely to have pleural adhesions, would increase the risk of hemorrhage[10]; consequently, avoidance of bypass, as far as it is feasible, would be desirable.

INDICATIONS FOR TRANSPLANTATION

The indication for lung transplantation is irreversible, progressively disabling, end-stage pulmonary disease and falls into four broad groups: restrictive, obstructive, infective, and pulmonary vascular. Cardiac function has to be satisfactory with no evidence of right or left ventricular failure. If clinical signs and symptoms of left and right ventricular failure are present, combined heart-lung transplantation is recommended.

Single-lung transplantation is recommended for patients who are less than 60 years of age and are not suffering from chronic infectious lung disease. The indication for single-lung transplantation in the majority of patients has been restrictive lung disease or pulmonary fibrosis. Experience up to 1989 suggested that patients suffering from obstructive lung disease with hyperinflation are not suitable for single-lung trans-

plants since postoperative ventilation-perfusion mismatch was considered highly likely. Stevens et al reported that in two emphysematous patients, perfusion of implants increased to 70 percent of total perfusion while ventilation and volume decreased to approximately 30 percent of total values.[11] Mal et al, in 1989, reported a successful case in an emphysematous patient; since then, several centers have successfully transplanted single lungs in this patient group.[12]

Patients suffering from pulmonary hypertension and cor pulmonale have traditionally undergone heart-lung transplantation. However, intervention with single-lung transplantation before the development of severe right heart failure may be an alternative approach. The primary consideration in these patients is the degree of reversibility of the right ventricular dysfunction. Experimental and clinical data suggest that a significant degree of right ventricular failure is reversible.[13,14] It is, therefore, suggested that single-lung transplantation be considered for patients with idiopathic pulmonary hypertension and for patients with pulmonary hypertension associated with congenital cardiac abnormalities. Total cardiopulmonary bypass is used with the latter group, while the former may be electively managed with partial bypass.[10]

Double-lung transplantation is indicated in patients with pulmonary disease that is infectious in character (eg, cystic fibrosis or bronchiectasis), because of the risk associated with leaving an infected lung after single-lung transplantation. According to Egan et al,[10] double-lung transplantation is, at the moment, recommended for patients with end-stage emphysema aged ≤ 50 years who have not previously undergone unilateral thoracotomy or pleurodesis, although others prefer the single-lung procedure.[12] A history of previous thoracotomy or pleurodesis is considered a serious relative contraindication to placing the patient on extracorporeal circulatory support for double-lung transplantation, and the unaffected side is operated on when single-lung transplantation is performed.[15,16]

PREOPERATIVE ASSESSMENT

Those accepted for transplantation have to fulfill the selection criteria (Table 20-1), which currently exclude patients on mechanical ventilators. In addition, systemic steroids should be discontinued before consideration for lung transplantation because of the adverse effects of steroids on bronchial healing.[3] It is often a lengthy and difficult process to wean these patients from steroids, and, in some cases, the patients were still on steroids.

TABLE 20-1. Selection Criteria for Lung Transplantation

End-stage progressive lung disease
No clinical evidence of right ventricular failure (ascites, hepatomegaly)
No evidence of left ventricular failure or coronary artery disease
No significant systemic disease
No contraindication to immunosuppressive medications
Psychological stability
Ambulatory and not mechanically ventilated
No steroidal medication

In addition to the regular assessment of the patient's condition, special emphasis is placed on an assessment of pulmonary and cardiac status. The investigations performed are listed in Table 20-2. The $\dot{V}/\dot{Q}$ scan is performed to decide on the comparative function of the two lungs and, thus, to make a selection of the worse lung to be transplanted. Unfortunately, the decision as to which lung is transplanted is determined more by which of the donor's lungs is considered to be in better shape, and by avoidance of the side previously operated on, than by the results of the $\dot{V}/\dot{Q}$ scan. There is also a surgical preference, as operating on the left side is technically easier.[10] The pulmonary function tests are often curtailed, as the patients are incapable of doing the full battery of tests.

Cardiac assessment is done by the use of echocardiography, radionuclide cardiac ejection scans, and coronary angiography in appropriate cases. Right-heart catheterization is only done electively in the exceptional case. This investigation was done in all of the initial cases assessed by the Toronto Group; however, 5 of 10 patients developed respiratory difficulties, three requiring ventilation. Arterial blood gases showed hypoxemia and/or hypercarbia and the chest radiogram was consistent with pulmonary edema. The reason for this complication is unclear, but suspicion has centered on air embolism during insertion of the pulmonary artery catheter, and pulmonary edema secondary to left ventricular dysfunction associated

TABLE 20-2. Lung Transplant Evaluation

Pulmonary assessment
  Pulmonary function test
  Ventilation-perfusion lung scan ($\dot{V}/\dot{Q}$)
  Treadmill exercise test
  Oxygen requirement at rest and exercise

Cardiac assessment
  Radionuclide angiographic ejection scans
  Two-dimensional echocardiogram
  Coronary angiography

with the various pulmonary vasodilator drugs used to assess reversibility of pulmonary hypertension.[17]

Radionuclide cardiac ejection scans are performed as a screening test to define, in conjunction with the echocardiogram, the level of functional competence of the right ventricle and, hence, to identify those patients who are likely to require femoral bypass and those who require heart-lung transplantation. The clinical usefulness of this test has been poor.

Finally, exercise testing is done to assess overall functional competence and the cardiac and pulmonary reserves. Various exercise tests have been suggested. The Toronto Group uses the treadmill exercise at 1 mph and a 4 percent gradient while oxygen saturation is monitored. As it is not unusual for patients to double their exercise tolerance during rehabilitation exercises prior to transplantation, the results relate to the best exercise time and saturation obtained (see Chapter 1).

OPERATIVE PROCEDURE

Single-Lung Transplantation

The operative intervention begins with a midline upper abdominal incision to mobilize the gastrocolic omentum off the transverse colon and to create a retrosternal tunnel through which it is passed.[15] The femoral artery and vein may then be exposed. While not performed routinely, this procedure may be dictated by results of preoperative investigations and by the response to clamping of the pulmonary artery during thoracotomy.

The first step in the thoracotomy is to collapse the lung to be transplanted. After the lung is removed, the pericardium is opened around the pulmonary veins and a left atrial clamp is placed as centrally as possible. The donor lung is then anastomosed, the left atrial cuff with the pulmonary veins attached being anastomosed to the recipient's left atrium. Next, the pulmonary artery anastomosis is completed, but left untied temporarily. Finally, the bronchial anastomosis is performed. The left atrial clamp is then gradually removed and the pulmonary artery anastomosis is observed for back bleeding, which usually occurs after 3 to 4 minutes. Lung inflation may assist the process by which back bleeding occurs. After several minutes, if no back bleeding results, the pulmonary artery clamp is gradually removed as the pulmonary artery suture is tied. The bronchial clamp is also removed and the anastomosis is tested for air leaks. Finally, the omentum is withdrawn from its position in the anterior mediastinum and is completely wrapped around the bronchus.

Double-Lung Transplantation

The double-lung transplant requires standard total cardiopulmonary bypass with a period of aortic cross-clamping and myocardial protection. Cardiopulmonary bypass should be available before induction of anesthesia. As the risk of bleeding during extraction of the diseased lung is higher, a low-dose heparin protocol, 1.5 to 2 mg/kg initially, to maintain an activated clotting time of 250 to 400 seconds is recommended. The omentum is mobilized as for a single-lung transplant.

The first anastomosis is an end-to-end tracheal anastomosis. The recipient trachea is transected just above the carina. On completion of the tracheal anastomosis, the omentum is wrapped around the suture line. As tracheal healing has been a problem after double-lung transplantation, Noiclerc et al have reported the use of bilateral bronchial anastomoses.[18] The atrial cuff and pulmonary artery anastomoses are performed as for the single-lung transplant.

ANESTHETIC TECHNIQUE

All operations are performed with extracorporeal bypass capabilities readily available. The anesthetic requirements are listed in Tables 20-3 and 20-4, and the technique used at Toronto General Hospital will be described.

Peripheral and arterial catheters are inserted prior to anesthesia. The pulmonary artery catheter was, at one time, inserted prior to anesthesia; however, since the patients are dyspneic, it is difficult to position them supine while awake. In addition, two single-lung transplant patients developed air embolism during insertion of the catheter while awake, with one of the two developing low-pressure pulmonary edema and hypoxemia late in the procedure, requiring bypass. In patients undergoing right lung transplant, who require the catheter to be placed in the left lung, catheter placement is accomplished by advancing the catheter from the right ventricle while the patient is on the left side. Placement of the catheter is verified with a chest x-ray.

TABLE 20-3. Anesthetic Equipment

ECG monitor
Arterial and pulmonary artery pressure monitors
Extracorporeal bypass machine with oxygenator
Pulse oximeter and end-tidal CO_2 monitor
Ventilators (anesthetic and constant-flow generators)
Right double- and single-lumen endotracheal tubes
14-Fr Fogarty venous catheter (bronchial blocker)
Peripheral intravenous, arterial, and pulmonary artery
  catheters

TABLE 20-4. Anesthetic Drugs

Fentanyl
Sodium thiopental
Succinylcholine/pancuronium
Isoflurane
Benzodiazepines
Dopamine, nitroglycerin, and phenylephrine in
  separate infusion systems

The patient is anesthetized with fentanyl (5 to 10 μg/kg) and incremental doses (25 mg) of sodium thiopental. Muscular paralysis is achieved with succinylcholine and/or pancuronium. If the right lung is to be transplanted, the patient is intubated with a right Robertshaw double-lumen tube. In left-lung transplants, a Fogarty venous catheter, to be used as a bronchial blocker, is inserted into the airway while the trachea is intubated with a single-lumen endotracheal tube. The patient is connected to a ventilator and an end-tidal CO_2 monitor, and is ventilated with 100 percent oxygen with a tidal volume of 8 to 10 mL/kg at a frequency of 12 to 20 breaths/min. The final settings are determined following blood gas analysis. The end-tidal CO_2 monitor provides inaccurate data at this stage due to high dead space ventilation.[16] In left-lung transplants, the Fogarty venous catheter is next positioned in the left mainstem bronchus, approximately 2 cm from the carina, under direct bronchoscopic control, and the volume required to block the bronchus is determined. Maintenance of anesthesia is with supplemental fentanyl or the addition of diazepam and/or isoflurane; ventilation is continued with oxygen or oxygen/air mixtures as required. The patient's status is monitored by blood gas analysis and hemodynamic measurements.

For double-lung transplantation, the anesthetic requirements are essentially the same, except that all cases are done on total cardiopulmonary bypass and the patients are intubated with a single-lumen endotracheal tube. The intraoperative management is the same as for any patient requiring bypass, although attention should be given to the hyperinflated condition of those with obstructive disease.

INTRAOPERATIVE MANAGEMENT

The major significant points in intraoperative management are pertinent to the single-lung transplants, and all data presented henceforth relate to these patients, who were operated on by the Toronto Group. The indications for operation are listed in Table 20-5. Of the 31 single-transplant patients, 10 had the right lung transplanted; one patient had sequential double-lung transplant done at the same operation, without bypass, using bronchial anastomoses. One of the 10

TABLE 20-5. Indications for Operation in the Toronto Lung Transplantation Experience

Pathology	Single-Lung Transplant		Double-Lung Transplant[a]
	No. of Cases	No. With Bypass	
Restrictive lung disease			
Idiopathic fibrosis	20	6	—
Eosinophilic granuloma-tous	1	0	1
Histoplasmic granuloma-tous[b]	1	0	—
Obstructive lung disease			
Emphysema	5	0	8
Bronchiolitis obliterans	—	—	—
Infective lung disease			
Cystic fibrosis	—	—	3
Bronchiectasis	—	—	1
Pulmonary vascular disease			
Primary pulmonary hypertension[b]	2	2	1
Eisenmenger's syndrome[b]	1	1	—
Retransplanted	1	0	

[a] Two separate single-lung transplants during the same operation.
[b] Total cardiopulmonary bypass.

right-lung transplant patients received a right lung following a previous double-lung transplant.

In total, there were 9 patients requiring bypass. The pulmonary hypertensive patients and the patient with Eisenmenger's syndrome had total cardiopulmonary bypass, a decision that was made preoperatively. They are excluded from the subsequent data and discussion. Six patients had femoral arteriovenous bypass established intraoperatively; none of the emphysematous patients undergoing single-lung transplantation required bypass.

Arteriovenous Bypass

The most significant decision that has to be made after anesthetizing the patient is whether femoral arteriovenous bypass may be required. If so, the femoral vessels on the side contralateral to the thoracotomy are exposed and prepared for possible cannulation. This decision is based on both the preoperative investigations and the response during one-lung ventilation of the blood gases, pulmonary artery pressures, and cardiac index. Thus, during the laparotomy stage of the operation, the lung to be removed is collapsed for 15 minutes and changes in the above parameters are monitored. The femoral vessels were exposed if, preoperatively, the right ventricular ejection fraction was < 25 percent and/or the patient could not exercise on the treadmill for a full 3-minute period and maintain an arterial saturation of > 85 percent. In-

traoperatively, on one-lung ventilation of $F_iO_2 = 1.0$, the vessels were exposed if arterial saturation was < 85 percent, the mean pulmonary artery pressure was > 38 mmHg, or cardiac index, on inotropic support, was ≤ 2.0 L/min/m². Exposure of the femoral vessels was carried out in 14 patients who fulfilled the above criteria.

The specific decision to place a patient on bypass is, however, based on the response to clamping of the pulmonary artery. Hemodynamic parameters and arterial and mixed venous gases are monitored at this time. In this series, if the patient's cardiac index was ≤ 2.0 L/min/m² and/or mixed venous oxygen saturation was < 65 percent, a nitroglycerin and/or dopamine (3.5 to 12 $\mu g/kg/min$) infusion was started, depending on sytemic blood pressure. If the arterial oxygen saturations were ≤ 90 percent on an F_iO_2 of 1.0 or, with the use of nitroglycerin and/or dopamine, the patient's cardiac index was ≤ 2.0 L/min/m² and/or systolic blood pressure was ≤ 90 mmHg, associated with a mixed venous oxygen saturation of ≤ 65 percent, the patient was placed on bypass.

Patient Data from the Series

The data presented relate to the first 22 patients (19 males, 3 females) with restrictive lung disease and 5 (1 male, 4 females) with obstructive lung disease. The average age was 43.7 ± 2.5 years (mean ± SD) for the combined group. Results are analyzed for those requiring bypass (B group) versus those who were not

TABLE 20-6. Pulmonary Function Tests (Percent Predicted)[a]

	Restrictive Disease	Obstructive Disease
Total lung capacity (%)	51.1	159.0
Forced vital capacity (%)	50.6	37.5
Forced expired volume in 1 second	55.4	17.5
Diffusion capacity (%)	31.6	35.0
PaO_2 (mmHg; mean ± SD)	53 ± 11	38.7 ± 7
$PaCO_2$ (mmHg; mean ± SD)	54 ± 11	48.0 ± 14

[a] $F_IO_2 = 0.21$.

placed on bypass (NB group). The pulmonary function tests (percent predicted) are indicated in Table 20-6. Femoral arteriovenous partial extracorporeal bypass was used in 6 patients, all with restrictive lung disease. In one of these patients, bypass was necessary late in the procedure as a consequence of low pulmonary capillary wedge pressure pulmonary edema thought to be secondary to air embolism on insertion of the pulmonary artery catheter. Therefore, only 5 patients were analyzed as requiring bypass directly due to the disease process. No useful data are available for the patient who was retransplanted.

The results of the analyses of the preoperative blood gas, initial pulmonary hemodynamic, and radionuclide angiographic data for the pooled patients are presented in Table 20-7. Highly significant differences are noted between the nonbypass and bypass patients in room air blood gases, pulmonary artery pressures, and cardiac index, while the ejection fractions of the right ventricle are not significantly different. The initial preclamping pulmonary artery pressures of the restrictive group were systolic, 51.7 ± 20 mmHg; diastolic, 27.0 ± 10 mmHg; and mean, 35.5 ± 10 mmHg, while for the obstructive group they were systolic, 37.2 ± 10.0 mmHg; diastolic, 23.6 ± 9.5 mmHg; and mean, 29.4 mmHg.

The exercise test data (Table 20-8) also showed significant differences. The nonbypass group showed a statistical difference in the amount of oxygen required to breathe to achieve a saturation of 95 percent at rest, in their saturation on exercise, and in their duration of exercise.

On clamping the pulmonary artery, the cardiac indices of the nonbypass and bypass groups were 3.10 ± .85 L/min/m² and 1.5 ±0.3 L/min/m², while the mixed venous saturations were 68 ± 3.5 percent and 41 ± 2.7 percent, respectively; both sets of data showed a probability value of ≤ .005. All of the bypass group had systemic hypotension, with a systolic blood pressure < 90 mmHg.

Seven patients in the nonbypass group required dopamine to maintain hemodynamic stability. Pulmonary vasodilators were not deemed to be helpful. Phenylephrine was used in all of the bypass patients, with no appreciable benefit.

Ventilation

The ventilation requirements during two-lung ventilation were a minute ventilation of 10.4 ± 1.8 L/min at a mean peak airway pressure of 41.3 ± 3 cmH₂O to achieve an acceptable PCO_2. During one-lung ventila-

TABLE 20-7. Results of Analysis of Data for Pooled Patients

	Nonbypass	Bypass	Significance[a]
Blood gases (room air)			
PO_2 (mmHg)	56.2 ± 8.8	39.8 ± 5.6	≤ .0005
PCO_2 (mmHg)	42.3 ± 8.0	37.0 ± 9.5	NS
Pulmonary artery pressure (mmHg)			
Systolic	42.3 ± 8.0	78.8 ± 19	≤ .0005
Diastolic	22.9 ± 7.0	41.6 ± 9.6	≤ .0005
Mean	30.7 ± 6.5	56.6 ± 12.8	≤ .0005
Cardiac index (L/min/m²)	3.8 ± 1.0	2.5 ± 0.6	≤ .0005
Radionuclide angiography (%)			
First pass	32.6 ± 4.8	38.0 ± 9.5	NS
Equilibrium at rest	30.3 ± 9.2	34.7 ± 11.5	NS
Equilibrium on exercise	30.3 ± 13.0	28.0 ± 12.7	NS

Abbreviation: NS, not significant.
[a] Student's *t*-test.

TABLE 20-8. Exercise Test Results

	Nonbypass	Bypass	Significance (NB vs B)
Oxygen required (L/min)	3.4 ± 2.2	6.25 ± 1.25	$\leq .005$
Resting O_2 saturation (%)	95.0	94.5	NS
Exercise O_2 saturation	89.5 ± 3.2	80.75 ± 4.3	$\leq .0005$
Duration exercise (min)	4.6 ± 1.4	1.57 ± 1.2	$\leq .0005$

Abbreviations: NB, nonbypass; B, bypass; NS, not significant.

tion, the mean peak airway pressure increased to 52 ± 4.5 cmH$_2$O and the minute ventilation increased to 12.5 ± 4.5 L/min to achieve a mean PCO$_2$ of 51.5 ± 2.7 mmHg. One patient had a PCO$_2$ of 75 mmHg, which was difficult to control because of the functional characteristics of the anesthetic ventilator; a constant-flow generator ventilator is recommended in such cases.

The alveolar-arterial oxygen differences (A-aDO$_2$) on one-lung ventilation before clamping of the pulmonary artery were 483 ± 126 mmHg for the nonbypass group and 606 ± 9.6 mmHg for the bypass group. The differences postclamping were 261.6 ± 43.4 mmHg for the nonbypass group and 608 ± 15.6 mmHg for the bypass group, $P < 0.0005$. Following establishment of the anastomoses and unclamping of both the bronchus and pulmonary artery, the peak airway pressure was 31 ± 3.5 cmH$_2$O while the A-aDO$_2$ was 366 ± 72 mmHg. In the first five cases, the pulmonary artery was unclamped before the bronchial anastomosis was completed to minimize the ischemic time. This resulted in a shunt being established with a marked increase in A-aDO$_2$.

COMMENTARY BASED ON THE TORONTO LUNG TRANSPLANT GROUP EXPERIENCE

Patients with terminal lung diseases of various etiologies can be helped with lung transplantation. Those with fibrotic lung disease are considered to be the ideal candidates for single-lung transplantation, while the best operation for patients with obstructive lung disease, ie, emphysema, is still being evaluated. It is notable that none of the emphysematous patients of the Toronto group and none of those reported by Mal et al[12] and Stevens et al[11] required bypass. Two transplants described by Veith and Koerner were performed with bypass, but these investigators were of the opinion that all lung transplants should be done with bypass control.[7] Single-lung transplantation for patients with hypertensive lung disease is still undergoing evolution and evaluation.

The major anesthetic aspect in the management of single-lung transplantation is the level of right ventricular competence and the support of the right ventricle subjected to an acute increase in afterload on clamping of the pulmonary artery. The data for the patients presented suggest that information useful in predicting the likelihood of bypass can be obtained from the patients' oxygen requirements, exercise tolerance, and pulmonary artery pressures. The management of the right ventricle that fails following clamping of the pulmonary artery is an area that requires additional research.

The literature is not conclusive as to which cardioactive drugs, inotropic and/or vasodilator, are best in sustaining right ventricular function in the face of long-standing pulmonary hypertension or acute cor pulmonale. Vasodilation of the pulmonary vasculature with a decrease in right ventricular afterload does not seem to be the only determinant of right ventricular function. The responsiveness of the pulmonary vasculature in pulmonary hypertension is unpredictable,[17] and those studies showing responsiveness were uncontrolled.[19]

In acute cor pulmonale, Rosenberg et al, using isoproterenol in experimental pulmonary embolism, reported 100 percent mortality, possibly due to decreased myocardial perfusion secondary to a decrease in mean arterial pressure.[20] Others demonstrated a significant improvement in survival and hemodynamic parameters using norepinephrine in experimental pulmonary embolism in anesthetized ventilated dogs.[21] In clinical studies of shock due to pulmonary embolism, Jardin et al evaluated the use of dobutamine and showed significant decreases in right atrial pressure and pulmonary and systemic vascular resistance with no change in mean arterial and pulmonary arterial pressures.[22] Boudrias et al, using dopamine in the same clinical setting, showed increases in mean arterial pressure, cardiac index, and heart rate, in addition to a significant rise in mean pulmonary arterial pressure.[23] Dopamine resulted in a greater increase in systemic blood pressure than equipotent doses of dobutamine.[24]

Salisbury demonstrated that right ventricular failure could be improved by aortic constriction, suggesting that myocardial perfusion may influence the ability of the right ventricle to pump against increased afterload.[25] Vlahakis et al showed improvements in right ventricular function, coronary perfusion, and myocardial metabolic parameters in an animal model of acute right ventricular failure through the use of phenylephrine, an alpha agonist.[26] These data suggest that the optimal pharmacologic goal in the management of acute right ventricular failure is maintenance of right ventricular perfusion and, hence, mean aortic blood pressure.

REFERENCES

1. Hardy JD, Webb WR, Dalton ML, et al: Lung homotransplantation in man. JAMA 186:1065–1074, 1963
2. Derom F, Barbier F, Ringoin S, et al: Ten month survival after lung homotransplantation in man. J Thorac Cardiovasc Surg 61:835–846, 1971
3. Lima O, Cooper JD, Peters WJ, et al: Effects of methylprednisolone and ALA thioprime following lung transplantation. J Thorac Cardiovasc Surg 82:211–215, 1981
4. Lima O, Goldberg M, Peters WJ, et al: Bronchial omentopexy in canine lung transplantation. J Thorac Cardiovasc Surg 83:418–421, 1982
5. Borel JF, Feurer C, Magnee C, et al: Effect of the new antilymphocyte peptide cyclosporin in animals. Immunology 32:1017–1025, 1977
6. Wildevuur CR, Benfield JR: A review of 23 human lung transplantations by 20 surgeons. Ann Thorac Surg 9:489–515, 1970
7. Veith FJ, Koerner SK: The present status of lung transplantation. Arch Surg 109:734–740, 1974
8. White JJ, Tanjer PH, Anthonisen NR, et al: Human lung homotransplantation. Can Med Assoc J 94:1199–1209, 1966
9. Rolly G, Malcolm-Thomas B, Verschraegen R, et al: Anaesthesia during human lung transplantation and early postoperative respiratory treatment. Int Anaesthesiol Clin 10:79–92, 1972
10. Egan TM, Kaiser L, Cooper JD: Lung transplantation. Curr Probl Surg October, 1989
11. Stevens PM, Johnson PC, Bell RL: Regional ventilation and perfusion after lung transplantation in patients with emphysema. N Engl J Med 282:245–249, 1970
12. Mal H, Andreassian B, Pamela F, et al: Unilateral lung transplantation in end-stage pulmonary emphysema. Am Rev Respir Dis 140:797–801, 1989
13. Daly PO, Dembitisky WP, Peterson KL, et al: Modifications of techniques and early results of pulmonary thromboendarterectomy for chronic pulmonary embolism. J Thorac Cardiovasc Surg 93:221–233, 1987
14. Hsieh CM, Mishkel G, Rakowski H, et al: Production and reversibility of right ventricular hypertrophy and right ventricular failure in dogs. J Surg Res 47:304–308, 1989
15. Cooper JD, Pearson FG, Patterson GA, et al: Technique of successful lung transplantation in humans. J Thorac Cardiovasc Surg 93:173–181, 1987
16. Nunn JF, Hill DW: Respiratory dead space and arterial to end-tidal CO_2 tension difference in anaesthetized man. J Appl Physiol 15:383–387, 1960
17. Packer M: Vasodilator therapy for primary pulmonary hypertension. Ann Intern Med 103:258–270, 1985
18. Noiclerc M, Metras D, Vaillant A, et al: Technique chirurgicale de la transplantation bi pulmonaire. J Lyon Chir 84:247–251, 1989
19. Packer M: Is it ethical to administer vasodilator drugs in patients with primary pulmonary hypertension? Chest 95:1173–1174, 1989
20. Rosenberg JC, Hussain R, Lenaghan R: Isoproterenol and norepinephrine therapy for pulmonary embolism. J Thorac Cardiovasc Surg 62:144–148, 1971
21. Angle MR, Molloy DW, Penner B: Cardiopulmonary and renal hemodynamic effects of norepinephrine in canine pulmonary embolism. Chest 95:1333–1337, 1989
22. Jardin F, Genevray B, Brun-Ney D, et al: Dobutamine: a hemodynamic evaluation in pulmonary embolism shock. Crit Care Med 13:1009–1013, 1985
23. Boudrias JP, Dubourg O, Gueret P, et al: Inotropic agents in treatment of cardiogenic shock. Pharmacol Ther 22:53–58, 1983
24. Stoner JD, Bolen JC, Harrison DC: Comparison of dobutamine and dopamine in treatment of severe heart failure. Br Heart J 39:536–571, 1977
25. Salisbury PF: Coronary artery pressure and strength of right ventricular contraction. Circ Res 3:633–640, 1955
26. Vlahakis GJ, Turley K, Hoffman JI: The pathophysiology of failure in acute right ventricular hypertension: hemodynamic and biochemical correlations. Circulation 63:87–95, 1981

21

MANAGEMENT OF PAIN AFTER THORACIC SURGERY

Donald S. Stevens, M.D.
W. Thomas Edwards, Ph.D., M.D.

It is common for a "routine" dose of narcotic administered postoperatively to fail to relieve pain. It is logical to think that a much better job of providing analgesia is being done today than 25 or 30 years ago; however, as can be seen in Table 21-1, this does not seem to be the case. In the 1950s, 33 percent of patients reported insufficient analgesia after surgery.[1-3] Multiple reports 20 and 30 years later showed 31 to 41 percent of patients had the same complaint.[4-11] Donovan et al also showed that 58 percent of medical-surgical patients had experienced "excruciating pain" during their hospitalization and that 43 percent were in pain at the time of the interview.[10]

There are many reasons for the undertreatment of postoperative pain. The behaviors that result from inappropriate attitudes about pain management are those of providers, patients, and payers (Table 21-2).[12,13] The treatment of pain following thoracic surgery, as in most other clinical settings within a hospital, has traditionally rested on the judgment of the nurse caring for the patient about how much pain a patient is experiencing and how much risk there is to treating pain with the standard "morphine, 1 to 2 mg, IV, q1h PRN," or "meperidine, 50 to 100 mg, IM, q3–4h PRN pain." Ultimately, the entire treatment plan rests on attitudes formed in physicians and nurses during their early professional training. As in other medical-surgical areas,[14-17] pain following thoracotomy and pain in patients following blunt chest trauma have frequently gone undertreated because of fears of inducing physiologic instability in the critically ill patient, fears of depressing ventilation in the spontaneously breathing patient, or fears of inducing narcotic dependence. In addition, little attention has been paid to developing appropriate evaluative and treatment skills during the basic clinical education of physicians and nurses.[18] As a result, assessment of pain, aggressive treatment, and the consequences of effective pain management have been poorly understood and post-thoracotomy pain has been handled in a very routine and perfunctory way.[12,13,19-25]

Correct treatment begins with a proper understanding of the source of the patient's complaint, proceeds through the development of a rational plan, and culminates in satisfactory treatment of the problem. Ultimately, this leads to a resolution—the appropriate relief of postsurgical pain, which in turn facilitates recovery.

Much of what is said regarding adults, particularly with regard to attitudes surrounding the treatment of pain, applies to children. Children experience serious and undertreated postoperative pain just as adults do. Efforts at understanding and quantifying children's pain may require application of some different tech-

TABLE 21-1. History of Provision of Analgesia

Reference	No. of Patients	Insufficient Analgesia with Moderate or Severe Pain (%)
Papper et al[1]	286	33
Lasagna & Beecher[2]	122	33
Keats[3]	?	26–53
Keeri-Szanto & Heaman[4]	106	20
Cronin et al[5]	100	42
Banister[6]	437	12–26
Tammisto[7]	100	24
Cohen[8]	109	75
Tamsen et al[9]	56	38
Donovan[15]	200	31
Sriwatanakul et al[11]	81	41

(From Harmer et al,[219] with permission.)

niques, but, fortunately, the pharmacology of acute pain management in children over approximately 6 years of age is not dramatically different from adults. Many of the same therapeutic approaches can be used with children as with adults, including patient-controlled analgesia (PCA) and intraspinal narcotics.[26] However, to treat pain successfully, it is necessary to believe the patient's report. When the patient says "*I hurt,*" it must be considered true, regardless of whether the observer feels there should or should not be the amount of pain the patient reports. Although anxiety and fear are important components of the acute pain experience in children, aggressive analgesia is still important.

DEFINITIONS

1. *Acute pain:* pain that has an identifiable temporal and causal relationship to the occurrence of an injury. This is in contrast to chronic pain, which persists beyond the time of healing of an injury and for which there may not be any clearly identifiable cause.[27]
2. *Noxious stimulus:* a stimulus the intensity of which is harmful or potentially harmful to the integrity of tissue.[28]
3. *Nociception:* the process of detection and signalling the presence of a noxious stimulus.[28]
4. *Pain:* an unpleasant sensory and emotional experience associated with actual or potential tissue damage, or described in terms of such damage (International Association for the Study of Pain definition).[29]

TABLE 21-2. Barriers to Appropriate Postoperative Pain Management

	Deficits in Knowledge/Skills	Resultant Attitude	Inappropriate Resultant Behavior
Health care professionals	Anatomy, physiology, and psychology of postoperative pain Pharmacology of opioid drugs Understanding how to assess pain and response to therapy	The "pain well," fear of physiologic fallout tolerance, respiratory depression, cardiovascular instability; "it doesn't make any difference"	PRN Rx; too little, too infrequently
	Knowledge of spectrum of existing drugs	Conventional approaches	Wrong drug; wrong route of administration
	Understanding existing modern pain Rx technology including advantages/disadvantages of PCA, etc	Patients cannot determine own needs or self-medicate safely	Rx determined by patient's ability to convince staff of sincerity; the adversarial stance
Patients and families	Knowledge of availability of modern pain control	Expect pain around a procedure; should not burden staff	Grin and bear it
	Understanding of "signals" and language to make the system respond to pain control needs	Staff is cruel, uncaring; does not understand—the *enemy*	Cajole, argue, demand—the adversarial approach
System and administrators	Knowledge of role of pain control in marketing services	Pain management team/equipment too expensive	Stonewall requests for personnel/equipment
	Knowledge of potential for reduction of surgical complications/length of stay versus expense of providing service	Service is "unnecessary"	Stonewall requests for payment

Abbreviation: PCA, patient-controlled analgesia.

5. *Suffering:* the reaction of an organism to the experience of pain.[28]
6. *Pain-related behavior:* behavior that leads an observer to conclude that pain and suffering are being experienced.[27]

Acute Pain Mechanisms, Pathways, and Natural History

The anatomy of the "pain pathway" is presented in schematic form in Figure 21-1. Acute pain begins with interruption of integumentary structures. Algogens (pain-causing substances), including small peptides and the prostaglandins, are locally elaborated or released and stimulate peripheral nociceptors. These are "pain-specific," small, thinly myelinated or unmyelinated fibers. The signal generated is projected along these nociceptor fibers into the dorsal horn of the spinal cord (or into the sensory nuclei in cranial nerves). There, modulation (either amplification or deamplification) of the signal can take place before it is projected into pain-specific areas of the deep brain structures and cerebral cortex, resulting in a variety of possible responses.

All along the pain pathway, reflexes are generated that result in responses that are both beneficial (eg, withdrawal from the noxious stimulus) and deleterious (sympathetic discharge and certain neuroendocrine changes characteristic of the stress response) to the injured organism.[30,31] Segmental reflex responses associated with surgery or trauma, for example, include increased skeletal muscle tone and localized spasm with associated increases in oxygen consumption and lactic acid production. Stimulation of sympathetic neurons causes tachycardia, increased stroke volume, cardiac work, and myocardial oxygen consumption. Tone is decreased in the gastrointestinal and urinary tracts. Suprasegmental reflex responses to pain result in increased sympathetic tone, hypothalamic stimulation, increased catecholamine and catabolic hormone secretion (cortisol, corticotropin, antidiuretic hormone, growth hormone, cyclic adenosine monophosphate, glucagon, aldosterone, renin, angiotensin II), and decreased secretion of anabolic hormones (insulin, testosterone). The effects of these changes include sodium and water retention and increased blood glucose, free fatty acids, ketone bodies, and lactate. Oxygen consumption is also increased. Metabolic substrates are mobilized from storage depots, and the postsurgical catabolic state and negative nitrogen balance can be aggravated if the process continues.

The natural history of acute pain ends in spontaneous remission. Pain intensity is greatest at the onset. As healing and stabilization of the injured part take place, there is a reduction in the amount of algogens released while the intrinsic pain modulation system continues to be active. This results in a gradual reduction in the pain sensation. This is true of most types of "simple" acute pain such as postsurgical, trauma, or burn pain. With activation of various pathways during different stages of the recovery, the character of

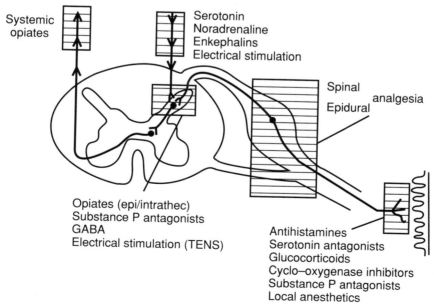

Fig. 21-1. A "map" of the path of nociceptive information from the periphery to the central nervous system. Modification of that information can be effected at any point of information transfer. (From Kehlet,[201] with permission.)

the pain may also change from sharp or cutting to deep and aching, with a concomitant change from being well-localized myotomal or dermatomal pain to poorly localized pain.

THE CONCEPTUAL FRAMEWORK OF POSTOPERATIVE PAIN THERAPY

The representation that best characterizes the relationship among the components of acute pain is shown in Figure 21-2. It does not matter to the observer what the relative sizes of the circles are because all that can be seen is the pain-related behavior. Certainly, a more extensive surgical dissection or trauma resulting in greater tissue damage will lead to the release of greater quantities of the various components of the inflammatory response and other algogens. It would be expected, therefore, that the patient who has a more extensive tissue-damaging operation will always have more pain than one who has a less extensive operation. In fact, in the case of a thoracotomy, some therapies for pain are significantly less effective than when they are used for less tissue-damaging operations.[32] It is common, however, to see two patients who have undergone similar operations with similar anesthetics, one of whom seems to experience great pain while the other appears to have little pain. Often, this difference is described in pejorative terms applied to the patient who seems to have the greater pain, but it is fully understandable if the definitions and the experiential nature of pain are understood. It is important to recall that pain is much more than the sum of its antecedent parts.

Nociception is modulated by many things, including ethnocultural backgrounds and learned behaviors, as well as the meaning of the particular experience for the individual.[22] It is the result of this combination of modulating factors, some ameliorating and some augmenting, that can lead to confusing and apparently paradoxical situations in pain control. Their existence must be accounted for in the process of making an appropriate judgment about a method of treatment. It is understandable that a patient who has undergone a thoracotomy for resection of a potentially metastatic squamous cell carcinoma may experience more pain than a similar patient who has had the same operation for a benign lesion, simply because of the difference in the meaning of the situations to the two patients. In general, a unidimensional approach to treatment will not be as successful as the application of both pharmacologic and nonpharmacologic approaches. Any approach that fails to account for individual patient variability in all aspects of the pain experience will result in a patchwork of treatment results.

Four principles of acute pain management on which

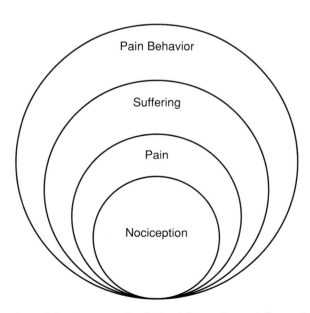

Fig. 21-2. The multifaceted model of acute pain derived from the multifaceted model of pain originally presented by J. Loeser. (Adapted from Loeser,[167] with permission.)

a therapeutic approach must be based can be identified[28]:

1. Correct *diagnosis* of the source and magnitude of nociception
2. *Understanding* of the relationship of ongoing nociception and other components of pain, including anxiety, ethnocultural components, meaning, prior experience, etc.
3. *Treatment* by establishment and maintenance of drug levels at active sites to achieve and maintain analgesia and anxiolysis as appropriate
4. Continued *re-evaluation* of the therapy and refinement of the approach

Some Questions to Ask Before Finalizing a Treatment Plan

Where does it hurt?

Is the location of the pain appropriate for the surgery performed and the patient's current position in bed, or is it in another location entirely? If nociception is not accounted for by the surgical procedure, or by deep visceral or referred pain as applicable, then a secondary process must be investigated and treated, and any one of several causes of postsurgical pain unrelated to the surgical procedure may be involved. The pain may result from intraoperative malpositioning and be myofascial in origin. It may arise as a deafferentation phenomenon (pain arising from the interruption of peripheral nerve fibers) subsequent to intercostal nerve injury. It may have nothing to do with surgery or anesthesia as in patients who have ongoing pain problems, such as underlying chronic pain, or other sources of acute pain, such as those that occur in multiple trauma victims.

What does it feel like?

The quality of the sensation is important. If it is sharp, it is probably direct nociception associated with the incision. Dull aching sensations, well responsive to narcotics, are typical of incisional pain arising from deeper tissue. Pulling or tugging is in keeping with the stitches in the wound and with some visceral stimulation.

Buzzing, stinging, or a sensation of electricity indicate abnormal neural function. These sensations are minimal following regional anesthesia. They are more indicative of neural compression and re-establishment of neural function when they occur in the acute postoperative setting. Painful dysesthesias, as in peripheral neuropathies, may also occur as part of a pre-existing medical condition.

TABLE 21-3. Technique for Grading Pain before and after Treatment

Five-point global scale	None = 0 A little = 1 A lot = 3 The worst = 4
Verbal quantitative	0..........5..........10 none worst imaginable
Visual pain analog scale (VPAS)	No Worst Pain Pain "Place a mark on the line to show where your pain is now."

How much pain?

Each patient should be asked to try to quantify the pain level using a system that was taught before surgery. The visual[33] or verbal pain analog scales (VPAS) are of use here (Table 21-3). It must be remembered that each patient serves as his or her own control, and response is best measured in changes from baseline values. A numerical scale without the visual analog can also be used effectively. The patient need only be asked to try to assign a "number from 0 to 10 to the pain, where 0 = no pain at all and 10 = the worst pain you could possibly imagine." This type of scale is not as accurate as a VPAS, but requires only that there be some preoperative teaching that can occur even while putting in a patient's intravenous catheter preoperatively.

During the patient's postoperative course, be it in the intensive care unit or on the floor, other scales can be added. Sensory and affective components of pain can be assessed using the short-form McGill Pain Questionnaire.[34] Intubated patients can still be assessed even if they are unable to communicate. Restlessness, sweating, tachycardia, lacrimation, pupil dilatation, and blood pressure can all be graded as signs of pain intensity, although any one of these markers of sympathetic activity is not an adequate measurement of pain intensity by itself.[35] It is crucial that pre- and post-treatment measurements be made and recorded in the chart. An accurate assessment of changes in this pain level with therapy can then be made.[20]

Approaches to Therapy—Formulating a Plan

The therapeutic approaches to treatment of acute thoracic pain that are applied at various levels in the pain pathway include the following (Fig. 21-1):

1. Techniques that interfere with nociception in the *periphery*, including the use of nonsteroidal anti-inflammatory drugs given systemically, local infiltration of the wound, intercostal nerve blocks, cryoanalgesia, and interpleural analgesia
2. Techniques that interfere with the first integration of the nociceptive information at the spinal cord level, including epidural and intrathecal infusion of local anesthetics, narcotics, or a combination
3. Techniques that modify nociceptive information broadly throughout the nervous system, particularly the use of systemic narcotics by bolus depot injection (intramuscularly or subcutaneously), bolus or continuous intravenous techniques, and PCA

The choice of a therapeutic modality should be based on a balance of availability of knowledge, skills, equipment, personnel, and drugs; the expected advantages to a particular patient; and the anticipated risks.[27]

LOCAL AND REGIONAL ANALGESIA TECHNIQUES—PERIPHERAL

Intercostal Blocks

Repeated intermittent intercostal nerve blocks have been recommended and used for many years to provide analgesia for chest injuries, such as fractured ribs, as well as for treatment of postoperative pain following surgery. Advantages to this technique include analgesia without widespread sympathetic blockade and analgesia without weakness of major muscle groups, such as can be seen with use of epidural local anesthetics. In addition, analgesia can be obtained without sedation or respiratory depression, as can be seen with narcotics administered either epidurally or parenterally.[36,37] Disadvantages of the intercostal block technique include the need for repeated procedures,[38] the risk of pneumothorax (0.073 to 19 percent),[39] and the potential for systemic toxic reactions to the anesthetic if excessive amounts of local anesthetic are used. Use of this technique may also not be appropriate in anticoagulated patients because of the risk of bleeding and hematoma formation subsequent to laceration of an intercostal artery or vein.[40]

Although pneumothorax from percutaneous injection is not problematic in the presence of a chest tube following thoracotomy, the presence of dressings and the problems of positioning have led to intercostal nerve blocks being performed under direct vision in-

traoperatively by the surgeon.[41,42] The intercostal nerve at the level of the incision, along with one or two nerves both above and below this level, are usually injected with either 4 or 5 mL of local anesthetic. The injection is usually performed where the nerves first appear visible through the parietal pleura. Additionally, one or two levels may be blocked at the level of the thoracostomy tube. There are mixed opinions regarding the effectiveness of this method of treatment. Some investigators feel that intraoperative intercostal blocks help postoperative patients from both an analgesic and a pulmonary function standpoint,[42] while other authors do not.[41] The controversy stems mostly from the transient nature of the relief provided by these procedures.

In an effort to decrease the number of injections required to provide long-lasting analgesia, a continuous technique has been developed for intercostal nerve blocks.[43–45] This is performed by inserting a plastic catheter into a single intercostal space through a Tuohy needle. Up to 20 mL of local anesthetic is then injected through the catheter to provide analgesia to several intercostal segments. Drawbacks include difficulty in placing the catheter correctly[46] and chest wall hematoma formation.[47,48]

Anatomic studies have been performed to locate the site of action responsible for intercostal blockade. Various substances have been injected to delineate the flow to various anatomic sites, including india ink,[49–51] x-ray contrast material,[52,53] liquid latex,[52] and radioactive tracer.[54] Two routes of spread appear to be involved. Injection of material into an intercostal space causes spread both peripherally and centrally along that same intercostal space. If sufficient volume is injected, spread to the paravertebral space can be demonstrated. Alternatively, spread may take place between the parietal pleura and the internal aspect of the ribs (Fig. 21-3). Spread of injected material into the epidural space,[54] as well as into the contralateral paravertebral space,[46] has also been seen. Such spread would explain the appearance of bilateral blocks.[54] Paravertebral spread of local anesthetic has also been suggested as the cause of the development of Horner's syndrome following an intercostal block at the level of the ninth rib. Rostral spread of the local anesthetic in the paravertebral space to the level of the cervicothoracic sympathetic ganglion is the presumed mechanism.[55]

Analgesia through use of intercostal blocks, whether by multiple injections or by placement of a continuous catheter, has been judged to be excellent as compared with traditional methods of parenteral narcotic administration.[56,57] Analgesia produced by continuous intercostal blockade may offer improved pulmonary function relative to treatment with sys-

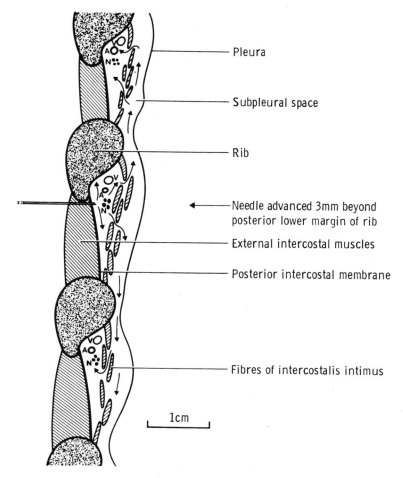

— Pleura

— Subpleural space

— Rib

— Needle advanced 3mm beyond
posterior lower margin of rib

— External intercostal muscles

— Posterior intercostal membrane

— Fibres of intercostalis intimus

1cm

Fig. 21-3. Schematic diagram showing the pattern of spread of solution injected 3 mm beyond the lower edge of the rib. The fascial sheath on the internal aspect of the external intercostal was impermeable to india ink. (From Nunn and Slavin,[49] with permission.)

temic narcotics in patients following thoracotomy, but this is still uncertain.[45,57–59] This technique is most appropriate for treatment of unilateral thoracic or upper abdominal pain.

Paravertebral Blocks

Regional analgesia for postoperative pain in the thorax can be provided by paravertebral nerve blocks, which also can be performed either as a single injection of local anesthetic or as a continuous block.[60] The technique is performed with the patient in the lateral position, with the side to be blocked uppermost. Injection should be performed at the intercostal space through which the incision was made, if possible. The point of injection is located 3 cm lateral to the top edge of the posterior spinous process of the appropriate vertebrae. Either a 3.5-in 22-gauge spinal needle or an appropriate-sized Tuohy needle can be used. The needle is introduced perpendicular to the skin in all planes, and is advanced until bone is contacted, at a depth of 1 to 1.5 in. When bone is contacted, a syringe filled with air is attached to the needle, which is then redirected cephalad. The needle is advanced to pass above the bone, which should be either the rib or the transverse process. A loss of resistance to an injection of air should be felt as the needle passes into the paravertebral space, through the superior costotransverse ligament[60] (Fig. 21-4). The needle must not be directed medially or the epidural space can be entered. The needle should also be aspirated to make sure that it has not entered pleura, lung, blood vessel, or a dural cuff.

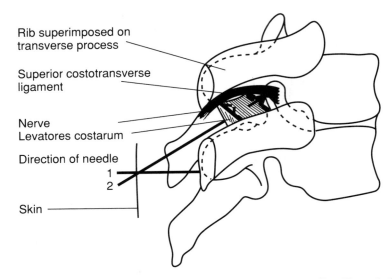

Fig. 21-4. Direction of needle: (*1*) initial to strike transverse process or rib; (*2*) angled to pass through superior costotransverse ligament. (From Eason and Wyatt,[60] with permission.)

X-ray contrast studies explain the effectiveness of this block.[61] Injection into a paravertebral catheter appears to cause flow into one intercostal space, and also up and down the paravertebral space ipsilaterally. This would allow several intercostal nerves to be bathed with anesthetic and would give analgesia over several dermatomal levels. However, epidural and interpleural spread may also be seen,[61] the results of which would be indistinguishable from spread in the paravertebral space.

If a single injection is to be performed, a recommended dose of local anesthetic would be 15 mL of 0.375 percent bupivacaine.[60] If a Tuohy needle is used, a catheter may be advanced through the needle 1 to 3 cm into the paravertebral space. It may be necessary to rotate the needle if the catheter cannot be passed beyond the end of the needle. Initial doses ranging from 25 to 30 mL of 0.25 percent bupivacaine with epinephrine, 1 : 200,000, have been used.[60]

The advantages of paravertebral blocks are similar to those for a continuous intercostal technique. Analgesia can be obtained without the physiologic effects of widespread sympathetic blockade because only unilateral sympathetic blockade is produced. Several levels can be covered by one injection. Because the injection is performed medial to the scapula, it may be performed more easily at high thoracic levels than intercostal blocks. Finally, a nerve block done this far posteriorly almost certainly blocks the posterior primary ramus of the intercostal nerve, which would provide analgesia to the posterior spinal muscles and the costovertebral ligaments, thus providing better analgesia than the routine intercostal block.

Risks of this technique include pneumothorax, epidural blockade, and inappropriate catheter placement.[62] Use of a loss-of-resistance technique should minimize the chance of pneumothorax, and gradual injection of the local anesthetic should minimize complications due to epidural blockade.

An alternative approach is intraoperative placement of a paravertebral catheter.[63] The approach is basically the same, except that it is performed at the end of the surgical procedures, prior to closing the incision. Normal saline is used for the loss-of-resistance test. After the loss of resistance has been obtained, the surgeon should be able to see a subpleural bubble of saline in the chest. Ten milliliters of saline can be injected at that time to allow easier threading of the catheter. Visualization of the catheter apparently helps with making this a successful technique.

Interpleural Block

Interpleural regional analgesia is a technique that has received a large amount of attention in the recent medical literature. It was originally described as a continuous technique using a catheter.[64,65] The approach has been to place an epidural catheter into the interpleural space (between the parietal and visceral pleurae) using a Tuohy needle. The point of injection is at the angle of the rib, approximately 8 to 10 cm from the midline, posteriorly. The needle is walked off the superior border of the rib, with the bevel directed cephalad. Entry into the interpleural space is detected by having a well-lubricated glass syringe containing air attached to the needle. Because pressure in the interpleural space is below atmospheric pressure (often called *negative pressure*), the plunger of the syringe is drawn inward. An epidural catheter is then advanced from 5 to 10 cm into the interpleural space. Alternate techniques involve using an anterior approach similar to the posterior approach, and the use of a "hanging drop" technique in which the syringe filled with air is replaced by a column of saline in the needle. Intermittent injections of local anesthetic into the catheter can be performed, or a continuous infusion may be used.

This technique has been used successfully to manage pain from surgical procedures, including renal surgery,[64] unilateral mammary surgery,[64–66] cholecystectomy[64,65] and thoracotomy.[67] There are case reports describing the use of interpleural analgesia following cholecystectomy in patients with cystic fibrosis,[68] following surgical procedures in children during which a subcostal incision was used,[69] and following thoracotomy in children.[70] It has also been used to provide analgesia for patients with multiple rib fractures.[71]

Intra-abdominal pain may also be controlled using this technique. Pain due to chronic pancreatitis[72] and pain from pancreatic cancer[73,74] have both been treated using this technique. Pain due to hepatic metastatic disease has also been controlled by this technique,[73] all indicating its potential usefulness following thoracoabdominal operations.

The exact mechanism of action is still uncertain. Possible explanations include diffusion of the anesthetic through the parietal pleura to block the intercostal nerves, diffusion of the local anesthetic posteromedially to the paravertebral area to block nerve roots and sympathetic ganglia, and direct action on pleural nerve endings.[75,76] Injection of x-ray contrast along with the local anesthetic through an interpleural catheter has shown spread throughout the entire pleural space. However, there does appear to be some influence of position in that a denser block tends to occur in dependent areas.[65,77,78] Blockade of intercostal nerves does seem to occur,[77] but it appears to be less dense than with standard percutaneous intercostal techniques.[75] Sympathetic blockade has also been seen to occur, with the development of Horner's syndrome and an increase in ipsilateral upper extremity temperature.[78,79] Relief of visceral pain may also indicate that sympathetic block is at least partially responsible for the analgesia seen.[72,73]

A major problem with interpleural analgesia has been inaccurate catheter placement. Use of a loss-of-resistance technique rather than a method to detect negative pressure initially resulted in a high incidence of incorrect catheter placement.[80] However, even use of a technique to detect negative pressure can result in placement of the catheter in the extrapleural space,[81] and a "hanging-drop" technique has been suggested as potentially improving the accuracy of catheter placement.[82] The authors tend to agree with this position. Pneumothorax can also occur, but has been described as being easily evacuated through the catheter.[81] Placement of the catheter into lung tissue has also been reported.[80] Some attempts at continuous intercostal catheter placement have resulted in interpleural catheter placement.[83]

Optimum concentration and total dose of local anesthetic to be used, as well as the preferred method of delivery (ie, intermittent bolus injection versus continuous infusion), remain controversial. Bupivacaine has been the local anesthetic most commonly used to provide analgesia.

Systemic toxicity has been seen when a continuous interpleural infusion of 2 percent lidocaine and epinephrine, 1 : 200,000, at 15 to 20 mL/h was used.[84] The pharmacokinetics of interpleural bupivacaine in various concentrations, with and without epinephrine, are still being evaluated. It appears that bupivacaine is absorbed very rapidly from the pleural space,[64,67] but it is unclear if epinephrine slows this absorption.[67,85,86] Intermittent doses ranging from 20 to 30 mL of 0.25 to 0.75 percent bupivacaine have been used, both with and without epinephrine. Variable analgesic effects have been obtained, but longer duration of action does appear to occur with higher concentrations for any given volume.[87] Much concern has been voiced regarding potential toxic levels of bupivacaine resulting from interpleural administration.

Central nervous system toxicity is generally associated with plasma levels of bupivacaine above 4 μg/mL,[88] but seizure activity has been reported with levels of 2.3 μg/mL[89] and 3.0 μg/mL.[90] Maximum plasma bupivacaine concentrations during interpleural infusions commonly are between 1.7 and 2.4 μg/mL, without seizure activity.[91,92] Individual concentrations as high as 4.2 μg/mL have been reported without toxic side effects.[70]

There is one case report of a patient who developed a toxic level of bupivacaine following a single interpleural injection of 30 mL of 0.5 percent bupivacaine with 1 : 200,000 epinephrine.[92] This patient had a pleural effusion that was noted on placement of the interpleural catheter. The patient had a history of pneumonia that had been treated and resolved 4 weeks preoperatively. A contraindication to the use of this technique may be a recent thoracic infection with concomitant pleuritis, since more rapid absorption of the local anesthetic than usual may take place under these circumstances.

Continuous interpleural infusion of bupivacaine has also been used. Conflicting opinions about the relative efficacy and safety of this approach[70,71,93] leave the question "to infuse or not to infuse" unanswered at this time. Certainly, an infusion of bupivacaine that exceeds 1.5 mg/kg/h should be closely monitored for early evidence of systemic toxicity.

It is necessary to be alert to the risk of inadequate analgesia with interpleural block. This is especially true in thoracotomy patients, because a large amount of the anesthetic agent may be removed through thoracostomy tube drainage.[94] Alternatively, inadequate analgesia may indicate that the tip of the catheter was not placed close enough to the appropriate neural structures for the block to be effective.[70]

One alternative to interpleural catheter placement for post-thoracotomy analgesia has been the use of an indwelling thoracostomy tube for the same purpose.[95] Local anesthetic can be injected and the thoracostomy tube clamped for a few minutes to keep the medication in the interpleural space. Of course, the risks of clamping a thoracostomy tube pertain in this situation.

Contraindications to interpleural analgesia include fibrosis of the pleura, which may create difficulties in identifying the pleural space using the "detection of negative pressure" technique; blood or fluid within the pleural space, which may either dilute the local anesthetic or be an indicator of inflammation of pulmonary tissue; and recent pulmonary infection, which may cause a more rapid absorption of the local anesthetic than is usually seen. Other usual contraindications, such as patient refusal, anticoagulation, or localized infection at the sight of injection also apply. As with other analgesic techniques, the risk of interaction with other intercurrent medical and surgical problems must be considered. One patient has been reported in whom the early symptoms of splenic rupture may have been masked by the use of an interpleural block.[93]

This technique is relatively new, and many questions still remain regarding its use.[96] It may prove to be most useful in certain circumstances that contraindicate the use of other regional analgesia techniques, such as the patient with severe vertebral injuries who requires analgesia for rib fractures, or the patient with pancreatic pain for whom epidural analgesia is difficult or contraindicated.

LOCAL AND REGIONAL ANALGESIA TECHNIQUES—CENTRAL

Alteration of afferent nociceptive information may also be effected at a central level. Small-fiber afferent conduction can be blocked at the nerve root or spinal cord level with local anesthetics, and nociceptive impulses can be down-modulated centrally by the action of intraspinal narcotics at the level of the dorsal horn of the spinal cord. Centrally applied regional analgesia techniques include epidural or subarachnoid intraspinal administration of local anesthetics, opiates, or mixtures of local anesthetics and opiates. Any of these techniques can be used with intermittent dosing or with continuous infusion of the analgesic agent.

Use of spinal anesthesia alone for pain relief during thoracotomy is not adequate, although subarachnoid block could be chosen for operation on the chest wall. Thoracic intrathecal opioids, however, are potentially useful and have been suggested as a method of providing postoperative analgesia for Cesarean section.[97] With the recent introduction of extremely small catheters for continuous spinal anesthesia,[98] placement of an intrathecal catheter that will remain in place for several days for intermittent intrathecal narcotic administration is a possibility. This cannot currently be recommended as a routine approach for post-thoracotomy pain, however.

Epidural anesthesia (combined with general anesthesia) and postoperative epidural analgesia are effective methods of providing pain relief to patients undergoing thoracotomy. Placement of a continuous epidural catheter can be quickly accomplished either preoperatively or prior to emergence from general anesthesia. Properative placement is preferable, because problems encountered during catheterization of the epidural space may not be detected if the patient is under general anesthesia. Paresthesias will not be detected, nor will early symptoms of intravascular injection of local anesthetics. Also, it will not be certain that the epidural catheter has been placed correctly until the patient awakens sufficiently to describe a decrease in sensation in the anesthetized area.

The loss-of-resistance technique may be the most frequently used method for locating the thoracic epidural space. Air and saline have both been used to detect the loss of resistance to injection. The use of saline is recommended because problems can develop with the use of air. In patients who are having combined regional/general anesthesia, nitrous oxide can diffuse into the bubble injected and could potentially cause mechanical compression of intraspinal structures. Also, use of air for loss of resistance has been implicated in producing a spotty epidural blockade.[99] It is also of note that air is not sterile and should certainly not be used for an immunocompromised patient.

The level of placement of the epidural catheter should be carefully considered. If local anesthetic is to be used, either alone or in a mixture with an opioid, the epidural catheter should be placed at an interspace close to the center of the dermatomal segments needing analgesia. If opioids alone are used, then a lumbar approach may be adequate, particularly if morphine is the opioid chosen. More lipid-soluble opioids should be given through a catheter placed as for segmental anesthesia. That is, thoracic analgesia may not be reliable if any opioid except morphine is used through a lumbar epidural catheter.

Placement of a thoracic epidural catheter should be done only by an anesthesiologist well experienced in epidural techniques.[100] Location of the epidural space between T_3 and T_7 is difficult because of the extreme caudad angulation of the long posterior spinous processes at these levels. A paramedian approach to the epidural space is easier than a midline approach at T_3 through L_1 because of the length and angulation of the overlying posterior spinous processes, but this technique should first be mastered in the lumbar interspaces. A paramedian approach may also allow for easier threading of the epidural catheter, once the epidural space has been located. From T_8 to L_2, the epidural space gradually becomes easier to locate, because the posterior spinous processes gradually angle to a more cephalad orientation; however, above L_2, the epidural space gradually becomes smaller because of the size of the spinal cord.[101]

Any epidural catheter that is placed, even solely for the provision of postoperative pain relief, must be properly tested for correct placement.[102] Care must be taken to have available the appropriate fluid and pharmacologic treatment to deal with the sympathectomy that can result from even small doses of local anesthetic given into the thoracic epidural space. A significant segmental block and associated sympathectomy may result from the usual 4 or 5 mL of 1.5 percent lidocaine plus epinephrine, 1 : 200,000, used for the test dose.

Local Anesthetic Infusions

Once a functioning catheter has been placed into the epidural space, adequate postoperative analgesia can be provided by the continuous infusion of local anesthetics. Rapid onset of analgesia can be obtained by use of 1 percent lidocaine, or more long-lasting analgesia can be obtained by use of 0.25 percent bupivacaine. An initial dose of 5 mL of either medication is recommended if the catheter tip is located at T_7 or above. If adequate analgesia is not obtained with this dose, it can be repeated after at least 20 minutes have passed. If no analgesia is obtained after the second dose, a definite decreased reaction to pinprick or cold sensation should be demonstrated to confirm correct placement of the epidural catheter. If it is not functioning correctly, it should be replaced.

Once adequate analgesia is obtained, the patient can be maintained on a continuous infusion of local anesthetic for prolonged analgesia. Use of a low concentration of bupivacaine is preferable, because of the relative sparing of motor function when this agent is used. A routine starting point would be the use of 0.125 percent bupivacaine (without epinephrine) at 6 to 8 mL/h through an infusion pump. The infusion should be started only after analgesia has been achieved by carrying out a conventional differential block.

Tachyphylaxis to bupivacaine is relatively common. This can be handled by increasing the volume infused each hour or by increasing the concentration of the bupivacaine infused. Escalation of the volume by 2 mL/h steps to a maximum of 14 to 16 mL/h is the usual practice. At this level, if there is inadequate analgesia, the bupivacaine concentration is increased to 0.25 percent and the infusion rate slowed to 8 mL/h. Further escalation in bupivacaine dosage can be made as just described, with the next step in concentration being to 0.375 percent. The maximum dose infused should not exceed 30 mg/h, however, and each increase in infusion rate should be preceded by reinforcement of the block as at the outset.

Use of such a continuous infusion technique allows prolonged analgesia,[103,104] but hypotension is frequently seen.[105,106] Blockade of the cardiac sympathetic supply has been suggested as the cause of this hypotension. Upper thoracic epidural block has been shown to decrease cardiac output, primarily by decreasing heart rate, but also by decreasing contractility.[107,108] Hypotension would presumably be due to this decrease in cardiac output coupled with a decrease in systemic vascular resistance from further thoracic sympathetic block. The hypotension can usually be treated by infusion of an adequate volume of fluid.[103] The occurrence of hypotension may limit the mobility of the patient, though, and may limit the usefulness of this technique.[109]

It is of note that the continuous epidural infusion of local anesthetics has been associated with a reduction in postoperative complications.[110] Other studies of the use of thoracic epidural analgesia for patients with unstable angina pectoris[108] or acute myocardial infarction[109] indicate that hypotension does occur in almost every case, but that there is not an unfavorable effect on myocardial perfusion, even in these patients. Therefore, if appropriate care is used for the routine postoperative patient, hypotension should not cause any undue complications if it is appropriately treated.

Intraspinal Opioids

Among techniques that have improved the use of opioids in acute pain management, nothing can compare with the efficiency with which intraspinal opioids produce analgesia. Comparison in one animal model showed that epidural morphine was 40 times more efficacious than subcutaneously administered morphine. Other narcotics showed increases in efficacy relative to their subcutaneous administration, but the ratio was lower than with morphine.[111]

Intraspinal opioids have been delivered in several ways:

1. Single-shot intrathecal
2. Single-shot epidural
3. Intermittent epidural by timed injection through a catheter
4. Intermittent epidural on demand through a catheter
5. Continuous infusion epidural without local anesthetic
6. Continuous infusion epidural with local anesthetic.

Single doses of intrathecal morphine and/or fentanyl have been given at the time of lumbar puncture to provide analgesia postoperatively, but the analgesia does not extend beyond 24 hours. Daily lumbar punctures to administer intrathecal morphine for analgesia following rib fractures have been used with success.[112] A similar series did not have good analgesic success with this technique, and instead reported unacceptable side effects from the use of intrathecal morphine.[113] In one comparison of intrathecal morphine, with epidural morphine for analgesia after thoracotomy,[114] both study groups received good analgesia, but a single intrathecal dose of morphine lasted only approximately 16 hours. A follow-up report from this same group describing the use of lumbar intrathecal morphine in a dose of 10 μg/kg again underscored the limited duration of this technique.[115] Note that the doses in these studies were small compared with the early reports, in which 1 to 2 mg of morphine were used. Even 10 μg/kg may prove to be larger than is necessary.

Overall, the use of a single intrathecal dose of morphine has been recommended for postoperative analgesia because of the ease and simplicity of administration.[116] However, the limited duration of analgesia often makes epidural opioid analgesia preferable. The advent of extremely small catheters for intrathecal placement could solve this limitation by allowing the development of continuous intrathecal techniques. There may also be an approach available in the future in which a dual-lumen 18- and 22-gauge, epidural-spinal needle allows passage of a 29-gauge spinal needle to administer an intrathecal dose of opioid, at the same time that an epidural catheter is placed.[117] Such an approach would allow the best points of both techniques to be used.

The use of epidural opiates for postoperative analgesia is recognized to be very effective in decreasing pain in the clinical setting as well as in the laboratory. The basic concept is to administer an opiate close to its site of action, the dorsal horn of the spinal cord.

The amount of opiate required to provide adequate analgesia depends on a number of factors, including the spinal level of administration, the location of the pain, the age of the patient, and the lipid solubility of the opioid involved.[118,119]

Morphine has been the opioid most commonly used. Because of its relatively low lipid solubility, morphine tends to stay dissolved in the cerebrospinal fluid (CSF) instead of being absorbed by the spinal cord structures or being taken up into the circulation. There is much more rostral migration of morphine sulfate than is seen with more lipid-soluble opioids such as fentanyl. Morphine can, therefore, be administered at lumbar levels for thoracic analgesia.[120–122] In fact, caudal epidural morphine has also been used to give post-thoracotomy analgesia.[123]

Rostral spread may also cause the side effects peculiar to epidural opioids. These include nausea, pruritus, and urinary retention as well as the phenomenon of so-called *late respiratory depression*. Use of lower doses in the thoracic region is recommended to limit the amount of rostral spread and, therefore, to limit the side effects that are all dose-related.

Use of a continuous catheter technique with intermittent bolus dosing of epidural narcotics allows for a relatively fast onset of analgesia, if a lipid-soluble opioid such as fentanyl is used. Rostral spread is limited by the high lipid solubility, so that fentanyl would be quickly bound to the tissues and not remain in the CSF to migrate toward the medulla. A subsequent (or simultaneous) dose of epidural morphine can be given to allow for the slower onset of the analgesia from the morphine. Analgesia is then maintained only with bolus doses of morphine.

Dosing schedules should be dependent on the patient's response to the medication. Dosing with the suggested amount given a second time approximately 6 hours after surgery is not uncommon. Dosing every 8 hours may be needed for the first 1 to 2 days. Dosing every 12 hours is the usual requirement, but, occasionally, patients will need only one dose per day for good analgesia. Timed reinjection (rather than when required) is preferable, and the dosing interval can usually be determined within the first 24 hours. Tables 21-4 and 21-5 provide dosing guidelines for the most commonly used intraspinal opioids, as well as suggestions for dose adjustment necessary to account for patient age and catheter position.

Catheters usually remain in place approximately 2 to 3 days in most patients. After this time, patients have usually had a marked decrease in their postoperative pain, are taking fluids orally, and can be switched to oral analgesics without problem. However, epidural catheters can be left in place indefinitely if there are no signs of inflammation and there is a need for continued aggressive analgesia.

TABLE 21-4. Intraspinal Opioids for Post-Thoracotomy Pain[a]

Drug	Single-Dose	Infusion	Onset	Duration
Epidural				
Morphine	1– 6 mg	0.1–1.0 mg/h	30 min	6–24 h
Meperidine	20–150 mg	2–20 mg/h	5 min	6–8 h
Fentanyl	25–150 μg	25–100 μg/h	5 min	3–6 h
Sufentanil	10–60 μg	10–50 μg/h	5 min	2–4 h
Subarachnoid				
Morphine	0.1–0.3 mg		15 min	8–24 h
Fentanyl	5–25 μg		5 min	3–6 h

[a] Doses must be carefully adjusted for age and catheter position (epidural)—see Table 21-4. Duration of analgesia is variable—tends to increase with dose and patient age.
For accuracy and convenience of administration, adjust concentration to allow approximately 10 mL/h for infusion.
For infusion with bupivacaine, use 0.0625 percent bupivacaine solution.

Comparisons of the analgesic effectiveness of intravenous or intramuscular opioids, intercostal block, epidural morphine, and epidural local anesthetics have been performed.[124–126] Segmental epidural block with local anesthetic resulted in patients being most mobile and alert, but the potential for hypotension required close monitoring and occasional use of vasopressors.[124] Epidural narcotic use allowed easier ambulation, and also did not impair bowel or bladder function. The duration of analgesia was greater, even for a single dose of epidural morphine, than for a single intercostal block.[125] There is evidence, too, that epidural morphine may provide not only better analgesia, but better preservation of pulmonary function in post-thoracotomy patients, as compared with routine parenteral morphine.[126]

The minor side effects of nausea, pruritus, and urinary retention, although symptomatically distressing, are not usually life-threatening to the patient. They can be treated with symptom-specific medication (such as metoclopramide or prochlorperazine for nausea, or diphenhydramine for pruritus), or they can be treated with parenteral opioid antagonists, such as naloxone.[32] Alternatively, systemic (*not* intraspinal) use of a mixed agonist/antagonist drug such as nalbuphine has been shown to be effective in some cases to reverse side effects without reversing analgesia.[127]

Respiratory depression is a potentially serious side effect of epidural opioids. It is obvious that much has been learned regarding this potential problem. However, what is its true incidence? How does this compare with the incidence of respiratory depression seen with intramuscular opioids as routinely prescribed?

Respiratory depression has been evaluated by determining the frequency and severity of oxyhemoglobin desaturation in patients receiving opioids.[128] Forty-nine postcesarean patients received either intramuscular meperidine, epidural morphine, or meperidine by PCA. Although physicians regard intramuscular meperidine as relatively safe and benign, in this study, 63 percent of patients had episodes of desaturation to $\leq$ 85 percent. In the epidural group, 71 percent of patients had similar episodes of desaturation to $\leq$ 85 percent. Both of these groups had what was known as "more frequent episodes of severe desaturation" compared with the PCA group, which had "prolonged periods of mild desaturation". The conclusion of the study was that "cesarean section patients receiving opioids by any of the methods studied may be at risk for respiratory depression." The authors did not recommend the use of intensive respira-

TABLE 21-5. Starting Doses—Epidural Morphine for Thoracic Pain[a]

Patient Age (years)	Catheter Tip at T_4-T_{11} Level	Catheter Tip at T_{12}-L_4 Level
15–44	4 mg	6 mg
45–65	3 mg	5 mg
66–75	2 mg	4 mg
76+	1 mg	2 mg

[a] Careful consideration must be given to the presence of other diseases and to the response to these suggested initial doses.

tory monitoring of patients who had received epidural opioids. The true incidence of respiratory depression with intramuscular narcotics is undoubtedly much higher than is commonly assumed. Adverse outcomes can indeed happen with intramuscular narcotics, just as well as with epidural or PCA narcotics. Assessment of patient condition remains the most important factor in averting potential problems, regardless of the method of administration of the analgesic.

The incidence of clinically significant, treatable respiratory depression associated with epidural morphine is very small—0.9 percent in one review[32] and 4 of 623 patients, or 0.6 percent, in another.[118] The onset is quite similar in most circumstances. There appears to be two peak times of onset, one within 1 to 2 hours and another again 6 to 12 hours later. The early peak appears to correspond with systemic absorption of the opioid from the epidural space. The later peak appears to correspond to rostral spread of the opioid. Most reports describe the gradual onset of respiratory depression, which corresponds to rostral migration. Most patients have become sedated prior to developing respiratory insufficiency. With the gradual accumulation of experience, it has become clear that use of epidural or intrathecal opioids requires observation of the patient for sedation, rather than for a decrease in respiratory rate, as the earliest sign of respiratory depression.[118]

Guidelines have been established by some institutions for whether respiratory monitoring should be instituted; these are described in Table 21-6.[118] However, it has become clear that intraspinal narcotics can be safely used in ward settings if the proper guidelines for selection of patients, dosing, and monitoring are used.[129,130]

TABLE 21-6.   Criteria for Determining When to Use a Respiratory Monitor[a]

A respiratory monitor is not required
  A. When all the following criteria are met:
    1. Age < 50 yr
    2. ASA physical status is I or II
    3. Surgical site is other than the thorax or upper abdomen.
    4. Duration of surgery is < 4 h
    5. Little or no narcotics or other long-acting central nervous system depressants are used before or during surgery
    6. Epidural morphine dose is 6 mg or less or the subarachnoid morphine dose is 0.5 mg or less
                         or
  B. When the postoperative care location provides continuous nursing surveillance

  [a] These are only guidelines. A respiratory monitor may be ordered for any patient at the discretion of the operating room anesthesiologist, the acute pain service, or the unit charge nurse.
  (From Ready et al,[118] with permission.)

Overall, prevention is better than treatment.[131,132] The use of a planned dosage scale based on location of the catheter, location of the surgical site, and age of the patient may prevent respiratory depression. It is especially important that no additional systemic opioids be given without discussion with a pain management specialist familiar with the use of epidural narcotics. Summation of the gradually increasing central effect with the systemic effect may cause severe respiratory depression. Other medications, such as sedatives and tranquilizers like the benzodiazepines, may also interact with epidural narcotics.

Treatment of clinically important respiratory depression should be with titrated doses of a narcotic antagonist. Divided doses of naloxone, 0.1 to 0.2 mg, can be given intravenously. Alternatively, 0.4 to 0.8 mg of naloxone can be given intramuscularly by nursing personnel if they are not cleared for intravenous administration. An ampule of naloxone should be left at the bedside at all times. It has been suggested that a continuous intravenous infusion of naloxone can prevent respiratory depression from epidural opioids.[133,134] An infusion of up to 5 μg/kg/h can be used without reversing the analgesic effect of the epidural opioid, but reversing the signs of respiratory depression (hypercarbia, decrease in respiratory rate, decrease in minute volume). Alternatively, use of a continuous intravenous infusion of nalbuphine has been described as antagonizing the respiratory depression without decreasing the analgesia.[135] A bolus of 200 μg/kg of nalbuphine, followed by an infusion of 50 μg/kg/h, was used to prevent respiratory depression.

Intermittent bolus dosing of epidural morphine is the most common way that epidural narcotics are used at present. However, in an effort to provide smoother analgesia, continuous infusion techniques using various opiates have been described. Morphine was the first opioid so used.

One series evaluated the relative effect of bolus dosing with bupivacaine, bolus dosing with morphine, and a continuous morphine infusion at 0.1 mg/h in post-thoracotomy patients with epidural catheters.[136] Use of 0.5 percent bupivacaine was associated with severe hypotension in 23 percent, urinary retention in 100 percent, and sensorimotor block in the upper extremities in 40 percent of patients. Bolus dosing with morphine, 5 mg, also resulted in urinary retention in 100 percent of patients, with pruritus in 40 percent and depressed consciousness in 27 percent. Low-dose continuous morphine infusion resulted in good analgesia with a much lower incidence of side effects. Additional 2 mg IV doses of morphine were also available to these patients. None showed a depressed level of consciousness. Only 7 percent developed urinary retention and only 3 percent developed pruritus. The first postoperative day, mean total dose was 2.4 mg/ 24 h by continuous epidural infusion and 5.7 ± 2.4 mg/24 h by intravenous supplement.

This study has been faulted because in the bolus group, with T_4-T_5 catheter placement, 5 mg boluses were given with a first postoperative day mean total dose of morphine sulphate, 21.7 ± 5.7 mg/24 h, which is far beyond the doses currently recommended.[118] Also, the dose of bupivacaine was large in the group treated with local anesthesia, and 0.5 percent bupivacaine can be expected to produce surgical anesthesia. The use of a continuous morphine infusion appears to be a viable technique, however, and fewer side effects may result if this technique is used compared with intermittent bolus dosing.[136] Continuous infusion of 0.1 mg/h of morphine has recently been shown to improve pain relief and markedly decrease intensive care unit stay in a group of patients with blunt chest trauma.[137]

Continuous infusion of fentanyl into an epidural catheter has also been used to treat postoperative pain. The greater lipid solubility of fentanyl compared with morphine should limit rostral migration of fentanyl and fewer side effects should occur.[138] One series compared continuous fentanyl epidural infusion with intramuscular papaveretum.[139] These patients had upper abdominal surgery performed. An epidural catheter was placed at the seventh thoracic interspace, and 6 mL/h of 10 μg/mL of fentanyl was used. Patients receiving the epidural fentanyl had better analgesia than the patients receiving the intramuscular narcotic preparation, and they were more alert. Respiratory function, as measured by forced expiratory volume at 1 second (FEV_1) and forced vital capacity (FVC), was significantly better in the epidural group. There were more complaints of nausea in the epidural group, but no urinary retention was observed. There was a 20 percent incidence of pruritus in the epidural group.

A continuous epidural fentanyl infusion has been used for post-thoracotomy pain, and its analgesic effect compared with cryoanalgesia of the intercostal nerves.[140] A continuous epidural catheter was placed in the epidural space close to the level of incision between T_6 and T_9. A bolus dose of 1.5 μg/kg of fentanyl diluted into 10 mL with normal saline was given, and was followed with a continuous epidural infusion of 0.6 μg/kg/h of fentanyl, using a solution of 12.5 μg/ mL. Bolus doses of epidural fentanyl and gradual increases in the epidural infusion rate were used if analgesia was inadequate. The cryoanalgesia group had six or seven intercostal nerves frozen, and had intramuscular papaveretum available for additional analgesia. Pruritus was more common in the epidural fentanyl group (44 percent versus 8 percent), but there

was no significant difference between the groups with regard to drowsiness, urinary retention, or nausea. The patients receiving epidural fentanyl had a trend for lower pain scores that was significant at 32 and 40 hours postoperatively.

It might seem that a continuous infusion of a highly lipid-soluble opioid could help avoid the risk of respiratory depression associated with intraspinal narcotics, but such does not appear to be the case. Epidural fentanyl, whether given by bolus dose or by continuous infusion, appears to cause some respiratory depression.[141,142] This appears to be rapid in onset, such as may be caused by systemic absorption. However, this depression does not appear to be statistically significant in most studies. Use of a CO_2 rebreathing test in one study did show an insignificantly diminished response to a CO_2 challenge.[141]

Combined Local Anesthetic-Opioid Infusions

More recently, a combined approach has been tried. Combining a local anesthetic and an opioid may give the benefits of each medication without the severity of side effects were the individual drugs used to full effect. One approach has been to use epidural doses of morphine for analgesia and to add intermittent bolus doses of bupivacaine to allow for greater movement.[143] One series of 50 patients with chest trauma showed that excellent analgesia was obtained in 96 percent of patients by using this technique.

Continuous infusions of local anesthetics mixed with opioid have also been used. Initial studies were performed with morphine and bupivacaine. One study evaluated the effectiveness of this technique in patients after major abdominal surgery.[144] This study showed that a continuous infusion of 0.5 percent bupivacaine provided no analgesia in 90 percent of patients after 16 hours, presumably due to tachyphylaxis. The addition of 0.5 mg/h of epidural morphine to the same infusion gave excellent analgesia in 100 percent of the study patients at 16 hours after surgery. A comparison of continuous epidural infusion of bupivacaine, morphine, or a mixture of bupivacaine and morphine for analgesia in post-thoracotomy patients found no difference demonstrable between the morphine and the combined morphine and bupivacaine groups regarding amount of analgesia, but there was a tendency (although not statistically significant) for the morphine group to have more complete analgesia than the bupivacaine group.[145] All three groups were far better than a control group that received "traditional" intramuscular morphine on an "as needed" basis.

Most of the work comparing bupivacaine and morphine infusions with bupivacaine and fentanyl infusions has been done in obstetric patients, but the principles can be extended to thoracotomy patients.[146] In one group of postcesarean patients, both infusions gave good analgesia, but the patients who received bupivacaine and fentanyl infusion had a lower incidence of nausea and pruritus. Adequate analgesia should be obtainable in the post-thoracotomy patient with fentanyl-bupivacaine mixtures using similar infusion techniques.

Continuous infusion of bupivacaine and sufentanil has also been compared in post-thoracotomy patients with bupivacaine and nicomorphine.[147] Only one patient of 40 (2.5 percent) had orthostatic hypotension. The serum bupivacaine level gradually increased over the 3 days of infusion, but remained well below toxic levels at all times. Respiratory depression was evidenced only by a slight rise in the arterial CO_2 on postoperative day 1 in the nicomorphine group, but not on later days. No elevation of CO_2 was seen in the sufentanil group. There was excellent analgesia to movement (forced expiration, coughing, pulmonary physiotherapy) in 80 percent of the sufentanil group, but in only 15 percent of the nicomorphine group. Sufentanil has also been infused without local anesthetic at a dose equalling approximately 0.1 μg/kg/h by high thoracic epidural with good effect.[148]

Overall, the use of combinations of local anesthetics with opioid for continuous epidural infusion appears to be an effective technique for postoperative analgesia. There seem to be fewer side effects with this technique compared with the use of either local anesthetics alone (hypotension) or opioid alone (pruritus, nausea, potential respiratory depression). However, there is some question whether the main site of action of opioid given in this fashion is intraspinal, since the circulating levels of fentanyl are the same and pain ratings are the same whether fentanyl is infused into the epidural space or intravenously.[149] Slow continuous infusions may be administering the opioid into another parenteral location. Absorption of opioid can occur from many locations, and still give analgesia—including from the interpleural space.[150] However, there may well be a combined effect, in that both intraspinal receptors close to the site of injection and other central opioid receptors may be involved in the production of analgesia.

SYSTEMIC ANALGESIA

Logical approaches to pain control need not be unduly complicated or time and personnel intensive. Such schemes begin with the choice of an appropriate drug and route of administration, but must always proceed with appropriate understanding of pharmacokinetics.

Nonopioid Systemic Analgesics

Because there are definite potential complications in the use of high doses of opioids, the use of systemic nonnarcotics in conjunction with opioids or alone is an attractive therapeutic alternative. The analgesic efficacy of some of these agents is, however, small enough that they are not useful without opioid. Some agents that have been suggested as "adjuvants to analgesia" actually have no analgesic properties and cannot be used without opioid.

Subanesthetic doses of anesthetic agents have been used in various clinical situations to provide analgesia. Examples of this are the use of nitrous oxide in patients with tetanus[151] and the use of methoxyflurane in patients in labor.[152] However, prolonged exposure to low levels of anesthetic agents also has its complications. Bone marrow suppression from the action of nitrous oxide inhaled over long intervals has been well documented.[151] Potential teratogenesis related to subanalgesic concentrations of nitrous oxide is also of concern to personnel working in the area where it is being administered.[153] Also, the metabolism of inhaled volatile anesthetic agents is being recognized as a potential problem, even for more recently developed agents.[154] The use of such agents in the post-thoracotomy patient would be limited.

Benzodiazepines, barbiturates, phenothiazines, and butyrophenones have all been used in conjunction with opioids.[155] They should be used for anxiolysis, sedation, and production of amnesia, but not for analgesia, because they have no analgesic properties. In the production of anxiolysis, however, they may depress consciousness and ventilation sufficiently that endotracheal intubation and mechanical ventilation are necessary. Their main use may well be for patients who will need prolonged ventilatory assistance and in whom sedation will be helpful during the first 24 to 48 hours postoperatively.

Nonsteroidal anti-inflammatory agents can also act as adjuvants to opioid analgesics. They interfere with the production of prostaglandins, which are compounds that can produce hyperalgesia.[156] As such, nonsteroidal anti-inflammatory agents may diminish the inflammatory response to surgery and may also diminish nociceptive input by this route. A number of these compounds have been used parenterally, including acetylsalicylate,[157] diclofenac,[158] dipyrone,[159] indoprofen,[160] and ketorolac.[161] The latter drug is currently available in the United States in parenteral form and is undergoing widespread evaluation for the managment of postoperative pain.

Indomethacin can be used to augment opioid analgesia in the postoperative period. It has been shown to provide improved analgesia after lower extremity surgery, when given intravenously,[162,163] but side effects such as gastrointestinal upset and hypotension may result. Rectal indomethacin has also been shown to provide improved analgesia after major abdominal surgery.[164] Indocin (indomethacin) suppositories (100 mg tid) were shown to provide better analgesia during the first 3 postoperative days, with less respiratory depression noted on the first postoperative day than with opioid alone. No difference was noted in this study between the control group and the study group with regard to gastrointestinal side effects. Indocin suppositories (100 mg tid) given to post-thoracotomy patients have been shown to reduce opioid requirements relative to controls.[165]

Systemic Opioid Analgesia

Opioids used for systemic administration must be front-loaded to achieve a minimum effective analgesic concentration (MEAC). From this pharmacologic vantage point it is much easier to maintain analgesia. The administration of narcotic without front-loading will not result in the achievement of MEAC for at least three elimination half-lives,[166] and subjects the patient to a needless period of unrelieved pain. Table 21-7 provides simple guidelines for front-loading of popular opioid drugs used in postoperative pain management.[12] Figure 12-2 is a model for acute pain, derived from Loeser's model,[167] in which the source of nociception is a known and potentially quantifiable noxious stimulus. In a postsurgical setting, this stimulus is the amount of tissue damage incurred as a result of the surgery. Greater tissue damage sometimes suggests the use of very potent drugs, but the choice of opioid is often dictated by convenience or familiarity to the care team. Even under those circumstances, a rational application of the chosen drug's pharmacologic profile in the clinical situation will improve the quality of pain management.

If depot drugs (intramuscular, subcutaneous, or transdermal) must be used, they should be administered on a time-contingent basis that is consistent with their uptake, redistribution, and elimination kinetics. This route of administration is not recommended in the intensive care unit, however, because of the extreme hysteresis in drug levels (and therefore in pain relief) that results from the nature of depot techniques. Continuous intravenous infusion of opioid is a relatively simple technique that is often overlooked as a possibility for non-intensive care unit patients when more sophisticated technology is not available. With this technique, it is recommended to front-load into the therapeutic window (Table 21-6) and then to maintain a therapeutic blood level of opioid by a continuous infusion. The rate of infusion can be determined by using a fairly simple calculation based on some elementary bits of information; it requires that front-loading be carried out using stepwise titration to analgesia[28]:

TABLE 21-7. Guidelines for Front-Loading Intravenous Analgesics

Drug	Total Front-Load Dose	Increments	Cautions
Morphine	0.08–0.12 mg/kg	0.03 mg/kg q 10 min	Histamine effects; nausea; biliary colic; reduce dose for elderly
Meperidine	1.0–1.6 mg/kg	0.30 mg/kg q 10 min	Reduce dose or change drug for impaired renal function
Codeine	0.5–1.0 mg/kg	1/3 total q 15 min	Nausea
Methadone	0.08–0.12 mg/kg	0.03 mg/kg q 15 min	Do not administer maintenance dose after analgesia is achieved; accumulation; sedation
Levorphanol	0.02 mg/kg	50–75 μg/kg q 15 min	Similar to methadone
Hydromorphone	0.02 mg/kg	25–50 μg/kg q 10 min	Similar to morphine
Pentazocine	0.5–1.0 mg/kg	1/2 total q 15 min	Psychomimetic effects; may cause withdrawal in narcotic-dependent patients
Nalbuphine	0.08–0.15 mg/kg	0.03 mg/kg q 10 min	Less psychomimetic effect than pentazocine; sedation
Butorphanol	0.02–0.04 mg/kg	0.01 mg/kg q 10 min	Sedation; psychomimetic effects like nalbuphine
Buprenorphine	up to 0.2 mg/kg	1/4 total q 10 min	Long-acting like methadone, levorphanol; may precipitate withdrawal in narcotic-dependent patients; safe to give subcutaneous maintenance after analgesia—different from methadone

1. Most conventionally used opioid drugs have an elimination half-life of approximately 3 hours.
2. The dose required to maintain the level achieved during front-loading will be one-half the dose required to produce analgesia during front-loading.
3. The hourly requirement is based on steps 1 and 2 and is infused continuously to maintain the therapeutic effect.

Example: A patient requires 7.5 mg IV of morphine sulfate to be rendered analgesic following a hysterectomy. A continuous infusion is to be used: 7.5 mg/2 = 3.75 mg eliminated in one elimination half-life. A total of 3.75 mg is eliminated every 3 hours, or 3.75 mg/3 h = 1.25 mg/h required.

This approximation tends to underestimate hourly requirements because the elimination half-life is actually less than 3 hours. As a first approximation, however, it usually yields fairly good results and makes the calculation of continuous infusion rates more than a guess.

The rational application of pharmacology states that simply increasing the infusion rate in a patient who has experienced breakthrough will leave the patient with nontherapeutic levels for at least three drug half-lives, and the achievement of a therapeutic effect requires that the estimate of the new infusion rate actually brings the individual patient into the therapeutic range. This is not necessarily the case. Breakthrough pain must be dealt with as new onset pain and opioid must be titrated to effect before the new infusion rate is established.

Patient-Controlled Analgesia

Patient-controlled analgesia is nothing but a technique for the administration of small doses of opioid intravenously on a demand basis. This is truly the ideal melding of the continuous intravenous infusion principle with a "need-driven" demand. Two major differences exist between conventional PRN regimens and PCA.[12] The first difference is that the route of administration is intravenous. This bypasses the lag induced in the feedback loop by uptake and redistribution from a subcutaneous or intramuscular depot. The second difference is the elimination of the complicated and time-consuming ritual (Fig. 21-5), that ensues when the nurse must be located, obtain the narcotic keys, draw up and chart medication, double-check patient drug administration records, and administer the medication. The elimination of these two delays by the use of a fixed prescription delivered by a

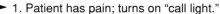

1. Patient has pain; turns on "call light."
2. Secretary answers; responds, "I'll get your nurse."
3. Nurse is located at far end of corridor, returns to station, checks med sheet and cardex.
4. Nurse looks for narcotic keys.
5. Narcotic cupboard unlocked, drug drawn up and charted.
6. Nurse administers drug to patient by IM SC injection.
7. Drug uptake and redistribution begin.
8. MEAC is achieved, but drug elimination begins.
9. Period of analgesia ensues.

A — 10. Circulating level drops out of therapeutic range.

1. Patient has pain; presses "demand switch."
2. Microprocessor checks Rx against most recent administration time.
3. MEAC achieved.
4. Period of analgesia ensues.

B — 5. Circulating level drops out of therapeutic range.

Fig. 21-5. The feedback loops for **(A)** PRN depot administration and **(B)** PCA administration of opioid. The interval from the first response to a patient's request for treatment until the achievement of analgesia, even if enough drug is prescribed and administered, may be as much as 80 minutes of every treatment cycle. MEAC, minimum effective analgesic concentration. (From Edwards,[12] with permission.)

microprocessor-controlled pump may eliminate as much as 80 minutes of every 4-hour cycle, which a patient could spend in pain even if enough opioid has been prescribed.[168]

Inasmuch as PCA is basically a modified intravenous infusion technique, many of the same principles apply as in determining intravenous infusion rates. The problem both with PCA and with continuous infusions is that requirements for narcotic are highest at the beginning of therapy. Even front-loading does not cover all eventualities in this regard because of such things as diminishing effects of general anesthetic agents and redistribution of analgesic drug, which take place most dramatically during the first 24 hours after surgery. In establishing the upper limit for PCA (the 1- or 4-hour limit that the instrument requires be set as an alarm condition), it is best to take account of as much as a fivefold increase in need during the early postoperative period.[169,170] If it is predicted that 1.5 mg/h should be infused to maintain MEAC for morphine in a particular patient, the 1-hour limit should be set at 7.5 mg/h, which allows patients to titrate their own increased requirement during the early phase. Maintenance doses should generally not exceed 0.02 mg/kg of morphine equivalent or the equivalent of 1.5 mg/dose in most adult patients. Lockout intervals of 5 to 10 minutes are usual and take account of the time required for a new concentration to be established at the active site. Breakthrough needs to be dealt with as with a continuous infusion in that an additional front-load will be necessary before a new prescription is started. It should be remembered that PCA can easily *keep* a patient comfortable; it is very difficult to *make* a patient comfortable with PCA alone.

What about relative overdose? The wonderful feature of PCA that makes overdose such a low-risk problem is that patients tend to titrate themselves into the therapeutic range and to keep themselves out of the toxic range. Most patients choose not to eliminate pain entirely, but maintain a satisfactory level of analgesia that is individually determined.[171–174] If an overestimate of the maintenance dose is made, the patient will become sleepy with each dose and the level will decrease during the sleeping period. Overdose is a more significant risk if a background infusion is added to PCA. Some machines do not allow such background infusion, but if one is used in an effort to provide longer pain-free periods, no more than one-half of the predicted hourly requirement (PHR) should be supplied in this way. *This is not the 1- or 4-hour limit.* Recall that those alarm limits are set deliberately high. Because patients do not control the infusion background, accumulation is possible. Therefore, if the PHR determined by calculation averages 2 mg

of morphine equivalent/h, no more than 1 mg should be given by background continuous infusion to PCA.

Problems do exist with PCA, as with any therapeutic technique. Lack of adequate analgesia results from inadequate dosing. This can arise from a failure of the patient to understand the technique, equipment malfunction, or programming errors. Overdose can occur, too, because of equipment malfunction or programming error.[175] An unusual problem is the administration of drug by someone other than the patient. This occurs primarily in pediatric patients for whom patient-controlled analgesia has become "parent-controlled," but also has been reported as "spouse-controlled" analgesia.[176]

The very nature of PCA requires that patients be awake and cooperative. The drowsy or uncooperative patient is not suitable for this technique. Pediatric patients can be very cooperative and learn quickly how to use the demand button. Certainly, patients as young as 6 years can use the technique effectively.[177,178] Most centers restrict general use of PCA to patients over 10 years of age, however. It is still unknown whether patients with a history of drug abuse can use PCA effectively.

Transdermal Approach

A conventional approach to opioid administration has been the deposition into some tissue of a bolus of drug that is taken up and redistributed according to many variables, including blood flow to the tissue in which the depot has been deposited and the intrinsic chemistry of the drug. One relatively new approach to opioid delivery has been the development of transdermal fentanyl (TTS-fentanyl).

In this approach, a patch containing a store of opioid is worn on the skin and functions as a depot from which it is metered to and absorbed through the skin. Various rates of delivery can be chosen by selecting different patches because the drug is slowly deposited into the skin from which it is taken up. Rather than being transdermal, it is functionally intradermal. One recent study examined the usefulness of this type of system after upper abdominal surgery.[179] Use of the transdermal fentanyl patch decreased demand for additional opioid, which was provided by a PCA device. Peak expiratory flow rates were improved when compared with control patients, who used just the PCA device.

Use of a transdermal delivery system may avoid underdosing a patient, due either to nursing delays or to the patient not requesting the medication soon enough. This would resemble a continuous opioid infusion without the need for an intravenous catheter. Potential dangers include error in choosing the dose required, giving the patient too much medication. The real problem with this error is that because there is a fairly large store of drug in the skin, it will continue to be taken up into the circulation for an extended period of time.[180] Usual side effects of opioid excess would then gradually occur and persist. Another caution should be noted if this system is used in patients with multiple medical problems or multisystem failure. Cancer patients became severely obtunded using transdermal fentanyl when they developed other unrelated medical complications.[181]

INFLUENCE OF PAIN CONTROL ON SURGICAL COMPLICATIONS, OUTCOME, AND COST

With the availability of the many different methods of analgesia described, there exists the potential remedy for the type of anguish described at the beginning of this chapter. Ethical issues aside, however, any technique must have benefits that outweigh its associated risks, so that it becomes financially rational to use it. There is evidence that appropriate postoperative pain control has a salutary effect on several specific areas. These include pulmonary function, pulmonary complications, endocrine and metabolic stress response, gastrointestinal function, hemodynamic stability, and length of hospital stay.

Pulmonary Function and Pulmonary Complications

Prevention of postoperative pulmonary complications is one of the major goals of providing adequate postoperative analgesia. The major pulmonary complications usually considered are atelectasis, lung infections, and arterial hypoxemia.[182] These have been related to decreases in vital capacity and reduced ability to cough and clear secretions.[183] Decreases in FVC and in FEV_1 have been documented to occur with different sites of surgical incision.[184] The decreases in FVC and FEV_1 are the same regardless of the preoperative pulmonary function test values; post-thoracotomy patients experience a drop in both FVC and FEV_1 to 25 percent of preoperative values on the first postoperative day.

Overall, reduction in functional residual capacity (FRC) is the most important mechanical abnormality affecting pulmonary complications.[185] This leads to atelectasis, because the FRC falls below closing volume (the lung volume at which small airway closure occurs), which causes arterial hypoxemia. Stasis of

secretions occurs, which also leads to greater potential for pulmonary infections.[186]

One relatively simple maneuver that improves FRC is changing the posture of the patient from supine to sitting. FRC is higher in the sitting position than in the supine position, and changing to the sitting position raises FRC above the closing volume. Oxygenation then improves.[187] One great advantage of the analgesic techniques described in this chapter is that they provide enough analgesia to allow patients greater mobility in their postoperative course. This allows the sitting position to be attained earlier and, therefore, it is possible to avoid pulmonary complications from airway closure and atelectasis. This has been demonstrated to be true for morbidly obese patients undergoing gastroplasty.[188] Fewer pulmonary complications resulted from the earlier mobility seen with epidural narcotic analgesia compared with the intramuscular route.

Splinting due to pain from the incision site definitely decreases FRC, and relief of incisional pain partially restores pulmonary function. Intercostal nerve blocks have been shown to limit the decreases in FVC and FEV_1 seen after thoracotomy.[189] This effect has been seen to last for the entire first week after thoracotomy.[190] The use of interpleural bupivacaine has also been shown to have a favorable effect on limiting decreases in FVC and FEV_1 after cholecystectomy.[191] The use of epidural local anesthetics has been shown to improve FVC relative to controls, in that there was a drop in FVC of only 30 to 45 percent after upper abdominal surgery, compared with a drop of 50 to 60 percent in control patients.[192,193] Also, there may be a lower incidence of atelectasis in patients using epidural local anesthetics when they are compared with patients receiving traditional intramuscular narcotics for analgesia.[194] Analgesia with epidural morphine also leads to significantly smaller decreases in FVC and FEV_1 than are seen in post-thoracotomy patients receiving intravenous morphine for analgesia.[126] Patient-controlled analgesia has also been found to produce higher FVCs compared with traditional intramuscular PRN narcotic regimens in patients after gastric bypass surgery.[195]

The use of analgesic techniques such as intercostal block, interpleural analgesia, epidural analgesia with local anesthetics and/or opioids, and PCA seems to produce some improvement in pulmonary function when compared with controls. However, some studies do not show any statistically significant decrease in complications after surgery, even if aggressive analgesia is provided.[196,197] Is there any definite evidence that the overall outcome is improved by aggressive analgesia? Certainly in patients with multiple rib fractures, such techniques are advantageous.[137]

Twenty-eight patients with multiple rib fractures were prospectively evaluated. Continuous throracic epidural morphine was used in 15 patients, and standard morphine parenteral analgesia was used in 13. With the use of epidural morphine, there was a significant decrease in ventilator-dependent time, intensive care unit stay, hospital stay, and a lower incidence of tracheostomy than there was in the control group. There is a strong case to be made, therefore, that more aggressive pain management techniques can benefit overall outcome, at least in patients with severe chest trauma. It is not clear that this response is specific to intraspinal opioids. Comparisons have been made between the various central regional analgesic techniques and intramuscular morphine, PCA morphine, and continuous infusion morphine.[198,199] The use of other aggressive analgesic techniques appears to produce almost the same effect on the prevention of decreases in FVC, FEV_1, and FRC as do epidural techniques. Therefore, if epidural techniques are contraindicated or technically impossible, the other techniques described in this chapter, if properly applied, may well have the same beneficial effect on postoperative pulmonary function.

The Endocrine-Metabolic Stress Response

When the body is injured, it responds both locally and generally. Surgical trauma is a form of injury, and both local and systemic responses to the injury are seen.[200] The local inflammatory reaction is considered beneficial for healing and for defense against infection. The generalized systemic response is an endocrine-directed metabolic activation. A hypermetabolic state follows the surgical insult, and there is an increase in both substrate mobilization and in the rate of most biochemical reactions. This is referred to as the *stress response.*

The stress response may be beneficial to the body by providing the best potential chance for healing and survival. However, if prolonged, that same stress response may be detrimental because of its devastating nutritional consequences. Much has been done to define what comprises the stress response and what effect different types of anesthesia have on that response. The reader is referred to recent reviews for an in-depth analysis of the individual hormonal responses involved.[200–202]

Overall, it appears that only major regional anesthesia is beneficial in preventing or diminishing the stress response to a surgical procedure.[200] General anesthesia, even very deep levels, does not appear to have much effect on the stress response to surgery.

Even high-dose narcotic techniques have shown only a very mild, short effect in diminishing the endocrine and metabolic stress response.

The beneficial effects of regional anesthesia can persist into the postoperative period, when a regional technique with local anesthetic is used to provide postoperative analgesia. This has been shown to be true for lower abdominal procedures and for procedures on the lower extremities.[200] One recent study indicated that there was a definite nitrogen-sparing effect when epidural analgesia was used during and after lower abdominal surgery.[203] However, it appears that regional techniques are much less successful in blocking the endocrine and metabolic stress response to surgery when the procedure is performed on either the upper abdomen or thorax. There is some evidence that epidural bupivacaine may block this response during the 24 hours after upper abdominal surgery[204] and that intercostal blocks may block the rise in glucose seen after thoracotomy.[205] However, the data obtained from most studies indicate a great degree of variability in obtaining any blockade of the metabolic and stress response, when the surgical site is cephalad to the lower abdomen.

Why is this the case? One partial answer may be that there is a limited blockade of fast-conducting afferent nerve fibers with thoracic epidural analgesia using 0.5 percent bupivacaine.[206] Incomplete blockade of somatic sensory fibers may allow the endocrine and metabolic stress responses to occur. Because it is easier to achieve a more complete somatosensory block in a more caudad location (fewer cardiovascular and respiratory complications follow such dense block of the lower thoracic to sacral segments), more complete interruption of the sensory afferent triggers of the stress response is possible with regional anesthesia for lower abdominal surgery than for thoracic surgery. Failure to block either the sympathetic or parasympathetic efferents may also allow the stress response to proceed unabated.[200]

Use of parenteral narcotic analgesics in the postoperative period has almost uniformly shown no benefit in reducing the stress response.[200] This has also been examined in post-thoracotomy patients, using continuous epidural infusion of dilute bupivacaine with either morphine or sufentanil.[207,208] Although the quality of analgesia was much better in the patients given the epidural infusion, there was no difference in the endocrine and metabolic stress responses to surgery in these patients when compared with controls.

Other medications do have potential for reducing the stress response. A preliminary study indicates that epidural clonidine may provide a method of blockade of the cortisol response to abdominal surgery.[209] If this medication can be used in the post-thoracotomy patient without side effects, then control of the stress response may well be possible along with use of an epidural catheter to provide postoperative analgesia.

Gastrointestinal Function

The slowing of gastrointestinal function, "postoperative ileus," is a routine postoperative finding. Return of normal gastrointestinal function is necessary for patient recovery. Opioids are well known to inhibit normal propulsive gastrointestinal motility. This is expected with parenteral opioids,[210,211] but can be seen with epidural opioids as well.[210-212] Are there methods of providing analgesia that are better than traditional methods, but that cause less slowing of gastrointestinal function?

One recent study examined the effect, after hysterectomy, of postoperative epidural analgesia with bupivacaine on postoperative paralytic ileus.[213] Study patients were given epidural bupivacaine for intraoperative anesthesia as well as for postoperative analgesia for the first 26 to 30 hours. A control group that received intramuscular ketobemidone was used for comparison. A significantly shorter duration of ileus was seen in the patients who received epidural bupivacaine when compared with controls.

Overall, it appears that analgesia with epidural local anesthetics may produce the least amount of gastrointestinal slowing. Longer duration of ileus is seen with epidural opioids than with epidural local anesthetics, but this is still better than the duration seen with parenteral narcotic analgesic therapy.[212] Patient-controlled analgesia would be expected to provide the same amount of gastrointestinal slowing as an equivalent dose administered parenterally elsewhere.

Hemodynamic Stability

Painful stimuli evoke a generalized sympathetic response.[214] With sympathetic stimulation, the major determinants of myocardial oxygen consumption, namely, heart rate, contractility (inotropy), and wall stress (afterload), are all increased. This can set the stage for myocardial ischemia. Treatment of the underlying pain is necessary to reverse this situation.

As discussed previously, use of analgesic techniques other than major regional anesthesia will not prevent the endocrine and metabolic stress response to surgery. However, there is good evidence that intraoperative use of epidural opioids can blunt the sympathetic response following major surgery. One recent study examined the effect of epidural morphine on plasma catecholamine levels and on the incidence of hypertension in patients undergoing operations on the ab-

dominal aorta.[215] Control patients received epidural saline. Study patients received one dose of intraoperative epidural morphine. All patients were given intravenous morphine for analgesia in the postoperative period. Patients who received epidural morphine received 50 percent less parenteral morphine in the 24 hours following surgery, and had lower analog pain scores as well. Plasma epinephrine levels were not different, but plasma norepinephrine levels were lower in the epidural morphine group. Most importantly, once the patients were normothermic, there was a lower incidence of hypertension needing treatment in the epidural morphine group (33 percent) than in the control group (75 percent). It appears that even though the stress response to surgery may not be eliminated by epidural opioids, there may be enough of a reduction in sympathetic nervous system activation to make this analgesic technique worthwhile for improving hemodynamic stability.

Length of Hospital Stay

Recent changes in reimbursement make the duration of hospital stay a very important consideration in patient care. It is, of course, best to avoid potential complications that can prolong a patient's recovery. Are there any data that show a benefit in reduction of hospital stay with these newer analgesic methods? One early study examined the effect of repeated intercostal blocks on the recovery time of patients undergoing cholecystectomy.[216] The control group received intramuscular meperidine for analgesia. Patients who received only intercostal blocks for analgesia were found to ambulate more quickly, and were discharged from the hospital sooner than the control group.

When the effect of PCA on hospital stay in postthoracotomy patients was investigated,[217] the use of PCA was found to shorten the length of hospitalization by 22 percent compared with the control group, which was treated with conventionally administered parenteral analgesics. More recent work has continued to verify these early observations. One study showed an average decrease of 4.6 hospital days (25 percent of time of hospitalization) in post-thoracotomy patients treated with PCA compared with non-PCA-treated patients.[218]

Role of Therapy Versus Role of Therapist

It appears that advanced techniques for analgesia can make a significant difference in overall patient outcome. Totally apart from the issue of providing better patient comfort, these techniques appear able to shorten the length of recovery time for post-thoracotomy patients. The implication of the finding that improvement in outcome may not be technique-specific is that it is the intervention of the care providers who are skilled at and aggressive about effective pain management that makes the difference. That is, the improvement in outcome may not be therapy-specific but therapist-specific. There is no current information to substantiate this position. At this institution, however, and in several others that use the acute pain service concept,[118] it is rare that following major chest surgery or chest trauma patients do not receive a consultation from and intervention by the acute pain management service at the request of the responsible surgeon. The clinical impression of both the surgeons and the pain management specialists is that in this group of patients, those who are treated aggressively for acute pain do markedly better than those who are not. This is, perhaps, one of the strongest arguments for the development of high levels of pain management skills in anesthesiologists, since the overall goals of postoperative pain management must always remain as follows:

1. To provide maximum patient comfort consistent with well being
2. To hasten recovery by reducing rates of complication
3. To perform the first two goals in the most efficient, cost-effective manner possible

Anesthesiologists are in a unique position to influence the postoperative course of patients following chest surgery, because their knowledge of pharmacokinetics and of block procedures, as well as their experience with the clinical pharmacology of analgesics, prepares them better than any other members of the health care team to carry out these goals.[219,220]

REFERENCES

1. Papper EM, Brodie BB, Rovenstine EA: Postoperative pain: its use in the comparative evaluation of analgesics. Surgery 32:107, 1952
2. Lasagna L, Beecher H: The optimal dose of morphine. JAMA 156:230, 1954
3. Keats AS: Postoperative pain: research and treatment. J Chronic Dis 4:72, 1965
4. Keeri-Szanto M, Heaman S: Postoperative demand analgesia. Surg Gynecol Obstet 134:647, 1972
5. Cronin M, Redfern PA, Utting JE: Psychometry and postoperative complaints in surgical patients. Br J Anaesth 45:879, 1973
6. Banister EHD: Six potent analgesic drugs. A double-blind study in postoperative pain. Anaesthesia 29:158, 1974
7. Tammisto T: Analgesics in postoperative pain relief. Acta Anaesthesiol Scand, suppl. 70:47, 1978
8. Cohen FL: Postsurgical pain relief: patients' status and nurses' medication choices. Pain 9:265, 1980
9. Tamsen A, Hartvig P, Fagerlund C, et al: Patient-controlled analgesic therapy: clinical experience. Acta Anaesthesiol Scand, suppl. 74:157, 1982
10. Donovan M, Dillon P, McGuire L: Incidence and characteristics of pain in a sample of medical-surgical inpatients. Pain 30:69, 1987
11. Sriwatanakul K, Weis OF, Alloza JL, et al: Analysis of narcotic usage in the treatment of postoperative pain. JAMA 250:926, 1983
12. Edwards WT: Optimizing opioid treatment of postoperative pain. J Pain Symptom Manage, suppl. 5:S24, 1990
13. Oden RV: Acute postoperative pain: incidence, severity, and etiology of inadequate treatment. Anesthesiol Clin North Am 7:1, 1989
14. Marks RM, Sachar EJ: Undertreatment of medical inpatients with narcotic analgesics. Ann Intern Med 78:172, 1973
15. Donovan BD: Patient attitudes to postoperative pain relief. Anaesth Intensive Care 11:125, 1983
16. Chapman PJ, Ganendran A, Scott RJ, Basford KE: Attitudes and knowledge of nursing staff in relation to management of postoperative pain. Aust N Z J Surg 57:447, 1987
17. Dudley SR, Holm K: Assessment of the pain experience in relation to selected nurse characteristics. Pain 18:179, 1984
18. Pilowsky I: An outline curriculum on pain for medical schools. Pain 33:1, 1988
19. Fields HC: Sources of variability in the sensation of pain. Pain 33:195, 1988
20. Egan K: Psychological issues in postoperative pain. Anesthesiol Clin North Am 7:183, 1989
21. Austin KL, Stapleton JV, Mather LE: Multiple intramuscular injections: a major source of variability in analgesic response to meperidine. Pain 8:47, 1980
22. Bates MS: Ethnicity and pain, a biocultural model. Soc Sci Med 24:47, 1987
23. Wallace LM: Preoperative state of anxiety as a mediator of psychological adjustment to and recovery from surgery. Br J Med Psychol 59:253, 1986
24. Parkhouse J, Lambrechts W, Simpson BRJ: The incidence of postoperative pain. Br J Anaesth 33:345, 1961
25. Benedetti UC, Bonica J, Bellucci G: Pathophysiology and therapy of postoperative pain; a review. Adv Pain Res Ther 7:373, 1984
26. Berde CB: Pediatric postoperative pain management. Pediatr Clin North Am 36:921, 1989
27. Ready LB, Edwards WT: IASP Task Force on Acute Pain. The management of acute pain, a practical manual. Pain, suppl. (in preparation)
28. Edwards WT, Breed RJ: The treatment of acute postoperative pain in the post-anesthesia care unit. Anesthesiol Clin North Am 8:235, 1990
29. Merskey H, Albe-Fessard DG, Bonica JJ, et al: Pain terms: a list with definition and notes on usage. Pain 7:249, 1979

30. Kehlet H: The stress response to anaesthesia and surgery: release mechanism and modifying factors. Clin Anaesth 2:215, 1984

31. Bent JM, Paterson JL, Mashiter, et al: Effects of high-dose fentanyl anaesthesia on the established metabolic and endocrine response to surgery. Anaesthesia 39:19, 1984

32. Stenseth R, Sellevold O, Breivil H: Epidural morphine for postoperative pain: experience with 1085 patients. Acta Anaesthesiol Scand 29:148, 1985

33. Huskisson EC: Visual analog scales. p. 33. In Melzack R (ed): Pain Measurement and Assessment. Raven Press, New York, 1983

34. Melzack R: The short form McGill Pain Questionnaire. Pain 30:191, 1987

35. Rawal N, Tandon B: Epidural and intrathecal morphine in intensive care units. Intensive Care Med 11:129, 1985

36. Rawal N, Sjostrand U, Christofferson E, et al: Comparison of intramuscular and epidural morphine for postoperative analgesia in the grossly obese: influence on postoperative ambulation and pulmonary function. Anesth Analg 63:583, 1984

37. Faust RG, Nauss LA: Post-thoracotomy intercostal block: comparison of its effects on pulmonary function with those with intramuscular meperidine. Anesth Analg 55:542, 1976

38. Gibbons J, James O, Quail A: Relief of a pain in chest injury. Br J Anaesth 45:1136, 1973

39. Moore DC: Intercostal nerve block for postoperative somatic pain following surgery of thorax and upper abdomen. Br J Anaesth 47:284, 1975

40. Nielsen CH: Bleeding after intercostal nerve block in a patient anticoagulated with heparin. Anesthesiology 71:162, 1989

41. Galway JE, Caves PK, Dundee JW: Effect of intercostal nerve blockade during operation on lung function and the relief of pain following thoracotomy. Br J Anaesth 47:730, 1975

42. Delilkan AE, Lee CK, Yong NK, et al: Postoperative local analgesia for thoracotomy with direct bupivacaine intercostal blocks. Anaesthesia 28:560, 1973

43. O'Kelly E, Garry B: Continuous pain relief for multiple fractured ribs. Br J Anaesth 53:989, 1981

44. Murphy DF: Intercostal nerve blockade for fractured ribs and postoperative analgesia, description of a new technique. Reg Anesth 8:151, 1983

45. Murphy DF: Continuous intercostal nerve blockade for pain relief following cholecystectomy. Br J Anaesth 55:521, 1983

46. Mowbray A, Wong KKS, Murray JM: Intercostal catheterization. Anaesthesia 42:958, 1987

47. Baxter AD, Flynn JF, Jennings FO: Continuous intercostal nerve blockade. Br J Anaesth 56:665, 1984

48. Moore DC: Intercostal blockade. Br J Anaesth 57:543, 1985

49. Nunn JF, Slavin G: Posterior intercostal nerve block for pain relief after cholecystectomy, anatomical basis and efficacy. Br J Anaesth 52:253, 1980

50. Moore DC: Intercostal nerve block: spread of india ink injected to the rib's costal groove. Br J Anaesth 53:325, 1981

51. Murphy DF: Continuous intercostal nerve blockade: an anatomical study to elucidate its mode of action. Br J Anaesth 56:627, 1984

52. Moore DC, Bush WH, Scurlock JE: Intercostal nerve block: a roentgenographic anatomic study of technique and absorption in humans. Anesth Analog 59:815, 1980

53. Hosie HE, Crossley AWA: A radiographic study of intercostal nerve blockade in healthy volunteers. Br J Anaesth 58:129P, 1986

54. Middaugh RE, Menk EJ, Reynolds WJ, et al: Epidural block using large volumes of local anesthetic solution for intercostal nerve block. Anesthesiology 63:214, 1985

55. Brown RH, Tewes PA: Cervical sympathetic blockade after thoracic intercostal injection of local anesthetic. Anesthesiology 70:1011, 1989

56. Rawal N, Sjostrand UH, Dahlstrom B, et al: Epidural morphine for postoperative pain relief: a comparative study with intramuscular narcotic and intercostal nerve block. Anesth Analg 61:93, 1982

57. Baxter AD, Jennings FO, Harris RS, et al: Continuous intercostal blockade after cardiac surgery. Br J Anaesth 59:162, 1987

58. Murphy DF: postoperative intercostal block. Br J Anaesth 61:370, 1988

59. Lyles R, Skurdal D, Stene J, Jaberi M: Continuous intercostal catheter techniques for treatment of post-traumatic thoracic pain. Anesthesiology 65:A205, 1986

60. Eason NJ, Wyatt R: Paravertebral thoracic block—a reappraisal. Anaesthesia 34:638, 1979

61. Conacher ID, Kokri M: Postoperative paravertebral blocks for thoracic surgery. Br J Anaesth 59:155, 1987

62. Purcell-Jones G, Pither CE, Justins DM: Paravertebral somatic nerve block: a clinical, radiographic, and computed tomographic study in chronic pain patients. Anesth Analg 68:32, 1989

63. Govenden V, Mattews P: Percutaneous placement of paravertebral catheters during thoracotomy. Anaesthesia 43:246, 1988

64. Kvalheim L, Reiestad F: Interpleural catheter in the management of postoperative pain. Anesthesiology 61:A231, 1984

65. Reiestad F, Stromskag KE: Interpleural catheter in the management of postoperative pain, a preliminary report. Reg Anesth 11:89, 1986

66. Schlesinger TM, Laurito CE, Bauman VL, Carranza CJ: Interpleural bupivacaine for mammography during needle localization and breast biopsy. Anesth Analg 68:394, 1988

67. Symreng T, Gomez MN, Rossi N: Intrapleural bupivacaine *v* saline after thoracotomy—effects on pain and lung function. A double-blind study. J Cardiothorac Anesth 3:144–149, 1989

68. Bruce DL, Gerken MV, Lyon GD: Postcholecystectomy pain relief by intrapleural bupivacaine in patients with cystic fibrosis. Anesth Analg 66:1187, 1987

69. McIlvaine WB, Chang J, Jones MA, et al: Intrapleural bupivacaine for analgesia after subcostal incision in children. Reg Anesth, suppl. 1. 13:31, 1988

70. McIlvaine WB, Knox RF, Fennessey PV, Goldstein M: Continuous infusion of bupivacaine via intrapleural catheter for analgesia after thoracotomy in children. Anesthesiology 69:261, 1988

71. Rocco A, Reiestad F, Gudman J, McKay W: Intrapleural administration of local anesthetics for pain relief in patients with multiple rib fractures, preliminary report. Reg Anesth 12:10, 1987

72. Sihota MK, Ikuta PT, Holmblad BR, et al: Successful pain management of chronic pancreatitis and postherpetic neuralgia with intrapleural technique. Reg Anesth, suppl. 2. 13:40, 1988

73. Durrani Z, Winnie AP, Ikuta P: Interpleural catheter analgesia for pancreatic pain. Anesth Analg 67:479, 1988

74. Waldman SD, Allen ML, Cronen MC: Subcutaneous tunneled intrapleural catheters in the long-term relief of right upper quadrant pain of malignant origin. J Pain Symptom Manage 4:86, 1989

75. Covino BG: Interpleural regional analgesia. Anesth Analg 67:427, 1988

76. Raj P: Intrapleural anesthesia—applications and contraindications. Anesthesiol Alert 1:1, 1988

77. Riegler FX, Pelligrino DA, VadeBoncoeur TR: An animal model of intrapleural analgesia. Anesthesiology 69:A365, 1988

78. Sihota MK, Holmblad BR: Horner's syndrome after intrapleural anesthesia with bupivacaine for postherpetic neuralgia. Acta Anaesthesiol Scand 32:593, 1988

79. Parkinson SK, Mueller JB, Rich TJ, Little WL: Unilateral Horner's syndrome associated with interpleural catheter injection of local anesthetic. Anesth Analg 68:61, 1989

80. Symreng T, Gomez MN, Johnson B, et al.: Intrapleural bupivacaine—technical considerations and intraoperative use. J Cardiothorac Anesth 3:139–143, 1989

81. Brismar B, Pettersson N, Tokics L, et al: Postoperative analgesia with interpleural administration of bupivacaine-adrenaline. Acta Anaesthesiol Scand 31:515, 1987

82. Squire RC, Morrow JS, Roman R: Hanging-drop for intrapleural analgesia. Anesthesiology 70:2, 1989

83. Graziotti PJ, Smith GB: Multiple rib fractures and head injury—an indication for intercostal catheterization and infusion of local anaesthetics. Anaesthesia 43:964, 1988

84. El-Baz N, Faber LP, Ivankovich AD: Intrapleural infusion of local anesthetic: a word of caution. Anesthesiology 68:809, 1988

85. Denson D, Sehlhorst CS, Schultz REG, et al: Pharmacokinetics of intrapleural bupivacaine: effects of epinephrine. Reg Anesth, suppl. 1. 13:47, 1988

86. Kambam JR, Hammond J, Parris WCV, Lupinetti FM: Intrapleural analgesia for postthoractomy pain and blood levels following bupivacaine intrapleural injection. Can J Anaesth 36:106, 1989

87. Stromskag KE, Reiestad F, Holmqvist ELO, Ogenstad S: Intrapleural administration of 0.25%, 0.375%, and 0.5% bupivacaine with epinephrine after cholecystectomy. Anesth Analg 67:430, 1988

88. Jorfeldt L, Lofstrom B, Pernow B, et al: The effect of local anaesthetics on the central circulation and respiration in man and dog. Acta Anaesthesiol Scand 12:153, 1968

89. Ryan DW: Accidental intravenous injection of bupivacaine: a complication of obstetrical epidural anaesthesia. Br J Anaesth 45:907, 1973

90. Yamashiro H: Bupivacaine-induced seizure after accidental intravenous injection, a complication of epidural anesthesia. Anesthesiology 47:472, 1977

91. El-Nagger MA, Raad C, Yogaratnam G, et al: Intrapleural intercostal nerve block using 0.75% bupivacaine. Anesthesiology 67:A258, 1987

92. Seltzer JL, Larijani GE, Goldberg ME, Marr AT: Intrapleural bupivacaine—a kinetic and dynamic evaluation. Anesthesiology 67:798, 1987

93. Pond WW, Somerville GM, Thong SH, et al: Pain of delayed traumatic splenic rupture masked by intrapleural lidocaine. Anesthesiology 70:154, 1989

94. Chan VWS, Arthur GR, Ferrante FM: Intrapleural bupivacaine administration for pain relief following thoracotomy. Reg Anesth, suppl. 2. 13:70, 1988

95. Lee VC, Abram SE: Intrapleural administration of bupivacaine for post-thoracotomy analgesia. Anesthesiology 66:586, 1987

96. Rosenberg PH, Scheinin BMA, Lepantalo MJA, Lindfors O: Continuous intrapleural infusion of bupivacaine for analgesia after thoracotomy. Anesthesiology 67:811, 1987

97. Chadwick HS, Ready LB: Intrathecal and epidural morphine sulfate for postcaesarean analgesia—a clinical comparison. Anesthesiology 68:925, 1988

98. Hurley RJ: Continuous spinal anesthesia. Int Anesthesiol Clin 27:46, 1989

99. Dalens B, Bazin J, Haberer J: Epidural bubbles as a course of incomplete analgesia during epidural anesthesia. Anesth Analg 66:679, 1987

100. Cousins MJ, Bromage PR: Epidural neural blockade. p. 253. In Cousins MJ, Bridenbaugh PO (eds): Neural Blockade in Clinical Anesthesia and Management of Pain. 2nd Ed. JB Lippincott, Philadelphia, 1988

101. Blomberg RG, Jaanivald A, Walther S: Advantages of the paramedian approach for lumbar epidural analgesia with catheter technique. Anaesthesia 44:742, 1989

102. Moore DC, Batra MS: The components of an effective test dose prior to epidural block. Anesthesiology 55:693, 1981

103. Griffiths DPG, Diamond AW, Cameron JD: Postoperative extradural analgesia following thoracic surgery: a feasibility study. Br J Anaesth 47:48, 1975

104. Shuman RL, Peters RM: Epidural anesthesia following thoracotomy in patients with chronic obstructive airway disease. J Thorac Cardiovasc Surg 71:82, 1976

105. Conacher ID, Paes ML, Jacobson L, et al: Epidural analgesia following thoracic surgery. Anaesthesia 78:546, 1983

106. James EC, Kolberg HL, Iwen GW, Gellatly TA: Epidural analgesia for post-thoracotomy patients. J Thorac Cardiovasc Surg 82:898, 1981

107. Otton PE, Wilson EJ: The cardiopulmonary effects of

upper thoracic epidural analgesia. Can Anaesth Soc J 13:541, 1966

108. Blomberg S, Emanuelsson H, Ricksten SE: Thoracic epidural anesthesia and central hemodynamics in patients with unstable angina pectoris. Anesth Analg 69:558, 1989

109. Toft P, Jorgensen A: Continuous thoracic epidural analgesia for the control of pain in myocardial infarction. Intensive Care Med 13:388, 1987

110. Yeager MP, Glass DD, Neff RK, Brinck-Johnsen T: Epidural anesthesia and analgesia in high-risk surgical patients. Anesthesiology 66:729, 1987

111. Edwards WT, White MJ, Xiao CS: A comparison of epidural and systemic narcotics in modification of vocalization behavior in the guinea pig. Pain 4:347, 1987

112. Kennedy BM: Intrathecal morphine and fractured ribs. Br J Anaesth 57:1266, 1985

113. Dickson GR, Sutcliffe AJ: Intrathecal morphine and multiple fractured ribs. Br J Anaesth 58:1342, 1986

114. Fromme GA, Gray JR: A comparison of intrathecal and epidural morphine for treatment of post-thoracotomy pain. Anesth Analg 64:214, 1985

115. Gray JR, Fromme GA, Nauss LA, et al: Intrathecal morphine for post-thoracotomy pain. Anesth Analg 65:873, 1988

116. Stoelting RK: Intrathecal morphine—an underused combination for postoperative pain management. Anesth Analg 68:707, 1989

117. Campbell C: Epidural opioids—the preferred route of administration. Anesth Analg 68:710, 1989

118. Ready LB, Oden R, Chadwick HS, et al: Development of an anesthesiology-based postoperative pain management service. Anesthesiology 68:100, 1988

119. Klinck JR, Lindop MJ: Epidural morphine in the elderly. Anaesthesia 37:907, 1982

120. Fromme GA, Steidl LJ, Danielson DR: Comparison of lumbar and thoracic epidural morphine for relief of post-thoracotomy pain. Anesth Analg 64:454, 1985

121. Larsen VH, Iversen AD, Christenson P, Anderson PK: Postoperative pain treatment after upper abdominal surgery with epidural morphine at thoracic or lumbar level. Acta Anaesthesiol Scand 29:566, 1985

122. Hakanson E, Bengtsson M, Rutberg H, Ulrick AM: Epidural morphine by the thoracic or lumbar routes in cholecystectomy. Effect on postoperative pain and respiratory variables. Anaesth Intensive Care 17:166, 1989

123. Brodsky JB, Kretzschmar KM, Mark JBD: Caudal epidural morphine for post-thoracotomy pain. Anesth Analg 67:409, 1988

124. Bromage PR, Camporesi E, Chestnut D: Epidural narcotics for postoperative analgesia. Anesth Analg 59:473, 1980

125. Rawal R, Sjostrand UH, Dahlstrom B, et al: Epidural morphine for postoperative pain relief: a comparative study with intramuscular narcotic and intercostal nerve block. Anesth Analg 61:93, 1982

126. Shulman M, Sandler AN, Bradley JW, et al: Postthoracotomy pain and pulmonary function following epidu-

ral and systemic morphine. Anesthesiology 61:569, 1984

127. Henderson SK, Cohen C: Nalbuphine augmentation of analgesia and reversal of side effects following epidural hydromorphone. Anesthesiology 65:216, 1986

128. Brose WG, Cohen SE: Oxyhemoglobin saturation following caesarean section in patients receiving epidural morphine, PCA, or IM meperidine analgesia. Anesthesiology 70:948, 1989

129. Ready LB, Edwards WT: Postoperative care following intrathecal or epidural opioids II. Anesthesiology 72:213, 1990

130. Mott JM, Eisele JH: A survey of monitoring practices following spinal opiate administration. Anesth Analg 65:S105, 1986

131. Morgan M: The rational use of intrathecal and extradural opioids. Br J Anaesth 63:165, 1989

132. Etches RC, Sandler AN, Daley MD: Respiratory depression and spinal opioids. Can J Anaesth 36:165, 1989

133. Rawal N, Wattwil M: Respiratory depression after epidural morphine—an experimental and clinical study. Anesth Analg 63:8–14, 1984

134. Rawal N, Schott U, Dahlstrom B, et al: Influence of naloxone infusion on analgesia and respiratory depression following epidural morphine. Anesthesiology 64:194, 1986

135. Baxter AD, Samson B, Penning J, et al: Prevention of epidural morphine induced respiratory depression with intravenous nalbuphine infusion in post-thoracotomy patients. Can J Anaesth 36:503, 1989

136. El-Baz NM, Faber LP, Jensik RJ: Continuous epidural infusion of morphine for treatment of pain after thoracic surgery: a new technique. Anesth Analg 63:757, 1984

137. Ullman D, Fortune SB, Greenhouse BB, et al: The treatment of patients with multiple rib fractures using continuous thoracic epidural narcotic infusion. Reg Anesth 14:43, 1989

138. Cousins MJ, Mather LE: Intrathecal and epidural administration of opioid. Anesthesiology 61:276, 1984

139. Welchew EA, Thornton JA: Continuous thoracic epidural fentanyl. Anaesthesia 37:309, 1982

140. Gough JD, Williams AB, Vaughan RS, et al: The control of post-thoracotomy pain. A comparative evaluation of thoracic epidural fentanyl infusions and cryo-analgesia. Anaesthesia 43:780, 1988

141. Renaud B, Brichant JF, Clergus F, et al: Continuous epidural fentanyl: ventilatory effects and plasma kinetics. Anesthesiology 63:A234, 1985

142. Ahuja BR, Strunin L: Respiratory effects of epidural fentanyl. Anaesthesia 40:949, 1985

143. Rankin APN, Comber REH: Management of fifty cases of chest injury with a regimen of epidural bupivacaine and morphine. Anaesth Intensive Care 12:311, 1984

144. Hjortso NC, Lund C, Mogensen T, et al: Epidural morphine improves pain relief and maintains sensory analgesia during continuous epidural bupivacaine after abdominal surgery. Anesth Analg 65:1033, 1986

145. Logas WG, El-Baz N, El-Ganzouri A, et al: Continuous

thoracic epidural analgesia for postoperative pain relief following thoracotomy: a randomized prospective study. Anesthesiology 67:787, 1987

146. Fischer RL, Lubenow TR, Liceaga A, et al: Comparison of continuous epidural infusion of fentanyl-bupivacaine and morphine-bupivacaine in management of postoperative pain. Anesth Analg 67:559, 1988

147. Hasenbos M, Eckhaus MN, Slappendel R, Gielen M: Continuous high thoracic epidural administration of bupivacaine with sufentanil or nicomorphine for postoperative pain relief after thoracic surgery. Reg Anesth 14:212, 1989

148. Stanton-Hicks MDA, Gielen M, Hasenbos M, et al: High thoracic epidural with sufentanil for post-thoracotomy pain. Reg Anesth 13:62, 1988

149. Loper KA, Ready LB, Downey M, et al: Epidural and intravenous fentanyl infusions are clinically equivalent after knee surgery. Anesth Analg 70:72, 1990

150. Fineman SP: Long-term post-thoracotomy cancer pain management with interpleural bupivacaine. Anesth Analg 68:694, 1989

151. Lassen HC, Henriksen E, Neukirch F: Treatment of tetanus: severe bone marrow depression after prolonged nitrous oxide anaesthesia. Lancet 1:527, 1956

152. Marx GF, Chen LK, Tabora JA: Experience with a disposable inhaler for methoxyflurane analgesia during labor: clinical biochemical results. Can Anaesth Soc J 16:66, 1969

153. Corbett TH, Cornell RG, Endres JL, Lieding K: Birth defects among children of nurse-anesthetists. Anesthesiology 41:341, 1974

154. Truog RD, Rice SA: Inorganic fluoride and prolonged isoflurane anesthesia in the intensive care unit. Anesth Analg 69:843, 1989

155. Mather LE, Phillips GD: Opioids and adjuvants: principles of use. p. 77. In Cousins MJ, Phillips GD (eds): Acute Pain Management. Churchill Livingstone, New York, 1986

156. Ferreira SH: Prostaglandin hyperalgesia and the control of inflammatory pain. p. 107. In Bonta IL, Bray MA, Parham MJ (eds): Handbook of Inflammation: The Pharmacology of Inflammation. Vol. 5. Elsevier Science Publishing, New York, 1985

157. Tammisto T, Tigerstedt I, Korttila K: Comparison of lysine acetylsalicylate and oxycodone in postoperative pain following upper abdominal surgery. Ann Chir Gynaecol 69:287, 1980

158. Tigerstedt I, Janhunen L, Tammisto T: Efficacy of diclofenac in a single prophylactic dose in postoperative pain. Ann Clin Res 19:18, 1987

159. Lal A, Pandey K, Chandra P: Dipyrone for treatment of post-operative pain. Anaesthesia 28:43, 1973

160. Rigamonti G, Zanella E, Lampugani R: Dose-response with indoprofen as an analgesia in postoperative pain. Br J Anaesth 55:513, 1983

161. Gillies GW, Kenny GN, Bullingham BE: The morphine-sparing effect of ketorolac tromethamine. Anaesthesia 42:727, 1987

162. Yrjola H, Silvennoian T, Vilppula E, Ahstrom-Bengs E: Intravenous indomethacin for postoperative pain: A double-blind study of ankle surgery. Acta Orthop Scand 59:43, 1988

163. Mattila MAK, Ahlstrom-Bengs E, Pekkola P: Intravenous indomethacin in prevention of postoperative pain. Br Med J 287:1026, 1983

164. Reasbeck PG, Rice MI, Reasbeck JC: Double-blind controlled trial of indomethacin as an adjunct to narcotic anesthesia after major abdominal surgery. Lancet 2:115–118, 1982

165. Kolker A, Patel U, Shah N, et al: Impact of indocin on postoperative opioid requirement following thoracotomy. Anesthesiology 71:A670, 1989

166. Stanski DR, Watkins DW: Drug Disposition in Anesthesia. Grune & Stratton, Orlando, FL, 1982

167. Loeser JD: Concepts of pain. p. 146. In Stanton-Hicks M, Boas R (eds): Chronic Low Back Pain. Raven Press, New York, 1982

168. Ferrante FM, Orav EJ, Rocco AG, Gallo J: A statistical model for pain in patient-controlled analgesia and conventional intramuscular opioid regimens. Anesth Analg 67:457, 1988

169. Mather LE, Owen H: The pharmacology of patient-administered opioids. p. 27. In Ferrante FM, Ostheimer GW, Covino BG (eds): Patient-Controlled Analgesia. Blackwell Scientific Publications, Cambridge, 1990

170. White PF: Patient-controlled analgesia: a new approach to management of postoperative pain. Semin Anesth 4:255, 1985

171. Thompson CC, Bailey MK, Conroy JM, et al: Patient-controlled analgesia—advances in the last five years. Anesthesiol Rev 3:14, 1989

172. Tamsen A: Patient characteristics influencing pain relief. p. 30. In Harmer M, Rosen M, Papper EM (eds): Patient-Controlled Analgesia. Blackwell Scientific Publications, Oxford, 1985

173. Johnson LR, Magnani B, Chan V, Ferrante FM: Modifiers of patient-controlled analgesia efficacy, 1. Locus of control. Pain 39:17, 1989

174. Bennett RL, Batenhorst RL, Graves DA: Morphine titration in postoperative laparotomy patients using patient-controlled analgesia. Curr Ther Res 32:45, 1982

175. White PF: Patient-controlled analgesia. Probl Anesth 2:339, 1988

176. Wakerlin G, Larson CP, Jr: Spouse-controlled analgesia. Anesth Analg 70:119, 1990

177. Dodd E, Wang J: Patient controlled analgesia for post-surgical pediatric patients ages 6–16 years. Reg Anesth, suppl. 2. 13:41, 1988

178. Broadman LM, Brown RE, Rice LJ, et al: Patient controlled analgesia in children and adolescents: a report of postoperative pain management in 150 patients. Anesthesiology 71:A1171, 1989

179. Rowbotham DJ, Wyld R, Peacock JE, et al: Transdermal fentanyl for the relief of pain after upper abdominal surgery. Br J Anaesth 63:56, 1989

180. Bell SD, Goldberg ME, Lerigani GE, et al: Evaluation of transdermal fentanyl for multi-day analgesia in postoperative patients. Anesth Analg 68:S22, 1989

181. Miser AW, Narang PK, Dothage JA, et al: Transdermal fentanyl for pain control in patients with cancer. Pain 37:15, 1989

182. Ali J, Weisel RD, Layug AB, et al: Consequences of postoperative alterations in respiratory mechanics. Am J Surg 128:376, 1974

183. Egbert LD, Laver MB, Bendixen HH: The effect of site of operation and type of anesthesia upon the ability to cough in the postoperative period. Surg Gynecol Obstet 44:161, 1964

184. Johnson WC: Postoperative ventilatory performance: dependence upon surigcal incision. Am Surg 41:615, 1975

185. Craig DB: Postoperative recovery of pulmonary function. Anesth Analg 60:46, 1981

186. Bishop MJ, Cheney FW: Respiratory complications of anesthesia and surgery. Semin Anesth 2:91, 1983

187. Craig DB, Wahba WM, Don HF, et al: "Closing volume" and its relationship to gas exchange in seated and supine position. J Appl Physiol 31:717, 1971

188. Rawal N, Sjostrand U, Christoffersson E, et al: Comparison of intramuscular and epidural morphine for postoperative analgesia in the grossly obese: influence on postoperative ambulation and pulmonary function. Anesth Analg 63:583, 1984

189. Kaplan JA, Miller ED, Gallagher EG: Postoperative analgesia for thoracotomy patients. Anesth Analog 54:773, 1975

190. Toledo-Pereyra LH, DeMeester TR: Prospective randomized evaluation of intrathoracic intercostal nerve block with bupivacaine on postoperative ventilatory function. Ann Thorac Surg 27:203, 1979

191. VadeBoncouer TR, Riegler FX, Gautt RS, Weinberg GL: A randomized, double-blind comparison of the effects of intrapleural bupivacaine and saline on morphine requirements and pulmonary function after cholecystectomy. Anesthesiology 71:339, 1989

192. Simpson BR, Parkhouse J, Marshall R, et al: Extradural analgesia and the prevention of postoperative respiratory complications. Br J Anaesth 33:628, 1961

193. Wahba WM, Craig DB, Don HF: Postoperative epidural analgesia: effect on lung volumes. Can Anaesth Soc J 22:519, 1975

194. Hasenbos M, van Egmond J, Gielen M, Crul JF: Postoperative analgesia by high thoracic epidural versus intramuscular nicomorphine after thoracotomy, part III. The effect of pre- and post-operative analgesia on morbidity. Acta Anaesthesiol Scand 31:608, 1987

195. Bennett R, Batenhorst RL, Foster TS, et al: Postoperative pulmonary function with patient-controlled analgesia. Anesth Analg 61:171, 1982

196. Pflug AE, Murphy TM, Butler Sh, Tucker GT: The effects of postoperative peridural analgesia on pulmonary therapy and pulmonary complications. Anesthesiology 41:8, 1974

197. Hjortso NC, Neumann P, Frosig F, et al: A controlled study on the effect of epidural analgesia with local anesthetics and morphine on morbidity after abdominal surgery. Acta Anaesthesiol Scand 29:790, 1985

198. Cheng EY, Wang-Cheng RW: Postoperative analgesia and respiratory function. Anesthesiology 71:A663, 1989

199. Cuschieri RJ, Morran CG, Howie JC, McArdle CS: Postoperative pain and pulonary complications: comparison of three analgesic regimens. Br J Surg 72:495, 1985

200. Kehlet H: Modification of responses to surgery by neural blockade: clinical implications. p. 145. In Cousins MJ, Bridenbaugh PO (eds): Neural Blockade in Clinical Anesthesia and Pain Management. 2nd Ed. JB Lippincott, Philadelphia, 1988

201. Kehlet H: Pain relief and modification of the stress response. p. 49. In Cousins MJ, Phillips GD (eds): Acute Pain Management. Churchill Livingstone, New York, 1986

202. Kehlet H: Surgical stress: the role of pain and analgesia. Br J Anaesth 63:189, 1989

203. Vedrine C, Vedrinne JM, Guiraud M, et al: Nitrogen-sparing effect of epidural administration of local anesthetics in colon surgery. Anesth Analg 69:354, 1989

204. Rutberg H, Hakanson E, Andenberg B, et al: Effects of the extradural administration of morphine, or bupivacaine, on the endocrine response to upper abdominal surgery. Br J Anaesth 56:233, 1984

205. Pother CE, Bridenbaugh LK, Reynolds F: Preoperative intercostal nerve block: effect on the endocrine metabolic response to surgery. Br J Anaesth 60:730, 1988

206. Lund JC, Hansen OB, Mogensen T, Kehlet H: Effect of thoracic epidural bupivacaine on somatosensory evoked potentials after dermatomal stimulation. Anesth Analg 66:731, 1987

207. Scott NB, Mogensen T, Bigler D, et al: Continuous thoracic extradural 0.5% bupivacaine with or without morphine: effect on quality of blockade, lung function and the surgical stress response. Br J Anaesth 62:253, 1989

208. Zwarts SJ, Hasenbros MAMW, Gielen MJM, Kho H: The effect of continuous epidural analgesia with sufentanil and bupivacaine during and after thoracic surgery on the plasma cortisol concentration and pain relief. Reg Anesth 14:183, 1989

209. Arnold DE, Coombs DW, Yearger MP, Brinck-Johnsen T: Single-blend comparison of epidural clonidine, epidural morphine, and parenteral narcotic analgesia upon postabdominal surgery neuroendocrine stress response (cortisol). Anesth Analg 68:S11, 1989

210. Scheinin B, Asantila R, Orko R: The effect of bupivacaine and morphine on pain and bowel function after colonic surgery. Acta Anaesthesiol Scand 31:161, 1987

211. Konturek SJ: Opiates and the gastrointestinal tract. Am J Gastroenterol 74:285, 1980

212. Thoren T, Wattwil M: Effects on gastric emptying of thoracic epidural analgesia with morphine or bupivacaine. Anesth Analg 67:687, 1988

213. Wattwil M, Thoren T, Hennerdal S, Garvill JE: Epidural analgesia with bupivacaine reduces postoperative paralytic ileus after hysterectomy. Anesth Analg 68:353, 1989

214. O'Gara PT: The hemodynamic consequences of pain and its management. Intensive Care Med 3:3, 1988

215. Breslow MJ, Jordan DA, Christopherson R, et al: Epidural morphine decreases postoperative hypertension by attenuating sympathetic nervous system hyperactivity. JAMA 261:3577, 1989

216. Bridenbaugh PO: Anesthesia and influence on hospitalization time. Reg Anesth 7:S151, 1982

217. Finley RJ, Kerri-Szanto M, Boyd D: New analgesic agents and techniques shorten postoperative hospital stay. Pain, suppl. 2:S397, 1984

218. Ross EI, Perumbetti P: PCA: is it cost effective when used for postoperative pain management? Anesthesiology 69:A710, 1988

219. Harmer M, Rosen M, Vickers MD: Patient-Controlled Analgesia. Blackwell Scientific Publications, Cambridge, 1985

220. Conacher I: Pain relief after thoracotomy. Br J Anaesth 65:806–812, 1990

22
ROUTINE POSTOPERATIVE RESPIRATORY CARE

John B. Downs, M.D.
Robert A. Smith, M.S.

Patients who require thoracotomy often have pre-existing pulmonary disease, which, when combined with the operative procedure itself, is likely to result in significant pulmonary dysfunction, the leading cause of postoperative morbidity. This likely explains the vigor with which clinicians have developed, initiated, and sustained numerous respiratory care treatment regimens, often in spite of sparse evidence supporting their efficacy. This chapter will review overall clinical considerations of post-thoracotomy respiratory care.

It is important to quantitate the degree of preoperative pulmonary insufficiency. Only with such information can attempts be made to restore and maintain the preoperative level of pulmonary function in the postoperative period. To achieve this goal, it is imperative that staff and equipment be used in an efficient manner. Patient-initiated, self-administered respiratory care techniques that create the least amount of patient discomfort should be used. Tasks that utilize expensive ancillary equipment, are time-consuming, or cause patient discomfort are not necessarily beneficial.

Respiratory therapy is often directed at prevention and treatment of atelectasis, the most common post-operative complication. Arterial hypoxemia, a reduction in arterial oxygen tension, is secondary to pulmonary venous admixture and is present to some degree in all patients who undergo thoracotomy. Successful prevention and treatment of arterial hypoxemia may be approached from several radically different directions, aspects of which will be discussed. Post-thoracotomy pleural drainage is frequently poorly understood by paramedical personnel, house officers, and, occasionally, staff surgeons. Such misunderstanding may cause life-threatening complications. A myriad of drugs aimed at altering postoperative respiratory function may be administered both topically and systemically with varying degrees of success. The rationale for use of several of these drugs will be discussed. Finally, the decision of whether to reintubate the trachea remains subjective and emotional. All these considerations are important to the successful care of patients who undergo operative procedures involving the thorax. A physiologic approach to the prophylaxis and treatment of such patients is likely to result in the most efficient utilization of equipment and personnel. In addition, such an approach is likely to result in patient cooperation and therapeutic benefits.

PREVENTION AND TREATMENT OF POSTOPERATIVE PULMONARY COMPLICATIONS WITH EMPHASIS ON ATELECTASIS

Individuals who have significant preoperative pulmonary dysfunction have an increased incidence of postoperative pulmonary insufficiency. Therefore, an accurate preoperative history and physical examination are necessary to identify such patients. When indicated, laboratory data should be obtained to provide supporting information. When patients with significant pulmonary dysfunction are identified preoperatively, an effective prophylactic regimen should be instituted. Such practice may decrease postoperative morbidity and mortality[1] (see Chapters 1 and 3).

Atelectasis, the most significant cause of postoperative morbidity, has been reported to occur in up to 84 percent of patients undergoing cardiopulmonary bypass for operative procedures on the heart and in 100 percent of patients undergoing thoracotomy for pulmonary resection. There is some disagreement concerning the frequency with which the left and right lungs are affected, but there is general agreement that atelectasis occurs more frequently in the basal lobes than in the middle and apical lung regions. Although some authors have attempted to correlate intraoperative fluid administration with the incidence of atelectasis, it is most commonly believed that restriction of normal respiratory effort secondary to pain, intrathoracic blood and fluid accumulation, and decreased lung compliance lead to rapid, shallow, and constant tidal volumes. Such a respiratory pattern may cause small airway closure and obstruction with inspissated mucus, both of which result in resorption of alveolar air and terminal airway collapse.

Diagnosis of atelectasis may be confirmed by chest roentgenogram, clinical findings, and arterial blood analysis for oxygen tension. However, there is a low positive correlation among these three methods. The reported incidence of atelectasis, therefore, may vary considerably, depending on the criteria used for diagnosis. Patients who undergo thoracotomy have a significant reduction in arterial oxygen tension. Clinical signs of atelectasis, such as increased respiratory rate, decreased tidal volume, increased body temperature, and increased heart rate, may be absent. Even though clinical, roentgenographic, and laboratory evidence of atelectasis may not agree, removal of airway obstruction will lead to resolution of all symptoms of atelectasis in many cases. In contrast, symptomatic treatment, such as administration of antibiotics, which may prevent the increase in body temperature and improve the roentgenographic picture, will not relieve arterial hypoxemia. Similarly, the administration of oxygen may improve the arterial oxygen tension, but may promote the loss of lung volume and cause deterioration of the roentgenographic picture. A chest roentgenogram obtained during deep inspiration may show resolution of atelectasis, but a return to normal shallow tidal breathing will rapidly cause recollapse, arterial hypoxemia, and clinical signs of atelectasis. Only when therapy is directed at the underlying problem will complete resolution be obtained. Successful prophylaxis and treatment of postoperative respiratory problems require an understanding of the disease process and treatment regimens. Therefore, consideration will be given to the physiology of respiration, airway collapse, and airway re-expansion.

Atelectasis, or loss of expiratory lung volume, can be resolved only if there is an increase in the resting lung volume, that is, an increase in functional residual capacity (FRC). Inflation of the lung is dependent on only two variables: lung compliance (C_L) and the distending pressure across the lung or the transpulmonary pressure (P_L), which is the difference between airway and intrapleural pressures (Fig. 22-1). Any change in lung volume must equal the product of C_L and ΔP_L. Therefore, an increase in FRC can occur only if there is an increase in P_L, an increase in C_L, or both. In evaluating any therapeutic maneuver, the clinician should question the ability of the maneuver to increase either of these two variables. Similarly, potentially undesirable side effects may be predicted following analysis of the effects of a maneuver on P_L and C_L.

It is extremely important that the reader avoid the common error of equating transpulmonary pressure with airway pressure. For example, increasing airway

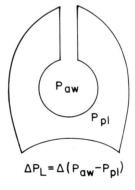

$$\Delta P_L = \Delta (P_{aw} - P_{pl})$$

Fig. 22-1. Lung volume is directly proportional to the difference between airway pressure (P_{aw}) and intrapleural pressure (P_{pl}), which is defined as the transpulmonary pressure (P_L).

pressure to 50 cmH$_2$O with a mechanical ventilator will increase lung volume, whereas an increase in airway pressure to 50 cmH$_2$O during a cough or use of a blow bottle system will cause a marked decrease in lung volume. By considering the change in intrapleural pressure, the effect of each maneuver on lung volume is easily explained. Mechanical ventilation will raise airway pressure and, to a lesser extent, intrapleural pressure; therefore, it will also increase transpulmonary pressure. Forced expiratory maneuvers, such as coughing and use of blow bottles, cause intrapleural pressure to increase to a greater extent than airway pressure, so that transpulmonary pressure and lung volume must decrease. The effects of respiratory equipment and maneuvers on lung compliance and on airway, intrapleural, and transpulmonary pressure must be considered in order to assess their physiologic effects. The following sections examine some of the maneuvers and devices suggested for the prevention and treatment of postoperative atelectasis.

Prolonged Postoperative Endotracheal Intubation and "Prophylactic" Mechanical Ventilation

The advent of extracorporeal blood oxygenators during the late 1950s and early 1960s to sustain life for complex operative procedures on the heart led to the widespread belief that postoperative mechanical ventilatory support for 1 to 2 days was a safe and desirable procedure to reduce metabolic demands in the early postoperative period. Such beliefs, although widely held, were not based on the findings of well-controlled prospective investigations. Recent information suggests that the practice is fraught with complications. An endotracheal tube renders the glottis incompetent, making an elective cough nearly impossible. Even a sterile suctioning procedure induces a degree of mucosal trauma, which may set the stage for pulmonary infection. Reflex airway closure may occur, causing widespread loss of lung volume and atelectasis. Also, sedation, which may be required to aid the patient's tolerance of the endotracheal tube and mechanical ventilator, will cause respiratory depression. Current practice in many institutions dictates that the patient's trachea be extubated as soon as possible following all types of thoracic operations to reduce the need for narcotics and sedation, to reduce the risk of tracheal contamination and trauma, and to allow better humidification of inspired gases by the patient's natural airway. Occasionally, a patient may have a significant reduction in body temperature postoperatively. In this instance, inspired gas may be heated to 40°C and humidified to 100 percent, allowing the lungs to act as a heat sink to effectively increase body temperature. This remains a valid indication for prolonged postoperative endotracheal intubation.

Pain Relief

Pain significantly impairs pulmonary function and delays early ambulation unless properly controlled. Vigorous chest physiotherapy, deep breathing exercises, and coughing should be encouraged only after administration of analgesic agents. More than 30 years ago, Burford and Burbank recommended that intercostal nerve blocks be used to control pain in patients with thoracic trauma to prevent compromise of respiratory function.[2] Subsequent investigators have documented a marked decrease in respiratory function secondary to post-thoracotomy pain, which may last up to 2 weeks. Numerous methods have been used in an attempt to reduce pain and improve pulmonary function after thoracotomy. These include intercostal nerve blocks, transcutaneous electrical nerve stimulation (TENS), cryoanalgesia, epidural blocks using local anesthetics, epidural narcotic analgesia, systemic analgesia using intermittent and/or continuous narcotic infusion, and patient-controlled narcotic analgesia (PCA) (see Chapter 21). Epidural and intercostal nerve blocks provide good pain relief and may sustain near-normal postoperative lung volumes. Intercostal blocks are uncomfortable and pneumothorax is a realistic complication; thus, they should be performed intraoperatively. Some authors have documented a marked decrease in the requirement for systemic pain medication in the immediate postoperative period and others have claimed a decrease in required length of hospital stay. However, there is also a fear that bilateral intercostal nerve blockade may decrease cough effectiveness. TENS is a simple, noninvasive method of pain relief. However, it requires a separate unit for each patient, changing of electrodes every 48 hours, and the training of patients, house staff, and nurses in its use. It may also cause 60-cycle interference with ECG monitoring and pacemaker function. An alternative approach is intraoperative nerve freezing (cryoanalgesia). The cryoprobe ($-20°C$) is placed on the intercostal nerve close to the intercostal foramen proximal to the collateral branch for 30 seconds.[3] The intercostal nerve at the thoracotomy incision and two intercostal nerves above the space are frozen. Cryoanalgesia produces effective pain relief with subsequent axonal regeneration. Cutaneous sensation usually returns in 2 to 4 weeks.

Injection of local anesthetic agents into the epidural space appears to be an efficient and effective means of decreasing postoperative pain and improving pulmonary function. Many studies have documented a marked increase in FRC and vital capacity when epidural analgesia is used in the postoperative period. However, epidural local anesthetics may cause hypotension and motor blockade of the lower extremities. Injection of 2 to 10 mg of preservative-free morphine sulfate into the epidural space has produced marked decreases in thoracotomy pain. Vital capacity and expiratory flow rates are increased significantly, so that cough effectiveness is improved following epidural morphine injection. Since patients have a decreased level of pain, but are without significant systemic depressing effects of morphine, they are more mobile and should have improvement in pulmonary function secondary to early ambulation. The technique appears to be safe, with only a few reports of respiratory depression following epidural morphine injection. Each injection produces significant pain relief for 12 to 24 hours; therefore, the technique is more efficient for producing postoperative pain relief than other methods.

Patient-controlled analgesia is an attractive alternative to systemic analgesia with intermittent and/or continuous infusion of narcotic.[4] PCA is based on the rationale that only the patient is cognizant of when and how much pain occurs. PCA incorporates a drug-dispensing system that administers a preselected dose of analgesic on patient demand. The patient can titrate analgesia in small doses initiated by depressing a hand-held switch. Thus, PCA can provide individualized pain control while reducing nursing time requirements.

Positioning

It has been realized by pulmonary physiologists that changes in body position alter the distribution of gas within the lungs during inspiration. For example, dependent lung regions receive the majority of gas flow during inspiration; similarly, gravity directs the majority of pulmonary blood flow to dependent lung regions. Therefore, ventilation and perfusion are relatively well matched in spontaneously breathing individuals. Knowledge of these effects may be used to explain various clinical observations and to promote resolution of some pathologic respiratory conditions. For example, the patient with atelectasis of the right lung will have a significant decrease in arterial blood oxygen tension. In the right lateral decubitus position, it would be anticipated that the arterial oxygen tension would be even lower, secondary to increased blood flow to areas of lung that are poorly ventilated. Placing the individual in the left lateral decubitus position might be expected to produce an increase in arterial oxygen tension. In addition, drainage of the

collapsed right lung would be promoted. On the other hand, were the patient to be placed in a right lateral decubitus position, increased ventilation would be directed toward the collapsed right lung, promoting reexpansion. Depending on the immediate goal, different positions might be encouraged. Piehl and Brown found that altering the position of five patients with severe respiratory distress, requiring high levels of positive end-expiratory pressure (PEEP), caused a significant increase in arterial oxygen tension.[5]

In an editorial, Al-Jurf questioned the efficacy of the time-honored cough.[6] He suggested that the cough is important only in promoting a precough deep breath and that frequent turning of the patient to alter regional ventilation, in combination with deep breathing to cause lung expansion, would be efficient postoperative therapy in the majority of patients. As mentioned previously, assumption of the upright position by patients will allow the diaphragm to descend and lung volume to increase. Ultimately, matching of ventilation and perfusion will be improved.

Chest Physiotherapy

Physical therapy, or physiotherapy, is one of the oldest and best-accepted forms of therapy aimed at the prevention and treatment of various pathologic respiratory conditions. Techniques include postural drainage, breathing exercises, vibration, deep breathing, coughing, and percussion. Most clinicians feel that chest physiotherapy is beneficial despite insufficient data to support the clinical impression.

Postural drainage depends greatly on gravity for its beneficial effects. Although postural drainage is often ordered as routine postoperative treatment following thoracic operative procedures, there is little rationale for its use in patients who do not have difficulty with increased secretions or who have an effective cough mechanism. However, postural drainage is effective in aiding in the clearance of secretions of patients with severe chronic obstructive lung disease or in patients who have an ineffective cough following their operation. In patients who incur atelectasis secondary to retained secretions, postural drainage should be directed toward the affected segments (Fig. 22-2). Often, postural drainage is combined with percussion, also known as tapotement. Recently, there have been conflicting reports regarding the efficacy of percussion in accelerating the central movement of peripheral secretions.

The thoracic surgical patient may also need assistance with coughing in the postoperative period. Pressure may be applied to specific chest regions to increase the expiratory flow of gas and, thus, assist the cough mechanism in moving secretions from the pe-

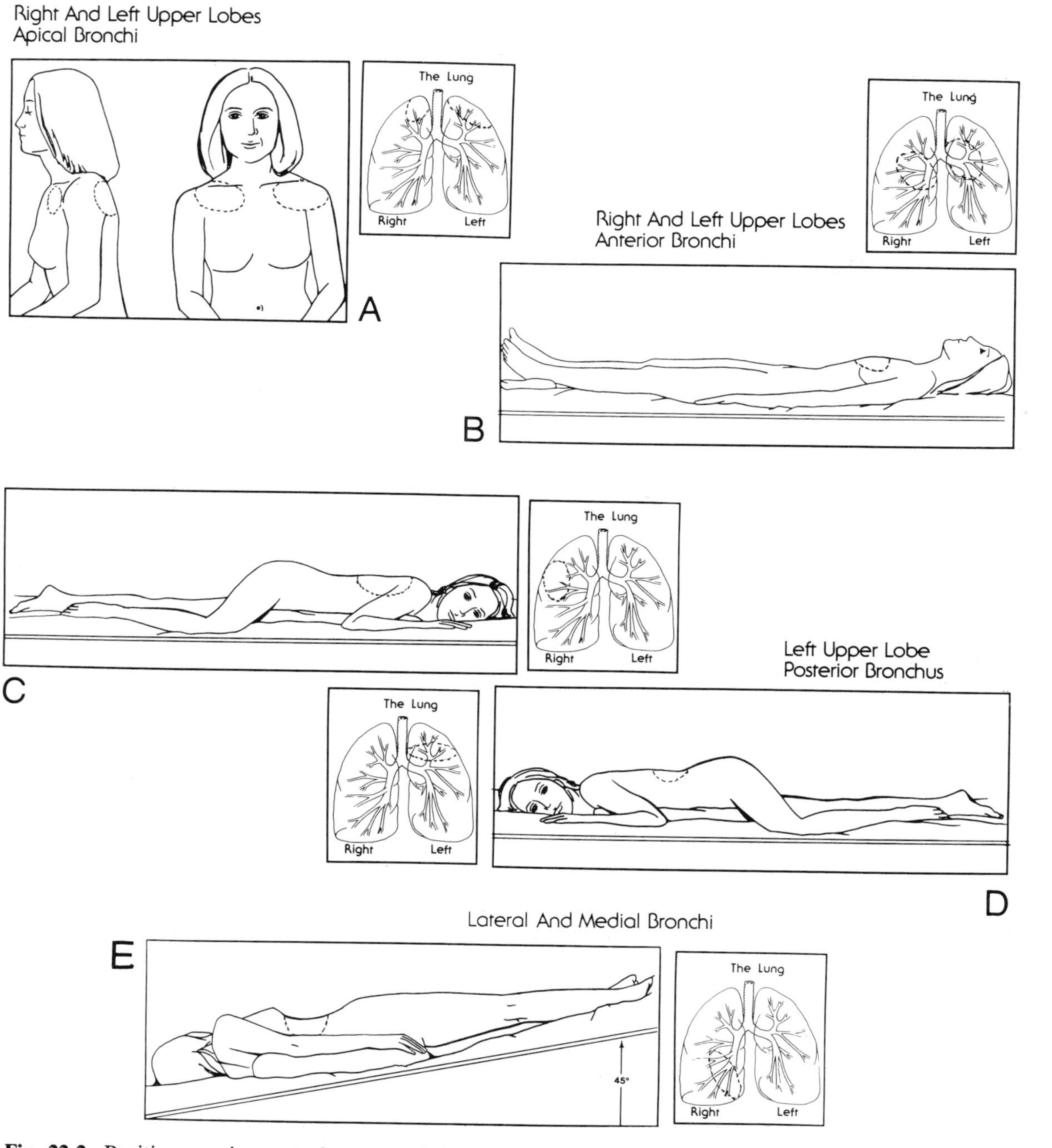
Right And Left Upper Lobes
Apical Bronchi
The Lung
Right
Left
A
Right And Left Upper Lobes
Anterior Bronchi
The Lung
Right
Left
B
The Lung
Right
Left
C
Left Upper Lobe
Posterior Bronchus
The Lung
Right
Left
D
Lateral And Medial Bronchi
E
45°
The Lung
Right
Left

Fig. 22-2. Position requirements for postural drainage of various lung regions. (Drawings by Mark Friedman.) **(A)** The patient sits upright and leans slightly backward with percussion anteriorly, then slightly forward with percussion posteriorly. **(B)** The patient lies on his or her back. **(C)** The patient lies on the left side with the right side of the body turned forward to an angle of approximately 45 degrees. The bed is flat. A pillow is placed in the left armpit and under the left chest for support. **(D)** The patient lies on the right side with the left side of the body turned forward to an angle of approximately 45 degrees. The bed is flat. The pillow is placed under the right armpit and under the left chest for support. **(E)** The pillow is placed under the right shoulder to the right hip, elevating the right side of the body slightly. The foot of the bed is elevated to approximate a 45-degree angle. (*Figure continues.*)

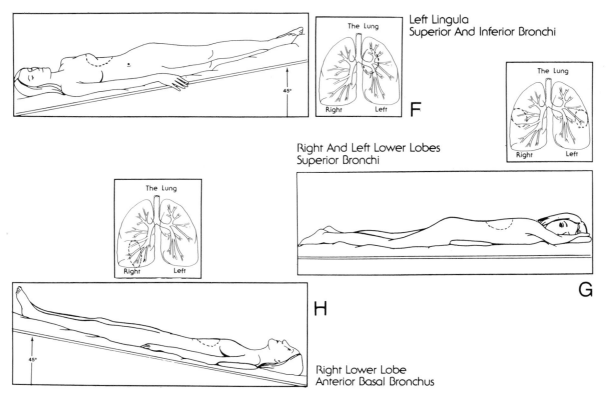

Fig. 22-2 (*Continued*). **(F)** The patient lies flat on his or her back. A pillow is placed under the left shoulder to the left hip, elevating the left side of the body slightly. The foot of the bed is elevated to approximate a 45-degree angle. **(G)** The patient lies facing downward with a pillow under the abdomen to flex the trunk. The bed is flat. **(H)** The patient lies on his or her back turned slightly onto the left side. The foot of the bed is elevated to approximate a 45-degree angle. (*Figure continues.*)

riphery. Application of hand pressure to the thoracic cage during exhalation is claimed to be particularly effective for removing peripherally retained secretions in intubated patients who are receiving mechanical ventilatory support. Some clinicians feel that a vibratory movement may be added to free tenacious secretions. However, there is no significant evidence that vibration is of benefit.

As early as 1928, Sante realized that atelectasis may be more effectively treated by allowing the patient to lie on the affected side, thus increasing ventilation to the atelectatic lung.[7] It was Sante's feeling that this maneuver, combined with an effective cough, usually would be more effective than bronchoscopy for resolving atelectasis. Soon thereafter, Winifred Linton, the superintendent physiotherapist at Brompton Hospital, developed the previously discussed physiotherapeutic techniques for patients with chest diseases (Fig. 22-2). Recently, some critical reviews have questioned the efficacy of chest physiotherapy in preventing or resolving atelectasis. However, Marini et al

found that chest physiotherapy was as effective as fiberoptic bronchoscopy for this purpose.[8] Although there is likely to be no improvement in oxygenation following chest physiotherapy, there has been documented improvement in lung-thorax compliance, indicating expansion of previously nonventilated lung regions. Stein and Cassara found that application of chest physiotherapy to a group of "poor-risk" patients during the pre- and postoperative periods significantly reduced morbidity and mortality due to pulmonary complications.[1] Chest physiotherapy has been shown to be ineffective in patients who have pneumonia; however, this finding was not unexpected, since pneumonia usually does not cause retention of sputum and atelectasis.[9]

Literature reviewing the physiologic effects of chest physiotherapy is sparse. However, there is a general consensus that chest physiotherapy is beneficial in selected patients, especially those who have difficulty in clearing copious secretions. In other patients, chest physiotherapy appears to offer no benefit when com-

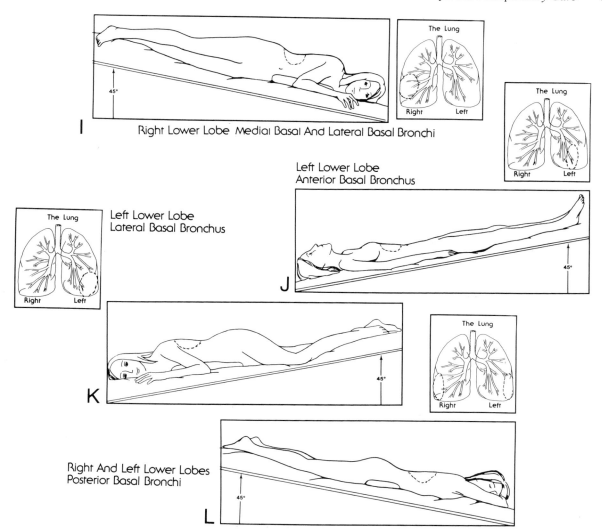

Fig. 22-2 (*Continued*). **(I)** The patient lies on the left side and hugs the pillow. The foot of the bed is elevated to approximate a 45-degree angle. **(J)** The patient lies on his or her back with the body turned slightly onto the right side. The foot of the bed is elevated to approximate a 45-degree angle. **(K)** The patient lies on the right side and hugs the pillow. The foot of the bed is elevated to approximate a 45-degree angle. **(L)** The patient lies on his or her abdomen with a pillow under the hips. The foot of the bed is elevated to approximate a 45-degree angle or higher.

pared with other, less time-consuming maneuvers, such as blow bottles and incentive spirometry. In view of the expense involved in supplying a chest physiotherapist to patients who require postoperative therapy, chest physiotherapy should be administered only to select patients.

Transtracheal Catheterization

In 1960, Radigan and King suggested the percutaneous placement of a small polyethylene tube for instillation of irritant materials into the trachea.[10] They found that atelectasis could then be eliminated in their postoperative patients and suggested that all patients who undergo thoracotomy should have a transtracheal catheter inserted. Subsequent investigators have suggested injecting pancreatic dornase or mucolytic agents through a transtracheal catheter. However, few studies have documented the effectiveness of the technique. Injection of irritant materials through a transtracheal catheter will stimulate vigorous coughing for 24 to 48 hours. However, following that period of time, patients seem to grow tolerant of the injections and they become less effective.

With time, evidence of significant complications began to appear in the literature. Subcutaneous emphysema, pneumomediastinum, hemoptysis, peritracheal abscess, fatal dysrhythmia, hematoma, air emboli, bleeding, and aspiration pneumonitis have all been reported. In view of the significant complications that may occur and the lack of documented efficacy, transtracheal catheterizations cannot be recommended as a routine postoperative procedure.

Tracheobronchial Suction

Occasionally, patients may be unable to clear secretions from their airways and may require tracheal suction with a small-bore plastic catheter. This maneuver is performed to ensure adequate removal of secretions from large airways and to maintain airway patency. Several considerations are important for proper tracheobronchial suctioning. The procedure should be performed in a sterile manner to prevent contamination of the patient's airway, which may lead to antibiotic-resistant bacterial pneumonia in susceptible patients. After the procedure has been carefully explained, the patient's head should be placed in a "sniffing" position and preoxygenation performed with one of several devices, which will be discussed below. A sterile glove is placed on the right hand, which is used to grasp a sterile, appropriately sized suction catheter. A light coating of sterile lubricant is placed on the distal third of the catheter, which is slowly advanced through the nose during inspiration. During exhalation, the vocal cords are more closely approximated, making advancement into the trachea less likely. Increasing loudness of breath sounds may be detected through the suction catheter as the tip approaches the larynx. If the catheter slips into the esophagus or coils in the oropharynx, breath sounds will diminish or disappear, indicating that the catheter should be retracted slightly and readvanced. Grasping the patient's tongue may prevent the patient from swallowing the catheter. Once the catheter is in place, humidity will be seen to precipitate within the tube during exhalation and will clear during subsequent inspiration. Vigorous coughing may be stimulated by advancing the catheter into the oropharynx. Therefore, gagging and coughing cannot be used as definitive signs of proper placement of the suction catheter. Once the proper position of the suction catheter is verified, oxygen tubing should be connected to the proximal end of the catheter and oxygen should be administered to the patient at a rate of 2 to 5 L/min to continue preoxygenation.

Following 2 to 5 minutes of preoxygenation, intermittent suction should be applied to the catheter, which may be alternately advanced and withdrawn 1 to 2 inches. If this is not productive of sputum, consideration should be given to the injection of 5 mL of sterile normal saline into the suction catheter to stimulate coughing and central movement of secretions. Suction should be applied to the catheter intermittently; it should not be applied continuously for more than 10 seconds, as doing so might cause a decrease in lung volume and severe arterial hypoxemia. It has been suggested that clinicians exhale and hold their breath while applying suction to the patient's trachea. The sensation of dyspnea will indicate when the procedure should be terminated.

A similar procedure is used for tracheal suctioning through an endotracheal tube. When an endotracheal tube is in place, preoxygenation of the patient may proceed more rapidly. If the patient is breathing spontaneously, the F_IO_2 should be increased to 0.8 to 1.0 for 2 to 5 minutes. A sterile suction catheter should then be advanced through the endotracheal tube and suction applied intermittently. Lavage with 5 mL of sterile normal saline may be performed during the period of preoxygenation. In patients who are receiving mechanical ventilatory support, the rate of the mechanical ventilator should be adjusted to 10 to 12 breaths/min and the F_IO_2 increased to 0.8 to 1.0. Following 2 to 5 minutes of preoxygenation and ventilation, suctioning may proceed. Some clinicians have advocated that manual compression of a 5 L anesthesia bag with a continuous flow of oxygen be used to provide positive-pressure breaths with a high F_IO_2. Such systems are readily contaminated and have no documented beneficial effects that cannot be duplicated by the patient's mechanical ventilator. Also, some patients may not require mechanical ventilation with a large tidal volume and high F_IO_2 for preoxygenation. For example, patients with severe chronic obstructive lung disease may require only a moderate increase in F_IO_2 and ventilator rate prior to the suctioning procedure.

Haight described the use of nasotracheal suctioning in the management of postoperative atelectasis in 1938.[11] Since that time, the procedure has been extremely popular among clinicians in order to stimulate deep breathing and coughing. Some investigators have suggested that it be performed routinely at least once in order to use the technique as an ongoing threat to the less cooperative patient. Thus, the procedure has been suggested as punitive as well as therapeutic. Many investigators have suggested different maneuvers to ensure entry by the catheter into the left mainstem bronchus. Recent investigations have suggested that turning the head to the opposite side or using the contralateral nostril will not increase the success rate of left mainstem catheterization. It is likely that the best way to ensure a left mainstem bronchus cannulation is to use a catheter with a curved tip with the patient in a left lateral decubitus position. A fiberoptic bronchoscope may be used to ensure that the left lung is suctioned if it is important to aspirate secretions from the left mainstem bronchus.

Sackner et al suggested that tracheal suction may produce significant mucosal trauma, which may subsequently act as a nidus for infection.[12] They claimed that catheter design is one of the major offending problems in producing mucosal damage. Later, Jung and Gottlieb suggested that mucosal damage did not occur secondary to catheter design fault; rather, it was secondary to repetition, vigor, and amount of applied suction.[13] Regardless of the immediate etiology, it is evident that tracheal suction may cause significant mucosal damage, contamination of the patient's airway, and, therefore, morbidity. Vigorous suctioning has also been shown to cause a significant reduction in lung volume, especially in infants, severe arterial hypoxemia secondary to deoxygenation of the lung, and severe cardiac dysrhythmia in a high percentage of patients when preoxygenation is not used. Many of these complications may not be readily reversible. For example, the loss of lung volume following suctioning in infants may take 30 to 60 minutes to resolve. Because of the potential risks of nasotracheal suction and the largely undocumented potential benefits, some authors feel that the technique should never be applied. However, nasotracheal suction may be indicated on occasion; but other methods are more likely to produce beneficial results with less risk of complications.

Bronchoscopy

Some researchers have suggested that bronchoscopy be performed immediately after thoracotomy in any patient with roentgenographic evidence of atelectasis. This will ensure the absence of any occluding foreign body and will allow removal of any obstruction. The hypoxemic individual is likely to suffer progressive arterial hypoxemia during the procedure; therefore, the clinician should be prepared to ventilate the patient with a high F_1O_2. Frequently, anesthesia personnel are requested to stand by for the procedure to provide such assistance. It should be kept in mind that bronchoscopy is effective at removing only secretions found in the large airways. Peripheral secretions are not obtainable with a bronchoscope. Furthermore, bronchoscopy is almost always unpleasant for the patient, is time-consuming for the clinician, and, therefore, cannot be frequently repeated.

Some authors have suggested that fiberoptic bronchoscopy is less traumatic for the patient and less likely to cause a decrease in arterial oxygen tension than nasotracheal suction; it also allows aspiration of secretions from distal lung regions. However, ventilation during fiberoptic bronchoscopy is more difficult than during rigid bronchoscopy. Although there is some debate concerning the ability of fiberoptic bronchoscopy to cause resolution of atelectasis, there are sufficient reports that document the efficacy of this technique, indicating that fiberoptic bronchoscopy must be considered to be beneficial for a large percentage of patients with atelectasis.

Following aspiration of secretions through a rigid bronchoscope, positive airway pressure may be applied to promote reinflation of a collapsed lung. In 1974, Bowen et al described the use of a rigid bronchoscope with a balloon cuff at its distal end and manual compression of an anesthesia bag for generation of positive pressure.[14] Thus, increased airway pressures could be applied to specific areas of lung to encourage re-expansion. Several years later, Millen et al described the use of a balloon-tipped fiberoptic bronchoscope to accomplish the same result.[15] Thus, although there is some disagreement, it is clear that bronchoscopy will provide a controlled means of aspirating secretions from the airway and will permit application of positive pressure to specific regions of the lung to promote lung inflation. When conservative respiratory therapy techniques fail, fiberoptic or rigid bronchoscopy should be used.

Sustained Inflation

During thoracotomy, sustained hyperinflation of the lung is manually accomplished by vigorous compression of the anesthesia reservoir bag. All surgeons and anesthesiologists have observed recruitment of collapsed lung units, which may occur during a 5- to 10-second period of sustained lung inflation. Surprisingly, this treatment has not been routinely applied in the postoperative period. It is likely that the difficulty of placing an endotracheal tube in the awake, tachypneic, agitated, and uncooperative postoperative patient with atelectasis is responsible for the lack of popularity of this technique.

Commonly, pediatric patients who have undergone thoracotomy and who have recurrent right upper lobe atelectasis may benefit from periodic endotracheal intubation for application of positive airway pressure, immediately followed by endotracheal extubation. Unfortunately, the psychologic and physiologic trauma to the patient and the time required by the clinician are factors that are likely to prevent routine application of this treatment modality.

Rebreathing

In the past, some clinicians have recommended that patients be instructed to rebreathe exhaled gas from a reservoir. By so doing, the patient will have an increase in physiologic deadspace and will require an increase in minute ventilation to maintain a normal arterial carbon dioxide tension. Thus, deep and rapid breathing may be promoted. Although early investigations suggested a beneficial effect of such therapy, it is now realized that significant arterial hypoxemia may occur during rebreathing. Most patients who are able to cooperate for rebreathing treatments should be able to take and sustain a deep breath, a maneuver that should produce the same beneficial effect. Therefore, rebreathing of exhaled gas can no longer be recommended.

Blow Bottles

Decades ago, clinicians felt that forced exhalation against a resistance would create an increase in airway pressure and cause inflation of the lung. Thus, water-filled bottles with submerged tubing were designed, and patients were instructed to blow vigorously into a water-filled bottle in order to displace fluid into a second bottle. Once accomplished, the task was to be repeated several times. Several investigators found the use of blow bottles to be associated with an increase in FRC. Since blow bottles are cheaper than many other forms of respiratory therapy, they have been advocated and widely applied, especially on thoracic surgical services. In 1973, Bartlett et al suggested that blow bottles are useful only because of the deep inspiration preceding the forced exhalation, and are less efficient than incentive spirometry.[16] Nunn et al found that vigorous forced exhalation caused a significant decrease in arterial oxygen tension; this effect was even more significant when oxygen was added to the inspired air.[17] Physiologically, a forced exhalation will decrease expiratory transpulmonary pressure and lung volume, which suggests that blow bottles should be avoided in postoperative patients. Not only is the maneuver fatiguing, but it may have a detrimental effect on pulmonary blood flow, cardiac output, FRC, and arterial oxygen tension. If there is any benefit from blow bottles, it is likely secondary to the deep breath that must precede the forced expiratory maneuver.

Intermittent Positive-Pressure Breathing

For more than three decades, intermittent positive-pressure breathing (IPPB) has been used for the prevention and treatment of postoperative atelectasis. Surprisingly, few, if any, studies have established the benefits of this form of therapy, and the results of numerous studies have been negative. Advocates of IPPB state that such investigations failed to provide proper administration techniques, equipment, etc; opponents claim that IPPB is used primarily because

of the financial rewards attendant on its application. As stated by Gold, "the overwhelming evidence against IPPB therapy in the surgical patient calls for its abandonment and the substitution of other (less harmful and expensive) approaches. . . ."[18] Since chest physiotherapy, incentive spirometry, blow bottles, and standard conservative respiratory therapy are less expensive in terms of equipment and personnel than IPPB, most investigators agree with Gold and have recommended discontinuation of IPPB.

There is general agreement that for IPPB to be effective, adequate volumes must be delivered to the patient's lungs. Recent investigations reporting beneficial effects of IPPB have used higher peak inflation pressures, sustained inspiratory airway pressure, and greater inspired volumes than earlier investigations. Currently, it is recommended that if IPPB is used, it should be volume limited rather than pressure limited, as is common in practice. Thus, IPPB should be administered to a preset tidal volume rather than to a preset airway pressure.

In addition, several investigations have indicated that IPPB may produce harmful side effects. Iverson et al found that patients who received IPPB therapy had an increased incidence of pulmonary complications (30 percent) compared with a similar group of patients who received incentive spirometry or blow bottle therapy (16 percent and 9 percent, respectively).[19] Browner and Powers found that postoperative patients receiving IPPB experienced a significant subsequent fall in FRC,[20] while Lareau,[21] Wright et al,[22] and Shim et al[23] observed a significant fall in PaO_2 following IPPB. The observations of Paul and Downs may explain the decrease in FRC and PaO_2 observed following IPPB.[24] Patients who underwent major thoracic operative procedures each had a pleural catheter inserted in the right hemithorax. Postoperatively, each patient had expiratory transpulmonary pressure measured during and following 15 minutes of IPPB. Each patient was observed to hyperventilate during treatment and to hypoventilate following treatment. During hypoventilation following IPPB, the expiratory transpulmonary pressure decreased in each patient. Presumably, hypoventilation was accompanied by absorption of oxygen from small airways, resulting in a decrease in FRC and a significant fall in PaO_2.

Since even properly administered IPPB with large tidal volumes may result in hypoventilation and associated ill effects, it may be contraindicated for the majority of postoperative patients. A conservative recommendation would be to apply IPPB only to patients who cannot generate an inspiratory transpulmonary pressure of sufficient magnitude to significantly increase lung volume, who require assistance in the clearance of secretions, and who require delivery of topical medications. Certainly, IPPB should not be applied routinely to postoperative patients.

Incentive Spirometry

In 1966, Ward et al suggested that a prolonged deep breath is the most efficient way for postoperative patients to prevent and reduce atelectasis.[25] These researchers equated this maneuver with a sigh or yawn. Subsequently, Bartlett et al described a device to encourage such activity.[26] Several other investigators have performed prospective comparisons of incentive spirometers with IPPB, blow bottles, chest physiotherapy, and other maneuvers and have found that incentive spirometry is associated with a lower complication rate and less atelectasis than other treatment regimens. Several investigators have found that patients who have a decreased FRC and arterial hypoxemia, presumably secondary to ventilation-perfusion mismatching, will experience a significant increase in PaO_2 following several deep breath maneuvers. Similarly, some investigators have found a reduction in atelectasis as diagnosed by chest roentgenogram following incentive spirometry. Bartlett et al performed a prospective investigation in patients who had undergone thoracotomy and provided the first sound physiologic basis for incentive spirometry.[26] They were able to show that the deep breath maneuver created an increase in inspiratory transpulmonary pressure, indicating an increase in lung volume. Similar measurements during IPPB failed to reveal a significant increase in transpulmonary pressure, which indicated lack of a deep breath during IPPB. Based on these results, incentive spirometry has become more popular than IPPB for the prevention and treatment of postoperative atelectasis. It is important to note that Bartlett et al failed to report expiratory transpulmonary pressures during either IPPB or incentive spirometry. Therefore, it was not possible to determine whether an increase in FRC was likely to have occurred in their patients. Rather, it has been assumed that a large inhaled volume will cause expansion of an atelectatic lung and that the expanded areas will remain open. Although this is a reasonable assumption, it represents the same presumptive thinking that led to the popularity of IPPB during the last two decades and it may not be correct. Future studies should be directed toward resolution of this question.

Since the introduction of the incentive spirometer, several different types of devices have been developed. Originally, the incentive spirometer required the patient to inhale deeply and sustain the inhalation for several seconds. A breath counter was incorporated into the design of the spirometer so the clinician could ensure patient cooperation.

Most incentive breathing devices currently used do not require that a preset inhaled volume be taken and do not ensure that the deep breath will be sustained. These devices encourage a rapid inspiratory flow rate rather than a large inhaled volume. These devices are technically simpler and less expensive than volume-directed devices (Fig. 22-3). Lederer et al compared three currently used devices and found no significant

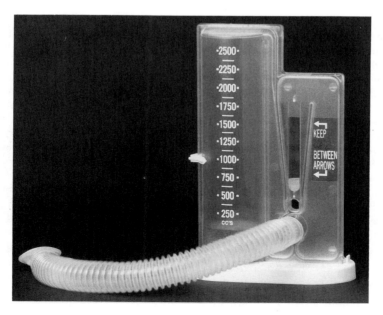

Fig. 22-3. A flow rate-sensitive incentive breathing device.

difference in their effects.[27] It is difficult to determine from available evidence whether measurement of the inhaled volume is necessary or desirable. However, it is likely that devices designed to ensure a large inspired volume are preferable.

Several investigations have failed to find a beneficial effect of incentive spirometry. It is likely that uncooperative patients or patients who are experiencing significant postoperative pain will not cooperate to perform a deep-breath maneuver. In such instances, it is foolish to expect that a bedside device will prevent atelectasis. Similarly, if patients are not given adequate instruction or if they misuse the device, it is unlikely that the device will be effective. Although some patients may be sufficiently self-motivated to not require supervision at all times, many will require immediate bedside attention. In such instances, incentive spirometry will be no more economic than IPPB or other respiratory care devices and maneuvers.

Continuous Positive Airway Pressure

As stated earlier, the goal in the treatment of atelectasis is to increase the FRC of the lung and to prevent small airway collapse. Such an increase in lung volume can occur only if there is an increase in lung compliance or an increase in expiratory transpulmonary pressure. It is unlikely that any respiratory therapy maneuver will directly increase lung compliance. Therefore, an increase in FRC is most likely to occur following an increase in expiratory transpulmonary pressure. Clinically, it is possible to increase transpulmonary pressure in two ways. Whenever airway pressure remains constant, a decline in intrapleural pressure will cause an increase in transpulmonary pressure and an increase in lung volume. A decrease in expiratory intrapleural pressure may be created by relieving abdominal distention, by reducing tension in abdominal and thoracic musculature, and by having patients assume a more upright position, causing abdominal contents to provide traction on the diaphragm.

Surgeons have known for decades that assumption of the upright position often causes improvement in postoperative pulmonary function. For that reason, early postoperative ambulation is a goal of most surgeons. Unfortunately, patients who undergo thoracotomy may not tolerate immediate ambulation postoperatively. In such patients, other means of preventing pulmonary complications must be provided. Application of positive pressure to the airway will cause intrapleural pressure to increase, but to a lesser extent than the increase in airway pressure. Therefore, transpulmonary pressure will increase as will lung

volume. This, of course, is the rationale for IPPB. During IPPB, the lung will sustain an increase in volume only during the inspiratory phase of the respiratory cycle. If an individual is assumed to inhale for 1 second and to do so 12 times/min, 80 percent of the patient's respiratory cycle will be spent in exhalation, during which there is no significant increase in airway pressure. Therefore, if there is an increase in FRC, it must be secondary to a residual effect of positive pressure applied during inspiration. Since the goal is to increase expiratory lung volume, a more logical approach would be to apply positive pressure to the airway during the expiratory phase of respiration. As a result, expiratory transpulmonary pressure will be increased, as will FRC.

Application of PEEP to the ventilatory pattern of patients with the adult respiratory distress syndrome (ARDS) who require mechanical ventilatory support has been commonly used for many years. Continuous application of positive pressure to the airway (CPAP) of spontaneously breathing patients throughout the respiratory cycle was practiced in the 1930s and 1940s for the treatment of congestive heart failure and "traumatic wet lung" and has recently been used in infants with idiopathic respiratory distress syndrome, as well as in some adults with ARDS.[2] However, CPAP has not been commonly used to prevent atelectasis in postoperative patients. Physiologically, this would seem a most reasonable approach to the prevention of atelectasis. Using methodology similar to that described by Bartlett et al,[28] Paul and Downs measured transpulmonary pressure of patients who underwent myocardial revascularization operations.[24] Expiratory transpulmonary pressure was measured before, during, and every 5 minutes after treatment with an incentive spirometer, IPPB, or CPAP applied with a face mask. They found that IPPB and CPAP both increased expiratory transpulmonary pressure during treatment. Because of pain, patients refused to inhale deeply during incentive spirometry and expiratory transpulmonary pressure was not increased, even during treatment. Following IPPB, there was a significant decrease in expiratory transpulmonary pressure. Presumably, this was secondary to a period of hypoventilation following treatment. Following CPAP, there was a significant decrease in expiratory transpulmonary pressure, but it remained above baseline levels for the ensuing 30 minutes. Not surprisingly, there was no significant alteration in expiratory transpulmonary pressure following incentive spirometry. In a similar group of patients, Downs and Mitchell determined that 6 cmH$_2$O CPAP was required to maintain FRC at preoperative levels.[29] Fowler et al reported data from four patients who had atelectasis unresponsive to chest physiotherapy, tracheobronchial suction, and fiberoptic bronchoscopy, and in whom 5 to 15 cmH$_2$O PEEP was effective in causing resolution of atelectasis in all patients in 24 hours or less.[30] Similar cases have been reported.

Early reports expressed fear that continuous application of positive pressure to the airway might force distal migration of secretions and worsen atelectasis secondary to small airway obstruction. However, evidence suggests that collateral channels to ventilation may be recruited during application of CPAP, causing inflation of previously unventilated lung regions.[31] If so, positive pressure distal to small airway obstruction may cause central migration of offending secretions and improvement in pulmonary function.

CPAP applied by face mask was originally described by Barach in the mid-1930s. Subsequently, CPAP was applied clinically during the next two decades. However, this form of treatment fell into disuse as a result of facial trauma induced by hard rubber, ill-fitting face masks, fear of gastric distention, vomiting, aspiration, and poor understanding of the dangers of endotracheal intubation. Greenbaum et al used a transparent, cushioned mask to treat 14 patients with significant arterial hypoxemia with up to 14 cmH$_2$O CPAP.[32] For eight patients, endotracheal intubation was avoided. Subsequent to this report in 1976, many patients have been treated with CPAP without significant complications and endotracheal intubation has been avoided. Andersen et al applied an average of 15 cmH$_2$O CPAP and chest physiotherapy with postural drainage to a group of postoperative patients with atelectasis.[33] CPAP was applied once an hour for 25 to 35 respirations with the highest tolerable airway pressure and, within 12 hours, most patients had improved dramatically. In contrast, a control group who received chest physiotherapy, postural drainage, and endotracheal suction had insignificant resolution of atelectasis. These investigators concluded that CPAP applied with a face mask could be used to treat atelectasis. Stock et al showed that CPAP by mask is more effective than incentive spirometry for the prevention of postoperative atelectasis.[34] There is uniform agreement that when CPAP is applied with a mask, the clinician must ensure that gastric distention, regurgitation, and aspiration do not occur. In addition, proper equipment must be used, including a soft, self-sealing face mask that will not induce facial trauma.

Presently, CPAP applied continuously, or periodically, appears to be the most physiologically sound approach to the prevention and treatment of postoperative atelectasis. The technique requires little patient cooperation and will not induce fatigue, as will many other respiratory therapy techniques. In fact, CPAP may be applied to the sleeping patient, unlike any other noninvasive form of respiratory therapy.

Further prospective evaluation of this technique will be required, but preliminary investigations indicate greater efficacy for face mask CPAP than for other forms of treatment.

RESPIRATORY MUSCLE TRAINING

Strength training of the respiratory muscles can reasonably be considered for patients with respiratory muscle weakness, except when muscle fatigue is the cause of the weakness. Then, the respiratory muscles require rest, not training. Clinically, it may be difficult to distinguish between muscle weakness and fatigue. Respiratory muscle weakness is suggested by chronic reduction in strength and a chronic elevation of PaCO$_2$. Respiratory muscle fatigue is suggested by an abrupt decrease in muscle strength, an abrupt increase in PaCO$_2$, and/or the acute development of paradoxical abdominal wall motion.

Respiratory muscle endurance training has much wider potential clinical application than respiratory muscle strength training, because the respiratory muscles must remain continuously active, even when placed under added loads. Because the respiratory muscles are most likely to fail when placed under the added load, training regimens should be designed to prepare them to withstand such conditions.

Two commonly used forms of respiratory muscle endurance training are inspiratory resistance loading[35] and inspiratory threshold loading.[36] During the former, resistive loads are applied for 5 to 15 minutes. Progress is measured by an increase in the maximal tolerable resistance over a specified period of time or an increase in the time a given load is tolerated.

The inspiratory pressure load is determined by the amount of weight applied to the inspiratory port of a unidirectional valve during inspiratory threshold loading training. The response is assessed by the increase in the amount of time a patient can breathe against a given load. Inspiratory threshold loading training has been shown to improve respiratory muscle endurance in patients with obstructive lung disease. The advantage of threshold loading over resistive loading is that the patient is obliged to generate a high inspiratory pressure with every breath.

PREVENTION AND TREATMENT OF POSTOPERATIVE HYPOXEMIA

It is not the purpose of this section to discuss in detail the physiology of postoperative oxygenation. However, some basic principles must be covered to arrive at a rational treatment plan for the postoperative patient. Too frequently, a low arterial oxygen tension is presumed to be secondary only to right-to-left intrapulmonary shunting of blood. Although this is a frequent cause of deficient arterial oxygenation, it is by no means the only major factor. Frequently, patients who require thoracotomy have pre-existing pulmonary disease, with areas of lung with low, but finite, ventilation/perfusion ratios. Most patients with severe chronic obstructive lung disease have a low arterial oxygen tension for this reason, and not because of significant fibrotic lung disease, which may produce low arterial oxygenation by causing a diffusion block to oxygen transfer from the alveolar space to the pulmonary capillary blood. However, all three mechanisms may explain the presence of inadequately oxygenated blood in the arterial circulation of some patients. That is, venous blood may pass through the lung without becoming fully oxygenated, which is the so-called venous admixture. Whether inadequate oxygenation of arterial blood occurs because of a diffusion defect, low, but finite, ventilation/perfusion ratio, or absolute right-to-left intrapulmonary shunting of blood, other variables may also have a significant influence on the ultimate arterial oxygen tension. For example, either an increase in oxygen consumption secondary to a marked increase in metabolic rate or a decrease in cardiac output may cause returning venous blood to have a decreased oxygen content. When venous blood oxygen saturation is low, arterial blood will have a much lower oxygen tension than might be explained on the basis of venous admixture alone. Similarly, a low hemoglobin concentration will result in a decrease in mixed venous oxygen saturation and amplification of arterial hypoxemia.

Such factors must be considered in evaluating the patient with arterial hypoxemia; otherwise, inappropriate therapy may be instituted. For example, a patient with a low cardiac output secondary to intravascular hypovolemia may be hypoxemic in the absence of elevated levels of intrapulmonary shunting of blood. Application of PEEP and/or vigorous diuresis in an attempt to improve arterial oxygenation could impede thoracic venous inflow of blood, resulting in further depression of cardiac output and, thereby, further deterioration of systemic oxygenation. Because the arterial oxygen tension is so greatly dependent on the arterial-venous oxygen content difference, it is imperative that mixed venous oxygen content and saturation be evaluated in patients with significant arterial hypoxemia in the postoperative period. In the absence of any clinical evidence to indicate deficient cardiac output or increased metabolic rate, a decrease in arterial oxygen tension may be considered to be secondary to venous admixture. However, if there is any

doubt, a pulmonary artery catheter should be inserted and a mixed venous blood sample obtained for analysis. Assumption of a fixed arterial-venous oxygen content difference in calculating right-to-left intrapulmonary shunting of blood is likely to lead to significant error in a large portion of postoperative thoracic surgical patients and, therefore, is not recommended.[37] This is especially the case in patients who have undergone cardiopulmonary bypass procedures, in whom a low cardiac output, decreased hemoglobin concentration, and increased oxygen consumption are likely to occur.

Evaluation of arterial oxygenation is complicated further by the effect of the inspired oxygen concentration on venous admixture and calculated right-to-left intrapulmonary shunting of blood (Fig. 22-4). For example, individuals with low, but finite, ventilation/perfusion ratios will have significant arterial hypoxemia when breathing room air. It is not unusual for individuals with severe chronic obstructive lung disease to have arterial oxygen tensions between 40 and 50 mmHg. However, when the F_iO_2 is elevated slightly, there is a dramatic increase in arterial oxygen tension. When right-to-left intrapulmonary shunting of blood is calculated before and after the administration of oxygen, a dramatic decrease in the calculated shunt fraction secondary to a masking effect of oxygen on low, but finite, ventilation/perfusion ratios is observed. The same effect will occur when a diffusion defect contributes to arterial hypoxemia.

It has long been felt that oxygen has little or no effect on absolute right-to-left intrapulmonary shunting of blood. However, some investigations have disclosed a significant increase in right-to-left intrapulmonary shunting of blood when high inspired oxygen concentrations are administered.[38] Although several mechanisms have been postulated in an attempt to explain this observation, it is likely that a high F_iO_2 will lead to rapid resorption of gas from terminal airways in areas of lung with low, but finite, ventilation-to-perfusion ratios. This phenomenon has been termed *absorption atelectasis* and was described by Lansing and Jamieson in 1963.[39] Subsequent investigators have observed significant atelectasis when 100 percent oxygen is inspired. It is likely that the presence of nitrogen in the inspired gas will prevent this effect, but application of positive pressure to the airway, even to 25 cmH_2O, is unlikely to prevent it. Therefore, the prevalent opinion that high F_iO_2 may be safely used for up to 24 hours because it may not cause oxygen toxicity should be considered inaccurate. Oxygen should be viewed as any other drug, and should be applied only when clinically indicated and in an amount required to produce the clinically desired effect.

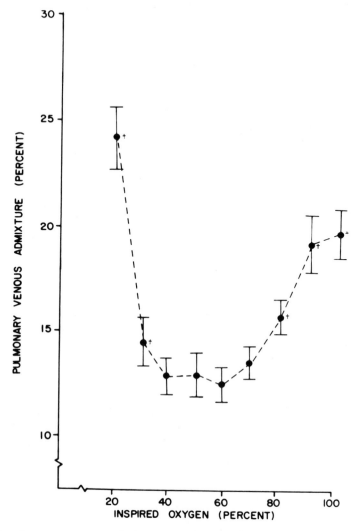

Fig. 22-4. Calculated pulmonary venous admixture depends greatly on the fractional concentration of inspired oxygen (F_IO_2). When the F_IO_2 is low, venous admixture may be elevated as a result of ventilation-to-perfusion mismatching, diffusion impairment, and right-to-left intrapulmonary shunting of blood. When the F_IO_2 is increased, venous admixture is greater, owing to increased intrapulmonary shunting of blood. [†], significantly greater than $F_IO_2 = 0.5$.

Postoperatively, many clinicians have administered an elevated F_IO_2 in an attempt to provide a safety margin, in case of unforeseen mishaps. Register et al determined that such a practice is ineffective and may cause significant hypoxemia following tracheal extubation.[40] Patients who received 50 percent oxygen postoperatively for 16 to 24 hours demonstrated a progressive fall in PaO_2. Following extubation, their PaO_2 levels were lower than those of patients who had received no more than 30 percent oxygen for the same period of time.

The response of venous admixture to changes in inspired oxygen concentration may be altered by different therapeutic regimens. For example, Douglas et al found that patients who had undergone cardiopulmonary bypass and who breathed room air had a significant decrease in right-to-left intrapulmonary shunting of blood if steroids were administered intravenously prior to bypass (Fig. 22-5).[41] However, when these patients breathed pure oxygen, the degree of right-to-left intrapulmonary shunting of blood was increased compared with that in patients who had re-

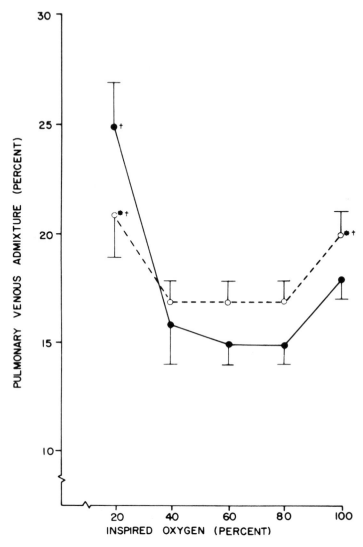

Fig. 22-5. Pretreatment with steroids may decrease venous admixture when inspired oxygen is low. However, an elevated F_IO_2 may cause increased right-to-left intrapulmonary shunting of blood following the administration of steroids. ○‑‑‑○, steroids; ●———●, placebo. (From Douglas et al,[41] with permission.)

ceived placebo. It is possible that steroids cause an increase in perfusion to poorly ventilated lung regions, which thus explains the increase in calculated shunt fraction when patients breathed pure oxygen. Steroids may decrease small airway resistance, thus improving the ventilation/perfusion ratio in other lung regions. Such an effect would cause an increase in arterial oxygen tension when patients breathe room air. Douglas et al also found that application of CPAP significantly decreased calculated shunt fraction regardless of the inspired oxygen concentration (Fig. 22-6).[41] Thus, when patients received steroids

and CPAP, arterial oxygen tension was increased from 52 ± 2 mmHg to 62 ± 3 mmHg (mean ± SEM, $P <$ .05). The significant increase in arterial oxygen tension appeared to be due to an additive effect of steroids and CPAP on areas of lung with low, but finite, ventilation/perfusion ratios (Fig. 22-7).

Patients who undergo thoracotomy often require oxygen administration in the immediate postoperative period, usually to maintain the arterial oxygen tension greater than 60 to 80 mmHg. Numerous devices have been described for the administration of oxygen to these patients, including face shields, face

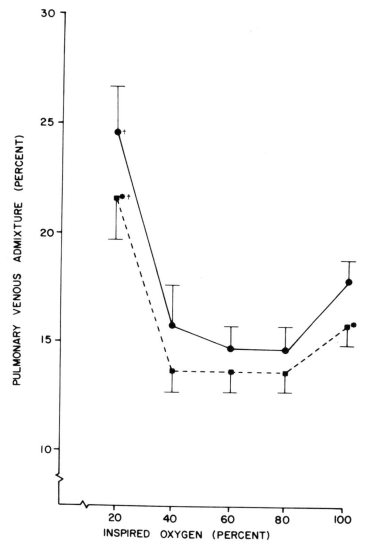

Fig. 22-6. Application of continuous positive airway pressure (CPAP) will reduce pulmonary venous admixture at all inspired oxygen concentrations following cardiopulmonary bypass. ●---●, CPAP; ●——●, no CPAP. (From Douglas et al,[41] with permission.)

masks, rebreathing masks, Venturi masks, oxygen tents, and nasal prongs. Available information suggests that no currently available device will give an accurate concentration of inspired oxygen at all times. Therefore, the device used to administer oxygen to the postoperative patient should be chosen with consideration of the desired objectives. If the clinician is concerned with limiting the inspired oxygen concentration to prevent depression of the patient's hypoxic drive to breathe, a Venturi mask would be the most logical choice. If the objective is merely to increase the inspired oxygen concentration to ensure

that the patient does not become hypoxemic, a device should be used that will remain in place and will increase the inspired oxygen concentration at most times, especially when the patient is active, eating, or ambulating. In these instances, face masks and face shields are less likely to remain in proper position than nasal prongs. It has been determined that oxygen administration at 3 L/min through nasal prongs will provide the patient with an F_IO_2 of 0.25 to 0.30. When a higher inspired oxygen concentration is desired, a face mask is used to deliver high flows of oxygen-enriched gas to the patient's face. Special care must

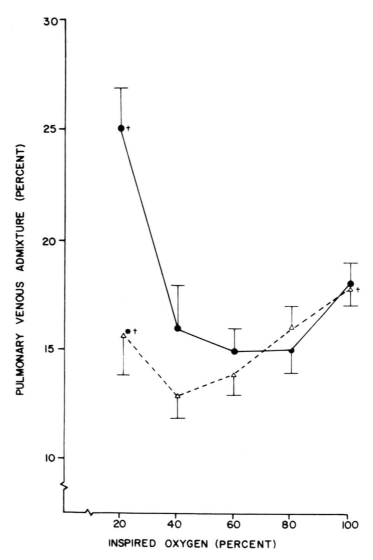

Fig. 22-7. Following cardiopulmonary bypass, steroids and CPAP appear to have different modes of action and may have additive effects. Therefore, pulmonary venous admixture is markedly decreased when the patient is breathing room air and remains unchanged at high inspired oxygen concentrations. △---△, CPAP and steroids; ●——●, control. (From Douglas et al,[41] with permission.)

then be taken to ensure that the device remains in place at all times. Usually, when 30 percent oxygen is inadequate to create a satisfactory arterial oxygen tension, other means, such as CPAP, are used.

A marked decrease in arterial oxygen tension may be secondary to a significant increase in right-to-left intrapulmonary shunting of blood due to small airway closure. If so, therapy should more appropriately be directed at increasing lung volume than at increasing the inspired oxygen concentration. Oxygenation of pulmonary capillary blood occurs predominantly

during the expiratory phase of respiration. Therefore, it is the expiratory lung volume, the FRC, that is responsible for the efficiency of arterial oxygenation. As discussed previously, an increase in FRC can occur most efficiently when expiratory transpulmonary pressure is increased. Therefore, it is not surprising that CPAP has been found to be efficacious for increasing arterial oxygen tension in many patients with small airway closure. Although many clinicians have suggested that PEEP and CPAP be applied only if the patients otherwise require "toxic" levels of inspired oxygen, CPAP can be applied early in a patient's treatment regimen, even when a face mask is used. Often, the increase in lung volume that occurs with low levels of CPAP may increase lung compliance and cause a dramatic increase in FRC. This frequently is indicated clinically by a sharp fall in the patient's respiratory rate, which is evidence that the work of breathing has been significantly reduced. Furthermore, arterial oxygen tension is often increased. When increasing inspired oxygen concentration and application of CPAP by face mask are inadequate to provide the desired arterial oxygen tension, consideration must be given to endotracheal intubation and mechanical ventilation.

PLEURAL DRAINAGE

Drainage of the pleural cavity was first described by Hewett in 1876 for the treatment of empyema.[42] In 1911, Kenyon described the use of an underwater seal system, a rather simple means of maintaining a closed pleural space.[43] As time progressed, thoracostomy tubes became routine after thoracotomy for many operative procedures; they are often placed as a means of treating pneumothorax, hemothorax, empyema, and pleural effusion. Because of the frequency with which pleural drainage is applied and because of the serious nature of complications, it is essential that all personnel dealing with pleural drainage systems be familiar with the mechanics and physiology involved. Although simple in concept, the underwater seal system for maintaining negative pressure within the pleural space is frequently misunderstood. The different systems for accomplishing pleural drainage are too numerous to discuss individually. The configuration of bottles, application of suction, and daily management of pleural drainage systems are based more on local custom than on precise physiologic principles. Therefore, only the basic principles will be discussed in any detail.

Thoracostomy Tubes

Thoracostomy tubes are frequently placed to treat various pathologic conditions; however, placement of thoracostomy tubes is occasionally recommended for prophylactic reasons. Insertion of a thoracostomy tube should not be considered a benign procedure and should be accomplished only by, or under the supervision of, an individual with considerable experience and judgment. Misplacement of the tube, especially when using the trocar technique, may cause laceration of the lung, liver, spleen, diaphragm, stomach, colon, and kidney. If the tube is too large, too stiff, or

is placed too superficially, the pleural space may not be sufficiently separated from the atmosphere, and recurrent pneumothorax may result. Often, subcutaneous emphysema results from thoracostomy tube insertion, and infection of the ribs has been reported. Intercostal artery and vein laceration may occur, resulting in significant bleeding. Almost universally, significant pain at the insertion site limits respiratory excursion. If possible, chest roentgenograms should be obtained to confirm the presence of significant pneumothorax or effusion, and thoracostomy tubes should be inserted only when necessary.

Drainage System

In an attempt to improve pleural drainage, various modifications of the basic underwater seal system, consisting of one-, two-, and three-bottle arrangements (Figs. 22-8 and 22-9), have been suggested. Recently, disposable plastic systems have been devised that circumvent many of the problems inherent in locally assembled systems, such as breakage and restrictive flow. However, inadequate suction may cause significant problems even with the disposable systems. If the flow rate of the suction system cannot exceed the rate of leakage of air into the pleural space, a tension pneumothorax will occur. In this instance, the patient would be safer with a simple underwater

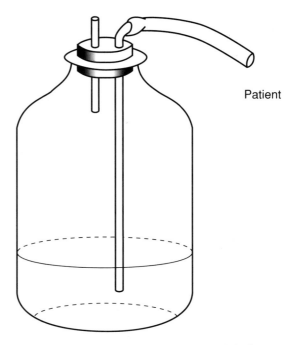

Patient

Fig. 22-8. Standard underwater seal pleural drainage system.

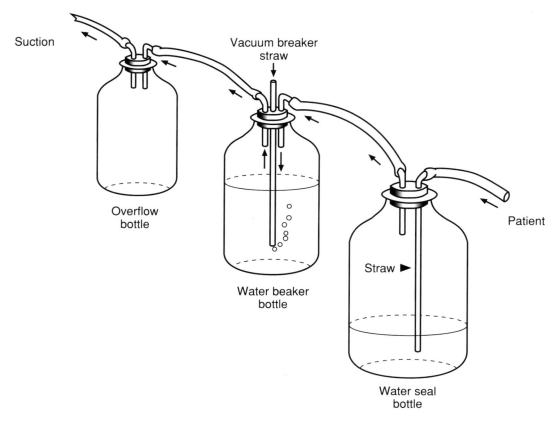

Suction

Vacuum breaker
straw

Overflow
bottle

Water beaker
bottle

Straw ▶

Water seal
bottle

Patient

Fig. 22-9. Three-bottle pleural drainage system.

seal system than with applied wall suction. Complications such as these have been discussed in detail by Emerson and McIntyre[44] and by Van Way.[45] In general, it is best to have negative pressure generated by a variable-control turbine pump rather than by a diaphragm regulator, which may have limited flow capability.

Munnell and Thomas polled 442 members of the Southern Thoracic Surgical Association and 48 nonmember thoracic surgeons to determine which drainage systems they used: 53 percent used a system with a single bottle, and 36 percent used a two-bottle system.[46] A dry trap first bottle may allow reverse air flow, especially when the suction gradient is low. Therefore, many practitioners use an underwater seal bottle first and a dry trap bottle second to protect the suction source from frothing and spillover. The three-bottle system uses a dry trap, a low negative-pressure water limiter bottle, and a water seal, usually in that order (Fig. 22-9). The most commonly applied disposable systems use this principle. Since there is a low negative-pressure limiter, usually set at 15 cmH$_2$O, there is no point in applying flow in excess of that necessary to create bubbling throughout the respiratory cycle. Any further negative pressure or flow ap-

plied to the system will result only in further entrainment of atmospheric air.

Management

Management of the pleural drainage system is fraught with confusion and often inappropriate action. For example, Heimlich stated that the chest drainage tube must be clamped during transport, even though he recognized that air and blood could accumulate in the chest, causing lung collapse.[47] Munnell and Thomas found that 35 percent of respondents clamped the thoracostomy tube during transport of the patient.[46] It should be apparent that if the underwater seal bottle is held above the patient, fluid may be siphoned from the underwater seal bottle into the patient's chest. Hence, the bottle must be kept below the level of the patient's chest at all times. Only during the brief period when it is necessary to elevate the chest tube drainage bottle above chest level should the tube be clamped. Therefore, the classic instruction given to nurses and other paramedical personnel to clamp chest tubes whenever the system is broken or the patient is moved should be condemned.

Suction applied to the thoracostomy drainage system is *never* lifesaving. On the contrary, limited flow by the suction system may prevent adequate drainage of air from the pleural space. Whenever there is doubt regarding the adequacy of drainage, the suction system should be disconnected and a simple underwater seal system instituted. Such a system will prevent significant buildup of pressure within the pleural space and will allow drainage of fluid as long as the tubing is patent. To ensure patency of the tubing, "milking" the chest tube (pushing air and fluid back into the chest) and "stripping" the tube (a distal movement to create vacuum within the tubing to suck fluid and/or air from the chest) have been recommended to be performed at regular intervals. In individuals who have significant drainage and/or bleeding, these maneuvers may be required every 5 minutes. If the temperature of the tubes approaches body temperature, it is likely that bleeding is active and there is an increased risk of clotting of the thoracostomy tube.

The thoracostomy drainage system should not be broken for routine procedures. For example, the bottle should not be emptied for intake and output measurements. Such procedures are likely to result in contamination of the system and may cause recurrent pneumothorax. Once the thoracostomy tube is positioned, a dry sterile dressing should be left in place for 24 to 48 hours. When removing the tube, the clinician should ensure that pleural pressure is above atmospheric pressure to prevent air entrainment and pneumothorax. Therefore, the patient should be instructed to take a deep breath and to perform a Valsalva maneuver during removal of the tube. A sterile occlusive dressing should be placed over the thoracostomy insertion site and should remain in place for at least 24 hours to ensure closure of the tube tract.

Thoracostomy tube drainage may be lifesaving. However, complications and errors in treatment may cause significant morbidity and mortality. Therefore, all physicians, nurses, and other personnel dealing with patients in whom thoracostomy tube drainage is necessary should have a good understanding of the mechanics and physiology involved. Several texts are available that describe the physiology of thoracostomy drainage in detail, and the reader is urged to consult these for further information.[48]

DRUG THERAPY

Perhaps surprisingly, drug therapy plays a small role in the routine respiratory care of the postoperative patient following thoracic surgery. For years, respiratory stimulants were administered to patients in an effort to reverse the respiratory depressant effects of anesthesia. However, such stimulants are not without untoward side effects and may cause significant increases in cardiac output, apprehension, and short-ness of breath. Careful administration of general anesthesia should ensure insignificant depression of respiratory drive in the postoperative period. There is no evidence that administration of respiratory stimulants will decrease the incidence of postoperative pulmonary complications, and postoperative respiratory depression can be treated in more appropriate ways. Therefore, the administration of respiratory stimulants is rarely, if ever, necessary. However, an occasional patient may require reversal of a narcotic with naloxone.

Some patients who undergo thoracotomy may have reactive airway disease with significant postoperative bronchospasm. Most patients will have had pulmonary testing prior to their operation to document the existence of bronchospastic disease and its reversibility with topical bronchodilators. Occasionally, patients may be operated on without acquisition of such preoperative data, and may require the administration of bronchodilators in the postoperative period. If so, racemic epinephrine, isoproterenol, isoetharine, metaproterenol, terbutaline, and salbutamol may be administered topically to promote bronchodilatation. Racemic epinephrine also may decrease mucosal edema secondary to airway trauma and has often been used in the postoperative period. The pharmacologic action of these drugs is reviewed in Chapter 9. All can be administered easily with a hand-held nebulizer, although in patients who are unable to inhale sufficiently, intermittent positive-pressure breathing may be a more efficient means of delivery. Table 22-1 lists the drugs and inhaled doses.

Parenteral bronchodilators such as the methylxanthines and catecholamines may also be administered to patients in the postoperative period. Increased levels of cyclic adenosine monophosphate (AMP) may cause relaxation of bronchial smooth muscles. Therefore, drugs such as the methylxanthines, which inhibit phosphodiesterase, the enzyme responsible for breakdown of cyclic AMP, may be useful. Additionally, drugs such as the catecholamines may stimulate adenylate cyclase, which will increase the production of cyclic AMP. Such drugs will have an additive effect and may be used in combination.

The administration of bronchodilators should not be routine practice. Only when objective evidence of increased airway resistance is present, such as wheezing and prolonged exhalation, should bronchodilators be administered. Commonly, bronchodilators stimulate the myocardium and may cause dysrhythmias. Furthermore, most of these drugs reverse hypoxic pulmonary vasoconstriction and may cause rapid and significant right-to-left intrapulmonary shunting of blood and arterial hypoxemia. Therefore, most patients who require the administration of bronchodilators should also receive supplemental oxygen.

TABLE 22-1. Respiratory Inhalant Products

Trade Name (Manufacturer)	Active Constituents	Usual Dosage
Sympathomimetics		
Vaponephrine (Fisons)	Racemic epinephrine, 2.25%	0.25–0.5 mL[a] 4–6 times daily
Medihaler-Epi (3M Riker)	Epinephrine, 0.7%	1–2 metered inhalations (0.16–0.32 mg) 4–6 times daily
Bronkaid Mist (Winthrop)	Epinephrine, 0.5%	1–2 metered inhalations (0.25–0.5 mg) 4–6 times daily
Primatene Mist (Whitehall)	Epinephrine, 0.55%	1–2 metered inhalations (0.22–0.44 mg) 4–6 times daily
Alupent (Boehringer Ingelheim) Metaprel (Dorsey)	Metaproterenol sulfate as a micronized powder in an inert propellant	2–3 metered inhalations (1.30–1.95 mg) not to exceed 12 inhalations daily
Alupent (Boehringer Ingelheim) Metaprel (Dorsey)	Metaproterenol sulfate, 0.5%	0.2–0.3 mL[a] 4–6 times daily
Poventil Inhaler (Schering)	Albuterol sulfate, 0.5%, 0.083%	2.5 mg 3–4 times daily[a]
Aerolone (Lilly)	Isoproterenol HCl, 0.25%	0.25–1.0 mL[a] 4–6 times daily
Ventolin (Allen & Hanburys)	Microcrystalline suspension of albuterol in propellants	2 metered inhalations (90 μg) 4–6 times daily
	Albuterol sulfate, 0.5%	2.5 mg[a] 3–4 times daily
Isuprel (Breon)	Isoproterenol HCl, 0.5% or 1%	0.25–0.5 mL[a] of 0.5% solution 4–6 times daily
Norisodrine Aerotrol (Abbott)	Isoproterenol HCl, 0.25%	1–2 metered inhalations (120–240 μg) 4–6 times daily
Isuprel Mistometer (Breon)	Isoproterenol HCl, 0.25%	1–2 metered inhalations (125–250 μg) 4–6 times daily
Medihaler-Iso (3M Riker)	Isoproterenol HCl, 2 mg/mL	1–2 metered inhalations (75–150 μg) 4–6 times daily
Norisodrine Sulfate Aerohalor (Abbott)	10% Aerohalor cartridges (powder)	2–4 Aerohalor inhalations (0.090–0.180 μg) 4–6 times daily

(continued)

In patients with known bronchospastic disease, consideration should be given to the administration of steroids prior to, during, and following operation. There is some evidence that topical steroids, such as beclomethasone, may be effective in preventing bronchospasm in the postoperative period. Similarly, cromolyn sodium may be useful when administered prophylactically to patients who have known bronchospastic disease. It should be emphasized that cromolyn sodium is not a bronchodilator and has no role in the treatment of active bronchospasm.

For several years, some clinicians have recommended the administration of mucolytic agents to the respiratory tract. However, most studies of the effectiveness of topically administered mucolytics have found that they have no significant influence on the incidence of postoperative atelectasis. There is no question that the administration of mucolytic agents will cause an increase in the production of sputum of some patients. However, it is not clear that mucolytic-enhanced sputum production is therapeutic. For example, most mucolytics are sufficiently irritating to the respiratory tract that increased production of sputum may occur in reaction to the irritant. In patients who have difficulty clearing secretions, administration of a mucolytic agent may cause deterioration in pulmonary function. Furthermore, if an individual has difficulty in raising secretions, further liquification of the secretions may cause them to run distally into peripheral airways rather than causing them to be cleared more easily. Since these agents are irritating, expensive, and potentially dangerous, they should not be used without very specific indications. Certainly, they cannot be recommended as a routine prophylactic measure.

Topical application of antibiotics to the respiratory tract has been recommended by various investigators. Amphotericin-B, bacitracin, polymyxin, neomycin,

TABLE 22-1 (*continued*).   Respiratory Inhalant Products

Trade Name (Manufacturer)	Active Constituents	Usual Dosage
Norisodrine Sulfate Aerohalor (Abbott)	20% Aerohalor cartrides (powder)	2–4 Aerohalor inhalations (0.180–0.360 μg) 4–6 times daily
Bronkosol (Breon)	Isoetharine HCl, 1%	0.25–0.5 mL^a 4–6 times daily
Bronkometer (Breon)	Isoetharine mesylate, 0.61%	1–2 metered inhalations (340–680 μg) 4–6 times daily
Maxair Inhaler (3M Riker)	Pirbuterol acetate	2 metered inhalations (0.4 mg) 4–6 times daily
Anticholinergics		
Atrovent (Boehringer Ingelheim)	Ipratropium bromide	2 metered inhalations (36 μm) 4 times daily
Corticosteroids		
Vanceril (Schering)	Beclomethasone dipropionate	1–2 metered inhalations (42–84 μg) 3–4 times daily
Beclovent (Glaxo)	Beclomethasone dipropionate	1–2 metered inhalations (42–84 μg) 3–4 times daily
Azmacort Inhaler (Rorer)	Triamcinolone acetonide	2 metered inhalations (400 μg) 3–4 times daily
Mucolytics		
Mucomyst (Mead Johnson)	Acetylcysteine, 10% or 20%	2–4 mL^b of 10% solution 4–6 times daily
Cromolyn sodium		
Intal Spinhaler (Fisons)	Cromolyn sodium as a micronized powder	One capsule (20 mg) via Spinhaler 4 times daily

^{a} Dilute with 2 to 5 mL diluent and give over 10 to 15 minutes by IPPB or compressor.

^{b} By IPPB or compressor. Simultaneous bronchodilator administration will decrease possible increased airway resistance caused by acetylcysteine.

and mycostatin (nystatin) are antibiotic agents that have been recommended for topical administration, since their systemic toxicity would be far greater if administered parenterally. In addition, carbenicillin, gentamicin, and kanamycin have also been recommended for topical use. Initially, topical administration was accomplished by nebulization. However, evidence has accumulated to indicate that nebulization of potent antibiotics leads to rapid creation of resistant bacteria in the environment. Furthermore, these antibiotics are just as effective when instilled directly into the trachea. Subsequently, several investigators have found no beneficial effect of either prophylactic or therapeutic administration of topical antibiotics. Finally, the topical administration of drugs such as polymyxin may lead to significant bronchospasm in susceptible individuals. Therefore, in the absence of information demonstrating a beneficial effect of topically administered antibiotic agents, their use should be restricted to the occasional case in which other modes of therapy have failed.

REINTUBATION OF THE TRACHEA

Following operation, if a patient's respiratory status deteriorates significantly, consideration must be given to reintubation of the trachea. Pediatric thoracic surgeons have used the technique of reintubation for many years in the treatment of atelectasis, especially of the right upper lobe. In such infants, the endotracheal tube is usually placed without anesthesia or muscle relaxation, and a small amount of saline solution is instilled through the tube; this is followed by vigorous manual ventilation and suction. Following repetition of this sequence three or four times, extubation is accomplished and the infant is allowed to breath spontaneously. This treatment has not gained favor in adult respiratory care, probably because of the difficulty involved with intubating awake adults. It may be necessary to produce a brief period of anesthesia and muscle relaxation in patients who require reintubation. This can usually be accomplished with a short-acting intravenous barbiturate anesthetic agent and a short-acting muscle relaxant.

Some patients ventilate inadequately in the postoperative period and may have significant elevation of their arterial carbon dioxide tension. Fortunately, hypoventilation resulting in hypercarbic acidosis is an infrequent postoperative problem. The individual with postoperative carbon dioxide retention may be somnolent, with shallow tidal breathing and a decreased respiratory rate. In such cases, respiratory depression is usually the result of parenteral administration of respiratory depressant drugs, such as narcotics or barbiturates, or is secondary to the insidious onset of hypercarbia causing decreased respiratory drive. The latter problem usually exists only in patients who have a hypoxic drive for respiration and who receive an excessive concentration of oxygen in the postoperative period. Analysis of arterial blood for carbon dioxide tension and pH is the most accurate means of diagnosing this problem. However, clinical observation of the patient is the only efficient means of knowing when to analyze arterial blood samples. Routine orders for blood sampling often will not be adequate for detecting or preventing this problem. A high degree of suspicion based on preoperative assessment is essential.

Numerous authors have detailed clinical tests to be used in determining when an individual requires reintubation and institution of mechanical ventilatory support. However, Browne and Pontoppidan found that only two clinical measurements correlated significantly with a patient's ability to maintain adequate spontaneous respiration, namely, vital capacity and the negative pressure created by an inspiratory effort against a closed airway.[49] The peak negative pressure generated against a closed airway is a direct reflection of the patient's muscular ability to generate negative intrapleural pressure and, therefore, the neuromuscular ability to breathe spontaneously. In contrast, the vital capacity maneuver requires adequate lung compliance in addition to muscular strength. For example, a patient may have normal respiratory muscle strength to breathe, but the lung may be so stiff that adequate spontaneous respiration cannot occur. Therefore, the combination of a peak negative pressure measurement and vital capacity measurement likely will indicate to the clinician if a patient has deficient respiratory muscle strength and/or decreased lung compliance. If an individual is able to generate a vital capacity of 15 mL/kg and a peak negative pressure of -20 cmH$_2$O or greater, the ability to support spontaneous ventilation should exist. The clinician should be careful to note that these maneuvers are independent of respiratory drive. An individual may have sufficient strength and compliance to support spontaneous ventilation, but if respiratory drive is inadequate, respiratory failure and acidosis will ensue.

Failure of the patient to support adequate spontaneous respiration, resulting in respiratory acidosis, is much less frequent than the problem of inadequate postoperative oxygenation. Patients with arterial hypoxemia may require intubation, but ventilation is infrequently required to treat postoperative arterial hypoxemia (Fig. 22-10). If CPAP cannot be adequately delivered by mask, the patient may require endotracheal intubation for consistent delivery of higher levels of CPAP. When necessary, this should be done early and prior to the administration of an excessive inspired oxygen concentration.

Once a decision is made to reintubate the patient, mechanical ventilator settings should be appropriate to treat and prevent further respiratory acidosis. In addition, some care should be taken to ensure that respiratory alkalosis does not occur. Prior investigations have revealed that an alveolar ventilation of approximately 4 L/min will provide a normal arterial carbon dioxide tension in the majority of postoperative patients. During mechanical ventilatory therapy, physiologic dead space is elevated and the dead space-to-tidal volume ratio approaches 0.50. Therefore, a minute ventilation of approximately 8 L/min is required for most postoperative adult patients.[50]

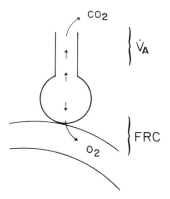

Fig. 22-10. Maintenance of functional residual capacity (FRC) is necessary to ensure optimum oxygenation of arterial blood, thus preventing right-to-left intrapulmonary shunting. Bulk flow of gas into and from the alveolar spaces is unnecessary to maintain this function. In contrast, efficient carbon dioxide excretion from alveolar spaces depends on bulk flow of gas from the lung. Therefore, alveolar ventilation ($\dot{V}_A$) may be manipulated to ensure maintenance of proper arterial carbon dioxide tension, and a continuous positive pressure may be applied to the airway to maintain approximate FRC and arterial oxygenation.

A ventilator rate of up to 10 breaths/min and a tidal volume of 8 to 12 mL/kg may be necessary to prevent respiratory acidosis and a further decrease in FRC. Intermittent mandatory ventilation is used to maintain a normal arterial blood pH. Care should be taken to ensure that adequate humidity is supplied to the patient at all times. Even short exposure to cool, unhumidified gas may cause significant tracheal mucosal damage and inspissation of secretions, with further compromise of respiratory function.

Once the patient is reintubated, care should be taken to maintain the sterility of the patient's airway. Therefore, the connection between the endotracheal tube and the breathing circuit should be broken only for necessary maneuvers. For example, suctioning of the tracheobronchial tree should occur only when auscultation of the patient's chest reveals the need for such treatment. Routine suctioning should be avoided. The patient's position should be changed frequently to prevent atelectasis and retention or secretions in dependent airways. The endotracheal tube should be equipped with a high residual volume, low-pressure cuff, and cuff pressure should be documented to be less than 20 mmHg. Inflation of the cuff should occur with no more air than is required to prevent an air leak. Intubation of the trachea is fraught with complications and should not be considered a benign form of therapy. Finally, once the patient is intubated, thought should be given to weaning the patient from oxygen, mechanical ventilation, and CPAP, and to extubating as soon as possible.

REFERENCES

1. Stein M, Cassara EL: Preoperative pulmonary evaluation and therapy for surgery patients. JAMA 211:787–790, 1970
2. Burford TH, Burbank B: Traumatic wet lung. J Thorac Surg 14:415–424, 1945
3. Maiwand MO, Makey AR, Rees A: Cryoanalgesia after thoracotomy: improvement of technique and review of 600 cases. J Thorac Cardiovasc Surg 92:291–295, 1986
4. Burns JW, Hodsman BA, McLintock TTC, et al: The influence of patient characteristics on the requirements for postoperative analgesia. Anaesthesia 44:2–6, 1989
5. Piehl MA, Brown RS: Use of extreme position changes in acute respiratory failure. Crit Care Med 4:13–14, 1976
6. Al-Jurf AS: Turn, cough and deep breaths (editorial). Surg Gynecol Obstet 149:887–888, 1979
7. Sante L: Massive (atelectatic) collapse of the lung. Ann Surg 88:161–171, 1928
8. Marini J, Pierson DJ, Hudson LD: Acute lobar atelectasis: a prospective comparison of fiberoptic bronchoscopy and respiratory therapy. Am Rev Respir Dis 119:971–978, 1979
9. Graham WGB, Bradley DA, Kleczek R, et al: Efficacy of chest physiotherapy and intermittent positive-pressure breathing in the resolution of pneumonia. N Engl J Med 299:624–627, 1978
10. Radigan LR, King RD: A technique for the prevention of postoperative atelectasis. Surgery 47:184–187, 1960
11. Haight C: Intratracheal suction in the management of postoperative pulmonary complications. Ann Surg 107:218–228, 1938
12. Sackner MA, Landa JF, Robinson MJ, et al: Pathogenesis and prevention of tracheobronchial damage with suction procedures. Chest 64:284–290, 1973
13. Jung RC, Gottlieb LS: Comparison of tracheobronchial suction catheters in humans. Chest 69:179–181, 1976
14. Bowen TE, Fishback ME, Green DC: Treatment of refractory atelectasis. Ann Thorac Surg 18:584–589, 1974
15. Millen JE, Vandree J, Glauser FL: Fiberoptic bronchoscopic balloon occlusion and reexpansion of refractory unilateral atelectasis. Crit Care Med 6:50–55, 1978
16. Bartlett RH, Gazzaniga AB, Geraghty TR: Respiratory maneuvers to prevent postoperative pulmonary complications—a critical review. JAMA 224:1017–1021, 1973
17. Nunn JF, Coleman AJ, Sachithanandan T, et al: Hypoxaemia and atelectasis produced by forced expiration. Br J Anaesth 37:3–12, 1965
18. Gold MI: Is intermittent positive-pressure breathing therapy (IPPB Rx) necessary in the surgical patient? Ann Surg 1844:122–123, 1976
19. Iverson LIG, Ecker RR, Fox HE, et al: A comparative study of IPPB, the incentive spirometer, and blow bottles: the prevention of atelectasis following cardiac surgery. Ann Thorac Surg 25:197–200, 1978
20. Browner B, Powers SR, Jr: Effect of IPPB on the functional residual capacity and blood gases in postoperative patients. Surg Forum 26:96–98, 1975
21. Lareau S: The effect of positive-pressure breathing on the arterial oxygen tension in patients with chronic obstructive pulmonary disease receiving oxygen therapy. Heart Lung 5:449–452, 1976
22. Wright FG, Jr, Foley MF, Downs JB, et al: Hypoxemia and hypocarbia following intermittent positive-pressure breathing. Anesth Analg 55:555–559, 1976
23. Shim C, Bajwa S, Williams MH, Jr: The effect of inhalation therapy on ventilatory function and expectoration. Chest 73:798–801, 1978
24. Paul WL, Downs JB: Postoperative atelectasis. Arch Surg 116:861–863, 1981
25. Ward RJ, Danziger F, Bonica JJ, et al: An evaluation of postoperative respiratory maneuvers. Surg Gyncol Obstet 123:51–54, 1966
26. Bartlett RH, Krop P, Hanson EL, et al: Physiology of yawning and its application to postoperative care. Surg Forum 21:222–224, 1970
27. Lederer DH, Van de Water JM, Indech RB: Which deep breathing device should the postoperative patient use? Chest 77:610–613, 1980
28. Bartlett RH, Brennan ML, Gazzaniga AB, et al: Studies on the pathogenesis and prevention of postoperative pulmonary complications. Surg Gynecol Obstet 137:925–933, 1973

29. Downs JB, Mitchell LA: Pulmonary effects of ventilatory pattern following cardiopulmonary bypass. Crit Care Med 4:295–300, 1976

30. Fowler AA III, Scoggins WG, O'Donohue WJ, Jr: Positive end-expiratory pressure in the management of lobar atelectasis. Chest 74:497–500, 1978

31. Stone DR, Downs JB: Collateral ventilation and PEEP in normal and edematous lungs of dogs. Anesthesiology 53:S186, 1980

32. Greenbaum DM, Millen JE, Eross B, et al: Continuous positive airway pressure without tracheal intubation in spontaneously breathing patients. Chest 69:615–620, 1976

33. Andersen JB, Olesen KP, Eikard B, et al: Periodic continuous positive airway pressure, CPAP, by mask in the treatment of atelectasis—a sequential analysis. Eur J Respir Dis 61:20–25, 1980

34. Stock MC, Downs JB, Gauer PK, et al: Prevention of postoperative pulmonary complications with CPAP, incentive spirometry, and conservative therapy. Chest 87:151–157, 1985

35. Aldrich TK, Karpel JP: Inspiratory muscle resistive training in respiratory failure. Am Rev Respir Dis 131:461–462, 1985

36. Clanton TL, Dixon G, Drake J, et al: Inspiratory muscle conditioning using a threshold loading device. Chest 87:62–66, 1985

37. Mitchell LA, Downs JB, Dannemiller FJ: Extrapulmonary influences on A-aDO$_2$$^{1.0}$ following cardiopulmonary bypass. Anesthesiology 43:583–586, 1975

38. Douglas ME, Downs JB, Dannemiller FJ, et al: Change in pulmonary venous admixture with varying inspired oxygen. Anesth Analg 55:688–695, 1976

39. Lansing AM, Jamieson WG: Mechanisms of fever in pulmonary atelectasis. Arch Surg 87:184–190, 1963

40. Register SD III, Downs JB, Stock MC, et al: Is 50% oxygen harmful? Crit Care Med 15:598–601, 1987

41. Douglas ME, Downs JB, Shook D: Response of pulmonary venous admixture. A means of comparing therapies? Chest 77:764–770, 1980

42. Hewett C: Drainage for empyema. Br Med J 1:317, 1876

43. Kenyon JA: A preliminary report on a method of treatment of empyema in young children. Med Rec 80:816, 1911

44. Emerson DM, McIntrye J: A comparative study of the physiology and physics of pleural drainage systems. J Thorac Cardiovasc Surg 52:40–46, 1966

45. Van Way CW III: Persisting pneumothorax as a complication of chest suction. Chest 77:815–816, 1980

46. Munnell ER, Thomas EK: Current concepts in thoracic drainage systems. Ann Thorac Surg 19:261–268, 1975

47. Heimlich HJ: Valve drainage of the pleural cavity. Dis Chest 53:282–287, 1968

48. von Hippel A: Chest Tubes and Chest Bottles. Charles C Thomas, Springfield, IL, 1970

49. Browne AGR, Pontoppidan H, Chang H, et al: Physiological criteria for weaning patients from prolonged artificial ventilation. Abstracts of scientific papers. pp. 69–72. Annual Meeting of the American Society of Anesthesiologists, 1972

50. Downs JB, Marston AW: A new transport ventilator: an evaluation. Crit Care Med 5:112–114, 1977

23
ETIOLOGY AND TREATMENT OF RESPIRATORY FAILURE

T. James Gallagher, M.D.

ETIOLOGY OF ACUTE RESPIRATORY FAILURE

The term *acute respiratory failure* (ARF) serves as a catchall phrase for many different changes occurring in the lung. The pathophysiology, precipitating event, presentation, and treatment of ARF differ tremendously depending on whether the lungs were otherwise healthy or already had some pre-existing underlying disease. However, considerable insight and understanding of ARF have been acquired, and effective treatments, resulting in dramatically decreased morbidity and mortality, have been developed during the last decade.

The terminology of this disease has varied greatly over the years. *Shock lung* was a very early term, and was based on the assumption that hemorrhagic or hypovolemic shock was a major causative factor. It is now known that shock by itself, while responsible for some ultrastructural changes of the pulmonary architecture, does not directly contribute to the development of respiratory failure.[1,2] More likely, the injuries commonly associated with hypovolemia, such as multisystem trauma, are the true culprits.

Pump lung was another early term, indicating the close association of postoperative respiratory failure with cardiopulmonary bypass. With continued equipment improvement, this problem has become rare; in fact, today, most postcardiopulmonary bypass patients are extubated the night of or the morning following surgery.[3] The term *congestive atelectasis* often appeared in the literature.[4] At one time, many felt the atelectasis that developed during ARF was a major contributor to or precursor of the phenomenon. However, as will be described, atelectasis develops late in the course of the entire process and plays an insignificant role in the early alterations of blood gas exchange. At autopsy, the lung maintains its shape and form surprisingly well, and very little collapse can be detected.[5] Although it may develop in response to other pathologic events, atelectasis is not a major precipitator of the adult respiratory distress syndrome (ARDS).

The *wet lung syndrome* was first described during World War II.[6] This surprisingly accurate clinical description later gave way to such terms as *Da Nang lung*. During the Vietnamese conflict, ARF often developed after resuscitation with large amounts of balanced electrolyte-containing solutions. Some felt that the ensuing hemodilution and reduction of colloid on-

619

cotic pressure caused the fluid accumulation in the pulmonary interstitial space. This debate centering on the appropriate resuscitation fluid still rages and will be discussed in detail later.

Today, the most frequently used descriptive terms include *acute respiratory insufficiency*, *ARDS*, and *ARF*. Within limits, these terms are quite interchangeable, but ARF will still be primarily used.

Clinical Characteristics and Diagnosis

The earliest, most subtle changes of ARF are first detected by blood gas analysis. Depending on the precipitating event, it may be as long as 48 hours before these abnormalities actually begin to manifest themselves (Table 23-1). The arterial oxygen tension (PaO_2) will be less than expected for the inspired oxygen concentration (F_IO_2); moreover, it does not respond to an increase in the administered oxygen percentage. For example, in most patients, a PaO_2 of 65 mmHg on 40 percent inspired oxygen is less than normally expected. The patient with ARF may then have the PaO_2 rise to only 80 mmHg, despite an increase in the inspired oxygen concentration to 80 or 90 percent. Normally, the PaO_2 should be over 600 mmHg when the F_IO_2 reaches 0.9.

The second characteristic of ARF includes failure to improve oxygenation despite the addition of mechanical ventilation. Contrary to what might be expected, positive-pressure ventilation by itself does not markedly improve the poor oxygenation characteristic of respiratory failure.

In contrast to the neonate who develops hyaline membrane disease, maintenance of $PaCO_2$ is usually not a problem in the adult with ARF.[7,8] Only in the late stages of the disease process does CO_2 retention become significant. Spontaneous respiratory rates of 40 to 50/min contribute to hypocapnia and a resultant respiratory alkalosis early in the disease. Arterial PCO_2 commonly averages 30 to 35 mmHg. Close inspection may reveal nasal flaring as well as involvement of the accessory muscles of respiration.[9]

Radiographic changes contribute little to the diagnosis of ARF. In the very early stages, severe blood gas derangements may occur, yet the chest radiograph may still be interpreted as entirely normal. Only later, usually as a preterminal event, are interstitial or alveolar infiltrative changes routinely present. Actually, at any stage of ARF, very little correlation exists among the patient's clinical course, blood gas exchange, and radiologic presentation.

Pulmonary mechanics also deteriorate during ARF. Lung volumes, including functional residual capacity (FRC), routinely decrease. At the same time, pulmonary compliance worsens and the lungs become stiffer. This means it will take an increasingly greater transpulmonary pressure gradient to deliver the same tidal volume.[7] Since transpulmonary pressure is the difference between airway and intrapleural pressure, during mechanical positive-pressure ventilation the respirator will need to develop higher inflation pressures during inspiration in order to deliver the same tidal volume.

Later, some minimal atelectasis may occur, but is usually not evident on chest radiography. Most often, the major pathophysiologic change involves a ventilation-perfusion mismatch. Perfusion remains largely unaltered while significant hypoventilation develops in many lung units. Characteristically, venous admixture or intrapulmonary shunt increases. Severe defects in oxygenation may accompany an almost completely normal chest film. Therefore, failure to document radiographic deterioration does not rule out the syndrome. In the very late stages of the disease, the familiar bilateral, fluffy infiltrates indicative of interstitial and alveolar fluid accumulation appear. At this so-called preterminal stage, CO_2 retention is more likely than hypocapnia. By this time, significant changes in compliance have already developed.

A variety of heterogeneous events may eventually result in or cause the ARF syndrome. Regardless of the precipitating event, the pulmonary response appears to be both nonspecific and predictable. The clinical features and the pathophysiologic changes of ARF are quite reproducible.

The clinical scenario just described always produces a very high mortality rate, and an autopsy reveals several significant findings. The lungs usually weight approximately three to four times normal. When they are excised and cut in cross-section, pink-tinged fluid flows out of both the alveolar and interstitial spaces. It is extremely difficult to specifically identify either space, let alone normal areas. The lung takes on a beefy red appearance, a so-called hepatization. Light microscopy reveals alveolar infiltration by red and white blood cells, including granulocytes, eosinophils, and other debris. Hyaline membranes may be seen both in the terminal airways and in the interstitial space. Significant interstitial edema can be demonstrated.[10] In fact, the untrained eye may fail to recognize the specimen as pulmonary tissue.

A more detailed inspection by electron microscopy

TABLE 23-1. Early Signs of ARF

Hypoxemia
Hypocarbia
Tachypnea
Decreased compliance
Increased venous admixture

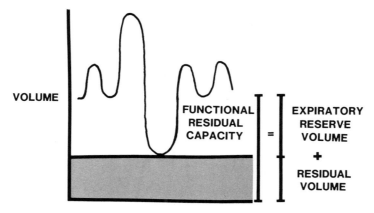

Fig. 23-1. A normal spirogram tracing. The small upward represent normal tidal volume excursions followed by a vital capacity maneuver. The shaded area at the bottom represents the residual volume, which remains constant. The expiratory reserve volume and the FRC are also illustrated.

indicates further derangement.[11] Normally, the alveolar epithelium and capillary endothelium are in very close juxtaposition, separated only by a very thin basement membrane. With ARF, significant swelling of the interstitial space separates the two surfaces. Edema of the alveolar walls can also be easily recognized and, when the walls are engorged, they may actually bulge into the terminal airways. Perivascular cupping also develops in response to the edema.

Pathophysiology

Characterization of the pathologic changes in ARF is begun by a study of lung volumes. Figure 23-1 depicts a typical, normal spirogram tracing.[12] The tracing demonstrates normal tidal volume changes and a vital capacity maneuver—maximal inhalation followed by maximal exhalation. Despite this maximal effort, some gas, known as the *residual volume*, always remains in the lung. No matter how much a person exhales, that volume remains and for this discussion it can be considered as relatively constant. The difference between the lung volume at end-tidal ventilation and residual volume is the *expiratory reserve volume*. Together, the expiratory reserve volume and the residual volume make up the FRC. However, since residual volume is more or less constant, changes ascribed to FRC principally relate to changes in the expiratory reserve volume (see Chapter 1).

Closing volume (Fig. 23-2) represents the lung volume required to prevent small airway or alveolar collapse. Closing volume is not actually a volume that is routinely measured, but, in fact, can be better appreciated as a concept.[13] It includes the lung volume necessary to balance any extra-alveolar forces tending to cause alveolar collapse. In normal circumstances,

closing volume approximately equals the residual volume. This means that a vital capacity maneuver will not lead to airway collapse.

Several disease processes contribute to or require an increase in closing volume. Obstructive pulmonary disease, the aging process, chronic smoking, ventilation-perfusion mismatch, and interstitial water accumulation cause an increase in closing volume. Not only interstitial water but also increased interstitial pressure secondary to the water requires an increased closing volume. As might be expected, inactivation or loss of surfactant contributes to the same types of changes in closing volume.

During respiratory failure, alterations can affect both FRC or, more precisely, expiratory reserve volume and closing volume. Most causes of decreased FRC are familiar (Table 23-2). Massive obesity and the supine and lithotomy positions contribute to a reduced FRC. Obesity can prevent adequate chest wall expansion; the supine and lithotomy positions both move the diaphragm cephalad, contributing to a loss of lung volume. Intra-abdominal manipulations, including surgical packing, peritonitis, and pancreati-

TABLE 23-2. Origins of Decreased FRC

Obesity
Smoking
Supine position
Lithotomy position
Upper abdominal surgery
Thoracic surgery
Peritonitis
Aspiration syndrome
Lung contusion

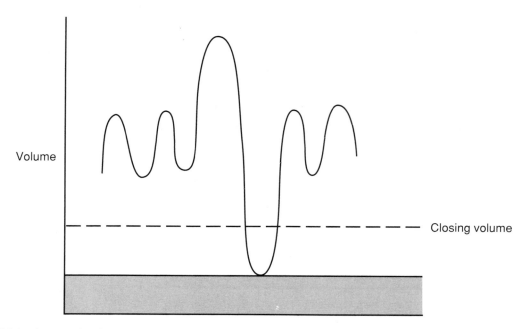

Fig. 23-2. A normal spirogram tracing. Closing volume, illustrated here, is greater than residual volume. If this patient were to exhale to residual volume, airway collapse might begin to occur.

tis, as well as aspiration or near drowning, can severely decrease FRC.

Therefore, the reduction of FRC for the reasons listed in Table 23-2 and an increase in lung closing volume will combine to produce small airway collapse, a major reason for blood gas derangement in ARF (Table 23-3). A change in one parameter alone would require significantly greater volume shifts. When both volumes are altered, the degree of change in each does not have to be as significant to cause severe pulmonary dysfunction.

The loss of FRC or residual volume means that pulmonary gas volumes are diminished at the end of tidal ventilation. If, at the same time, closing volume has been elevated, airway collapse will occur when the changes are great enough that, at end exhalation, resting lung volume remains less than the closing volume (Fig. 23-3).

To recapitulate, in respiratory failure lung volume changes occur. Expiratory reserve volume decreases while closing volume moves in the opposite direction. Airway collapse takes place when both changes are large enough to produce a resting lung volume that is less than closing volume. The resultant airway collapse produces hypoxemia, as documented by blood gas analysis.

Fluid Flux across the Lung

To better appreciate the lung volume changes in ARF, a detailed, in-depth understanding of the anatomic derangements commonly present in ARF is needed. In reality, the alveolus is surrounded by the blood in much the same way a ball might sit in a bucket of water. The perivascular interstitial space separates the alveolar and capillary epithelial and endothelial linings, and blood gas exchange takes place across these membranes. The interstitial space behaves more as a potential than as a real space. The larger arterioles and venules, as well as the lymphatics, reside in the central or peribronchiolar interstitial compartment.

The lymphatics drain any excess or accumulated fluid back into the central circulation.[14] The lymph flows to the thoracic duct, which in turn empties into

TABLE 23-3. Predisposing Factors for ARF

Multiple-system trauma
Pancreatitis
Peritonitis
Abdominal sepsis
Prolonged intra-abdominal or thoracic surgery
Pneumonia
Near drowning
Aspiration of gastric contents
Inhalation of noxious agents
Fat embolism
Flail chest
Pulmonary embolism

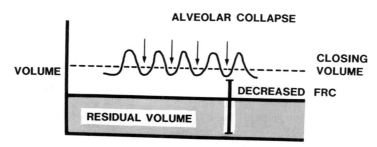

Fig. 23-3. While expiratory reserve volume has decreased, closing volume has increased. At the end of normal tidal ventilation, the closing volume exceeds gas volume left in the lungs. Therefore, airway collapse and hypoxemia begin to develop.

the azygous system. Lymph flow removal operates under the control of several different mechanisms. Elevated interstitial or capillary pressures accelerate flow, while the intrinsic motion of the lung during spontaneous respiration also encourages lymphatic drainage. The lymphatic vessels also have their own peristaltic motion, which contributes to maintaining the parenchyma in essentially a dry state.

The alveolar capillary interface actively participates in many of the derangements occurring during ARF.[15] A series of endothelial cells line the capillary wall. These elongated cells are not tightly bound to each other, but are actually separated by junctions on the order of 40 Å in diameter. Albumin molecules normally measure approximately 80 to 100 Å, which permits the cleft to act as a filtering mechanism to inhibit most albumin movement across the membrane.[16] The epithelial cells lining the alveoli form a very tight boundary and render that structure watertight to any fluid from the interstitial space.

Water can move across the capillary membrane by active transport, by vesicle movement, or directly through the interendothelial clefts. In ARF, the major fluid shifts principally take place by fluid fluxes through the aforementioned endothelial junctions. The remaining mechanisms do not play a major role. Because of the pore size, only water and small protein molecules can pass, while, under normal circumstances, most of the albumin remains in the vascular compartment.

The perivascular interstitial space is more a potential than a real space and fluid does not usually accumulate in it, but instead moves to the central or peribronchiolar space and eventually finds it way into the lymphatic circulation. Mucopolysaccharides reside primarily in central interstitial areas, and their osmotic properties help draw any fluid to that area. The lymphatics then clear water and any protein, including albumin, that might accumulate.[17]

Several opposing factors influence the fluid flux across the alveolar capillary-endothelial junctional clefts.[18] The pulmonary capillary hydrostatic or microvascular pressure tends to move fluid in the direction of the interstitial space. Capillary pressure should not be confused with pulmonary capillary wedge pressure (PCWP), since capillary pressure cannot be measured clinically and must be estimated. Several different formulas have been proposed and most authorities accept an estimate of approximately 40 to 50 percent of the difference between PCWP and pulmonary venous pressure. Additionally, the pressure changes with position. When the lung is upright, apical microvascular pressures are close to zero, while capillary pressures at the bases are usually much higher than alveolar pressures. The low-pressure pulmonary circulation distribution changes in response to gravity and, therefore can vary markedly from one area of the lung to the next, depending on position.[19]

The interstitial space itself usually contains a small amount of fluid and albumin or other small protein molecules. An oncotic pressure develops, primarily dependent on the albumin concentration. That oncotic pressure exerts its influence to draw fluid from the capillary to the interstitial space. Methods to sample interstitial fluid oncotic pressure are not readily available to the clinician. Therefore, this factor cannot be accurately determined during any particular illness. Obviously, a large movement of non-protein-containing fluid into the interstitial space would reduce tissue oncotic pressure.

Two other forces act to oppose fluid egress from the capillary bed. Most protein remains in the plasma, where it exerts a large oncotic effect tending to prevent water from moving out of the capillary compartment. Several devices are now available that permit clinical determinations of oncotic pressure. Normal values range up to 20 to 25 mmHg.[20]

Any fluid tending to accumulate in the interstitial portions of the lung will obviously develop its own hydrostatic pressure. While interstitial pressure normally has a slightly negative value, very small accumulations of fluid will rapidly convert that pressure to positive.[21] The pressure elevation then acts to oppose further fluid shifts. Like oncotic pressure, interstitial hydrostatic pressure remains extremely difficult to determine. Various techniques, including use of micropipets or implanted capsules, markedly alter this delicate space and make any pressure determinations unreliable, especially during changing conditions. The best estimates and extrapolations from chronic animal implantations indicate that human hydrostatic pressure usually remains subatmospheric, at approximately -7 cmH$_2$O. The negative pressure results in part from lung expansion and deflation during spontaneous ventilation.[22]

Fluid flux across the capillary also depends on the filtration coefficient ($K_{F,C}$).[23] The filtration coefficient varies in response to permeability changes if such changes do indeed exist. Permeability will be discussed later, but the mechanism appears to involve an alteration of the endothelial pore size or diameter, and most likely represents a reversible phenomenon. This evidence comes from laboratory animals that were infused with so-called permeability substances and eventually returned to normal without other than supportive care.[24] Since flow correlates with the fourth power of the radius, even small changes in radius have quite pronounced effects on fluid fluxes. If the radius were to double, flow would increase by a factor of 16. Therefore, any fluid changes are much more pronounced when permeability has been altered.

The reflection coefficient (O_c) reflects solute movement across a membrane.[22] A solute that cannot cross has a value of 1; if the solute can freely cross, then O_c approaches a value of zero. The value of O_c changes in each vascular bed in any species and probably equals approximately 0.9 in human lung. This means that, normally, very little protein moves across the alveolar-capillary membrane.

These effects are described by the Starling equation (sometimes referred to as *Starling forces*):

$$J_uW = K_{F,C}(P_c - P_t) - 0_c(\pi C - \pi T)$$

where J_uW = net volume movement
$K_{F,C}$ = filtration coefficient
P_c = capillary hydrostatic pressure
P_t = tissue hydrostatic pressure
0_c = reflection coefficient
πC = capillary oncotic pressure
πT = tissue oncotic pressure

The Starling equation *describes the forces present*; it, of course, does not itself influence or cause net fluid flow. It mathematically expresses the interrelationship of the various forces present.

Lung Water and Disease States

Under normal circumstances, the balance of all the forces produces a slow but continuous fluid movement into the perivascular interstitial space at a rate of approximately 10 to 20 mL/h. This slow influx permits easy removal by the lymphatics. Acute respiratory failure develops when other events alter this delicate balance.

Several different events can influence microvascular pressure.[25] A simple example is an obstructive phenomenon such as a pulmonary embolus. Vascular occlusion precedes cessation of flow, and capillary pressure soon increases. If none of the other Starling forces were to change, the equilibrium would be unbalanced and fluid movement across the capillary membrane would accelerate.

Left ventricular failure can also increase microvascular pressure. Forward flow diminishes and the eventual backup in the pulmonary vascular bed elevates microcapillary pressures. These changes do not occur immediately, since, as previously described, the pulmonary bed is never fully patent. Therefore, before any pressure increase secondary to congestive heart failure might develop, vascular bed recruitment must be maximized. Increases in flow or cardiac output do not usually elevate capillary pressure because of the recruitment phenomenon. Not until flow exceeds 250 percent of baseline values does pressure increase.[26]

Intense vasoconstriction from the release of vasoactive amines or secondary to hypoxic pulmonary vasoconstriction can also locally affect microvascular pressure.[27,28] These localized changes explain some of the infiltrates that develop after pulmonary embolus and that were previously ascribed to pulmonary infarction. In fact, these infiltrates represent fluid accumulation caused by the high pressures.

Serum oncotic pressure relates to serum albumin levels. If oncotic pressure alone decreases while all the other Starling factors remain unchanged, then fluid flux into the interstitium increases. Massive hemodilution secondary to infused balanced electrolyte solutions will reduce serum oncotic pressure. Hypoalbuminemia also develops during chronic illness when albumin production diminishes and fails to replace the eventual loss of circulating molecules. The stress of illness and surgery, combined with inattention to the suddenly increased nutritional needs, quickly worsens the problem. Unfortunately, exogenously administered albumin has little or no effect on restoring serum levels to normal since most of the protein moves out of the circulating volume and into various storage depots.[29,30]

Some reports have indicated that an increased fluid flux and eventual water accumulation in the interstitium occurred whenever the serum oncotic pressure or the serum oncotic-PCWP gradients were reduced.[31] However, despite total elimination of the gradient, several clinical trials have failed to show any derangement in pulmonary function as judged by PaO_2, venous admixture, or intrapulmonary shunt (Q_{SP}/Q_T).[32]

Until recently, interstitial or extravascular lung water accumulation could not be clinically measured. However, with the advent of a microprocessor to measure extravascular lung water by the thermal dye technique, these data should be forthcoming. Early reports have demonstrated a very poor correlation between extravascular lung water and blood gas exchange.[33,34]

The thermal dye method uses fluid at 0°C to equilibrate rapidly with all lung water during one circuit through the pulmonary bed. Since transit time and concentration are known, total lung water can be calculated. Indocyanine green dye combines with albumin and, therefore, permits the measurement of vascular water. Subtracting vascular from total lung water gives extravascular or interstitial water.

It is not feasible to predict lung water changes based on information from a single parameter (Fig. 23-4). A change of one Starling factor while all others remain fixed would obviously lead to a major imbalance. The rate and direction of any fluid shift will be dependent on its degree and on the particular factor affected. However, alteration of only one force rarely happens. A decreased colloid oncotic pressure tends to produce more water movement into the lung parenchyma. However, as water begins to move in that direction and accumulate, other changes simultaneously occur. The increased water in the interstitium elevates tissue hydrostatic pressure, which then opposes further fluid egress from the vascular compartment. Simultaneously, the water dilutes the albumin already present, decreasing the tissue oncotic effect; this further opposes fluid accumulation and movement across the capillary membrane. Finally, loss of intravascular water lowers pulmonary blood volume and microvascular pressure. The reduced vascular pressure also opposes further interstitial water accumulation. It remains virtually impossible to change one aspect of the Starling equation without affecting all or most of the others.

Since accurate measurement of any parameter except serum oncotic pressure is not possible, predictions of lung water accumulation are difficult. As previously shown, when one factor changes, its eventual influence on all the others cannot yet be accurately determined. All the numbers may change, but when placed back into the equation they may balance, so that no net increase in fluid actually takes place. It is not difficult to see that predictions of pulmonary function or extravascular lung water based only on serum oncotic pressure could be quite inaccurate.

A third major factor influencing lung water changes is pulmonary capillary permeability. Most investigators believe that significant alterations of capillary integrity can occur at the previously described endothelial junctions. Any increase in size dramatically affects fluid movement, including albumin leakage.[5] Alterations of pulmonary capillary permeability occur primarily during sepsis.[34] Either direct bacterial action or secondary endotoxin release can initiate the events. The bacteria or toxin apparently interact with the capillary endothelium. Damage to the vessel wall causes platelets to accumulate and adhere to the injured surface. Serotonin released from the platelets can locally alter the capillary integrity as well as elevate microvascular pressure.

Histamine can be released by stimulated pulmonary mast cells. Histamine also has the ability to alter permeability, and its effects can be reversed by the administration of antihistamines. Other factors influencing permeability include the toxic substances inhaled after combustion, and other chemical agents too numerous to list here.[24,35] These substances affect both capillary and alveolar integrity.

Some authorities have questioned the existence of permeability alterations.[22] If permeability changes are a real phenomenon, then, compared with the effects of pressure elevations, fluid flux should dramatically increase. Since flow relates directly to the radius, any increase will measurably affect the fluid flux rate. If they are not different from pressure-related

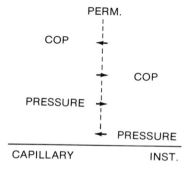

Fig. 23-4. The Starling forces balanced across the capillary membrane. Change of one factor will not influence a fluid shift unless all others remain unchanged.

changes, the fluid flux rate should be about equal, given the same circumstances.

Fluid flux across the lung cannot be directly measured, but pulmonary lymph flow rate acts as an excellent indirect indicator of both quantity and quality of the fluid movement. The greater the protein in lymph, the more likely are permeability changes.

In laboratory studies in sheep, lymph flow rate and lymph protein concentration were measured at the same pulmonary microvascular pressure.[36,37] The lymphatics draining the lung were cannulated to collect all lymph flow. One group of sheep received a supposed permeability-altering substance (live *Pseudomonas* vaccine) while the other did not. Microvascular pressures were kept identical in both groups. Marked differences in flow rate and albumin concentration at the same pressure occurred in the *Pseudomonas* group compared with the control group, and these differences were ascribed to permeability changes.[38] However, some of the data have been questioned, and it is still unclear to some authorities whether permeability is a real factor.

Treatment of so-called permeability alteration remains mostly nonspecific. As previously mentioned, antihistamines may be of benefit in the treatment of histamine-induced changes. Prostaglandin E_1 appears to have a nonhemodynamic influence on the changes occurring after pulmonary emboli.[39] However, no other modalities for specifically interfering with capillary membrane alterations are available. Although steroids have been advocated to restore capillary integrity to normal, there is very little evidence to substantiate such claims.[40] In fact, there are such contradictory data regarding the efficacy of steroid usage in respiratory failure that readers are urged to make their own determination.

Interstitial fibrosis and hyaline membranes develop in relation to the amount of protein flux. Fibrosis first begins approximately 6 days after the onset of interstitial water accumulation.[5] The pathologic alterations are primarily in the interstitial space and consist of increased collagen deposition. The more severe forms of fibrosis occur in those cases categorized as having altered permeability. Once it occurs, pulmonary interstitial fibrosis is irreversible. It probably is responsible for the radiographic changes and altered pulmonary function in some patients after recovery from ARF. Fibrosis can also account for chronic, fixed alterations of compliance.

Hyaline membrane formation does not result from alteration of type I alveolar histiocytes, but instead appears to correlate with the appearance of increased permeability.[5] The greater the protein leakage, the more likely hyaline membrane formation. The chemical makeup of hyaline membranes consists of al-

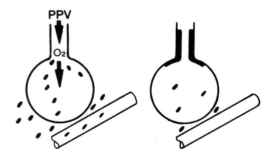

Fig. 23-5. Hyaline membrane formation. Protein in the alveolus is dried. Hyaline membranes form at the terminal air space and alter ventilation.

bumin, globulin, and fibrin. The first step most likely includes leakage of protein-laden edema fluid into the alveoli. This may explain the reduced incidence following cardiogenic pulmonary edema. If mechanical ventilation with high inflation pressure commences, drying, denaturation, coagulation, and inspissation of the secretions will accelerate deposition of hyaline membranes in the terminal airways.

Hyaline membrane lining of the terminal airways narrows the lumen (Fig. 23-5). This may contribute to a decrease in pulmonary compliance and prolongation of the ventilatory time constant of the involved units.

Not every imbalance of the Starling forces leads to interstitial fluid accumulation or ARF (Fig. 23-6). In fact, only the few extremes ever require therapy. The lung functions with at least three protective or safety valve mechanisms, the pulmonary lymphatics being the first line of defense. Conflicting evidence at this time makes evaluation of lymphatic efficiency difficult since it varies in different species.[41] However, in

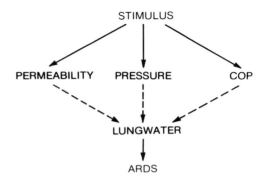

Fig. 23-6. The factors leading to acute respiratory failure. Either alone or in combination, capillary permeability, microvascular pressure, and/or serum colloid oncotic pressure are altered. When lung safety mechanisms fail, lung water increases. COP, capillary osmotic pressure.

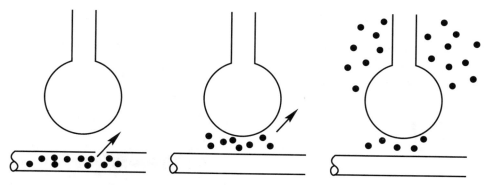

Fig. 23-7. When water moves into the lung, it first collects in the perivascular space and then moves to the peribronchiolar areas.

humans, flow can increase at least 5 to 7 times over basal rates to aid in the removal of any excess fluid accumulation. As might be expected, protein and excess water are removed equally effectively.

Once the lymphatic mechanism exhausts itself, the interstitial space bears the major burden for ensuring continued normal gas exchange (Fig. 23-7). The pulmonary interstitial space functions as a two-compartment model consisting of the perivascular and peribronchiolar compartments. The peribronchiolar area, as previously mentioned, contains the lymphatics as well as the larger venules and arterioles.

The explanation of water accumulation in the lung can be extrapolated from various animal and laboratory data, including work on the isolated intact hind limb of the dog.[21] The analogy is based on intact parietal and visceral pleurae. When alterations of the Starling forces occur, fluid first leaks into the perivascular areas, but the volume of this potential space is apparently quite limited. At rest, alveolar expansion helps maintain a slightly negative pressure. The perivascular areas connect to the peribronchiolar space via high-resistance pathways. Slightly increased peri-

vascular volume increases the negative pressure to approximately 0 cmH$_2$O, and the connecting channels to the peribronchiolar compartment begin to open.

Once fluid begins to move into the peribronchiolar areas, little further increase in interstitial pressure is detected (Fig. 23-8). The lung acts as a reservoir to soak up the increased fluid, increasing its capacity by a factor of 8, while blood gas exchange remains essentially unaffected.[41] However, pressure-sensitive receptors in the interstitium detect the slight changes, and hyperventilation ensues. Careful measurement may determine a decrease in pulmonary compliance, and larger transpulmonary pressure gradients (the difference between intrapleural and airway pressure) are required to deliver the same tidal volume.

Once the interstitial absorptive capacity exhausts itself, the interstitial pressure begins to increase. At this stage, gas exchange deteriorates and becomes clinically detectable. The increased pressure does not change alveolar geometry, but first impinges on the terminal airways. These untethered units are not really attached to any other nearby structure and are easily influenced by any increase of interstitial pres-

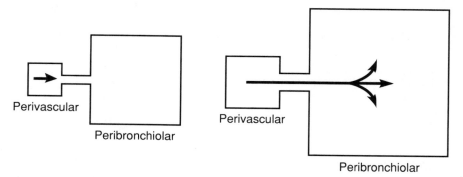

Fig. 23-8. Small amounts of fluid in the perivascular space overcome the high-resistance pathways and fluid moves into the peribronchiolar areas.

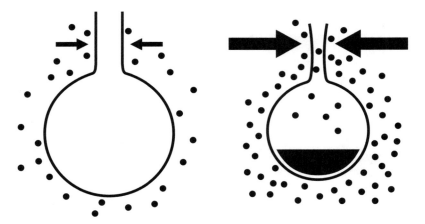

Fig. 23-9. The effects of pulmonary interstitial water. High interstitial pressure begin to narrow terminal airways and alter ventilation. Eventually, fluid accumulates in the alveoli.

sure. The elevated pressure constricts the airways and relative hypoventilation ensues, while perfusion simultaneously continues unimpaired (Fig. 23-9).[5]

A significant ventilation-perfusion imbalance occurs at this point.[42] The narrowed terminal airways cause an increase in the time constant required to ventilate or move oxygen molecules into the alveoli. Since any oxygen already present in the alveolus rapidly moves into the capillary blood, that unit may at least momentarily be devoid of oxygen while perfusion continues unchanged and blood departs that alveolar-capillary unit not completely saturated. In the pulmonary venous system, this blood combines with blood having normal amounts of oxygen coming from unaffected areas. The net effect is a dilution of the overall oxygen concentration. Clinically, arterial PO_2 decreases and venous admixture or intrapulmonary shunt increases.

If interstitial pressure continues to increase, the terminal airway may occlude and alveolar collapse follow. However, it should be stressed again that atelectasis does not reflect the primary pathologic changes occurring in ARF. The process is a continuum that begins with ventilation-perfusion alterations. Even at autopsy, true segmental atelectasis represents a rare finding. Obviously, compliance and resistance further deteriorate as interstitial pressure continues to increase.

The third pulmonary safety valve mechanism involves the alveoli themselves. Eventually, with continued increases in interstitial pressure secondary to fluid inflow, water and protein make their way into the alveoli. Although the alveolar walls themselves become edematous, the epithelial lining remains intact. Water most likely makes its way through the terminal airways and not the alveolar wall. Alveolar

fluid accumulation appears to be an all-or-none phenomenon, with the entire lung filling almost at once.[43] The various interconnecting channels, such as the pores of Kohn, provide an easy access route for this process.[44] At this stage, pulmonary water increases by over 1,500 mL, and the easily recognizable clinical signs of pulmonary edema, rales, and frothy sputum are detectable.

The accumulated water inactivates the alveolar surfactant as well as the type I cells responsible for its production (Fig. 23-10). Since surfactant normally reduces surface tension, its inactivation causes a decreased alveolar volume. The water already present prevents complete collapse. However, lung volume, including FRC, measurably decreases, and blood gas function deteriorates further. The water also obviously interferes with gas exchange.

Causes of Acute Respiratory Failure

Multiple factors have been identified as potential mediators of ARDS. However, it must be emphasized that it is still unclear as to their exact roles. Some may

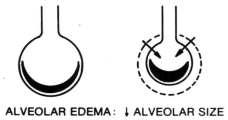

ALVEOLAR EDEMA: ↓ ALVEOLAR SIZE

Fig. 23-10. Fluid in the alveoli interferes with surfactant. Surface tension increases, causing a decrease in alveolar volume and FRC.

have more involvement as initiators of the events rather than any active involvement on an ongoing basis.

Complement activation has been studied more than any other single factor.[45] Activation of complement leads to white blood cell aggregation along the endothelial cells within the pulmonary vasculature. Complement activation follows as a result of trauma or sepsis.[46] Once neutrophil aggregation has occurred, activation must follow. This results in the release of oxygen radicals and various peroxidases, all of which affect capillary permeability and lead to water leakage and accumulation within the lung interstitium.[47]

Neutrophil aggregation may follow as a result of endotoxin activation or phagocytosis by other cells. Substances released include elastase, peroxidase, and collagenases.[48] The peroxidase, in particular, leads to the release of toxic oxygen radicals. These, in turn, are mediated by such factors as catalase and superoxide dismutase. The elastase, peroxidase, and collagenases can all activate complement to keep the entire process in action.

Cell membranes can be stimulated secondary to shock, trauma, or sepsis to release arachidonic acid. When metabolized by cyclo-oxygenase, thromboxanes and prostacyclins result. Thromboxane A_2 results in pulmonary vasoconstriction as well as bronchoconstriction. The prostacyclins are primarily vasodilators and also lend themselves to some membrane stabilization. Prostaglandin E_2 can depress lymphocyte function. It is unclear if the metabolites of arachidonic acid mediated through the lipoxygenase pathway and resulting in leukotrienes have a major role in ARDS. The leukotriene (LTE_4) can cause neutrophil adherence.

The neutrophil release of toxic oxygen radicals includes superoxide (O_2-), peroxide (H_2O_2), and hydroxyl radicals ($OH-$). Peroxide is mediated by superoxide dismutase. Catalase scavenges peroxide. These radicals, when available in abundance, can lead to cell membrane damage and may also interfere with hyaluronic acid. This latter alteration interferes with pulmonary interstitial function.

The pulmonary macrophages or monocytes are responsible for the release of interleukin-1 and tissue necrosis factor (TNF). Interleukin-1 causes neutrophil degranulation and adherence to the capillary endothelium.[49] TNF is thought to be responsible for the fever, malaise, and hypotension seen in septic patients.[50]

The neutrophils are known to migrate across the capillary endothelium and are found in both the alveolar and interstitial spaces. These cells, which are responsible for both lysosome and oxygen radical release, are mediated by complement and endotoxin as well as antigen-antibody reactions. Macrophages or monocytes are found primarily in the alveoli. They are known to release the prostanoids, leukotrienes, oxygen radicals, elastase, and monokines. Platelet aggregation may also play a role. Platelets are known to release serotonin, a potent vasoconstrictor. Platelets also release lysosomes, responsible for elastase, collagenase, and thromboxane activation.

Clinical situations associated with a high incidence of ARF (Table 23-3) include major, multiple-system trauma, especially when associated with direct chest injuries.[51–53] Obviously, the resultant chest contusion can cause major disruption of the pulmonary gas exchange system. The response to generalized trauma is not often predictable. Most times, unlike direct penetrating injuries, blunt trauma invariably affects more than one organ system. The exact mechanism of pulmonary involvement remains unclear but may include a number of factors, such as interference with normal clotting mechanisms and release of free fatty acids from both long bone fractures and soft tissue injuries. Both responses may work alone or synergistically. Coagulation deficits may result in multiple peripheral thrombi in the pulmonary vascular bed. The pulmonary circulatory bed primarily acts as an efficient filtering system. At any one time, a large percentage of the vascular channels have little or no flow. Obliteration secondary to clots or thrombi in the patent vessels does not initially result in hypertension, but instead results in recruitment of previously nonpatent pathways. In fact, 70 percent of the pulmonary vascular bed must be occluded before any increase in pulmonary artery pressure occurs.

Once microvascular pressure does increase, pulmonary interstitial water accumulation is much more likely to occur. In fact, some authorities feel that the most important effect of Starling forces on water movement involves alteration of pulmonary microvascular pressure.[54,55] All other alterations appear to be of secondary importance. The release of free fatty acids after soft tissue injuries leads to the same type of alterations in the pulmonary circulatory bed as might be expected in the fat embolism syndrome.

Acute peritonitis from any cause, including perforation of large or small bowel, or pancreatitis with or without abscess formation can cause a very severe form of ARF.[56–59] Again, the precise factors have not been well elucidated. Release of endotoxin, live bacteria, and/or viruses may interfere with capillary integrity, cause permeability alterations, and eventually increase lung water.

Additional changes take place during acute peritoneal inflammation. The small and large intestine develop marked distention from both the secondary ileus and bowel gas retention, as well as bowel wall edema. The abdominal inflammation and bowel distention produce significant diaphragmatic elevation, with decreases in FRC and pulmonary compliance.

Many investigators still feel that endotoxin release operates as a primary cause of ARF, although this has never been well documented. The endotoxin not only alters capillary permeability, but also leads to intense vasoconstriction and marked pulmonary hypertension.[60]

Respiratory failure may develop after major surgery, especially upper abdominal or intrathoracic procedures. Risk factors identified include smoking, morbid obesity, abnormal pulmonary function testing, and length of operation. These predictors are useful for problems involving alveolar hypoventilation and CO_2 retention, but are not nearly as useful for predicting hypoxic difficulties.[61]

Oxygenation can deteriorate because of patient refusal or inability to make maximal sustained inspiratory efforts. Failure to cough and take deep breaths leads to progressive partial and, eventually, complete atelectasis.[62] Since perfusion remains unchanged, PO_2 decreases. Although adequate documentation is lacking, protracted surgical manipulation, especially of the small bowel, may possibly lead to progressive hypoxemia. Since no other causes have been described, some have felt this response resulted from release of endogenous substances that affect the integrity of the alveolar capillary membrane.

Respiratory failure can also appear during an acute pneumonic process.[63] The familiar lobar pneumonia of bacterial origin is relatively easy to distinguish and has little bearing on the variety of ARF described here. However, the interstitial form of either viral or bacterial origin presents an entirely different picture. The invasion of bacteria or viruses may affect the alveolar capillary membrane, and the gradient for fluid movement may shift in the direction of the interstitial compartment. If lymphatic involvement develops, the ability to rapidly remove any accumulating water may be severely compromised. The interstitial inflammation can affect fluid flux rates, which may increase in proportion to the relative effectiveness of the various safety valve mechanisms. That, plus the inflammatory process itself, contributes to ultrastructural derangements and the eventual increased interstitial pressure. The clinical picture appears similar to other causes of respiratory failure—hypoxemia and tachypnea develop while lung mechanics deteriorate. The usual mechanical disruptions include altered compliance and loss of lung volume.

The changes brought about by lobar pneumonia are not only different, but do not respond to the same treatment modalities as the more common forms of respiratory failure. In these circumstances, the alveoli fill with proteinaceous debris and the ventilation-perfusion alterations occur because of alveolar rather than interstitial derangements. Until that clears, the patient is unlikely to respond to the usual treatment modalities so effective in ARF. In fact, increased airway pressures during unilateral lung disease may actually cause deterioration of pulmonary function. The pressure will be directed to the noninvolved, more compliant lung and will not affect the diseased portion. The high airway pressures may interfere with the pulmonary circulation. Being a low-pressure system, the pulmonary circulation is responsive to both gravitational and alveolar pressure. Flow can, therefore, be directed away from the noninvolved healthy lung to the poorly ventilated, involved side, producing the very worst matching of ventilation to perfusion. Most gas is delivered to the noninvolved healthy lung, while perfusion redirects itself to the diseased portion. A radiographically significant lobar pneumonia may have minimal influence on gas exchange. Both alveolar ventilation and perfusion may alter to such a degree that significant ventilation-perfusion changes do not take place.

Alterations of the alveolar side of the alveolar-capillary membrane interface also contribute to the development of ARF. Aspiration of fresh- and saltwater, as well as of gastric contents, represents common problems.[64] Saltwater drowning very closely mimics fulminant pulmonary edema, since the fluid-filled alveoli cannot enter into gas exchange. Fortunately, in time, the saltwater is absorbed and the alveoli generally do not suffer any long-term ill effects. The major clinical challenge is to provide adequate support until resolution begins. The water absorbed may cause some increase in intravascular volume; however, this is usually not of clinical importance. Likewise, hemolysis or electrolyte disturbances are not major factors in saltwater drowning. The immediate and most important lifesaving function involves early restoration of blood gas exchange using mechanical ventilation and positive end-expiratory pressure (PEEP). After near drowning, attempts to remove water are not very successful since aspirated volumes are usually not large and alveolar absorption begins almost immediately.

Freshwater drowning represents a more difficult clinical problem. Not only are the alveoli filled with fluid, but the freshwater inactivates the surfactant lining the alveoli. The surfactant produced by the type II alveoli cells lines the alveolar surface and reduces surface tension, preventing cell collapse. The type II cells are also inactivated or destroyed by the freshwater. Since those cells must regenerate, the period of dysfunction is markedly lengthened. All these factors serve to make freshwater drowning a more difficult clinical problem to treat than saltwater drowning. When compared with saltwater drowning, the unstable alveoli after freshwater aspiration are more likely to require both mechanical ventilatory support and PEEP/continuous positive airway pressure (CPAP) for an increased interval.[65] As in saltwater drowning, electrolyte and hemolytic disturbances are actually of secondary importance. If they are severe enough to present a problem, the patient has usually already had an early, overwhelming hypoxic insult.

Aspiration of gastric contents can lead to several different sequelae.[66,67] Large particulate matter can become lodged in and obstruct the airway at any level. The gastric fluid can fill the alveoli in a manner similar to that in drowning and interfere with oxygenation and CO_2 elimination. Aspiration of fluid with a pH less than 2.5, as well as a large volume, has been associated with both high morbidity and high mortality. The acid causes severe damage to the alveolar capillary membrane, with loss of integrity and eventual interstitial fluid accumulation. Since Mendelson's description of acid aspiration, ingestion of antacids has become a popular prophylactic measure against acid aspiration, especially in the preanesthetic period.[68] However, alkali aspiration can have clinical effects as severe as those after acid aspiration.[69]

Aspiration may occur after active vomiting or silent regurgitation. Reports have demonstrated the appearance of gastric contents in the lung despite protection of the airway with a cuffed endotracheal tube. During the induction of anesthesia, cricoid pressure and the head-up position have been recommended to prevent aspiration. However, these are not 100 percent effective and the clinician must always be on the alert. As in the case of drowning, removal of the aspirate does not affect outcome unless large particulate material obstructs the airway.

ARF may also develop after the inhalation of various substances, including the products of combustion. Toxic substances are often released, owing to burning of synthetic materials in closed spaces. The major pathologic disruptions occur either to the alveolar-capillary membrane or to the alveoli themselves. Identification or listing of all such toxic products is not possible, but the severity of the problems usually relates to both the particular substance and the inspired concentration. The inflammation of the alveolar walls and destruction of the surfactant in general are not dissimilar to the changes after aspiration. However, certain substances can have very specific actions, such as interference with particular aspects of cellular function.

Some pulmonary changes may develop as a direct result of the hypoxia due to carbon monoxide inhalation.[70] This may account for some of the capillary membrane changes that disrupt the normal pathways of fluid movement in and out of the lung. Most likely, the immediate deaths in these instances are due to the hypoxia. Poisoning of the cytochrome oxidase system rapidly destroys most cellular respiration. Fat embolism syndrome can also contribute to or act as a precursor of ARF.[71] Patients most at risk include those with long bone fractures or major soft-tissue injuries. It can also occur in conjunction with major orthopedic surgery of the femur, hip, or pelvis. In all these circumstances, large fat globules are released from the marrow into the venous circulation and make their way to the pulmonary circulatory bed.

The fat itself is not the major problem; rather, the free fatty acids that are released are the actual culprits.[72] After arrival in the pulmonary artery, they may begin to alter and interfere with the normal capillary wall architecture. Platelets are then attracted to the injured area of the capillary, where they agglutinate and release serotonin. Not only do the fatty acids directly increase pulmonary vascular permeability, but the serotonin also alters capillary integrity and, in addition, promotes an intense pulmonary vasoconstriction. The resulting alteration of the previously balanced Starling forces means that conditions now favor water movement across the capillary bed into the pulmonary interstitium. If the pulmonary safety valve mechanisms are overwhelmed, interstitial water accumulates and the fine reticular pattern characteristic of interstitial edema will become evident on the chest radiographs.

Diagnosis of the fat embolism syndrome is difficult.[73] The reputed characteristic findings do not appear with any regularity. Hypoxia, in association with the previously mentioned events, predominates as the most consistent finding. The chest radiograph may have the ground-glass appearance due to interstitial water. The mental confusion, often present, develops as a result of either the hypoxia or the petechial hemorrhages present in the cerebral cortex. The free fatty acids interfere with the normal clotting mechanisms, and petechiae can also develop in the eye grounds and nail beds. However, these changes are not always present and the diagnosis may require correlation of a history of long bone fractures with unexplained hypoxia. Even fat globules in the urine are not a common finding.

Special therapeutic maneuvers, including the administration of heparin and intravenous alcohol, appear to have no specific benefits. Both supposedly help clear the fat, one by decreasing and the other by increasing serum lipase activity. Neither has been very successful in ameliorating the course of the disease. The traditional methods of treatment for ARF work as well in this circumstance as in any of the others.[74] Perhaps the most helpful ancillary measure includes immobilization of the involved extremity to prevent further release of fat particles.

Flail chest represents another specialized form of ARF. Direct blunt trauma to the thorax usually causes the injury.[75] A flail chest has at least two consecutive ribs fractured in at least two places. Each rib section between the two fracture sites essentially floats free. During normal spontaneous breathing, as the diaphragm moves down and the chest wall out, intrathoracic pressure, which at rest is between −3 and −5 cmH$_2$O, becomes even more negative. This difference between intrathoracic and ambient or airway pressure permits gas to move freely into the lungs. With a flail chest, however, each time intrathoracic pressure becomes more negative, the free segment moves inward instead of out with the rest of the chest wall. This is the often-described paradoxical motion. Since the chest wall moves inward, pulmonary expansion may be altered or decreased in the area underlying the injury site.

Not all cases of flail chest result in hypoxia.[76] Oxygenation deteriorates not because of the flail, but because of the underlying pulmonary contusion resulting from the same impact originally causing the flail. The contusion is an area of edema and hemorrhage. If, as is usually the case, the edema interferes more with ventilation than with perfusion, a ventilation-perfusion mismatch may develop and hypoxemia follows. The rapid shallow respirations and chest wall splinting occur in response to the decreased oxygenation and interstitial fluid accumulation as well as to the pain.

This respiratory pattern accentuates the flail. Early observers interpreted this finding as evidence that the altered oxygenation resulted directly from the flail. The use of PEEP and/or CPAP with intermittent mandatory ventilation (IMV) has helped delineate the problem.[77] As end-expiratory pressure increases independently of any ventilator rate changes, the tachypnea subsides owing to the improved oxygenation. Once the spontaneous rate decreases, the flail becomes much less pronounced. Decreasing PEEP/CPAP and recurrence of hypoxemia cause a resumption of the hyperventilation, and the paradoxic motion resumes anew.

It is clear that any therapy must concentrate first and most importantly on the lung contusion and not on the flail. Measures to internally or externally stabilize the chest wall are not required. These methods have previously included wire fixation, towel clips, and controlled mechanical ventilation. Prolonged, controlled mechanical ventilation and patient paralysis neither improve nor alter the course of the disease.

Spontaneous respiration will not interfere with the healing process of the fractured ribs, provided the hypoxia secondary to the contusion is adequately corrected with expiratory positive pressure. This appreciation of the important pathologic changes can measurably shorten the time of ventilatory support. The normalization of blood gas exchange responds to appropriate PEEP or CPAP therapy and can usually be discontinued within 5 to 7 days. Mechanical support can then be easily weaned. Even after withdrawal of all ancillary support, some flailing may still be clinically detectable but will have no effect on blood gas exchange provided hypoxemia is no longer present. When cases of flail chest are described as not requiring mechanical ventilation, no doubt any underlying parenchymal damage is only minimal and hypoxemia does not constitute a major problem.

Pulmonary embolism may also lead to the development of ARF; however, the major changes are vascular in origin and are not directly germane to the present discussion.

With an understanding of the basic pathophysiologic changes occurring in ARF, the rationale behind the various treatment modalities can more readily be understood. In summary, respiratory failure develops secondary to disruption of the Starling forces. When the lung safety valve mechanisms are overwhelmed, water accumulation produces alterations in normal ventilation-perfusion relationships. Lung volumes decrease and, in the final stages, the alveoli are overwhelmed by the sudden inflow of water and protein.

TREATMENT OF RESPIRATORY FAILURE

Effective treatment of ARF presumes the correct diagnosis has been made. All other causes of reduced PaO$_2$ or increased intrapulmonary shunt must have been evaluated and, if present, appropriately treated. These include copious pulmonary secretions, altered F$_I$O$_2$, pneumothorax, atelectasis, right mainstem intubation, severe bronchospasm, pneumonia, increased oxygen consumption, decreased cardiac output, and other similar events.[78,79]

Oxygen Therapy

Once the basic pathophysiologic derangements present in ARF are understood, the clinician can plan a specific treatment regimen. The initial therapeutic response to the hypoxia includes supplemental oxygen therapy. This will usually correct or prevent severe hypoxemia and buy time until events can be sorted out and the patient begun on the most efficacious therapy. However, prolonged high inspired oxygen concentrations might eventually prove detrimental. Sufficient data exist that demonstrate an actual increase in intrapulmonary shunt when breathing oxygen at close to 100 percent concentrations.[80,81]

A major alteration in ARF is ventilation-perfusion mismatching secondary to narrowing of the terminal airways. In essence, the time constants are extended, which means it requires a finitely longer time to deliver the same gas volume in the alveoli. At an F_IO_2 of 0.5 or less, nitrogen comprises a large component of the alveolar gas mixture. Nitrogen acts as an inert gas and, at ambient pressure, blood and tissues are already saturated with nitrogen molecules. Although nitrogen continually moves between the alveoli and the blood and between blood and tissue, no net accumulation occurs in any of the compartments. Hence the label *inert gas*. During ARF, elevated interstitial pressures increase the likelihood of airway and eventually alveolar collapse. Sufficient lung volume will prevent or oppose those effects; when adequate nitrogen is in the mixture, there are no real problems.[82] Although oxygen rapidly exits from the alveoli via capillary perfusion, enough of the inert nitrogen remains behind to act as a splint and maintain alveolar patency by preventing collapse due to the elevated interstitial pressures.

When the ARF patient breathes 100 percent oxygen, blood perfusing the alveoli rapidly extracts all the oxygen present. The increased time constants mean a prolongation of the time the alveoli contain little if any gas. The alveoli, now devoid of any gas, cannot continue to oppose the elevated interstitial pressure and begin to collapse, and the calculated intrapulmonary shunt increases. Unfortunately, these changes are not prevented by the application of PEEP or CPAP.

When this mechanism is operative, the increase in intrapulmonary shunt is accompanied by a reduction in lung volume, specifically FRC. Therefore, a therapeutic maneuver originally designed to increase oxygenation may actually contribute to a further deterioration of pulmonary function.

High inspired oxygen concentrations can also blunt the protective mechanism of hypoxic pulmonary vasoconstriction (HPV).[27] Normally, a low alveolar oxygen pressure (P_AO_2) represents alveolar hypoventilation secondary to ventilation-perfusion mismatch or alveolar collapse. Capillary perfusion continues basically unaltered despite the ventilation changes resulting from events such as terminal airway narrowing. A major ventilation-perfusion mismatch is prevented by the protective HPV response. The vasoconstriction diverts blood from altered areas of ventilation to noninvolved areas. The reduced flow to the hypoventilated areas helps preserve $\dot{V}/\dot{Q}$ relationships and maintains

oxygenation, thus preventing deterioration of the shunt fraction. A high F_IO_2 blunts this response; localized tissue hypoxia remains minimal and perfusion continues or increases to the involved areas.[83] Intrapulmonary shunt may actually increase. Since the amount of pulmonary vascular smooth muscle is minimal, a large intrapulmonary blood volume, indicated by high capillary wedge pressure, can ablate the entire HPV mechanism.[84,85]

High inspired oxygen concentrations may also lead to pulmonary oxygen toxicity.[86] Most available evidence indicates that lung changes begin after breathing 100 percent oxygen for as little as 6 hours. The pathophysiology resembles ARF. In fact, the two conditions are often indistinguishable, particularly if extremely high O_2 concentrations are delivered for any length of time during respiratory failure. The derangements develop in response to the accumulation of superoxide, hydrogen peroxide, and other toxic radicals. Alveolar infiltration, interstitial edema, and hyaline membrane formation are all demonstrable. The changes at atmospheric pressure are related to both the exposure time and concentration of inspired oxygen. Most authorities agree that at an F_IO_2 of less than 0.5, the risk of O_2 toxicity is minimal. At an F_IO_2 above 0.6, changes may appear after 48 hours, whereas substantial chest pain may begin as early as 6 hours after breathing 100 percent oxygen. The earliest detectable findings include a reduction of vital capacity.

A high inspired oxygen concentration can be excluded as a helpful adjunctive maneuver in ARF. Not only does it have its own peculiar problems, as previously described, but oxygenation does not markedly improve despite the increase in delivered concentration.

Oxygen can improve the hypoxia secondary to $\dot{V}/\dot{Q}$ mismatch.[87] The effective therapeutic range appears to include an F_IO_2 between 0.21 and 0.35. The increased oxygen concentration has the effect of converting hypoventilated units to more normally ventilated areas apparently by minimizing the amount of time the alveoli are devoid of oxygen. Alveoli always have some gas present so that perfusion to totally unoxygenated units does not develop. If ventilation is absent altogether, as eventually happens in most units, an increased F_IO_2 cannot significantly alter the ventilation-perfusion relationships and thereby improve oxygenation.

Adjuvant Therapy

Is there any role for steroid therapy in the treatment of ARF? Recent evidence has demonstrated that complement activation, particularly C_5A, may play a direct role.[40] Conditions associated with ARF such as sepsis, pancreatitis, and multiple-system trauma can all activate the complement system.

The specific complement factor, C_5A, interacts with leukocytes to cause plugging of the pulmonary vascular bed. Steroids may have a role in decreasing the effects of C_5A. The key may be early dosage since the white blood cell plugging occurs only transiently, being dissipated in less than 1 hour.

Both diuretic therapy and albumin infusions have been extensively used as treatment modalities during ARF.[88–90] Proponents have argued that since the diuretics increase free water clearance and decrease intravascular volume, the eventual reduction of intravascular pressure and concomitant elevation of colloid oncotic pressure will influence the Starling forces so that the direction of any fluid shift will be from the pulmonary interstitial to the intravascular space.[91] Unfortunately, these methods have been uniformly unsuccessful in reversing the clinical syndrome and have not improved mortality rate. The events originally responsible for the imbalance in the Starling forces are apparently still active. Neither diuretics nor albumin, even in high doses, have enhanced oxygenation; presumably, therefore, they cannot change the gradient for fluid movement.

Much has been written about the relationship of ARF and pulmonary hypertension.[92,93] When present, pulmonary hypertension does represent a severe form of respiratory dysfunction. However, not all severe cases of ARF necessarily involve pulmonary hypertension.[94] Therefore, the cause-effect relationship of pulmonary hypertension remains unclear. Pulmonary hypertension has several detrimental aspects. The elevated pressures contribute to changes in the Starling forces favorable to fluid movement into the interstitium. Additionally, elevated pulmonary artery pressure may severely affect right ventricular afterload and, ultimately, cardiac output.

Specific therapy aimed at the reduction of pulmonary hypertension has had mixed or unpredictable results. The most popular agent, sodium nitroprusside, has been found to increase intrapulmonary shunt. However, when shunt does change, it appears to relate to reductions in cardiac output rather than to direct alterations of pulmonary artery pressure.[95,96] If cardiac output increases with nitroprusside, as hoped for, intrapulmonary shunt does not necessarily change. Nitroprusside, as well as all other vasodilators, does not have specific effects on the circulation. Unfortunately, while used in attempting to lower pulmonary artery pressure, it also profoundly affects the systemic circulation.

Respiratory alkalosis theoretically acts as a pulmonary vasodilator and reduces pulmonary artery pressure.[19] However, the mechanical rate needed to achieve significant alkalosis may itself have detrimental effects.

As previously indicated, clinical data have demonstrated that interstitial lung water accumulation, while often responsible for ARF, does not correlate with the hypoxemia.[97–99] Therefore, even if some decrease in lung water occurs after diuretic and albumin therapy, it is probably not of sufficient magnitude to influence gas exchange.[100]

Ventilator Therapy

The initial response after lung water begins to accumulate includes tachypnea and hyperventilation. However, because of the interstitial derangements, including altered compliance, spontaneous breathing cannot increase ventilation to most of the affected lung units. The patient cannot generate a large enough transpulmonary pressure gradient to overcome the extra-alveolar forces or pressures that were originally responsible for the total or partial terminal airway collapse. As terminal airway narrowing worsens, the units become essentially devoid of all gas, and alveolar collapse ensues. Even combined diaphragmatic and chest wall movement cannot develop a pressure gradient large enough to expand the collapsed units. The patient continues to hyperventilate, but to no avail. The newly collapsed units remain nonventilated while perfusion and the intrapulmonary shunting and ventilation-perfusion mismatch continue.[101] While oxygenation does not improve, the linear carbon dioxide dissociation curve permits easy removal of that gas via the remaining ventilated units and accompanying increase in minute ventilation. In fact, CO_2 elimination proceeds without difficulty until actual alveolar infiltration develops.

The next logical step in the development of an effective treatment regimen for ARF includes the addition of the mechanical ventilator. Since the primary problem was one of breathing or respiration, the use of such a device seems logical. However, the mechanical ventilator by itself does not enhance oxygenation.

Consideration of the lung as a two-unit model can improve understanding of the problem. The positive-pressure ventilation will significantly increase airway pressure. If the pressure generated is sufficient to open the collapsed units, then gas will move into those areas during the mechanical inspiratory phase. Since perfusion continues unchanged throughout the entire process, some improvement in blood gas exchange would be expected. However, oxygenation does not significantly increase. This is due to the fact that when the mechanical ventilator cycles into the

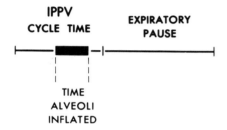

IPPV CYCLE TIME

EXPIRATORY PAUSE

TIME
ALVEOLI
INFLATED

Fig. 23-11. During intermittent positive-pressure ventilation (IPPV), the airway pressure sufficient to keep alveoli expanded accounts for only a small portion of the inspiratory phase of ventilation.

exhalation phase, airway pressure rapidly reverts to the baseline or ambient level. Any distending force on the affected alveolar units is removed and the terminal airways or alveoli recollapse. Perfusion continues and once again marked alterations of ventilation-perfusion relationships persist.

Examination of the entire inspiratory-expiratory cycle illustrates why positive-pressure ventilation does not alleviate the problem (Fig. 23-11). Gas exchange can only improve when alveoli are both ventilated and perfused. Mechanical ventilation re-expands the collapsed alveoli only during mechanical inspiration and even then not during the entire time of inspiration. In fact, evaluation of the entire inspiratory-expiratory cycle indicates that alveolar re-expansion occupies only a small portion of the entire ventilatory cycle. Under those circumstances, no real improvement in gas exchange can be expected.

To provide better understanding of these events, an explanation of some aspects of pulmonary physiology is in order. The reasoning can apply to the lung as a whole or to an individual alveolus. During a condition of increased interstitial pressure, the lung requires elevated airway pressures to maintain full expansion. As airway pressure diminishes, so does lung volume. Eventually a pressure is reached below which complete collapse occurs. This point represents the critical closing pressure (CCP). Efforts to re-expand the involved portion require airway pressure application in excess of the closing pressure. The critical opening pressure refers to that point when the alveoli begin to re-expand.[102] That pressure usually exceeds the CCP. Once it is reached, expansion proceeds quite easily with further pressure increases.

With the patient attached to a mechanical ventilator, the following scenario takes place. During mechanical inspiration, the respirator develops an airway pressure greater than the terminal airway units' critical opening pressures. With alveolar recruitment,

blood gas exchange begins. However, during exhalation, the airway pressure drops below opening pressure; no further blood gas exchange takes place in the affected units. However, if airway pressure is not permitted to reach CCP, collapse will not recur and blood gas exchange will be markedly enhanced. Positive end-expiratory pressure prevents airway pressure from falling below CCP and oxygenation continues improved.[103] PEEP and mechanical ventilation appear to work in tandem. The ventilator generates significantly high airway pressures to overcome the interstitial pressure effects and re-expands the collapsed alveoli while PEEP prevents their recollapse. The overall effect includes sustained improvement in gas exchange as well as restoration of resting lung volume.[104] Neither PEEP nor mechanical ventilation alone can successfully reverse the changes described. Rather, both must function in tandem, one to recruit and the other to sustain the acquired changes.

PEEP Versus CPAP

Confusion still exists regarding the difference between PEEP and CPAP. Comparison of spontaneous breathing patterns demonstrates the differences (Fig. 23-12). Both have an elevated baseline or resting airway pressure. During CPAP, the spontaneous effort reduces airway pressure. However, at no time does the inspiratory airway pressure reach atmospheric or become subambient. The amount of reduction in pressure depends on the patient's breathing effort and the type of spontaneous breathing system.

PEEP implies that during spontaneous breathing, airway pressure does reach ambient or subambient levels. Positive pressure develops only at end-expiration, hence the designation *positive end-expiratory pressure.*

Attachment to a mechanical ventilator does not alter the terminology. If during mechanical ventilation the baseline pressure is elevated and the patient does not breathe spontaneously, CPAP is in effect. This has previously been designated *continuous positive-pressure breathing.* When mechanical ventilation and spontaneous breathing coexist, as with IMV, then either CPAP or PEEP may be operative. If the spontaneous effort reduces airway pressure to ambient or subambient levels, then IMV with PEEP is the appropriate terminology. On the other hand, if airway pressure does not reach ambient levels, then the system is IMV with CPAP. Depending on the patient's respiratory effort, the mode may actually change from breath to breath.

During spontaneous breathing, the greater the reduction in airway pressure, the greater the enhance-

CPAP

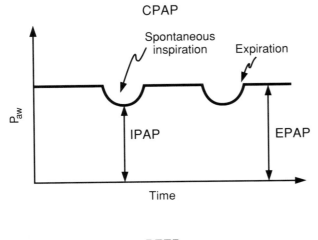

PEEP

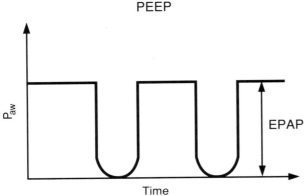

Fig. 23-12. PEEP and CPAP spontaneous breathing patterns. With CPAP, despite negative deflections, airway pressure remains positive during the entire cycle. PEEP maintains positive airway pressure only during the exhalation phase. Inspiratory positive airway pressure (IPAP) refers to the lowest positive airway pressure. It is determined by the inspiratory effort. Expiratory airway pressure (EPAP) represents the baseline pressure. P_{AW}, airway pressure.

ment of venous return.[105,106] However, the greater the airway pressure change, the greater the work of breathing.[107] Clinically, an attempt is made to reach a middle ground, maximizing venous return but not at the cost of a markedly increased work of breathing.

When using PEEP or CPAP, the clinician must initially select an appropriate end point. Various plans have been proposed.[108,109] Many have advocated PEEP/CPAP levels that restore PaO_2 to a level consistent with adequate oxygen saturation while the patient breathes less-than-toxic concentrations of oxygen. At a normal pH, a PaO_2 of 70 mmHg or higher indicates a hemoglobin saturation of 90 percent or

more. Pulmonary oxygen toxicity has not been reported with an F_1O_2 of 0.5 or less.

The usual clinical response to developing hypoxia almost always includes an increase in supplemental oxygen. Once all the other causes of a reduced PaO_2 have been ruled out and ARF appropriately diagnosed, PEEP/CPAP therapy is begun; initial levels of 3 to 5 cmH_2O are incrementally increased.[110] As PaO_2 improves, the F_1O_2 can be concurrently reduced. Once the end point (an arterial saturation of 90 percent on an F_1O_2 of less than 0.5) is reached, therapy is considered complete. Any further increase in PaO_2 will require an appropriate increase in PEEP/CPAP. At times, the disease process will further deteriorate, requiring another upward adjustment of the end-expiratory pressure.

As will be discussed, high levels of PEEP/CPAP may interfere with cardiac function. Therefore, some clinicians advocate arbitrary upper limits for CPAP/PEEP, arguing that high levels may seriously impair cardiac function. The usual limits prescribed are 15 to 18 cmH_2O. However, at least one clinical study has demonstrated that a substantial number of patients with apparently severe forms of ARF did not respond to PEEP/CPAP levels up to 15 cmH_2O. Not until PEEP was increased, in some cases far in excess of 15 cmH_2O, did any real improvement in oxygenation occur.[111] If those patients had been arbitrarily maintained at the recommended lower levels, they would not have experienced any improvement in oxygenation. The choice should be predicated on physiologic parameters rather than on arbitrary selection of an end point. The parameters may vary with the clinician, but the eventual PEEP/CPAP levels will more nearly relate to the underlying disease process.

Another proposed end point has been pulmonary compliance.[112] Compliance is calculated as the volume delivered divided by the airway pressure differential required to deliver that volume. Either dynamic or static compliance can be chosen. Static compliance includes changes in both lung and chest wall. Clamping the expiratory limb of the circuit after delivery of the breath while performing an inflation hold helps determine static compliance. Dynamic compliance uses the peak inflation pressure developed during mechanical inspiration, including airway resistance.

Several studies have attempted to demonstrate a correlation between compliance and oxygen delivery, which includes cardiac output and arterial oxygen content. When compliance is maximized, oxygen delivery also appears maximal. However, further increases in PEEP/CPAP, while demonstrating a reduction in both compliance and oxygen delivery, result in marked improvement in other parameters of oxygenation, namely, PaO_2 and intrapulmonary shunt. Oxygen delivery decreases in response to a reduction in cardiac output. It is now known that appropriate cardiovascular interventions will maintain cardiac output, which further emphasizes the lack of correlation between compliance and other factors. In fact, other studies have also failed to show any consistent relationship between oxygenation and compliance.

Optimal PEEP/CPAP

Gallagher et al popularized the concept of optimal PEEP/CPAP.[113] Intrapulmonary shunt or venous admixture reduction to 15 percent identified the optimal therapeutic goal. For critically ill patients, it is recommended to calculate shunt rather than to follow PaO_2 since many patients have multisystem failure. Either increased oxygen consumption, decreased cardiac output, or a combination of both can cause a reduction in mixed venous or pulmonary artery oxygen content. With any degree of pulmonary dysfunction, only a fixed amount of oxygen is delivered to the blood. Therefore, the amount of oxygen in blood returning to the lungs will determine the PaO_2.[79]

Intrapulmonary shunt or venous admixture, on the other hand, changes only in relation to pulmonary changes. Shunt indicates the portion of cardiac output not oxygenated during flow through the lungs. Cardiac output has less influence on shunt fraction, and, therefore, intrapulmonary shunt more directly reflects only pulmonary changes.

Certain errors may develop when calculating intrapulmonary shunt.[101] Occasionally, researchers have advocated calculating shunt by the modified shunt equation. Since this method assumes a constant oxygen consumption, it should not be used in critically ill patients, who often have a continually changing rate of oxygen consumption. The shunt equation assumes 100 percent saturation in the pulmonary capillary bed; therefore, the inspired oxygen concentration must exceed 30 percent to guarantee total saturation.

Venous admixture or intrapulmonary shunt accounts for all disruptions of blood gas exchange in the lung. These include true anatomic shunting, such as lack of perfusion after a pulmonary embolus. True anatomic shunt may develop during high-altitude pulmonary edema when profound arteriolar constriction directs blood away from ventilated areas. Shunting may also develop when ventilation is completely impaired while some perfusion continues. Atelectasis exemplifies this type of change. Most times, the major pathophysiology events in ARF relate not to true shunting but rather to ventilation-perfusion mismatch in areas where ventilation is less than normal in comparison with the degree of alveolar perfusion.

Major alterations in cardiac output can directly influence the shunt fraction. Since shunt varies with ventilation-perfusion relationships, any large change in pulmonary blood flow might conceivably alter the shunt calculation. In fact, various vasoactive agents, including dopamine and nitroprusside, have been implicated in these changes.[114] Most of the changes occur with alteration of cardiac output. The patency of the pulmonary vascular system depends more on flow than on pressure. As cardiac output varies, flow and, hence, ventilation-perfusion relationships also change. If cardiac output does not markedly change, shunt remains the same.

The goal of a reduction of intrapulmonary shunt to 15 percent developed because it corresponds to most authorities' definitions of respiratory failure.[115] An alveolar-arterial oxygen gradient [$P(A - a)O_2$] of 300 to 350 mmHg ($F_IO_2 = 1.0$) approximately equals a 15 percent shunt when cardiac output is undisturbed. Since most have advocated initiating therapy at a $P(A - a)O_2$ of 350 mmHg, it does not seem unreasonable to initiate treatment that could restore pulmonary function to that level. The results indicate that the goal can be easily achieved without any untoward risk to the patient. The incidence of pulmonary barotrauma and cardiac depression is similar to that with other ventilatory modes, and the vast majority of patients require less than 25 cmH_2O PEEP or CPAP. The mortality rates strictly from respiratory failure equal or are less than those with other methods. To date, there is no definitive evidence indicating the best method to treat respiratory failure, since mortality rates do not appear to differ. However, more subtle differences may relate to such things as duration of therapy, complications from the therapy, and length of hospital stay. Until questions of this type are settled, a clear-cut answer as to the preferred treatment regimen does not exist.

When all patients are treated to the same end point, for example, shunt reduction to 125 percent of normal, there are means of comparing the severity of the illness. Since the criteria remain the same, those requiring greater levels of raised-airway-pressure therapy to attain the same therapeutic end point must have a more significant pulmonary injury. In addition, other interventions, including adjustment of the rate and duration of IMV, can also be applied on the basis of objective criteria and, thus, used to compare ARF in different patient populations.

Once PEEP/CPAP has attained a therapeutic end point, how long should the modality remain in effect at that particular level? There is no known correct answer. Clinicians usually select some arbitrary minimal time. In general, the longer it takes to reach a preselected level or the higher that level, the longer

TABLE 23-4. Indications for CPAP Mask

Mild ARF
Spontaneous respiration
Normocarbia
Awake and cooperative

the time before attempting to reduce PEEP/CPAP. When levels of over 20 cmH$_2$O are in effect, each 24-hour period may see the original level reduced by only one-third to one-half. Weaning from PEEP/CPAP should proceed in the same organized, incremental manner as titration to optimal levels, provided shunt remains within the same acceptable range. Blood gas exchange continues to act as a more sensitive indicator than any other method, including radiography or pulmonary mechanics.

Face-mask CPAP can be used for mild forms of ARF.[116] Essentially, the method provides continuous distending pressure to the airway while avoiding the necessity of intubation. A continuous flow of gas at a specified F$_I$O$_2$ through a system similar to a ventilator circuit constitutes all that is necessary. However, the ventilator itself is not actually required. The patient must have adequate spontaneous respiration (PaCO$_2$, 45 mmHg) and be alert and cooperative (Table 23-4).

Detrimental effects of the CPAP mask include patient discomfort and gastric distention. Air does accumulate in the stomach and a nasogastric tube should always be placed during facemask CPAP therapy (see Chapter 22).

When levels above 10 cmH$_2$O are required, intubation and mechanical ventilation at low rates may be more efficacious. The ventilator delivers the higher pressures necessary to reach critical opening pressures, while CPAP maintains the levels that prevent airway closure. If CPAP alone is used, high levels will be required to open the airway units, while actually lower pressure levels could be maintained with an occasional higher pressure during the inspiratory phase of mechanical ventilation.

Complications of PEEP/CPAP

Major problems identified with PEEP/CPAP therapy include interference with cardiac output.[117,118] Several factors appear to operate at different points in the circulation. With the initiation of positive airway pressure therapy, any degree of hypovolemia frequently causes a reduced cardiac output. In reality, the patient may be normovolemic, but the raised airway pressure imparts some reduction of venous return to the right heart. The elevated airway pressures are transmitted across the pulmonary parenchyma to the intrathoracic space. The normally negative intrathoracic pressure may become positive and interfere with superior and inferior vena cava blood return. Dye studies during positive-pressure mechanical inspiration have demonstrated actual narrowing of both structures during their intrathoracic course.[119] Stroke volume decreases and cardiac output falls. The arterial blood pressure trace on the oscilloscope may indicate the onset of the problem. Soon after the mechanical breath, the amplitude of the arterial trace markedly diminishes, eventually returning to baseline levels before the next breath. Further evidence of the problem often includes a low central venous pressure or PCWP. Spontaneous breathing reduces intrathoracic pressure and can enhance venous return and restore cardiac output.

During positive-pressure breathing, the high airway pressures can also influence pulmonary artery pressure.[120–122] As before, each positive-pressure breath elevates all intrathoracic pressures, including pulmonary artery pressure. Pulmonary vascular resistance increases, and right ventricular afterload also subsequently rises. Radionuclide scanning has demonstrated unsuspected changes. Normally, the right ventricle, a thin-walled chamber, operates at low pressures and generates only approximately one-tenth the work of the left ventricle. In response to increased pulmonary vascular pressure and resistance, right ventricular dilatation ensues and the intraventricular septum begins to bulge into the left ventricle.[123,124] At this point, right and left ventricular end-diastolic pressures must equilibrate.[125] The left ventricle, being a much thicker muscle, cannot dilate nearly so easily and is also constrained by the rigid pericardium. The septum bulges into the left ventricular outflow tract, interfering with stroke volume. Appropriate therapy should include positive inotropic support, primarily to support right ventricular function. Spontaneous ventilation in lieu of positive-pressure mechanical breaths will also limit those pressure effects by reducing the number of intrusions each hour on the pulmonary artery.[126–128]

Distention by PEEP/CPAP of terminal airway units can eventually influence the pulmonary vascular bed. As lung volume increases, especially with overdistention, several changes occur in the pulmonary capillary bed. Again, positive-pressure breathing further complicates the problem. Each mechanical breath can trap blood in the pulmonary circulation, leading to decreased left ventricular preload and, eventually, decreased stroke volume. Overdistention of the airway may impinge on capillary diameter and flow. Pulmonary vascular resistance increases, and right ventricular function can deteriorate.

One laboratory study has demonstrated the probable release of endogenous cardiac depressants.[118] After one animal was placed on mechanical ventilation with PEEP, cardiac output decreased. Blood from that first animal was then cross-circulated to a second animal not mechanically ventilated, and the cardiac output of the second animal also decreased. The evidence points to release of some endogenous substance, perhaps secondary to lung expansion.

Data also suggest possible altered ventricular compliance. Again in animals, cardiac output fell after the introduction of PEEP/CPAP and mechanical ventilation. Despite the return of transmural PCWP (wedge pressure minus intrathoracic pressure) to original values, stroke volume remained less than before the institution of mechanical ventilation.[122] This suggests altered ventricular contractility or compliance. The investigators postulate that pulmonary parenchyma overdistention could cause the lung to come in close contact with the left ventricle, perhaps changing compliance and interfering with ventricular function (Fig. 23-13).

Another clinical problem associated with PEEP/CPAP therapy involves accurate PCWP measurements. By convention, pressures are recorded at end-expiration and the catheter tip zeroed to the right atrium. As previously stated, alveolar overdistention interferes with and constricts the pulmonary circulation. Therefore, any measurement of pulmonary vascular pressure can reflect both intra- and extravascular forces. Reports have appeared indicating that the position of the catheter tip itself influences the pressures recorded. If the tip lodges in zone I, where alveolar pressure is normally higher than vascular pressure and where there is little actual blood flow, PCWP readings can be meaningless. In zone II, alveolar pressure is less than pulmonary arterial pressure but greater than venous pressure. Alveolar pressure changes still exert an influence on recorded wedge pressure. The same interrelationships are operative, but less so in the dependent zone III areas, where vas-

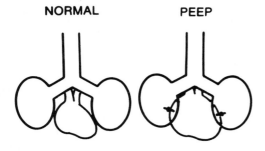

Fig. 23-13. One effect of PEEP on ventricular function. Overdistention of the lung may compress and interfere with left ventricular function and/or compliance.

cular pressures are usually greater than alveolar pressure. High airway pressures can obviously impact here and, at times, change these relationships. Fortunately, clinical studies have demonstrated that, at most times, the catheter tip is in either zone II or zone III.[129] Also, in the supine position most, if not all, of zone I is eliminated. Therefore, provided the catheter is properly zeroed, the tip location does not constitute a major problem.

The problem still remains of how to measure PCWP during mechanical ventilatory support. To remove all effects of PEEP and give true vascular pressures, some clinicians have advocated disconnecting the patient from the ventilator. However, sudden removal of PEEP can trigger a large influx of blood into the pulmonary vascular bed. This effect can be imagined as similar to the opening of a dam in the intrathoracic superior and inferior vena cava. In the space of one or two heart beats, a massive inflow of blood dramatically increases the pulmonary vascular volume.

It should be apparent to the reader that any interpretation of wedge pressure during mechanical ventilation and expiratory positive pressure risks error. At times, little correlation exists between left ventricular end-diastolic volume and wedge pressure, especially with pre-existing myocardial disease. Clinical evaluation in light of all data will be required to determine the meaning of a wedge pressure of 20 mmHg recorded during 15 cmH_2O of raised airway pressure therapy. The values change and do not always accurately reflect the true hemodynamic relationships during PEEP/CPAP.

Various mathematical formulas have been proposed to predict the effect of the various PEEP/CPAP levels on wedge pressure. However, since the data for these calculations come from a small series of patients, they usually cannot be accurately applied to any individual case.

A different approach involves subtracting intrathoracic from measured wedge pressure to calculate transmural or true intravascular capillary wedge pressure. An esophageal balloon catheter can estimate intrathoracic pressure. However, real doubt exists about the validity of the measurement obtained in the supine position because of the influence of the mediastinal structures. Direct catheterization of the intrathoracic space to measure intrapleural pressure, while feasible, does increase patient morbidity and cannot be advocated as standard therapy.[130] In addition, the location of the catheter may preclude measurement of overall intrathoracic pressure.

Recent data have called into question the entire validity of the PCWP during mechanical ventilatory support.[131] Normally, it is assumed that wedge pressure reflects left ventricular end-diastolic pressure

(LVEDP). Studies on animals treated with mechanical ventilation and CPAP demonstrate even a marked discrepancy between transmural wedge pressure and LVEDP. In all instances, transmural wedge pressure was significantly higher than transmural LVEDP. It appears that in the absence of spontaneous breathing, airway pressure neither is equally transmitted nor equally impinges on all the intrathoracic pressures. Left heart filling pressures are not nearly as high as would be indicated by wedge pressure. This study may explain some of the difficulty encountered when assessing cardiac function during raised airway pressure therapy. The reported low cardiac outputs may actually indicate inadequate left ventricular filling pressures and volume. Whether blood has remained trapped in the lungs is not clear.

A further complication of raised airway pressure therapy includes the changes in renal function.[132,133] Clinically, these most often manifest themselves as a decrease in urine flow.[134] Further laboratory determinations may indicate an elevated vasopressin level as well as changes in urinary sodium excretion.[135] Glomerular filtration rate also falls during positive-pressure therapy.

The clinical alterations are clear, but the responsible mechanisms are not. Also, spontaneous breathing may mitigate some of the responses. Very few attempts have been made to investigate the apparent differences in renal function when continuous positive-pressure therapy is replaced by a method permitting spontaneous breathing.

When animals have no spontaneous respiratory efforts, positive airway pressure decreases carotid sinus and aortic arch baroreceptor activity, and all of the above-mentioned changes in renal function take place. When animals breathe spontaneously, changes in sodium excretion and vasopressin are not as large as in the group without spontaneous breathing. These differences may be explained by a greater transmural inferior vena cava pressure in the spontaneous group. It is probably safe to conclude that more than one mechanism operates to produce these observed variations in renal physiology.

Intermittent Mandatory Ventilation

While raised airway pressures can be applied in connection with any form of mechanical ventilation, there may be particular reasons to primarily use IMV.[136] IMV promotes spontaneous breathing while simultaneously limiting the number of positive-pressure breaths. Spontaneous breathing has several theoretic and proven benefits.

Mechanical positive-pressure breathing, in addition to recruitment and re-expansion of collapsed airway units, primarily determines alveolar ventilation. Clinically, the $PaCO_2$ indicates the adequacy or level of the ventilatory process. As stated previously, CO_2 elimination during ARF does not ordinarily present a problem. However, in preterminal situations in which alveolar infiltration is present with fluffy infiltrative changes on the radiograph, hypercapnia may be more prone to develop. Earlier, $PaCO_2$ is usually low, 30 to 32 mmHg, with its straight-line dissociation curve facilitating its elimination.

In view of this concept, an understanding of gas exchange suggests that controlled positive-pressure breathing is not the ideal therapeutic approach. The philosophy of IMV relates to delivering mechanical ventilation only at a rate necessary to supplement the patient's own spontaneous activities. It limits the mechanical impact on the system.

Arbitrary criteria of the appropriateness of the spontaneous ventilatory efforts include a $PaCO_2$ of 35 to 45 mmHg, a pH of greater than 7.35, and a spontaneous rate of fewer than 30 breaths/min. A pH of 7.35 provides a more reasonable basis of evaluation in normally hypercapnic patients. Attempts to lower their $PaCO_2$ to the previously indicated range might result in apnea. Some patients also compensate for metabolic alkalosis by retaining CO_2, and again pH becomes a more useful clinical tool.[137] A spontaneous breathing rate above 30/min indicates an unnecessarily high level of work to maintain $PaCO_2$. While $PaCO_2$ and pH may be normal, these levels are at the cost of a marked increase in the work of breathing. Somewhere at rates above 40 breaths/min, exhalation changes from a passive to an active maneuver, markedly increasing the physiologic cost.

Studies on healthy subjects indicate that during spontaneous ventilation, gas distribution is primarily to the dependent lung portions.[138] In the upright position these are the basilar units, while in the supine position they are the posterior aspects. Several factors are responsible for this distribution pattern (see Chapter 8).

Both the weight of lung parenchyma and the pulmonary blood volume act to compress the lung segments or alveoli. In the upright position, the basilar alveoli are more compressed than those in the apex. However, compared with the apical units, the volumes of the basilar alveoli are such that they are on a much more favorable portion of the pressure-volume curve. Smaller changes in transpulmonary pressure gradients result in larger volume changes than in their less-dependent counterparts, which are already at maximal volume and in which large pressure changes are required to effect any volume increase.

Similarly, position also influences pulmonary blood flow. The pulmonary circulation, being a low-pressure system, remains quite gravity-dependent. The majority of the right ventricular outflow goes to dependent lung portions. In comparison, ventilation to those same areas does not match the amount of blood flow; an average ventilation-to-perfusion ratio approaches approximately 0.6. However, both the volume of blood flow and ventilation to the dependent lung portions exceed that to any other lung area. Therefore, the dependent units, basilar in the upright position and posterior in the supine position, are those most involved in blood gas exchange.

Studies in healthy volunteers have demonstrated that in a supine, spontaneously breathing subject, more diaphragmatic motion occurs in the posterior or dependent position.[139] The radius of curvature of the diaphragm promotes more excursion in that plane, which enhances the ventilation already directed to those areas. During paralysis and controlled mechanical ventilation, diaphragmatic motion involves the anterior nondependent portion. The passive diaphragmatic motion responds secondarily to increases in intrathoracic pressure. Simultaneously, the abdominal contents push upward on the diaphragm and provide resistance to any movement of the posterior-dependent portion. Therefore, controlled ventilation results in poor matching of ventilation-perfusion, since ventilation flows to the anterior or nondependent lung units while blood remains in the basilar segments.[140] In fact, the redistribution of blood flow contributes to an increase in calculated physiologic dead space, and units are greatly overdistended in proportion to the amount of circulation. Normally, with controlled, positive-pressure breathing, tidal volumes of 10 to 15 mL/kg are delivered. These represent at least twice the volumes used during spontaneous efforts, and such large volumes contribute to a spillover effect. Once the nondependent areas are filled, gas moves into the dependent units, which are better situated to participate in gas exchange. Without this hyperventilation during mechanical breathing, $PaCO_2$ would increase and atelectasis would soon develop.

IMV, since it promotes spontaneous breathing activity, exemplifies a theoretically sounder method of ventilation. It provides the best matching of ventilation to perfusion and should, therefore, maximize oxygenation while optimizing ventilation-perfusion relationships.

Since IMV allows for spontaneous breathing and also limits the number of positive-pressure breaths, interference with cardiac function remains minimal. In fact, an almost linear relationship exists between cardiac output and the mechanical ventilator rate. Spontaneous breathing reduces intrathoracic pressure, enhancing venous return, and also reduces overall mean airway pressure (Fig. 23-12).[141] Both effects minimize cardiovascular deterioration. Limiting the number of ventilator breaths also contributes to a lowered mean airway pressure, since the reduced number of positive-pressure inflations limits the number of transient increases in pulmonary artery pressure (Figs. 23-14 and 23-15). Therefore, interference with right ventricular afterload is minimized.

Newer evidence indicates that pulmonary barotrauma, including pneumothorax, pneumomedia-

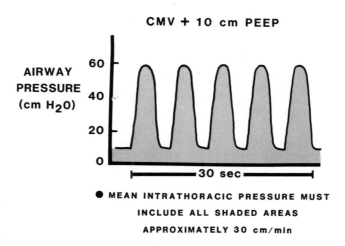

Fig. 23-14. Controlled mechanical ventilation and 10 cmH$_2$O PEEP/CPAP. The area under the curve represents a mean airway pressure of 30 cmH$_2$O. CMV, controlled mechanical ventilation.

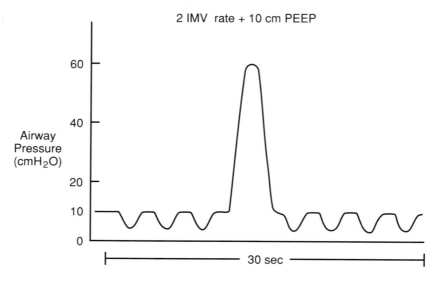

2 IMV rate + 10 cm PEEP

Airway Pressure (cmH₂O)

30 sec

Mean Intrathoraic Pressure
• 1/5 Inspiratory peaks
• Subtract all spontaneous deflections
• Approximately 12 cm/min

Fig. 23-15. IMV and 10 cmH₂O PEEP. Negative deflections of the baseline represent spontaneous breathing. The number of mechanical breaths per minute is also decreased. The result is a much lower mean airway pressure than seen in Figure 23-14. Cardiac output has less impairment.

stinum, and pneumoperitoneum, correlates with both the frequency and the absolute peak inflation pressure of the positive-pressure breath; limiting the ventilator frequency should have a favorable influence. In fact, the incidence of barotrauma with IMV and high PEEP levels is equal to that obtained when controlled mechanical ventilation and low-level PEEP are used.

Since the patient can breathe spontaneously on IMV, the need to control respiratory effort by paralysis, sedation, or hypocapnia does not arise. The patient does not "fight" the ventilator. Respiratory alkalosis, with its attendant problems of cardiac dysrhythmias and increased oxygen consumption, does not develop. Since the patient no longer requires paralysis, accidental disconnection from the ventilator does not pose quite the same hazard as it would if controlled ventilation were used.

IMV was originally proposed as a weaning technique (Table 23-5). However, in that aspect, it is not superior to any other technique. Patients will be weaned from mechanical support when ready, regardless of the method. However, weaning with IMV requires fewer direct nursing interventions. On controlled ventilation, weaning involves transferring a patient receiving 100 percent machine support of respiration to a continuous flow T-piece system. Weaning

usually is based on some objective criteria, which might include a negative inspiratory force of more than -25 cmH₂O, a vital capacity of at least 1.0 to 1.5 L, and/or a dead space-to-tidal volume ratio (V_D/V_T) less than 0.6. The actual choices will vary with the physician. The patient must abruptly supply 100 percent of the ventilatory requirements. The patient remains off the ventilator for a very short period the first time and, if all goes well, is then taken off the machine for progressively longer periods. Ventilatory support alternates continually between 100 and 0 percent. Obviously, this method requires close, continual nursing supervision.

With IMV, on the other hand, weaning proceeds in a smooth, stepwise fashion from total mechanical ventilatory support to complete self-support over a time course determined by the patient's physiologic response. Those parameters measured include the aforementioned pH, PaCO₂, and spontaneous breathing rate. Other values, such as (V_D/V_T), are not required.

TABLE 23-5.   IMV Weaning Criteria

pH > 7.35
PaCO₂ 35–45 mmHg
Spontaneous rate < 30/min

As a general rule, patients who develop ARF and who are promptly treated can be weaned in the first 24 hours to a ventilator rate of 2 to 3 breaths/min. As long as the patient meets the criteria, the rate can be incrementally reduced by 1 to 2 breaths/min. The patient usually begins at an IMV rate of 8/min. With a 12 mL/kg tidal volume, faster rates are normally not required. Periodic hyperinflation or sighs are not used because low-level PEEP/CPAP (< 5 cmH$_2$O) ensures that the lung always remains at least at FRC. Discontinuation of all mechanical ventilatory support requires a functional return to normal of all systems. Adequate oxygenation implies an F$_I$O$_2$ below 0.5 and at least a 90 percent hemoglobin saturation with less than 5 to 6 cmH$_2$O PEEP/CPAP. Also, on totally spontaneous breathing, the respiratory rate remains less than 30/min while pH exceeds 7.35, and PaCO$_2$ remains at the original baseline levels. Obviously, patients must be able to maintain their own airway, and all other criteria for extubation must be satisfied. At this juncture, extubation can be safely performed.

Pressure-Support Ventilation

Pressure-support ventilation represents a new form of spontaneous respiration.[142] The methodology takes advantage of the microprocessors now built into the newer mechanical ventilators. In essence, when the patient initiates a spontaneous breath, the ventilator senses the effort and delivers a high flow of gases to develop an airway pressure above the baseline pressure. In effect, a positive-pressure breath is delivered to the patient. The ventilator controls the level of pressure support desired above the baseline. The ventilator then delivers sufficient flow during the inspiratory phase of ventilation to maintain that pressure. Various algorithms are used to sense when the patient's inspiratory effort stops and when the patient finishes the inspiratory effort. However, the ventilator flow then cycles off and the pressure returns to baseline. The length of the pressure-support breath is dependent on the duration of the patient's spontaneous effort. This will vary on a breath-to-breath basis. Therefore, while the level of pressure support remains fixed, tidal volume will vary on a breath-to-breath basis. The number of these breaths per minute varies based on the patient's own spontaneous respiratory rate.

Pressure-support ventilation minimizes the inspiratory work of breathing. The patient generally initiates an inspiratory effort of less than 0.5 cmH$_2$O. During the remainder of the inspiratory phase, lung and chest expansion are passive. This method minimizes respiratory work. A decrease in the patient's spontaneous rate represents indirect evidence of that reduction.

The clinician should attempt to adjust the level of pressure support to that consistent with a reduction of the patient's own spontaneous respiratory rate. The method may also be combined with mandated positive-pressure breaths to ensure that the patient receives some ventilation in the event apnea ensues. Pressure-support levels generally range between 5 and 30 cmH$_2$O.

Pressure-support ventilation has been advocated as a technique to wean patients from mechanical ventilation. However, there is no evidence to suggest that this method is superior to any other currently described technique. In the author's opinion, the method is more one to minimize respiratory work during mechanical ventilation than to actually wean a patient. In fact, if used for protracted periods of time, its ability to reduce the work of breathing may actually lead to a form of respiratory muscle disuse atrophy.

Pressure support is usually added in 5 cmH$_2$O increments until the desired reduction in respiratory rate takes place. Discontinuation of pressure support can be conducted in reciprocal fashion. If dysynchronous breathing develops during IMV or other forms of ventilation, transition to pressure support may be of benefit. Individuals may be so weak that the inspiratory work required during IMV therapy may be overwhelming. The clinician should recognize that pressure-support ventilation is a form of positive-pressure breathing. The resultant increase in mean airway pressure means that the usual complications can develop. These include barotrauma and reduction of venous return and, ultimately, cardiac output.

Airway Pressure-Release Ventilation

Airway pressure-release ventilation has been introduced recently in the United States and is still undergoing therapeutic evaluation.[143] In effect, a level of CPAP is applied to hold the lung at a static lung volume. The patient is able to breathe spontaneously. Intermittently, the airway pressure is reduced to a lower level for a varying period of time. The amount of pressure release, or reduction, as well as its duration and frequency, are variable. Reduction in pressure results in a decrease in lung volume and a so-called exhalation phase.

Advocates of this technique maintain that it results in lowered mean airway and peak airway pressures. They therefore presume that less barotrauma should occur. There is no evidence yet to support the potential reduction in barotrauma or enhancement on cardiac performance compared with other methods of ventilatory support. The methodology requires that the patient be normocapneic. The author's experience has indicated that the technique has been successful in mild forms of respiratory failure. However, in true ARDS, requiring not only positive pressure to improve oxygenation, but also mechanical ventilation to remove carbon dioxide, the technique has not been of any benefit.

REFERENCES

1. Fowler AA, Hamman RF, Good JT, et al: Adult respiratory distress syndrome: risk with common predispositions. Ann Intern Med 98:593, 1983
2. Petty TL: Adult respiratory distress syndrome: historical perspective and definition. Respir Med 2:99, 1981
3. Shapiro BA, Cane RD, Harrison RA: Positive end-expiratory pressure therapy in adults with special reference to acute lung injury: a review of the literature and suggested clinical correlations. Crit Care Med 12:127–140, 1984
4. Jenkins MT, Jones RF, Wilson B, et al: Congestive atelectasis: a complication of intravenous infusion of fluids. Ann Surg 175:657–664, 1950
5. Teplitz C: The core pathobiology and integrated medical science of adult acute respiratory insufficiency. Surg Clin North Am 56:1091–1133, 1976
6. Brewer LA, Burbank B, Sampson PC, et al: The "wet lung" in war casualties. Ann Surg 123:343–362, 1946
7. Pontoppidan H, Geffin B, Lowenstein E: Acute respiratory failure in the adult. N Engl J Med 287:626–698, 743–752, 799–806, 1972
8. Farrell P, Avery ME: Hyaline membrane disease. Am Rev Respir Dis 111:654–688, 1975
9. Taylor RW, Norwood SH: The adult respiratory distress syndrome. pp. 1057–1068. In Civetta JM, Taylor RW, Kirby RR (eds): Critical Care. Philadelphia, JB Lippincott, 1988
10. Sibbald WJ, Short AK, Warshawski FJ, et al: Thermal measurements of extravascular lung water in critically ill patients: intravascular Starling forces in extravascular lung water in the adult respiratory distress syndrome. Chest 87:585–591, 1985
11. Sachneeberger-Keeley EE, Karnovsky MJ: The ultrastructural basis of alveolar capillary membrane permeability to peroxidase used as a tracer. J Cell Biol 37:781–793, 1968
12. West JB: Respiratory Physiology. Williams & Wilkins, Baltimore, 1974
13. Craig DB, Wabba WM, Don HF, et al: "Closing volume" and its relationship to gas exchange in seated and supine position. J Appl Physiol 31:717–721, 1971
14. Nieman GF: Current concepts of lung fluid balance. Respir Care 30:1062–1076, 1985
15. Demling RH: The role of mediators in human ARDS. J Crit Care 3:56–72, 1988
16. Teplitz C: The ultrastructural basis for pulmonary pathophysiology following trauma—pathogenesis of pulmonary edema. J Trauma 8:700–703, 1968
17. Parker CJ, Parker RE, Granger DN, et al: Vascular permeability and transvascular fluid and protein transport in the dog lung. Circ Res 48:549–561, 1981
18. Tranbaugh RF, Lewis FR: Mechanisms and idiologic factors of pulmonary edema. Surg Gynecol Obstet 158:193–206, 1984
19. Robin ED: Some basic and clinical challenges in the pulmonary circulation. Chest 81:357–363, 1982
20. Layon AJ, Gallagher TJ: Five percent human albumin in lactated Ringer's solution for resuscitation from hemorrhagic shock: efficacy and cardiopulmonary consequences. Crit Care Med 18:410–413, 1990
21. Guyton AC: Interstitial fluid pressure. II. Pressure-volume curves of interstitial space. Circ Res 26:452–460, 1965
22. Gabel JC: Relationship of pressure and permeability in the pulmonary vasculature. In: Annual Refresher Course. American Society of Anesthesiology, San Francisco, 1976
23. Fishman AP, Hecht HH: The Pulmonary Circulation and Interstitial Space. University of Chicago Press, Chicago, 1969
24. Pietra GG, Szidon JP, Leventhal MM, et al: Histamine and interstitial pulmonary edema in the dog. Circ Res 24:325–337, 1971
25. Demling RH: Correlation of changes in body weight and pulmonary vascular pressures with lung water accumulation during fluid overload. Crit Care Med 7:153–156, 1979
26. Muller WH: Observations on the pathogenesis and management of pulmonary hypertension. Am J Surg 135:302–311, 1976
27. Fishman AP: Hypoxia on the pulmonary circulation: how and where it works. Circ Res 38:221–237, 1976
28. Scanlon TS, Benumof JL, Wahrenbrock EA, et al: Hypoxic pulmonary vasoconstriction and the ratio of hypoxic lung to perfused normoxic lung. Anesthesiology 49:117–181, 1978
29. Rothschild MA, Oratz M, Schreiber SS: Extravascular albumin. N Engl J Med 301:497–498, 1979
30. Rowe MI, Arango A: The choice of intravenous fluid in shock resuscitation. Pediatr Clin North Am 22:269–274, 1975
31. Guyton AC: A concept of negative interstitial pressure based on pressures in implanted capsules. Circ Res 16:452–460, 1963
32. Virgilio RW, Smith DE, Zarins CK: Balanced electrolyte solutions: Experimental and clinical studies. Crit Care Med 7:98–106, 1979
33. Hopewell PC: Failure of positive end-expiratory pressure to decrease lung water content in alloxan-induced pulmonary edema. Am Rev Respir Dis 120:813–819, 1979
34. Hill SL, Elings VB, Lewi FR: Changes in lung water and capillary permeability following sepsis and fluid overload. J Surg Res 28:140–150, 1980
35. Fein A, Leff A, Hopewell PC: Pathophysiology and management of the complications resulting from fire and inhaled products of combustion. Review of the literature. Crit Care Med 8:911–998, 1980
36. Vreim CE, Snashall PD, Demling RH, et al: Lung lymph

and free interstitial protein composition in sheep with edema. Am J Physiol 23-L1650–1653, 1976

37. Bowers RE, Brigham KL, Owen PJ: Salicylate pulmonary edema: the mechanism in sheep and review of the clinical literature. Am Rev Respir Dis 115:261–268, 1977

38. Brigham KL, Woolverton WC, Blake LH, et al: Increased sheep lung vascular permeability caused by *Pseudomonas* bacteremia. J Clin Invest 54:792–804, 1974

39. Weir EK, Grover RF: The role of endogenous prostaglandins in the pulmonary circulation. Anesthesiology 48:201–212, 1978

40. Jacob HS: Damaging role of activated complement in myocardial infarction and shock lung: ramifications for rational therapy. Crit Care State of Art 1:1–18, 1980

41. Taylor AE, Granger DN, Brace RA: Analysis of lymphatic protein flux data. I. Estimation of the reflection coefficient and surface area product for total protein. Microvasc Res 13:297–313, 1977

42. West JB: Ventilation-perfusion relationships. Am Rev Respir Dis 116:919–943, 1977

43. Parker JC, Guyton AC, Taylor AE: Pulmonary interstitial and capillary pressures estimated from intra-alveolar fluid pressures. J Appl Physiol 44:267–276, 1978

44. Macklem PT: Collateral ventilation. N Engl J Med 298:49–50, 1978

45. Demling RH: The role of mediators in human ARDS. J Crit Care 3:56–72, 1988

46. Craddock PR, Fehr J, Kronenberg R, et al: Complement and leukocyte-mediated pulmonary dysfunction in hemodynamics. N Engl J Med 296:769–774, 1977

47. Rinaldo JE: Mediation of ARDS by leukocytes: clinical evidence and implications of therapy. Chest 89:590–593, 1986

48. Slade R, Stead A, Graham J, et al: Comparison of lung antioxidant levels in human and laboratory animals. Am Rev Respir Dis 131:742–746, 1985

49. Dunn CJ, Flemming WE: The role of interleukin 1 in the inflammatory response with particular reference to endothelial cell leukocyte adherence. J Leukocyte Biol 37:745–746, 1985

50. Abraham E: Tumor necrosis factor. Crit Care Med 17:590–591, 1989

51. Gallagher TJ, Civetta JM, Kirby RR, et al: Post-traumatic pulmonary insufficiency: a treatable disease. South Med J 70:1308–1313, 1977

52. Walker L, Eiseman B: The changing pattern of post-traumatic respiratory distress syndrome. Ann Surg 181:693–697, 1975

53. Demling RH, Selinger SL, Bland RL, et al: Effect of hemorrhagic shock on pulmonary microvascular fluid filtration and protein permeability in sheep. Surgery 77:512–519, 1975

54. Staub NC: Pulmonary edema. Physiol Rev 54:678–811, 1974

55. Robin ED, Cross CE, Zelis R, et al: Pulmonary edema. N Engl J Med 288:239–246, 292–304, 1973

56. Anderson RR, Holliday RL, Driedger AA, et al: Documentation of pulmonary capillary permeability in

adult respiratory distress syndrome accompanying human sepsis. Am Rev Respir Dis 119:869–876, 1979

57. Craddock PR, Fehr J, Brigham KL, et al: Complement and leukocyte-mediated pulmonary dysfunction in hemodialysis. N Engl J Med 296:769–774, 1977

58. Bachofen M, Weibel ER: Alterations of gas exchange apparatus in adult respiratory insufficiency associated with sepsis. Am Rev Respir Dis 116:589–615, 1977

59. Clowes GHA, Hirsch MFE, Williams L, et al: Septic lung and shock lung in man. Ann Surg 181:681–692, 1975

60. Sibbald W, Peters S, Lindsay RM: Serotonin and pulmonary hypertension in human septic ARDS. Crit Care Med 8:490–494, 1980

61. Tisi GM: Preoperative evaluation of pulmonary function. Validity indications and benefits. In Murray J (ed): Lung Disease. American Lung Association, New York, 1980

62. Bartlett RH, Brennan MI, Gazzaniga AB, et al: Studies on the pathogenesis and prevention of postoperative pulmonary complications. Surg Gynecol Obstet 137:925–933, 1973

63. Powner DJ, Eross B, Grenvik A: Differential lung ventilation with PEEP in the treatment of unilateral pneumonia. Crit Care Med 5:170–172, 1977

64. Modell JH: The Pathophysiology and Treatment of Drowning and Near Drowning. Charles C Thomas, Springfield, IL, 1971

65. Modell JH, Graves SA, Ketover A: Clinical course of 91 consecutive near-drowning victims. Chest 70:231, 1971

66. Stewardson RH, Nyhus IM: Pulmonary aspiration: an update. Ann Surg 112:1192–1197, 1977

67. Marx GF: Aspiration pneumonitis. JAMA 201:129–130, 1967

68. Mendelson CL: The aspiration of stomach contents into the lungs during obstetric anesthesia. Am J Obstet Gynecol 52:191–205, 1946

69. Gibbs CP, Schwartz DJ, Wynne JW, et al: Antacid pulmonary aspiration in the dog. Anesthesiology 51:380–388, 1979

70. Goldbaum LR, Rami Rez RG, Absalom KB: What is the mechanism of carbon monoxide toxicity? Aviat Space Environ Med 46:1289–1291, 1975

71. Grossling HR, Ellison LH, Degraff AC: Fat embolism: the role of respiratory failure and its treatment. J Bone Joint Surg 56:1327–1337, 1974

72. Nixon JR, Brock-Utne JG: Free fatty acid and arterial oxygen changes following major injury: a correlation between hypoxemia and increased free fatty acid levels. J Trauma 18:23–26, 1978

73. Murray DG, Racz GB: Fat embolism syndrome: a rationale for treatment. J Bone Joint Surg 56:1338–1349, 1974

74. Kusajima K, Webb WR, Parker FB, et al: Pulmonary response of unilateral positive end expiratory pressure (PEEP) on experimental fat embolism. Ann Surg 181:676–680, 1975

75. Jensen NK: Recovery of pulmonary function after crushing injuries of the chest. Dis Chest 22:319–346, 1952

76. Trinkle JK, Richardson JD, Franz JL, et al: Management of flail chest without mechanical ventilation. Ann Thorac Surg 19:355–363, 1975

77. Cullen P, Modell JH, Kirby RR, et al: Treatment of flail chest: use of intermittent mandatory ventilation and positive end-expiratory pressure. Arch Surg 110:1099–1103, 1975

78. Cheney FW, Colley PS: The effect of cardiac output on arterial blood oxygenation. Anesthesiology 52:496–503, 1980

79. Prys-Roberts C, Kelman GR, Greenbaum R: The influence of circulatory factors on arterial oxygenation during anesthesia in man. Anaesthesia 22:257–275, 1967

80. Turaids T, Nobrega FT, Gallagher TJ: Absorptional atelectasis breathing oxygen at simulated altitude: prevention using inert gas. Aerospace Med 38:189–192, 1967

81. Oliven A, Abinader E, Bursztein S: Influence of varying inspired oxygen tensions on the pulmonary venous admixture (shunt) of mechanically ventilated patients. Crit Care Med 8:99–101, 1980

82. Dubois AB, Turaids T, Mammen RE, et al: Pulmonary atelectasis in subjects breathing oxygen at sea level or at simulated altitude. J Appl Physiol 21:828–836, 1966

83. Suter PM, Fairley HB, Schlobohm RM: Shunt, lung volume, and perfusion during short periods of ventilation with oxygen. Anesthesiology 43:617–627, 1975

84. Benumof JL, Rogers SN, Moyce PR, et al: Hypoxic pulmonary vascular pressures with lung water accumulation during fluid overload. Crit Care Med 7:153–156, 1979

85. Benumof JL, Wahrenbrock EA: Blunted hypoxic pulmonary vasoconstriction by increased lung vascular pressures. J Appl Physiol 38:846–950, 1975

86. Winter PM, Smith G: The toxicity of oxygen. Anesthesiology 37:210–241, 1972

87. Douglas ME, Downs JB, Dannemiller FJ, et al: Change in pulmonary venous admixture with varying inspired oxygen. Anesth Analg 55:688–695, 1976

88. Bone RC: Treatment of adult respiratory distress syndrome with diuretics, dialysis, and positive end-expiratory pressure. Crit Care Med 6:136–139, 1978

89. Richardson JD, Franz JL, Grover FL, et al: Pulmonary contusion and hemorrhage—crystalloid versus colloid replacement. J Surg Res 16:330–336, 1974

90. Granger DN, Gabel JC, Drake RE, et al: Physiologic basis for the clinical usage of albumin solutions. Surg Gynecol Obstet 146:97–114, 1978

91. Puri VK, Weil MH, Michaels S, et al: Pulmonary edema associated with a reduction in plasma oncotic pressure. Surg Gynecol Obstet 151:344–348, 1980

92. Zapol W, Snider MT: Pulmonary hypertension in severe acute respiratory failure. N Engl J Med 296:476–480, 1977

93. Sibbald WJ, Patterson NAM, Holliday RL, et al: Pulmonary hypertension in sepsis. Crit Care Med 73:583–591, 1975

94. Gallagher TJ, Civetta JM: Normal pulmonary vascular resistance during acute respiratory insufficiency. Crit Care Med 9:647–650, 1981

95. Colley PS, Cheney FW, Hlastala MP: Ventilation-perfusion and gas exchange effects of sodium nitroprusside in dogs with normal edematous lung. Anesthesiology 50:489–495, 1979

96. Gallagher TJ, Etling T: Failure to alter intrapulmonary shunt with sodium nitroprusside. p. 90. In Abstracts of Scientific Papers. Society of Critical Care Medicine, 1978

97. Hill SL, Elings VB, Lewis FR: Changes in lung water and capillary permeability following sepsis and fluid overload. J Surg Res 28:140–150, 1980

98. Hechtman HB, Weisel RD, Vito L, et al: The independence of pulmonary shunting and pulmonary edema. Surgery 74:300–306, 1973

99. Demling RH, Staub NC, Edmunds LH, Jr: Effect of end-expiratory airway pressure on accumulation of extra-vascular lung water. J Appl Physiol 38:907–912, 1975

100. Tranbaugh RF, Lewis FR, Christensen JM, et al: Lung water changes after thermal injury: the effects of crystalloid resuscitation and sepsis. Ann Surg 192:479–490, 1980

101. Cane RD, Shapiro BA, Harrison RA, et al: Minimizing errors in intrapulmonary shunt calculations. Crit Care Med 8:294–297, 1980

102. Ashbaugh DG, Petty TL: Positive end-expiratory pressure: physiology, indications and contraindications. J Thorac Cardiovasc Surg 65:165–170, 1973

103. Powers SR: The use of PEEP for respiratory support. Surg Clin North Am 54:1125–1136, 1974

104. Dueck R, Wagner PD, West JB: Effects of positive end-expiratory pressure on gas exchange in dogs with normal and edematous lungs. Anesthesiology 47:359–366, 1977

105. Downs JB, Douglas ME, Sanfelippo, et al: Ventilatory pattern, intrapleural pressure and cardiac output. Anesth Analg 56:88–96, 1977

106. Sturgeon CL, Douglas ME, Downs JB, et al: PEEP and CPAP: cardiopulmonary effects of high positive end expiratory pressure. Anesthesiology 43:533–539, 1975

107. Gherini S, Peters RM, Virgilio RW: Mechanical work on the lungs and work of breathing with positive end-expiratory pressure and continuous positive airway pressure. Chest 76:251–256, 1979

108. Demers RR, Irwin RS, Braman SS: Criteria for optimum PEEP. Respir Care 22:596–601, 1977

109. Powers SR, Mannal R, Neclerio M, et al: Physiologic consequences of positive end-expiratory pressure (PEEP) ventilation. Ann Surg 178:265–271, 1973

110. Downs JB, Klein EF, Jr, Modell JH: The effect of incremental PEEP on PaO₂ in patients with respiratory failure. Anesth Analg 52:210–215, 1973

111. Kirby RR, Downs JB, Civetta JM, et al: High-level positive end-expiratory pressure (PEEP) in acute respiratory insufficiency. Chest 67:156–163, 1975

112. Suter PM, Fairley HB, Isenberg MD: Optimum end expiratory airway pressure in patients in acute pulmonary failure. N Engl J Med 292:284–289, 1975

113. Gallagher TJ, Civetta JM, Kirby RR: Terminology update: optimal PEEP. Crit Care Med 6:323–326, 1978

114. Berk JL, Hagen JF, Tong RK, et al: The use of dopamine to correct the cardiac output resulting from positive end-expiratory pressure. A two-edged sword. Crit Care Med 5:269–271, 1977

115. Gallagher TJ, Civetta JM: Goal-directed therapy of acute respiratory failure. Anesth Analg 59:831–834, 1980

116. Smith RA, Kirby RR, Gooding JM, et al: Continuous positive airway pressure (CPAP) by face mask. Crit Care Med 8:483–485, 1980

117. Quist J, Pontoppidan H, Wilson RS, et al: Hemodynamic responses to mechanical ventilation with PEEP: the effect of hypervolemia. Anesthesiology 42:45–55, 1975

118. Patten M, Liebman PR, Hechtman HB: Humorally mediated decreases in cardiac output associated with positive end-expiratory pressure. Microvasc Res 13:137–139, 1977

119. Natori H, Tamaki S, Kira S: Ultrasonographic evaluation of ventilatory effect on inferior venal caval configuration. Am Rev Respir Dis 120:421–427, 1979

120. Howell JBL, Permutt S, Proctor DF, et al: Effect of inflation of the lung on different parts of pulmonary vascular bed. J Appl Physiol 16:71–76, 1961

121. Hobelmann CF, Smith DE, Virgilio RW, et al: Hemodynamic alterations with positive end-expiratory pressure: the contribution of the pulmonary circulation. J Trauma 15:951–958, 1975

122. Robotham JL, Lixfeld W, Holland L, et al: The effects of positive end-expiratory pressure on right and left ventricular performance. Am Rev Respir Dis 121:677–683, 1980

123. Manny J, Patten MT, Liebman PR, et al: The association of lung distention, PEEP and biventricular failure. Ann Surg 187:151–157, 1978

124. Cassidy SS, Gaffney FA, Johnson RL: A perspective on PEEP. N Engl J Med 304:421–422, 1981

125. Laver MB, Strauss HB, Pohost GM: Right and left ventricular geometry: adjustments during acute respiratory failure. Crit Care Med 7:509–519, 1979

126. Kirby RR, Perry JC, Calderwood HW, et al: Cardiorespiratory effects of high positive end-expiratory pressure. Anesth Analg 56:88–96, 1977

127. Jardin F, Farcot JC, Bosiante L, et al: Influence of positive end-expiratory pressure on left ventricular performance. N Engl J Med 304:387–392, 1981

128. Banner MJ, Gallagher TJ, Bluth LI: A new microprocessor device for mean airway pressure measurement. Crit Care Med 9:51–53, 1981

129. Kronberg GM, Quan SF, Schlobohm RM, et al: Anatomic location of tips of pulmonary artery catheters in supine patients. Anesthesiology 51:467–469, 1979

130. Downs JB: A technique for direct measurement of intrapleural pressure. Crit Care Med 8:285–290, 1980

131. Downs JB, Douglas ME: Assessment of cardiac filling pressure during continuous positive-pressure ventilation. Crit Care Med 8:285–290, 1980

132. Fewell JE, Bond GC: Role of sinoaortic receptors in initiating the renal response to continuous positive-pressure ventilation in the dog. Anesthesiology 52:383–386, 1979

133. Laver MB: Dr. Starling and the ventilator kidney. Anesthesiology 52:383–386, 1979

134. Marquez JM, Douglas ME, Downs JB, et al: Renal function and cardiovascular responses during positive airway pressure. Anesthesiology 50:393–398, 1979

135. Ueda H, Neclerio M, Leather RP, et al: Effects of positive end-expiratory pressure ventilation on renal function. Surg Forum 23:209–211, 1972

136. Downs JB, Klein EF, Jr, Desautels D, et al: Intermittent mandatory ventilation: a new approach to weaning patients from mechanical ventilators. Chest 64:331–335, 1973

137. Gallagher TJ: Metabolic alkalosis complicating weaning from mechanical ventilation. South Med J 72:766–787, 1979

138. Milic-Emili J, Henderson AM, Dolovich MB, et al: Regional distribution of inpired gas in the lung. J Appl Physiol 21:749–759, 1966

139. Froese AB, Bryan AC: Effects of anesthesia and paralysis on diaphragmatic mechanism in man. Anesthesiology 44:247–255, 1974

140. Weinstein ME, Rich CL, Peters RM, et al: Hemodynamic and respiratory response to varying gradients between end expiratory pressure in patients breathing continuous positive airway pressure. J Trauma 18:231–235, 1978

141. Douglas ME, Downs JB: Cardiopulmonary effects of intermittent mandatory ventilation. Int Anesthesiol Clin 18:97–121, 1980

142. MacIntyre N: New modalities of ventilation: pressor-support ventilation. pp. 219–230. In Stoelting RK, Barash PG, Gallagher TJ (eds): Advances in Anesthesia. Vol. 6. Year Book Medical Publishers, Chicago, 1989

143. Stock MC: Alternate modes of ventilatory support in adults. pp. 357–384. In Stoelting RK, Barash PG, Gallagher TJ (eds): Advances in Anesthesia. Vol. 5. Year Book Medical Publishers, Chicago, 1988

24

TECHNIQUES OF VENTILATION AND OXYGENATION

James R. Hall, M.D.

Support of breathing will be divided into two categories: support of oxygenation and support of ventilation. Since the underlying physiologies of oxygenation and ventilation are different, although interrelated, support of oxygenation and ventilation must be considered separately when therapy for either or both must be undertaken in a patient.

Support of ventilation is based on mechanical ventilatory provision of part or all of the alveolar ventilation, since this is the means by which carbon dioxide is eliminated, thereby determining alveolar carbon dioxide tension:

$$P_ACO_2 \; \alpha \; (\dot{V}CO_2/\dot{V}_A)$$

Support of oxygenation is achieved by providing supplemental oxygen (increasing the fraction of oxygen inspired, F_IO_2) or improving ventilation-perfusion relationships by increasing resting lung volume. The use of supplemental oxygen can improve the state of oxygenation by increasing the driving pressure for oxygen to enter the blood, ie, increasing alveolar oxygen tension:

$$P_AO_2 = (P_{BAR} - P_{H_2O}) \times F_IO_2 - (k \times P_ACO_2)$$

where

$$k = (F_IO_2 + (1 - F_IO_2)/R) \approx 1.2$$

Note that lowering P_ACO_2 by mechanical ventilation has very little *direct* effect on P_AO_2, especially as F_IO_2

increases above 0.21. The mechanisms by which alteration in resting lung volume and functional residual capacity (FRC) may improve oxygenation are elucidated in Chapters 22 and 23. Techniques for this form of therapy are discussed in this chapter.

FEATURES COMMON TO OXYGENATION AND VENTILATION

Although many technical aspects of the support of oxygenation and ventilation differ, including the breathing circuits, there are three features common to both: (1) provision of fresh gas, including gas flow rate and inspired oxygen concentration; (2) provision of water vapor to the airways; and (3) provision of drugs via the airways. Since these three features are applicable to systems used for support of oxygenation or ventilation, they will be covered in this introductory section.

Provision of Fresh Gases Into Circuits

A flow of fresh gases can be provided into breathing circuits by using either flowmeters or demand valves. Selection of the flow-metering device depends on applications of the circuit and economy. For circuits in which continuous or intermittent gas flow rates are high, the use of demand valves may provide savings in oxygen and air costs. Some ventilators have demand valves incorporated into their circuits to provide gas flow for mechanical breaths or for the patient's spontaneous breaths. Appropriateness of their use is discussed later in the chapter.

The provision of different concentrations of inspired oxygen (F_IO_2) can be attained in three ways: (1) relative flow metering; (2) air-oxygen blending; or (3) air entrainment devices.

Relative Flow Metering

Relative flow metering uses one flowmeter for oxygen and one for air. The outputs of these flowmeters are mixed in a proximal part of the breathing circuit, and adjustment of their relative flow rates provides the desired concentration of oxygen. There are two distinct disadvantages to this system: (1) analysis of the gas mixture and adjustment of flow rates are performed by skilled personnel, an expensive endeavor; and (2) changes in total circuit flow require adjustment of both flowmeters and repeat analyses of the oxygen concentration of the gas mixture, which is time consuming and expensive. For these reasons, relative flow metering is not the method of choice for providing accurate fractional inspired oxygen concentrations.

Air-Oxygen Blenders

Air-oxygen blenders are commercially available devices that permit delivery of known concentrations of oxygen by adjustment of a single control. The flow rate of the resulting gas mixture then can be adjusted by using a single flowmeter. Although the inspired oxygen concentration from this device or any device

should be measured periodically (eg, during each 8-hour shift), adjustments in gas flow from the blender can be made without repeat oxygen analysis, thus effecting considerable savings in personnel time and cost. Air-oxygen blenders, even though they represent an initial capital investment, are the means of choice for oxygen delivery into circuits that need high and/or temporally varying flow rates.

Air Entrainment Devices

Air entrainment devices, which operate on the Venturi principle (Fig. 24-1), are used to provide different oxygen concentrations. The concentrations of oxygen may be provided at several preset levels or over a wide range, depending on the type of entrainment mechanism in the device. The type of entrainment mechanism may also limit the measurement accuracy of the oxygen concentration delivered. Air entrainment devices are suitable for providing different concentrations of inspired oxygen to simple oxygen delivery devices (eg, face masks and face shields), but are not suitable for use with ventilator breathing circuits or nonrebreathing circuits used with distending airway pressure therapy.

Provision of Water Vapor

The provision of adequate humidification is important for two reasons: (1) prevention of excessive water loss via the airways with subsequent inspissation of secretions; and (2) prevention of excess heat loss via the airways (heat of vaporization of water requires 540 cal/g). The point in the conducting airways at which the inspired gases reach the patient's body temperature and reach 100 percent relative humidity at that temperature is the isothermal saturation

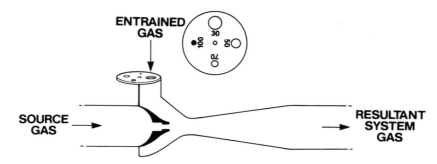

Fig. 24-1. The Venturi principle. The gas source, which generally is oxygen, provides the driving flow for a Venturi device. The entrained gas is generally room air, which has an oxygen concentration of 21 percent. The resultant system gas is a mixture of the source gas and the entrained gas, and its flow rate is the sum of the source gas and entrained gas flow rates. Many devices operating on the Venturi principle permit selection of the resultant F_IO_2 by adjustment of a variable orifice, which limits inflow of the entrained gas.

boundary (ISB).[1] Since many patients undergoing various forms of breathing support will have had much of their natural air conditioning system bypassed with use of an artificial airway, it is important that adequate humidification and heat be provided with the inspired gases in order that the ISB remain as proximal as possible in the airways.

Water vapor is provided by humidifiers. Particulate water is provided by nebulizers, but this is not the primary form desired for routine provision of water via the airways (see below). The amount of water contained in an air sample compared with the capacity of that sample for water vapor is the relative humidity of the sample. To minimize heat and water loss during support of breathing, it is ideal to deliver the gases at a temperature very near the patient's body temperature and 100 percent relative humidity.

Water vapor content, as delivered by humidifiers, is a function of three factors: (1) temperature of the system; (2) surface area for water-gas contact within the system; and (3) duration of time for that contact. Although commercially available humidifier systems for use with breathing circuits vary these three factors in many different ways, they basically can be grouped into four categories: (1) pass-over humidifiers; (2) bubble and jet humidifiers; (3) aerosol-generating humidifiers; and (4) wick humidifiers. The principle for each type of humidifier is illustrated in Figures 24-2 to 24-5. Each of the four types may or may not be heated. Since heating can improve humidification (Fig. 24-6), this is a desirable feature on all systems used for long-term breathing support in adults and on all systems used with neonates and children.

The efficiency of available systems varies widely. Some systems cannot maintain adequate heat pro-

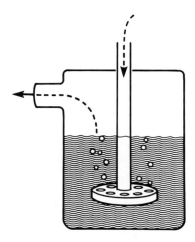

Fig. 24-3. Bubble humidifier. Water content of the respiratory gases is determined by the air-water interface, duration of contact, and temperature of the system, all of which may be variable. Increased surface area for air-water contact increases this system's efficiency above that of the pass-over humidifier.

duction and/or produce sufficient relative humidity to provide satisfactory performance for long-term patient care. Wick humidifiers with a heater incorporated into the system are the most efficient type available.[2] Less efficient systems, even those without heaters, may be used when the patient's natural air conditioning system is not bypassed (eg, face masks, nasal cannulae, and face shields).

The position of the humidifier in the breathing circuit has an important effect both in minimizing heat and water vapor losses before the inspired gases reach the patient and in decreasing and controlling rain-out of water in the circuit tubing. To minimize heat and water losses, the distance between the humidifier and

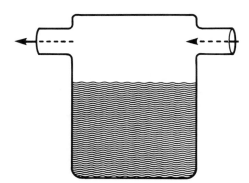

Fig. 24-2. Pass-over humidifier. Water content will vary depending on duration of gas-water contact, temperature of the system, and surface area for contact, which is fixed by the manufacturing design, but may vary in some systems depending on water level. Heating the system is an option used by several manufacturers.

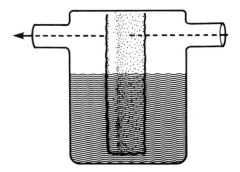

Fig. 24-4. Wick humidifier. Respiratory gases pass through a water-saturated wick, which provides a large surface area for evaporation. The system may be heated to further improve efficiency.

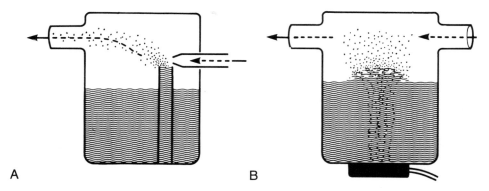

A   B

Fig. 24-5. Aerosol-generating humidifiers. Each of these aerosol generators functions as a humidifier in that the particulate water serves as a source of evaporation for water in the respiratory tract. (**A**) Aerosol is generated by the breakup of water emanating from the capillary tube. (**B**) Particulate water is generated by an ultrasonic transducer, which is below and physically separated from the water within the system.

the patient should be as short as safety and patient care practices permit. Heat also can be maintained by heating the inspiratory limb of the circuit with a heating element, although this may produce additional costs and safety problems. Rain-out of water in the breathing circuit may pose a problem, especially with very efficient systems and with systems in which there is also an aerosol generator. For this reason it is best to maintain the proximal end of the inspiratory limb, including the humidifier, more dependent than the distal end's connection to the patient. Water traps provide means of collecting condensate in the inspiratory limb. Water traps should always be placed in breathing circuits when moderate-to-high levels of distending airway pressure are used so that the circuit is never opened to ambient pressure for the removal of condensate.

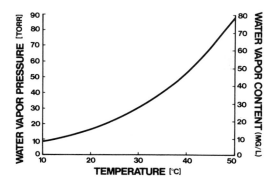

Fig. 24-6. Water vapor pressure and content. Water vapor pressure is a function of system temperature. Water vapor content is shown for saturated conditions (100 percent relative humidity). (Data from Hall and Brouillard.[116])

Provision of Medication Via the Airways

Drugs may be administered via the airways by using *nebulizers* inserted into the breathing circuit. Deposition of drugs, like that of water which is nebulized, will depend on particle size as well as particle density and physical characteristics of the breathing gas mixture.[3,4] Deposition of solute-containing particles will also depend on their hygroscopicity. Particles larger than 1 μm will be deposited primarily in the nasopharyngeal airways, and particles larger than 50 μm may rain out into the breathing circuit. Particles between 0.3 and 1 μm will be deposited in the small airways. For many of the bronchoactive and vasoactive drugs that are nebulized for the nonintubated patient, action will not be limited by "loss" in the upper airways since there is uptake from mucosa and respiratory tract epithelium. Loss in the breathing circuit, however, is not acceptable.

The location of the nebulizer is important to optimize delivery of as much of the prescribed drug dose as possible. The ideal location for the nebulizer is between the breathing circuit and the patient's airway. This is especially important with breathing circuits in which there are high gas flows. If the nebulizer is inserted in the inspiratory limb and continuous nebulization is used, a significant portion of the drug then may be lost out of the expiratory limb. Use of an in-line nebulizer between the breathing circuit and the patient will prevent this (Fig. 24-7). The gas driving this nebulizer may be air or oxygen, as dictated by patient needs. Care must be taken in using certain types of nebulizers to make sure the chamber containing the drug remains in a dependent position throughout the period of nebulization.

Orders for administration of drugs via the airways should include the name of the drug, amount to be

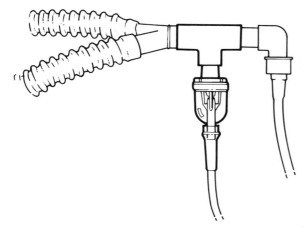

Fig. 24-7. Medication via the airways. An aerosol generator, which can be driven with either air or oxygen, is applied by using a T-connector between the breathing circuit and the connection to the patient's airway. Note the dependent position required for this aerosol generator.

administered, and total volume to be administered or duration of administration. Drugs should never be ordered or administered by volume or concentration alone.

Extreme caution must be exercised when in-line nebulization is performed in circuits providing pressure support ventilation (PSV). The increased pressure in the circuit produced by nebulization can adversely affect the sensing mechanism controlling the PSV gas flow.[5]

SUPPORT OF OXYGENATION

Support of oxygenation can be undertaken by two different means. The simpler of the two is the provision of supplemental oxygen via any one of several devices. The second, more complex, method is an alteration in resting lung volume, ie, FRC, by application of distending airway pressure. Each approach may produce an increase in arterial oxygen tension, but only the distending airway pressure therapy is directed at the underlying pathophysiology of an oxygenating disability.

Provision of Supplemental Oxygen

Oxygen Delivery Devices

Increasing the inspired oxygen concentration can be achieved with any one of several commercially available devices. This approach to improving arterial oxy-gen tension and content, however, does have limits. The constraints placed on this technique include necessity for gas flows high enough to meet inspiratory needs, an adequate reservoir to meet inspiratory needs, and maintenance of the device consistently on the patient. This last constraint is one that must be met in each and every patient for whom it is desired to have a guaranteed minimum inspired oxygen concentration greater than that of room air. Patients will remove masks and face shields because of discomfort, for suctioning, for eating, to be out of bed, etc. Therefore, a device that can be applied easily and will remain continuously in place is desirable. This describes the nasal cannula, but none of the mask devices in routine use. Fourteen devices used routinely for the provision of supplemental oxygen are considered separately and are summarized in Table 24-1.

Nasal Cannula

Nasal cannulae, which are applied easily, deliver 100 percent oxygen via two nasal prongs. The flow from each nasal prong is directed posteriorly, and the nasal passages serve as oxygen reservoirs. A rough rule of thumb for the inspired oxygen fraction (F_IO_2) provided using this technique is an increment of 3 percent/L/min of oxygen flow.[6] The oxygen can be humidified prior to delivery through the small-bore tubing of the device, although care must be taken that water droplets do not accumulate in the tubing and occlude the flow of oxygen. Although these cannulae can be used at flow rates up to 7 to 8 L/min, patient comfort generally dictates a limit on flow of 3 to 4 L/min. Complications related to the use of cannulae, especially at high flow rates, include drying of mucous membranes with subsequent pain and epistaxis. These cannulae, when applied properly, will provide supplemental oxygen continuously while allowing the patient freedom to eat, be suctioned, be out of bed, etc, all without removal of the oxygen delivery device. The facial discomfort with the cannulae, in general, is less than with face masks and face shields.

Nasal Catheter

The nasal catheter is a device placed within one nasal passage, its distal end residing in the nasopharynx. The proximal end of the catheter must be secured outside the anterior naris with tape or other device. These two reasons, along with the fact that this technique requires a moderately large-bore catheter in the nasal passage, make this method for oxygen supplementation less desirable than the nasal cannula.

TABLE 24-1.   Oxygen Delivery Devices[a]

Device	Applications	Approximate Attainable F_IO_2	Gas Flow Rate to Device	Comments
Nasal cannula	General use: adult and pediatric	≤ 0.40	1–6 L/min*	$F_IO_2 \simeq 0.40$ at 6 L/min recommended maximum
Nasal catheter	Not recommended			See text
Simple mask	General use: adult and pediatric	≤ 0.60	6–12 L/min*	Uses small-bore delivery tubing; provides less humidity than aerosol mask
Aerosol mask	General use: adult and pediatric	≤ 0.60	6–12 L/min**	Uses large-bore delivery tubing
Face shield	General use: adult and pediatric	≤ 0.40	6–12 L/min**	Uses large-bore delivery tubing
Partial rebreathing mask	Limited use: adult and pediatric	≤ 0.80	Sufficient to maintain reservoir bag inflation*	Higher F_IO_2 values and humidity available with modification of aerosol face mask (see text)
Non-rebreathing mask	Limited use: adult and pediatric	≤ 1.00	Sufficient to maintain reservoir bag inflation*	Higher F_IO_2 values and humidity available with modification of aerosol face mask (see text)
Venturi mask	Limited use: adult and pediatric	0.24, 0.28, 0.30, 0.35, 0.40	2–8 L/min*	High total gas flow results from lower F_IO_2 settings
Tracheostomy collar	General use: adult and pediatric	≤ 0.60	6–12 L/min**	Preferred oxygen/humidification source for tracheostomies
T tube	Not recommended			See text
Hood	Limited Use: neonatal	≤ 1.00	4–8 L/min**	Delivered temperature and humidity are very important
Tent	Limited use: pediatric	≤ 0.50	10–20 L/min**	Flow requirements dependent on size of tent; F_IO_2 should be monitored continually
Incubator	General use: neonatal	≤ 0.40	5–12 L/min**	F_IO_2 should be monitored continually
Mask for closed system	Limited use: adult	≤ 1.00	Sufficient to maintain reservoir bag inflation**	Application and observation as if the patient were intubated (see text)

[a] *Limited use* and *not recommended* are explained under Comments or in the text. Attainable F_IO_2 is an approximate maximum under ideal conditions, including appropriate maintenance of the device on the patient. Gas flow rate to the device may be oxygen (*) or an air-oxygen mixture obtained with oxygen driving a Venturi device (**).

Face Masks

Oxygen masks are available commercially in several forms. All but the continuous positive airway pressure (CPAP) mask are applied in such a manner that they can be removed readily by the patient.

Simple Mask. The simple mask is supplied with small-bore delivery tubing. Gas flow is unidirectional within the tubing, and washout of the patient's exhalate is dependent on fresh gas flow. Washout of the exhalate occurs through side ports in the body of the mask. This mask is suitable only for use with nonheated, bubble-type humidifiers, since aerosol particles or high humidity can produce water rain-out in the small-diameter tubing, thereby blocking oxygen flow to the mask.

Aerosol Mask. In the aerosol mask, gas flow is unidirectional within the large-bore delivery tubing, and washout of the patient's exhalate through mask side ports is dependent on fresh gas flow. The large-diameter delivery tubing permits use of heated humidifiers and aerosol generators with the mast and, therefore, makes it more suitable than the simple mask for the recently extubated patient. Maximum F_IO_2 attainable with this make is limited by room air entrainment through the side ports of the mask. Higher delivered F_IO_2 values can be achieved with reservoirs ("tusks") placed in the side port holes (Fig. 24-8). Use of good facial mask fit, higher delivered gas flows (driving oxygen flow rate equal to or exceeding 20 L/min), and side port reservoirs will permit delivery not only of higher F_IO_2 but also of higher humidity.

Face Shield. This variation of the simple mask, which supplies oxygen in the vicinity of the face, permits suctioning, mouth care, etc, without removal of the supplemental oxygen source from the patient. It is bulkier and heavier than the face mask and, therefore, is not as useful for the mobile patient.

Partial Rebreathing Mask. With this mask, the patient's fresh gas source is both from a gas reservoir and directly from the fresh gas flow. Since the fresh gas flow is directed both into the reservoir bag and into the volume under the mask itself without the use of valves, exhalate can re-enter the reservoir or be washed out through the side ports in the mask. The amount of exhalate entering the reservoir bag will be dependent on fresh gas flow, which must be adjusted so the patient does not rebreathe exhaled carbon dioxide.

Non-Rebreathing Mask. The non-rebreathing mask is similar to the partial rebreathing mask in construction, with the addition of a valve between the body of the mask and the fresh gas flowing into the reservoir bag, so that all of the exhalate is directed out through the side ports in the body of the mask and cannot enter the reservoir bag. This mask also has one-way flap valves on the exhalation ports to prevent room air entrainment. Fresh gas flow, therefore, must always be adjusted so that the reservoir bag never collapses.

Tracheostomy Collar. The tracheostomy collar is a device with large-bore delivery tubing for application above tracheostomy tubes, tracheostomy buttons, and laryngectomy tubes. The device is not connected directly to the tube and, therefore, its manner of operation is similar to that of the aerosol mask. Unless the application of distending airway pressure is required, no oxygen delivery device should be connected directly to a tracheostomy tube, since traction from the connected circuit may lead to tracheal damage.

T Tube. The T tube is connected directly to an endotracheal tube or tracheostomy tube. Even though a distal reservoir ("tail") may be used to provide higher

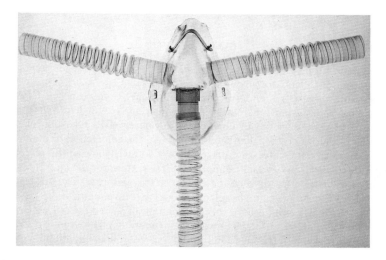

Fig. 24-8. Aerosol mask with reservoirs. This modification of an aerosol mask with "tusk" reservoirs in the exhalation ports provides an additional 100 mL reservoir for increasing F_IO_2 as well as humidity. Modification merely requires the use of 10 cm sections of disposable breathing circuit tubing (2 cm in diameter).

F_IO_2 values, the system is open to ambient pressure and thereby promotes loss of lung volume (decreased FRC). Therefore, the simple T tube system is not recommended for either short-term or long-term use. Maintenance of supplemental oxygen concentrations and appropriate levels of distending airway pressure can be achieved with the breathing circuit shown in Figure 24-9.

Venturi Mask. The Venturi mask is a combination of mask and air entrainment mechanism that, depending on the setting of the mechanism, will provide different delivered concentrations of oxygen. The device operates on the Venturi principle, which is illustrated in Figure 24-1. The mask operates at relatively low driving flows of pure oxygen. The total gas flow in this device or any device operating on the Venturi principle can be calculated as shown in Figure 24-10.

Hoods, Tents, and Incubators. These devices surround the head or body of the patient, generally an infant or small child. The oxygen concentration provided within any one of these devices is a function of oxygen concentration delivered, tightness of all fittings and seals for the device, frequency and duration of personnel entry into the device, and gas flow rate into the device. Since large leaks associated with any of these devices may lower the desired oxygen concentration, fresh gas flow rate will have to be increased accordingly. Each time the device is opened to the room, the desired oxygen concentration will not be reached again until the diluting gases are washed out. These devices, therefore, are not optimum for oxygen delivery if they must be entered frequently for patient care. However, they do provide supplemental oxygen in their contained atmosphere without noxious devices being applied directly to pediatric patients. Another

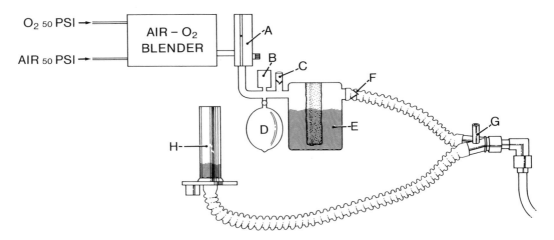

Fig. 24-9. Breathing circuit for distending airway pressure. This circuit, which is similar to the patient circuit component of the intermittent mandatory ventilation circuit (see Fig. 24-20), is used for patients receiving distending airway pressure therapy via endotracheal tube, tracheostomy tube, or CPAP mask. The sources for fresh gas flow are oxygen and air (each at 50 psi), which are blended to give the desired F_IO_2. Other components of the circuit are as follows: (**A**) a high-flow flowmeter; (**B**) a pressure relief valve for preventing pressure buildup in the circuit to greater than 5 cmH$_2$O above the selected expiratory airway pressure level (this should be a threshold resistor valve set approximately 5 cmH$_2$O above the selected expiratory airway pressure level); (**C**) an air entry valve, which is another safety feature for the circuit that provides a fresh gas source (room air) for the inspiratory limb of the circuit if the high-pressure fresh gas sources fail; (**D**) a reservoir bag (a 3-L reservoir bag is generally selected—see text for modifications); (**E**) a humidifier (a wick humidifier, which is the most efficient type for this application, is placed distal to the preceding three circuit components in order that humidity not interfere with their functions); (**F**) a one-way valve, which is located distal to the humidifier so that the potential compressible gas volume of the humidifier is excluded from the actual compressible gas volume of the respiratory limb (note that this also pertains to the preceding circuit components); (**G**) a port for connecting airway pressure monitoring system; and (**H**) an exhalation and distending airway pressure valve, which serves to prevent room air entrainment via the expiratory limb during the patient's inspiration and also to provide the desired expiratory level of airway pressure (an Emerson Exhalation PEEP valve is illustrated).

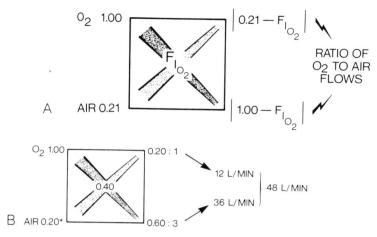

Fig. 24-10. Simplified air entrainment calculation. The entrainment ratio and total gas flow for any device operating on the Venturi principle can be easily calculated. (**A**) Oxygen (oxygen = 100 percent oxygen) is depicted in the upper left corner of the box, and air (air = 21 percent oxygen) is depicted in the lower left corner. The F_IO_2 selected for the system is entered into the box, and oxygen and air are *absolutely* subtracted diagonally across the box, providing $|0.21 - F_IO_2|$ in the upper right corner and $|1 - F_IO_2|$ in the lower right corner. This is the ratio of flows of oxygen (upper) to air (lower). (**B**) A mathematical example for $F_IO_2 = 0.40$ illustrates the Venturi principle: the oxygen-to-air ratio is 1 : 3; if oxygen is set at 12 L/min on the flowmeter, then the flow rate for the entrained air is 36 L/min, giving a resultant system flow of 48 L/min. (For ease of subtraction in this example, air is shown as 20 percent oxygen.)

undesirable and potentially dangerous feature of these devices can be excessive noise. Care must be taken to assure that the oxygen delivery system, including humidifier (as well as all other devices applied on or near an incubator, tent, or hood), do not generate excessive noise levels that can result in subsequent hearing impairment in infants and small children.

Masks for Closed Systems. These masks permit F_IO_2 values up to 1.0 and the application of low levels of distending airway pressure. They fit occlusively so that there is no leak of delivered gases or room air entrainment, but they should be applied so that patient comfort is optimum. An occlusive seal can be achieved with masks having a compliant, air-filled rim (Vital Signs facemask, Vital Signs, Inc., Fig. 24-11) or a J-shaped lip (Bird CPAP mask, Bird/3M Corporation, Fig. 24-12). The mask can be applied using a mask strap so that it will exert minimum pressure on the face of the patient. The mask and the breathing circuit cannot be removed readily by the patient, who must, therefore, be under close observation at all times, just as when intubated. The mask should be clear so that vomitus may be easily seen. The rim of the mask should be lifted periodically to observe the patient's face, especially the bridge of the nose, for any pressure-related injury, although this generally is

not a problem if the mask has been applied properly. The fresh gas flow for delivery of air and oxygen in this type of system may emanate from a demand valve or from a flowmeter and reservoir, which must never empty completely. This circuit, although applicable for delivery of high known concentrations of oxygen,

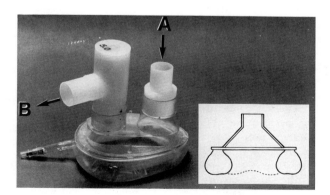

Fig. 24-11. Vital Signs facemask, which is suitable for application of distending airway pressure therapy (see text). Fresh gas enters through port *A* and exhaled gases are removed to the atmosphere via port *B*. The air-filled rim provides a soft, cushioned seal with the patient's face. Mask straps can be applied by using the pegs on the front of the mask.

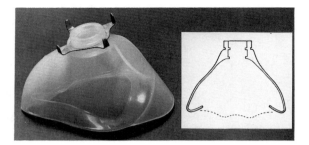

Fig. 24-12. Bird CPAP mask, which is suitable for distending airway pressure therapy (see text). Note the J shape of the lips of the mask (insert). Mask straps can be attached by using the strap ring on the front of the mask.

generally is reserved for the application of distending airway pressure.

Distending Airway Pressure Therapy

Distending airway pressure therapy is the application of positive airway pressure to promote an increase in resting lung volume, or FRC. The increase in FRC is achieved by increasing the volume of alveoli already open and by recruiting alveoli that were closed prior to the application of this therapy. In the spontaneously breathing patient, the application of distending airway pressure may be made in the inspiratory phase as well as in the expiratory phase; both the expiratory level and the inspiratory level have titratable therapeutic end points. In the apneic patient, the application of distending airway pressure can be made during the expiratory phase, and the mechanical ventilator increases airway pressure above the expiratory distending airway pressure level during delivery of the mechanical breath. In the spontaneously breathing patient who is also receiving mechanical ventilatory support, distending airway pressure can be applied during the patient's inspiration and expiration; the delivery of a mechanical breath increases airway pressure above the expiratory airway pressure level (see Chapters 22 and 23).

Varied nomenclature has been applied to this therapy over the years. One form of nomenclature is based on the airway pressures generated by the therapy and another is based on the type of breathing circuit involved with generation of the positive airway pressure. The simplest approach, and the one in which the most information is transmitted concerning this form of therapy, is that in which the *actual airway pressure* is indicated and no differing forms of nomenclature are used. The use of the term *distending airway pressure* is not an attempt to add yet another name for this therapeutic modality, but it is an effort to direct con-

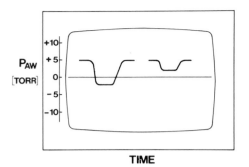

Fig. 24-13. Airway pressure monitoring. Two different airway pressures (P_{aw}) are shown as they might appear in a calibrated oscilloscopic display of airway pressure. Time is shown on the x-axis, a function of oscilloscopic sweep speed. Airway pressure is shown on the y-axis over the -10 to $+10$ mmHg range. Note the difference that would be seen with $P_{aw} = (+5)/(-2)$ mmHg versus $P_{aw} = (+5)/(+2)$ mmHg.

sideration toward use and quantitation of the therapy and away from acronymic confusion.

A better understanding of the therapy and its quantitation can be achieved by considering an example. By convention, pressure during spontaneous breathing will be indicated as expiratory/inspiratory; units of measurement may be either cmH_2O or mmHg.* For example, a spontaneously breathing patient with an airway pressure of $(+5)/(-2)$ mmHg is depicted in the left side of Figure 24-13. If the inspiratory airway pressure level were increased to $(+2)$ mmHg without any change in the expiratory pressure level, the airway pressure now would appear as depicted in the right side of Figure 24-13. These examples appear as they would in an oscilloscopic display. Since both the inspiratory pressure level and the expiratory pressure level are titratable, it is important that the airway pressure be routinely monitored.

Circuit for Distending Airway Pressure Therapy

The breathing circuit for providing distending airway pressure therapy has several essential components. The circuit may or may not be a part of the circuit attached to a mechanical ventilator, since support of ventilation and support of oxygenation are separate functions. A circuit that is independent of a mechanical ventilator is shown in Figure 24-9. This circuit would be used for the application of all levels of dis-

---

* If airway pressure is monitored on a vascular pressure monitoring system where the unit of measure is *mmHg*, measurements can be converted to *cmH_2O*: mmHg $\times$ 1.36 = cmH_2O.

tending airway pressure, ranging from low maintenance pressures (eg, P_{aw} = 5/0 cmH$_2$O) to very high
therapeutic pressure (eg, P_{aw} = 38/34 cmH$_2$O).

Before each circuit component is considered separately, it should be noted that the expiratory (maximum) and inspiratory (minimum) levels of airway
pressure basically are functions of the expiratory
valve and the fresh gas flow rate, respectively. Although different equipment is available for delivering
each, provision of distending airway pressure therapy
consists merely of the selection and variation of these
two system variables.

Fresh Gas Source

The fresh gas source for the circuit can be either a
high-flow source and reservoir bag or a demand valve.
When a fresh gas source and reservoir bag are used,
the flowmeter through which the fresh gas source is
provided must have the capability for metering high
flow rates, which may exceed 60 L/min. The reservoir
bag must be compliant enough to provide net movement of several hundred millimeters of gas, but not so
compliant as to become markedly distended at higher
airway pressures; generally, a 3 L anesthesia bag is
selected. For higher levels of distending airway pressure, where the less-compliant anesthesia bags are too
small for tidal excursion of adult patients, a 3 L bag
can be encased within a pliable netting, eg, women's
hosiery. With the reservoir bag in the circuit, the fresh
gas flow rate is adjusted to attain the desired inspiratory level of the distending airway pressure. When a
demand valve is used in this circuit, the demand flow
rate must be adjusted to provide the desired inspiratory pressure level for the distending airway. Selection of an appropriate demand valve is critical since
lack of sensitivity can lead to increased work of
breathing and impairment in the breathing pattern.[7–9]

Humidifier

Since distending airway pressure therapy generally is
provided via an endotracheal or tracheostomy tube,
the natural air conditioning system of the patient is
bypassed and adequate humidification is of paramount importance. The location of the humidifier in
relation to the one-way valve of the inspiratory limb is
also important. If the gaseous volume within the humidifier is large, it is desirable to locate the humidifier proximal to a one-way valve in the inspiratory
limb. The one-way valve must not become partially or
completely dysfunctional because of the collection of
condensate; to avoid such problems, another valve
may have to be placed between the fresh gas source or
reservoir and the humidifier. Heated wick humidifiers
provide the most efficient humidification for these
high-flow applications.[2]

Connection to Patient

The distending airway pressure circuit may be applied to the patient's airway via mask or via endotracheal or tracheostomy tube. The use of a mask for safe
and efficient application of distending airway pressure therapy has been reported in adults and infants.[10–13] The use of a mask does have several limitations: (1) the patient must be conscious and alert, and
should be able to remove the device if vomiting occurs; (2) there must be no serious facial injuries; (3)
the applied distending airway pressure should not exceed 10 to 12 cmH$_2$O (7 to 9 mmHg), which is less than
the opening pressure of the esophagus; and (4) the
duration of the distending airway pressure therapy
should not exceed approximately 72 hours. Application of distending airway pressure therapy by mask
may not necessitate placement of a nasogastric tube,
although if one is used, it can be passed through a
small sealed opening made in the mask. Distending
airway pressure therapy is more commonly provided
by applying the circuit described to the patient's airways via an endotracheal tube.

Expiratory Valve

For the patient receiving distending airway pressure
therapy, the expiratory level of the airway pressure is
determined by selection of either an expiratory valve
with a fixed pressure setting or a variable valve requiring pressure adjustment. The expiratory valve
that delivers the distending airway pressure should
function as a threshold resistor, not as a flow resistor.[14] That is, the valve should open at the desired
level of expiratory airway pressure and maintain that
pressure regardless of the flow rate through the valve
(Fig. 24-14). If a valve has flow-resistive characteristics, then high gas flows generated within the circuit
(eg, by an attempted cough by the patient) may produce back pressure great enough to cause pulmonary
barotrauma. Also, when a flow-resistive valve is used,
expiratory gas flow may be retarded so that mean
airway pressure becomes elevated, resulting in
impedance to venous return and decreases in cardiac output and systemic arterial blood pressure[15]
(Fig. 24-15).

The expiratory valve not only provides the expiratory pressure level, but also may serve as a one-way
valve in the expiratory limb, preventing entrainment
of room air into the circuit. If the expiratory valve is
part of a mechanical ventilator circuit, then the valve

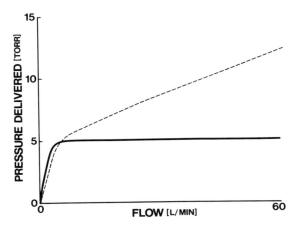

Fig. 24-14. Resistances with threshold resistor versus flow resistor. The performances of a threshold resistor (———) and a flow resistor (- - - -) are illustrated for a flow range of 0 to 60 L/min. Once the threshold resistor valve has reached its preset pressure, the delivered pressure (airway pressure) does not rise. The flow resistor valve will produce a continuing increase in pressure over the entire flow range.

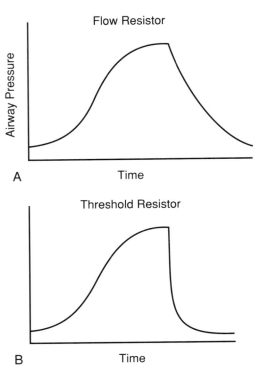

Fig. 24-15. Threshold versus flow resistor valves. The difference between (**A**) a threshold resistor and (**B**) a flow resistor is seen in the expiratory phase of the airway pressure curve. The threshold resistor permits near-instantaneous return to baseline pressure level, whereas the flow resistor impedes gas flow, thereby delaying return of airway pressure to baseline. These differences can be observed easily by using airway pressure monitoring techniques.

also may serve the function of stopping gas flow from the expiratory limb during the mechanical breath to the patient. Several commercial valves, which are available for application in any breathing circuit, will be considered, as will an underwater seal.

Boehringer PEEP Valve. Boehringer PEEP valves (Boehringer Laboratories, Inc.) are weighted-ball systems that can also serve as one-way valves for the expiratory limb. These devices are available for several pressure levels (2.5, 5, 10, and 15 cmH$_2$O) and can be stacked serially to provide higher levels, including intercalated values of expiratory airway pressure. They must be maintained in an upright position, since their function and integrity are gravity dependent.

Emerson Exhalation PEEP Valve. The Emerson Exhalation PEEP valve (J.H. Emerson Co.) is a water-weighted diaphragm. It functions as a one-way valve in the expiratory limb and also can function to close the expiratory limb during mechanical ventilation when the valve is part of a mechanical ventilator circuit. This valve must be maintained in an upright position since it is water-filled and since the integrity of function as a one-way valve is dependent on seating of the diaphragm over the expiratory port in the base of the valve.

Siemans-Elema PEEP Valve. The Siemens-Elema PEEP valve (Siemans-Elema AB) is a spring-loaded platen that opposes the port connected to the expir-

atory limb of the breathing circuit. Tension on the spring and, therefore, opening pressure on the expiratory limb are variably adjustable.

Vital Signs PEEP Valves. Vital Signs PEEP valves (Vital Signs, Inc.) also have a spring-loaded platen, although the physical configuration of the springs is different from that in the Siemans-Elema valve. The pressure applied by each valve is preset, and several different valves with different pressures are available (5, 7.5, 10, and 12.5 cmH$_2$O).

Underwater Seal. Underwater seal is the oldest means for applying distending airway pressure therapy. A rigid extension of the expiratory limb is placed beneath water, with the depth of placement determining the pressure generated within the expiratory circuit. The diameter of this extension should equal the diameter of the expiratory limb itself, since this will prevent flow-resistive pressure generation.

SUPPORT OF VENTILATION

The purpose of ventilation is the maintenance of the body's acid-base homeostasis by the excretion of carbon dioxide. This is accomplished in the spontaneously breathing individual by the titration of alveolar ventilation against several feedback variables, including carbon dioxide tension, hydrogen ion concentration, and arterial oxygen tension. Ventilation must be supported mechanically when a patient cannot maintain sufficient alveolar ventilation to eliminate the carbon dioxide being presented each minute to the lungs by the pulmonary arterial circulation.

Many patients who need ventilatory support also have metabolic acid-base disturbances, predominantly metabolic alkalosis.[16] Since to make these patients eucapnic with the mechanical ventilatory support would exacerbate their metabolic alkalosis and prolong weaning from mechanical ventilation, the support of mechanical ventilation is directed primarily at assisting the body in defense of the arterial pH. Carbon dioxide tension is used as a secondary determinant unless some overriding disease process dictates otherwise (eg, increased intracranial pressure with a need to maintain hypocapnia).

An arterial pH within a normal range (7.35 to 7.40) is maintained by mechanical ventilatory support of carbon dioxide elimination, since arterial carbon dioxide tension is proportional to alveolar carbon dioxide tension, which in turn is related to alveolar ventilation:

$$P_aCO_2 \propto P_ACO_2 \propto (\dot{V}CO_2/\dot{V}_A)$$

The amount of alveolar ventilation needed is determined by the amount of carbon dioxide being produced and presented to the lungs each minute. A practical approach to mechanical ventilatory support in defense of arterial pH is presented below; this section will develop the background reasons for the amount of support predicted on carbon dioxide production. If carbon dioxide production equals 200 mL/min, then to make the patient eucapnic ($P_aCO_2 = P_ACO_2 = 40$ mmHg) would require the following level of alveolar ventilation:

$$\dot{V}_A = \dot{V}CO_2/F_ACO_2$$
$$\dot{V}_A = (200\ mL/min)/(40\ mmHg/713\ mmHg)$$
$$\dot{V}_A = 3,565\ mL/min$$

Since the alveolar space of the lungs is in series with the conducting airways, a volume greater than the alveolar ventilatory volume must be provided to eliminate carbon dioxide. This is the volume of the conducting airways, or the anatomic dead space (V_{DANAT}), which is approximately 2.2 mL/kg. Anatomic dead space ventilation ($\dot{V}_{DANAT}$) in a 70-kg individual with a respiratory rate of 8 breaths/min would be:

$$\dot{V}_{DANAT} = 2.2\ mL/kg \times 70\ kg \times 8/min$$
$$\dot{V}_{DANAT} = 1,232\ mL/min$$

The total volume of gases moved in and out of the lungs in 1 minute is the minute ventilation ($\dot{V}_E$), which is the sum of alveolar ventilation and dead space ventilation (taken here as anatomic dead space ventilation):

$$\dot{V}_E = \dot{V}_A + \dot{V}_{DANAT}$$
$$\dot{V}_E = 3,565\ mL/min + 1,232\ mL/min$$
$$\dot{V}_E = 4,797\ mL/min$$

Mechanical ventilatory support is basically the provision of the minute ventilation based on a knowledge of the patient's measured or estimated dead space and an estimation of the need for the level of support of the alveolar ventilation. In practice, this entails selection of a delivered tidal volume of 12 to 15 mL/kg at a mechanical frequency sufficient to support carbon dioxide excretion in defense of arterial pH.

The volume delivered by a mechanical breath is a result of the pressure difference generated between the airway* of the patient and the alveoli, since gas flow in a tubular system is the result of a pressure difference. The flow of gases into the lungs is opposed by the resistance of the patient's airways and endotracheal or tracheostomy tube and the compliance, or stiffness, of the patient's lungs. Increased resistance, either in the airways or in some portion of the mechanical system, will oppose delivery of the intended gas volume. Likewise, decreased compliance (increased stiffness) will oppose delivery of the mechanical breath. Since various pathophysiologic processes of pulmonary disease, as well as mechanical components of the ventilator system, may produce increased resistance and/or decreased compliance, the resultant effect that this will have on delivered tidal volume should be appreciated for each mechanical ventilatory system (Fig. 24-16).

Mechanical Ventilators

More than 100 mechanical ventilators are available commercially in the world today.[17] When this total is combined with the number of commercially available breathing circuits and individually constructed breathing circuits, some of which are described in the literature, there are several hundred conceivable systems that could be used to provide mechanical venti-

---

* *Airway* indicates the point of connection of the patient to the breathing circuit.

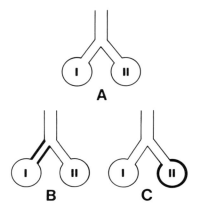

Fig. 24-16. Impedance of lung compartments. (**A**) Compartments I and II are shown with equal resistances and compliances; gas flow would be evenly distributed between the two compartments. (**B**) The resistance of compartment I exceeds that of compartment II; gas flow within a finite time period would be less into compartment I than into compartment II, although, over an infinite inspiratory time, gases would be evenly distributed, since the compliances of I and II are equal. (**C**) The compliance of compartment II is decreased; gas distribution will be uneven no matter what the duration of inspiration, compartment I receiving proportionately more gas than compartment II.

lation. Since it would not be reasonable to undertake detailed consideration of all of these, an overview of mechanical ventilators will be provided.

Mechanical ventilators can be classified into negative-pressure and positive-pressure devices. Within each category, characterization and classification of different ventilators can be made, depending on several of their mechanical or operational features.

Negative-Pressure Ventilators

The iron lung, which was one of the earliest forms of mechanical ventilatory support available, was described in 1929 by Drinker and McKhann[18] and by Drinker and Shaw.[19] Although negative-pressure ventilators are not used for routine postoperative care today, they are being used for long-term ventilatory support, including home care.[20–23] Two types of currently available negative-pressure ventilators, the iron lung and the cuirass, will be described.

Iron Lung

The iron lung, a large, rigid box, encloses the entire body of the patient except for the head. Ventilation of the patient occurs when an electrically driven motor

powering a bellows generates negative pressure within the box surrounding the patient. Since part of this negative pressure around the patient's chest is transmitted through the chest wall into the distal airways, a pressure gradient is produced between the patient's mouth (atmospheric pressure) and the lung parenchyma so that gas flows into the lungs. The amount of negative pressure generated within the iron lung is the primary mechanical determinant of the patient's tidal volume and is a function of the extent of the bellows' movement, which is controlled by the position of the drive arm on the drive shaft. The rate of ventilation is a function of the rotational speed and gear reduction in the drive assembly, which is controlled by a variable resistor. The advantages of this type of ventilatory support include the patient's continuing ability to speak and eat, as well as the lack of need to artificially maintain the airway in the awake patient, who can protect the airway. Its disadvantages include the inaccessibility of the patient for nursing care and the need to pass all forms of tubing and monitor wiring required by the patient into the iron lung through specially sealed ports.

Cuirass Ventilator

Another form of negative-pressure mechanical ventilator is the cuirass, or chest shell, ventilator. This unit surrounds only the trunk of the patient, leaving the head, neck, and extremities free and accessible. The anterior and lateral portions of the shell are rigid, and the remainder of the trunk is sealed into the ventilator with a plastic wrap. A negative pressure is produced within this shell by a negative pressure-generating device, which is attached via a noncompliant hose. This type of mechanical ventilatory support has advantages similar to those of the iron lung, as well as improved access for patient care. Its disadvantages include the continued limited access to the trunk of the patient, the difficulty in attaining a satisfactory seal in some patients, and the relative immobility to which the patient must be subjected to be ventilated by the unit. A triggering mechanism has been described for the cuirass ventilator that permits assisted negative-pressure ventilation (U-Cyclit, J.H. Emerson Co.).

Positive-Pressure Ventilators

The usual function of a positive-pressure ventilator is to move a volume of gas into a patient's lungs and then to permit passive expulsion of the exhalate by the patient. Since gas flow in any system of tubes occurs in response to a difference in pressure, the tidal volume delivery will occur when the pressure at the patient's airway exceeds the pressure in the alveoli. Gas flow during the inspiratory phase will be opposed by the resistance of the airways and by the resistance of components of the ventilator system, as well as by the compliance of the lung-thorax unit. Expiratory gas flow occurs when the alveolar pressure exceeds the pressure at the airway. Gas flow out of the lungs is a function of the lung-thorax compliance and is opposed by airway resistance and resistance of components of the expiratory limb of the ventilator system. To promote understanding of how this volume of gas is generated and driven into the lungs, including the frequency with which this is done, several characteristics of positive-pressure ventilators will be considered. These characteristics are also the basis of classification of positive-pressure ventilators, and include their power source, mechanism for volume delivery, cycling mechanisms, modes of ventilation, breathing circuits, safety, and other technical features.

Power Source

The power provided for delivery of volume by a positive-pressure mechanical ventilator is either electric or pneumatic. Pneumatic sources may have their flows directly or indirectly converted into the volume provided. Electric power generally is translated into delivered volume, with an electric motor driving a direct volume-displacement device or powering a gas compressor. In the latter case, the primary power source is electric, while the actual power used as the mechanism for volume delivery is pneumatic.

Mechanism for Volume Delivery

The characteristic of mechanical ventilators that describes the mechanism for volume delivery generally is considered in terms of pressure or flow generation.[17,24] A mechanical ventilator is described as a flow generator or pressure generator, depending on which characteristic of volume delivery remains constant or relatively constant throughout the inspiratory phase. The *flow generator* maintains a constant flow rate (Fig. 24-17) or constant flow pattern (Fig. 24-18) during the inspiratory phase while airway pressure changes. Changes in lung or thoracic compliance or in airway resistance will have less effect on delivery of respiratory gases with ventilators that are flow generators than with ventilators that are pressure generators.[25] Ventilators that function as *pressure generators* maintain a constant amount of pressure or a constant pressure pattern during the inspiratory phase. Flow rate is variable, decaying exponentially during inspiration with a true pressure generator (Fig. 24-19). It should be noted that few ventilators function as pure pres-

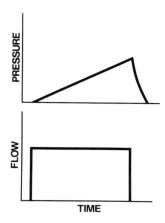

Fig. 24-17. Constant-flow generator. A mechanical ventilator that performs as a constant-flow generator will produce a constant gas flow rate into the patient's airways, while airway pressure will rise linearly until the end of inspiration.

sure or pure flow generators. It also should be appreciated that this distinction does not correspond to the cycling or limiting mechanisms by which ventilators are classified (see below).

Cycling Mechanisms

Considerations of cycling mechanisms include cycling from expiration to inspiration (ie, beginning of the mechanical breath) and cycling from inspiration to expiration (ie, ending the mechanical breath).

Cycling the ventilator for the cessation of the inspiration phase (beginning of the expiratory phase) may

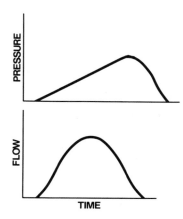

Fig. 24-18. Variable-flow generator. A mechanical ventilator functioning as a variable-flow generator will have a constant flow pattern into the patient's airways, eg, sine wave illustrated here. Pressure will rise in a curvilinear manner until the end of inspiration.

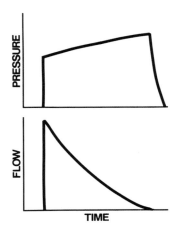

Fig. 24-19. Constant-pressure generator. A mechanical ventilator that functions as a constant-pressure generator will produce a rapidly rising, then constant, pressure on the patient's airways, while flow decreases exponentially until the end of inspiration.

be controlled by time, volume, pressure, flow, or a combination of these. When ventilators are classified by a cycling mechanism, the changeover from inspiration to expiration is the referred cycling mechanism. If the ventilator is *time-cycled*, the duration of the inspiratory phase is determined by a timing mechanism and is independent of the volume delivered, the inspiratory pressure attained, the inspiratory flow characteristics, and the patient's pulmonary condition. Time cycling may be accomplished with electronic, electromechanical, pneumatic, or fluidic techniques.

For the *volume-cycled* ventilator, the volume delivered is the independent variable; the inspiratory phase ends when this volume has been attained. It should be noted that this volume is the volume *delivered* by the system, but may not be the volume *received* by the patient. The duration of inspiration, inspiratory gas flow pattern, and peak inspiratory pressure are variables dependent on the patient's pulmonary condition or other system conditions. Mechanisms for volume cycling include a full excursion of a preset volume displacement device, integration of flow, and detection of an electrical signal that has characteristics proportional to volume displaced. The last two mechanisms provide feedback to interrupt or redirect volume delivery.

With *pressure-cycled* ventilators, the inspiratory phase ends when a preset pressure is reached. Dependent variables are the absolute inspiratory time, delivered volume, and inspiratory gas flow; the normal or disease characteristics of the patient's lungs will be the primary determinant for these variables.

For the *flow-cycled* ventilator, the inspiratory phase ends when the delivered gas flow has reached a preset level. Dependent variables include delivered volume and absolute time of the inspiratory phase. The mechanism used is the inspiratory valve (Bennett valve) developed for this type of cycling, changing from the inspiratory to the expiratory position when a predetermined low flow rate is reached (approximately 1 L/min).[17]

Some ventilators have the capacity for selecting the cycling mode. Other ventilators have a built-in primary cycling mechanism with a different secondary, or backup, cycling mechanism. Other ventilators have combination cycling mechanisms, although most of these have a designated primary cycling mechanism.

Cessation of the expiratory phase (beginning of the inspiratory phase) may be initiated automatically or by the patient. Automatic cycling, or primary ventilator control, generally is accomplished with a timing mechanism. This form of cycling is independent of the pressure, expiratory volume, and expiratory gas flow rate or pattern. The time-cycling mechanisms are the same as those that end the inspiratory phase.

Inspiration may be cycled by the patient ("patient-triggered"). The inspiratory phase begins when a preset negative pressure has been generated by the patient. Most ventilators with this form of cycling have a variable sensitivity control, which can be adjusted to meet the needs of different inspiratory efforts by the patient. This also describes a mode of ventilation, assist-mode ventilation (see below).

Modes of Ventilation

Modes of ventilation fall into one of three categories or combinations thereof; control-mode ventilation (CMV), assist-mode ventilation (AMV), and intermittent mandatory ventilation (IMV). CMV is the oldest form of mechanical ventilatory support and encompasses the function of the negative-pressure ventilators, as well as of the earlier models of positive-pressure ventilators. AMV was developed as an option for CMV ventilators and used the same circuits with modifications to detect the patient's inspiratory effort and alter subsequent cycling. IMV is a newer form of ventilation, requiring a circuit different from those for CMV and AMV.

Control-Mode Ventilation. CMV provides mechanical breaths with equal time intervals between each. A circuit exclusively for CMV has no provision for delivery of gas volume when a patient attempts spontaneous breathing: the effort will only generate negative pressure within all or part of the breathing circuit, depending on how the circuit's valves are arranged. These patient efforts, while not contributing to effective alveolar ventilation, can markedly increase the patient's work of breathing. True CMV is only suitable for the apneic patient, and a circuit exclusively for CMV is not recommended for general use in an intensive care unit, since ventilators and circuits that provide IMV can perform the CMV function as well (see below).

Assist-Mode Ventilation. Ventilators operating as AMVs will sense patient effort to inspire and will follow with a mechanical breath. The detection of the patient's inspiratory effort can be made via electronic, magnetic, or pneumatic transduction, the last being the most common method. AMV circuits have no means for providing volume during a patient's spontaneous ventilatory effort other than positive-pressure delivery of gas. Since no beneficial effects of ventilatory support with AMV have been found when compared with CMV, and since ventilators and circuits exclusively for CMV are not recommended, circuits designed exclusively for AMV are also not recommended.[26]

Assist-Control-Mode Ventilation. Assist-control-mode ventilation is a combination mode wherein the ventilator will provide assisted breaths in response to patient effort and will also provide a set rate of mechanical breaths to the patient each minute. Again, since this circuit has no provision for supporting the patient's spontaneous ventilatory effort with other than positive-pressure gas delivery, it is not a recommended means of support.

Intermittent Mandatory Ventilation. IMV is a means of ventilatory support whereby the patient may breathe spontaneously in an unimpeded, unassisted manner *and* receive a set number of mechanical breaths per minute in support of alveolar ventilation.[27] The patient breathes at the rate and depth selected through normal physiologic mechanisms, but also receives the number of mechanical breaths selected for the IMV rate. This rate may be zero, at which point the patient could be on the IMV circuit of a mechanical ventilator or on a spontaneous breathing circuit independent of a mechanical ventilator (see the section *Circuit for Distending Airway Pressure Therapy*).

Figure 24-20 is a schematized presentation of an IMV circuit. The ventilator circuit can be considered

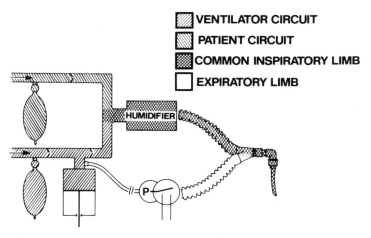

Fig. 24-20. Intermittent mandatory ventilation circuit. This simplified schematic representation of an IMV circuit shows the patient circuit component and the ventilatory circuit component. Depending on the actual ventilator used, the fresh gas sources may be at 50 psi or less; the circuit illustrated has a premixed air-oxygen source (*arrows*) for each circuit subcomponent. The patient circuit (*top*) has its own reservoir as well as a one-way valve providing unidirectionality of flow. The ventilator circuit (*bottom*) also has a reservoir bag and one-way valve, as well as a means for volume generation, which is illustrated with a piston in this example. The one-way valve distal to the piston prevents any gas flow from the inspiratory limb or the patient circuit subcomponent. Both circuits enter a common humidifier, which serves the inspiratory limb. The expiratory limb ends in a combination valve, which serves to prevent room air entrainment (one-way valve function), provide the desired expiratory pressure level for distending airway pressure therapy, and occlude the expiratory limb during mechanical inspiration. The last function is accomplished by the charging line, which is shown between the piston of the ventilatory circuit and the expiratory valve (*P*).

as having two component circuits, one serving the mechanical ventilator and one serving the patient's spontaneous breathing. Each component of the circuit has a fresh gas source, a reservoir bag, and one-way valving to provide unidirectional gas flow. It is most efficacious to use a blender to provide the F_IO_2 setting prior to flowmetering the fresh gas into either circuit. Although separate humidifiers could be used for the ventilator circuit and for the patient circuit, it is more common to combine the two circuits prior to their entry into a single humidifier, which then serves the inspiratory limb of the breathing circuit. The humidifier that serves the breathing circuit must be capable of efficiently warming and humidifying a high continuous gas flow; this would be a wick-type humidifier.[2]

The gas source for the ventilator circuit must have a flow rate sufficient to accommodate the tidal volume and minute ventilation settings for mechanical ventilation. When the ventilator circuit is supplied from a fresh gas source with a reservoir bag, the flow rate must be sufficient to prevent collapse of the reservoir bag. The flowmeter for the ventilator circuit can have a low maximum flow rate capability (15 L/min). The gas source for the patient circuit must have a flow rate capability sufficient to maintain inspiratory airway pressure at the desired level. Adequacy of the flow rate is assessed by continuously monitoring airway pressure, ie, inspiratory level, and adjusting the flow rate to the patient circuit accordingly. The flowmeter for the patient circuit must have a high maximum flow rate capability (75 L/min; eg, the High-Flow Oxygen Flow Meter, Timeter Instrument Corporation, Lancaster, PA). The inspiratory flow rate for the ventilator circuit has to be adjusted only when a change is made in set tidal volume or mechanical frequency. The gas flow rate into the patient circuit has to be adjusted to accommodate the patient's inspiratory needs while maintaining the desired level of inspiratory airway pressure. Expiratory gas flow proceeds via the expiratory limb through the exhalation valve and the valve for providing distending airway pressure; these two valve functions may be combined into one valve serving both purposes (Fig. 24-21).

To provide distending airway pressure therapy and mechanical ventilatory support concomitantly, it is necessary to have a ventilator and breathing circuit capable of meeting the needs for both forms of support. It is *not* satisfactory to use a ventilator or a breathing circuit in which the demand valve or flow rate control is used simultaneously for both the ventilator circuit and the patient circuit. Since the flow rate control or demand valve may be an integral part of either the inspiratory timing or the mechanism controlling tidal volume, this will lead to undesired changes in mechanical ventilatory parameters when

the flow rate for the patient's spontaneous circuit is changed, or vice versa. *Flow rate controls for the fresh gas sources must be separate for the patient circuit and the ventilator circuit.* When a ventilator is designed to use one flow source for both the patient circuit and the ventilator circuit, it is necessary to provide a spontaneous breathing circuit for the patient that is separate from the ventilator circuit. This is accomplished easily by adapting a circuit as described above to a mechanical ventilator. The ventilator circuit then serves mechanical ventilatory needs, and the externally applied circuit provides fresh gas flow during the patient's spontaneous breathing.

Two modifications of the originally described IMV technique have been proposed in order that the delivery of mechanical breaths may be in phase with the patient's inspiratory effort. Although no exact convention exists for their nomenclature, they are known as synchronized IMV (SIMV) and intermittent demand ventilation (IDV). Each of these two modifications of IMV delivers the positive-pressure mechanical breath immediately after a patient's spontaneous inspiratory effort occurs. SIMV provides a set number of mechanical breaths each minute, and each of these breaths is synchronized with patient effort, if present. If the patient is apneic, mechanical ventilatory support is provided at the rate set for the SIMV. IDV provides synchronized mechanical breaths at a preset ratio to the number of spontaneous breaths the patient is taking. That is, if IDV is set for 1 mechanical breath for every 6 patient breaths and the patient is breathing 18 times per minute, 3 mechanical breaths will be provided each minute. However, if the patient becomes apneic, there will be no mechanical breaths provided, and alveolar ventilation will be zero. If IDV is used, some back-up mechanism for mechanical ventilation should be provided.

Pressure Support Ventilation

Pressure support ventilation (PSV) is a newer form of ventilatory support that augments the patient's inspiratory efforts with pressure applied at a selected value. PSV is applied throughout the inspiratory phase during spontaneous ventilation. The PSV technique differs from the *modes* of ventilation (discussed above) and from distending airway pressure therapy. PSV can be used for patients who are breathing completely spontaneously or who are being supported with IMV; it can also be used for patients receiving distending airway pressure therapy.

PSV, which is an adjunct form of ventilatory support, is controlled with a microprocessor incorporated into the mechanical ventilator's circuit. When the patient makes the initial inspiratory effort, the

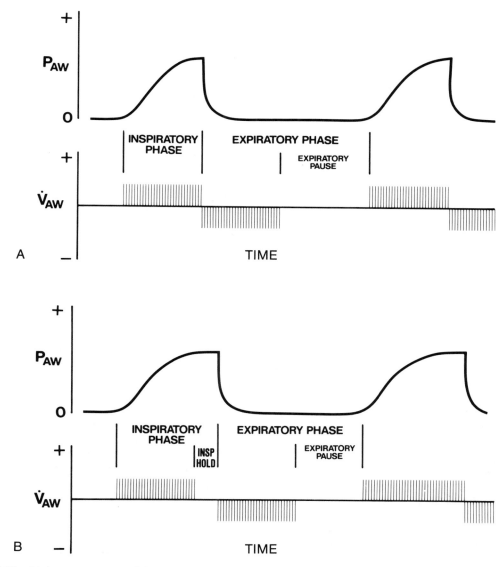

Fig. 24-21. Airway pressure and flow during mechanical ventilation. (**A**) Relationship between airway pressure and flow in the airway is depicted for positive-pressure ventilation. Note that the expiratory pause is part of the expiratory phase; the inspiratory-to-expiratory ratio is the ratio of time for the inspiratory phase and the expiratory phase. (**B**) Airway pressure and flow are shown with an end-inspiratory hold (note the no-flow condition). The inspiratory phase includes the end-inspiratory pause, and the inspiratory-to-expiratory ratio is still the ratio of time for the inspiratory phase and the expiratory phase. P_{AW}, airway pressure; V_{AW}, airway ventilation.

slight negative pressure change is detected by a very sensitive pressure transducer, and application of a constant, support pressure is begun. Pressure is applied continuously throughout inspiration at the value selected by the clinician (Fig. 24-22).

Since the initial reports of PSV in 1984 and 1985,[28,29] several benefits have been demonstrated for this technique. Larger tidal volumes are achieved with lower peak airway pressures.[30] Work of breathing is less, as demonstrated by measurements of work and oxygen consumption.[29,31–33] Spontaneous breathing patterns improve with application of PSV, including decreased respiratory rate, longer expiratory phase, and better synchrony with positive-pres-

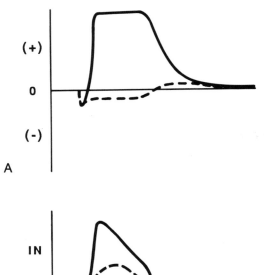

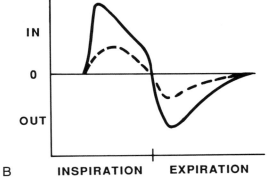

Fig. 24-22. Pressure and flow during pressure support ventilation (PSV [———]) versus spontaneous ventilation (SV [---]). Changes are depicted for (**A**) airway pressure and (**B**) gas flow as they would be measured at the proximal airway (see Fig. 24-23). The patient's negative-pressure inspiratory effort, which initiates PSV gas flow, is followed immediately by a rapidly increasing, then sustained, airway pressure. Note that PSV gas flow initially increases rapidly, then tapers during the inspiratory phase. As the inspiratory (tidal) volume is approached, PSV gas flow ceases.

sure mechanical breaths when they are being applied.[30,32,34] Electromyographic studies have shown that PSV can reduce respiratory muscle fatigue.[35,36] For these reasons, PSV has promoted weaning from mechanical ventilatory support in patients unable to be weaned using other forms of ventilatory support.[35,37,38] PSV has been used successfully with other types of pulmonary pathophysiology, including bronchopleural fistula and chronic obstructive pulmonary disease with air trapping.[39,40]

As with all other forms of positive-pressure support, monitoring airway pressure continuously is necessary, especially since problems attendant to the application of PSV can be detected more readily with such monitoring (see Chapter 23).[7,41]

Mechanical Dead Space

Mechanical dead space results from two sources within the breathing circuit: (1) the common physical volume through which both inspiratory and expiratory gases flow, and (2) the volume amount lost with each mechanical breath due to gas compression and system expansion that occurs during positive-pressure ventilation. The gas compression system compliance dead space can easily be calculated. This form of dead space is readily compensated for in breathing circuits for adult patients by increasing delivered ventilation. However, in breathing circuits for neonates and children, this form of dead space is decreased by using less-compliant breathing circuit components, especially tubing.

Elbow Connectors

Use of an elbow with an occlusively sealing port provides the means for suctioning and for the introduction of a fiberoptic bronchoscope without completely disconnecting the circuit from the patient. This will prevent deleterious pressure losses within the circuit during the application of distending airway pressure therapy.

Mechanical Ventilatory Patterns

The mechanical ventilatory cycle, as shown in Figure 24-21A, is divided into the inspiratory phase and the expiratory phase. The inspiratory phase is that period during which positive airway pressure is generated and inspiratory gas flow is occurring; it ends as airway pressure begins to become more negative and gas flow begins in the opposite direction. The expiratory phase occurs over the remainder of the ventilatory cycle, including that time during which gas flow moves out of the patient and that time during which there is no net gas flow, the expiratory pause. If an inspiratory hold (see below) is used, it is part of the inspiratory phase even though no gas is flowing into the patient's lungs (Fig. 24-21B).

Several aspects of the mechanical ventilatory pattern are important when considered in view of normalcy or disease of patients' lungs. The fundamental pulmonary features are lung and thoracic compliances and airway resistance. In many pathophysiologic lung conditions, the regional differences in compliance and resistance, producing areas with different time constants, will be considerations equally as important as the absolute abnormality in either compliance or resistance. Important attributes of the mechanical ventilatory pattern include inspiratory pressure pattern and flow rate, inspiratory time, inspiratory hold, expiratory pressure pattern, expiratory time, and inspiratory/expiratory time relationship.

Since few mechanical ventilators function as pure flow or pure pressure generators, and since inspiratory flow and pressure patterns are dependent on the patient's compliance and resistance, consideration of a mechanical ventilator based on the concept of a constant-flow or a constant-pressure generator is more theoretical than practical. However, the type of flow pattern actually produced may have important effects depending on the presence or absence of lung pathology and, if present, the type of pathophysiology. The inspiratory phase of the mechanical breath must occur over a finite time. If there is no regional resistive impedance to inspiratory gas flow, the distribution of inspiratory gases will be even. If, however, one or more compartments have increased resistance, inspiratory gases will be distributed unevenly, more going to the compartment with the lower resistance (Fig. 24-16B). An improvement in distribution with this type of pathophysiology can potentially be achieved by several means. Lower inspiratory flow rate will allow more time for even gas distribution in the face of high resistive compartments.[42] Lower inspiratory flow rates will require a longer inspiratory time to attain the desired delivered tidal volume, and this time generally should be maintained at 1 second or longer.[43] Since the expiratory phase should not be shortened so that the inspiratory phase may be longer, the total ventilatory time must be increased. That is, respiratory rate may have to be decreased, a factor that in and of itself has been shown to improve gas distribution in obstructive airways pathology.[44]

The different rates and patterns of inspiratory gas flow, accelerating, decelerating, or constant inspiratory gas flows, may improve distribution.[42,45] However, the efficiency of the pattern may depend on the presence or absence of turbulence, with accelerating flow being more advantageous if inspiratory gas flow is turbulent.[42] No one inspiratory flow pattern is ideal, and, in the design or selection of mechanical ventilatory patterns, the waveform is not as important as other features that lead to effective alveolar ventilation.[46,47] The use of excessively high flow rates is detrimental, leading to increasing dead space production and decreased efficiency of alveolar ventilation.[43,46,48]

The provision of an end-inspiratory pause (inspiratory hold, inspiratory plateau) may improve gas distribution, which may be better than increasing inspiratory time alone or decreasing inspiratory flow rate alone.[42,45,47,49] The pause generally is on the order of 0.6 to 1.2 seconds, and its application may be of benefit with several types of inspiratory flow patterns.[49,50] The use of inspiratory hold increases mean airway pressure, and, in so doing, may have adverse effects on cardiovascular function. Increasing mean airway pressure with different ventilatory patterns can decrease cardiac output.[15] Inspiratory hold has also been shown to decrease arterial blood pressure, decrease ventricular stroke work, and increase pulmonary vascular resistance.[51] As with many other aspects of support of breathing, the beneficial potential of inspiratory hold must be balanced against its potentially detrimental cardiovascular effects. With the advent and appropriate use of distending airway pressure therapy, inspiratory hold is no longer used routinely.

The relative timing of inspiration and expiration is important, but the factors to be considered should be inspiratory and expiratory time rather than the inspiratory-to-expiratory ratio alone. Even in patients with normal lungs, the distribution of the tidal volume will require a finite period of time, which should be a minimum of one second.[43]

Expiration must also occur over a finite period of time. The phase of the ventilatory period allotted to expiration includes that time during which expiratory gas flow is occurring and that time during which no gas flow is occurring, the expiratory pause (Fig. 24-21). Increases or decreases in mechanical ventilatory rate may change the time relationship for the expiratory pause, shortening it with increasing mechanical frequency and lengthening it with decreasing mechanical frequency. The mechanical frequency or changes in inspiratory and expiratory timing should not be executed in such a way that the period for the patient's expiratory gas flow is compromised.

Airway pressure during the expiratory phase of the ventilatory cycle may return to zero (ie, to equilibrium with the atmospheric pressure), or it may return to some preset expiratory pressure level that is being used to promote an increase in the resting lung volume (FRC). A complete consideration of this therapeutic modality is presented in the section *Distending Airway Pressure Therapy*.

In the past, a negative pressure has been applied to the airways during the expiratory phase with the intention of "assisting" the patient's expiratory gas flow. However, this has been shown to increase physiologic dead space and decrease lung compliance.[43,52] Therefore, negative airway pressure should not be used during the expiratory phase.

Selection of a Mechanical Ventilator

Selection of a mechanical ventilator should be based on the specific ventilatory support needs of the patient. Routine postoperative care will exclude negative-pressure ventilators. Since there is great disparity in the efficiency of humidifiers, the selection of an efficient, safe humidifier is very important. Nebulizers, valves for distending airway pressure therapy, instruments for measuring airway pressure, and alarms for airway pressure and oxygen concentration may be selected separately with some basic ventilators. However, more recently developed ventilators incorporate most of these functions into their overall design. Selection of a mechanical ventilator also should be based on overall economy, efficiency, safety, and service. Ease of use and safety are important since the ventilator will be used by many different individuals.

Safety features associated with mechanical ventilators are very important. The ventilator circuit and the breathing circuit should be supplied with a maximum pressure relief ("pop-off") valve or flow diversion mechanism so that excessively high pressures do not build up in the breathing circuit and the patient's airways. A high-pressure alarm should be included in the circuit for detection and notification of this problem. The breathing circuit or ventilator circuit should be supplied with an alarm device that detects circuit disconnection, which would result in no ventilatory support for the patient. These devices generally are low-pressure alarms with time delays. Direct airway pressure monitoring serves as an integral safety feature for mechanical ventilatory support. If the airway pressure trace is continuously displayed, it will provide an ever-present visual monitor for mechanical ventilation or malfunction thereof (Fig. 24-23). The ventilator circuit should have continuous monitoring of inspired oxygen concentration. This can be accomplished by any one of several in-line monitors with alarms.

Routine Application and Weaning of Support

In the routine postoperative patient, several aspects of support of breathing should be provided. For support of ventilation, these include tidal volume and mechanical frequency, and, for support of oxygenation, F_IO_2 and distending airway pressure.

For support of ventilation, tidal volume should be delivered at 12 to 15 mL/kg. The exception to this is the postoperative pneumonectomy or lobectomy patient, in whom tidal volume should be set at 8 to 12 mL/kg. To support ventilation so that initially apneic patients are eucapnic and have a normal arterial pH, mechanical frequency is set at 7 to 8 breaths/min.[53] For the initial support of oxygenation, F_IO_2 is set at 0.80 and distending airway pressure is provided at 5/0 cmH$_2$O (see Chapters 22 and 23).

Routine weaning begins initially with F_IO_2. If good oxygenation has been obtained at $F_IO_2 = 0.80$, F_IO_2 may be decreased to 0.40. If oxygenation has not been completely satisfactory at the initial setting, the change in F_IO_2 should be decremental, the first step lowering it perhaps to 0.60. For routine application and weaning of oxygenation support, the distending airway pressure of 5/0 cmH$_2$O remains unchanged.

During weaning of support of ventilation, tidal volume remains unchanged throughout the weaning pro-

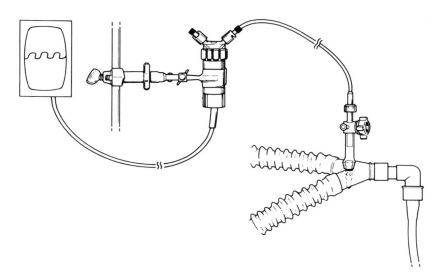

Fig. 24-23. Airway pressure monitoring system. Air airway pressure monitoring system can be constructed by using a circuit Y-connector with one port attached to pressure tubing, which leads to a pressure transducer. Airway pressure is displayed on a calibrated oscilloscope. An in-line stopcock permits zeroing of the system. Note that the breathing circuit and pressure tubing are lower than the transducer to prevent entry of condensate into the pressure monitoring system, since the system should be air-filled and fluid-free.

cess. Weaning of mechanical frequency begins after muscle relaxants and their reversal, narcotics and their reversal, and patient temperature have been assessed. Weaning proceeds with decrements of 1 to 2 breaths/min as long as arterial pH remains above an acceptable level. Since arterial PCO_2 is a secondary determinant of adequacy of ventilation, no changes are made for slight variations in arterial carbon dioxide tension. Weaning proceeds until a mechanical frequency of 0, 1, or 2 breaths/min is reached. Clinical assessment is then made of the level of consciousness and adequacy of airway protective function in the patient prior to extubation. Since a decrement in mechanical frequency from 2 to 1 breath/min represents a 50 percent reduction in support and a decrement from 1 to 0 breaths/min represents termination of mechanical ventilatory support, an adequate clinical assessment is very important if the patient is to be extubated before a rate of zero is reached.

SPECIAL TECHNIQUES

Mechanical Ventilation with Interrupted Airways Disease

Interrupted airways disease occurs when a conducting airway or airways at the exchange level of the lung become open to the tissues surrounding it, thus permitting gas flow without the lungs through an abnormal pathway. The underlying pathophysiology with interrupted airways disease is that of a bronchopleural fistula. This may result from traumatic interruption (gunshot or stab wound), surgical interruption (wedge resection, lobectomy, pneumonectomy), or pulmonary infection with subsequent airways interruption. The patient already has been or will soon be treated with a chest tube placed in the affected side, with application of negative pressure through a chest-bottle system in an attempt to aspirate the leaking air and maximally expand the affected lung. The problem of hypoventilation generally occurs when the patient is undergoing positive-pressure mechanical ventilation, which is not effective in supporting partially or completely the elimination of carbon dioxide. This is due to the loss of part of the tidal volume through the bronchopleural fistula, which is now being evacuated through the chest-bottle system. In many cases, an attempt to improve alveolar ventilation by increasing either mechanical frequency or tidal volume results in worsening of the patient's overall ventilatory status, producing a rise in $PaCO_2$ and a fall in arterial pH. The attempt to increase minute ventilation by increasing mechanical rate or tidal volume leads not only to increasing gas loss through the fistula, but also to increasing alveolar dead space as a result of the greater mean pressures being generated throughout the remaining good portion of the patient's lungs (see Chapter 15).

The underlying problem is one of gas flow and, therefore, gas loss across the bronchopleural fistula. Increasing negative pressure in the chest-bottle system will exacerbate the problem, just as does increasing ventilatory rate or volume, since this, too, increases flow through the fistula.

The goal in the treatment of the bronchopleural fistula is to reduce flow through the fistula, thereby promoting its closure. In the nonpneumonectomy patient who has lung remaining on the affected side, an additional goal is to maximally expand the lung and eliminate the gaseous volume in the pleural space. Since either increasing negative pressure within the chest-tube system or increasing positive pressure via mechanical ventilation only worsens the situation, an effort must be made to reduce one or both of these pressures. Even though it may appear contradictory to the supportive goal in the patient, a reduction in mechanical ventilatory rate or tidal volume should initially be tried. If this fails, several additional supportive techniques are available.

Since this is generally a unilateral lung problem, selective bronchial intubation and differential treatment of the lungs may permit diminution or ablation of flow through the bronchopleural fistula on the affected side while promoting adequate support of ventilation on the unaffected side. This can be accomplished in adult patients with an endobronchial tube appropriate for long-term airway management (Broncho-Cath, National Catheter Co.). For the patient who requires continued support of ventilation after the selective bronchial intubation, dual ventilatory circuits may have to be used. This is accomplished more easily by using separate ventilators with separate circuits than by attempting to use a split or dual breathing circuit with one mechanical ventilator. If it is necessary to ventilate both lungs synchronously, an adaptation of the electrical timing system for two mechanical ventilators in simultaneous use is available (J.H. Emerson Co.). Once the side with the bronchopleural fistula has been isolated by selective bronchial intubation, it may be necessary to use only the unaffected side for the partial or complete support of ventilation needed for the patient.

If selective bronchial intubation is not possible in the patient with a bronchopleural fistula, a technique can be used whereby gas flow through the fistula is diminished or stopped during the mechanical ventilator's inspiratory cycle. This technique uses the interruption of the vacuum-breaker bottle's aspiration of the water-seal bottle in the chest-bottle system during the positive-pressure phase of mechanical inspiration, which can be accomplished by inserting an expiratory valve (Emerson Exhalation Valve, J.H. Emerson Co.) in-line between the two bottles and activating the valve with a line teed from the charging line that activates the expiratory valve of the breathing circuit (Fig. 24-24). Therefore, when the expiratory valve is closed as the mechanical inspiratory phase begins, the vacuum applied to the chest-tube system will be interrupted and a no-flow system will be temporarily established. Since no gas flow from the pleural space is being promoted during this phase, the delivered tidal volume will enter and be distributed throughout the patient's lungs. Since the resistance in the bronchopleural fistula compartment is now increased above its previous near-zero value, gas distribution will occur depending on relative compartmental resistances. Some leak through the fistula into the pleural space may occur, resulting in a small reduction in lung size (ie, increase in pleural air space), but this gas will be evacuated during the expiratory phase of mechanical ventilation when once again the vacuum aspiration of the chest-tube system is applied to the pleural space.

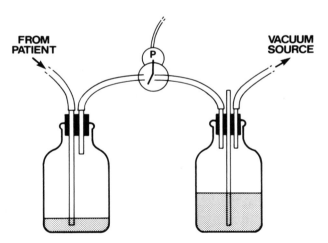

FROM PATIENT

P

VACUUM SOURCE

Fig. 24-24. "Charging" the chest-bottle system. To stop aspiration from the pleural space during mechanical inspiration, a valve is interposed between the underwater-seal bottle and the vacuum-breaker bottle in a two-bottle system. The line that activates closure of the expiratory valve of the breathing circuit is teed to activate the valve, which stops flow between the two bottles. Pressure in the vacuum-breaker bottle remains at the level preset by the depth of the vacuum-breaker straw; pressure in the water-seal bottle may increase during the mechanical breath. During the expiratory phase of mechanical ventilation, flow will resume within the system and will evacuate in a conventional manner any gas that has accumulated in the pleural space.

Technical considerations with this form of therapy for interrupted airways disease include the use of a two-bottle chest-tube system, wherein gas flow through the bronchopleural fistula is diminished or stopped by interrupting the vacuum aspiration during the inspiratory phase of mechanical ventilation. The vacuum-interrupting valve should be placed between the water-seal bottle and the vacuum-breaker bottle, not between the patient and the water-seal bottle, for infection-control purposes. The valve's activation must be timed with the closure of the expiratory valve of the breathing circuit. Therefore, the length of tubing that is teed from the charging line of the ventilator must provide pressure transmission for simultaneous closure of each valve. The use of self-contained single-unit chest-bottle systems (eg, Pleurevac, DeKnatel) is not appropriate for this form of therapy. More frequent radiographic monitoring of the patient may be required.

High-Frequency Ventilation

High-frequency ventilation is uniquely applicable to the treatment of the patient with interrupted airways disease. Rhythmic movement of gases into and out of the lungs has been appreciated for centuries and, throughout this time, support of breathing has been directed at emulating the cyclic movement of the respiratory gases. Quantitation of this movement, including measurement of the conducting airways' volume (anatomic dead space), was achieved at approximately the turn of this century.[54]

However, in 1909, Meltzer and Auer described a nonrhythmical means of supporting respiration in which they used a continuous fresh gas flow delivered to the airways at a pressure of approximately 15 to 20 mmHg.[55] They studied the respiratory and cardiovascular function of their dog model over several hours, inferring good oxygenation from color and satisfactory ventilation from cardiovascular stability. They recognized specific problems associated with the establishment and maintenance of the airways for these studies and used three different techniques: (1) tracheostomy tube through a large stoma, with gas inflow via the tracheostomy tube and gas outflow via the stoma; (2) side-by-side tubes through tracheal incisions; and (3) a catheter through an oral endotracheal tube. The conclusions from their study were anticipatory of the developments of today in that they believed this nonrhythmic support could provide adequate respiration and, more important, could provide a means for performing cardiovascular studies without the overlay of respiratory variation. In fact, almost 60 years later, other noncyclic forms of support of ventilation were developed in conjunction with cardiovascular studies. To eliminate respiratory variation in carotid sinus blood pressure studies in dogs, Sjostrand et al developed and used high-frequency positive-pressure ventilation (HFV).[56] For measuring transmyocardial pressure transmission, Lunkenheimer et al developed a high-frequency oscillatory technique that also effectively ventilated dogs.[57] The ventilatory frequencies in these early studies were 60 to 100/min (Sjostrand et al[56]) and 23 to 40 Hz (Lunkenheimer et al[57]). In both studies, the dogs' airways were maintained with oral endotracheal tubes: an intraluminal catheter was inserted for provision of HFV in the series of Sjostrand et al, and the high-frequency oscillator was applied at the proximal end of an endotracheal tube in the series of Lunkenheimer et al. Work at the same time by Heijman et al introduced the first human applications of HFV[58]; this study was conducted in normal surgical patients in whom Heijman et al reported good ventilation and oxygenation as well as cardiovascular stability during the application of HFV.

The technique used by Heijman et al should not be confused with the technique of apneic oxygenation, which has been studied by several groups, including Frumin et al, who reported in 1959 adequate oxygenation for periods up to 55 minutes with the provision of a low fresh gas flow and no rhythmic support of ventilation.[59] However, in their eight patients, the carbon dioxide tensions rose as high as 250 mmHg, with ventricular ectopy progressing to ventricular tachycardia in two of their eight patients, obviously not a suitable form of long-term ventilatory support.

Principles of High-Frequency Ventilation

The basic difference between HFV and conventional mechanical ventilation is in the means by which respiratory gases are transferred in the conducting airways. During spontaneous respiration and conventional mechanical support of ventilation, transfer of respiratory gases through the conducting airways is accomplished by bulk flow of the gases into and out of the lungs. The carbon dioxide that is presented via the pulmonary arterial circulation to the gas compartment of the gas exchange unit is transferred from whole blood into the gas phase by diffusion. The transfer of respiratory gases within the gas exchange portion of the lung also occurs by molecular diffusion, which terminates at about the level of the terminal bronchiole, or 17th airway generation. Convective movement, or bulk flow, is then responsible for the transfer of carbon dioxide out of and oxygen into the lungs through the conducting airways.

In the HFV technique, molecular diffusion is still the primary process responsible for transfer of respiratory gases at the exchange level in the lung parenchyma. However, it is *augmented diffusion* that is primarily responsible for transfer of these gases through the conducting airways. This was originally described in soils by Scotter et al when they were able to enhance the diffusivity of oxygen 4.5- to 50-fold with the application of a 5 mL volume above the soil at a 1 Hz frequency.[60] Application of this principle of augmented diffusion has been described for airways by Fredberg,[61] Slutsky et al,[62] and Lehr et al.[63]

Techniques of High-Frequency Ventilation

Two general considerations are relevant for any HFV technique: (1) *airway management*, including flow pathways; and (2) the *system* for the delivery of the HFV. For airway management and gas flow patterns, essentially two types of systems exist: open and closed. With the open system, there is control over only the gas inflow, not the gas outflow. With the closed system, there is control over both gas inflow and outflow. For example, with the closed system, the potential for the application and control of distending airway pressure exists, whereas it may not with the open system.

One example of an *open system* is the percutaneous placement of a transtracheal catheter, eg, 14-gauge Angiocath, for elective or emergency airway management for application of HFV.[64] A similar open system is one in which a catheter is placed via the nose or mouth with its distal end residing in the trachea above the carina. Inflow is intraluminal* and outflow is extraluminal with this technique, which has been used by Erickson and Sjostrand in the development of laryngoscopic HFV.[65] These investigators reported satisfactory ventilation and oxygenation with 60 breaths/min using this technique, which allows a virtually unobstructed view by the endoscopist. Another open system would be that using an uncuffed endotracheal tube or endotracheal tube without cuff inflation.[66,67]

When open systems are used, the gas outflow pathway is not established mechanically and, therefore, depends on natural airway patency for adequate gas egress. Outflow can be compromised by head and neck position, cross-sectional area of the endotracheal tube exceeding an acceptable maximum cross-sectional area of the trachea, secretions in the airways, airway edema, or other airway pathology. Aspiration is a potential problem with open systems and may occur during HFV, depending on the type and position of the gas inflow pathway.[68] Although it has been reported not to occur during the actual administration of HFV with certain techniques, it has been

---

* *Lumen* in this section refers to an artificial airway device, for example, endotracheal tube lumen or tracheostomy tube lumen.

shown to occur immediately after cessation of the HFV.[69,70]

For long-term ventilatory support, a better system would be one that guarantees airway protection and patency for gas outflow, the *closed system*. With a closed system, the pathways for inflow and outflow are established physically by an artificial airway device. The two paths may exist simultaneously within the same part of the system, providing bidirectionality of gas flow within the system. A closed system has been used by Jonzon et al in much of their later HFV work, in which they have placed a catheter within a short segment of an endotracheal tube for delivery of the HFV.[71] Another double-lumen technique is the use of an endobronchial tube in which the side-by-side lumens provide separate inflow and outflow tracts. A quadruple-lumen endotracheal tube has been designed specifically for the provision of HFV (Hi-Lo Jet Tracheal Tube, National Catheter Co.). In more widespread use today is a circuit elbow specifically modified for HFV (Jet Ventilator Adaptor, Portex Inc.). Since this elbow can be used with any endotracheal or tracheostomy tube that has a standard 15-mm outside diameter connector, the need for special airway management or special equipment is eliminated.

The different variables related to the provision of HFV are outlined in Table 24-2. Gas inflow and outflow have been discussed above. Each of the other variables will be discussed below.

Ventilators for HFV basically include four types, as shown in Table 24-3, which also lists references to representative studies or case reports. The volume displacement pump can be a piston within a cylinder that is driven by an electric motor. Systems have been described with displacement volumes of 1 to 100 mL and frequencies of 1 to 100 Hz.[66] One of the first volume-displacement HFV ventilators was the airways vibrator developed and patented by John H. Emerson in 1959.

Flow interruption can be achieved with magnetic valves and slotted ball bearings. The electromagnetic valve is available as the AGA Bronchovent (AGA Medical AV, Lidingo, Sweden), described by Borg et al.[72] The slotted ball-bearing device (J.H. Emerson Co.) is a

TABLE 24-2. Variables Related to Provision of High-Frequency Positive-Pressure Ventilation

Volume-frequency source
Fresh gas flow
Inspiratory and expiratory timing
System compliance
Gas inflow pathway (inspirate)
Gas outflow pathway (expirate)
Patient

TABLE 24-3. Volume-Frequency Sources for High-Frequency Ventilation

Devices	References
Volume displacement pumps	57, 66
Flow interruption devices	
Electromagnetic valves	56, 58, 65, 67, 71, 72, 79, 81, 82, 84, 92, 117, 118
Slotted ball bearings	96, 97
Fluidic ventilators	64, 73, 75, 80
High-fidelity speakers	62

flow interrupter that has a frequency determined by the speed of an electric motor attached to the ball bearing.

Several fluidic ventilators have been used with the HFV technique; the rates attained have been between 60 and 900/min.[64,73] Fluidic ventilators are uniquely suited to HFV because of their rapid response times and their lack of moving parts for delivery of gases, very important considerations when ventilatory rates may exceed 15 Hz. The applications of fluidic technology has been described by Klain and Smith[74] and by Smith et al.[75]

Another volume-frequency source for HFV can be provided by high-fidelity speakers. This technique can produce a wide range of frequencies and variable volume displacement. The frequency range in which HFV is accomplished is shown in Table 24-4, along with the conventional mechanical ventilatory range of 1 to 20 breaths/min (0.02 to 0.3 Hz).

Humidification is available with some HFV techniques, but not with others. When available, it varies from actual humidification of all or part of the fresh gas flow to aerosolization of a drip irrigant in the inflow pathway. Efficiency of humidification with HFV technology has not been studied extensively, although the deleterious effects of using dry gases with HFV have been reported.[76]

The timing of gas inflow and outflow can be of critical importance with the HFV technique. This has been recorded in different studies as inspiration-to-expiration ratio or as inspiratory time. The capability of varying the inspiration-to-expiration ratio is available on some ventilators, but not on others. When this has been studied as an independent variable, an inspiratory time equal to 22 to 32 percent of the ventilatory cycle has been found to be most efficacious.[58,71]

In Table 24-5, the various forms of airway management, including applicable breathing circuit components, are listed under the classification of open and closed systems, with selected references. As with all forms of positive-pressure ventilatory support, monitoring airway pressure is very important, not only for adjusting therapy, but also to detect and prevent adverse effects.[77,78]

TABLE 24-4.   Frequency Range for High-Frequency Ventilation[a]

Designation	Hz	Min	Selected References
Conventional mechanical ventilation	0.02–0.3	1–20	71, 81, 118
Low-frequency HFV	1–2.5	60–150	56, 58, 64–67, 71–76, 79–84, 92, 117, 118
Medium-frequency HFV	2.5–6	150–360	62, 75, 80
High-frequency HFV	6–16	360–960	57, 62, 66, 75
Ultra-high-frequency HFV	>16	>960	57, 62

[a] Frequencies are given in rates *per second* (Hz) and *per minute* (Min). Suggested designations are for ranges extant in the current literature. The breakpoint of 2.5 Hz represents the upper limit of the range currently accepted for clinical (nonresearch) applications by the Food and Drug Administration. Selected references are provided for each range.

Physiologic Effects of High-Frequency Ventilation

Different neural effects in terms of control of breathing have been reported by different groups of investigators. Apnea has been produced in several models, sometimes immediately on application of the HFV, with spontaneous ventilation returning immediately

TABLE 24-5.   Airway Management for High-Frequency Ventilation

System	References
Open systems	
Percutaneous transtracheal catheter	64, 75, 80
Nasotracheal catheter (for laryngoscopy)	65, 72
Endotracheal tube with cuff	66, 67
Fiberoptic bronchoscope with inflow via suction port	87
Closed systems	
Endotracheal tube with cuff inflated	58, 81
Tracheostomy with cuff inflated	62, 92
Endotracheal or tracheostomy tube with circumferential ligation of tube in trachea	67, 117, 118
Catheter in endotracheal tube lumen	56, 71
Endobronchial tube with both lumens in trachea	
Endobronchial tube with selective lung ventilation	83
Rigid bronchoscope with side arm attachment[a]	72, 82, 84
Uncuffed endotracheal tube in infants and children[b]	79

[a] Listed as closed system even without tight airway seal because outflow path is established.

[b] Listed as closed system even without use of endotracheal tube cuff because outflow path is intraluminal and because cuffed endotracheal tubes are not used routinely in patients of this age group.

following its discontinuation.[56,79] Others have reported that patients or animals have continued spontaneous ventilatory activity during application of HFV.[57,75,80] Continued spontaneous ventilatory activity has several advantages for improving cardiovascular function, but has disadvantages in terms of a quiet operative field for thoracic surgery. Therefore, several groups have used muscle relaxants during HFV for animal studies and for patient applications.[57,58,62,64–66,75,76,79–84]

The cardiovascular effects of HFV are the result of the lower airway pressure produced with this technique of ventilatory support and, in some series, they are also the result of the production of apnea associated with the technique. A lower mean airway pressure with HFV results in a lower pleural pressure, which can result in increased venous return, thereby improving cardiac output. For patients who do not become apneic during HFV, the continued contribution of the intrathoracic pump mechanism to venous return also will enhance cardiac output.

Respiratory effects related to HFV compared with conventional CMV include lesser mean and peak airway pressures and more negative pleural pressures.[81] The lower peak and mean airway pressures may reduce the incidence of pulmonary barotrauma with HFV compared with control mode ventilation, although no series has yet been reported.

Improvement in pulmonary oxygenating ability has been demonstrated with HFV, including a reduced shunt fraction and a reduced alveolar-arterial PO_2 difference.[85] Given the potential increase in cardiac output and the potential for improved pulmonary oxygenating ability, oxygen transport certainly may be enhanced, as has been reported by Eriksson et al.[81]

Applications for High-Frequency Ventilation

Since the introduction of HFV, several patient series have been reported. These have included the use of HFV in elective adult surgical patients and in infants and children undergoing surgery.[58,79] Use of HFV in patients with normal lungs has proved to be advantageous for ventilation during bronchoscopy, laryngoscopy, otolaryngologic surgery, microscopic neurovascular surgery, and surgery on the upper airway.[65,72,81,86] HFV has been applied during fiberoptic bronchoscopy as well as during rigid bronchoscopy.[87,88]

Several series have demonstrated benefits with HFV in neonates with acute respiratory insufficiency.[89–91] Cases and small series of HFV in adults with adult respiratory distress syndrome (ARDS) have been reported, but no large series has yet demonstrated therapeutic benefit of HFV for ARDS.[92–94] In fact, there is evidence that HFV alone will not provide adequate therapy for ARDS without the concomitant application of distending airway pressure therapy.[93,95]

Many of the case reports of the application of HFV in acute lung injury have been related to interrupted airways disease—traumatic, surgical, or related to infection.[96,97] The low peak and mean airway pressures, along with the ability to provide support for carbon dioxide elimination without convective gas movement, makes HFV an improved technique for interrupted airways disease.

Extracorporeal Membrane Oxygenation

Development of means for artificial support of heart and lung functions was directed primarily at needs related to open heart surgery prior to the early 1960s.[98] The use of extracorporeal membrane oxygenation (ECMO) for support of patients acutely ill with respiratory failure began in the late 1960s, and early efforts in adults had a low survival rate (10 percent).[99]

The earliest comprehensive study of the pathophysiology and treatment of ARDS was undertaken under the auspices of the National Heart, Lung, and Blood Institute of the National Institutes of Health. During the 7 years of the study (1971 to 1977), nine medical centers compiled data on more than 500 patients, including 90 who were entered into an ECMO study (42 ECMO patients and 48 conventional therapy patients). There was no difference in survival between the two groups. Conclusions were that ECMO did not improve survival or affect the progress of the pulmonary pathophysiology when compared with conventional therapy.[100]

ECMO was studied because it held several potential benefits, including "resting the lung" while supporting other organs during lung reparation. ECMO has the advantage of avoiding administration of high inspired oxygen concentrations while still providing satisfactory tissue and organ oxygenation as well as removal of carbon dioxide. Using ECMO while reducing conventional ventilatory support also produces reduced pulmonary barotrauma and decreased pulmonary arterial pressure.

Although the original NIH study did not realize these benefits in ARDS patients, subsequent applications in neonates have proven more successful. Beginning in the early 1970s, several series have reported marked improvement in outcome with meconium aspiration syndrome, persistent pulmonary hypertension of the newborn, congenital diaphragmatic hernia, and infant respiratory distress syndrome.[101–106] Data analyzed from a national registry series of 715 neonatal ECMO patients (1980 to 1987) demonstrated an overall survival of 81 percent,[107] which, in earlier series, had been the overall mortality rate with conventional therapy.[108] As neonatal ECMO has evolved, entry criteria have been used,[102,103,106,109] and experience with ECMO technology has been shown to improve survival.[107] ECMO is now a proven support modality for neonatal respiratory failure of several causes, and additional neonatal ECMO centers are being established to meet national needs.

In the past decade, ECMO generally has been used in adults for two reasons: as a bridge to heart transplantation or as support during acute respiratory failure. As a bridge to heart transplantation, ECMO has had limited success. Several small series of pretransplant patients have included ECMO, but no statistically significant evidence exists at present supporting the efficacy of ECMO as a definitive bridge to heart transplantation.[110–112] ECMO also has been suggested as an adjunct supportive measure to lung transplantation.[113] Small series of ECMO support for acute respiratory failure in adults have been reported since the original NIH series.[114,115] No outcome data from any large series have yet contradicted the findings of the original study.

The potential for improved outcome with application of ECMO in adults must be weighed against newer support techniques that already have enhanced outcome. These advances include an appreciation that the underlying pathophysiology of ARDS is primarily an oxygenation disability and *not one of ventilatory failure*. Therefore, simultaneous application of support of ventilation with support of oxygenation (ie, mechanical ventilation and distending airway pressure) is unnecessary and in many cases may actually result in worse cardiovascular function and increased pulmonary barotrauma. The use of distending airway pressure therapy has been studied extensively, and it is now known that this is a therapeutic modality that should be titrated against physiologic end points and not applied at empirically selected levels. These advances in conventional support and the commitment of substantial resources (people, equipment, support services, time) to each patient undergoing ECMO precludes its being a cost-effective, clinical tool for supporting respiratory failure in adults today. However, outcome and experience with neonatal ECMO may militate against the current restrictions imposed by cost containment and limited reimbursement, and ECMO technology must again be evaluated for adult respiratory failure.

REFERENCES

1. Dery R: Determination of the alveolar humidity and temperature in the dog. Can Anaesth Soc J 18:145–151, 1977
2. Poulton TJ, Downs JB: Humidification of rapidly flowing gas. Crit Care Med 9:59–63, 1981
3. Bates DV, Fish BR, Hatch TF, et al: Deposition and retention models for internal dosimetry of the human respiratory tract. Health Phys 12:173–207, 1966
4. Beekmans JM: The deposition of aerosols in the respiratory tract. Can J Physiol Pharmacol 43:157–172, 1965
5. Beaty CD, Ritz RH, Benson MS: Continuous in-line nebulizers complicate pressure support ventilation. Chest 96:1360–1363, 1989
6. Oberlin DC, Nishimura TG: Tracheal oxygen concentrations using nasal prongs. Anesthesiology 53:S384, 1980
7. Martin LD, Rafferty JF, Wetzel RC, Gioia FR: Inspiratory work and response times of a modified pediatric volume ventilator during synchronized intermittent mandatory ventilation and pressure support ventilation. Anesthesiology 71:977–981, 1989
8. Gibney RTN, Wilson RS, Pontoppidan H: Comparison of work of breathing on high gas flow and demand valve continuous positive airway pressure systems. Chest 82:692–695, 1982
9. Christopher KL, Neff TA, Bowman JL et al: Demand and continuous flow intermittent mandatory ventilation systems. Chest 87:625–630, 1985
10. Smith RA, Kirby RR, Gooding JB, et al: Continuous positive airway pressure (CPAP) by face mask. Crit Care Med 8:483–485, 1980
11. Greenbaum DM, Millen JE, Eross B, et al: Continuous positive airway pressure without tracheal intubation in spontaneously breathing patients. Chest 69:615–620, 1976
12. Hoff BH, Flemming DC, Sasse F: Use of positive airway pressure without endotracheal intubation. Crit Care Med 7:559–562, 1979
13. Buck JB, McCormack WC: A nasal mask for premature infants. J Pediatr 66:123–125, 1965
14. Hall JR, Rendelman DC, Downs JB: PEEP devices: flow-dependent increaes in airway pressure. Crit Care Med 6:100, 1978
15. Cournand A, Motley HL, Werko L, et al: Physiological studies of the effects of intermittent positive-pressure breathing on cardiac output in man. Am J Physiol 152:162–174, 1948
16. Hodgkin JE, Soeprono FF, Chan DM: Incidence of metabolic alkalemia in hospitalized patients. Crit Care Med 8:725–728, 1980
17. Mushin WW, Rendell-Baker L, Thompson PW, et al: Automatic Ventilation of the Lungs. Blackwell Scientific Publications, Oxford, 1980
18. Drinker P, McKhann C: The use of a new apparatus for the prolonged administration of artificial respiration. JAMA 92:1658–1660, 1929
19. Drinker P, Shaw LA: An apparatus for the prolonged administration of artificial respiration. J Clin Invest 7:229–247, 1929
20. Splaingard ML, Frates RC, Jr, Jefferson LS, Harrison GM: Home pressure ventilation: report of 20 years of experience in patients with neuromuscular disease. Arch Phys Med Rehabil 66:239–242, 1985
21. Hill NS: Clinical applications of body ventilators. Chest 90:897–905, 1986
22. Levy RD, Bradley TD, Newman SL, et al: Negative pressure ventilation. Effects on ventilation during sleep in normal subjects. Chest 95:95–99, 1989
23. Mohr CH, Hill NS: Long-term follow-up of nocturnal ventilatory assistance in patients with respiratory failure due to Duchenne-type muscular dystrophy. Chest 97:91–96, 1990
24. Hunter AR: The classification of respirators. Anaesthesia 16:213–234, 1961
25. Mapleson WW: The effect of changes of lung characteristics on the functioning of automatic ventilators. Anaesthesia 17:300–314, 1962
26. Downs JB, Douglas ME, Ruiz BC, et al: Comparison of assisted and controlled mechanical ventilation in anesthetized swine. Crit Care Med 7:5–8, 1979
27. Downs JB, Klein EF, Desautels D, et al: Intermittent mandatory ventilation: a new approach to weaning patients from mechanical ventilators. Chest 64:331–335, 1973
28. MacIntyre NR: Pulmonary mechanics and gas exchange during pressure support ventilation. Chest 86:A285, 1984
29. Kanak R, Fahey PJ, Vanderwaarf C: Oxygen cost of breathing: changes dependent upon mode of ventilation. Chest 87:126–127, 1985
30. Tokioka H, Saito S, Kosaka F: Comparison of pressure support ventilation and assist control ventilation in patients with acute respiratory failure. Intensive Care Med 15:364–367, 1989
31. Brochard L, Harf A, Lorino H, Lemaire F: Inspiratory pressure support prevents diaphragmatic fatigue during weaning from mechanical ventilation. Am Rev Respir Dis 139:513–521, 1989
32. Tokioka H, Saito S, Kosaka F: Effect of pressure support ventilation on breathing patterns and respiratory work. Intensive Care Med 15:491–494, 1989

33. Viale JP, Annat GJ, Bouffard YM, et al: Oxygen cost of breathing in postoperative patients: pressure support ventilation vs continuous positive airway pressure. Chest 93:506–509, 1988

34. Fassoulaki A, Eforakopoulou M: Cardiovascular, respiratory, and metabolic changes produced by pressure-supported ventilation in intensive care patients. Crit Care Med 17:527–529, 1989

35. Brochard L, Harf A, Lorino H, Lemaire F: Inspiratory pressure support prevents diaphragmatic fatigue during weaning from mechanical ventilation. Am Rev Respir Dis 139:513–521, 1989

36. Brochard L, Pluskwa F, Lemaire F: Improved efficacy of spontaneous breathing with inspiratory pressure support. Am Rev Respir Dis 136:411–415, 1987

37. Hurst JM, Branson RD, Davis K, Barrette RR: Cardiopulmonary effects of pressure support ventilation. Arch Surg 124:1067–1070, 1989

38. MacIntyre NR: Respiratory function during pressure support ventilation. Chest 89:677–683, 1986

39. Gagnon L, Blouin A, Cormier Y: Bronchocutaneous fistula in dogs: influence of fistula size and ventilatory mode on air leak. Crit Care Med 17:1301–1305, 1989

40. Conti G, Bufi M, Antonelli M, et al: Pressure support ventilation (PSV) reverses hyperinflation induced isorhythmic A-V dissociation. Intensive Care Med 15:319–321, 1989

41. Black JW, Grover BS: A hazard of pressure support ventilation. Chest 93:333–335, 1988

42. Lyager S: Influence of flow pattern on the distribution of respiratory air during intermittent positive-pressure ventilation. Acta Anaesthesiol Scand 12:191–211, 1968

43. Watson WE: Observations on physiological deadspace during intermittent positive-pressure respiration. Br J Anaesth 34:502–508, 1962

44. Sabar EF, Norlander O, Osborn JJ, et al: Gas distribution studies in experimental unilateral bronchial constriction using an accelerating flow, volume-controlled respirator. Surgery 58:713–719, 1965

45. Jansson L, Jonson B: A theoretical study on flow patterns of ventilators. Scand J Respir Dis 53:237–246, 1972

46. Bergman N: Effects of varying respiratory waveforms on gas exchange. Anesthesiology 28:390–395, 1967

47. Dammann JF, McAslan TC: Optimal flow pattern for mechanical ventilation of the lungs. Crit Care Med 5:128–136, 1977

48. Fairley HB, Blenkarn GD: Effect on pulmonary gas exchange on variations in inspiratory flow rate during intermittent positive-pressure ventilation. Br J Anaesth 38:320–328, 1966

49. Fuleihan SF, Wilson RS, Pontoppidan H: Effect of mechanical ventilation with end-inspiratory pause on blood-gas exchange. Anesth Analg 55:122–130, 1976

50. Dammann JF, McAslan TC, Maffeo CJ: Optimal flow pattern for mechanical ventilation of the lungs: 2. the effect of a sine versus square wave flow pattern with and without an end-inspiratory pause on patients. Crit Care Med 6:293–310, 1978

51. Nordstrom L: Haemodynamic effects of intermittent positive-pressure ventilation with and without an end-inspiratory pause. Acta Anaesthesiol Scand, suppl. 47:29–56, 1972

52. Watson WE: Some observations of dynamic lung compliance during intermittent positive pressure respiration. Br J Anaesth 34:153–157, 1962

53. Downs JB, Marston AW: A new transport ventilator: an evaluation. Crit Care Med 5:112–114, 1977

54. Haldane JS, Priestley JG: The regulation of the lung-ventilation. J Physiol 32:225–266, 1905

55. Meltzer SJ, Auer J: Continuous respiration without respiratory movements. J Exp Med 2:622–625, 1909

56. Sjostrand U, Jonzon A, Sedin G, et al: High-frequency positive-pressure ventilation (discussion). Opuscula Medica 18:74–75, 1973

57. Lunkenheimer PP, Rafflenbeul W, Kellr H, et al: Application of transtracheal pressure oscillations as a modification of "diffusion respiration." Br J Anaesth 44:627, 1972

58. Heijman K, Heijman L, Jonzon A, et al: High-frequency positive-pressure ventilation during anaesthesia and routine surgery in man. Acta Anaesthesiol Scand 16:176–187, 1972

59. Frumin MJ, Epstein RM, Cohen G: Apneic oxygenation in man. Anesthesiology 20:790–798, 1959

60. Scotter DR, Thurtell GW, Taats PAC: Dispersion resulting from sinusoidal gas flow in porous materials. Soil Sci 104:306–309, 1967

61. Fredberg JJ: Augmented diffusion in the airways can support pulmonary gas exchange. J Appl Physiol Respir Environ Exercise Physiol 49:232–238, 1980

62. Slutsky AS, Drazen JM, Ingram RH, Jr, et al: Effective pulmonary ventilation with small-volume oscillations at high frequency. Science 209:609–611, 1980

63. Lehr J, Barkyoumb J, Drazen JM: Gas transport during high frequency ventilation (HFV). Fed Proc 40:384, 1981

64. Smith RB, Cutaia F, Hoff BH, et al: Long-term transtracheal high frequency ventilation in dogs. Crit Care Med 9:311–314, 1981

65. Eriksson I, Sjostrand U: A clinical evaluation of high-frequency positive-pressure ventilation (HFPPV) in laryngoscopy under general anaesthesia. Acta Anaesthesiol Scand, suppl. 64:101–110, 1977

66. Bohn DJ, Miyasaka K, Marchak BE, et al: Ventilation by high-frequency oscillation. J Appl Physiol Respir Environ Exercise Physiol 48:710–716, 1980

67. Jonzon A, Sedin G, Sjostrand U: High-frequency positive-pressure ventilation (HFPPV) applied for small lung ventilation and compared with spontaneous respiration and continuous positive airway pressure (CPAP). Acta Anaesthesiol Scand, suppl. 53:23–26, 1973

68. Szele G, Keenan RL: Does percutaneous transtracheal high-frequency ventilation prevent aspiration? A word of caution! Crit Care Med 9:163, 1981

69. Keszler H, Klain M, Nordin U: High-frequency jet ventilation prevents aspiration during cardiopulmonary resuscitation. Crit Care Med 9:161, 1981

70. Klain M, Keszler H, Nordin U: Aspiration: a danger during high-frequency ventilation? Crit Care Med 9:163, 1981

71. Jonzon A, Oberg PA, Sedin G, et al: High-frequency positive-pressure ventilation by endotracheal insufflation. Acta Anaesthesiol Scand, suppl. 43:1–43, 1971

72. Borg U, Eriksson I, Sjostrand U: High-frequency positive-pressure ventilation (HFPPV): a review based upon its use during bronchoscopy and for laryngoscopy and microlaryngeal surgery under general anesthesia. Anesth Analg 59:594–603, 1980

73. Carlon GC, Howland WS, Klain M, et al: High-frequency positive ventilation for ventilatory support in patients with bronchopleural fistulas. Crit Care Med 7:128, 1979

74. Klain M, Smith RB: Fluidic technology. Anaesthesia 31:750–757, 1976

75. Smith RB, Klain M, Babinski M: Limits of high-frequency percutaneous transtracheal jet ventilation using a fluidic logic controlled ventilator. Can Anaesth Soc J 27:351–356, 1980

76. Nordin U, Keszler H, Klain M: How does high-frequency jet ventilation affect the mucociliary transport? Crit Care Med 9:160, 1981

77. Saari AF, Rossing TH, Solway J, Drazen JM: Lung inflation during high-frequency ventilation. Am Rev Respir Dis 129:333–336, 1984

78. Black JW, Grover BS: A hazard of pressure support ventilation. Chest 93:333–335, 1988

79. Heijman L, Nilsson LG, Sjostrand U: High-frequency positive-presure ventilation (HFPPV) in neonates and infants during neuroleptal analgesia and routine plastic surgery, and in postoperative management. Acta Anaesthesiol Scand, suppl. 64:111–121, 1977

80. Klain M, Smith RB: High-frequency percutaneous transtracheal jet ventilation. Crit Care Med 5:280–287, 1977

81. Eriksson I, Jonzon A, Sedin G, et al: The influence of the ventilatory pattern on ventilation, circulation and oxygen transport during continuous positive-pressure ventilation. Acta Anaesthesiol Scand, suppl. 64:149–163, 1977

82. Borg U, Eriksson I, Lyttkens L, et al: High-frequency positive-pressure ventilation (HFPPV) applied in bronchoscopy under general anaesthesia. Acta Anaesthesiol Scand, suppl. 64:69–81, 1977

83. Benjaminsson E, Klain M: Intraoperative dual-mode independent lung ventilation of a patient with bronchopleural fistual. Anesth Analg 60:118–119, 1981

84. Eriksson I, Sjostrand U: Experimental and clinical evaluation of high-frequency positive-pressure ventilation (HFPPV) and the pneumatic valve principle in bronchoscopy under general anesthesia. Acta Anaesthesiol Scand, suppl 64:83–100, 1977

85. Malina JR, Nordstrom SG, Sjostrand UH, et al: Clinical evaluation of high-frequency positive-pressure ventilation (HFPPV) in patients scheduled for open chest surgery. Anesth Analg 60:324–300, 1981

86. Rouby JJ, Viars P: Clinical use of high frequency ventilation. Acta Anaesthesiol Scand, suppl. 90:134–139, 1989

87. Ramanathan S, Sinha K, Arismendy J, et al: Bronchofiberscopic high frequency ventilation. Anesthesiology 55:A352, 1981

88. MacIntyre NR, Ramage JE, Follett JV: Jet ventilation in support of fiberoptic bronchoscopy. Crit Care Med 15:303–307, 1987

89. Bland RD, Kim MH, Light MJ, et al: High-frequency mechanical ventilation of low-birth-weight infants with respiratory failure from hyaline membrane disease: 92% survival. Pediatr Res 2:531, 1977

90. Pagani G, Rezzonico R, Marini A: Trials of high-frequency jet ventilation in preterm infants with severe respiratory disease. Acta Paediatr Scand 74:681–686, 1985

91. Cornish JD, Gerstmann DR, Clark RH, et al: Extracorporeal membrane oxygenation and high-frequency oscillatory ventilation: potential therapeutic relationships. Crit Care Med 15:831–834, 1987

92. Bjerager K, Sjostrand U, Wattwil M: Long-term treatment of two patients with respiratory insufficiency with IPPB/PEEP and HFPPV/PEEP. Acta Anaesthesiol Scand, suppl. 64:55–68, 1977

93. Gallagher TJ, Banner MJ: High-frequency positive-pressure ventilation for oleic acid induced lung injury. Crit Care Med 8:232, 1980

94. Gallagher TJ, Boysen PG, Davidson DD, et al: High-frequency percussive ventilation compared with conventional mechanical ventilation. Crit Care Med 17:364–366, 1989

95. Schuster DP, Klain M: High-frequency ventilation during acute lung injury. Anesthesiology 55:A70, 981

96. Hoff B, Smith RB, Wilson E, et al: High-frequency ventilation (HFV) during bronchopleural fistula. Anesthesiology 55:A71, 1981

97. Kuwik R, Glass DD, Coombs DW: Evaluation of high frequency positive-pressure ventilation for experimental bronchopleural fistula. Crit Care Med 9:164, 1981

98. Pierce EC II: Extracorporeal Circulation for open heart Surgery. Charles C Thomas, Springfield, IL, 1969

99. Gille JP: World census of long-term perfusion for respiratory support. pp. 525–530. In Zapol W, Qvist J (eds): Artificial Lungs for Acute Respiratory Failure. Hemisphere Publishing, New York, 1976

100. Extracorporeal Support for Respiratory Insufficiency. A Collaborative Study. National Heart, Lung, and Blood Institute: US Department of Health, Education & Welfare, Washington, DC, 1979

101. Graves ED III, Loe WA, Redmond CR, et al: Extracorporeal membrane oxygenation as treatment of severe meconium aspiration syndrome. South Med J 82:698, 1989

102. Moront MG, Katz NM, Keszler M, et al: Extracorporeal membrane oxygenation for neonatal respiratory failure. A report of 50 cases. J Thorac Cardiovasc Surg 97:706–714, 1989

103. Weber TR, Pennington DG, Connors R, et al: Extracorporeal membrane oxygenation for newborn respiratory failure. Ann Thorac Surg 42:529–535, 1986

104. Bartlett RH, Gazzaniga AB, Toomasian J, et al: Extracorporeal membrane oxygenation (ECMO) in neonatal respiratory failure. Ann Surg 204:236–245, 1986

105. Trento A, Griffith BP, Hardesty RL: Extracorporeal membrane oxygenation experience at the University of Pittsburgh. Ann Thorac Surg 42:56–59, 1986

106. Krummel TM, Greenfield LJ, Kirkpatrick BV, et al: Clinical use of an extracorporeal membrane oxygenator in neonatal pulmonary failure. J Pediatr Surg 17:525–531, 1982

107. Toomasian JM, Snedecor SM, Cornell RG, et al: National experience with extracorporeal membrane oxygenation for newborn respiratory failure. Data from 715 cases. ASAIO Trans 34:140–147, 1988

108. Zwischenberger JB, Cilley RE, Hirschl RB, et al: Life-threatening intrathoracic complications during treatment with extracorporeal membrane oxygenation. J Pediatr Surg 23:599–604, 1988

109. Nading JH: Historical controls for extracorporeal membrane oxygenation in neonates. Crit Care Med 17:423–425, 1989

110. Pennington DG, McBride LR, Kanter KR, et al: Bridging to heart transplantation with circulatory support devices. J Heart Transplant 8:116–123, 1989

111. Bolman RM III, Spray TL, Cox JL, et al: Heart transplantation in patients requiring preoperative mechanical support. J Heart Transplant 6:273–280, 1987

112. Kanter KR, Pennington DG, McBride LR, et al: Mechanical circulatory assistance after heart transplantation. J Heart Transplant 6:150–154, 1987

113. Bartlett RH, Kolobow T, Cooper JD, et al: Extracorporeal gas exchange, lung transplantation, and the artificial lung. ASAIO Trans 30:679–681, 1984

114. Egan TM, Duffin J, Glynn MF, et al: Ten-year experience with extracorporeal membrane oxygenation for severe respiratory failure. Chest 94:681–687, 1988

115. Gattinoni L, Pesenti A, Mascheroni D, et al: Low-frequency positive-pressure ventilation with extracorporeal CO_2 removal in severe acute respiratory failure. JAMA 256:881–886, 1986

116. Hall JR, Brouillard RG: Water vapor pressure calculation. J Appl Physiol Respir Envir Exercise Physiol 58:2090, 1985

117. Borg U, Lyttkens L, Nilsson LG, et al: Physiologic evaluation of the HFPPV pneumatic valve principle and PEEP. Acta Anaesthesiol Scand, suppl. 64:37–53, 1977

118. Jonzon A: Phrenic and vagal nerve activities during spontaneous respiration and positive-pressure ventilation. Acta Anaesthesiol Scand, suppl. 64:29–35, 1977

25

NUTRITIONAL CARE OF THE THORACIC SURGICAL PATIENT

Eldar Søreide, M.D.
Bjørn Skeie, M.D.
Jeffrey Askanazi, M.D.

Traditionally, care of the thoracic surgical patient has involved a great deal of attention to the circulatory and respiratory systems, with nutritional support relegated to a minor role. This is not surprising given the emergency nature of cardiorespiratory physiology versus the long-term implications of nutritional support. However, it is increasingly recognized that chronic respiratory disease and surgical illness are accompanied by malnutrition, which again is associated with a poorer prognosis in these patients. Thus, nutritional support is now receiving increasing attention both because the specific effects of nutrients on general organ function and immunologic function are better understood and because more knowledge about the interaction between nutrition and the respiratory system has been accumulated. This review aims to improve understanding of the interactions among illness, metabolism, and nutritional support. The discussion includes a brief review of commonly used terminology, followed by a discussion of the general effects of perioperative nutritional support, and the specific effects of nutrition on the respiratory system. Finally, theoretical and practical considerations of enteral versus parenteral nutrition will be addressed.

BASIC TERMS AND DEFINITIONS

Energy Metabolism

The main goal of nutritional support is to provide protein and energy for all the biochemical processes taking place in the body and to maintain and restore body proteins. However, excessive energy intake, particularly when given as carbohydrate, may cause respiratory and hepatic side effects.[1-4] When deciding on how much energy to provide it is, therefore, important to know how much energy the patient is consuming. Different methods have been developed to measure total body energy consumption. The term *basal metabolic rate* (BMR) refers to energy consumption in the absence of activity and food intake.[5] *Resting energy expenditure* (REE) (Figs. 25-1 and 25-2) refers to energy consumption measured during rest at any time,[5] and therefore includes, among other things, the effect of nutrients to increase energy expenditure, termed *thermic effect* or *diet-induced thermogenesis* (DIT) (Fig. 25-2). On average, DIT increases the energy expenditure close to 10 percent,[1] and several studies have shown that DIT is enhanced in already hypermetabolic patients.[6,7] For both research and clinical pur-

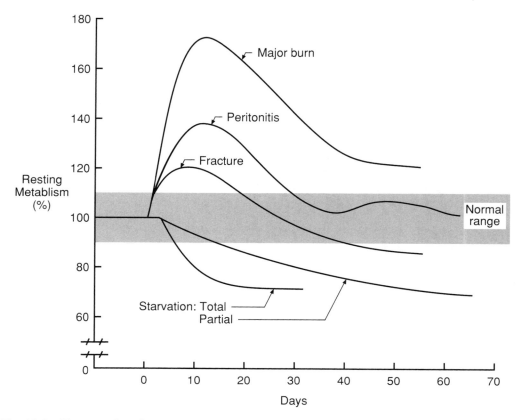

Fig. 25-1. Changes of resting energy expenditure in different pathologic states over 60 days. (From Long,[166] with permission.)

poses, the use of REE as a parameter for energy consumption is preferred to BMR.

When the total amount of energy to be given is determined, the actual composition of nutrients must also be determined. In this connection, it is important to know the caloric content of different nutrients, which are as follows: glucose, 3.75 kcal/g; fat, 9.3 kcal/g; and protein, 4.3 kcal/g. Different nutrients not only have different caloric content, but also have different effects on gas exchange in the human body when oxidized.[5] In studies of metabolism, the relationship between O_2 consumption and CO_2 production is often expressed as the *respiratory quotient* (RQ). The RQ for oxidation of carbohydrate, fat, and protein is, respectively, 1.0, 0.71, and 0.81.[5] Naturally, the RQ is a reflection of oxidation of all three substrates, and any given substrate intake may produce a different RQ under different clinical conditions (Fig. 25-3).[8] The highest observed whole-body RQ in humans would not be expected to be greater than 1.2 or lower than 0.69, and values outside this range should be considered as errors in measurement.

Measured Versus Predicted Resting Energy Expenditure

The most frequently used method of measuring REE is indirect calorimetry, which uses data for oxygen consumption ($\dot{V}O_2$) and CO_2 production ($\dot{V}CO_2$) to calculate actual energy consumption of the body.[5] Measurements of $\dot{V}CO_2$ are easily disturbed by changes in ventilation, independent of metabolic production of CO_2.[5] Therefore, gas exchange measurements must be performed in a steady-state manner without causing the patient's breathing pattern to be altered.[9] In mechanically ventilated patients, $\dot{V}CO_2$ may be a more reliable indicator of the metabolic situation.[5] The main problem with metabolic studies in intensive care patients is that the accuracy of $\dot{V}O_2$ measurements may decrease with increasing oxygen enrichment (F_IO_2), especially when F_IO_2 exceeds 0.6.[10,11] Liggett et al used the indirect Fick method to determine REE for patients who had thermodilution pulmonary artery catheters in place.[12] They calculated REE by multiplying $\dot{V}O_2$ by the caloric value for oxygen, and

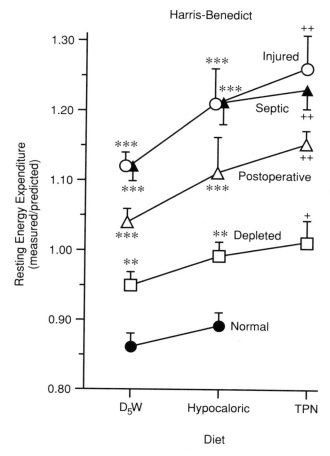

Fig. 25-2. Effect of disease and diet. D_5W = 5 percent dextrose alone, energy intake 0.31 × REE; Hypocaloric = dextrose and amino acids, energy intake < 0.8 × REE; TPN = total parenteral nutrition, energy intake > 0.8 × REE. Differs from normal: *$P < 0.05$, **$P < 0.01$, ***$P < 0.01$; differs from dextrose (D_5W): +$P < 0.05$, ++$P < 0.01$. 1 kcal = 4.2 kJ. (From Shaw-Delanty et al,[6] with permission.)

TABLE 25-1. Harris Benedict Formula for Predicting Basal Metabolic Rate

Males: 66 + (13.8 W) + (5 H) − (6.8 A)
Females: 655 + (9.6 W) + (1.8 H) − (4.7 A)

Abbreviations: W, weight in kilograms; H, height in centimeters; A, age in years.
(From Harris and Benedict,[167] with permission.)

ited value in the individual patient. Studies of surgical patients have also shown that using simple mean values for kilocalorie per kilogram per day are as good as or even better than the traditional formulas that estimate REE on the basis of age, sex, height, and other parameters.[6,14] In critically ill patients on mechanical ventilation, values for measured REE varying from 70 to 140 percent of estimated REE have been found.[19,24] Some of the variation in REE may be explained by the coexistence of malnutrition and stress in intensive care patients. REE in these patients will be the algebraic result of malnutrition-reducing and stress-increasing REE,[25] but clinical observation may unfortunately give little indication of which patients are hypermetabolic and which are hypometabolic.[19] The coexistence of malnutrition and surgical disease (eg, cancer) may also explain why measured REE levels in malnourished patients were higher than in normal individuals and postoperative patients (Fig. 25-2) but lower than in normal individuals (Fig. 25-1).[26,27] A drawback of measuring REE is that changes may occur from day to day in any given patient.[16–18,28] Thus, a single measurement may be misleading.[16] The variation of REE during the course and treatment of different clinical conditions is also illustrated in Figure 25-1.

Protein Metabolism

To prevent loss of muscle mass and other important tissues, it is essential to provide not only calories, but also proteins (amino acids). The standard for measuring losses and gains in body proteins has been *nitrogen balance*.[5] The reason is that approximately 95 percent of total body nitrogen is found in protein. Nitrogen balance refers simply to the measuring of all nitrogen intake and subtracting nitrogen losses (N-balance = N-intake − N-excretion). Since changes in nitrogen excretion occur mainly as urinary urea, the nitrogen loss can be calculated using a measurement of 24-hour urinary urea excretion.[5] When nitrogen balance is negative, it means that the patient has a net loss of body proteins (*catabolic phase*). A positive nitrogen balance, on the other hand, indicates that restoration

found an excellent agreement when comparing results obtained with the thermodilution method with those obtained from gas exchange measurements.

Indirect calorimetry has been widely used to study metabolic changes relating to malnutrition, injury, and sepsis.[1,2,13–24] This method is also gaining acceptance for clinical monitoring, although it remains hampered by all the time-consuming labor involved.[5] In clinical practice, REE is most often estimated (Table 25-1), but the usefulness of formulas to estimate REE in critically ill patients is still debated.[6,14,19,23] Several studies[14,19,24] have found estimated REE reliable when it comes to groups of patients, but of limited

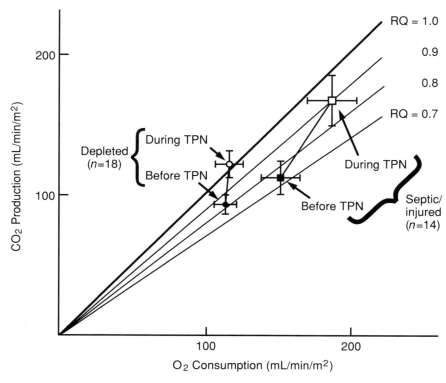

Fig. 25-3. Alterations in gas exchange in depleted or septic/injured patients when 5 percent dextrose infusions are replaced by glucose and amino acid-based TPN. (From Askanazi et al,[8] with permission.)

of body proteins and, therefore, tissue is taking place (*anabolic phase*).

Body Composition

Besides the use of nitrogen balance, depletion and repletion of body mass have, traditionally, been described in terms of weight loss and weight gain. Recently, more precise and direct techniques (multiple isotope dilution and gamma-neutron activation) to study body composition have been developed and applied in studies of surgical patients.[5,29,30] Several studies have shown that changes in body weight are not always good parameters of changes in the nutritional status of patients and that, in connection with the clinical effects of nutritional depletion and repletion, the changes in body composition are better parameters than weight changes alone.[29-33]

Body fat and *lean body mass* (LBM) constitute the two major compartments of the body.[5,34] LBM is composed of an extracellular component (the *extracellular mass* [ECM]) and an intracellular component (the *body cell mass* [BCM]). The BCM represents the total mass of living, functioning, oxygen-consuming, and work-performing cells, and approximately two-thirds

of the body protein store is located intracellularly. Since the BCM, unlike the ECM, is metabolically active, it represents an important parameter that may be used under conditions in which metabolic activity must be defined as a function of body size.[34]

Total body water accounts for approximately 60 percent of body weight; the extracellular water accounts for approximately one-third of the total body water. The interaction between dislocation of body compartments and nutritional status has important implications for the surgical patient. It has been shown that malnutrition in surgical patients is associated with both a relative and an absolute increase in extracellular water.[29,30,32] This means that a BCM loss can be masked by an increase in extracellular water so that clinically important losses of BCM are not identified through measured weight loss. The increased extracellular water, which is also found in lung and gut tissue, may also explain why malnourished surgical patients are susceptible to postoperative respiratory failure and mechanical complications like wound dehiscence.[29,32,35,36] This dislocation of body fluid compartments should also be taken into consideration in connection with perioperative fluid management.[29] Another important clinical observation made with body composition studies is that short-term changes in weight in surgical patients are due to either increases or decreases in extracellular water and not to changes in body proteins.[29,30,32] The synthesis of new LBM protein proceeds at such a slow rate that weight gain due to changes in LBM protein take place only over a week or so. On the other hand, weight loss due to breakdown of tissue (LBM) occurs much more rapidly than weight gain due to its synthesis.[5] These data imply a theme that will be repeatedly stressed in this review: preventing LBM loss is easier than restoring LBM.

PREOPERATIVE NUTRITIONAL SUPPORT

General Effects of Malnutrition

Metabolic Changes

In an otherwise healthy, fasting subject, fat oxidation is the main energy source.[5] Ongoing glucose requirements for the central nervous system, renal medulla, and white blood cells are initially met by glycogen consumption. Following this, amino acids from muscle proteins, as well as glycerol from hydrolysis of triglycerides, are mobilized for the production of glucose (gluconeogenesis). However, several adaptive mechanisms that promote energy and protein conservation soon develop. In his classic study of prolonged fasting, Benedict found that weight loss was rapid the first week, mainly due to initial water loss, but then continued at a decreasing rate throughout the first month.[37] A reduction in REE up to 35 percent develops.[5] Another important adaptive mechanism is that as more ketones become available, the brain progressively uses more ketones as an energy source instead of oxidizing only glucose. The increased ketone oxidation results in decreased glucose requirements, with a concomitant reduction in protein losses. Even small intakes of carbohydrate in late starvation markedly suppress gluconeogenesis and have a large protein-sparing effect.[38] Interestingly, if total fasting is continued long-term, fat stores are more limiting for survival than the protein stores, and fasts of 60 days usually end in death.[5]

It is important to understand that if patients with surgical disease undergo fasting or semistarvation, the metabolic situation will be quite different from that of fasting or semistarvation in otherwise healthy subjects. For instance, it has been shown that both in patients with surgically treatable cancer[39] and in injured and septic patients,[40] prolonged starvation does not induce a reduction in gluconeogenesis from amino acids, as it does in normal individuals. Furthermore, the hypermetabolism found in injured and septic patients,[40,41] as well as in many surgical cancer patients,[26,27,42] increases energy and protein requirements. Therefore, in surgical patients, underfeeding will add to the catabolic stress induced by the disease itself, causing a more rapid deterioration of nutritional status. From this, it is clear that malnutrition carries a different significance in surgical patients and that nutritional support is important to avoid rapid decreases in body stores of fat and proteins.

Clinical Effects of Malnutrition

Postoperative complications like sepsis, pneumonia, respiratory failure, and impaired healing of the wound (fistula, wound dehiscence, wound infection, anastomotic leakage) have been described in 20 to 50 percent of patients undergoing major intra-abdominal and intrathoracic surgery.[31,35,43] Numerous studies have shown a correlation between malnutrition and adverse surgical outcome in patients undergoing major surgery,[31,35,44–46] and several studies from both Europe and the United States have found evidence of moderate-to-severe protein-calorie malnutrition in as many as 30 to 50 percent of surgical patients.[47–49]

Bronchogenic cancer is a common diagnosis among patients undergoing thoracic surgery, and many of the general aspects of cancer and nutritional status therefore apply to the thoracic surgical patient. Cancer is frequently associated with malnutrition, and the extent of the malnutrition is mainly related to the type and site of the tumor. In the early stages of disease, malnutrition is most pronounced in patients with cancer of the esophagus and stomach.[50] Weight loss in patients with various types of cancer correlates with decreasing performance and a decreased median survival time.[50] Besides the anatomic extent of lung cancer and histologic characteristics of the tumor, the immunologic and nutritional status of the patient is also believed to be important to survival.[51] Fatzinger et al used serum albumin, an often-used nutritional marker, to predict survival in stage III non-oat cell lung cancer.[52] They found that in patients with unresectable or resectable primary tumors, a serum albumin level of less than 3.4 g/dL indicated a poor prognosis (Fig. 25-4). They concluded that hypoalbuminemia signaled the onset of an end-stage metabolic effect of the tumor on the host's protein metabolism, and that the presence of hypoalbuminemia had an irreversible effect on survival, despite artificial feeding and the removal or destruction of the tumor by a combination of irradiation, operation, and chemotherapy.

In a recent Canadian study of 1,076 consecutive pa-

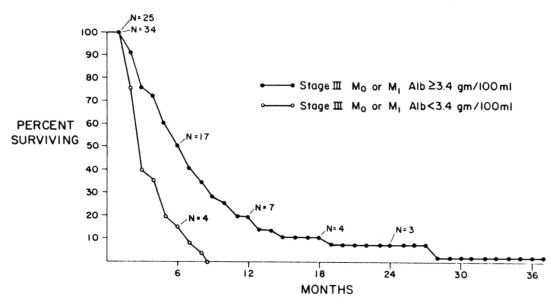

Fig. 25-4. Actuarial survival curves for 59 patients with unresectable non-oat-cell lung cancer divided on the basis of preadmission serum albumin (Alb) levels. (From Fatzinger et al,[52] with permission.)

tients undergoing pulmonary resection for lung cancer, nonfatal major complications occurred in 9.8 percent.[46] The overall operative death rate was 3.2 percent, and weight loss was found to be a significant risk factor for major complications and death. Hill showed that protein depletion in patients undergoing major surgery is associated with a measurable impairment of respiratory function and is in itself a significant risk factor in the development of postoperative pneumonia.[29] From this background, it is clear that an understanding of both the effects of malnutrition and refeeding in thoracic surgical patients is important for the clinician.

The Diagnosis of Malnutrition

Historically, the diagnosis of malnutrition has mainly been based on the occurrence and degree of weight loss.[29,53,54] More than 10 percent weight loss during a recent illness is considered to be clinically significant. To better correlate nutritional status with surgical outcome, the use of parameters other than weight loss has been advocated. Better correlation between weight loss and prognosis in surgical patients has been obtained by adding anthropometric, biochemical, and immunologic measurements to the nutritional assessment.[35,55–57] Anthropometric measurements quantify the effect of malnutrition and refeeding on body fat and LBM, but their accuracy and usefulness in individual patients has been questioned.[30] The most frequently used biochemical test

has been the serum level of albumin.[31,47,58,59] However, it has been documented that nonnutritional factors, such as severity of the illness, influence serum levels of albumin to a much greater extent than the nutritional status alone.[32,59] This is presumably because serum albumin levels are determined to a large degree by capillary leakage to the extracellular space.[32,59,60] Nonetheless, several studies have been able to show increased morbidity and mortality in surgical patients with depressed levels of serum albumin.[31,35,55] The importance of albumin as an indicator of operative complications seems to be due primarily to the extent to which albumin reflects alterations in body-water compartments rather than actual protein status.[32]

Various other tests, including tests of immunocompetence, have also been used as prognostic indicators in malnourished surgical patients.[56,57] Although to some extent able to predict postoperative outcome, tests of immunocompetence, like serum albumin, appear to be rather nonspecific and related to many other factors besides nutritional status.[61] Muscle wasting is prominent in severe malnutrition, and studies have shown that skeletal muscle function is indeed a very sensitive parameter of nutritional deprivation and restoration.[62,63] Mullen et al[55,58,64] used anthropometric, biochemical, and immunologic parameters to improve the ability to predict an adverse clinical event in the individual patient. A prognostic nutritional index (PNI) was established, and it was found that the index could clearly identify the patient at risk. Several other investigators,[31,54,65,66] on the other hand, have found that a detailed history and a proper physical examination are as good as any objective test in defining patients at risk of postoperative complications. Windsor and Hill compared a formalized clinical assessment with objective assessments of weight loss and physiologic functions.[31] They differentiated between malnourished patients with and without clear evidence of dysfunction in two or more organ systems. Their results indicate that only those patients who have impairment of important bodily functions in addition to significant loss of body weight are at high risk of postoperative complications.

Refeeding Malnourished Patients

Clinical Effects of Refeeding

Although several studies[44,45,55] have established the association of malnutrition and a high incidence of operative complications, these studies did not reveal whether malnutrition was a cause of complications or whether the increased complication rate and malnutrition merely occurred concurrently due to advanced primary disease or nonnutritional comorbidities.[35,43] Several studies have, therefore, tried to determine whether preoperative nutritional support could positively influence nutritional status and reduce postoperative morbidity and mortality in patients undergoing major intrathoracic and intra-abdominal surgery.

Starker et al[32,33,36,67] investigated the use of serum albumin as an index of nutritional support. In the initial study, measurements of sodium balance were used to indicate alterations in the extracellular fluid (ECF) compartment.[32] By examining concurrent alterations in plasma levels of albumin, body weight, and sodium balance, the relationship of serum albumin concentration to the status of the ECF, as well as to hepatic synthesis and nitrogen balance, was established (Figs. 25-5 and 25-6). All patients had a positive nitrogen balance. These investigators further showed that in nutritionally depleted patients receiving 2 weeks of total parenteral nutrition (TPN) prior to a major abdominal operation, the postoperative course correlated with the preoperative response to nutritional support.[33] Patients who exhibited the characteristic response to preoperative TPN, diuresis of the expanded ECF with a resultant loss of weight and increase in serum albumin, developed significantly fewer complications in the postoperative period than patients who did not exhibit this response. In a follow-up study, it was demonstrated that patients who do not diurese and show a rise in serum albumin after 2 weeks may respond with diuresis and a decrease in serum albumin if TPN is maintained for 4 to 6 weeks,

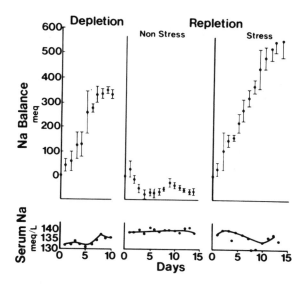

Fig. 25-5. The effect of nutritional support on sodium balance in a nonstressed versus a stressed group of patients. (From Starker et al,[32] with permission.)

with a consequent fall in postoperative morbidity and mortality.[67] Increases in BCM occurred in all patients, and it seemed that although restoration of BCM occurred primarily in muscle, the contraction of extracellular fluid occurred in other tissues, possibly the gut and lung.[36] This reduction in tissue edema could explain the decrease in surgical wound complications. A TPN-induced reduction of the ratio of extracellular and intracellular water has also been associated with an improvement in immune function.[57]

Using their PNI,[55,58] Mullen et al were able to correlate malnutrition, preoperative TPN, and outcome.[64] In the high-risk group (PNI ≥ 50 percent), adequate (≥5 days) preoperative nutritional support was asso-

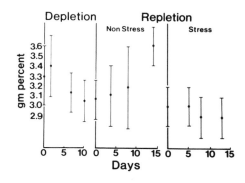

Fig. 25-6. Serum albumin levels rise in the nonstressed group of patients versus the stressed group of patients, in whom a slight decline occurred. (From Starker et al,[32] with permission.)

ciated with a sevenfold reduction in major sepsis and a fivefold reduction in mortality, but, interestingly, with little change in PNI. Hill and Haydock were able to show that the wound healing response in malnourished patients was impaired at an earlier stage of nutritional depletion than had previously been supposed.[29] Furthermore, their studies emphasized the importance of nutritional repletion, particularly of recent adequate food intake to restore the wound-healing response.[29,68]

Randomized, prospective trials of preoperative TPN in patients undergoing intrathoracic and intra-abdominal surgery have produced conflicting results,[43,69] and only a few studies have demonstrated significant reduction in overall operative complications and mortality. The results of controlled trials in preoperative enteral nutrition have been similar to TPN, with approximately half showing substantive improvement in clinical outcome.[69] Two recent large prospective studies of preoperative TPN failed to document a significantly reduced mortality.[43,45,70] Preliminary results revealed that preoperative TPN significantly reduced nonseptic complications, but with the cost of significantly more septic complications, including both pneumonia and wound infections.[69,70] Based on earlier studies,[33,64,67] the increased infection risk and lack of significant benefits in patients receiving preoperative TPN were surprising. However, no definite reason for the increased septic complication rate was detected, and preoperative nutritional support is still advocated to correct overt deficiencies in severely malnourished patients undergoing major surgery and to prevent in-hospital starvation in patients when surgery is delayed for several days.[69,71] In clinical practice, the remaining problems seem to be how to identify high-risk patients who could benefit from preoperative nutritional support and how to undertake nutritional support with a minimum of risk to the patient and without extensive costs and use of manpower.[54,69]

Nutritional Requirements

REE has been shown to be approximately 25 kcal/kg/d in malnourished surgical patients.[6,15] Elwyn showed that to restore lost BCM in these patients, energy intake should exceed 30 kcal/kg (Fig. 25-7).[53] For optimal restoration of BCM, the nitrogen intake should be at least 300 to 350 mg/kg/d.[25,72] A confusing factor when deciding how much energy to provide is whether to include the energy derived from proteins. Including protein calories in total energy intake has been advocated by some authors,[73] while others[41,74] use only nonprotein calories in recommendations of caloric intake. The argument for not including pro-

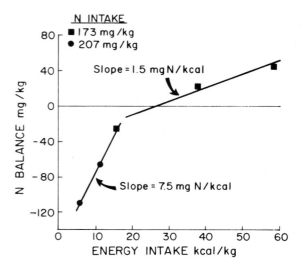

Fig. 25-7. Nitrogen balance at various levels of energy (glucose) intake in postoperative (●) and depleted (■) patients. (From Elwyn,[53] with permission.)

tein-derived energy seems to be that the exogenous protein is primarily meant to be a source of nitrogen and not of energy. However, it seems illogical not to incorporate the caloric value derived from protein since it does provide energy. Proteins can be administered in amounts ranging from 15 to 30 percent of REE,[73] providing approximately 500 kcal/d in patients with normal liver and renal function.

Although not generally agreed on, many authors think that the nonprotein calories can be given as fat and glucose in a 50:50 ratio.[25,74–76] With low-calorie intake, the nitrogen-sparing effect of glucose is definitely greater than fat, but when energy intake exceeds 500 kcal, fat and glucose have the same effects on nitrogen balance.[72,75] Further, prolonged use of high loads of glucose as the sole energy source carries the risk of inducing the essential fatty acid deficiency (EFAD) syndrome which, among other things, causes an increased susceptibility to infections.[77] The EFAD syndrome has only been described in connection with TPN using high loads of glucose. The reason is that continuous high-rate infusions of glucose almost completely inhibit release of fatty acids from adipose tissue. It may only take 2 weeks of hyperalimentation with glucose to produce EFAD. Thus, it is important to recognize that while the role of fat as a calorie source is disputed, there is an absolute necessity for lipid emulsion in order to provide essential fatty acids.

When commencing artificial nutrition in severely malnourished patients (weight loss ≥ 35 percent), caution must be taken not to overload the metabolic and physiologic capacity.[53] Most of the complications associated with refeeding seem to be caused by TPN-induced hypophosphatemia.[53,78,79] The manifestations may be neuromuscular, neurologic, hematologic, and cardiovascular. To avoid these potentially life-threatening complications, energy and nitrogen intake should be increased step by step over several days, and all electrolytes, including phosphate, should be carefully monitored and supplemented in appropriate amounts.[53,79]

Vitamins and trace elements are often referred to as micronutrients.[61,76] Deficits in trace elements may cause various symptoms, and trace elements should, therefore, be included in nutritional protocols from the first day. The general guideline for vitamin administration is, therefore, to include all vitamins in nutritional protocols from the first day.[61,76] In Table 25-2, daily requirements for electrolytes, trace elements, and vitamins are given, while Table 25-3 shows a suggested standard TPN formula for refeeding a 70 kg patient.

TABLE 25-2. Daily Intravenous Electrolyte, Trace Element, and Vitamin Requirements in Adults

	Amount
Sodium	60 or more mEq
Potassium	60 or more mEq
Calcium	10–15 mEq
Phosphate	20–50 mEq
Magnesium	8–20 mEq
Zinc	2.5–4.0 mg (additional 2.0 mg in acute catabolic stress[a])
Copper	0.5–1.5 mg
Chromium	10–15 μg
Manganese	0.15–0.8 mg
Selenium	40–120 μg
Molybdenum	20–30 μg
Iodide	70–140 μg
Iron	1–7 mg
Vitamin A	4,000–5,000[b] IU
Vitamin D	400 IU
Vitamin E	12–15 IU
Ascorbic acid	45 mg
Folic acid	400 μg
Niacin	12–20 mg
Riboflavin	1.1–1.8 mg
Thiamin	1.0–1.5 mg
Vitamin B₆ (pyridoxine)	1.6–2.0 mg
Vitamin B₁₂ (cyanocobalamin)	3 mg
Pantothenic acid	5–10 mg
Biotin	150–300 μg

[a] Frequent monitoring of blood levels in these patients is essential to supply proper dosage.
[b] Assumes 50 percent intake as carotene, which is less available than vitamin A.
(Data from Weinsier and Butterworth[168,169] and Krey and Murray.[170,171])

TABLE 25-3. Suggested Nutrient Regimen for the Standard 70 kg Man Following Weight Loss Aiming at Nutritional Repletion

Regimen	Content
Nutrient mixture	
Protein	110 g (= 440 kcal)
Nonprotein calories	1,500–2,000 kcal
Distribution	50% glucose and 50% fat
Parenteral solutions[a]	
1,000 mL	11% amino acids (440 kcal)
1,000 mL	20% glucose (800 kcal)
500 mL	20% fat emulsion (1,000 kcal)

[a] The parenteral solutions can be mixed in one bag and infused over 24 hours (100 mL/h). Electrolytes, trace elements, and vitamins are added in the same bag.

POSTOPERATIVE NUTRITIONAL SUPPORT

Metabolic Aspects in Postoperative, Injured, and Septic Patients

Hypermetabolism and Hypercatabolism

The two most prominent metabolic responses to injury, accelerated breakdown of skeletal muscle and increased oxygen consumption, were first described by Cuthbertson.[40] Subsequently, it has been demonstrated that a similar hypercatabolic state occurs with established sepsis.[80] The extent to which net catabolism of body protein takes place depends both on severity and type of insult and on dietary intake. In general, accidental injuries, like burns and multiple fractures, produce a much more pronounced metabolic response than surgical procedures.[6,21,81] Although the metabolic consequences of sepsis and injury are different in some aspects, they bear similarities that allow for simultaneous discussion of both.

Shock and Flow Phase

Originally, Cuthbertson divided the metabolic response of injury into an initial hypometabolic ebb (or shock) phase and a subsequent hypermetabolic flow phase.[40] In the shock phase, there is an outpouring of catecholamines and other hormones,[40,41] and the most prominent metabolic finding due to the hormonal changes in hyperglycemia, which correlates with the severity of injury.[82] The subsequent flow phase is characterized by both hypermetabolism and that of hypercatabolism.[8,21,40,81] The degrees of hypermetabolism and hypercatabolism tend to be parallel, although in the individual patients, the correspondence may be poor. The increased REE of injury is partly due to a resetting of the hypothalamic "thermostat" and is accompanied by an increase in core temperature.[80] Another component of the higher REE is increased substrate cycling seen with injury and sepsis.[80,83]

Carbohydrate and Fat Metabolism

As mentioned above, glucose metabolism in the early stages of injury and sepsis is characterized by hyperglycemia primarily due to glycogenolysis.[82] The hyperglycemia that occurs in the flow phase is related to increased production of glucose from amino acids, glycerol, and lactate.[41,80,83] In contrast to the situation in normal subjects, hepatic glucose production is maintained at normal or elevated rates despite hyperglycemia.

Teleologically, the excessive level of circulation glucose can be viewed as a successful adaptation to the requirements of a new situation.[80] The wound, regenerating tissue, and white blood cells use large amounts of glucose, primarily for glycolysis to lactate. The lactate returns to the liver for reconversion to glucose. Since wounds are poorly vascularized, a high glucose gradient between plasma and tissue facilitates a high glucose extraction.[80] The increased conversion of glucose to lactate may also be important for the provision of the 5-carbon sugar, ribose, via the hexose monophosphate shunt (Fig. 25-8), as well as providing NADPH for biosynthetic processes.[84] The ribose molecules are essential for nucleic acid synthesis, which again is required for cell reparative processes.

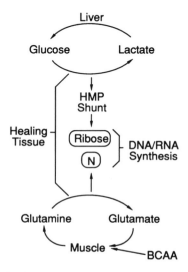

Fig. 25-8. The hexose-monophosphate (HMP) shunt. N, nitrogen; BCAA, branch-chain amino acids.

Lipolysis and fat oxidation are also enhanced in traumatized and septic patients,[21,41,83] and a low RQ indicates that fat is the preferred substrate for oxidation in insulin-resistant tissues.[8,83] All organs, except the brain, contribute to the protein loss in hypercatabolic patients. However, the bulk of proteolysis occurs in skeletal muscle, which is the biggest protein source in the body.[80] The net rates of protein loss in injury are much higher than protein losses associated with simple starvation or bed rest.

Nutritional Implications in Postoperative, Injured, and Septic Patients

Nutritional Goals

The hypercatabolic response to accidental injury, sepsis, and surgical procedures will cause loss of LBM, primarily including the vitally important body compartment BCM. Therefore, to preserve the cardiorespiratory, immunologic, and working capacity of the patient, nutritional support in postoperative and septic/injured patients should aim at the prevention of extensive BCM loss without adding metabolic stress.[8,25,53] The hypercatabolic response in the early flow phase can be ameliorated, although not completely overcome, with nutritional support.[25,80,83] This is not unexpected since both the metabolic stress response and the muscle atrophy induced by immobility[83] may contribute to a net negative nitrogen balance despite apparently adequate nutrition in these patients.

While the beneficial clinical effects of nutritional support in severely injured and septic patients is self-evident, the role of immediate TPN in otherwise uncomplicated postoperative patients is still not clarified. As shown in Figure 25-7, hypocaloric infusions of glucose and amino acids have significant nitrogen-sparing effects compared with fasting in postoperative patients. However, in a prospective and randomized trial of 122 patients undergoing major thoracoabdominal procedures and total cystectomy, Woolfson and Smith did not find a significant improvement in morbidity, mortality, or duration of hospital stay in patients receiving immediate postoperative TPN compared with 5 percent glucose.[85] On the other hand, Askanazi et al retrospectively studied the effect of nutritional support on duration of hospital stay in patients undergoing major surgery (radical cystectomy).[86] A significantly shorter length of hospital stay was found for patients receiving immediate postoperative TPN (Fig. 25-9), and surgical complications did not explain this difference. There is some indirect evidence that immediate postoperative nutritional support may be beneficial. Russell et al demonstrated

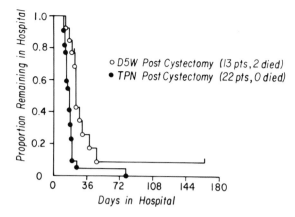

Fig. 25-9. Duration of hospitalization. The group receiving TPN had a shorter median duration of hospitalization than the group receiving 5 percent dextrose (D5W) (17 versus 24 days; *P* < 0.002). The tick mark (′) indicates last follow-up (ie, death). (From Askanazi et al,[86] with permission.)

that hypocaloric diet and fasting induced skeletal muscle fatigue accompanied by structural and biochemical changes in muscle, and these changes may contribute to the phenomenon of fatigue commonly seen after surgery.[87,88] Christensen and Kehlet further found that there was a significant correlation between the postoperative fatigue and catabolic changes such as loss in body weight and total body fat.[89] They concluded that therapeutic measures should involve a conversion of postoperative catabolism to anabolism, and that enteral or parenteral nutrition should be used to achieve this goal since many patients only have a limited intake of nutrients in the late postoperative period. Many researchers therefore think that the possible beneficial effects of immediate nutritional support after major surgery, preferentially using peripheral catheters or gastroenteral feeding tubes, outweigh the costs and risks in postoperative patients either malnourished preoperatively or not able to return to adequate oral intake within a few days.[25,53,71]

Nutritional Requirements

Some early recommendations for nutritional support in injured and septic patients did not take into account possible side effects of excessive energy intake, and based the amounts of calories to be delivered mainly on the effect of the nitrogen balance.[1–4] They therefore tended to be high, varying from 1.75 to 3.0 times REE, or even higher.[90,91] However, several studies have shown that, with the exception of the most severely injured patients, zero or close to zero nitro-

gen balance can be achieved by providing approximately 1.33 times REE.[74,75,92] Present recommendations are, therefore, generally aimed at lower energy intakes. Bursztein et al recommend that calories in the amount of 1.33 times REE be provided.[25] Several studies[6,75] have found REE to be between 25 and 30 kcal/kg/d in most septic and injured patients, and 1.33 times this value would give 35 to 40 kcal/kg/d. However, others have suggested daily energy requirements of 30 to 40 kcal/kg in moderately stressed injured and septic patients and 40 to 50 kcal/kg in severe sepsis and extensive trauma patients.[76] As previously stated, otherwise uncomplicated postoperative patients are less hypermetabolic than accidentally injured or septic patients (Fig. 25-2) and have been found to have an REE between 20 and 25 kcal/kg.[6]

The recommended calorie-to-nitrogen ratio in septic and injured patients is approximately 150 kcal : 1 g nitrogen.[25] The effect of increasing nitrogen intake on nitrogen balance seems to level off at values above 200 mg nitrogen/kg/d (Fig. 25-10).[74,92,93] Nonetheless, many investigators recommend higher nitrogen intake (270 to 500 mg nitrogen/kg/d) to assure optimal condition for preserving BCM.[25,53] In Figure 25-11, the energy metabolism in a severely injured patient given TPN is illustrated.

NUTRITION AND THE RESPIRATORY SYSTEM

Coexisting lung disease is an important determinant of medical operability in lung cancer patients.[46] During the presurgical workup, special consideration is given to pulmonary function and extent of resection. The interaction between nutritional status and lung function is, therefore, of clinical interest in the thoracic surgical patient. In this section, the respiratory implications of malnutrition and refeeding patients and the specific respiratory effects of different nutrients will be reviewed. The importance of nutrition in connection with acute respiratory failure and mechanical ventilation will then be discussed.

Respiratory Effects of Malnutrition and Refeeding

Respiratory Muscle

It was first thought that the body had a mechanism by which it could spare certain critical muscles, such as the diaphragm and the myocardium, during starvation. However, it has been shown that the respiratory

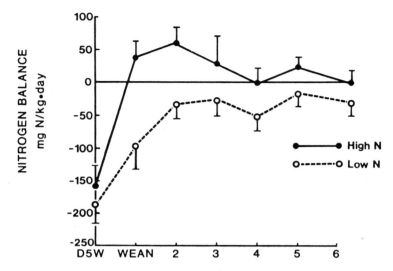

Fig. 25-10. Nitrogen balance in septic patients receiving low (approximately 200 mg nitrogen/kg) or high (approximately 350 mg nitrogen/kg) nitrogen TPN for each day of a 6-day study period. (From Windsor and Hill,[31] with permission.)

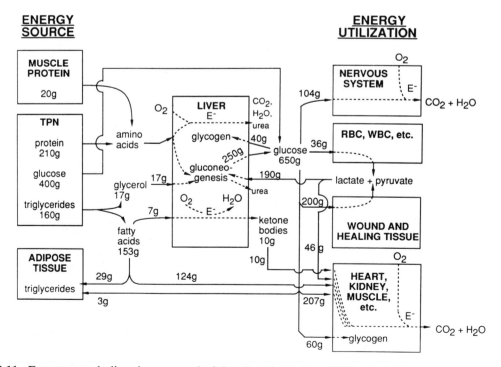

Fig. 25-11. Energy metabolism in a severely injured patient given TPN at 1.2 times energy expenditure. Measured energy expenditure was 3,250 kcal (13,598 kJ) per day. Nonprotein calories were provided as glucose and fat in a 50:50 ratio. (From Bursztein et al,[5] with permission.)

muscles are subject to the same catabolic changes as other skeletal muscles during starvation and stress.[94] The diaphragm, the principal muscle of respiration, is often used to exemplify the entire respiratory system. The relationship between malnutrition and the respiratory system has been widely studied by Arora and Rochester.[94–96] These investigators found that for a body weight loss of 32 percent, the corresponding loss of diaphragm was 43 percent.[95] The respiratory muscle weight loss was associated with loss of respiratory muscle strength to 37 percent, vital capacity to 63 percent, and maximum voluntary ventilation to 41 percent of normal values.[96] Several researchers have examined the relationship between BCM and respiratory function in malnourished surgical patients.[29,97] Kelly et al examined the relationship between BCM and inspiratory muscle strength in surgical patients requiring nutritional support.[97] Prior to nutritional repletion, there was a significant positive relationship between maximal inspiratory pressure and BCM. Hill divided 80 patients awaiting major gastrointestinal surgery into two groups based on the degree of protein depletion.[29] Approximately half the patients had experienced a small protein loss (mean, 2 percent), while the others had a mean protein loss of 36 percent. There were no differences between these two groups with regard to age, surgical diagnosis, presence of chronic lung disease, smoking, degree of obesity, proportion of thoracic and upper abdominal incisions, duration of anesthesia, or use of prophylactic physiotherapy and antibiotics. Before surgery, there was a highly significant difference between these two groups for respiratory muscle strength, vital capacity, and peak expiratory flow rate. The protein-depleted patients also had a significantly higher incidence of postoperative pneumonia and longer hospital stay. These results indicate that malnutrition is associated with a measurable impairment of respiratory function, and is, of itself, a significant risk factor in the development of postoperative pneumonia.

The impairment in respiratory muscle function exceeds the loss of muscle mass.[94,98] This suggests that diaphragmatic pressure is reduced in part because there is less muscle, and also because the remaining muscle is weaker. Malnourished patients undergoing nutritional repletion have been found to improve muscle strength function within 2 weeks, long before BCM is completely restored.[87,90,99] This may indicate that an increase in cellular energy levels contributes more to improved muscle strength over the short term than does an increase in BCM.[88] The effects of nutritional repletion on respiratory muscles seem to be biphasic.[100] Initially, there is a rapid restoration of biochemical functions that results in functional improvement. This is followed by a period of repletion of actual muscle tissue (BCM). However, improvement of respiratory muscle mass is a slow process requiring one to several weeks to obtain significant results.[101]

Respiratory Drive and Pulmonary Defense Mechanisms

Malnutrition also influences lung function by altering the ventilatory response to hypoxia. Doekel et al found that clinical semistarvation in normal volunteers for 10 days reduced ventilatory response to hypoxia by 42 percent.[102] Refeeding restored the depressed ventilatory drive. Weissman et al showed that semistarvation significantly decreased both ventilatory drive and REE (Fig. 25-12).[103] Using mean inspiratory flow as an index of neuromuscular drive, they noted a 26 percent decrease following 7 days of hypocaloric glucose feeding. Refeeding with amino acids was found to restore the depressed ventilatory drive. The effects of individual nutrients on ventilatory drive and ventilation will be discussed in the next section.

The effects of protein-calorie malnutrition on the immune system are most profound for cell-mediated immunity,[56] but the humoral system may also be affected with abnormal immunoglobulin turnover and reduced levels of secretory immunoglobulin A.[104] The specific effects of malnutrition on pulmonary defense mechanisms have not been well characterized. Pulmonary defense mechanisms depend on the integrity of the respiratory epithelium as well as on the immune system, but there are limited data on the effects of malnutrition on the respiratory epithelium or ciliary function.[105]

Alveolar macrophages play an important role in the defense against bacteria in the lung, and are important to both cell-mediated and humoral immunity.[105] Hence, the influence of malnutrition on immune function may have a direct impact on alveolar defenses. Alveolar phagocytic function and the clearance of various micro-organisms have been found to be impaired in malnourished animal models.[106] Niederman et al did a study of lower respiratory tract bacterial binding in patients with chronic tracheostomies.[107] Because airway colonization by *Pseudomonas aeruginosa* is common in these patients, this organism was used in the adherance assay, and its pattern of recovery from cultures of respiratory mucosa was serially followed. Patients with greater degrees of nutritional impairment had more tracheal cell adherance and were more frequently colonized by *Pseudomonas*. This suggests that nutritional impairment alters resistance of airway mucosa to infections and, thus, may precipitate nosocomial lung infections and sepsis.

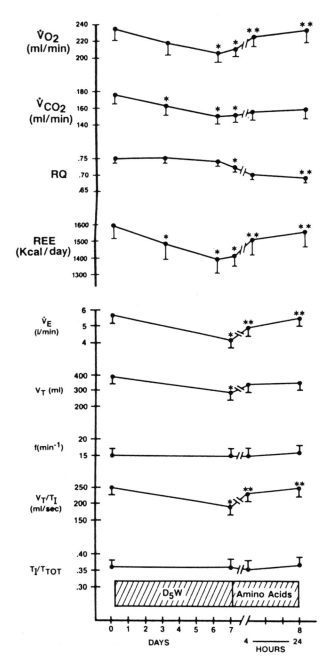

Fig. 25-12. Effects of semistarvation with 5 percent dextrose (D_5W) and subsequent amino acid infusion on oxygen consumption ($\dot{V}O_2$), carbon dioxide production ($\dot{V}CO_2$), respiratory quotient (RQ), resting energy expenditure (REE), minute ventilation ($\dot{V}_E$), tidal volume (V_T), frequency (f), mean inspiratory flow (V_TT_I), and inspiratory duty cycle (T_I/T_{TOT}). *, Significantly different from day 0 ($P < 0.05$); **, significantly different from values obtained after 7 days of 5 percent dextrose infusion ($P < .05$). (From Weissman et al,[103] with permission.)

Chronic Obstructive Pulmonary Disease

Several reports have documented the common occurrence of weight loss in patients with chronic obstructive pulmonary disease (COPD).[108–110] Patients with COPD are normally divided into two subgroups: those suffering primarily from emphysema ("pink puffers") and those suffering primarily from chronic bronchitis ("blue bloaters"). It is important to recognize that although both groups may experience severe respiratory impairment, it is the emphysematic patients who experience weight loss. Openbrier et al surveyed a large number of patients with chronic bronchitis (30 patients) and emphysema (77 patients).[110] In the former group, they identified only one patient with body weight of less than 90 percent of ideal body weight (IBW); this patient had bronchogenic carcinoma. In the emphysema group, 43 percent of the patients weighed less than 90 percent of IBW; in this group, there were significant correlations between the presence of malnutrition and a greater degree of airflow obstruction and respiratory muscle weakness, a finding supported by other studies.[111,112] The cause of weight loss in COPD patients seems to be multifactorial.[101,105] Several studies[110,113] have found apparently adequate calorie intake in these patients; therefore, it has been suggested that the main cause of weight loss is an increased energy demand resulting from the underlying disease state.[89,101] Resting energy expenditures of 15 to 40 percent above predicted values have been reported in malnourished COPD patients.[99,101] Recently, Morrison et al found that whole-body protein synthesis was depressed in emphysema, and their findings indicate that a fall in muscle protein synthesis contributes significantly to the weight loss seen in these patients.[114] Further, it has been shown that the diaphragm may atrophy in patients with COPD uncomplicated by malnutrition.[111] Therefore, the adverse effects of malnutrition may be additive to an already existing muscle weakness, thus making COPD patients particularly vulnerable to nutritional depletion.

It has been suggested that the weight loss in COPD patients may be beneficial because metabolic demands are reduced and this leads to lower ventilatory requirements, alleviating the overworked respiratory muscles. This is true in overweight hypercapnic COPD patients (chronic bronchitis, "blue bloater"), in whom a low intake of calories and carbohydrates with concomitant weight loss will decrease arterial PCO_2 and improve respiratory muscle strength.[115] In normal or underweight COPD patients (emphysema, "pink puffer"), however, weight loss is associated with negative effects on lung function, increased incidence of heart failure, and increased mortality.[108,116] Further, Driver et al compared stable COPD patients and COPD patients with acute respiratory failure, and were able to show that, unlike the stable COPD patients, body protein and fat stores were markedly depleted in almost half the patients with respiratory failure.[117]

The clinical short-term effects of refeeding malnourished COPD patients have also been studied. Goldstein et al investigated the effects of 2 weeks of hypercaloric diets using either fat or glucose as the main nonprotein energy source.[101] They found that patients with emphysema and weight loss had a pattern of energy metabolism and fuel oxidation distinctly different from that of malnourished patients without lung disease. The results showed that although these patients were hypermetabolic, unlike other groups of hypermetabolic patients, they were not hypercatabolic. Further, the COPD patients, also unlike other hypermetabolic patients, did not demonstrate preferential fat oxidation. Two weeks of refeeding in these patients was associated with both weight gain, accompanied by a contraction of body water (Fig. 25-13), and improved respiratory and skeletal muscle function; there was no deterioration in blood gas values. The finding of both improved skeletal and respiratory muscle strength after refeeding COPD patients is in accordance with other studies of malnourished patients.[87,97,118] In two follow-up studies, the ventilatory and metabolic effects of fat versus carbohydrate-based refeeding were compared in malnourished patients with and without emphysema.[7,119] The results demonstrated that malnourished patients with emphysema have an enhanced

thermic response (DIT) to nutrients (Fig. 25-14), a phenomenon that was accentuated by a moderately high carbohydrate diet. The authors also found a lower exercise efficiency in the emphysema patients and that a hypercaloric carbohydrate regimen placed a greater stress on the respiratory system during exercise than did the fat regimen (Fig. 25-15). As can be seen, all these data are of importance in the design of nutritional support regimens for COPD patients, the goal being to improve muscular function and minimize the nutrient-related increases in metabolic and ventilatory demand.[101,105]

Respiratory Effects of Specific Nutrients

The major function of the respiratory system is to meet the body's demand for oxygen and to eliminate CO_2. In patients with acute and chronic respiratory diseases, it is crucial to understand the effects of various nutrients on the respiratory system. Administration of nutrients will not only improve respiratory muscle function, but may also influence the gas exchange through their specific physiologic and pharmacologic properties.[120–122]

Carbohydrates

The characteristic response to increased hypercaloric intakes of carbohydrates in both normal subjects and patients is increased CO_2 production ($\dot{V}CO_2$).[123] The extent to which this occurs, however, differs among

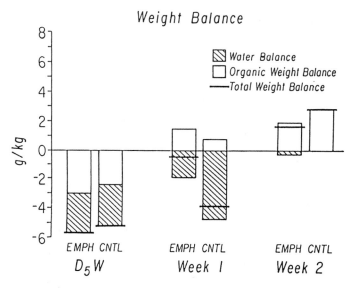

Fig. 25-13. Water, organic weight (based on protein, fat, and carbohydrate balance), and total weight balance in 10 emphysema patients (EMPH) and in six control patients (CNTL). D_5W, 5 percent dextrose. (From Goldstein et al,[101] with permission.)

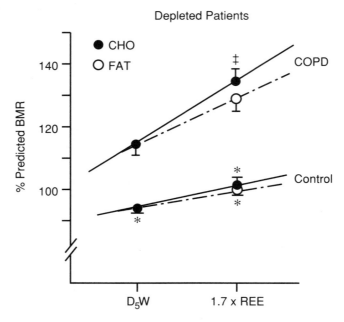

Fig. 25-14. Energy expenditure during 5 percent dextrose solution (D_5W) and during refeeding with a carbohydrate-based regimen (CHO) and a fat-based regimen (FAT) in malnourished patients with and without COPD, expressed as percent of predicted basal metabolic rate. $P < 0.001$ compared with COPD patients, same diet; $P < 0.05$ compared with the fat-based (55 percent fat) diet. (From Goldstein et al,[7] with permission.)

various groups of patients (Fig. 25-3). With the shift from fat oxidation to glucose oxidation, an increase in RQ occurs; if sufficient glucose is given, lipogenesis occurs, with a dramatic rise in the level of CO_2 production (Fig. 25-16). Due to the increased CO_2 production, high intakes of carbohydrate stimulate ventilation. It is possible for a small patient to double CO_2 production, going from approximately 500 kcal/d to 3,000 kcal/d of glucose-based TPN.[5] For normal subjects, such as increase in minute ventilation has no noticeable effect on breathing. However, it may be impossible for patients with impaired lung function to meet this increase in ventilation. Askanazi et al first reported that the large increase in CO_2 production seen with administration of excessive amounts of glucose could precipitate respiratory distress in hypermetabolic patients.[1,2] This finding was later confirmed by others.[124] Weaning from mechanical ventilatory support may also be difficult if glucose is administered as the only nonprotein calorie source.[125,126]

The effect of carbohydrates like glucose on O_2 consumption seems to depend on the amount of glucose given and the rate of infusion,[123] whether protein is given simultaneously,[8,120,123] and what patient population is under study (Fig. 25-3). Studies of patients

with stable COPD[127] and patients given TPN, including amino acids, have shown a rise in O_2 consumption and REE in response to increased glucose intake.[120] On the other hand, Rodriguez et al did not find an increase in O_2 consumption when continuous infusions of glucose in hypercaloric amounts were given to healthy volunteers and moderately stressed surgical patients.[123]

Lipids

Substitution of fat emulsions for glucose lowers the RQ, reducing minute ventilation and ventilatory demand.[120] Intravenous fat emulsions (IVFEs) are, therefore, a useful substrate in providing nutritional support in the patient with reduced pulmonary reserve. However, numerous studies have suggested varying degrees of pulmonary dysfunction when IVFEs are given.[128,129] The lung dysfunction is evidenced by a decrease in PaO_2, and studies from the pediatric literature suggest that parenteral lipid emulsions interfere with pulmonary diffusing capacity in premature infants.[130,131] In adults, these changes have generally not been of sufficient magnitude to carry much clinical significance, but are of interest in understanding the relationship between IVFEs and the lung.[121]

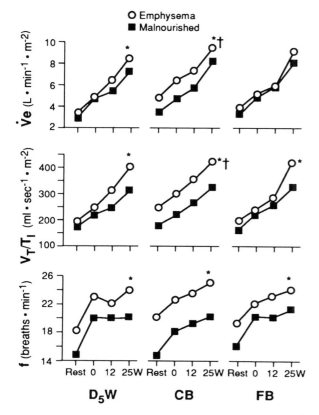

Fig. 25-15. Minute ventilation (V_E), inspiratory flow (V_T/T_I), and breathing frequency (f) in eight malnourished patients with emphysema and eight without emphysema at rest and at three exercise intensities (0, 12, and 25 W) during 5 percent dextrose (D_5W), carbohydrate-based (CB), and fat-based (FB) diets. *, Different from malnourished at rest and all exercise intensities: $P < 0.025$; †, different from FB diet, same group: $P < 0.005$. (From Goldstein et al,[119] with permission.)

In a study of adults, both healthy volunteers and ventilator-dependent critically ill patients, Jarnberg et al found no significant changes in values for blood gases and diffusing capacity during infusion of a 20 percent fat emulsion.[132] Recently, Venus et al studied the cardiopulmonary effects of a fat emulsion, 20 percent Intralipid, 500 mL given over 8 to 10 hours, in critically ill patients requiring ventilatory support to augment spontaneous breathing and in patients with full-blown adult respiratory distress syndrome (ARDS), with and without sepsis.[133,134] They found that the lipid infusion increased mean pulmonary artery pressure (MPAP) and pulmonary venous admixture (Q_s/Q_T) in all groups studied, particularly in ARDS patients with sepsis. The hemodynamic changes resolved when the lipid infusion was terminated. The hemodynamic changes in the ARDS patients were associated with a significant decrease in the PaO_2/F_IO_2 ratio, a sign of worsened oxygenation. In a follow-up study of nonseptic mechanically ventilated intensive care unit patients, the effects of the rate of infusion of gas exchange parameters and central hemodynamics were tested.[135] When 500 mL of 20 percent Intralipid were given over 24 hours, no effects on Q_s/Q_T or MPAP were found. If the same amount was infused over 6 hours, these parameters increased significantly. It is important to recognize that these investigators did not conclude that fat emulsion should be abandoned in critically ill patients, but rapid infusions should be avoided and adequate oxygenation verified for patients with compromised pulmonary function receiving intravenous fat.[133–135]

The pulmonary dysfunction seen with fat emulsion has been attributed to the associated hyperlipemia.[128] However, the polyunsaturated fatty acids in the IVFEs serve as precursors to the eicosanoids (prostaglandins, thromboxanes, leukotrienes), and several authors now attribute the decrease in PaO_2 to ventilation/perfusion inequalities caused by IVFE-related changes in the production of eicosanoids.[121,129,133] In oleic-damaged rabbit lungs, Hageman et al found an increased pulmonary production of vasodilatory prostaglandins together with a decrease in PaO_2 in the lung injury group (Fig. 25-17).[129] Although this hypothesis has not yet been thoroughly tested in humans, it helps explain why different effects of parenteral fat emulsion are seen in different patient populations with different rates of infusion, and why the actual composition of different fat emulsions may be important.[121] The eicosanoids also modulate many of the events in inflammatory processes and immune functions.[136] The possibility of modifying eicosanoid synthesis through rate and type of dietary PUFAs, thereby influencing the inflammatory and immunologic response, has considerable potential therapeutic consequences for different lung diseases and has received much attention.[121,136] Long-term home TPN has produced dramatic improvement in lung function in some patients with cystic fibrosis,[137,138] but more studies are needed to determine the exact role of different fat emulsions in the treatment of this and other inflammatory lung diseases.

Proteins

Administration of TPN consisting of glucose and amino acids has been shown to cause abrupt increases in minute ventilation.[1] Such an increase in minute ventilation has been reported to have resulted in respiratory distress in a patient with compromised pul-

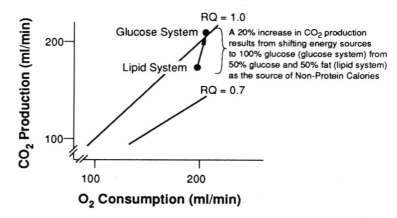

Fig. 25-16. Gas exchange and breathing patterns during TPN. The figure shows the reduction of CO_2 production in substituting a part of the carbohydrate intake (glucose system) by fat intake (lipid system). (Data from Askanazi et al.[120])

monary function,[2] and the increased ventilatory demand has been ascribed to increases in CO_2 production. However, some of the TPN-induced increase in ventilation is actually due to the amino acids.[103,122,123] Weissman et al gave eight normal subjects an infusion of 5 percent dextrose for 7 days (semistarvation), followed by an infusion of 3.5 percent amino acids for 24 hours (Fig. 25-12).[103] During the period of semistarvation there were decreases in metabolic rate and central neuromuscular ventilatory drive, represented by a significant decrease in mean

inspiratory flow. Infusion of amino acids in amounts commonly used in clinical practice, 400 kcal/d, caused a rise in resting minute ventilation and ventilatory drive (Fig. 25-12) and in the ventilatory response to CO_2. These observations may be important for patients with marginal respiratory function unable to increase their minute ventilation. To avoid respiratory distress, caution should be used not only when administering large glucose loads, but also when infusing amino acids in acutely ill patients.

To further examine the effects of protein intake on

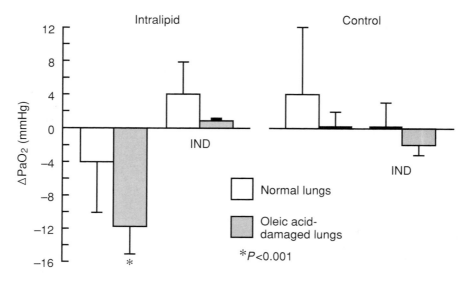

Fig. 25-17. Changes in PaO_2 occurring as a result of infusion over 1 hour of 4 mL/kg of Intralipid. The only significant P_ACO_2 decrease occurred in the lung injury group. IND, indomethacin. (From Hageman et al,[129] with permission.)

ventilation, Askanazi et al studied the ventilatory response to protein intake in malnourished patients.[122] They found that when the amino acid component of a fixed caloric intake was increased, arterial CO_2 (PaCO$_2$) significantly decreased and an enhanced ventilatory response to CO_2 stimulus, seen as a leftward shift of the minute ventilation to PaCO$_2$ regression, was found (Fig. 25-18). Most of this effect was believed to be due to increased ventilatory chemosensitivity, and the increase in minute ventilation at any given PaCO$_2$ reflected a markedly increased mean inspiratory flow and tidal volume, while respiratory timing was less affected.

In a recent study, Takala et al demonstrated that the effects of amino acid infusions on respiration were also influenced by the amino acid profile.[139] They compared a 4-hour infusion of an amino acid solution consisting primarily of branched-chain amino acid (BCAA) (leucine, isoleucine, and valine) to a standard amino acid solution in healthy subjects. Both solutions significantly increased minute ventilation and mean inspiratory flow, but only the BCAA infusion caused a significant increase in O_2 consumption, a significant decrease in PaCO$_2$, and a major increase in the ventilatory response to CO_2 inhalation (Fig. 25-19). In this study, amino acids were infused at rates corresponding to those in routine clinical use. Whether these effects of BCAA are salutary depends on the clinical setting. In patients with normal ventilatory reserve, the difference between the ventilatory response to the two amino acid solutions is unlikely to be of clinical significance. However, the increase in ventilatory demand may theoretically increase the risk of respiratory failure in critically ill patients with already increased respiratory work and drive[139] and, on the other hand, be beneficial to patients with reduced respiratory drive (COPD, sleep apnea syndromes).[126] In this connection, it seems important to recognize that animal studies indicate that in chronic starvation, BCAA becomes an extremely important energy substrate for the main respiratory muscle, the diaphragm, as the rate of utilization is 10- to 20-fold

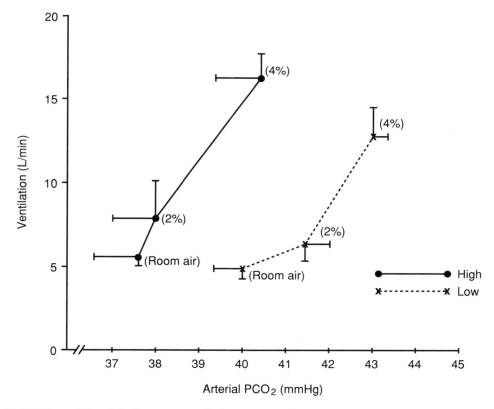

Fig. 25-18. The relationship between ventilation and arterial PCO$_2$. With increasing nitrogen intake, there was a leftward shift of the regression curves. The concentration of administered CO_2 is noted in parentheses. (From Askanazi et al,[122] with permission.)

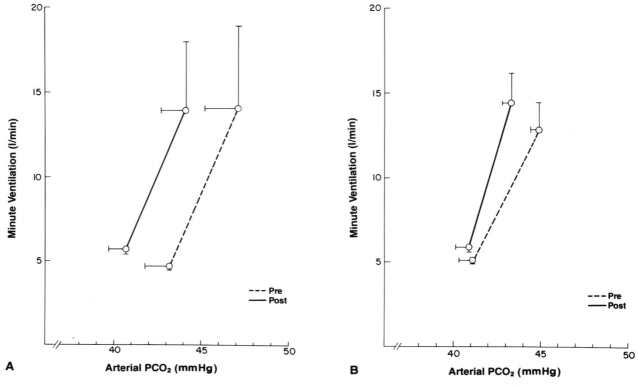

Fig. 25-19. Ventilatory responses to CO_2 before and after 4 hours of infusion. The points of each line represent the mean values of V_E and the corresponding $PaCO_2$ while breathing room air and 4 percent CO_2. **(A)** BCAA solution; **(B)** standard amino acid solution. (From Takala et al,[139] with permission.)

greater than normal.[140] All of these respiratory effects need to be considered, together with the protein-saving effects of increasing nitrogen intake, particularly in connection with the use of BCAA in hypermetabolic patients.[141]

Electrolytes

Inorganic nutrients may also influence the ventilatory function. Among the multisystem effects of hypophosphatemia, skeletal dysfunction and ventilatory failure have been reported.[79] Aubier et al studied the effect of hypophosphatemia on diaphragmatic contractility in artificially ventilated patients.[142] Diaphragmatic function was evaluated before and after correction of the deficiency. Increases in serum phosphorus were accompanied by marked increases in transdiaphragmatic pressure, indicating improved contractility of the diaphragm. These results emphasize the importance of maintaining normal serum phosphate levels to achieve successful weaning from a ventilator. Hypomagnesemia may also induce abnormalities of respiratory muscle strength that disappear

with magnesium replacement.[143] To avoid respiratory problems, the possibility of magnesium deficiency should be considered in patients at risk (diuretic therapy, severe malabsorption, alcoholism).

Nutritional Aspects of Mechanical Ventilation

Pingleton and Eulberg evaluated the nutritional status of 80 patients admitted consecutively to the intensive care unit with acute respiratory failure.[144] Body weight of less than 80 percent of IBW was noted in 24 percent of these patients. Driver and LeBrun found that patients with malnutrition who required mechanical ventilation had a significantly higher mortality than well-nourished patients on mechanical ventilation.[145] Mechanically ventilated patients, although they may begin with normal BCM, often undergo progressive malnutrition.[100] The study of Bassili and Deitel indicated an increased ability to wean patients from ventilators when they receive appropriate nutritional support as opposed to those receiving dextrose only.[146] The improvement of muscle function seen with nutritional repletion is, therefore, of clinical importance in artificially ventilated patients.[63,100] Further, Larca and Greenbaum found that ventilator-dependent patients who responded to nutritional support with an increase in serum albumin were more likely to be weaned from mechanical ventilation than those who did not.[125] Nutritional support during weaning is mandatory for prompt replenishment of muscle glycogen during periods of rest.[100,143] However, excessive amounts of carbohydrates should be avoided since the associated increase in CO_2 production will hamper the weaning process.[100,143] To optimize nutritional support, it is helpful if energy expenditure is measured rather than predicted. It seems to be widely accepted that 35 to 50 percent of nonprotein calories should be provided as fat.[143] However, as previously stated, lipid emulsions should, due to their cardiopulmonary effects, be administered slowly and with caution in marginally oxygenated patients.[121,133–135] The effect of amino acid infusions to increase ventilatory drive must also be taken into consideration when weaning patients with marginal respiratory function.[122,139] While the increased ventilatory response to $PaCO_2$ may theoretically help in the weaning process, excessive amounts of amino acids may cause a feeling of breathlessness in patients unable to adequately increase minute ventilation in response to increased respiratory drive.[100] The issue that is probably most crucial to the success of nutritional support in these patients is that of timing, meaning that nutritional support should not be delayed since it is easier to prevent BCM loss than to restore BCM.

ENTERAL VERSUS PARENTERAL NUTRITIONAL SUPPORT

When the decision is made to provide nutritional support, many practical aspects have to be considered. In this section, the benefits and complications of parenteral and enteral nutrition will be reviewed.

Practical Considerations

Several studies have shown no significant metabolic differences between enteral nutrition (ENT) and TPN.[147,148] Although ENT, compared with TPN, is less costly, simpler to administer, and requires less laboratory monitoring, it has not achieved the popularity accorded to TPN. This may partly be due to real problems of ENT, such as absorption dysfunctions, diarrhea and danger of aspiration,[3,147] but lack of familiarity with the method may also be an important reason. For short periods a decompression gastric tube can be used for nutritional support.[25] Most often, however, soft, small-caliber, silastic tubes that can remain in place for prolonged periods are preferred.[3,148,149] The nasogastric method, which requires intact gastric motility to get the feeding into the small bowel, is the most frequently selected route of enteral therapy.[150] Placing the tube intraduodenally seems to have some advantages, including a reduced risk of aspiration and improved digestion of the nutrients provided. To facilitate placement of the tube intraduodenally, use of tubes with a weighted tip has been proposed, but Silk et al found that spontaneous transpyloric passage was unlikely to occur very frequently with any type of tube.[149] The main advantage of weighted tubes was found to be that they were easier to place in endotracheally intubated patients. Some authors consider the jejunum a better location for enteral feeding, and various techniques for placing jejunostomy tubes have been reported.[3]

Peripheral catheters can be used to provide short-term nutrition support, using isotonic solutions like 5 percent glucose.[25] In hypercatabolic patients, Massar et al showed with glucose and protein-based TPN that the calories supplied by peripheral veins are insufficient to meet the energetic requirements, even if they are previously well nourished.[151] The high blood flow in central veins allows the use of hypertonic solutions, and central venous catheterization has become a common practice for supplying parenteral nutrition.

Complications

Metabolic Complications

TPN, especially when given through central catheters, may produce dangerous concentrations of blood glucose, even in previously nondiabetic patients.[3] The hyperglycemia is usually transient and responds to reduction in caloric intake or substitution for some of the carbohydrate by a calorie-equivalent amount of fat. The regular use of insulin to get the blood sugar down is no longer recommended, but adding insulin to TPN is still a common practice in many hospitals. Blood sugar should be measured at least once a day, and urine sugar up to four times a day.

Abnormal liver function tests and fatty liver infiltration have also been associated with parenteral nutrition, especially when it is carbohydrate-based.[4] Fortunately, most cases are mild, self-limited, and require only a lower caloric intake and increased proportion of lipids. The use of fat emulsions must also be monitored,[73] especially in the most severely traumatized and septic patients, in whom fat emulsion may exceed the plasma capacity to remove fat from

TABLE 25-4. Suggested Monitoring Schedule during Total Parenteral Nutrition

Parameter	Frequency
Volume in	Daily
Volume out	Daily
Body temperature	Daily
Weight	Biweekly
Urine sugar and albumin	Four times daily
Electrolytes	Daily
BUN/creatinine	Biweekly
Ca^{++}, P, Mg	Weekly
Platelets	Biweekly
Blood sugar	Daily
Liver profile	Biweekly
Triglycerides, cholesterol, plasma fatty acids	Weekly

Abbreviation: BUN, blood urea nitrogen.
(Adapted from Robin and Greig,[73] with permission.)

the circulation.[152] However, several studies have shown that fat is easily cleared and metabolized in most patients.[8,57,83,153] Previous testing of lipid tolerance has included checking for aggregation of fat (creaming) when serum was incubated with the fat emulsion. However, the clinical significance of this test is probably minimal.[154] The most reliable way to follow the lipid metabolism and to check for fat intolerance is to measure plasma fatty acids, triglycerides, and cholesterol.

A rise in blood urea indicates that protein intake must be reduced. As described earlier, severe electrolyte disturbances, particularly hypophosphatemia,[155] may occur when refeeding severely malnourished patients.[78,79] Although originally described in connection with TPN, it is now clear that severe hypophosphatemia may develop following the institution of enteral feedings as well.[154] Table 25-4 outlines some suggestions on how to monitor enteral and parenteral nutrition. Once the patient is stable and tolerating a particular regimen, usually after 7 to 10 days, most of the blood tests described in Table 25-4 can be performed less frequently.[73]

Mechanical Complications

The main differences between TPN and ENT are the type and incidence of side effects.[3] Enteral feeding may be given as either continuous or intermittent infusions; however, whatever technique of administration is used, the most frequent problem encountered in ENT is diarrhea, with an incidence of 10 to 25 percent.[147,150,156] Formula dilution, continuous pump infusion, increasing the proportion of fat, and/or antidiarrhea medication will, in most cases, solve the problem.[3,150] A particular problem with gastroenteral tube feeding is the increased risk of aspiration into the

lungs. Although not a common complication, undetected insertion of feeding tubes into the lower airways with severe complications and fatal outcome has been described.[157] After the tubes have been properly installed, the risk of aspiration will continue to endanger the patient. When possible, the patient should be kept in a semisitting position or with the head elevated in the lateral decubitus position.

Catheter-Related Infections

A thorough review of all complications (pneumothorax, air embolism, thrombosis, arterial puncture, and wrong catheter placement) associated with the insertion of central venous catheters is beyond the scope of this chapter.[3,158] Instead, the clinical implications of catheter-related infection, one of the most common complications in long-term use of central venous catheters for nutritional purposes, will be reviewed.[159]

There seems to be little consensus on the definitions of catheter-related infections.[159] This has resulted in a wide range of reported incidences of infection and made it more difficult to provide practical guidelines to the clinician. Infection at the insertion site depends on aseptic precautions, the extent of local trauma, and the location of the insertion site.[159,160] Although inflammation at the catheter site has been associated with an increased incidence of infection, inflammation does not necessarily mean infection, as the catheter or infusate may act as an irritant to tissue.[159] Catheter-related sepsis has been reported in up to 15 percent of patients receiving TPN, but caution must be taken when interpreting the results of different studies since the applied methods, definitions, and populations studied vary.[158,159] Because a positive culture from blood drawn through a catheter may be due to bacteremia liberated from sources other than a colonized catheter, a different approach has been advocated, with the catheter tip being cultured along with the blood samples; the clinical features of infection should resolve after removal of the catheter.[158] By these criteria, however, catheter-related sepsis can only be proved by removing the catheter, which has been shown to be unnecessary in over 75 percent of these patients.[161] Such wastage of noninfected catheters can be avoided by using a new technique that entails culturing samples of blood drawn simultaneously through the catheter and a peripheral vein.[162] If the colony count in the catheter blood is five or more times that in the peripheral blood, the diagnosis of catheter-related sepsis is highly likely.

Different approaches to the management of catheter sepsis have been tried, including trying to salvage the catheter using antibiotics, antiseptics, and fibrinolytic agents.[158] Some investigators still recommend prompt removal of the catheter when the patient develops signs of catheter-related sepsis, even if the insertion site is not inflamed.[159] Controversy also exists as to whether to replace the catheter over a guidewire or use another site. Pettigrew et al have shown that infection of the new catheter is no more likely to occur if it is substituted for the infected catheter over a guidewire or placed at another site.[161]

Triple-lumen catheters are frequently used in critically ill patients and patients undergoing major surgery. Several studies have found an increased risk of catheter sepsis when these catheters are used for parenteral nutrition.[163,164] Pemberton et al found no difference in catheter exit infection and, therefore, suggested that the infections were introduced into the multi-lumen catheter during sampling, monitoring, and administration of drugs.[163] On the other hand, Lee et al found no statistically significant difference in the rate of bacterial contamination or sepsis in patients receiving TPN through triple-lumen catheters versus single-lumen catheters.[165] These researchers concluded that triple-lumen catheters may be used for short-term administration of TPN. Since an indwelling catheter is a potential source of dangerous infection, both multi-lumen and single-lumen catheters should be removed as soon as clinically feasible.[159]

REFERENCES

1. Askanazi J, Rosenbaum SH, Hyman AI, et al: Respiratory changes induced by the large glucose loads of total parenteral nutrition. JAMA 243:1444–1447, 1980
2. Askanazi J, Elwyn DE, Silverberg PA, et al: Respiratory distress secondary to a high carbohydrate load: a case report. Surgery 87:596–598, 1980
3. Berger R, Adams L: Nutritional support in the critical care setting (part 2). Chest 96:372–380, 1989
4. Baker AL, Rosenberg IH: Hepatic complications of total parenteral nutrition. Am J Med 82:489–497, 1987
5. Bursztein S, Elwyn DH, Askanazi J, Kinney JM: Energy Metabolism, Indirect Calorimetry and Nutrition. Williams & Wilkins, Baltimore, 1989
6. Shaw-Delanty SN, Elwyn DH, Askanazi J, et al: Resting energy expenditure in injured, septic, and malnourished adult patients on intravenous diets. Clin Nutr (in press)
7. Goldstein S, Askanazi J, Weissman C, et al: Energy expenditure in patients with chronic obstructive pulmonary disease. Chest 91:222–224, 1987
8. Askanazi J, Carpentier YA, Elwyn DH, et al: Influence of total nutrition on fuel utilization in injury and sepsis. Ann Surg 191:40–46, 1980
9. Spencer JL, Zikria AB, Kinney JM, et al: A method for

10. Ultman JS, Bursztein S: Analysis of error in determination of respiratory gas exchange at varying F_IO_2. J Appl Physiol 50:210–216, 1981
11. Takala J, Keinanen O, Vaisanen P, et al: Measurement of gas exchange in intensive care: laboratory and clinical validation of a new device. Crit Care Med 17:1041–1047, 1989
12. Liggett SB, St John RE, Lefrak SS: Determination of resting energy expenditure utilizing the thermodilution pulmonary artery catheter. Chest 91:562–566, 1987
13. Bursztein S, Saphar P, Singer P, et al: A mathematical analysis of indirect calorimetry measurements in acutely ill patients. Am J Clin Nutr 50:227–230, 1989
14. Hunter DC, Jaksic T, Lewis D, et al: Resting energy expenditure in the critically ill: estimations versus measurement. Br J Surg 75:875–878, 1988
15. Chikenji T, Elwyn DH, Gil KM, et al: Effects of increasing glucose intake on nitrogen balance and energy expenditure in malnourished adult patients receiving parenteral nutrition. Clin Sci 72:489–501, 1987
16. Van Lanschot JJB, Feenstra BWA, Vermeij CG, et al: Accuracy of intermittent metabolic gas exchange recordings extrapolated for diurnal variations. Crit Care Med 16:737–742, 1988
17. Weismann C, Kemper M, Damask MC, et al: The effect of routine intensive care interactions on metabolic rate. Chest 86:815–818, 1984
18. Weismann C, Kemper M, Hyman AI: Variation in the resting metabolic rate of mechanically ventilated critically ill patients. Anesth Analg 68:457–461, 1989
19. Weismann C, Kemper M, Askanzazi J, et al: Resting metabolic rate of the critically ill patient: measured versus predicted. Anesthesiology 64:673–679, 1986
20. Elwyn DH, Gump FE, Munro HN, et al: Changes in nitrogen balance of depleted patients with increasing infusions of glucose. Am J Clin Nutr 32:1597–1611, 1979
21. Askanazi J, Carpentier YA, Jeevandam M, et al: Energy expenditure, nitrogen balance, and norepinephrine excretion after injury. Surgery 89:478–484, 1981
22. Shaw S, Elwyn DH, Askanazi J, et al: Effects of increasing nitrogen on N balance and energy expenditure in nutritionally depleted adult patients receiving parenteral nutrition. Am J Clin Nutr 37:930–940, 1983
23. Van Lanschot JJB, Feenstra BWA, Vermeij CG, et al: Calculation versus measurement of total energy expenditure. Crit Care med 14:981–985, 1986
24. Carlsson M, Berkson J, Dunn HL: Clinical implications of continuous measurement of energy expenditure in mechanically ventilated patients. Clin Nutr 3:103–110, 1984
25. Bursztein S, Elwyn DH, Askanazi J, et al: Guidelines for parenteral and enteral nutrition. pp. 229–255. In: Energy Metabolism, Indirect Calorimetry, and Nutrition. Williams & Wilkins, Baltimore, 1989
26. Dempsey DT, Mullen JL: Macronutrient requirements in the malnourished cancer patient. Cancer 55:152–162, 1985
27. Knox LS, Crosby LO, Mullen JL, et al: Energy expendi-

ture in malnourished cancer patients. Ann Surg 197:152–162, 1983

28. Vermeij CG, Feenstra BWA, Van Lanschot JB, et al: Day-to-day variability of energy expenditure in critically ill surgical patients. Crit Care Med 17:623–626, 1989

29. Hill GL: Body composition research at the University of Auckland: some implications for modern surgical practice. Aust N Z J Surg 58:13–21, 1988

30. Forse RA, Shizgal HM: The assessment of malnutrition. Surgery 88:17–24, 1980

31. Windsor JA, Hill GL: Weight loss with physiological impairment: basic indicator of surgical risk. Ann Surg 207:290–296, 1988

32. Starker PM, Gump FE, Askanazi J, et al: Serum albumin levels as an index of nutritional support. Surgery 91:194–199, 1982

33. Starker PA, Lasala PA, Askanazi J: The response to TPN. A form of nutritional assessment. Ann Surg 198:720–723, 1983

34. Shizgal HM: Nutritional assessment with body composition measurements. J Parenter Enteral Nutr 11:42S–47S, 1987

35. Bozzetti F, Migliavaca S, Gallus G, et al: "Nutritional" markers as prognostic indicators of postoperative sepsis in cancer patients. J Parenter Enteral Nutr 9:464–470, 1985

36. Starker PM, Askanazi J, Lasala PA, et al: The effect of parenteral nutritional repletion on muscle water and electrolytes. Ann Surg 198:213–217, 1983

37. Benedict FG: A Study of Prolonged Fasting. Carnegie Institute, Washington, DC, Publ. No. 203, 1915

38. Gamble JL: Physiological information gained from studies on life raft ration. Harvey Lect 42:247–273, 1946

39. Daly JM, Thom AK: Neoplastic diseases. pp. 567–587. In Kinney JM, Jeejeebhoy KN, Hill GL, Owen OE (eds): Nutrition and Metabolism in Patient Care. Philadelphia, WB Saunders, 1988

40. Cuthbertson D: The metabolic response to injury and its nutritional implications. Retrospect and prospect. J Parenter Enteral Nutr 3:108–130, 1979

41. Douglas RG, Shaw JHF: Metabolic response to sepsis and trauma. Br J Surg 76:115–122, 1989

42. Shike M, Russel DM, Detsky AS, et al: Changes in body composition in patients with small cell lung cancer. The effect of total parenteral nutrition as an adjunct to chemotherapy. Ann Intern Med 101:303–309, 1984

43. Buzby GP, Williford WO, Peterson OL, et al: A randomized clinical trial of total parenteral nutrition in malnourished surgical patients: The rationale and impact of previous clinical trials and pilot study on protocol design. Am J Clin Nutr 47:357–365, 1988

44. Studley HO: Percentage of weight loss: a basic indicator of surgical risk in patients with chronic peptic ulcer. JAMA 106:458–460, 1936

45. Dempsey DT, Mullen JL, Buzby GP: The link between nutritional status and clinical outcome: Can nutritional intervention modify it? Am J Clin Nutr 47:352–356, 1988

46. Deslauris J, Ginsberg RJ, Dubois P, et al: Current operative morbidity associated with elective surgical resection for lung cancer. Can J Surg 32:335–339, 1989

47. Hill GL, Pickford I, Young Ga, et al: Malnutrition in surgical patients: an unrecognized problem. Lancet 1:689–692, 1977

48. Elwyn DH, Bryan-Brown CW, Shoemaker WC: Nutritional aspects of body water dislocations in postoperative and depleted patients. Ann Surg 182:76–85, 1975

49. Bistrian BR, Blackburn GL, Hallowell E, et al: Protein status of general surgical patients. JAMA 230:858–860, 1974

50. Bozzetti F, Migliavacca S, Scotti A, et al: Impact of cancer type, site, stage and treatment on the nutritional status of patients. Ann Surg 196:170–179, 1982

51. Nakahara K, Monden Y, Ohno K, et al: Importance of biological status to the postoperative prognosis of patients with stage III nonsmall-cell lung cancer. J Surg Oncol 36:155–160, 1987

52. Fatzinger P, DeMeester T, Darkjian H, et al: The use of serum albumin for further classification of stage III nonoat-cell lung cancer and its therapeutic implications. Ann Thorac Surg 37:115–122, 1984

53. Elwyn DH: Nutritional requirements of adult surgical patients. Crit Care Med 8:9–20, 1980

54. Hill GL: Surgical nutrition: time for some clinical common sense. Br J Surg 75:729–730, 1988

55. Mullen JL, Buzby GP, Waldman MT, et al: Prediction of operative morbidity and mortality by preoperative nutritional assessment. Surg Forum 30:80–82, 1979

56. Peck MD, Alexander JW: The use of immunological tests to predict outcome in surgical patients. Nutrition 6:216–219, 1990

57. Forse R, Christou N, Meakins JL, et al: Reliability of skin testing as a measure of nutritional state. Arch Surg 116:1284–1288, 1981

58. Buzby GP, Mullen JL, Matthews DC, et al: Prognostic nutritional index in gastrointestinal surgery. Am J Surg 139:160–167, 1980

59. McLaren DS: A fresh look a protein-energy malnutrition in the hospitalized patient. Nutrition 4:1–6, 1988

60. Fleck A, Raines G, Hawker F, et al: Increased vascular permeability: A major cause of hypoalbuminaemia in disease and injury. Lancet 1:781–784, 1985

61. Lemyne M, Jeejeebhoy N: Total parenteral nutrition in the critically ill patient. Chest 93:568–575, 1986

62. Klidjian AM, Archre TJ, Foster KG, et al: Detection of dangerous malnutrition. J Parenter Enteral Nutr 6:119–121, 1982

63. Russel DMcR, Leiter LA, Whitwell J, et al: Skeletal muscle function during hypocaloric diets and fasting. A comparision with standard nutritional assessment parameters. Am J Clin Nutr 37:133–138, 1983

64. Mullen JL, Buzby GP, Matthews DC, et al: Reduction of operative morbidity and mortality by combined preoperative and postoperative nutritional support. Ann Surg 192:604–612, 1980

65. Baker J, Detsky AS, Wesson DE, et al: Nutritional assessment. A comparison of clinical judgment and objective measurements. N Engl J Med 306:969–972, 1982

66. Pettigrew RA, Hill GL: Indicators of surgical risk and clinical judgment. Br J Surg 73:47–51, 1986

67. Starker PM, LaSala P, Askanazi J: The influence of preoperative total parenteral nutrition on morbidity and mortality. Surg Gynecol Obstet 162:569–574, 1986

68. Windsor JA, Knight GS, Hill GL: The wound healing response in surgical patients: recent food intake is more important than nutritional status. Br J Surg 75:135–137, 1988

69. Buzby G: Perioperative nutritional support. Snow Bird conference. J Parenter Enteral Nutr, suppl. 14:1975–1995, 1990

70. Cormack D, Moley J, Pass H, et al: Prospective randomized trial of parenteral nutrition in patients with upper GI cancer and weight loss undergoing surgical treatment. J Surg Res (in press)

71. Health and Policy Committee, American College of Physicians: Perioperative parenteral nutrition. Ann Intern Med 107:252–253, 1987

72. Shaw SN, Elwyn DH, Askanazi J, et al: Effects of increasing nitrogen intake on nitrogen balance and energy expenditure in nutritionally depleted adult patients receiving parenteral nutrition. Am J Clin Nutr 37:930–940, 1983

73. Robin AP, Greig PD: Basic principle of intravenous nutritional support. Clin Chest Med 7:29–39, 1986

74. Baker JP, Detsky AS, Stewart S: Randomized trial of total parenteral nutrition in critically ill patients: metabolic effects of varying glucose-lipid ratio as the energy source. Gastroenterology 87:53–59, 1984

75. Nordenstrom J, Askanazi J, Elwyn DH, et al: Nitrogen balance during total parenteral nutrition. Glucose vs fat. Ann Surg 197:27–33, 1983

76. Berger R, Adams L: Nutritional support in the critical care setting. Part 1. Chest 96:139–150, 1989

77. Wene JD, Connor WE, Den Besten L: The development of fatty acid deficiency in healthy man fed fat-free diet intravenously and orally. J Clin Invest 56:127–134, 1975

78. Weinsier RL, Krumdieck CL: Death resulting from overzealous total parenteral nutrition: the refeeding syndrome revisited. Am J Clin Nutr 34:393–399, 1981

79. Tucker SB, Schimmel EM: Postoperative hypophosphatemia: a multifactorial problem. Nutr Rev 47:111–116, 1989

80. Goldstein SA, Elwyn DH: The effects of injury and sepsis on fuel oxidation. Annu Rev Nutr 9:445–475, 1989

81. Kinney JM, Duke JH, Long CL, et al: Tissue fuel and weight loss after injury. J Clin Pathol, suppl. 44. 23:65–72, 1970

82. Stoner HB, Frayn KN, Barton RN, et al: The relationships between hormones and the severity of injury in 277 recently injured patients. Clin Sci 56:563–573, 1979

83. Shaw JHF, Wolfe RR: An integrated analysis of glucose, fat, and protein metabolism in severely traumatized patients. Ann Surg 209:63–72, 1989

84. Newsholme EA, Leech AR: pp. 623–626. In. Biochemistry for the Medical Sciences. John Wiley & Sons, Chichester, 1983

85. Woolfson AMJ, Smith JAR: Elective nutritional support

after major surgery: a prospective randomized trial. Clin Nutr 8:15–21, 1989

86. Askanazi J, Hensle TW, Starker PM, et al: Effect of immediate postoperative nutritional support on length of hospitalization. Ann Surg 203:236–239, 1986

87. Russell DM, Prendergast PJ, Darby H, et al: A comparison between muscle function and body composition in anorexia nervosa: the effect of refeeding. Am J Clin Nutr 38:229–237, 1983

88. Russell DM, Walker PM, Leiter LA, et al: Metabolic and structural changes in skeletal muscle during hypocaloric dieting. Am J Clin Nutr 39:503–513, 1984

89. Christensen T, Kehlet H: Postoperative fatigue and changes in nutritional status. Br J Surg 71:473–476, 1984

90. Wilmore DW, Long JM, Mason AD, et al: Catecholamines: mediator of the hypermetabolic response to thermal injury. Ann Surg 180:653–669, 1974

91. Rutten D, Blackburn GI, Flatt JP, et al: Determination of optimal hyperalimentation infusion rates. J Surg Res 18:477–483, 1975

92. Greig PD, Elwyn DH, Askanazi J, et al: Parenteral nutrition in septic patients: effect of increasing nitrogen intake. Am J Clin Nutr 46:1040–1047, 1987

93. Larsson J, Martenson J, Vinnars E: Nitrogen requirements in hypercatabolic patients. Clin Nutr, suppl. 4:0.4, 1984

94. Rochester DF: Malnutrition and respiratory muscles. Clin Chest Med 7:91–101, 1986

95. Arora NS, Rochester DF: Effects of body weight and muscularity on human diaphragm muscle mass, thickness and area. J Appl Physiol 52:64–70, 1982

96. Arora NS, Rochester DF: Respiratory muscle strength and voluntary ventilation in undernourished patients. Am Rev Respir Dis 126:5–8, 1982

97. Kelly SM, Rosa A, Field S, et al: Inspiratory muscle strength and body composition in patients receiving total parenteral nutrition therapy. Am Rev Respir Dis 130:33–77, 1984

98. Rochester DF, Braun NMT: Determinants of maximal inspiratory pressure in chronic obstructive pulmonary disease. Am Rev Respir Dis 132:43–47, 1985

99. Wilson DD, Rogers RM, Sanders MH, et al: Nutritional intervention in malnourished patients with emphysema. Am Rev Respir Dis 134:672–677, 1986

100. Weissmann S, Hyman AI: Nutritional care of the critically ill patient with respiratory failure. Crit Care Clin 3:185–203, 1987

101. Goldstein SA, Thomashow BM, Kvetan V, et al: Nitrogen and energy relationships in malnourished patients with emphysema. Am Rev Respir Dis 138:636–644, 1988

102. Doekel RC, Jr, Zwillich CW, Scoggin CH, et al: Clinical semistarvation: depression of hypoxic ventilatory response. N. Engl J. Med 295:358–361, 1976

103. Weissman C, Askanazi, J, Rosenbaum S, et al: Amino acids and respiration. Ann Intern Med 34:68–77, 1983

104. Stiehm ER: Humoral immunity in malnutrition. Fed Proc 39:3093–3097, 1980

105. Wilson DO, Rogers RM, Hoffman RM: State of the art:

nutrition and chronic lung disease. Am Rev Respir Dis 132:1347–1365, 1985

106. Shennib H, Chiu RCJ, Muldar DS, et al: Depression and delayed recovery of alveolar macrophage function during starvation and refeeding. Surg Gynecol Obstet 158:535–540, 1984

107. Niederman MS, Merill WW, Ferranti RD, et al: Nutritional status and bacterial binding in the lower respiratory tract in patients with chronic tracheostomies. Ann Intern Med 100:795–800, 1984

108. Vanderbergh E, Van de Woestijne KP, Gyselen A: Weight changes in the terminal stages of chronic obstructive pulmonary disease: relation to respiratory function and prognosis. Am Rev Respir Dis 95:556–566, 1967

109. Hunter AMB, Carey MA, Larch HV: The nutritional status of patients with chronic obstructive pulmonary disease. Am Rev Respir Dis 124:376–381, 1981

110. Openbrier DR, Irwin MM, Rogers RM, et al: Nutritional status and lung function in patients with emphysema and chronic bronchitis. Chest 83:17–22, 1983

111. Arora NS, Rochester DF: Effect of chronic pulmonary disease on diaphragm muscle dimension, abstracted. Am Rev Respir Dis 123:176, 1981

112. Campbell JA, Gughes RL, Sahgal V, et al: Alterations in intercostal muscle morphology and biochemistry in patients with obstructive lung disease. Am Rev Respir Dis 122:679–686, 1980

113. Braun SR, Keim NL, Dixon RM, et al: The prevalence and determinants of nutritional changes in chronic obstructive pulmonary disease. Chest 85:558–563, 1984

114. Morrison WL, Gibson JNA, Scrimgour C, et al: Muscle wasting in emphysema. Clin Sci 75:415–420, 1988

115. Tirlapur V, Afzal M: Effect of low calorie intake on abnormal pulmonary physiology in patients with chronic hypercapnic respiratory failure. Am J Med 77:987–994, 1984

116. Renzetti AD, McClement DH, Litt BD, et al: The Veterans Administration cooperative study of pulmonary function-mortality in relation to respiratory function in chronic obstructive pulmonary disease. Am J Med 41:115–129, 1966

117. Driver AG, McAlevey MT, Smith JL: Nutritional assessment of patients with chronic obstructive pulmonary failure. Chest 82:568–571, 1982

118. Wilson DO, Rogers RM, Sanders MH, et al: Nutritional intervention in malnourished patients with emphysema. Am Rev Respir Dis 134:672–677, 1986

119. Goldstein SA, Askanazi J, Elwyn DH, et al: Submaximal exercise in emphysema and malnutrition at two levels of carbohydrate and fat intake. J Appl Physiol 67:1048–1055, 1989

120. Askanazi J, Nordstrom J, Rosenbaum SH, et al: Nutrition for the patient with respiratory failure. Glucose versus fat. Anesthesiology 54:373–377, 1981

121. Skeie B, Askanazi J, Rothkopf M, et al: Intravenous fat emulsions and lung function: a review. Crit Care Med 16:183–194, 1988

122. Askanazi J, Weissman C, Lasala P, et al: Effects of increasing protein intake on ventilatory drive. Anesthesiology 60:106–110, 1984

123. Rodriquez JL, Askanazi J, Weissman C, et al: Ventilatory and metabolic effects of glucose infusions. Chest 88:512–518, 1985

124. Covelli HD, Black JW, Olsen MV, et al: Respiratory failure precipitated by high carbohydrate loads. Ann Intern Med 95:579–581, 1981

125. Larca L, Greenbaum DM: Effectiveness of intensive nutritional regimens on patients who fail to wean from mechanical ventilation. Crit Care Med 10:297–300, 1982

126. Askanazi J, Weissman C, Rosenbaum SH, et al: Nutrition and the respiratory system. Crit Care Med 10:163–172, 1982

127. Gieske T, Gurushanthaiah G, Glauser FL: Effects of carbohydrates on carbon dioxide excretion in patients with airway disease. Chest 71:55–58, 1977

128. Greene HL, Hazlett D, Demaree R: Relationship between Intralipid-induced hyperlipemia and pulmonary function. Am J Clin Nutr 29:127–135, 1976

129. Hageman JR, McCulloch K, Gora P, et al: Intralipid alterations in pulmonary prostaglandin metabolism and gas exchange. Crit Care Med 11:794–798, 1983

130. Percira GR, Fox WW, Stanley CA, et al: Decreased oxygenation and hyperlipemia during intravenous fat infusions in prenative infants. Pediatrics 66:26–30, 1980

131. Levene MI, Wigglesworth JS, Desai R, et al: Pulmonary fat accumulation after Intralipid infusion in the preterm infant. Lancet 2:815–819, 1980

132. Jarnberg P, Lindholm M, Eklund J: Lipid infusion in critically ill patients: acute effects on hemodynamics and pulmonary gas exchange. Crit Care Med 9:27–31, 1981

133. Venus B, Prager R, Patel CB, et al: Cardiopulmonary effects of Intralipid infusions in critically ill patients. Crit Care Med 16:587–590, 1988

134. Venus B, Smith RA, Patel C, et al: Hemodynamic and gas exchange alterations during Intralipid infusion in patients with adult respiratory distress syndrome. Chest 95:1278–1281, 1989

135. Kirvelä O, Venus B, Askanazi J, et al: The effects of different infusion rates of Intralipid on gas exchange, hemodynamics, and prostaglandin metabolism in acute respiratory failure. Anesthesiology, suppl. 3A. 71:A169, 1989

136. Kinsella JE, Lokesh B, Broughton S, et al: Dietary polyunsaturated fatty acids and eicosanoids: potential effects on the modulation of inflammatory and immune cells: an overview. Nutr Int 6:24–44, 1990

137. Askanazi J, Rothkopf M, Rosenbaum SH, et al: Treatment of cystic fibrosis with long-term home parenteral nutrition. Nutr Int 3:277–279, 1987

138. Skeie B, Askanazi J, Rothkopf M, et al: Improved exercise tolerance with long-term parenteral nutrition in cystic fibrosis. Crit Care Med 15:960–962, 1987

139. Takala J, Askanazi J, Weissman C, et al: Changes in respiratory control induced by amino acid infusions. Crit Care Med 16:465–469, 1988

140. Goldberg AL, Odessey R: Oxidation of amino acids by diaphragms from fed and fasted rats. Am J Physiol 223:1384–1391, 1972

141. Cerra FB, Mazuski JE, Chute E, et al: Branched-chain metabolic support: a prospective, randomized, double-blind trial in surgical stress. Ann Surg 199:286–291, 1984

142. Aubier M, Murciano D, Lecocguic Y, et al: Effect of hypophosphatemia on the diaphragmatic contractility in patients with acute respiratory failure. N Engl J Med 313:420–424, 1985

143. Benotti PN, Bistrian B: Metabolic and nutritional aspects of weaning from mechanical ventilation. Crit Care Med 17:181–185, 1989

144. Pingleton SK, Eulberg M: Nutritional analysis of acute respiratory failure patients, abstracted. Chest 83:343, 1983

145. Driver AG, LeBrun M: Iatrogenic malnutrition in patients receiving ventilatory support. JAMA 244:2195–2196, 1980

146. Bassili HR, Deitel M: Effect of nutritional support on weaning patients off mechanical ventilation. J Parenter Enteral Nutr 5:161–163, 1981

147. Grote AE, Elwyn DH, Takala J, et al: Nutritional and metabolic effects of enteral and parenteral feeding in severely injured patients. Clin Nutr 6:161–167, 1987

148. Fletcher JP, Little JM: A comparison of parenteral nutrition and early postoperative enteral feeding on nitrogen balance after major injury. Surgery 100:21–24, 1986

149. Silk DBA, Rees RG, Keohane PP, et al: Clinical efficiency and design changes of "fine-bore" nasogastric feeding tubes: a seven-year experience involving 809 intubations in 403 patients. J Parenter Enteral Nutr 11:378–383, 1987

150. Cataldi-Betcher EL, Seltzer MTI, Slochum BA, et al: Complications occurring during enteral nutritional support. A prospective study. J Parenter Enteral Nutr 7:546–551, 1983

151. Massar EL, Daley JM, Copeland EM, et al: Peripheral vein complications in patients receiving amino acid/dextrose solutions. J Parenter Enteral Nutr 7:159–162, 1983

152. Lindholm M, Rossner S: Rate of elimination of Intralipid fat emulsion from the circulation in ICU patients. Crit Care Med 10:740–746, 1982

153. Nordenstrom J, Carpentier YA, Askanazi J, et al: Metabolic utilization of intravenous fat emulsion during total parenteral nutrition. Ann Surg 196:221–231, 1982

154. Mayfield C, Nordenstrom J: Creaming and plasma clearance of intravenous fat emulsion in critically ill patients. Clin Nutr 3:93–97, 1984

155. Hayek ME, Eisenberg PG: Severe hypophosphatemia following the institution of enteral feedings. Arch Surg 124:1325–1328, 1989

156. Keohane PP, Attrill H, Love M, et al: Relation between osmolality of diet and gastrointestinal side effects in enteral nutrition. Br Med J 288:678–680, 1984

157. Hendry PJ, Akyurekli Y, McIntyre R, et al: Bronchopleural complications of nasogastric feeding tubes. Crit Care Med 14:892–894, 1986

158. Mughal MM: Complications of intravenous feeding catheters. Br J Surg 76:15–21, 1989

159. Plit ML, Lipman J, Eidelman J, et al: Catheter-related infection. A plea for consensus with review and guidelines. Intensive Care Med 14:503–509, 1988

160. Pinilla JC, Ross DF, Martin T, et al: Study of incidence of intravascular catheter infection and associated septicemia in critically ill patients. Crit Care Med 11:21–25, 1983

161. Pettigrew RA, Lang SDR, Haydock DA, et al: Catheter-related sepsis in patients on intravenous nutrition: a prospective study of quantitative catheter cultures and guidewire changes for suspected sepsis. Br J Surg 72:52–55, 1985

162. Mosca R, Curtas S, Forbes B, et al: The benefits of isolator cultures in the management of suspected catheter sepsis. Surgery 102:718–723, 1987

163. Pemberton LB, Lyman B, Lander J, et al: Sepsis from triple- vs single-lumen catheter during total parenteral nutrition in surgical or critically ill patients. Arch Surg 121:591–593, 1986

164. Hilton E, Haslett TM, Borenstein MT: Central catheter infections: single-versus triple-lumen catheters. Am J Med 84:667–672, 1988

165. Lee RB, Buckner M, Sharp KW: Do multi-lumen catheters increase central venous catheter sepsis compared to single-lumen catheters? J Trauma 28:1472–1475, 1988

166. Long CL: Energy balance and carbohydrate metabolism in infection and sepsis. Am J Clin Nutr 30:1301–1310, 1977

167. Harris JA, Benedict FG: Standard Basal Metabolism Constants for Physiologists and Clinicians. A Biometric Study of Basal Metabolism in Man. pp. 223–250. JB Lippincott, Philadelphia, 1919

168. Weinsier RL, Butterworth CE, Jr: p. 98. In: Handbook of Clinical Nutrition. CV Mosby, St. Louis, 1981

169. Weinsier RL, Butterworth CE, Jr: Guidelines for essential trace elements preparation for parenteral use. JAMA 241:2051–2054, 1974

170. Krey SH, Murray RL: Dynamics of Nutritional Support: Assessment, Implementation, Evaluation. Appleton-Century-Crofts, 1986

171. Krey SH, Murray RL: Invited review: multivitamin preparations for parenteral use. A statement by the nutrition advisory group. J Parenter Enteral Nutr 3:25, 1979

26
COMPLICATIONS OF THORACIC SURGERY

Aliasghar Aghdami, M.D.
Richard L. Keenan, M.D.

"The operation was a success, but the patient died" was an old adage that is unacceptable in the era of modern anesthesiology. Anesthesiologists as well as surgeons today recognize the need to anticipate operative and postoperative complications so that their occurrence is minimized or avoided entirely, and to provide prompt and effective treatment if and when they do occur. This chapter discusses some of the major complications of noncardiac thoracic surgery, with emphasis on those associated with pulmonary resection. Other complications are covered in chapters specifically related to them. Table 26-1 lists the major complications considered in this chapter.

MAJOR ANESTHETIC COMPLICATIONS

The most feared anesthetic complication, without doubt, is the patient not waking up. The incidence of death or permanent brain damage due solely to anesthesia is believed to be between 1 and 2 per 10,000 cases.[1] Most are the result of hypoxia of the brain suffered as a result of a cardiac arrest occurring during the operation or in the recovery room. Decreased oxygen delivery to the brain may occur as a result of ischemia of the brain, when blood flow stops as a result of myocardial depression from anesthetic overdose. It can also occur prior to arrest as a result of arterial hypoxemia, insufficient inspired oxygen, or inadequate ventilation; in this latter case, arrest occurs when the myocardium becomes hypoxic as well. The oxygen storage capacity of the brain is nil, with stores of high-energy phosphate sufficient to maintain tissue viability for only a few minutes.[2] Hypoxic brain damage will occur first in the most metabolically active areas, the cortical and subcortical gray matter. Consciousness is normally lost when cerebral venous oxygen tension (normally above 30 mmHg) falls below 20 mmHg; electroencephalographic activity ceases at this level as well. Irreversible damage is usually evident 1 or 2 minutes later.

Treatment consists of standard cardiopulmonary resuscitation methods,[3] which are successful in approximately 50 percent of intraoperative cases.[4] Postresuscitative care is currently under intense investigation[5]; evidence of a potentially preventable "reperfusion syndrome" involving cell damage possibly mediated by calcium or free oxygen radicals is exciting,[6] but as yet a specific postresuscitation therapy cannot be recommended. Intravenous barbiturate coma, the first to be tried, failed to show any advantage.[7]

The majority of anesthetic deaths reported in the past are now regarded as preventable, and most of these have been due to a failure to provide adequate ventilation.[4,8,9] Responding to this information, anesthesiologists in the United States have accepted monitoring standards that incorporate the routine use of pulse oximetry, by which oxygenation of the arterial

TABLE 26-1.   Complications of Noncardiac Thoracic Surgery

Major anesthetic complications
  Death, brain damage

Pulmonary complications
  Tracheobronchial obstruction
  Mediastinal shift
  Air leakage
  Lung torsion and infarction
  Bronchial stump disruption
  Pleural effusion, empyema, chylothorax

Chest wall problems
  Paradox
  Mediastinal and subcutaneous emphysema
  Hematoma
  Wound dehiscence
  Pain

Hemorrhage
  Postoperative bleeding into the pleura
  Bleeding into the tracheobronchial tree

Cardiac complications
  Dysrhythmias
  Pulmonary hypertension, right heart failure
  Cardiac herniation
  Pulmonary thromboembolism

Nerve injuries
  Intercostal nerves
  Phrenic nerve
  Vagus nerve
  Recurrent laryngeal nerve
  Brachial plexus injury

Complications of diagnostic procedures
  Bronchoscopy
  Mediastinoscopy
  Scalene node biopsy
  Needle biopsy and thoracentesis

blood can be followed, and capnography to monitor the adequacy of carbon dioxide removal. It is not unreasonable to expect that anesthetic mortality will decline significantly as a result of better respiratory monitoring. The liability insurance industry already has evidence that when oximetry and capnometry are used, fewer malpractice claims resulting from hypoxia are seen.[10] At the Medical College of Virginia, 11 intraoperative cardiac arrests due to unrecognized hypoxemia occurred in 163,240 cases over a 15-year period ending in 1983.[4] Following the introduction of routine monitoring with pulse oximetry in 1984, not a single such case has been recorded in the following 5 years involving over 60,000 cases of anesthesia.

In thoracic anesthesia, in which the organs of respiration are compromised, meticulous attention to oxygenation and carbon dioxide removal is doubly important in preventing cardiac arrest, permanent brain damage, and death.

PREVENTION OF POSTOPERATIVE COMPLICATIONS

Patients scheduled for pulmonary or chest wall resections require evaluation of their pulmonary status, and any deficiencies should be improved preoperatively. Respiratory problems, especially atelectasis and pneumonia, are the most frequent complications following thoracotomy, and are theoretically preventable.[11]

Prior to pulmonary resection, complete pulmonary function studies, including blood gas analysis, ventilation-perfusion scans, and a respiratory history, can provide insight into whether a patient can tolerate the loss of functional lung tissue.[12,13] The probability of postoperative pulmonary insufficiency can thus be minimized.

Infection is a common feature in patients with chronic obstructive pulmonary disease (COPD) who require thoracic surgery. Proper management of infection has long been recognized as an important means of preventing postoperative atelectasis and pneumonia.[14] Just as important is the clearance of secretions with active chest physiotherapy. Exercises for the chest wall, diaphragm, arm, and shoulder should be taught preoperatively and stressed twice daily postoperatively. Deep breathing, coughing, and, if necessary, tracheal suctioning are equally important both preoperatively and postoperatively.[15] Cigarette smokers have a higher incidence of pulmonary complications.[16] Cessation of smoking even a few days before surgery, combined with physiotherapy, can minimize postoperative atelectasis.

In the postoperative period, adequate pain control improves the ability to breathe and can facilitate coughing, although systemic and even epidural narcotic administration can centrally depress ventilation. Good pain control can minimize postoperative complications.

Fluid balance is especially important in patients undergoing pulmonary resectional surgery. While fluid overload can contribute to right heart failure, dehydration thickens secretions, making them difficult to remove. Thus, care must be taken to maintain an adequate but not excessive fluid balance.

PULMONARY COMPLICATIONS

Tracheobronchial Obstruction

Blood, blood clots, or thick secretions are the most common causes of airway obstruction following pulmonary resection. The use of a double-lumen endotracheal tube (Carlen's, Robertshaw; see Chapter 14) during anesthesia and surgery will help to prevent these postoperative problems.[17] By isolating the two bronchi, secretions and blood from the operative side will not spill to the opposite side and a cleaner functioning lung can be maintained during resection. Postoperatively, obstruction may occur if secretions are allowed to be aspirated into the tracheobronchial tree during recovery from anesthesia. Frequent postoperative bedside auscultation will reveal the early signs of airway obstruction, which consist of wheezing, rhonchi, and decreased breath sounds. Tachypnea and dyspnea will become evident; chest radiography will reveal air trapping, atelectasis, or pneumonia. Prompt aggressive use of tracheal suctioning is indicated, and bronchoscopy may be necessary.

Gastric dilation, as noted on physical examination postoperatively or by the presence of a large gastric air bubble on a radiograph, requires immediate gastric intubation and emptying to avoid regurgitation and aspiration. Chemical bronchitis is most effectively avoided rather than treated. Treatment should include bronchoscopy if solid material is suspected, followed by tracheal intubation and ventilation with positive end-expiratory pressure (PEEP) to avoid alveolar collapse.

Physiotherapy and postoperative suctioning are most important in patients after left upper lobectomy, because as the left lower lobe rises to fill the left hemithorax, the long left bronchus tends to kink as it passes under the aortic arch.

Mediastinal Shift

Following the removal of any pulmonary tissue, the mediastinum compensates for this volume loss by shifting toward the involved hemithorax. This compensatory process should not normally encroach on functioning lung tissue, but should obliterate empty space. Changes are most marked following pneumonectomy, in which the remaining lung expands and pushes the mediastinum to the operated side; elevation of the diaphragm and narrowing of the interspaces of the empty hemithorax also occur. Figure 26-1 demonstrates the progressive mediastinal shift in the days (Fig. 26-1A), months (Fig. 26-1B) and years (Fig. 26-1C) after pneumonectomy.

Excessive mediastinal shift in the immediate postoperative period following segmental or lobar resection is suggestive of loss of volume on the operated lung and is most often due to atelectasis. Aggressive physiotherapy, suctioning, and bronchoscopy are indicated in that case. If the secretions are excessive and thick and the amount of collapse is extensive, or if the lung does not re-expand, ventilatory support via an endotracheal tube should be considered. Less commonly, fluid accumulation or pneumothorax on the contralateral (nonoperative) side may also cause an

exaggerated mediastinal shift, and may be ruled out with a chest radiograph and physical findings.

Air Leakage

Air leakage from the site of resection of a pulmonary lobe or segment is common initially, since most pulmonary fissures are not complete and small air conduits are invariably transected. This does not pose a hazard, assuming that chest drainage tubes have been placed correctly at the time of surgery.[18] Two chest tubes placed in the pleura at the level of the diaphragm going to the apex, one anteriorly and one posteriorly, should effectively drain blood, pus, and air, and allow the lung to be fully expanded. Underwater drainage is normally supplemented by constant suction (see Chaper 22 for a more detailed description of chest drainage systems). Initial air leakage normally stops in 3 or 4 days.

Major segmental or bronchial air leaks typically do not occur early, and are dealt with below. Persistent moderate air leaks (beyond 7 days) often respond to removal of the chest tube, allowing the lung to collapse moderately, and then reinsertion of a new tube.

Mechanical ventilatory support is commonly used following pulmonary resection.[19] Usually, volume-limited ventilators can be made to cope with large air leaks; however, positive-pressure ventilation, especially with PEEP, may prolong air leaks and increase the risk of infection and pneumothorax.[20] High-frequency jet ventilation has been attempted as an alternative to conventional ventilation in the presence of large air leaks.[21,22] Clinical results have been mixed, and laboratory work continues in the search for optimum frequency and ventilator design (see Chapter 24).[23]

Torsion and Infarction of Lobe or Segment

After resection of pulmonary tissue, the vessels of a remaining lobe or segment may become twisted as the lung expands to occupy the cavity. Occasionally, torsion occurs in this process. Typically, the pulmonary and bronchial arteries remain open; however, the lower-pressured pulmonary veins collapse, compromising venous outflow. Engorgement causes massive enlargement of the lung area drained by the involved veins. Because of the threat of infarction, this complication must be recognized and promptly treated.[24]

Chest radiography will show a homogeneous density that enlarges on subsequent films. Hemoptysis is common. Dyspnea, elevated temperature, pulse, and respiratory rate are seen. On the posterolateral film, the outline of the blood supply can sometimes be helpful in diagnosis. With torsion, the vessels may be seen to travel toward the apex rather than the base, as is

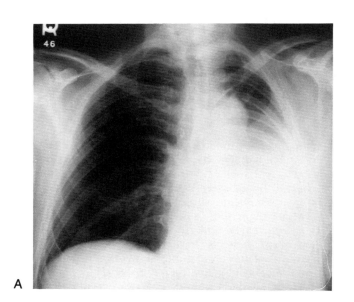

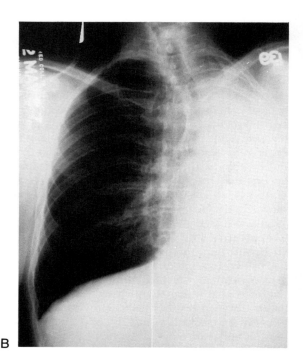

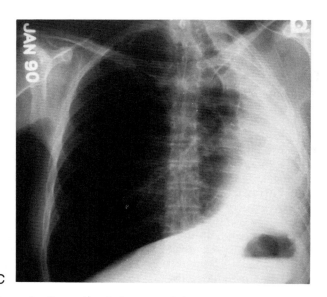

Fig. 26-1. (A) Chest radiograph of a patient 3 days post-left pneumonectomy. The heart shadow is almost completely in the left hemithorax. The space normally filled with the left lung is largely opaque from heart shadow and accumulated fluid. Note also that the intercostal spaces are narrower on the left than on the right. **(B)** The same patient 1 month post-left pneumonectomy. Note the flattened right hemidiaphragm and further mediastinal shift, with tracheal deviation, as a result of further expansion of the remaining lung. **(C)** The same patient nearly 3 years post-left pneumonectomy. Dramatic tracheal deviation toward the operative side is seen. The mediastinum completely fills a very diminished left hemithorax.

the usual pattern. Bronchoscopy will usually show closure of the affected bronchus.

Immediate repeat thoracotomy is indicated in an attempt to release the torsion. If lung tissue is already nonviable, lobectomy will be required. Infarction as a result of compromised blood supply not only further decreases the remaining pulmonary function, but also results in lung gangrene and infection if the problem is not promptly corrected.[25] Signs of sepsis, such as fever and chills, are occasionally observed with hemoptysis, and foul, purulent sputum may be present. Purulent chest drainage may also be seen and, as fluid accumulates in the hemithorax, thoracentesis will yield pus. Management requires thoracotomy with removal of the involved tissue, followed by generous drainage of the pleural space.

Bronchial Stump Disruption

Closure of the bronchial stump following pulmonary resection is an important surgical consideration, since a major bronchopleural fistula is associated with a mortality rate of greater than 20 percent.[26] Proper initial closure of the stump may be tested intraoperatively by having the surgeon fill the hemithorax with saline and providing 40 cmH$_2$O of pressure in the anesthesia breathing system. If no bubbles appear, the stump has been properly closed.[27] Fistulae appearing in the first few postoperative days are usually the result of improper closure and present as an abrupt increase in air leak from the chest tube, hemoptysis, and a change in the chest radiograph that may show increased pneumothorax or partial lung collapse on the involved side. Prompt reoperation with closure of the disruption is recommended.[28] Bronchopleural fistulae appearing after the first week are usually due to necrosis at the suture line from an inadequate blood supply, infection, or malignant tumor in the bronchial stump. Late bronchial breakdowns typically occur in patients whose general condition precludes immediate reoperation. Continued chest tube drainage will, therefore, be required until definitive surgical correction is possible, usually weeks later.[29] Figure 26-2 illustrates a bronchopulmonary fistula.

In providing anesthesia for patients with late bronchopleural fistulae, two problems must be considered, in addition to that of general debilitation. First, the air leak may be so great that positive-pressure ventilation with an anesthetic machine may not provide adequate alveolar ventilation, even with high gas flows. Clamping the chest tubes is no solution, since a tension pneumothorax will result. Thus, unless the leak is small, a double-lumen endotracheal tube is indicated. Consideration should be given to inserting the tube with the patient awake, under topical anesthesia, and

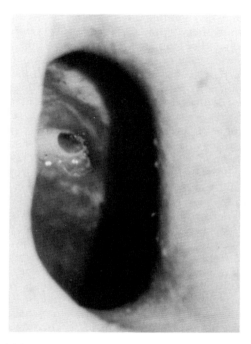

Fig. 26-2. Bronchopleural cutaneous fistula following postpneumonectomy empyema, as viewed through a Eloesser flap on the chest wall. Note the bubbles surrounding the opening of the bronchus.

breathing spontaneously. Alternatively, general inhalation anesthesia without the use of muscular paralysis and the maintenance of spontaneous ventilation may be used prior to insertion of the double-lumen tube.[30] Either way, 100 percent oxygen should be administered so that arterial oxygenation might be maintained even in the face of hypoventilation and hypercarbia. Second, pleural infection is present in many patients with persistent large bronchopleural fistulae, often with empyema. This, too, is an indication for the use of a double-lumen tube, to isolate and protect the contralateral lung. Prior to the insertion of the tube, the patient with an infected pleural space should be kept in a reverse Trendelenburg position to minimize spillage of infected pleural fluid through the fistula back into the tracheobronchial tree. For the same reason, placing the patient in the lateral position with the involved hemithorax uppermost should be avoided until after intubation with effective isolation of the infected side.

Pleural Effusion, Empyema, and Chylothorax

Accumulation of fluid in the hemithorax, particularly at the bases, is not unusual following pulmonary resection. The presence of a persistent or increasing effusion, when combined with clinical signs of sepsis, such as an otherwise unexplained fever, should lead to the suspicion of empyema. Postoperative infection in the pleural space is usually the result of a persistent air leak, failure of the remaining lung to fill the space, or significant operative contamination. Pre-existent pulmonary infection may be an important source; proper preoperative preparation is, therefore, most important in preventing postoperative infectious complications. If empyema does develop, the source of infection must be identified and treated. This might include bronchopleural fistula, chest wall infection, or communication with the gastrointestinal tract. While antibiotics play an important supportive role in the treatment of empyema, immediate drainage is essential.[31,32] In cases in which significant unfilled pleural space remains, such as after pneumonectomy, open pleural drainage will be required for 2 to 3 weeks after initial drainage. This will involve rib resection, and eventually even thoracoplasty in some cases.

Chylothorax occurs more commonly on the left than the right as a complication of thoracotomy for pulmonary resection. It is the result of surgical dissection between the aorta and esophagus.[33] Disruption of the thoracic duct or one of its major branches allows escape of chyle into the pleural space. Since chyle is bacteriostatic and sterile, infection is infrequent. While chest tubes are in place and the patient remains fasting, signs are few. However, removal of the tubes will result in dyspnea and effusion as chyle accumulates, and reinsertion of a chest drain is required. Alimentation of the patient results in an increased volume of thick, creamy drainage. Drainage can be minimized by a limited diet, supplemented by intravenous hyperalimentation. In most cases, drainage ceases within 1 or 2 weeks. If not, operative repair is required, since continuous loss of fat and fat-soluble vitamins is poorly tolerated.[34]

CHEST WALL COMPLICATIONS

Paradox

The dynamics of respiratory paradox are described in Chapter 8. Paradoxical chest wall motion is seen in postoperative, spontaneously breathing patients when bony elements of the thorax have been resected. The extent of paradox will depend on the amount of chest wall support removed at surgery. Its influence on the patient's ability to sustain adequate ventilation will depend also on the patient's preoperative pulmonary status; patients with chronic pulmonary disease will tolerate less paradox than those with normal pre-

operative pulmonary function. The state of the mediastinum also plays a role in determining the amount of paradox. Paradoxical air movement will be less in patients with a mediastinum fixed by fibrosis from pre-existent pleural pathology (tuberculosis is the classic example) than in patients with a normally supple mediastinum. All these factors must be considered preoperatively to determine the feasibility of chest wall resection and to anticipate the need for postoperative ventilatory support.

Surgical methods of stabilizing the chest wall are available that use musculocutaneous chest wall flaps, plastic mesh, and metal struts.[35–37] These methods are designed to stabilize the chest, thus minimizing the paradox and improving the function of remaining lung tissue.

Initial postoperative management of patients requiring chest wall resection includes continued tracheal intubation and mechanical ventilation, perhaps with some PEEP. Within 48 hours, stabilization of the chest wall will usually be sufficient to allow removal of ventilatory support. However, support may be continued for longer periods if necessary.

Mediastinal and Subcutaneous Emphysema

Air leakage from disrupted pulmonary tissue, either directly from the tracheobronchial tree or via the pleural space, into adjacent tissue ("emphysema") is common after pulmonary surgery. Air from disrupted alveoli and small bronchi may dissect along the pulmonary vessels and bronchial tree and enter the mediastinum. Alternatively, air in the pleural space may gain access to the mediastinum through surgically created disruptions in the pleura (Fig. 26-3). Air then dissects along the mediastinal structures and enters the subcutaneous tissues of the neck, chest, and head. Subcutaneous emphysema of the chest may also occur as a result of air leakage around the chest tube as it exits the thorax. Pneumoperitoneum is a recognized complication that sometimes follows pneumothorax.[38] Air in the mediastinum dissects distally into the retroperitoneum, ruptures into the peritoneal cavity, and presents on the radiograph as free air under the diaphragm.

Normally, well-placed chest tubes will prevent or minimize this problem. Mediastinal and subcutaneous emphysema are not normally harmful to the patient. However, their occurrence should prompt careful assessment for the presence of a persistent pulmonary air leak, and for the possibility of leakage from nonpulmonary structures, such as the esophagus, which could have been injured during surgery.

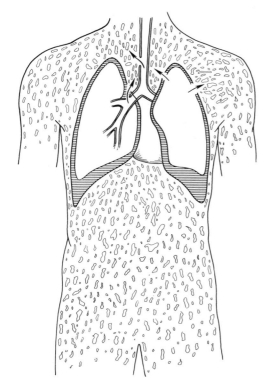

Fig. 26-3. Genesis of mediastinal and subcutaneous emphysema. Arrows denote routes by which air from the tracheobronchial tree may gain access to the mediastinum.

Wound Dehiscence

Because of the rich blood supply of the muscles of the chest wall, faulty wound healing with dehiscence is rare after thoracotomy. Hematoma and infection are typically the cause, and debilitated patients have a much higher incidence than do patients with good nutrition.[39,40] It is important, therefore, that hematomas of the chest wall be evacuated when discovered. Nutrition of debilitated patients should be optimized as well, as described in Chapter 25.

When a dehiscence occurs in the absence of infection, steps may be taken to close the wound, drain the pleural space, and re-expand the lung. Infection of the elements of the chest wall, when present, must be treated by laying open the wound and performing adequate debridement. Secondary closure is attempted at a later date.[41]

Postoperative Pain

The pain experienced following left or right thoracotomy is more severe than after most surgical procedures, including median sternotomy. The pain is largely due to musculoskeletal disruption occurring at the time of surgery. This includes the removal, cutting, and breaking of ribs; the tearing and stretching of the fibrous connections of ribs to the vertebral bodies posteriorly and sternal cartilage anteriorly; and the cutting of major chest wall muscles. Severe postoperative chest wall pain inhibits coughing and even breathing, thus interfering with the normal mechanism for removing tracheobronchial secretions. Good analgesia, therefore, is desirable to prevent atelectasis and pneumonia. This important consideration is discussed in detail in Chapter 21.

HEMORRHAGE

Postoperative Bleeding Into the Pleura

The blood lost following thoracotomy typically flows into the pleural space and is drained by the chest tubes. While some blood loss is expected, it normally should not exceed 500 mL in 24 hours following pulmonary surgery. Sustained loss at a rate of more than 100 to 200 mL/h is usually considered an indication for re-exploration with removal of clots and control of the bleeding site. Bleeding is almost always from the systemic circulation, often from vessels in the chest wall or in the mediastinum, pericardiophrenic vessels, branches of the azygous system, or branches of the bronchial arteries.

Bleeding from the pulmonary circulation rarely occurs, but is massive when it does, since the system carries a high flow, even though at low pressure. This complication is rare, in part, because surgeons are aware of its catastrophic nature and take special care in suturing pulmonary vessels.[42]

Blood loss following pulmonary resection can be monitored via chest tube drainage and postoperative chest radiography. It should be kept in mind that excessive bleeding invariably results in clot formation within the chest, which may obstruct the chest tubes; thus, lack of drainage alone is no guarantee that all is well. Careful attention must also be paid to changes in the radiograph, such as fluid accumulation and mediastinal shift, and signs of hypovolemia. Intravenous blood and fluid replacement should be ongoing in an attempt to restore and maintain normovolemia even as the loss continues. Evidence of excessive bleeding with clot formation suggests immediate thoracotomy to remove clots, stop the bleeding, and re-expand any lung tissue compressed by the accumulated blood.

Bleeding after the first 24 hours following thoracotomy is very unusual, and is likely the result of erosion by infection of a vessel at the point of suture or pressure from a rib or chest tube. Emergency thoracotomy is required.

Bleeding Into the Tracheobronchial Tree

With advanced tuberculosis now a rarity in developed countries, spontaneous massive hemoptysis is mostly of historic interest. Significant bleeding into the tracheobronchial tree is now seen largely as a complication of bronchoscopic biopsy. Most often it results from the biopsy of an adenoma or vascular malignancy, although it is possible to enter a bronchial artery or even a pulmonary vessel if the bite is too deep. It is also a rare complication of pulmonary artery catheterization.

With the onset of brisk bleeding, three goals must be kept in mind: (1) stop the bleeding; (2) keep the airway clear of blood; and (3) maintain ventilation. Tamponade of the bleeding site with pledgets, possibly soaked with a vasoconstrictor, is possible with a rigid bronchoscope. This will often suffice to stop the bleeding. It is important that all bleeding be controlled and that all blood and clots be removed bilaterally from the tracheobronchial tree before the bronchoscope is removed. If tamponade fails, immediate thoracotomy to control the bleeding site is necessary. This is a desperate situation in which speed in the control of bleeding is critical, and ventilation is less important than preserving patency of the airways. Ideally, a double-lumen endotracheal tube should be inserted while surgical preparations are made, so that the uninvolved lung can be ventilated without fear of obstruction with clots, and blood can be drained from the involved side. However, in the face of massive hemorrhage, this may not be feasible. Blockade of the involved bronchus with packing or a Fogarty catheter may then be attempted if rigid bronchoscopy has been used, followed by removal of the bronchoscope and immediate intubation with a single-lumen tube. In the case of flexible bronchoscopy, tamponade is maintained as best as possible while suctioning and ventilation continue through the endotracheal tube.

CARDIAC COMPLICATIONS

Dysrhythmias

Following pulmonary resection, significant supraventricular dysrhythmias are not unusual. They may include atrial fibrillation, atrial flutter, and paroxysmal tachycardia.[43,44] Occasionally, the resulting pulse rate disturbances will be great enough to interfere with hemodynamic function, especially in the elderly.[45] Likely causes of postpneumonectomy atrial rhythm disturbances include increased pulmonary vascular resistance leading to pulmonary hypertension and dilation of the right atrium and ventricle. Additionally, irritation of the right heart and pulmonary veins from surgical manipulation, mediastinal shift, and inflammation may contribute. Nonspecific additive factors may be hypoxemia, pain, and increased vagal tone.

Diagnosis of an atrial dysrhythmia postoperatively is relatively straightforward. Careful surveillance for the onset of a rapid or irregular pulse should be routine, with ECG confirmation when it occurs. Specific treatment of postpneumonectomy atrial fibrillation or flutter is often undertaken with digitalis. If the rhythm is not controlled, intravenous verapamil, propranolol, or esmolol may also be used. Rarely, and only if the patient's circulation is severely compromised, will electrical cardioversion be required. Treatment of nonspecific factors such as pain and fever are also important and must not be neglected.

Digitalis therapy instituted preoperatively or at the time of pneumonectomy has been widely used; it seems to lessen the severity of the dysrhythmia and makes it more manageable when it occurs.[46–48]

Pulmonary Hypertension and Right Heart Failure

Patients with COPD frequently have right ventricular dysfunction as a result of pulmonary hypertension.[49,50] Moreover, exercise increases pulmonary artery pressure further in these patients, suggesting that the pulmonary vascular bed's normal ability to expand with increased blood flow has been restricted, presumably by fibrotic obliteration of some alveolocapillary units, which is irreversible, as well as from hypoxic pulmonary vasoconstriction, which may be reversible. As pulmonary artery pressure increases during exercise in patients with COPD, right ventricular function deteriorates, as evidenced by a fall in ejection fraction.[51,52] Right ventricular contractility has also been observed experimentally to fall in association with an increase in pulmonary artery pressure, presumably due to subendocardial ischemia from ventricular wall stress as the chamber dilates.[53]

Surgical removal of all or part of a lung obviously decreases the cross-sectional area of the pulmonary tree. Normally, the remainder of functioning lung tissue is sufficient to accommodate the increase in pulmonary blood flow associated with moderate exercise without developing pulmonary hypertension. However, if the patient has pre-existent COPD with all the changes noted above, pneumonectomy may well result in severe pulmonary hypertension and right heart failure. This is a complication to be avoided, since the prognosis is poor in postpneumonectomy patients who develop right heart failure.[54,55]

Preoperative assessment of the pulmonary circulation is, therefore, an important element in the management of patients with known COPD who may require pulmonary resection. Measurement of pulmonary artery pressures preoperatively is advised, either with cardiac catheterization or with a flow-directed pulmonary artery catheter. If the mean pulmonary artery pressure at rest exceeds 25 mmHg, pulmonary hypertension is present and is considered an unfavorable sign.[56] An estimate of postoperative function can be made by obtaining pressures before and after occluding the pulmonary artery of the operative lung with an inflatable balloon on the catheter.[57,58] Pneumonectomy may not be advisable if the pulmonary artery pressure rises more than 5 mmHg with occlusion. Unfortunately, the pulmonary occlusion test has not proved to be as definitive of outcome as originally thought,[59] and clinical judgment continues to be required in deciding whether to proceed with pulmonary resection in some cases. Exercise testing with measurement of oxygen consumption currently seems promising and has recently been reviewed by Olsen (see Chapter 1).[60]

Patients at risk for right heart failure following pulmonary resection should be managed with a pulmonary artery catheter. The diagnosis of right heart failure may be made when (1) the right atrial pressure is elevated, (2) the pulmonary artery wedge (left atrial) pressure is normal, and (3) the cardiac output is low. As is typical of pulmonary hypertension, the pulmonary artery diastolic pressure is significantly higher than the wedge pressure. The classic signs of peripheral edema, hepatomegaly, and oliguria may appear.

Treatment should begin with the aggressive treatment of all possible causes of pulmonary vasoconstriction, such as hypoxemia and acidosis, and causes of increased pulmonary blood flow, such as pain and sepsis with fever. Inotropic support of the heart is recommended, particularly with agents that are pulmonary vasodilators, such as dobutamine and amrinone. Nitroprusside may also be of some value. Digitalis, except for the control of heart rate in atrial dysrhythmias, is less useful.

Volume loading is controversial in the treatment of right heart failure. Cardiac output may be improved by the administration of fluids to patients with right heart failure in the absence of pulmonary hypertension, as when the failure is due to ischemic heart disease.[61] However, in right heart failure following pulmonary resection, when the pulmonary vascular resistance is high, volume loading is unlikely to be of benefit. Indeed, fluid restriction guided by right atrial pressure monitoring may be the most effective course.

Cardiac Herniation

In humans, the mediastinum completely separates the right from the left pleura. More important, the pericardial sac not only contains the heart, but holds it in place within the mediastinum. Surgical disrup-

tion of the pericardium, which is sometimes required to facilitate hilar dissection during pulmonary surgery, may lead to later herniation of a portion of the heart through the defect.[62–64] Herniation occurs after chest closure, usually early in the postoperative course. It is probably caused by a differential pressure in the two hemithoraxes, and is most likely to follow pneumonectomy. Increased pressure from coughing or positive-pressure ventilation in the intact lung, or decreased pressure from suction on the operated side, or both, contribute to the heart being pushed (or pulled) through the defect.

Symptoms are sudden in onset, are dramatic, and vary in regard to which hemithorax is involved. Herniation following right pneumonectomy into the right pleural space results in rotation of the heart to the right with torsion of the heart's venous input, causing severe restriction in venous return and a fall in cardiac output.[65,66] Following left pneumonectomy, the heart does not rotate so much as it protrudes through the pericardial defect. However, the edges of the defect compress the myocardium, typically at the level of the atrioventricular groove,[67] leading to myocardial ischemia, dysrhythmias, obstruction to ventricular outflow, and myocardial infarction if not promptly reduced. In both cases, sudden cardiovascular collapse is typical and the mortality rate is high.

A chest radiograph showing protrusion of the heart shadow into the operative hemithorax (Fig. 26-4), coupled with sudden cardiovascular collapse, justifies a diagnosis of cardiac herniation. The ECG typically shows abnormal rotation of the electrical axis; dysrhythmias and ST-T wave abnormalities may be present.

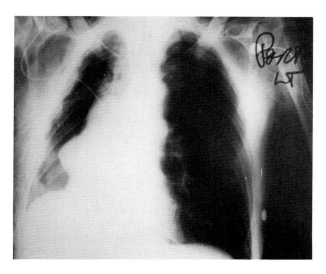

Fig. 26-4. Partial cardiac herniation following right pneumonectomy. (From Brooks,[90] with permission.)

Once the diagnosis of cardiac herniation is made, immediate surgery is required. While the patient is being prepared and transported to the operating room, steps to reverse the pressure differential that favors herniation may be taken in an attempt to reduce the hernia even before the chest is opened. Suction of the operative pleural space should be discontinued; air injection into the empty hemithorax might be considered. Meanwhile, spontaneous ventilation of the intact lung is desirable, with avoidance of coughing; if positive-pressure ventilation is used, rapid shallow ventilation, to minimize peak airway pressure, is desirable. Placing the patient in the lateral position with the operated hemithorax uppermost allows gravity to contribute to the reduction.

Pulmonary Thromboembolism

Pulmonary thromboembolism is a well-known surgical complication with a mortality rate solely from this complication as high as 0.5 percent of major adult operations. Venous thrombosis is the underlying cause, with foci in the deep veins of the legs accounting for the vast majority. However, thrombus formation in a long pulmonary artery stump following pulmonary resection can also occur and propagate back into the remaining pulmonary artery where flow is obstructed.[68,69]

Prophylaxis against venous thromboembolism is recommended for patients at high risk, which includes those over the age of 40 years who are obese, have malignant disease, or have a history of deep vein thrombosis. Subcutaneous "minidose" heparin,[70] intermittent pneumatic compression of the legs during and after surgery, and dextran[71] have been advocated.

The manifestations of pulmonary embolism are directly related to the amount of pulmonary arterial tree blocked by the embolus or emboli. Dyspnea and tachypnea are the most frequent manifestations. Apprehension and tachycardia also frequently occur. Pleural pain, cough, and an accentuated P_2 heart sound occur in 50 to 60 percent of cases. Hemoptysis and pleural rub are less common, and are probably signs of pulmonary infarction. Syncope and cardiovascular collapse occur when more than half of the pulmonary vascular bed has been blocked. Hypoxemia on arterial blood gas analysis is a hallmark of pulmonary embolism, as is pulmonary hypertension.[72] Hypoxemia probably occurs because of shunting to the remaining intact pulmonary tree and altered ventilation-perfusion relationships following the release of vasoactive substances from platelets.[73]

Diagnosis of pulmonary embolism is extremely difficult because of the nonspecific nature of the clinical manifestations. Differential diagnosis includes myocardial infarction, massive intrapleural hemorrhage, esophageal perforation, and septic shock. Because of the potentially catastrophic nature of any of these, an accurate diagnosis is required, despite the inherent difficulties. Lung scans using radioisotopes have been widely used; however, while they can be useful in following the course of therapy, they are of limited diagnostic value, particularly in post-thoracotomy patients in whom perfusion defects from atelectasis and pre-existent chronic lung disease are expected. Pulmonary arteriography is regarded as the most accurate diagnostic method. However, the procedure is invasive, requiring cardiac catheterization and injection of a bolus of dye, and carries its own morbidity.[74] Steps should also be taken to rule out each of the other entities on the differential list that might cause circulatory collapse.

Death within the first hour of pulmonary embolization is common, especially when the size of the embolus is large and cardiovascular collapse occurs. Emergency pulmonary embolectomy with cardiopulmonary bypass at this point may be lifesaving, but is associated with a very high mortality rate,[75] with uncontrollable intrapulmonary hemorrhage following restoration of flow being the most serious complication.[76] Therefore, if the patient survives the first hour, treatment is usually directed at stabilizing the patient's hemodynamics with inotropic drugs if necessary and preventing further episodes of embolization. Continuous intravenous heparin therapy is initiated, in a dose sufficient to prolong the partial thromboplastin time to twice normal. This may be followed later with oral anticoagulation with Coumadin preparations. Insertion of a vena cava filter may also be considered if the source of emboli is thought to be from the pelvis or lower extremity, especially if a contraindication to heparinization (such as peptic ulcer) exists.[77] Insertion of a caval filter can usually be accomplished through a transvenous approach not unlike that of jugular cannulation for central venous access, under local anesthesia.[78]

NERVE INJURIES

Intercostal Nerves

The intercostal nerves are most vulnerable to injury from lateral thoracotomy incisions. Direct interruption, crushing with retractors, laceration by fractured rib ends, stretching of nerve roots, and inclusion in sutures during closure can all occur. It is not uncommon, therefore, for the patient to experience an area of numbness or hypersthesia over the area of the fifth or sixth dermatome. Patients should be warned preoperatively of this possibility, and reassured that normally no disability results from it. However, in rare instances, intercostal nerve damage will result in chronic pain for which the patient will seek treatment.

The post-thoracotomy pain syndrome is defined as pain that recurs or persists along a thoracotomy scar at least 2 months following the surgical procedure.[79] It is a phenomenon of the chest wall, and can be of myofascial origin or a form of deafferentation pain. Myofascial pain presents with soreness of the incisional site that is aggravated by movement, often with "trigger-point" areas of sensitivity. Myofascial pain usually responds to injection of the points with local anesthetics. Physical therapy is also helpful, especially when the major trunk muscles, such as the trapezius, are involved.

Deafferentation pain occurs as a result of damage to nerves, and presents with causalgia-like symptoms, including sensory loss, burning, and evidence of sympathetic hyperactivity over the distribution of the nerve involved.[80] Treatment includes sympathetic or local nerve blockade with local anesthetics, transcutaneous electrical stimulation, and medication with antidepressant drugs. Improvement is seen in some patients, but not all. Surgical resection and cryoneurotomy have been tried, but with only occasional success.[81] Because interruption of the neural pathway proximal to the lesion may actually worsen deafferentation pain in some patients, it is not recommended. It should also be noted that a patient who has undergone thoracotomy for cancer may fear (with reason) the pain as a herald of recurrence. Careful evaluation for recurrence should be undertaken; if the results are negative, reassurance of the patient often alleviates the pain.

Phrenic Nerve

Because the phrenic nerve lies superficially beneath the mediastinal pleura, it is liable to be damaged during pulmonary resection, and might even be involved with malignant disease. Interruption of the phrenic nerve causes paralysis of the diaphragm on the side of operation, causing it to flail. This further decreases the patient's already limited ability to breathe postoperatively and delays recovery. Whenever possible, therefore, the phrenic nerve should be protected from damage during thoracotomy.

Phrenic nerve damage should be suspected when a patient with no apparent pulmonary compromise cannot be weaned from the ventilator postoperatively. Paradoxical diaphragmatic motion on fluoroscopy confirms the diagnosis. Following pneumonectomy, the hemidiaphragm will become fixed by fibro-

sis in an elevated position regardless of whether the phrenic nerve is intact. However, in a post-pneumonectomy patient with chronic pulmonary disease, a flail diaphragm can complicate management for 2 or 3 weeks postoperatively. Careful attention to detail will be required to clear the tracheobronchial tree of secretions, and mechanical support may be necessary for longer than usual to maintain adequate ventilation.

Vagus Nerve

The main trunk of the vagus nerve is readily identified at the time of surgery, and should be preserved. Unilateral interruption of the vagus normally does not produce immediate problems, but postoperative gastrointestinal atony and even pyloric obstruction occasionally result, requiring surgical intervention. Thus, if the vagus nerve is known to have been injured, careful surveillance of gastrointestinal function is warranted. Additionally, if the vagus nerve is damaged high in the chest proximal to the recurrent laryngeal nerve, ipsilateral vocal cord paralysis will result as well.

Recurrent Laryngeal Nerve

Damage to the recurrent laryngeal nerve at the time of thoracotomy is more likely on the left than on the right. The left recurrent laryngeal nerve branches from the vagus at the level of the aortic arch, passes beneath the arch near the ligamentum arteriosum, and ascends up the mediastinum to enter the neck, where it innervates the left vocal cord. Dissection of the hilum of the left lung normally includes identification and careful preservation of the nerve. However, the presence of malignant nodes may necessitate its sacrifice. The right recurrent laryngeal nerve leaves the vagus near the innominate artery and passes beneath it to ascend through the neck to the right vocal cord. Because of its more distant position, the right recurrent laryngeal nerve is rarely damaged during pulmonary resection.

Interruption of the recurrent laryngeal nerve results in paralysis of the ipsilateral vocal cord in adduction. Partial airway obstruction, decreased ability to cough, and aspiration from an incompetent glottis may be seen postoperatively. Hoarseness may also be noted, but is not diagnostic, since it also occurs with vocal cord edema following prolonged intubation. Direct or indirect laryngoscopy will differentiate edema from paralysis. Nerve repair is not feasible, although injection of a stiffening material into the involved vocal cord may improve its function. In some cases, return of function is seen after several days to weeks if the nerve was anatomically intact, but functionally impaired by edema or compression.

Brachial Plexus Injury

Injuries to the brachial plexus have been reported in association with thoracotomy.[82,83] These are typically stretch injuries, due to positioning. They can involve the "up" arm of a patient in the lateral position if the arm is suspended from the anesthesia screen too far cephalad, or if the shoulder is pulled cephalad by the full weight of an unsupported arm during thoracotomy. The prognosis of stretch injuries is usually good. Physical therapy of the involved extremity should be provided, and return of function within approximately 4 months can be expected. Brachial plexus stretch is best prevented by careful placement of the uppermost arm on a pillow overlying the opposite arm; in this way, the shoulder is free to be mobilized, but the arm does not hang freely.

COMPLICATIONS OF DIAGNOSTIC PROCEDURES

Bronchoscopy

Although serious complications following bronchoscopy are rare, hoarseness and sore throat are common. Typically, they abate within 24 hours and do not require specific therapy beyond mild nonnarcotic analgesics. Vocal cord edema can occur after unusually prolonged or traumatic procedures, especially in children. Steroid therapy can be helpful in this event. Care should be taken during the procedure to prevent the complications typical of laryngoscopy, such as damage to lips and teeth.

Tracheobronchial irritation, with an increase in coughing postoperatively, can be caused by bronchoscopy, particularly if brushings are performed. Postoperative fever is frequent, and a transient bacteremia is not unusual following bronchoscopy. If pulmonary infection is known to be present, preoperative antibiotic therapy is advised in an attempt to prevent septicemia. Similarly, antibiotic prophylaxis in patients with known intracardiac lesions (eg, mitral valve prolapse) should be undertaken preoperatively. Hemoptysis commonly follows bronchoscopy, but is usually not massive.

Mediastinoscopy

Mediastinoscopy is useful in the diagnosis and staging of pulmonary malignancy.[84–86] Through a small incision in the root of the neck, and after careful palpation of the vascular structures and abnormal masses, the mediastinoscope is inserted and passed into the mediastinum. The vessels of greatest concern include the innominate artery, the superior vena cava, and the pulmonary artery. The pleural space can also be entered, or the phrenic and recurrent laryngeal nerves damaged.[87]

Careful monitoring by the anesthesiologist of the carotid pulses is essential during the insertion of the mediastinoscope, since compression of the innominate or carotid artery can occur. Interruption of the carotid or superficial temporal pulse should be announced to the surgeon, and absence of pulse for longer than 1 minute should be avoided.

Pneumothorax may be treated when it occurs by chest tube insertion. Most local bleeding can be managed by electrocoagulation or application of a clip through the mediastinoscope. However, when a major structure such as the pulmonary artery or vena cava is involved, immediate thoracotomy is required, usually through a median sternotomy.

Scalene Node Biopsy

Scalene node biopsy is used in the staging of lung cancer and in the diagnosis of nonmalignant diseases such as sarcoidosis.[88,89] Structures of concern include the internal jugular vein, the subclavian artery and vein, the transverse cervical artery and vein, and the phrenic nerve. In addition, the thoracic duct must be considered on the left side.

Control of bleeding is generally possible without extending the incision or entering the chest. Air embolus is a possibility if the internal jugular vein has been entered. The anesthesiologist should be alert to this possibility and be prepared to lower the head of the table to place the wound at heart level. Thoracic duct damage occurring during the procedure may be controlled by suture ligature. If thoracic duct leak is discovered postoperatively, immediate reoperation and repair are required.

Thoracentesis and Pleural Needle Biopsy

Insertion of a needle for drainage of air or fluid from the pleura, or for obtaining a biopsy with a Cope's needle, can result in damage from the needle itself. Pneumothorax, hemothorax, and intercostal nerve injury can occur. Pneumothorax results when the needle perforates the visceral pleura and damages the lung. If pneumothorax allows the lung to collapse 1 cm or more from the chest wall a chest tube is required. Hemothorax is less common, and is usually the result of injury to an intercostal vessel or a major muscular branch. Excessive bleeding (eg, 500 mL or more) may require open incision for control.

Syncope can occur with thoracocentesis. Hypotension, pallor, and, occasionally, bradycardia may be seen. The procedure should be interrupted and the patient placed supine with the feet elevated. Syncope can be avoided with premedication with a narcotic and a vagolytic such as atropine.

REFERENCES

1. Keenan RL: Anesthesia disasters: incidence, causes, and preventability. Semin Anesth 5:175, 1986
2. Siesjo BK: Brain Energy Metabolism. John Wiley & Sons, Chichester, NY 1978
3. American Heart Association (AHA) and National Academy of Sciences–National Research Council (NAS-NCR): Standards for cardiopulmonary resuscitation (CPR) and emergency cardiac care (ECC). JAMA, suppl. 255:2841, 1986
4. Keenan RL, Boyan CP: Cardiac arrest due to anesthesia. A study of incidence and causes. JAMA 253:2373, 1985
5. Safar P: Resuscitation from clinical death: pathophysiologic limits and therapeutic potentials (review). Crit Care Med 16:923, 1988
6. Siesjo BK: Mechanisms of ischemic brain damage. Crit Care Med 16:954, 1988
7. Abramson NS, Safar P, Detre K, et al: Randomized clinical study of thiopental loading in comatose survivors of cardiac arrest. N Engl J Med 1986:314, 1986
8. Tinker JH, Dull DL, Caplan RA, et al: Role of monitoring devices in prevention of anesthetic mishaps: a closed claims analysis. Anesthesiology 71:541, 1989
9. Eichhorn JH: Prevention of intraoperative anesthesia accidents and related severe injury through safety monitoring. Anesthesiology 70:572, 1989
10. Pierce EC: Anesthesia: standards of care and liability. JAMA 262:773, 1989
11. Kirsh MH, Rotman H, Behrendt DM: Complications of pulmonary resection. Ann Thorac Surg 20:215, 1975
12. Block AJ, Olsen GN: Preoperative pulmonary function testing. JAMA 235:257, 1976
13. Gass GD, Olsen GN: Preoperative pulmonary function testing to predict postoperative morbidity and mortality. Chest 89:127, 1986
14. Churchill ED: The surgical treatment of carcinoma of the lung. J Thorac Cardiavasc Surg 2:254, 1933
15. Stein M, Cassara EL: Preoperative pulmonary evaluation and therapy for surgery patients. JAMA 211:780, 1970
16. Chalon J, Tayyab MA, Ramanthan S: Cytology of respiratory complications after operation. Chest 67:32, 1975
17. Carlens E: A new flexible double-lumen catheter for bronchospirometry. J Thorac Cardiovasc Surg 18:742, 1949
18. Symbas PN: Chest drainage tubes. Surg Clin North Am 69:41, 1989
19. Bjork VO, Engstrom CG: The treatment of ventilatory insufficiency after pulmonary resection with tracheostomy and prolonged artificial ventilation. J Thorac Cardiovasc Surg 30:356, 1955
20. Stein M, Ching N, Roberts EB, et al: Pneumothorax complicating continuous ventilatory support. J Thorac Cardiovasc Surg 67:17, 1974
21. Poelaert J, Mortier E, De Deyne C, Rolly G: The use of combined high-frequency jet ventilation in bilateral bronchopleural fistulae. Acta Anaesthesiol Belg 38:225, 1987
22. Roth MD, Wright JW, Bellamy PE: Gas flow through a bronchopleural fistula. Measuring the effects of high-frequency jet ventilation and chest-tube suction. Chest 93:210, 1988
23. Orlando R III, Gluck EH, Cohen M, Mesologites CG: Ultra-high-frequency jet ventilation in a bronchopleural fistula model. Arch Surg 23:591–593, 1988
24. Schuler JG: Intraoperative lobar torsion producing pulmonary infarction. J Thorac Cardiovasc Surg 65:951, 1973
25. Nullin MJ, Zumbro GL, Fishback ME, et al: Pulmonary lobar gangrene complicating lobectomy. Ann Surg 68:951, 1973
26. Hankins JR, Miller JE, Attar S, et al: Bronchopleural fistula: thirteen-year experience with 77 cases. J Thorac Cardiovasc Surg 76:755, 1978
27. Smith DE, Karish AF, Chapman JP, et al: Healing of the bronchial stump after pulmonary resection. J Thorac Cardiovasc Surg 46:548, 1963
28. Barker WL, Faber LP, Ostermiller WE, et al: Management of persistent bronchopleural fistula. J Thorac Cardiovasc Surg 62:393, 1971
29. Dorman JP, Campbell D, Grover FL, et al: Open thoracostomy drainage of postpneumonectomy empyema with bronchopleural fistula. J Thorac Cardiovasc Surg 66:979, 1973
30. Francis JG, Smith KG: An anaesthetic technique for the repair of bronchopleural fistula. Br J Anaesth 34:817, 1962
31. Adler RH, Plaut ME: Postpneumonectomy empyema. Surgery 71:210, 1972
32. Zumbro GL, Treasure R, Geiger JP, Green DC: Empyema after pneumonectomy. Ann Thorac Surg 15:615, 1973
33. Bessone LN, Ferguson TB, Burford TH: Chylothorax. Ann Thorac Surg 12:527, 1971
34. Milsom JW, Kron IL, Rheuban LS, Rodgers BM: Chylothorax: an assessment of current surgical management. J Thorac Cardiovasc Surg 89:211, 1985
35. Bjork VO: Thoracoplasty. A new osteoplastic technique. J Thorac Cardiovasc Surg 28:194, 1954
36. Graham J, Usher FC, Perry JL, et al: Marlex mesh as a prosthesis in the repair of thoracic wall defects. Ann Surg 151:469, 1960
37. LeRoux BT, Stemmler P: Maintenance of chest wall stability. A further report. Thorax 26:424, 1971
38. Glauser FL, Bartlett RA: Pneumoperitoneum in association with pneumothorax. Chest 66:536, 1974
39. Boyd AD, Gonzales LL, Altemeier WA: Disruption of

chest wall closure following thoracotomy. J Thorac Cardiovasc Surg 52:47, 1966

40. Maclean LD, Meakins JL, Taguchi K, et al: Host resistance in sepsis and trauma. Ann Surg 182:207, 1975
41. Williams CD, Cummingham JN, Falk EA, et al: Chronic infection of the costal cartilages after thoracic surgical procedures. J Thorac Cardiovasc Surg 66:592, 1973
42. Peterffy A, Henze A: Hemorrhagic complications during pulmonary resections: a retrospective review of 1428 resections with 113 hemorrhagic episodes. Scand J Thorac Cardiovasc Surg 17:283, 1983
43. Mowry F, Reynolds EF: Cardiac rhythm disturbances complicating resectional surgery of the lung. Ann Intern Med 61:1688, 1964
44. Ghosh P, Pakrashi BC: Cardiac dysrhythmias after thoractomy. Br Heart J 34:374, 1972
45. Breyer RH, Zippe C, Pharr WF, et al: Thoracotomy in patients over age seventy years: ten-year experience. J Thorac Cardiovasc Surg 81:187, 1981
46. Bergh NP, Dottori O, Malmberg R: Prophylactic digitalis in thoracic surgery. Scand J Respir Dis 48:197, 1967
47. Shields TW, Yjiki GT: Digitalization for prevention of arrhythmias following pulmonary surgery. Surg Gynecol Obstet 126:743, 1968
48. Burman SO: The prophylactic use of digitalis before thoracotomy. Ann Thorac Surg 14:359, 1972
49. Matthay RA, Berger HUJ: Cardiovascular performance in chronic obstructive pulmonary disease. Med Clin North Am 65:489, 1981
50. Jezek V, Schrijen F, Sadoul P: Right ventricular function and pulmonary hemodynamics during exercise in patients with chronic obstructive bronchopulmonary disease. Cardiology 58:20, 1973
51. Berger HJ, Matthay RA: Non-invasive radiographic assessment of cardiovascular function in acute and chronic respiratory failure. Am J Cardiol 47:950, 1981
52. Matthay RA, Berger HJ, Davies R, et al: Right and left ventricular exercise performance in chronic obstructive pulmonary disease, radionuclide assessment. Ann Intern Med 93:234, 1980
53. Cassidy SS, Robertson CH, Pierce AK, et al: Pulmonary hypertension in sepsis. Measurement of the pulmonary artery diastolic-pulmonary wedge pressure gradient and the influence of passive and active factors. Chest 73:583, 1980
54. Adams WE, Perkins JF, Flores A, et al: The significance of pulmonary hypertension as a cause of death following pulmonary resection. J Thorac Surg 26:407, 1952
55. Harrison RW, Adams WE, Long ET et al: The clinical significance of cor pulmonale in the reduction of cardiopulmonary reserve following extensive pulmonary resection. J Thorac Surg 36:352, 1958
56. Uggla L-G: Indications for and results of thoracic surgery with regard to respiratory and circulatory function tests. Acta Chir Scand 111:197, 1956
57. Sloan H, Morris JD, Figley M, et al: Temporary unilateral occlusion of the pulmonary artery in the preoperative evaluation of thoracic patients. J Thorac Surg 30:591, 1955

58. Wiederanders RE, White SM, Saichek HB: The effect of pulmonary resection on pulmonary artery pressures. Ann Surg 160:889, 1964
59. Olsen GN, Block AJ, Swenson EW, et al: Pulmonary function evaluation of the lung resection candidate: a prospective study. Am Rev Respir Dis 111:379, 1975
60. Olsen GN: The evolving role of exercise testing prior to lung resection. Chest 95:218, 1989
61. Coma Canella I, Lopez-Sendon J: Ventricular compliance in ischemic right ventricular dysfunction. Am J Cardiol 45:555, 1980
62. Deiraniva AK: Cardiac herniation following intrapericardial pneumonectomy Thorax 29:545, 1974
63. Dippel WF, Ehrenhaft JL: Herniation of the heart after pneumonectomy. J Thorac Cardiovasc Surg 65:207, 1973
64. Gates GF, Setle RS, Cope JA: Acute cardiac herniation with incarceration following pneumonectomy. Radiology 94:561, 1970
65. Kirchoff AC: Herniation of the heart: report of a case. Anesthesiology 12:774, 1951
66. McKleven JR, Urgena RB, Rossi NP: Herniation of the heart following radical pneumonectomy: a case report. Anesth Analg 51:680, 1972
67. Yacoub MH, Williams WG, Ahmad A: Strangulation of the heart following intrapericardial pneumonectomy. Thorax 23:261, 1968
68. Arciniegas E, Coates EO: Massive pulmonary arterial thrombosis after pneumonectomy. J Thorac Cardiovasc Surg 61:487, 1971
69. Chaung TH, Dooling JA, Conally JM, Shifts LM: Pulmonary embolization from vascular stump thrombosis following pneumonectomy. Ann Thorac Surg 2:290, 1966
70. Kakkar VV, Carrigan TP, Spindler JR, et al: Efficacy of low doses of heparin in prevention of deep vein thrombosis after major surgery: a double-blind, randomized trial. Lancet 2:101, 1972
71. Bonnar J, Walsh J: Prevention of thrombosis after pelvic surgery by dextran 70. Lancet 1:614, 1972
72. McIntyre KM, Sasahara SA: The hemodynamic response to pulmonary embolism in patients without prior cardiopulmonary disease. Am J Cardiol 28:288, 1971
73. Mlczoch J, Lucher S, Weir EK, et al: Platelet-mediated pulmonary hypertension and hypoxia during pulmonary microembolism. Chest 74:648, 1978
74. Allison PR, Dunhill MS, Marshall R: Pulmonary embolism. Thorax 15:273, 1960
75. Sautter KD, Myers WO, Ray JF, et al: Pulmonary embolectomy: review and current status. Prog Cardiovasc Dis 17:371, 1975
76. Brown S, Muller D, Buckberg G: Massive pulmonary hemorrhagic infarction following revascularization of ischemic lungs. Arch Surg 108:795, 1974
77. Greenfield LJ: Complications of venous thrombosis and pulmonary embolism. pp. 430–445. In Greenfield LJ (ed): Complications in Surgery and Trauma. 2nd Ed. JB Lippincott, New York, 1990
78. Greenfield LJ, Stewart JR, Crute S: Improved techniqued for Greenfield vena caval filter insertion. Surg Gynecol Obstet 156:217, 1983

79. Classification of chronic pain. Pain, suppl. 24:3. S138, 1986

80. Carlsson CA, Persson K, Peletieri L: Painful scars after thoracic and abdominal surgery. Acta Chir Scand 151:309, 1985

81. Conacher ID: Percutaneous cryotherapy for post-thoracotomy neuralgia. Pain 25:227, 1986

82. Clausen EG: Postoperative paralysis of the brachial plexus. Surgery 12:933, 1942

83. Ewing MR: Postoperative paralysis in the upper extremity. Lancet 1:99, 1950

84. Ashbaugh DG: Mediastinoscopy. Arch Surg 100:568, 1970

85. Pearson FG: Mediastinoscopy. Surg Annu 2:95, 1970

86. Goldberg EM, Glickman AS, Kahn FR, et al: Mediastinoscopy for assessing mediastinal spread in clinical staging of carcinoma of the lung. Cancer 25:347, 1970

87. Wildstrom A: Palsy of the recurrent nerve following mediastinoscopy. Chest 67:365, 1975

88. Blair CR, Hughes JH: Scalene node biopsy: a reevaluation. J Thorac Cardiovasc Surg 52:595, 1966

89. Baker NH, Hill L, Ewy HG, et al: Pulmonary lymphatic drainage. J Thorac Cardiovasc Surg 54:695, 1967

90. Brooks JW: Complications of thoracic and chest wall surgery. In Greenfield LJ (ed): Complications of Surgery and Trauma. 2nd Ed. JB Lippincott, Philadelphia, 1990

INDEX

Page numbers followed by f indicate figures; those followed by t indicate tables.

Abdominal muscles, function of, 166
Abscess, lung, 91
    computed tomography scan of, 59, 63f
    drainage, therapeutic bronchoscopy for, 325
    empyema with, radiologic findings with, 59
    in infant/neonate, anesthetic and perioperative considerations with, 516t
    one-lung ventilation with, 371
    radiologic findings with, 59
Absorption atelectasis, 606
Accessory muscles, 165
    function of, 166
Acetaminophen, for postoperative analgesia, in infant/neonate, dosage and administration of, 507t
Acetylcholine, physiologic pulmonary actions of, 128–129
Acetylcholine receptors, in myasthenia gravis, 402
Acetylsalicylate, as adjuvant to opioid analgesics, 578
Achalasia
    in infant/neonate, anesthetic and perioperative considerations with, 512t
    pathophysiology of, 394
    treatment of, 394
Achlorhydria, 260
Acid-base balance. See also Acidosis; Metabolic acidosis; Metabolic alkalosis; Respiratory acidosis; Respiratory alkalosis
    after massive transfusion of stored blood, 479

during volume infusion, in hemorrhagic shock, 476–477
Acidosis. See also Lactic acidosis; Metabolic acidosis; Respiratory acidosis
    effect on oxyhemoglobin dissociation, 148, 148t
Acquired immunodeficiency syndrome, 95–108
    in Africa, 96, 99
    anesthetic management with, 107–108
    AZT treatment, 105
    bronchoscopy in, 324
    causative organism, 96
    in children, 103
    clinical syndromes of, 100
    current incidence per 100,000 population, in U.S., 97t
    diarrhea in, 100–101
        treatment of, 105
    and duty to care, 109
    encephalopathy of, 101
        in children, AZT treatment, 105
    epidemiology of, 96–97
    first known case of, 95
    geographic prevalence, in U.S., 97
    harbingers of, 100
    hazards to health care workers, 105–107
    hazards to patients, 107
    high risk groups for, 98–99
    historical perspective on, 95–96
    in hospital setting, 105–108
    incidence of, among homosexuals, 99
    in utero transmission of, 103
    Kaposi's sarcoma of, 95–96, 101, 108
    nephropathy of, 102–103
    neurologic syndromes in, 101–102

nutritional therapy with, 107
    opportunistic infections in, 100–101
        treatment of, 104–105
    origin of, 96
    pathophysiology of, 97–98
    and polypharmacy of addiction, 107
    in pregnancy, 104
    prevention of, 103–104
    psychosis in, 102
    risk groups, 98t, 98–99
    seroprevalence rate, in U.S., 99
    therapy for, 103–105
    transfusion-related, 99–100, 103, 108
    in trauma victims, 478
    weight loss in, 101
Acute pain service, role of therapy versus therapist in, 584–585
Acute respiratory failure
    adjuvant therapy for, 633–634
    airway pressure-release ventilation in, 643–644
    with aspiration, 631
    clinical characteristics of, 620
    clinical situations associated with, 629
    definition of, 619
    diagnosis of, 620
    early signs of, 620, 620t
    etiology of, 619–620, 628–632
    extracorporeal membrane oxygenation during, 676
    factors leading to, 626f, 626–627
    with fat embolism syndrome, 631–632
    with flail chest, 632
    with inhalational injury, 631
    intermittent mandatory ventilation in, 640–643
    mortality rate for, 620
    oxygen therapy for, 632–633

Acute respiratory failure (*Continued*)
pathophysiology of, 621–622
PEEP/CPAP therapy, 636–637
optimal, 636–638
postoperative, 630
predisposing factors for, 622, 622t
pressure-support ventilation in, 643
with pulmonary embolism, 632
radiographic findings in, 620
selective positive-pressure ventilation during, 371–372
treatment of, 632–644
ultrastructural changes in, 620–621
ventilator therapy for, 634–644
Acyclovir, indications for, in AIDS, 104
Adenine nucleotides, handling of, in lungs, 115–116, 127–128
Adenoid cystic carcinoma, of trachea, 446t, 446–447
Adenopathy, in AIDS, 101
Adenosine
handling of, in lung, 119
receptors, in airway smooth muscle, 227
Adenosine diphosphate
action of, in lung, 129
handling of, by lung, 127–128
Adenosine monophosphate, handling of, by lung, 127–128
Adenosine triphosphatase, 128
in pulmonary endothelial cells, 118–119
Adenosine triphosphate
action of, in lung, 129
handling of, by lung, 127–128
Adenylate cyclase, 613
membrane-bound, 225
Adrenal hyperactivity, with lung cancer, 89
Adrenalin. *See* Epinephrine
Adrenergic receptors
in airways, 225, 225t
stimulation, 225–226
physiologic effects of, 225, 225t
Adrenocorticotropic hormone, in lung, 125
actions of, 127
Adult respiratory distress syndrome, 85.
See also Acute respiratory failure
clinical, radiographic, and pathologic findings in, 37–39, 40t
course of, 37–38
CPAP in, 604
diseases associated with or known to precipitate, 37, 39t

distending airway pressure therapy in, 676–677
effects of lipid infusion in, 697
etiology of, 619–620
high-frequency ventilation for, 676
leukotrienes in, 122
pathophysiology of, 676
radiographic findings with, 45
synonyms for, 39t
systemic oxygen uptake in, 154–155
typical radiographic progression in, 41f–43f
typical sequence of findings in, 37–39, 40t, 41f–43f
Affinity hypoxia, 143–144, 148
definition of, 163
AIDS. *See* Acquired immunodeficiency syndrome
AIDS dementia complex, 101–102
AIDS-related complex, 100
Air, radiographic density, 20, 20f–21f
Air bronchograms, 20, 27–28, 28f
Air entrainment calculation, 657f
Air entrainment devices, 650. *See also* Venturi injector; Venturi principle
Airflow
forces opposing, 169–172
production of, 169
Airflow obstruction. *See also* Airway obstruction
chronic. *See also* Chronic obstructive pulmonary disease
diseases associated with, 84–86
platelet-activating factor in, 125
in chronic obstructive pulmonary disease, 85
measurement of, 3
Airflow resistance. *See also* Airway resistance
imposed by endotracheal tubes, 174–175
Air leakage
postoperative, 711, 714
with tracheostomy, 70
Air-oxygen blenders, 650
Air tracheograms, 542
Airway(s)
adrenergic receptors of, 225
anatomy of, in infant/neonate, 489, 489t, 490f
assessment of, 322
bleeding. *See* Hemoptysis
caliber of, during general anesthesia, 173–174
collapse of, detection of, 3

connective tissue, 224
cross-sectional area of, 224
function of, 223–224
preoperative assessment and treatment of, 223
innervation of, 224, 348–349
management of, with AIDS, 108
mucosal layer, 224
pharmacology of, 225–227
provision of medication via, 652–653
smooth muscle of, 224
calcium in, 225–226
cyclic nucleotide function in, 225–226
function, 225–226
receptors in, 226t, 226–227, 348–349
structure of, 223–224
upper, surgery on, ventilation during, 676
Airway conductance, relationship of, to lung volume, 170, 171f
Airway fire, with laser therapy, 431, 436–437
Airway obstruction. *See also* Airflow obstruction
bronchoscopy with, 325
diagnostic evaluation of, 449–450
extrathoracic
anesthetic technique with, 339
signs and symptoms of, 322, 323f
history with, 449–450
identification of, measurement of airway resistance in, 176
intrathoracic
anesthetic technique with, 340
signs and symptoms of, 322, 323f
management of, 451–452
by mediastinal mass, 338–339, 397–400
in pediatric patient, 537, 539
physical examination with, 449–450
position-dependent, 338, 398–399, 447, 537
postoperative, after surgery for mediastinal mass, 399
preoperative evaluation for, 90
pulmonary function studies with, 450
signs of, 711
upper, in infant/neonate, management of, 511
Airway pressure, 594f, 594–595. *See also* Distending airway pressure
monitoring, 658, 658f

Airway pressure-release ventilation, in acute respiratory failure, 643–644

Airway resistance, 170, 348–350. *See also* Airflow resistance
  effects of anesthesia on, 174, 349–350
  effects of antimuscarinic drugs on, 265t
  and endotracheal intubation, 176–177, 177f
  measurement of, 170–171
    by body plethysmography, 6, 7f
    in identification of obstruction, 176
  relationship of, to lung volume, 170, 171f
  upper limits of normal for, 176–177

Alanine amino transferase, screening blood for, 109

Albumin
  infusion, in acute respiratory failure, 634
  serum
    in cancer patient, prognostic significance of, 685–686, 686f
    in diagnosis of malnutrition, 686
    factors affecting, 624–625
    as index of nutritional support, 687, 687f
    prognostic significance for operative complications, 686

Albuterol, 227
  dosage and administration of, 228t, 230
  duration of action, 228t, 230
  mechanism of action, 228t
  pharmacology of, 230
  postoperative administration of, 613
  relative potency of, 229
  structure of, 227f

Alfentanil
  effects of
    on airway resistance, 350
    on ventilatory control, 358
  intravenous route for, 275–276
  premedication, duration of action, 267f

Algogens, 565

Alkalosis. *See* Metabolic alkalosis; Respiratory alkalosis

Alpha-stat blood gas values, 311

Altitude, acclimatization to, 182–183

Alveolar air equation, 15–16

Alveolar-capillary membrane, 116. *See also* Capillary membrane

in acute respiratory failure, 630

Alveolar-capillary unit, cell organization of, 115–116

Alveolar carbon dioxide tension, 300
  determination of, 649
  and spontaneous ventilation, 357, 358f
  ventilation response to, and oxygen concentrations, 360f

Alveolar collapse, in acute respiratory failure, 623f, 628

Alveolar dead space, 301t, 301–302
  in upright position, 194

Alveolar ducts, cross-sectional area of, 224

Alveolar hypoventilation, 16

Alveolar macrophages, in immune defense, 693

Alveolar oxygen tension, 15–16
  determination of, 649
  in hypoxic pulmonary vasoconstriction, 352

Alveolar pressure, 3f
  in upright position, 194–196

Alveolar proteinosis, bronchopulmonary lavage for, 425

Alveolar rupture, due to barotrauma, 48–49

Alveolar-to-arterial carbon dioxide tension gradient, with ventilation-perfusion mismatch, 197

Alveolar-to-arterial oxygen tension gradient, 15
  in one-lung ventilation, 204–205, 350
  with ventilation-perfusion mismatch, 197

Ambenonium (Mytelase), for myasthenia gravis, 403, 403t

Amikacin, indications for, in AIDS, 104

Amine precursor uptake and decarboxylation cells, 117

Aminophylline
  dosage and administration of, 235–236
  effects on hypoxic pulmonary vasoconstriction, 207
  intravenous dosage, 235, 236t

Amnesia
  definition of, 256
  premedication for, 259, 259f

Amphetamine, metabolism, by lung, 131

Amphotericin, indications for, in AIDS, 104

Ampligen, 105

Amrinone, in treatment of right heart failure, 717

Anaerobic threshold, during exercise, prognostic signficance of, 14–15

Analgesia. *See also* Postoperative analgesia
  premedication and, 259

Anatomic dead space, 301, 301f, 661
  with atropine, 262
  effects of antimuscarinic drugs on, 265t
  with scopolamine, 263
  ventilation, 661

Anemia. *See also* Hemoglobin concentration
  oxygen delivery in, 150

Anesthesia. *See also* Induction technique
  death or brain damage due to, incidence of, 709
  effects of
    on airway resistance, 349–350
    on lung volumes, 348
    on respiratory control, 183–188
    on respiratory mechanics, 172–177
  management, with HIV-infected patients, 107–108
  pulmonary blood flow during, 350–357

Anesthetic complications, 709–710

Anesthetic drugs
  choice of, for intrathoracic surgery, 347
  effects of, 347
  and hypoxic pulmonary vasoconstriction, 207–210, 352–356
  respiratory effects of, 364t
  subanesthetic doses, for analgesia, 578

Anexate. *See* Ro 15-1788

Angiotensin, metabolism, in lung, 125

Angiotensin-converting enzyme, 125
  in pulmonary endothelial cells, 119, 119f

Angiotensin I, handling of, in lungs, 116, 119, 125

Angiotensin II
  actions of, in lung, 125, 127
  handling of, in lungs, 115
  synthesis and metabolism of, 125, 126f

Antacids, 391
  gastrointestinal actions of, 275
Anthropometry, 686
Antibiotic therapy
  in flail chest patient, 469
  perioperative, 92
  prophylactic
    with diagnostic procedures,
      720
    for nosocomial infections, 92
    preoperative, with chronic pul-
      monary disease, 88–89
    for prevention of bacterial endo-
      carditis, 542–544
  topical, for respiratory tract,
    614–615
Anticholinergics
  bronchodilator effects of, 237–238
  inhalant products, 615t
  premedication, 258
    for bronchoscopy, 334
    for infant/neonate, dosage and
      administration of, 497t
Anticholinesterases
  desensitization crisis with, 404
  for myasthenia gravis, 403, 403t
  overdosage, 403
  preoperative, for myasthenic
    patient, 411
Anticoagulation, with pulmonary
    thromboembolism, 718
Antidiuretic hormone, increase in, and
    lung cancer, 89
Antimuscarinic drugs
  comparison of, 265t
  pharmacology of, 261–262
  side effects of, 262, 265t
Antisialagogues, 259–260
Antiviral drugs, resistance to, 104
Anxiety, relief of, 258
Aortic aneurysms, magnetic resonance
    imaging of, 55, 56f
Aortic counterpulsation balloon
    catheter, malplacement of,
    80f
Aortic dissection, diagnosis, computed
    tomography and magnetic
    resonance imaging in, 55,
    57f
Aortic rupture
  diagnosis and management of, 475
  site of, 475t
Aortopulmonary artery stenosis
  anesthetic and perioperative consid-
    erations with, 524t
  description of, 524t

Apnea of prematurity, management of,
    492
Apneic oxygenation, 328, 673
Apneic threshold, 181, 184
Apparatus dead space, 301, 301f
Arachidonic acid
  action of, in lung, 129
  metabolism of, 119–120, 120f
    cyclo-oxygenase pathway, 120f,
      120–122, 121f
    cytochrome P-450 mono-oxyge-
      nase pathway, 120f, 122,
      124f
    lipoxygenase pathway, 120f, 122,
      123f
  metabolites, 120
ARF. *See* Acute respiratory failure
Argon laser, characteristics of, 430t
Arterial-alveolar pressure difference, in
    upright position, 194f,
    194–196
Arterial blood gas analysis, 15–16
  for infant/neonate, during thoracic
    operations, 502
  preoperative, 15
  in surgical repair of congenital
    diaphragmatic hernia, 532
Arterial blood pressure, monitoring, in
    infant/neonate, during tho-
    racic operations, 500–501
Arterial carbon dioxide content, 300
Arterial carbon dioxide tension, 145,
    300
  in acute respiratory failure, 620
  in differentiation of cardiac versus
    pulmonary impairment,
    14t
  as index of ventilatory controls, 180,
    180f
  measurement of, 302–303
  reciprocal relationship with ventila-
    tion, 177, 177f
  temperature-corrected versus uncor-
    rected, use of, 311
  and ventilation, 699f–700f
Arterial-end-tidal CO_2 difference, in
    thoracic surgery, 314
Arterial mixed venous oxygen satura-
    tion, monitoring of, 156
Arterial oxygenation
  deficient, causes of, 606
  in one-lung ventilation, 350
    effects of anesthetics on, 208
    versus two-lung ventilation,
      204–205
Arterial oxygen content, 145

  calculation of, 285–286
Arterial oxygen desaturation, 15
Arterial oxygen saturation, 145
  minimum safe level of, 156
Arterial oxygen tension
  with acute respiratory failure, 620
  decreased, effects on minute ventila-
    tion, 178, 178f
  effects of hypoxic pulmonary vaso-
    constriction on, 206, 206f
  with endobronchial intubation,
    312–314, 314f
  methods for increasing, with small
    airway closure, 610–611
  monitoring, applications in thoracic
    surgery, 312–313
  normal, 145, 147f
  postresection, prognostic evaluation
    of, 11
  upper and lower safety limits for,
    146
Arterial pH, ventilatory support in
    defense of, 661
Arterio-interstitial pressure difference,
    in upright position, 195
Arteriovenous bypass, for lung trans-
    plantation, 559
Arteriovenous malformations, hemop-
    tysis with, 428
Arteriovenous oxygen content differ-
    ence, and transfusion of
    stored blood, 144
Arthralgia, in AIDS, 103
Arthritic changes, radiographic findings
    with, 26
Aspiration
  after esophageal surgery, 397
  with esophagorespiratory tract fistu-
    la, 395
  in esophagoscopy, prevention,
    342–343
  prevention of, 273–274
  radiographic findings with, 26, 37,
    38f
  risk factors for, 273–274
    with enteral nutrition, 702
  sequelae of, 631
  therapeutic bronchoscopy for, 325
Aspiration pneumonitis, 85
Assist-control-mode ventilation, 665
Assist-mode ventilation, 664–665
Asthma
  association of sinusitis and nasal
    polyps with, 89
  cromolyn sodium therapy, 239–240
  leukotrienes in, 122

pathophysiology of, 239
and respiratory infections, 89
platelet-activating factor in, 125
pulmonary function testing in, 8–9
steroid therapy for
aerosolized (topical), 243–244
long-term, 245
systemic, 244–245
Ataractic drugs
and opioids, combined effects of,
268, 269f
premedication, 267–268
Atelectasis
in acute respiratory failure, 619, 628
chest physiotherapy for, 596–599
congestive, 619
in infant, reintubation technique for,
615
linear, 27, 27f
lobar, 27–28, 28f–29f
radiographic signs of, 28, 29f
localized, diagnostic significance of,
324
mediastinal shift with, 711
with overinserted endotracheal tube,
68
plate-like, 27, 27f
postoperative
causes of, 594
diagnosis of, 594
incidence of, 594
in infant/neonate, management
of, 510
prevention of, 594–605, 710
treatment of, 594–605
pulmonary blood flow distribution
in, mechanism of, 206–211
pulmonary vascular response to,
206, 351, 352f
radiographic findings with, 27–31,
45
simulating mediastinal widening, 28
total lung, 28
radiographic appearance of, 28,
29f, 31f
Atracurium
effects of, on airway resistance, 350
for myasthenic patients, 408
precautions for, in trauma patient,
467
Atrial dysrhythmia(s), postoperative,
716
Atrial fibrillation, postpneumonectomy,
716
Atrial flutter, postpneumonectomy, 716
Atrial natriuretic peptide

actions of, 126
in lung, 126–127
metabolism of, by lungs, 126
Atropine
antisialagogue activity, 259
bronchodilator effect, 263f
contraindications to, 452
dosage and administration of, 237
duration of action, 237
effects of, 265t
on airway resistance, 350
on cardiac rhythm, 260–261
on pulmonary mechanics, in
fiberoptic bronchoscopy,
327
indications for, 9f
induction, for infant/neonate, 498
intravenous route for, 275–276
mechanism of action, 237
pharmacology of, 261–262
premedication
for bronchoscopy, 334
dosage and administration of,
262
duration of action, 262
history of, 256
for infant/neonate, 498
dosage and administration of,
497t
pulmonary effect of, 262–263
side effects of, 237, 263
structure of, 238f
Atropine analog, indications for, 9f
Authority, definition of, 256
Autologous blood programs, 103, 109
Autotransfusion, 477
Awareness, in trauma patient, 467
Axillary artery catheterization, in
infant/neonate, for blood
pressure monitoring, 501
Azathioprine, for myasthenia gravis,
404
Azidothymidine, 105
AZT. *See* Azidothymidine

Bacterial endocarditis
antibiotic prophylaxis
pediatric doses for, 544, 544t
recommended protocols, for den-
tal/respiratory system procedures, 543t, 543–544
causative organisms, 543
prevention of, during diagnostic or
therapeutic surgical procedures, 542–544
Barbiturates, 256, 258

antianalgesic effect of, 260
effects of, on respiratory control, 185
indications for, 578
premedication, 267
ventilatory response to, 267, 268f
Barotrauma, 48
with IMV and PEEP, 641–642
interstitial air from, 48–49
Basal metabolic rate, 681
Harris Benedict formula for prediction of, 683, 683t
Base excess, 147
BCM. *See* Body cell mass
Beck's triad, 472–473
Beclomethasone diproprionate, 241
aerosolized (topical) therapy,
243
contraindication to, 244
dosage and administration of,
243–244
indications for, 614
pharmacology of, 243
structure of, 241f
Beer's law, 294–295, 295f, 297
Bellingham formula, 147
Benzo(a)pyrene, pulmonary damage
induced by, 131
Benzodiazepines
amnestic effect, 259, 259f
comparison of, 273t
indications for, 270–271, 578
oral, 276
in postoperative management of
infant/neonate, 507
premedication, 267, 270–273
for bronchoscopy, 334
effects on incidence of anesthetic
convulsions, 271
respiratory effects of, 362–363
side effects of, 273
Bernoulli's law, 329, 331f
Bert effect, 146
Beta-adrenergic agents, tachyphylaxis
with, 233
Beta$_2$-agonists, 227
effects on hypoxic pulmonary vasoconstriction, 207
nonbronchodilator actions of, 232t,
232–233
prolonged brochodilatory effects of,
mechanism of action, 232
Betamethasone, pharmacology of,
242t
Bias, definition of, 288
Bicarbonate. *See also* Sodium bicarbonate

Bicarbonate (*Continued*)
  blood or cerebrospinal fluid levels, and ventilatory response to CO_2, 177–178
Bicitra. *See* Sodium citrate
Biopsy
  bronchoscopic, 325
    bleeding after, 716
  thoracoscopy for, 340
Bird CPAP mask, 657, 658f
Bitolterol, 227
  dosage and administration of, 228t, 230–231
  duration of action, 228t
  indications for, 231
  mechanism of action, 228t
  side effects of, 230–231
  structure of, 227f
Blalock-Hanlon atrial septectomy
  anesthetic and perioperative considerations with, 523t
  description of, 523t
Blalock-Taussig shunt
  anesthetic and perioperative considerations with, 523t
  description of, 523t
Bleeding. *See also* Blood loss; Hemoptysis; Hemorrhage
  postoperative
    in infant/neonate, 509
    into pleura, 715
    into tracheobronchial tree, 716
Bleomycin, pulmonary toxicity of, 392
Blood
  storage, effect on oxyhemoglobin dissociation, 148, 148t
  stored, transfusion
    filtering during, 478
    management of, 479
  viscosity of, and hemodilution, 155
Blood distribution
  within microcirculation, control of, 144
  within organs, control of, 144
Blood donors, incidence of seropositivity among, 103
Blood gas analysis. *See* Arterial blood gas analysis; Pulse oximetry
Blood gas analyzer, development of, 302–303
Blood loss
  after pulmonary resection, 715
  after thoracotomy, 715

in infant/neonate, during thoracic operations, assessment of, 502–503
Blood pressure. *See also* Arterial blood pressure
  age- and size-related differences in, 486, 486t
  and oxygen delivery, 152–153
Blood substitutes, for volume infusion, in hemorrhagic shock, 477
Blood supply, safety of, 103
Blood transfusion
  cytomegalovirus transmission in, 478
  in hemorrhagic shock, 477–479
  hepatitis transmission in, 108, 478
  HIV transmission in, 99–100, 103, 108, 478
  mismatched, 478
  during pulmonary resection, 421
  in sickle cell disease, 150
Blood volume
  age- and size-related differences in, 486, 486t
  and oxygen delivery, 150–152
Blow bottles, 602
BMR. *See* Basal metabolic rate
Body cell mass, 684
  and respiratory function, 693
  restoration of, in malnourished patients, 688
Body composition, 684–685
Body fat, 684
Body plethysmography, 170
  for determining lung volume, 6, 7f
Body weight, as index of nutritional status, 684–685
Boehringer PEEP valve, 660
Bohr effect, 147
Bombesin, actions of, in lung, 127
Boyle's law, 6
Brachial plexus injury, 720
  with stretch, 720
Bradycardia
  with atropine, 262, 262f
  during induction, prevention of, 260–261
Bradykinin
  action of, in lung, 126, 129
  handling of, in lungs, 115–116, 119, 126
  synthesis and metabolism of, 125, 126f
Brain damage, hypoxic, 709

Branched-chain amino acid infusion, respiratory effects of, 699, 700f
Breathing. *See also entries under* Respiratory
  control of, normal variations with age, 182
  forces involved in, 169–172
Breathing patterns, during total parenteral nutrition, 698f
Brevital. *See* Methohexital
Bronchial artery(ies), 224
  injury, in mediastinoscopy, 340
Bronchial blockers, 372–374
Bronchial carcinoma. *See also* Bronchogenic carcinoma
  and myasthenic syndrome, 412–413
Bronchial compression, with mediastinal mass, 397–398
Bronchial injury, traumatic, 471–472
Bronchial lavage. *See also* Bronchopulmonary lavage
  in pediatrics, 525
Bronchial obstruction, with mucus plug, 28, 28f
Bronchial stump
  closure of, 713
  disruption of, 713
Bronchiectasis
  bronchopulmonary lavage for, 425
  hemoptysis with, 428
  in infant/neonate, anesthetic and perioperative considerations with, 512t
  one-lung ventilation with, 371
Bronchiole(s), structure and function of, 224
Bronchiolitis obliterans organizing pneumonia, in AIDS, 101
Bronchitis
  arachidic, 522
  asthmatic, bronchopulmonary lavage for, 425
  chemical, prevention, 711
  chronic
    and chronic cor pulmonale, 88
    and nutritional status, 694
    systemic steroid therapy for, 245
  pulmonary function testing in, 8–9
  vegetal, 522
Bronchobiliary fistula, in infant/neonate, anesthetic and perioperative considerations with, 512t
Bronchocath double-lumen endobronchial tube, 383, 384f

Bronchoconstriction, 349
reversible, of chronic obstructive
pulmonary disease, 85
Bronchodilation, 349
Bronchodilator(s)
anticholinergic, 237–238
effect on flow-volume loop, 9f
perioperative therapy with, 92
postoperative administration of,
613, 614t–615t
in spirometric examinations, 3
sympathomimetic, 227–233
xanthine, 233–237
Bronchogenic carcinoma. *See also*
Bronchial carcinoma
diagnosis of, 325
and nutritional status, 685
Bronchography, in children, anesthesia
for, 522–525
Bronchopleural fistula, 422, 713,
713f
anesthetic considerations with,
422–423
causes of, 422, 671
management of, 422–423
mechanical ventilation with,
671–672
one-lung ventilation with, 371, 374
radiographic evidence of, 62, 67f
Bronchopneumonia, 32, 33f
Bronchoprovocation
in asthmatics, 9
indications for, 90
Bronchopulmonary dysplasia, in
infant/neonate, anesthetic
and perioperative consid-
erations with, 512t
Bronchopulmonary lavage
anesthesia for, 425–428
complications of, 427
indications for, 425
one-lung ventilation with, 372
position for, 426–427
procedure for, 426–427
set-up for, 426, 426f
unilateral, flow manipulation in,
427
Bronchoscope(s)
for laser resection, 433
pediatric magnifying, 511
Bronchoscopy. *See also* Fiberoptic
bronchoscopy
anesthetic technique for, 333–334
for aspiration of secretions from airway, 601
in aware patient, 327

complications of, 325–326, 720
diagnostic, indications for, 324
in children, 511, 522
for esophagorespiratory tract fistula
identification, 395
in evaluation of resectability of cancer, 2
indications for, 91, 324–325, 449
for preoperative assessment of
pathology, 325
in infant/neonate, anesthesia for,
511, 522, 525
laser therapy with, 333, 432
with mediastinal mass, 398
in pediatric patient, 537–539
morbidity and mortality with, 326
physiologic changes with, 326
premedication for, 258, 333–334
rigid
advantages of, 325
anesthetic management for,
336–337
indications for, 325, 601
during laser therapy, 432–433
ventilation during, 433–434
ventilation in, methods of,
328–332
sympathetic response to, attenuation of, 326
therapeutic
indications for, 325
in children, 522
post-thoracotomy, 601
in tracheal reconstruction, 450–451,
453–454
with tracheobronchial injury,
471–472
ventilation during, 433–434, 676
methods of, 328–333
Bronchospasm
in asthmatics, 9
with bronchoscopy, 326
postoperative, treatment of, 613–614
Bronchospirometry, 10
Bronchus(i)
nutrient blood supply, 224
structure and function of, 224
Budesonide, 241
aerosolized (topical) therapy, 243
dosage and administration of, 244
pharmacology of, 244
structure of, 241f
Bullet wound(s). *See* Gunshot wound(s)
Bullous disease
complications of, 423
prognosis for, 424–425

radiographic appearance of, 423f
surgical management of
anesthetic considerations in,
423–424
indications for, 423
Bupivacaine
intrapleural administration of, 421,
571
in infant/neonate, 505–506
for postoperative analgesia,
508
and opioids, combined infusions of,
for postoperative analge-
sia, 578
pharmacology of, 571
pulmonary uptake of, 132
respiratory effects of, 361
spinal, for postoperative analgesia,
dosage and administration
of, 576–577
tachyphylaxis to, 573
toxicity, 571
Buprenorphine, front-loading, 579t
Butorphanol, front-loading, 579t

CaCO$_2$. *See* Arterial carbon dioxide content
Caffeine, structure of, 234f
Calcitonin gene-related peptide, action
of, in lung, 129
Calcium, and smooth muscle function,
225–226
Calcium balance. *See also*
Hypocalcemia
after massive transfusion of stored
blood, 479
Calcium channel(s)
receptor-operated, 226
voltage-operated, 226
Calcium entry blocking drugs, effects
on hypoxic pulmonary
vasoconstriction, 207
Caloric requirements, age- and size-
related differences in, 486,
486t
cAMP. *See* Cyclic adenosine monophosphate
Cancer. *See also* Esophageal cancer;
Lung cancer
and nutritional status, 685
Candidiasis
in AIDS, 95–96, 101
oral
and airway management, 108
with beclomethasone therapy,
243

CaO_2. *See* Arterial oxygen content
Capillary hydrostatic pressure, 623
 increased, 34–37
Capillary membrane. *See also* Alveolar-
 capillary membrane
 fluid transport across, 623–624
Capillary permeability
 alterations of, 625–626
 effects of sympathomimetics on,
  232–233
 factors affecting, 625
 increased, pulmonary edema secondary to, 37, 623–628
Capnogram
 camel, 309, 309f
 cardiogenic oscillations on, 309–310,
  310f
 clinical significance of, 302
 curare, 309, 309f
 with increased expiratory resistance,
  309f
 normal, 302, 302f
 phases of, 302, 302f, 308–311
Capnography, 301f, 301–302, 710
 for continuous carbon dioxide monitoring, 308–311
Capnometers
 aspiration-type, 306
 clinical
  design of, 306
  technologies for, 303
 gas sampling design, 306–307
 infrared absorption interference
  and, 307–308
 mainstream, 306–307, 307f
 sidestream, 306
  sampling sites for, 310, 310f
 zeroed, 310–311
Capnometry, for infant/neonate, during
 thoracic operations, 500
Carbohydrates
 metabolism, in response to injury or
  sepsis, 690
 oxidation, respiratory quotient for,
  682
 refeeding based on, ventilatory and
  metabolic effects of, 695,
  697f
 respiratory effects of, 695–696
Carbon dioxide
 continuous monitoring of, 308–311
 effect on oxyhemoglobin dissociation, 148, 148t
 elimination, in one-lung versus two-
  lung ventilation, 204–205
 measurement, in gas phase, 303–308

monitoring
 applications in thoracic surgery,
  311–314
 during endobronchial anesthesia,
  314–315
 production of
  effects of carbohydrates on,
   695–696
  effects of malnutrition and
   refeeding on, 694f
  measurement of, 682–683
  during total parenteral nutrition,
   698f
 ventilatory sensitivity to
  indices of, 180, 180f
  with inhalation anesthesia, 360f
  with local anesthesia, 361–362
  measurement of, 179, 357
   rebreathing method, 179,
    357
   steady-state method, 179,
    357
Carbon dioxide laser
 characteristics of, 429, 430t
 choice of endotracheal tube for,
  435–436
 methods of use, 432
Carbon dioxide optode, for continuous
 carbon dioxide monitor-
 ing, 308
Carbon dioxide retention, 15
Carbon dioxide tension, 285. *See also*
 Alveolar carbon dioxide
 tension
 in blood, measurement of, 302–303
 end-tidal, 311
 steady-state adjusted, 156
 and ventilatory support, 661
Carbon dioxide transport, monitoring,
 300–302
Carbon monoxide
 effect on oxyhemoglobin dissociation, 148, 148t
 poisoning, 148, 631
Carboxyhemoglobin, 294
 light absorbance spectrum of, 295f
Carbuterol, 227
 structure of, 227f
Carcinoid syndrome, 89
Carcinoid tumors, of lung, K cells in,
 117
Cardiac complications, 716–718
Cardiac contusions
 diagnosis and management of, 475
 signs and symptoms of, 475, 475t
Cardiac disease, surgery for, 257

Cardiac dysfunction, association with
 chronic pulmonary dis-
 ease, preoperative assessment, 91
Cardiac evaluation, prior to thoracic
 surgery, 91
Cardiac flow. *See* Cardiac output
Cardiac herniation, 717–718
 diagnosis of, 340
Cardiac index, 286
Cardiac injuries, penetrating. *See also*
  Cardiac tamponade
 mortality with, 472
 sites of, 472t
Cardiac output
 in hyperdynamic state, 154
 low, in infant/neonate, management
  of, 511
 monitoring of, 156
 in oxygen delivery, 286
 during PEEP/CPAP, 637–638
 pharmacologic support of, 153
 and regional blood flow, 153
Cardiac silhouette
 air collections around, 49
 progressive enlargement of, 59
Cardiac slowing. *See* Bradycardia
Cardiac tamponade
 anesthetic management with, 474
 diagnosis of, 472–473, 473t
 in infant/neonate, anesthetic and
  perioperative considerations with, 519t
 monitoring with, 473
 treatment of, 473
Cardiomegaly, 37
Cardiomyopathy, caused by doxorubicin, 391–392
Cardiopulmonary bypass, for lung
 transplantation, 558–559
Cardiovascular disease
 with concurrent congestive heart
  failure, and mortality, 83
 incidence, 83
Carina, resection and reconstruction of,
 459, 459f
Carlens double-lumen endobronchial
 tube, 377, 378t, 379–380
 alternate insertion technique for,
  380, 380f
Carotid bodies, chemoreceptors, and
 ventilatory responses, 178
Catecholamines
 dosage and administration of, 228t
 duration of action, 228t
 handling of, in lungs, 127

mechanism of action, 228t
pharmacology of, 229
postoperative administration of, 613
structure of, 227f, 229
Catechol-o-methyltransferase, 119, 229
  activity of, 127, 128f
Catheter(s). *See also* Central venous pressure catheters; Nasal catheter; Pulmonary artery catheterization; Swan-Ganz catheter; Transthoracic atrial catheters; Transtracheal catheterization
  multi-lumen, for nutritional support, 703
  peripheral, for nutritional support, 701
  radiographic monitoring of, 63
Catheter-related infections, with nutritional support, 702–703
Caudal block, for postoperative analgesia, in infant/neonate, 507–508
Caval injuries, traumatic, 475
CBF. *See* Cerebral blood flow
Cell-mediated immunity, 97
  effects of malnutrition on, 693
Cell-saver techniques, 477
Central Gortex shunt
  anesthetic and perioperative considerations with, 524t
  description of, 524t
Central nervous system, chemoreceptors, in ventilatory control, 177–178
Central venous catheterization
  for nutritional support, 701
    infection with, 702–703
  during tracheal reconstruction, 453
Central venous oxygen saturation, 156
Central venous pressure
  in hypovolemia, 151–152
  monitoring
    with cardiac tamponade, 473–474
    with hemothorax, 471
    in infant/neonate, during thoracic operations, 501–502
    in trauma patient, selection of cannulation site, 470
Central venous pressure catheters
  aberrant placement of, 72f
  complications of, 75

intracardiac positioning of, 75
location, radiographic evaluation of, 75
overinsertion of, 75
subclavian approach with, complications of, 75
Cerebral blood flow
  autoregulation of, 152
  effect of inhalation anesthetics on, 152–153
  regulation of, 152
Cerebral circulation, 152
Cerebral metabolic rate of oxygen, and inhalation anesthesia, 153
cGMP. *See* Cyclic guanosine monophosphate
Chemoreceptors
  in carotid body, and ventilatory responses, 178
  central nervous system, in ventilatory control, 177–178
  peripheral
    effects of inhalation anesthesia on, 184
    and ventilatory responses, 178
Chemosensitivity
  to carbon dioxide, testing, 179
  ventilatory indices of, 180–181
Chemotactic peptides, actions of, in lung, 127
Chest-bottle system(s)
  single-unit, 672
  two-bottle, 672, 672f
Chest drainage, with empyema, 341, 422
Chest drainage system(s), 711
  blood loss monitoring with, 715
Chest injury. *See also* Trauma, thoracic
  causes of, 463
Chest physiotherapy, 596–599, 710
  after left upper lobectomy, 711
Chest radiography, 19–80
  abnormalities found on, 25–26
  anatomy seen on, factors affecting, 22–25
  anteroposterior view, 22
  decubitus view, 48
  in diagnosis of cardiac herniation, 717, 717f
  film exposure, 22
  in infant, 494f–496f, 495
  lateral view, 19, 22, 23f, 48
  lordotic view, 22, 24f
  oblique view, 22, 24f
  peripheral pulmonary markings on, 50–51

portable examination, 19, 22, 48
  artifacts, 25, 25f, 51, 52f
  evaluating, 26–27
posteroanterior view, 19, 22, 23f, 48
postoperative, 711–712, 715
preoperative, 324
  evaluating, 26
rotational distortion in, 22, 24f
successful approach to, 78–80
with tracheal lesions, 450, 451f–452f
Chest tubes
  management of, in infant/neonate, 508–509
  placement of, radiographic evaluation of, 70, 70f–71f
Chest wall
  abnormalities in, 85
  complications, postoperative, 714–715
  dysfunction, during and after thoracotomy and upper abdominal surgery, 89
  elastic properties of, 167–168
  equilibrium position of, 167
  pressure across, 169
  relaxation pressure volume characteristics of, 167, 167f
  surgical stabilization of, 714
Chest wall pain, postoperative, 715
Children. *See* Infant/neonate; Pediatric patient
Chloral hydrate, 256
  premedication, for infant/neonate, dosage and administration of, 497t
Chloride, effect on oxyhemoglobin dissociation, 148, 148t
Chlorpromazine
  in hemorrhagic shock, 480
  premedication with, 268
Cholecystokinin, actions of, in lung, 127
Cholinergic crisis, in myasthenia gravis, 403–404
Cholinesterase inhibitors, respiratory effects of, 364t
Chronic obstructive pulmonary disease
  arterial blood gas analysis in, 16
  and bullae, 423
  bullous emphysema in, radiographic appearance of, 32, 34f
  and complications associated with surgery, 90
  and concurrent coronary artery disease, 1
  decreased hypoxic ventilatory response in, 182

Chronic obstructive pulmonary
disease (*Continued*)
effects of malnutrition and refeeding
on, 694–695, 695f
FEV_1/FVC ratio in, 3
infection in, 710
and lung cancer, 1
pathophysiology of, 85–86
preoperative assessment in, 716–717
preoperative preparation with, and
incidence of complica-
tions, 84
radiographic findings with, 27, 36f,
36–37
right ventricular dysfunction in,
716
ventilation in, during spinal anesthesia, 172
ventilatory responses in, 183
to midazolam, 363
weight loss in, 694
Chronic pulmonary disease. *See also*
Chronic obstructive pul-
monary disease
after adult respiratory distress syndrome, 39, 40t
cardiac dysfunction associated with,
86–88
categories of, 84
definition of, 84
incidence, 83
and increased risk of nosocomial
infections, 88–89
pathophysiologic features of, 85
patient counseling, 91–92
preoperative evaluation with, 90
preoperative preparation of patient
with, 83–92
smoking-related, 83
Chylothorax
in infant/neonate, anesthetic and
perioperative considera-
tions with, 512t
postoperative, 713–714
in infant/neonate, management
of, 509–510
Cimetidine
effects of, on airway resistance, 350
gastrointestinal actions of, 274–275
indications for, 391
Circulation, monitoring, 285
Circulatory function, regulation of, 152
Clara cell(s), 116–117, 224
cytochrome P-450 enzymes, 131
Clark PO_2 electrode, 287, 288f. *See also*
Transcutaneous oxygen

monitoring
applications in thoracic surgery,
312–313
in continuous monitoring of oxygen
tension, 287–290, 290f
Closing capacity, 186
during anesthesia, 348, 348f
Closing volume, 622f–623f
definition of, 621
Clotrimazol, indications for, in AIDS,
104
CO_2. *See* Carbon dioxide
Coagulopathy. *See also* Disseminated
intravascular coagulation
in acute respiratory failure, 629
after massive transfusion, 478–479
in AIDS, 108
Coarctation of the aorta, repair
anesthetic and perioperative considerations with, 512t, 523t
description of, 523t
Cocaine, anesthesia, for flexible
fiberoptic bronchoscopy,
334
Codeine
front-loading, 579t
for postoperative analgesia, in
infant/neonate, dosage and
administration of, 507t
Coeur en sabot, 496f
Collagen vascular disorders, and primary pulmonary hyperten-
sion, 86
Colloid osmotic pressure, during volume infusion, 476
Colterol, structure of, 227f
Complement, activation, in acute respiratory failure, 629,
633–634
Complement C5a, actions of, in lung,
127
Compliance, 169, 661, 662f
decrease in, in restrictive pulmonary
disease, 85
dynamic, 170
effective, 170
in normalcy and disease, in ventilatory support, 668–669
in PEEP/CPAP, for acute respiratory
failure, 636–637
quasistatic, 170
static, 170
Complications. *See also* Pulmonary
complications
of anesthesia, 709–710
of bronchoscopy, 325–326

cardiac, 716–718
chest wall, 714–715
of diagnostic procedures, 720
of esophageal surgery, 397
of nutritional support, 701–702
postoperative
correlation with nutritional status, 685–686
in infant/neonate, management
of, 506–511
prevention of, 710
of pulmonary resection for lung cancer, 686
of thoracic surgery, 709–720, 710t
Computed tomography
of chest tube positioning, 70, 70f
of mediastinal mass, 398
in pediatric patient, 537, 538f
of mediastinum, 55
of pleural fluids, 59, 62f–63f
pulmonary densities, during anesthesia, 172
Congenital diaphragmatic hernia. *See*
Diaphragmatic hernia,
congenital
Congenital heart disease. *See also*
Infant/neonate, cyanotic;
specific anomaly
associated anomalies, 495
and premedication, 497–498
preoperative evaluation with,
494–496
Congestive atelectasis, definition of, 619
Congestive heart failure, in patient with
chronic obstructive pul-
monary disease, 36–37
Conjunctival oxygen tension, measurement of, 293–294
Consciousness, level of, effects of
antimuscarinic drugs on,
265t
Constant-flow generator, 663, 663f
Constant-pressure generator, 663,
664f
Continuous positive airway pressure
(CPAP). *See also* One-lung
ventilation, differential
lung CPAP/PEEP; Positive
end-expiratory
pressure/CPAP
with bronchopleural fistula, 422
effects of, on venous admixture, 608,
609f–610f
face-mask, 605, 611
indications for, 638, 638t
side effects of, 638

for increasing arterial oxygen tension, with small airway closure, 610–611
indications for, 604
nonventilated-lung, 214–215
    system for, components of, 215, 215f
in one-lung ventilation, selective application of, 213f, 214–215, 217, 356
versus positive end-expiratory pressure, 635–637
in prevention and treatment of atelectasis, 604–605
for respiratory distress syndrome, 490
Controlled drugs, 256
Control-mode ventilation, 664–665
Convulsions, anesthetic-related, effects of premedication on, 271
Coronary artery injuries, traumatic, diagnosis and management of, 474–475
Coronary blood flow, autoregulation of, 153
Cor pulmonale, 85
acute, 87
after lung resection, predicting, 13
chronic, 87–88
lung transplantation for, 556, 561
manifestations of, 87
onset of, 87
pathophysiology of, 86–88
postoperative respiratory failure, prediction of, 11
preoperative assessment, 91
with sleep-related disturbances, 86
treatment of, 92
Corticosteroids
for acute respiratory failure, 633–634
aerosolized (topical) therapy, 243–244
for asthma, 241
dosage and administration of, 242–243
indications for, 614
for inflammatory lung disease, 241
inhalant products, 615t
metabolism of, 242
pharmacology of, 241–242, 242t
side effects of, 243
structures of, 241, 241f
systemic therapy with, 244–245
withdrawal from, before lung transplantation, 556–557

Cortisone, pharmacology of, 242t
Co-trimoxazole
indications for, in AIDS, 104
side effects of, 104
Coughing
diagnostic significance of, 324, 339
in postoperative period, for therapeutic purposes, 596–598
Crafoord's tampon, 372
Cricothyroidotomy, 443–444
Critical closing pressure, 635
Critical opening pressure, 635
Critical point, 144
definition of, 163
Cromolyn sodium
dosage and administration of, 239–240
indications for, 238, 614
inhalant product, 615t
mechanism of action, 239
pharmacology of, 239–240
side effects of, 240
structure of, 239f
Croup (infectious), in infant/neonate, anesthetic and perioperative considerations with, 513t
Cryoanalgesia, for pain relief, 595
Cryptococcosis, in AIDS, 101
Cryptosporidiosis, in AIDS, 101
Cuirass ventilator, 662
Curare
with cyclopropane, cardiorespiratory effects of, 174
effects of, on airway resistance, 350
Curare test, in myasthenia gravis, 403
Cutaneous blood flow
in hypovolemia, 151
monitoring of, 156
CVP. *See* Central venous pressure
Cyclic adenosine monophosphate
function in airway smooth muscle, 226, 613
as second messenger, 225–226
Cyclic guanosine monophosphate
function in airway smooth muscle, 226
as second messenger, 225–226
Cyclic nucleotides, and smooth muscle function, 225–226
Cyclophosphamide, for myasthenia gravis, 404
Cystic adenomatoid malformation, in infant/neonate, anesthetic and perioperative considerations with, 513t

Cystic fibrosis
bronchopulmonary lavage for, 425
long-term home TPN in, 697
in pediatrics, anesthetic and perioperative considerations with, 513t, 525
Cystic hygroma, in infant/neonate, anesthetic and perioperative considerations with, 513t
Cytochrome P-450 mono-oxygenase system
physiologic and pathophysiologic roles of, 131
pulmonary, 116–117, 131
Cytomegalovirus
in AIDS, 95–96, 101
ganciclovir-resistant, 104
transmission, in blood transfusion, 478

Dalton's law of partial pressure, 15
Da Nang lung, 619–620
Dead space. *See* Alveolar dead space; Anatomic dead space; Apparatus dead space; Physiologic dead space
Dead space-to-tidal volume ratio, 14–15
Deafferentation pain, of post-thoracotomy pain syndrome, 719
Death(s), anesthetic, 709–710
Deceleration injuries
impact, 464
momentum, 464
Demand valves, 649–650
Dementia, and AIDS, 101–102
Demerol. *See* Meperidine
Depolarizing relaxants, for myasthenic patients, 408
Depression, with chronic pulmonary disease, 92
Dermacare Laser Safety System, 431
Dermatomyositis, with lung cancer, 89
Desensitization crisis, in myasthenia gravis, 404
Dexamethasone, 241
pharmacology of, 242, 242t
structure of, 241f
Dextran, indications for, 718
Dextran 40, as plasma expander, in hemorrhagic shock, 477
Diagnostic procedures
anesthesia for, 321–343
complications of, 720
preoperative assessment for, 321–324

Diamorphine, epidural, respiratory effects of, 362
Diaphragm. *See also* Flail diaphragm contractility
    effect of hypophosphatemia on, 700
    effects of sympathomimetics on, 233
    effects of theophylline on, 236
  costal portion, 165
  crural portion, 165
  depression of, with tension pneumothorax, 52, 53f
  effects of malnutrition on, 693
  embryology of, 526
  eventration of, in infant/neonate, anesthetic and perioperative considerations with, 515t
  excursion of, 166
  motor innervation of, 165–166
  radiographic appearance of, 23f, 25
  tonic activity of, during anesthesia, 172–173
  traumatic rupture of, diagnosis and management of, 472
Diaphragmatic electromyography, 182
Diaphragmatic hernia, congenital
  anesthetic and perioperative considerations with, 513t, 526–534
  associated anomalies, 528–529, 529t
  classification of, 526, 533
  extracorporeal membrane oxygenation for, 533–534, 676
  incidence of, 526
  mortality with, 526, 529
  pathophysiology of, 526–530, 529f
  physiologic categories of, 529
  prenatal repair of, 534
  signs and symptoms of, 526–528
  sites of, 526, 528f
  surgical repair of
    monitoring during, 531
    outcome, and oxygenation, 533–534, 534f
    postoperative management for, 532–533
    preoperative stabilization for, 531–532
    survivors, follow-up studies of, 534
    technique, 531–532
    timing of, 531
Diarrhea, in AIDS, 101
  treatment of, 105

Diazepam
  amnestic effect, 259
  anxiolytic effect, 258, 260, 260f
  effects on incidence of anesthetic convulsions, 271t
  and hypoxic pulmonary vasoconstriction, clinical studies of, 355
  pharmacology of, 272
  in postoperative management of infant/neonate, 507
  premedication, 271–272, 273t
    dosage and administration of, 272
    for infant/neonate, dosage and administration of, 497t
  respiratory effects of, 363
  ventilatory response to, 271–272, 272f
Diclofenac, as adjuvant to opioid analgesics, 578
Dideoxycytidine, for HIV infection, 105
Diet-induced thermogenesis, 683f
  definition of, 681–682
  in malnourished patients with emphysema, 695
Diffusing capacity
  determination of, 6–7
  to predict postoperative lung function and survival, 10
Diffusion hypoxia, 361
Digitalis
  for atrial dysrhythmias, 716
  intoxication, 88
Digitalization
  perioperative, 716
  preoperative
    with esophageal surgery, 395
    indications for, 420
    risk vs. benefits, with chronic pulmonary disease, 88
    in treatment of right heart failure, 717
Dihydroergotamine, effect on distribution of blood, 153
Dihydroxyeicosatetraenoic acids, metabolism, in lungs, 122
2,3-Diphosphoglycerate, 147
  effect on oxyhemoglobin dissociation, 148, 148t
  in stored blood, 479
Dipyrone, as adjuvant to opioid analgesics, 578
Displacement, of carbon dioxide response curve, 180, 180f

Disseminated intravascular coagulation, 478–479, 479t
  diffuse alveolar pulmonary hemorrhage in, 40, 45f
Distending airway pressure
  breathing circuit for, 656, 656f, 658–660
    connection to patient, 659
    expiratory valve, 659–660, 660f
    fresh gas source, 659
    humidifier, 659
  for support of oxygenation, 658–660, 670, 676–677
DIT. *See* Diet-induced thermogenesis
Diuretic therapy
  in acute respiratory failure, 634
  in posttraumatic renal failure, 480–481
Dobutamine
  for heart failure, 561
  and hypoxic pulmonary vasoconstriction, 207, 357
  indications for, 153
  in treatment of right heart failure, 717
Dopamine
  for heart failure, 561
  in hemorrhagic shock, 480
  and hypoxic pulmonary vasoconstriction, 210, 357
  indications for, 153
Dor operation, 394
Double-lumen endotracheal tube(s). *See* Endotracheal tube(s), double-lumen
Down regulation, definition of, 163
Doxorubicin, cardiomyopathy caused by, 391–392
2,3-DPG. *See* 2,3-Diphosphoglycerate
Droperidol, 258
  premedication, 267–270
    for infant/neonate, dosage and administration of, 497t
  respiratory effects of, 363
Ductus arteriosus, 486–487. *See also* Patent ductus arteriosus
Ductus venosus, 486–487
Duty to care, 109
Dyphylline, 237
  structure of, 234f
Dysphagia, 338
Dysphoria, and opioids, 266–267
Dyspnea, diagnostic significance of, 338–339
Dysrhythmias
  with AIDS, 102

with antimuscarinic drugs, 262
with bronchoscopy, 326
with esophageal surgery, 395
with mediastinal lymphoma, 400
perioperative
    with chronic pulmonary disease,
        88
    with pulmonary resection,
        419–420
postoperative, 716
pathophysiology of, 88

Eaton-Lambert (myasthenic) syndrome,
    338, 412–413, 433
Echocardiography
indications for, 61, 91
with mediastinal mass, 398
ECM. *See* Extracellular mass
ECMO. *See* Extracorporeal membrane
    oxygenation
Ectopic bronchus, in infant/neonate,
    anesthetic and periopera-
    tive considerations with,
    513t
EDHF. *See* Endothelium-derived hyper-
    polarizing factor
Edrophonium. *See also* Tensilon test
effects of, on airway resistance, 350
EFAD. *See* Essential fatty acid deficien-
    cy syndrome
Egg-on-a-string appearance, 495f
Eicosanoids
and acute lung injury, 133
definition of, 119
processing of, in lungs, 115, 119–125
production of, effects of lipid infu-
    sion on, 697
Elastance, 169
Electrical alternans, with cardiac tam-
    ponade, 473, 473f
Electrocardiography
with cardiac tamponade, 473
in diagnosis of cardiac herniation,
    717
indications for, 91
for infant/neonate, during thoracic
    operations, 500
preoperative, 324
Electrolytes
analysis, for infant/neonate, during
    thoracic operations, 502
requirements for, in nutritional pro-
    tocols, 689, 689t
respiratory effects of, 700
Electromyography, in myasthenia
    gravis, 403

Emergence, rapid, facilitation of, 261
Emergency medicine, development of,
    463
Emerson Exhalation PEEP valve, 660
Emphysema
airflow obstruction in, 8, 85–86
bullous, surgical management of,
    423–424
effects of malnutrition and refeeding
    on, 694–695, 695f
functional residual capacity with,
    168
lobar, in infant/neonate
    acquired, anesthetic and periop-
        erative considerations
        with, 516t
    congenital, anesthetic and peri-
        operative considerations
        with, 516t
lung transplantation for, 556, 561
mediastinal, postoperative, 714, 715f
pulmonary, ventilatory effects of
    head-down position in,
    172
with recurrent or persistent atelecta-
    sis, in infant/neonate, 510f
refeeding in, ventilatory and
    metabolic effects of, 695,
    697f
subcutaneous
    with esophageal perforation, 393
    in infant/neonate, anesthetic and
        perioperative considera-
        tions with, 521t
    postoperative, 714, 715f
surgical, and pneumothorax, 469
systemic steroid therapy for, 245
weight loss with, 694
Empyema, 39
anesthetic considerations with,
    422–423
computed tomography scan of, 59,
    63f
drainage of, 341, 422
in infant/neonate, anesthetic and
    perioperative considera-
    tions with, 514t
with lung abscess, radiologic find-
    ings with, 59
postoperative, 713–714
Endobronchial intubation, 371–387
bronchial blockers, 372–374
with bronchopleural fistula, 671–672
with empyema, 422
with hemoptysis, 429
isolation techniques, 372–387

tube types for, 372t
left-sided, 375–376
oxygenation monitoring with,
    312–313, 314f
for pulmonary resection, 420
right-sided, 375–377
Endobronchial tubes
double-lumen, 377–384
    complications with, 384–387
    cuff seal
        bronchoscopic evaluation of,
            425, 425f
        testing adequacy of, 425,
            426f
    designs for, 383–384, 385f
    differential lung ventilation with,
        422
    in bullous disease, 424
    disposable, 383, 384f
    disposable connector for, 377,
        378f
    positioning, bronchoscopic deter-
        mination of, 425, 425f
    reusable Cobb connector for,
        377, 378f
    selection of, 383
malpositioning of, 384–387
single-lumen, 374–377
Endocarditis. *See* Bacterial endocarditis
Endothelial cells
cytochrome P-450-dependent mono-
    oxygenase activity, 131
growth factors produced by, 130
inhibition of antiproliferative fac-
    tors, 130
pulmonary
    metabolic functions, 115–116
    metabolism of humoral sub-
        stances at cell surface of,
        118–119
    secretory functions, 115–116
    surface projections of, 116,
        117f
    synthesis and release of cyclo-
        oxygenase products, 120
pulmonary capillary, 623
    caveolae in, 118f
Endothelin, 119, 130, 132
Endothelium. *See also* Pulmonary
    endothelium
cytochrome P-450 enzymes, 131
Endothelium-derived contracting fac-
    tor(s), 130
handling of, in lung, 119
Endothelium-derived hyperpolarizing
    factor, 130

Endothelium-derived relaxing factor, 132
  actions of, 129–130
  handling of, in lungs, 115–116, 119
  mechanism of action of, 129, 129f
  production or release from endothelial cell, 129
  synthesis of, 129f, 129–130
Endotoxin, in acute respiratory failure, 629–630
Endotracheal intubation
  adrenergic response to, premedication for, 261
  for application of positive airway pressure, 601
  awake, 343
  effects on respiratory mechanics, 174–177
  esophageal perforation in, 393
  in infant/neonate, 503–505
  with mediastinoscopy, 340
  with oral *Candida* infection, 108
  postoperative, prolonged, 595
  reintubation, 615–617
  in repair of esophageal atresia/tracheoesophageal fistula, 536–537
  tracheal injury in, 448f, 448–449
  in tracheal reconstruction, 454
Endotracheal tube(s)
  adapter for fiberoptic bronchoscope, 332, 332f–333f
  armored, 456, 457f
  with bronchoscope inserted, cross-sectional area of, 327, 327f
  for bronchoscopy, 329, 333, 334f
  Carden, 333
  cuff injuries, 448f, 448–449
  diameter of, 65
  double-lumen
    designs, 69
    for differential lung ventilation and PEEP, 216
    for esophageal surgery, 395–396
    in evaluation of split lung function, 10
    malplacement of, complications of, 69
    placement of
      correct, 69
      radiographic evaluation of, 69–70
      during tracheobronchial bleeding episode, 716

  in prevention of tracheobronchial obstruction, 710–711
  in provision of anesthesia in patient with bronchopleural fistula, 713
  for pulmonary resection, 420
  for selective PEEP, 202–203
  stimulation of carina and main bronchi with, premedication for, 261
  in surgical treatment of esophagorespiratory tract fistula, 397
  for esophageal surgery, choice of, 395–396
  as fixed inspiratory and expiratory resistor, 174–175
  for laser resection
    choice of, 435–436
    cuff inflation, safety precautions, 435
    flammability of, 435–436
    protection of, 434–435
  overinflation of balloon cuff, 65, 66f, 68f
  overinsertion of, 65–68
  position of
    assessment of, 324
    radiographic evaluation of, 65–69
  possible complications of, 65
  quadruple-lumen, for high-frequency ventilation, 674
  removal of, from pediatric patient, 552–553
  selection of, for infant/neonate, 503, 503t
  sizes of, 553t
    and airflow resistance, 175
    and PEEP, with bronchoscope inserted, 327–328, 328t
  use of Nd-YAG laser through, 434
End-tidal carbon dioxide tension, 311
Energy
  metabolism, 681–682
    in injured patient, 691, 692f
  requirements
    age- and size-related differences in, 486, 486t
    postoperative, 691
Enflurane
  effects of
    on airway resistance, 349–350
    on respiratory control, 184, 185t
    on ventilatory control, 358–361

  on ventilatory response to carbon dioxide, 360f
  on ventilatory response to hypoxia, 361f
  and hypoxic pulmonary vasoconstriction
    clinical studies of, 354–355
    in vitro studies, 353, 353f
    in vivo studies, 353–354
  neuromuscular effects of, in myasthenic patients, 406–407
ENT. *See* Enteral nutrition
Enteral nutrition
  malplacement of tubes for, 702
  mechanical complications of, 702
  versus parenteral nutrition, 701–703
  practical considerations with, 701
  preoperative, effect on clinical outcome, 688
Enzyme-linked immunosorbent assay, for HIV, 97
Epidural analgesia/anesthesia
  continuous thoracic, 469
  intravenous, for AIDS patients, 108
  placement of catheter for, 573
  for postoperative analgesia, 572, 595
    local anesthetic infusion for, 573
  respiratory effects of, 361–362
Epiglottitis, in infant/neonate, anesthetic and perioperative considerations with, 514t
Epinephrine, 229
  dosage and administration of, 228t, 229
  duration of action, 228t
  effects on hypoxic pulmonary vasoconstriction, 210
  indications for, 229
  mechanism of action, 228t
  pharmacology of, 229
  racemic, postoperative administration of, 613
  side effects of, 229
  structure of, 227f
Epithelial (type I) cells, 224, 628
Epoxyeicosatetraenoic acids, metabolism, in lungs, 122
EPP. *See* Equal pressure point
Equal pressure point, 3f
Erb-Duchenne palsy, in infant/neonate, anesthetic and perioperative considerations with, 514t
Esmolol
  for atrial dysrhythmias, 716

for hypercyanotic episodes with tetralogy of Fallot, 498
for intraoperative dysrhythmias, 420
Esophageal atresia
associated anomalies, 535
diagnosis of, 534–535
incidence of, 534
mortality with, 535
pulmonary complications of, 535–536
repair
anesthetic and perioperative considerations with, 534–537
complications of, 537
and tracheoesophageal fistula, anatomic combinations of, 535, 535f
Esophageal cancer
chemotherapy, 391–392
esophageal obstruction with, 391, 392f
fistula formation with, 394
radiation therapy, 392
surgical treatment of, 392–393
Esophageal dilatation, 394
anesthetic management for, 396
Esophageal duplication, in infant/neonate, anesthetic and perioperative considerations with, 514t
Esophageal injury
corrosive or caustic, in infant/neonate, anesthetic and perioperative considerations with, 513t
in mediastinoscopy, 340
Esophageal intubation, 68–69
Esophageal perforation
causes of, 393
during endoscopy, 342
iatrogenic, 393
in infant/neonate, anesthetic and perioperative considerations with, 514t
intrathoracic, 393–394
treatment of, 394
Esophageal resection. *See also* Esophageal surgery
with gastric pull-through or colonic interposition, radiographic appearance of, 55, 55f
Esophageal rupture, 49, 50f
causes of, 393
intrathoracic, 393–394
Esophageal stenosis, in infant/neonate,

anesthetic and perioperative considerations with, 514t
Esophageal stethoscope, in infant/neonate, 505
Esophageal stricture(s)
benign, 392, 393f
in infant/neonate, anesthetic and perioperative considerations with, 514t
surgical treatment of, 393
Esophageal surgery. *See also* Esophageal resection
anesthetic considerations, 395–397
diseases requiring, 390–395
induction for, 395
intraoperative considerations and management, 395
lung isolation in, 374
monitoring in, 395
postoperative complications of, 397
preoperative evaluation for, 395
Esophagectomy, indications for, 392, 394
Esophagitis, in infant/neonate, anesthetic and perioperative considerations with, 515t
Esophagomyotomy, 394
Esophagorespiratory tract fistula
causes of, 394
preoperative localization of, 395
surgical treatment of, 394
anesthetic management for, 396–397
Esophagoscope(s), 342f, 342–343
Esophagoscopy, 342–343
anesthetic management for, 342–343
in pediatrics, anesthetic and perioperative considerations with, 525–526
risk of aspiration in, 342–343
Esophagus
anatomy and anatomic relations of, 389, 390f
blood supply to, 389
innervation of, 389–390
peristalsis in, 390
surgical diseases and treatment of, 390–395
Essential fatty acid deficiency syndrome, 688
Ethambutol, indications for, in AIDS, 104
Ether, effects of, on hypoxic pulmonary vasoconstriction, 208
Etilofrine, effect on distribution of

blood, 153
Etomidate, effects of, on airway resistance, 349–350
Euphoria, and opioids, 266–267
Exercise, pulmonary artery pressure increases with, in chronic obstructive pulmonary disease, 716
Exercise protocol(s)
constant versus incremental, 12, 12f
end points, submaximal versus maximal, 12, 12f
Exercise reconditioning, 92
Exercise testing, 11–15
differentiation of cardiac versus pulmonary impairment by, 14t
for lung transplantation candidate, 557, 560, 561t
and post-thoracotomy complications, 14
protocol, 14–15
for thoracotomy patients, summary of data for, 13t
Exercise tolerance, in lung cancer patients, and post-thoracotomy hospital mortality, 14
Expiration, muscles of, 166
Expiratory positive airway pressure, 636f
Expiratory reserve volume, 621f, 623f
definition of, 621
External respiration, definition of, 163
Extra-alveolar air
iatrogenic causes of, 48
in nonsurgical or nontraumatized patients, 48
radiographic findings with, 48–52
traumatic causes of, 48
types of, 48
Extracellular fluid, and serum albumin levels, 687
Extracellular mass, 684
Extracorporeal membrane oxygenation, 676–677
with congenital diaphragmatic hernia, 533–534
neonatal, 676–677
Extrinsic ventilatory defects, 7–8
Extubation
accidental, 68
after pulmonary resection, 421
after tracheal reconstruction, 459
criteria for, for infant/neonate, 504–505, 505t

Face masks, for oxygen therapy, 654t, 654–658

Facial paralysis, in AIDS, 102

Familial primary pulmonary hypertension, 86

Famotidine, gastrointestinal actions of, 274–275

Fasting, adaptive mechanisms in, 685

Fat
caloric content of, 682
effects on nitrogen balance, 688
metabolism, in response to injury or sepsis, 690
oxidation, respiratory quotient for, 682
refeeding based on, ventilatory and metabolic effects of, 695, 697f

Fat embolism syndrome, 629, 631
diagnosis of, 631
management of, 631–632

FEF. *See* Forced expiratory flow

Fenoterol, 227
dosage and administration of, 228t, 231
duration of action, 228t
mechanism of action, 228t
pharmacology of, 231
relative potency of, 229
structure of, 227f

Fentanyl
and bupivacaine, combined infusions of, for postoperative analgesia, 578
effects of
on airway resistance, 349–350
on ventilatory control, 358
epidural
after thymectomy, 411
for postoperative analgesia
dosage and administration of, 575t
duration of action, 575t
and hypoxic pulmonary vasoconstriction, clinical studies of, 355
induction, for infant/neonate, 498
intrathecal, for postoperative analgesia, 574
for postoperative analgesia, in infant/neonate, 507
dosage and administration of, 507t
premedication, 265–267
for bronchoscopy, 334
duration of action, 267f

pulmonary uptake of, 132
respiratory effects of, 362
spinal, for postoperative analgesia, dosage and administration of, 577
subarachnoid, for postoperative analgesia
dosage and administration of, 575t
duration of action, 575t
for surgical repair of congenital diaphragmatic hernia, 532
transdermal, for postoperative analgesia, 581–582

Fentanyl/Althesin, for myasthenic patients, 409

Fentanyl/etomidate, for myasthenic patients, 409

Fetal circulation, 486–487. *See also* Persistent fetal circulation

Fetal hemoglobin, 298

Fetal respiration, 486

FEV_1. *See* Forced expiratory volume at 1 second

FEV_1/FVC ratio, 7–9, 9f
in asthmatics, 9
to predict postoperative lung function and survival, 10

Fiberoptic bronchoscopy
advantages of, 325
anesthetic management for, 334–336
for aspiration of secretions from airway, 601
for determination of cuff seal adequacy, 425f
for determination of endobronchial tube positioning, 387, 425f
in evaluation of resectability of cancer, 2
general anesthesia for, 336
indications for, 325
in intubated patient, 327–328
laser therapy with, 333, 432
with mediastinal mass, 398
in pediatrics, indications for, 525
ventilation during, 336
methods of, 332–333

Filtration coefficient, 624

F_IO_2. *See* Inspired oxygen tension

Flail chest, 632
criteria for intubation with, 468, 468t
diagnosis of, 467–468
management of, 468–469
mechanisms of, 467
monitoring with, 468–469

mortality rate with, 469
pain relief with, 469
prognosis for, 467, 469
radiologic findings with, 468

Flail diaphragm, 719

Flexible fiberoptic bronchoscopy. *See* Fiberoptic bronchoscopy

Flow generator(s), 663, 663f

Flowmeters, 649–650
for intermittent mandatory ventilation, 666
for relative flow metering, 650

Flow phase, of metabolic response to injury, 689–690

Flow-pressure-volume analysis, 171

Flow-volume curve(s). *See* Flow-volume loop(s)

Flow-volume loop(s), 4
with airway obstruction, 450
diagnostic utility of, 322f–323f, 324
effect of bronchodilator on, 9f
with extrathoracic obstruction, 5, 323f
with fixed obstruction, 5
with intrathoracic obstruction, 323f
with mediastinal mass, 398, 400f
in pediatric patient, 537–539
normal, 4f, 322f
with upper airway obstruction, 4f, 4–5

Flow-volume studies, indications for, 90

Fluid balance, postoperative, 710

Fluid management, perioperative, 684

Fluid overload, 35
cardiopulmonary effects of, 34
radiologic findings with, 47

Fluid requirements, age- and size-related differences in, 486, 486t

Flumazenil, 271
respiratory effects of, 363

Flunisolide, 241
aerosolized (topical) therapy, 243
dosage and administration of, 244
pharmacology of, 244
structure of, 241f

Fluorescence quenching, 287, 289f

Fluoroscopy, indications for, 91

Fluroxene, and hypoxic pulmonary vasoconstriction, in vivo studies of, 354, 354f

Fogarty catheter, as bronchial blocker, 373–374

Fome-Cuff tube, 435

Foramen ovale, 486–487
patent, potential, identification of, 92

Forced expiratory effort, forces acting on chest during, 3f
Forced expiratory flow, 2f
Forced expiratory volume at 1 second, 2f, 3–4, 4f, 324
  in fiberoptic bronchoscopy, 327
  postoperative, effects of postoperative analgesia on, 582–583
  post-thoracotomy, 582
  predicted postoperative calculation, 11
    compatible with long-term survival, 11
  in prediction of postoperative lung function and survival, 10
Forced oscillation, 170–171
Forced vital capacity, 2, 2f, 4, 4f, 324
  in fiberoptic bronchoscopy, 327
  postoperative, effects of postoperative analgesia on, 582–583
  post-thoracotomy, 582
  to predict postoperative lung function and survival, 10
Foreign bodies
  in airway, removal of, bronchoscopy for, 325
    in children, 522
  in esophagus, 342
  intrathoracic, removal of, 340
Formoterol, 227
  duration of action, 232
  mechanism of action, 232
  pharmacology of, 231
  relative potency of, 231
  structure of, 227f
Foscarnet, indications for, 104
Fractional hemoglobin saturation, 286, 294
  decreased, 287
FRC. *See* Functional residual capacity
Functional hemoglobin saturation, definition of, 294
Functional residual capacity, 167–168, 175, 594
  in acute respiratory failure, 620–622, 623f
  in asthma, 85
  changes with postural alterations, 168
  components of, 621
  decreased
    during anesthesia, 186, 200, 348, 348f
    pathophysiology of, 621t, 621–622
  determination of, 5–6

and general anesthesia, 172–173
  during intubation, 175–176, 176f
  maintenance of, 616f
  in obstructive lung disease, 168
  and oxygenation, 649, 653, 658
  postoperative, effects of postoperative analgesia on, 582–583
  post-thoracotomy, 582
  with pulmonary emphysema, 168
  in respiratory distress syndrome, 490
  in restrictive pulmonary disease, 85
FVC. *See* Forced vital capacity

Ganciclovir, indications for, in AIDS, 104
Gangrene, complicating lobectomy, 713
Gas exchange
  in acute respiratory failure, 627f, 627–628
  alterations in, in depleted or septic/injured patients, 684f
  efficiency, during and after thoracotomy and upper abdominal surgery, 89
  evaluation of, 15
  measurement of, 682–683
  in positive-pressure ventilation, 634–635, 635f
  during total parenteral nutrition, 698f
  in upright position, regional differences in, 197, 198f
Gastric dilatation/distention
  postoperative, 711
    in infant/neonate, management of, 510–511
    radiologic evaluation of, 62–63
  prevention, in infant/neonate, 505, 511
Gastric pH, pharmacologic manipulation of, 391
Gastroesophageal reflux (disease), 390–391, 393
  in infant/neonate, anesthetic and perioperative considerations with, 515t
Gastrostomy, in repair of esophageal atresia/tracheoesophageal fistula, 396–397, 536
General anesthesia
  in bullectomy, 424
  with cardiac tamponade, 474
  chest wall mechanics during, 173
  effects of

    on pulmonary gas exchange, 185–188
    on respiratory mechanics, 172–174
  for fiberoptic bronchoscopy, 336
  for laser therapy, 432–433
  for thoracoscopy, 342
  for thymectomy, 405–406
Glaucoma, with antimuscarinic drugs, 262
Glenn shunt
  anesthetic and perioperative considerations with, 524t
  description of, 524t
Glossopharyngeal nerve, blockade, 335, 335f
Glottis
  in determination of functional residual capacity, 175–176
  in infants, in respiratory mechanics, 175–176
Gluconeogenesis, 685
Glucose
  caloric content of, 682
  determinations, in infant/neonate, during thoracic operations, 502
  effects on nitrogen balance, 688
  metabolism, in response to injury or sepsis, 690
Glycolysis, in hyperdynamic state, 154
Glycopyrrolate
  anticholinergic effect, dose-response for, 264f
  antisialagogue effect, 259, 264f, 264–265
  bronchodilator effect, 263f
  dosage and administration of, 238
  duration of action, 238
  effects of, 265t
    on cardiac rhythm, 260–261
    on pulmonary mechanics, in fiberoptic bronchoscopy, 327
  pharmacology of, 261–262
  premedication
    for bronchoscopy, 334
    dosage and administration of, 263
    for infant/neonate, dosage and administration of, 497t
    pharmacology of, 263
  pulmonary effects of, 263–264
  structure of, 238, 238f
Goblet cell(s), 224

Gordon-Green right-sided single-lumen
  endobronchial tube, 375,
  376f, 376–377
Granuloma(s), suture, bronchial stump,
  therapeutic bronchoscopy
  for, 325
Gravitational effects. *See also*
  Pulmonary perfusion, distribution of
  on distribution of pulmonary blood
    flow, in lateral decubitus
    position, 198, 199f, 205
  on distribution of ventilation, in
    upright position, 196
Great vessels
  transposition of, radiographic find-
    ings with, 495f
  traumatic injuries to, diagnosis and
    management of, 475
Guanylate cyclase, activation, by
  endothelium-derived relaxing factor, 129f, 129–130
Gunshot wound(s)
  cardiac, 472
  destruction secondary to, calcula-
    tion of, 464
  evaluation of, 464

Hagen-Poiseuille relationship, 155
Halothane
  cerebrovascular effects of, 151–152
  effects of
    on airway resistance, 349–350
    on hypoxic pulmonary vasocon-
      striction, 207–208
    on lung metabolism, 132
    on respiratory control, 184, 185t
    on ventilatory control, 358–361
    on ventilatory response to carbon
      dioxide, 360f
    on ventilatory response to hypox-
      ia, 361f
  and hypoxic pulmonary vasocon-
    striction
    clinical studies of, 354–355, 356f
    in vitro studies of, 353, 353f
    in vivo studies of, 354, 354f
  induction, for infant/neonate, 498
  interference with transcutaneous
    oxygen monitoring, 293
  for myasthenic patients, 407
  ventilatory depression with, 173
Hamman's sign, 471
Harris Benedict formula, for prediction
  of basal metabolic rate,
  683, 683t

Health care workers
  hepatitis B virus infection in, 109
  occupational exposure
    to hepatitis B, 107
    to HIV, 105–106
Heart. *See also entries under* Cardiac
  abnormalities of, with AIDS, 102
  boot-shaped, 496f
  radiographic appearance of, 23f, 25
  size, radiologic evaluation of, 35–36,
    47
  transplantation, extracorporeal
    membrane oxygenation as
    bridge to, 676
Heart failure
  pleural effusion with, 56
  radiographic findings with, 35f,
    35–36, 47
  right, 35
  postoperative, 716–717
Heart rate
  age- and size-related differences in,
    486, 486t
  with atropine, 262, 262f
  effects of antimuscarinic drugs on,
    265t
Heart shadow, on chest radiography, 22
  changing density in, 28, 28f
Helium dilution technique, for determining lung volume, 5f
Helium/oxygen protocol, for laser therapy, 436, 436t
Heller's myotomy, 394
Hematocrit
  age- and size-related differences in,
    486, 486t
  and hemodilution, 155
  optimal, in postoperative patients,
    150
  in people living at high altitude, 150
Hematoma(s), chest wall, postthoracotomy, 715
Hemiparesis, after mediastinoscopy,
  340
Hemithorax, opacification of, in postoperative period, 57–59
Hemodilution
  contraindications to, 156
  effects of
    on oxygen delivery, 155
    on serum oncotic pressure, 624
  indications for, 156
  isovolemic, response to, 155
Hemodynamic response to surgery,
  effects of postoperative
  analgesia on, 584

Hemodynamics, during bronchopulmonary lavage, 427
Hemoglobin. *See also* Fractional
  hemoglobin saturation
  affinity for oxygen, regulation of,
    147–148
  analysis, for infant/neonate, during
    thoracic operations, 502
  reduced, 294
    light absorbance spectrum of,
      295f
  relaxed (R structure) form, 147
  tight (T structure) form, 147
Hemoglobin concentration
  and exercise capacity, 150
  and hematocrit, 149–150
  lower limits of, in surgical patients,
    149–150
  preoperative, 149–150
  in preterm infant with patent ductus
    arteriosus, 541
Hemoglobinometry, 145
Hemoglobin saturation, 286
  measurement of, 294–300
  monitoring
    invasive, 296
    noninvasive, 296–300
  versus oxygen saturation, 294
  and oxygen transport status, 300
Hemomediastinum, postoperative, in
  infant/neonate, manage-
  ment of, 509
Hemopneumothorax, in infant/neonate,
  anesthetic and perioopera-
  tive considerations with,
  515t
Hemoptysis
  after bronchoscopy, 720
  bronchoscopy for, 325
  diagnostic significance of, 324
  intubation with, 429
  with lobar torsion, 711–712
  management of, 428–429, 429f
  massive, causes of, 428, 428t
  mortality from, 428
  one-lung ventilation with, 371,
    373–374
  with tracheal tumors, 447
Hemorrhage. *See also* Hypovolemia;
  Mediastinal hemorrhage;
  Pulmonary hemorrhage
  airway, 428–429. *See also*
    Hemoptysis
  with bronchoscopy, 326
  in mediastinoscopy, 339–340
  postoperative, 715–716

Hemorrhagic shock
  autotransfusion in, 477
  blood replacement in, 477–478
  compensatory mechanisms in, 476
  definition of, 475
  fluid infusion in
    access for, 476
    technique, 476
  inotropes and vasodilators in, 480
  management of, 476–480
  massive transfusion in, 478–479
  rapid-infusion devices used in, 477
  resuscitation with, 476
  stages of, 475–476
  volume replacement in, 476, 477f
Hemothorax
  acute traumatic, 470–471
    classification by severity, 470
    diagnosis of, 470–471
    management of, 471
  in infant/neonate, anesthetic and perioperative considerations with, 515t
  with pleural needle biopsy, 720–721
  postoperative, in infant/neonate, management of, 509
  thoracotomy for, 471, 471t
Henderson-Hasselbalch equation, 156
Heparin, minidose, 718
Heparin therapy, with pulmonary thromboembolism, 718
Hepatic function, neonatal, 488
Hepatitis, 108–109
  risk to health care workers, 109
  transfusion-related, 108, 478
Hepatitis A, 108
  epidemiology of, 108
Hepatitis B
  epidemiology of, 108–109
  prevention, 109
    after exposure, 109
  risks to health care workers, 109
  transfusion-related, 109
  transmission, 109
  vaccine, 109
Hepatitis B immune globulin, 109
Hepatitis B virus, 108–109
  carriers, 109
Hepatitis C. *See* Non-A, non-B hepatitis
Hepatization, 620
Hernia(s). *See also* Diaphragmatic hernia; Hiatus hernia
  foramen of Bochdalek
    in infant/neonate, 526–528, 527f–528f

    anesthetic and perioperative considerations with, 513t
    signs and symptoms of, 526–528
    pathophysiology of, 529f, 529–530
  foramen of Morgagni, in infant/neonate, 526, 528f
    anesthetic and perioperative considerations with, 513t
Herpes simplex
  in AIDS, 101
  resistant to acyclovir, 104
Hetastarch, for volume replacement, in hemorrhagic shock, 477
Hexose-monophosphate shunt, 690, 690f
HFV. *See* High-frequency ventilation
Hiatus hernia, 526
  in infant/neonate, anesthetic and perioperative considerations with, 515t
  paraesophageal (type II), 391
  sliding (type I), 390–391
  surgical repair of, 391
High-frequency jet ventilation
  with air leakage, 711
  with bronchopleural fistula, 422–423
  in bullectomy, 424
  during rigid bronchoscopy, 332, 433–434
  in surgical treatment of esophagorespiratory tract fistula, 397
High-frequency ventilation, 672–676
  airway management and flow patterns in, 673–674, 675t
  closed system, 673–674
  frequency range for, 674, 675t
  humidification with, 674
  and hypoxic pulmonary vasoconstriction, 211
  indications for, 672, 676
  open systems for, 673–674
  physiologic effects of, 675
  principles of, 673
  techniques of, 673–674
  variables related to provision of, 674, 674t
  ventilators for, 674, 674t
Histamine
  effects of, 625
  in lung, 127
    action of, 129
  receptors, in airway smooth muscle, 226t, 227

    release, 625
    drugs causing, 349–350
Histamine$_1$ blockers, 227
Histamine$_2$ blockers
  effects of, on airway resistance, 350
  gastrointestinal actions of, 274–275
  indications for, 391
  premedication, 260, 278
Histotoxic anoxia, 154
HIV. *See* Human immunodeficiency virus
Hodgkin's disease, with AIDS, 101
Hopkins lens telescope, 329, 330f
Horner's syndrome, 568, 571
Hospitalization time, effects of postoperative analgesia on, 584
HTLV-III. *See* Human T-cell lymphotropic virus type III
Human immunodeficiency virus, 96
  antibodies, seronegativity for, 97–98
  antibody tests, limitations of, 97–98
  detection of, 97
  epidemiology of, 96–97
  forms of, 96
  infection, treatment of, 105
  origin of, 96
  screening for, 98
  transmission, 98–99
    heterosexual, 99
    methods of, 99–100
    occupational, 106
  type 1, 96
  type 2, 96
  vaccine development, 104
  virulent mutants, 96
Human T-cell lymphotropic virus type III, 96
Humidification
  with high-frequency ventilation, 674
  in oxygenation and ventilation, 650–652
Humidifier(s)
  aerosol-generating, 651, 652f
  bubble, 651, 651f
  for distending airway pressure therapy, 659
  pass-over, 651, 651f
  position of, in breathing circuit, 651–652
  wick, 651, 651f
Humoral immunity, effects of malnutrition on, 693
Hyaline membrane disease, in infant/neonate, anesthetic and perioperative considerations with, 515t

Hyaline membranes, formation of, 626, 626f

Hydralazine
effect on blood flow and oxygen delivery, 153
and hypoxic pulmonary vasoconstriction, 207, 357

Hydrocortisone, 241
intravenous, 244
pharmacology of, 242, 242t
structure of, 241f

Hydromorphone
front-loading, 579t
premedication, for bronchoscopy, 334

5-Hydroperoxyeicosatetraenoic acid, production of, 122

Hydropneumothorax
complicating bronchopulmonary lavage, 427
with esophageal perforation, 393–394

Hydrothorax, with esophageal perforation, 393–394

Hydroxyeicosatetraenoic acid, metabolism, in lungs, 122

Hydroxyl radicals, in acute respiratory failure, 629

5-Hydroxytryptamine
action of, in lung, 129
handling of, in lungs, 115–116, 127
metabolism, in pulmonary endothelium, 119
uptake
by lung, 127
in pulmonary endothelium, 119

Hydroxyzine
anxiolytic effect, 258, 260, 260f
and opioids, combined effects of, 270, 270f
premedication, 267–268, 270
for infant/neonate, dosage and administration of, 497t

Hyperbaric oxygenation, therapeutic, 146

Hypercapnia
effects on hypoxic pulmonary vasoconstriction, 210–211
ventilatory response to, 177–178, 361
with inhalation anesthesia, 184, 185t
normal variations with age, 182
ventilatory sensitivity to
indices of, 180, 180f
measurement of, 179

Hypercarbia, 15
with congenital diaphragmatic hernia, 530
and development of dysrhythmias, 88
postoperative, 616

Hypercatabolism, 689
nutritional support with, 690–691

Hypercortisonism, 243

Hyperdynamic state(s), 154–156
definition of, 154
systemic oxygen transport in, 154

Hyperglycemia, in response to injury or sepsis, 690

Hyperinflation, with chronic obstructive pulmonary disease, 86

Hypermetabolism, 689
in surgical patients, 685

Hyperoxia, pulmonary, 130

Hypertransfusion, 35
cardiopulmonary effects of, 34

Hyperventilation, in restrictive pulmonary disease, 85

Hypnosis, premedication for, 260

Hypnotics
antianalgesic effect of, 260
definition of, 256
premedication, 260
for infant/neonate, dosage and administration of, 497t
respiratory effects of, 363

Hypocalcemia, neonatal, 492–493

Hypocapnia
in acute respiratory failure, 620
effects on hypoxic pulmonary vasoconstriction, 210

Hypocarbia
and development of dysrhythmias, 88
in restrictive pulmonary disease, 85

Hypoglycemia, in newborn, 492

Hypoinflation, acute, radiographic findings with, 22, 25f, 27

Hypomagnesemia, effects on respiratory muscle strength, 700

Hyponatremia, and lung cancer, 89

Hypophosphatemia
monitoring for, 702
multisystem effects of, 700
TPN-induced, 689

Hypotension, in esophageal surgery, 396

Hypothermia
after massive transfusion of stored blood, 479
in infant/neonate, 493

in trauma patient, management of, 467

Hypoventilation, in bronchoscopy, 326

Hypovolemia
cardiovascular assessment with, 151
hemodynamic and metabolic effects of, 151
and hemoglobin concentration, 150
and hypoxia, 151
reaction of body to, 150–151
restoration of blood volume with, 150

Hypoxemia
anemic, 287
during anesthesia, 350
in bronchoscopy, 326
with congenital diaphragmatic hernia, 529–530
detection of. See also Pulse oximetry
clinical abilities in, 299–300
with endobronchial intubation, 387
in esophageal surgery, 396
hypoxemic, 287
in infant/neonate, 494–495
during one-lung ventilation, causes of, 211
postoperative
evaluation of patient with, 606
prevention and treatment of, 605–611
treatment of, 616–617
prevention of, 593
with pulmonary embolism, 718
in restrictive pulmonary disease, 85
with surgical manipulation, 630
toxic, 287
treatment of, 593
ventilatory response to, with halogenated anesthetics, 359, 361f

Hypoxia. See also Affinity hypoxia
anemic, 143, 148
during anesthesia, 709
anoxic, 143
with chronic obstructive pulmonary disease, 86
definition of, 287
and development of dysrhythmias, 88
hypoxemic, definition of, 287
ischemic, definition of, 287
with pulmonary emboli, 86, 86t
stagnant, 143
types of, 143
ventilatory response to, 178, 178f

effects of malnutrition and refeeding on, 693
indices of, 181, 181f
with inhalation anesthesia, 184, 185t, 361f
with nitrous oxide, 361
normal variations with age, 182
ventilatory sensitivity to, measurement of, 179–180
non-steady-state technique, 180
rebreathing technique, 358
steady-state technique, 179, 358
Hypoxic pulmonary vasoconstriction, 350–352
in atelectatic lung, during anesthesia, determinants of, 206–211, 207f
effect of diazepam on, 363
effect of midazolam on, 363
effects of, on arterial oxygen tension, 206, 206f
effects of anesthetics on
in vitro studies of, 352–353
in vivo studies of, 353–354
leukotrienes in, 122
and nitroglycerin, 205–206
pathophysiology of, 132
and sodium nitroprusside, 205–206
and vasodilators, 356–357

Ibuprofen, for postoperative analgesia, in infant/neonate, dosage and administration of, 507t
Ileus, postoperative, 584
effects of postoperative analgesia on, 584
Immune system, effects of malnutrition on, 693
Immunocompetence, tests of, prognostic significance of, 686
Immunosuppressive therapy, for myasthenia gravis, 404
Inapsine. *See* Droperidol
Incentive spirometry, 603–604
devices for, 603f, 603–604
Indirect colorimetry, 682–683
Indomethacin
as adjuvant to opioid analgesics, 579
for pharmacologic closure of patent ductus arteriosus, 540
Indoprofen, as adjuvant to opioid analgesics, 578
Induction technique
in asthma patient, 9
effects of

on airway resistance, 350
on functional residual capacity, 186, 200
on pulmonary resistance, 173
in esophageal surgery, 395
for infant/neonate, 498–499
for thymectomy, 405–406
for tracheal reconstruction, 453
in trauma care, 466
Inertance, 169
Infant/neonate. *See also* Premature infant
absent pericardium in, anesthetic and perioperative considerations with, 518t
achalasia in, anesthetic and perioperative considerations with, 512t
agenesis, aplasia, or hypoplasia of lung or lobes in, anesthetic and perioperative considerations with, 512t
airway anatomy in, 489, 489t, 490f
airway management in, intraoperative, 505
anesthetic management for, 498–506
arterial blood gas analysis for, during thoracic operations, 502
arterial blood pressure monitoring, during thoracic operations, 500–501
ASA physical status classification, 498
birth-related changes in, 486–489
blood loss, during thoracic operations, assessment of, 502–503
bronchiectasis in, anesthetic and perioperative considerations with, 512t
bronchobiliary fistula in, anesthetic and perioperative considerations with, 512t
bronchography in, anesthesia for, 522–525
bronchopulmonary dysplasia in, anesthetic and perioperative considerations with, 512t
bronchoscopy in, anesthesia for, 511, 522, 525
caloric requirements, 486t, 488
capnometry for, during thoracic operations, 500

cardiac tamponade in, anesthetic and perioperative considerations with, 519t
cardiovascular procedures in, not requiring cardiopulmonary bypass, 523t–524t
central venous pressure monitoring, during thoracic operations, 501–502
chest radiology in, 494f–496f, 495
chylothorax in
anesthetic and perioperative considerations with, 512t
management of, 509–510
coarctation of aorta in, anesthetic and perioperative considerations with, 512t, 523t
corrosive or caustic esophageal injury, anesthetic and perioperative considerations with, 513t
croup (infectious), anesthetic and perioperative considerations with, 513t
cyanotic
evaluation of, 494–496
induction technique for, 498–499
cystic adenomatoid malformation in, anesthetic and perioperative considerations with, 513t
cystic fibrosis in, anesthetic and perioperative considerations with, 513t, 525
cystic hygroma in, anesthetic and perioperative considerations with, 513t
diaphragmatic hernia in, anesthetic and perioperative considerations with, 513t
ectopic bronchus in, anesthetic and perioperative considerations with, 513t
electrocardiography for, during thoracic operations, 500
electrolyte analysis for, during thoracic operations, 502
electrolyte requirements, 488
empyema in, anesthetic and perioperative considerations with, 514t
endotracheal intubation in, 503–505
complications of, 504
effects on respiratory mechanics, 175

Infant/neonate (*Continued*)
  epiglottitis in, anesthetic and perioperative considerations with, 514t
  Erb-Duchenne palsy in, anesthetic and perioperative considerations with, 514t
  esophageal duplication in, anesthetic and perioperative considerations with, 514t
  esophageal perforation in, anesthetic and perioperative considerations with, 514t
  esophageal stenosis in, anesthetic and perioperative considerations with, 514t
  esophageal stricture in, anesthetic and perioperative considerations with, 514t
  esophagitis in, anesthetic and perioperative considerations with, 515t
  eventration of diaphragm in, anesthetic and perioperative considerations with, 515t
  extracorporeal membrane oxygenation for, 676
  extubation, criteria for, 504–505, 505t
  fluid requirements in, 486t, 488
  foramen of Bochdalek hernia in, anesthetic and perioperative considerations with, 513t
  foramen of Morgagni hernia in, anesthetic and perioperative considerations with, 513t
  functional residual capacity in, 175
  gastric distention in, management of, 510–511
  gastroesophageal reflux in, anesthetic and perioperative considerations with, 515t
  glucose determinations in, during thoracic operations, 502
  glucose requirements, 488, 492
  hemoglobin analysis for, during thoracic operations, 502
  hemomediastinum in, management of, 509
  hemopneumothorax in, anesthetic and perioperative considerations with, 515t
  hemothorax in

    anesthetic and perioperative considerations with, 515t
    management of, 509
  hepatic function in, 488
  hiatal hernia in, anesthetic and perioperative considerations with, 515t
  hyaline membrane disease in, anesthetic and perioperative considerations with, 515t
  hypocalcemia in, 492–493
  hypoglycemia in, 492
  immediate postoperative measures for, 505–506
  induction techniques for, 498–499
  Kartagener's syndrome in, anesthetic and perioperative considerations with, 516t
  lobar emphysema in
    acquired, anesthetic and perioperative considerations with, 516t
    congenital, anesthetic and perioperative considerations with, 516t
  low cardiac output in, management of, 511
  lung abscess in, anesthetic and perioperative considerations with, 516t
  lung cysts in
    bronchogenic, anesthetic and perioperative considerations with, 516t
    congenital, anesthetic and perioperative considerations with, 516t
  maintenance of anesthesia in, during thoracic operations, 505
  management of chest tubes in, 508–509
  mediastinal masses in, anesthetic and perioperative considerations with, 517t
  mediastinitis in, anesthetic and perioperative considerations with, 517t
  monitoring, during thoracic operations, 498, 499t, 499–503
  myasthenia gravis in, anesthetic and perioperative considerations with, 517t
  neuromuscular blockade for, during thoracic operations, 502
  oxygen delivery device for, 656–657

  pain perception in, 493–494
  pectus carinatum in, anesthetic and perioperative considerations with, 518t
  pectus excavatum in, anesthetic and perioperative considerations with, 518t
  pericardial cysts in, anesthetic and perioperative considerations with, 518t
  pericardial effusion in, anesthetic and perioperative considerations with, 519t
  pericarditis
    acute, anesthetic and perioperative considerations with, 518t
    chronic constrictive, anesthetic and perioperative considerations with, 518t
  phrenic nerve palsy in, anesthetic and perioperative considerations with, 519t
  pneumatocele in, anesthetic and perioperative considerations with, 519t
  pneumomediastinum in, anesthetic and perioperative considerations with, 517t
  pneumopericardium in, anesthetic and perioperative considerations with, 519t
  pneumothorax in
    anesthetic and perioperative considerations with, 519t
    management of, 508–509
  Poland's syndrome in, anesthetic and perioperative considerations with, 520t
  postanesthetic apnea in, 491–492
  postoperative analgesia for, 505–508
  postoperative atelectasis in, management of, 510
  postoperative complications in, management of, 506–511
  premedication for, 496–498
    dosage and administration of, 497, 497t
    guidelines for, 497t
  preoperative assessment of, 494–496
  preoperative orders for, 496
  preoxygenation, 498, 504
  pulmonary arteriovenous fistula in, anesthetic and perioperative considerations with, 520t

pulmonary artery sling in, anesthetic and perioperative considerations with, 520t, 542

pulmonary sequestration in, anesthetic and perioperative considerations with, 520t

pulse oximetry for, during thoracic operations, 500

renal function in, 488

respiratory insufficiency in, high-frequency ventilation for, 676

respiratory mechanics in, 168–169

right middle lobe syndrome in, anesthetic and perioperative considerations with, 520t

scimitar syndrome in, anesthetic and perioperative considerations with, 520t

sternal clefts in, anesthetic and perioperative considerations with, 520t

stress response, to surgery, 493–494

subcutaneous emphysema in, anesthetic and perioperative considerations with, 521t

subglottic stenosis in, anesthetic and perioperative considerations with, 521t

temperature monitoring, during thoracic operations, 502

tension pneumothorax in, anesthetic and perioperative considerations with, 521t

termination of operation in, 505

thermoregulation for, 493

thymus conditions in, anesthetic and perioperative considerations with, 521t

tracheal stricture in, anesthetic and perioperative considerations with, 521t

tracheomalacia in, anesthetic and perioperative considerations with, 521t

transitional circulation in, 487–488

transport to intensive care unit, 506

upper airway obstruction in, management of, 511

urinary output monitoring, during thoracic operations, 502

vascular rings in, anesthetic and perioperative considerations with, 522t, 524t, 542

ventilatory response to hypoxia, 182

ventilatory support for, postoperative, 506

vocal cord paralysis in, anesthetic and perioperative considerations with, 522t

Infective lung disease

lung transplantation for, 556, 559t, 561

physical signs of, 322

Infiltrate(s)

with acute respiratory failure, 620

alveolar, 27

from aspiration, radiology of, 37

changing, assessing, 48

definition of, 27

diffuse, 45–47

interstitial, 27

localized, 45–47

mediastinal shift with, 711

postoperative, clinical significance of, 31, 31f

from pulmonary embolus, 624

from pulmonary infarction, 44

radiographic findings with, 27–48

related to clinical picture, 45

Infrared absorption

collision-broadening interference, 307–308

interference, and capnometers, 307–308

Infrared absorption spectra, of anesthetic and respiratory gases, 305f, 307

Infrared absorption spectrometry, for carbon dioxide measurement, 304–306, 305f

Inhalation anesthesia

for fiberoptic bronchoscopy, 336

in provision of anesthesia in patient with bronchopleural fistula, 713

Inhalation anesthetics

for AIDS patients, 108

effects of

on cerebral blood flow, 152–153

on respiratory control, 184, 185t

on ventilatory control, 357–361

and hypoxic pulmonary vasoconstriction

clinical studies of, 354–356, 356f

in vivo studies of, 353–354

for thymectomy, 406–407

Inhalation injury, from radioactive dust, bronchopulmonary lavage for, 425

Injury

metabolic response to, 689–690

nutritional implications of, 690–691

nutritional support for, 690–691

Innominate artery, compression, in mediastinoscopy, 339–340

Innovar, effects on incidence of anesthetic convulsions, 271t

Inspiration, muscles of, 165–166

Inspiratory capacity, 6

Inspiratory duty cycle, effects of malnutrition and refeeding on, 694f

Inspiratory positive airway pressure, 636f

Inspired oxygen fraction, increases in, effects of, 146

Inspired oxygen tension

during bronchopulmonary lavage, 426–427

effects of

on arterial oxygen tension, 606–607

on hypoxic pulmonary vasoconstriction, 210

on venous admixture, 606–607, 607f

monitoring of, 156

in one-lung ventilation, 212

provision of different concentrations of, 650

range of, 145, 146t

for respiratory distress syndrome, 490

for support of oxygenation and weaning of support, 670

Intercostal block

effect on respiratory mechanics, 172

in infant/neonate, 505–506

for postoperative analgesia, 568–569, 595

Intercostal muscles, 165

actions of, 166

innervation, 166

reduced tone of, during anesthesia, 173

Intercostal nerve(s), injury, 718–719

with pleural needle biopsy, 720–721

Interface, between different tissues, 19–20

Interferon, recombinant, for AIDS, 105

Interleukin-1, in acute respiratory failure, 629

Intermittent demand ventilation, 666

Intermittent mandatory ventilation, 664–666

in acute respiratory failure, 640–643

Intermittent mandatory
ventilation (*Continued*)
circuit for, 665f, 665–666
with flail chest, 468
weaning, 642t, 642–643
Intermittent positive-pressure breathing, 602–603
side effects of, 602
Internal respiration, definition of, 163
Interpleural block
contraindications to, 572
in infant/neonate, 505–506
for postoperative analgesia, 570–572
Interrupted airways disease
definition of, 671
high-frequency ventilation for, 672,
676
mechanical ventilation with,
671–672
Interstitial air, 48
Interstitial edema, in acute respiratory
failure, 620–621
Interstitial fibrosis, development of, 626
Interstitial fluid. *See also* Lung water
effects of, 627–628, 628f
hydrostatic pressure, 623–624
oncotic pressure, 623
pressure, 623–624
in acute respiratory failure,
627–628
Interstitial pneumonitis, in AIDS, 101
Intramucosal pH, 156
Intrapleural pressure, 594, 594f
Intrapulmonary shunt
in acute respiratory failure, 620
in hypoxic pulmonary vasoconstriction, 351–352
during one-lung ventilation,
204–206, 205f, 208–209,
209f, 350, 355, 356f
postoperative, evaluation of, 606
reduction of, for treatment of acute
respiratory failure, 637
Intravenous anesthesia
effects of, on respiratory control,
185
and hypoxic pulmonary vasoconstriction, clinical studies
of, 354–355, 356f
Intravenous drug abusers, AIDS in, 99
Intravenous fat emulsions, respiratory
effects of, 696–697
Intrinsic ventilatory defect, 7–8
Intubation. *See also* Endobronchial
intubation; Endotracheal
intubation

complications associated with, 68
4-Ipomeanol, pulmonary damage
induced by, 131
Ipratropium bromide
bronchodilator effects of, 237–238
dosage and administration of, 237
duration of action, 237
indications for, 9f
pharmacology of, 237
structure of, 238f
Iron lung, 662
Isoetharine
dosage and administration of, 228t,
229
duration of action, 228t
mechanism of action, 228t
pharmacology of, 229
postoperative administration of, 613
relative potency of, 229
structure of, 227f
Isoflurane
cerebrovascular effects of, 151–152
effects of
on airway resistance, 349–350
on arterial oxygenation, during
one-lung ventilation, 208
on blood flow distribution, shunt
flow, and arterial oxygen
tension in one-lung ventilation, 209–210
on chest recoil, 348
on respiratory control, 184, 185t
on ventilatory control, 358–361
on ventilatory response to carbon
dioxide, 360f
on ventilatory response to hypoxia, 361f
and hypoxic pulmonary vasoconstriction
clinical studies of, 354–356, 356f
in vitro studies of, 353, 353f
in vivo studies of, 354, 354f–355f
neuromuscular effects of, in myasthenic patients, 406–407
Isoniazid, indications for, in AIDS, 104
Isoproterenol, 229
dosage and administration of, 228t
duration of action, 228t
intravenous, 229
mechanism of action, 228t
metabolism, by lung, 131
postoperative administration of, 613
relative potency of, 229
structure of, 227f
Isothermal saturation boundary,
650–651

Isovolume technique, 171

Kaposi's sarcoma
in AIDS, 95–96, 101
and airway management, 108
Karnofsky scale of performance, 90, 90t
Kartagener's syndrome, in
infant/neonate, anesthetic
and perioperative consid-
erations with, 516t
K cells, 117, 127
Kerley B lines, 35, 36f
Ketamine
antiarrhythmic properties, 474
with cardiac tamponade, 474
effects of
on airway resistance, 349–350
on functional residual capacity,
173
on incidence of anesthetic convulsions, 271t
on lung metabolism, 132
on respiratory control, 185
emergence phenomena with, 361
and hypoxic pulmonary vasoconstriction
clinical studies of, 354–355
in vivo studies of, 353
induction technique
in hypovolemic hemorrhagic
shock, 466
for infant/neonate, 499
myocardial contractility with, 474,
474t
nasal instillation, 276
respiratory effects of, 361, 364t
Ketorolac, as adjuvant to opioid analgesics, 578
Kidney. *See also* Renal
in hypovolemia, 151
Killer cells, 97
Kinetic halo, 50
Kinins, actions of, in lung, 127
Klebsiella pneumoniae, 31
Kussmaul's sign, 473

Lactic acidemia, 157
Lactic acidosis, in hyperdynamic state,
154
Lambert-Beer equation, 294–295
Lambert-Eaton myasthenic syndrome.
See Eaton-Lambert (myas-
thenic) syndrome
Laryngeal edema, in children, 522
Laryngeal injury, postintubation, 448
Laryngoscopy

with mediastinal mass, 398–399
sympathetic response to, 326
in tracheal reconstruction, 453
ventilation during, 676
Laryngospasm, with bronchoscopy, 326
Larynx
anesthesia of, 335–336
laser surgery of, ventilation for, 436
nerve supply of, 335f
Laser(s)
characteristics of, 429, 430t
critical volume for, 430
definition of, 429
extinction length of, 430
power density of, 430
Laser-Flex tube, 435
Laser-Guard endotracheal tube wrapping, 434–435
Laser Shield tube, 435
Laser therapy
aiming beam for, 432
airway fire with, 431, 436–437
for airway tumors, results of, 431
anesthesia for, 429–437
with bronchoscopy, 333, 432
choice of anesthesia gases for, 436
choice of laser, 432
complications of, 431
endotracheal tube protection during, 434–435
general anesthesia for, 432–433
hazards of, 431–432
helium/oxygen protocol for, 436, 436t
local versus general anesthesia for, 434
mortality in, 431
Lateral decubitus position
blood flow distribution in, with two-lung ventilation, factors affecting, 208
distribution of perfusion and ventilation in, 197–203, 205, 596
in anesthetized, closed chest conditions, 200–201
in anesthetized, open chest, paralyzed conditions, 201f, 201–202, 202f
in anesthetized, open chest conditions, 201, 201f
in awake patient, 197–200
effects on ventilation-perfusion matching, 187–188
physiology of, 197–203
Lateral position test, 10–11

LAV. *See* Lymphadenopathy virus
LBM. *See* Lean body mass
Lean body mass, 684
Left ventricular dysfunction, 87–88
with right ventricular hypertrophy, 88
Left ventricular end-diastolic pressure, 639–640
Left ventricular failure, 624
Left ventricular hypoplasia, with congenital diaphragmatic hernia, 529–530
Legs, intermittent pneumatic compression of, 718
Leukotriene(s)
actions, within lung, 122
and acute lung injury, 133
in acute respiratory failure, 629
bronchoconstrictor effect, 227
pulmonary metabolism of, 122
receptors, in airways, 227
release
cellular source of, 122
from lung, 122
Levorphanol, front-loading, 579t
Lidocaine
anesthesia, for flexible fiberoptic bronchoscopy, 334–335
effects of, on respiratory control, 185
plus epinephrine, for postoperative epidural analgesia, 573
pulmonary uptake of, 132
respiratory effects of, 361–362
toxic reaction to, 326
Life support devices
malplacement of, 63–78, 68f, 80f
position of, radiographic study of, 63–78
radiographic appearance of, 63–78
Light absorption
of hemoglobin species, 295f
through living tissue, 296f, 297
Lipids, respiratory effects of, 696–697
Lipid tolerance, testing, 701–702
Lipoxins
actions, in lungs, 125
formation of, by alveolar macrophages, 125
5-Lipoxygenase, 122
activities, in lungs, 125
15-Lipoxygenase, activities, in lungs, 125
Liver, during anesthesia, 151
Lobar torsion
postoperative, 711–713

radiographic findings with, 711–712
Lobectomy. *See also* Pulmonary resection
indications for, 712–713
predicted postoperative FEV_1 with, 11
radiographic findings after, 61–63
Local anesthesia
for flexible fiberoptic bronchoscopy, 334–336
for laser therapy, 434
respiratory effects of, 361–362
Local anesthetics
epidural, for postoperative analgesia, 595–596
in infant/neonate, 508
infusion, for postoperative epidural analgesia, 573
intrapleural, for postoperative analgesia, in infant/neonate, 508
lumbar administration of, for postoperative analgesia, in infant/neonate, 508
and opioids, combined infusions of, for postoperative analgesia, 577–578
paravertebral spread of, 568, 569f
thoracic administration of, for postoperative analgesia, in infant/neonate, 508
toxicity, with bronchoscopy, 326
Lorazepam
amnesic effect, 259
premedication, 271, 273t
dosage and administration of, 272
duration of action, 272
pharmacology of, 272, 272f
respiratory effects of, 363
Lordosis, on chest x-ray, 22, 24f
Lower esophageal sphincter
incompetent, 391
pressure
drugs affecting, 390, 390t
factors affecting, 390
Lung(s)
abscess in. *See* Abscess
agenesis, aplasia, or hypoplasia of, in infant/neonate, anesthetic and perioperative considerations with, 512t
alveolar region of, cellular composition of, 116t
bioactive peptides in, 125t, 125–127
cell types in, 115

Lung(s) *(Continued)*
    collapse, in open chest, 203f, 204
    cytochrome P-450-dependent
        metabolism in, 116
    elastic properties of, 167–168
    elastic recoil pressure of, 3f
    as endocrine organ, 119
    equilibrium position of, 167
    fluid fluxes across, 622–624
    gradient of pleural pressure in. *See*
        Pleural pressure, gradient
        of
    handling of biologically active com-
        pounds by, 115, 116t
    intrapulmonary gas distribution,
        effects of anesthesia on,
        186–188
    metabolic and hormonal functions
        of, 115–133
    metabolic and secretory components
        of, 115–118
    metabolic enzyme pathways present
        in, 131, 131t
    metabolic processes within, 118–119
    metabolism of humoral substances
        at cell surface within,
        118–119
    metabolism of xenobiotics in,
        116–117, 130–132, 131t
    microvascular permeability in,
        effects of sympathomimet-
        ics on, 232–233
    physiologic actions of peptides in,
        127
    preoperative examination of, 322
    pressure across, 169
    processing and action of specific
        factors in, 119–130
    radiographic appearance of, in
        intraoperative or postoper-
        ative period, 25–26, 44–
        48
    relaxation pressure volume charac-
        teristics of, 167, 167f
    septic emboli in, radiography of,
        32
    synthesis and release of vasoactive
        compounds, 118–119
    uptake mechanisms for humoral
        substances, 118–119
Lung cancer
    coexistent disease, 1
    extrapulmonary syndromes associat-
        ed with, 89
    histopathologic cell types, 1–2
    K cells in, 117

non-oat-cell, prognosis for, and
        serum albumin levels,
        685–686, 686f
    pulmonary resection for, complica-
        tions of, 686
    resectability, diagnosis and evalua-
        tion of, 2
    screening for, 1
    staging of, 91, 720
    surgery for, 257
Lung compartments, impedance of,
        662f
Lung cysts
    classification of, 423
    functional impairment with, 423
    in infant/neonate
        bronchogenic, anesthetic and
            perioperative considera-
            tions with, 516t
        congenital, anesthetic and peri-
            operative considerations
            with, 516t
Lung function, pulmonary metabolic
        processes as clinical indi-
        cators of, 133
Lung injury
    acute, pathophysiology of, 132–133
    metabolized xenobiotics associated
        with, 131, 131t
Lung resection. *See* Pulmonary resec-
        tion
Lung scans, with pulmonary embolism,
        718
Lung transplantation, 555–562
    anesthetic technique for, 558, 558t
    arteriovenous bypass for, 559
    cardiac assessment for, 557, 557t,
        560, 560t
    cardiopulmonary bypass for,
        558–559
    double-lung
        indications for, 556
        operative procedure, 558
        survival, 555
    exercise testing for, 557, 560, 561t
    history of, 555–556
    indications for, 555–556
    intraoperative management,
        558–561
    mortality after, 555
    operative procedure, 557–558
    outcome with, 561–562
    potential intraoperative problems,
        556
    preoperative assessment for,
        556–557

pulmonary assessment for, 557,
        557t, 560, 560t
    results, 559–560
    selection criteria for, 557t
    single-lung, 561–562
        indications for, 556, 558–559,
            559t
        operative procedure, 557
    survival, 555
    ventilation for, 560–561
Lung volume(s), 594, 594f
    in acute respiratory failure, 620–622
    determination of, 5–6
    effects of anesthesia on, 348
    end-expiratory, dynamically deter-
        mined, 168–169
    normal, 8f
    physiologic determinants of,
        166–169
    resting, alteration of, 649, 653
    with restrictive lung disease, 8f
Lung water
    and disease states, 624–628
    measurement of, 625
Lymphadenopathy virus, 96
Lymphatics, pulmonary, 622–623
    efficiency of, evaluation of, 626
Lymphoma, mediastinal, 400

MACH effect, 49
Macintosh-Leatherdale combined endo-
        bronchial tube and
        bronchial blocker, 376,
        377f
Macintosh-Leatherdale left-sided single-
        lumen endobronchial tube,
        375f, 375–376
Magill balloon-tipped bronchial block-
        er, 372–373, 373f
Magnetic resonance imaging, of medi-
        astinum, 55
Magnification, of x-rays, 22
Malnutrition. *See also* Refeeding
    clinical effects of, 685–686
    diagnosis of, 686–687
    effects of, 685–687
    and extracellular water, 684
    metabolic changes in, 685
    respiratory effects of, 691–695
    respiratory effects of proteins in,
        699, 699f
    and resting energy expenditure, 683
    and risk of infection, 91
Mannitol, effects on renal function in
        posttraumatic renal fail-
        ure, 480

Mass spectrometry, for carbon dioxide measurement, 303–304, 304f
Mast cell-derived mediators, 118t
  release, inhibition of
    by cromolyn sodium, 239
    by sympathomimetics, 232
    by theophylline, 236
Mast cells, pulmonary, 118
Maximal inspiratory pressure, 166, 167f
Maximal oxygen consumption, 14
  in differentiation of cardiac versus pulmonary impairment, 14t
Maximum expiratory pressure, 166, 167f
Maximum mid-expiratory flow rate, 3
Maximum voluntary ventilation, 3, 9–10
MCHC. *See* Mean corpuscular hemoglobin concentration
Mean corpuscular hemoglobin concentration, 147
  effect on oxyhemoglobin dissociation, 148, 148t
Mean inspiratory flow, effects of malnutrition and refeeding on, 694f
Mechanical ventilation, 257–258
  in acute respiratory failure, 634–644
  after near-drowning, 630
  airway pressure and flow during, 666, 667f
  with bronchopleural fistula, 671–672
  effects of, on lung volume, 595
  with interrupted airways disease, 671–672
  nutritional aspects of, 700–701
  postoperative
    evaluation of patient for, 616
    management of, 616–617
  prophylactic, 595
  for respiratory distress syndrome, 490
Mechanical ventilator(s), 661–671
  monitors and alarms with, 670
  negative-pressure, 662
  positive-pressure, 662–669
    automatic cycling, 664
    cycling mechanisms, 663–664
    elbow connectors, 668
    flow-cycled, 664
    mechanical dead space, 668
    mechanism for volume delivery, 663, 663f
    modes of ventilation, 664–666
    patient-triggered cycling, 664

power source, 663
    pressure-cycled, 664
    principle of, 662–663
    time-cycled, 664
    volume-cycled, 664
  safety features of, 670
  selection of, 669–670
Mechanical ventilatory pattern(s), 668–669
  and airway resistance, 668–669
  and compliance, 668–669
  expiratory phase, 668–669
  expiratory pressure pattern, 669
  expiratory time, 669
  frequency
    for support of ventilation, 670
    for weaning of support, 670–671
  inspiratory/expiratory time relationships, 669
  inspiratory hold, 668–669
  inspiratory phase, 668–669
  inspiratory pressure pattern and flow rate, 668–669
  inspiratory time, 669
Mechanomyography, 405, 407f
Meconium aspiration syndrome, extracorporeal membrane oxygenation in, 676
Median sternotomy
  bronchial isolation in, 374
  in bullectomy, 424
Mediastinal air
  in postoperative portable examinations, 49
  radiographic appearance of, 49–50, 50f
Mediastinal hemorrhage, postoperative, 52–55
  radiographic appearance of, 54f
Mediastinal mass
  anesthetic considerations with, 397–401
  cardiac involvement with, 400–401
  computed tomography of, in pediatric patient, 537, 538f
  diagnosis of, 338
  in pediatric patient
    anesthetic and perioperative considerations with, 517t, 537–539
    on chest x-ray, 537, 539t
    radiographic evaluation of, 537
    risk of airway obstruction or cardiovascular collapse during repair of, 539, 539t

preoperative assessment with, algorithm for, 398, 399f
  pulmonary arterial involvement with, 400–401
  radiation therapy for, effects on ventilatory function, 398, 400f
  superior vena cava syndrome with, 400–401, 401f
    postoperative complications with, 401
  tracheobronchial obstruction by, 397–400
    anesthetic management of, 397–400
Mediastinal shift, 30f–31f
  absence of, clinical significance of, 59
  after pneumonectomy, 711, 712f
  assessment of, 52
  excessive, 711
  postoperative, 711
  in spontaneously ventilating patient with open chest in lateral decubitus position, 203f, 203–204
  with tension pneumothorax, 52, 53f
Mediastinal widening, 55
  actual, 52
  after tracheostomy, 70
  apparent, 52
    on chest x-ray, 22
  with esophageal perforation, 393
  mass producing, computed tomography of, 55, 56f
Mediastinitis, 397
  in infant/neonate, anesthetic and perioperative considerations with, 517t
Mediastinoscope(s), 337, 337f
Mediastinoscopy
  anesthetic technique for, 339–340
  approaches to, 338
  complications of, 339–340, 720
  contraindications to, 338
  in diagnosis of tumors, 338
  diagnostic yield of, 340
  in evaluation of resectability of cancer, 2
  historical development of, 337–338
  indications for, 91, 338
  morbidity and mortality of, 340
  postoperative concerns with, 340
  premedication for, 258
  preoperative evaluation for, 338–339
  safety of, 340

Mediastinotomy, in evaluation of
        resectability of cancer, 2
Mediastinum
    radiology of, 52–55
    radiolucent halo around, 49–50
    role in paradox, 714
Mendelson's syndrome, 37
Meperidine
    effects of
        on airway resistance, 349–350
        on lung elastic recoil, 348
    epidural, for postoperative analgesia
        dosage and administration of,
            575t
        duration of action, 575t
    front-loading, 579t
    for postoperative analgesia, in
        infant/neonate, dosage and
        administration of, 507t
    premedication
        for bronchoscopy, 334
        for infant/neonate, dosage and
            administration of, 497t
    pulmonary uptake of, 132
Mestinon. *See* Pyridostigmine
Metabolic acidosis
    with congenital diaphragmatic her-
        nia, 530
    ventilatory response to, 178
    ventilatory sensitivity to, testing,
        180
Metabolic alkalosis
    prevention of, 273–274
    ventilatory response to, 178–179
    and ventilatory support, 661
Metaproterenol, 227
    dosage and administration of, 228t,
        230
    duration of action, 228t, 230
    mechanism of action, 228t
    pharmacology of, 230
    postoperative administration of, 613
    relative potency of, 229–230
    structure of, 227f
Metaraminol, metabolism, by lung,
        131
Methadone
    front-loading, 579t
    for postoperative analgesia, in
        infant/neonate, 507
        dosage and administration of,
            507t
Methemoglobin, 294
    light absorbance spectrum of, 295f
Methohexital
    effects of

    on airway resistance, 349
    on functional residual capacity,
        173
    and hypoxic pulmonary vasocon-
        striction, clinical studies
        of, 354
    premedication, for infant/neonate,
        dosage and administration
        of, 497t
Methoxyflurane, and hypoxic pul-
        monary vasoconstriction,
        in vitro studies of, 353
Methylprednisolone, 241
    intravenous, 244
    for myasthenia gravis, 404
    pharmacology of, 242, 242t
    structure of, 241f
Methylxanthines, postoperative admin-
        istration of, 613
Metoclopramide
    gastrointestinal actions of, 275
    indications for, 391
    premedication, 260, 278
Metocurine, effects of, on airway resis-
        tance, 350
Microatelectasis, radiographic picture
        of, 34
Microvascular pressure
    in acute respiratory failure, 629
    factors affecting, 624
Midazolam
    amnesic effect, 259, 273
    effects of, on airway resistance,
        350
    indications for, 271
    paradoxic response to, 273
    pharmacology of, 273
    in postoperative management of
        infant/neonate, 507
    premedication, 273, 273t
        duration of action, 273
        for infant/neonate, dosage and
            administration of, 497t
    respiratory effects of, 363
Minimum alveolar concentration, and
        effects of inhalation anes-
        thesia on respiration, 184,
        185t
Minitracheostomy, 445
Minute ventilation, 661
    effects of amino acid administration
        on, 697–699
    effects of malnutrition and refeeding
        on, 694f
    in ventilatory response to hypercap-
        nia, 180, 180f

Minute volume, during and after thora-
        cotomy and upper abdom-
        inal surgery, 89
Mitomycin C, pulmonary damage
        induced by, 131
Mitral stenosis, hemoptysis with, 428
Mitral valvular disease, radiographic
        findings with, 27, 37
Mixed venous blood sampling, 286
Mixed venous oxygen saturation, 286
Mixed venous oxygen tension
    during anesthesia, 350
    and hypoxic pulmonary vasocon-
        striction, 210, 353
    monitoring, clinical utility of, 296
Monitoring
    during anesthesia, 709–710
    with cardiac tamponade, 473
    in esophageal surgery, 395
    with flail chest, 468–469
    of infant/neonate, during thoracic
        operations, 498, 499t,
        499–503
    of oxygenation, importance of,
        285
    for pulmonary resection, 420
    of systemic oxygen transport during
        surgery, 156
    in thymectomy, 405
    during total parenteral nutrition,
        701–702, 702t
    during tracheal reconstruction,
        452–453
    during tracheostomy, 441
    in trauma care, 466
    of ventilation, 300–311
        importance of, 285
Monitoring devices
    malplacement of, 63–78, 68f, 80f
    position of, radiographic study of,
        63–78
    radiographic appearance, 63–78
Monoamine oxidase, 119
    activity of, 127, 128f
Morphine
    and bupivacaine, combined infu-
        sions of, for postoperative
        analgesia, 577–578
    caudal, for postoperative analgesia,
        in infant/neonate, 508
    effects of
        on airway resistance, 349–350
        on ventilatory control, 358
    epidural
        for postoperative analgesia, 575,
            596

dosage and administration of, 575t
duration of action, 575t
starting doses, 575t
respiratory effects of, 362
front-loading, 579t
for hypercyanotic episodes with tetralogy of Fallot, 497
intrathecal, for postoperative analgesia, 574
intravenous, for postoperative analgesia, in infant/neonate, 506–507
oral, 276
for postoperative analgesia, in infant/neonate, dosage and administration of, 507t
premedication, 258, 261, 265–267
for bronchoscopy, 334
dosage and administration of, 265–266
effects of, on respiratory control, 185, 186f
history of, 256
for infant/neonate, dosage and administration of, 497t
pulmonary uptake of, 132
spinal, for postoperative analgesia, dosage and administration of, 576–577
subarachnoid
for myasthenic patients, 409
for postoperative analgesia
dosage and administration of, 575t
duration of action, 575t
for thymectomy, 411
Motor vehicle accident(s)
alcohol-related, 463
chest injury in, 463
mortality rate, 463
numbers of, 463
Mucociliary clearance
with atropine, 237
with sympathomimetics, 233
with theophylline, 236
Mucolytics
indications for, 614
inhalant products, 615t
Mucus-producing cells, 224
Muscle relaxants
effects on respiratory mechanics, 174
for myasthenic patients, 407–408
respiratory effects of, 364t

MVV. *See* Maximum voluntary ventilation
Myasthenia gravis
autoimmune aspects of, 402
cholinergic crisis in, 403–404
clinical classification of, 402t
diagnosis of, 402–403
immunosuppressive therapy, 404
incidence of, 401
in infant/neonate, anesthetic and perioperative considerations with, 517t
medical treatment of, 403
versus surgical management of, 404
versus myasthenic syndrome, 413t
neuromuscular assessment in, 405
pathophysiology of, 401–402
plasmapheresis for, 404
preoperative, 411
postoperative ventilatory requirement in, 409–411
techniques to decrease, 411
prevalence of, 401
responses of patients in remission, 409
reversal of residual neuromuscular blockade in, 408–409
sensitivities to medications in, 409
steroid therapy, 404
thymus gland in, 404
treatment of, thymectomy for, 401, 404–405
effects of, 412
types of, 401
Myasthenic crisis, 403
Myasthenic syndrome, 412–413
versus myasthenia gravis, 413t
Mycobacterium avium-intracellulare, in AIDS, 101
Mycoplasma pneumoniae, 31
Myocardial depressant factor, 151
Myocardial dysfunction
with AIDS, 102
with congenital diaphragmatic hernia, 529–530
Myocardial perforation, with transvenous pacemaker, 79f
Myocarditis, with AIDS, 102
Myofascial pain, of post-thoracotomy pain syndrome, 719
Mytelase. *See* Ambenonium

Nalbuphine
front-loading, 579t

premedication, 265–267
Naloxone
effects of, on airway resistance, 349
for opioid-induced respiratory depression, 576
Narcotic analgesics, definition of, 255–256
Narcotics
definition of, 255–256
intravenous
for AIDS patients, 108
for postoperative analgesia, in infant/neonate, 506–507
premedication
for bronchoscopy, 334
for infant/neonate, dosage and administration of, 497t
respiratory effects of, 364t
spinal, for children, 564
Nasal cannula, for oxygen therapy, 653, 654t
Nasal catheter, for oxygen therapy, 653, 654t
Nasogastric intubation
with congenital diaphragmatic hernia, 530
in infant/neonate, 505, 511
Nasogastric tubes, placement of, radiographic evaluation of, 70
Nasotracheal intubation, in pediatric patient, 489, 553–554
for thoracic surgery, 503
Nasotracheal suction, 600–601
Near-drowning, 630–631
Nebulizers, 652–653
Necrotizing enterocolitis, and patent ductus arteriosus, 540
Nedocromil sodium
dosage and administration of, 240
mechanism of action, 240
pharmacology of, 240
structure of, 239f
Needle tracheostomy, 443
Nembutal. *See* Pentobarbital
Neodymium-yttrium-garnet laser
characteristics of, 429, 430t
choice of endotracheal tube for, 435–436
critical volume for, 430
mechanism of action, 432
methods of use, 432
use of, through endotracheal tube, 434
Neonate. *See* Infant/neonate; Pediatric patient

Neoplasms
   with AIDS, 101
   bronchial, signs and symptoms of, 324
Neostigmine (Prostigmin)
   effects of, on airway resistance, 350
   for myasthenia gravis, 403, 403t
Nerve injuries, surgical, 718–720
Neuroepithelial bodies, 117
Neurologic syndromes, in AIDS, 101–102
Neuromuscular blockade
   for infant/neonate, during thoracic operations, 502
   precautions with, in trauma patient, 467
   for surgical repair of congenital diaphragmatic hernia, 532
Neuromyopathic syndromes, with lung cancer, 89
Neuropathies, with AIDS, 102
Neurovascular surgery, ventilation during, 676
Neutrophil aggregation, in acute respiratory failure, 629
Neutrophils, in acute respiratory failure, 629
Nicardipine, and hypoxic pulmonary vasoconstriction, 357
Nicomorphine, and bupivacaine, combined infusions of, for postoperative analgesia, 578
Nifedipine
   effect on blood flow and oxygen delivery, 153
   and hypoxic pulmonary vasoconstriction, 357
Nissen fundoplication, 391
Nitrofurantoin, pulmonary damage induced by, 131
Nitrogen balance
   definition of, 683
   and energy intake
      in malnourished patients, 688, 688f
      in surgical patients, 688, 688f
   in nutritional support for septic patient, 691, 692f
Nitrogen washout, for determining lung volume, 5, 6f
Nitroglycerin
   effects on blood flow and oxygen delivery, 153
   and hypoxic pulmonary vasoconstriction, 207, 357

nasal instillation, 276
transdermal, 276
Nitroprusside
   effects on hypoxic pulmonary vasoconstriction, 207
   in treatment of right heart failure, 717
Nitrous oxide, 173
   effects of
      on hypoxic pulmonary vasoconstriction, 208
      on lung metabolism, 132
      on ventilatory control, 361
      on ventilatory response to carbon dioxide, 360f
   in esophageal surgery, 396
   respiratory effects of, 364t
   subanesthetic doses, for analgesia, 578
Nociception
   definition of, 564
   modulation of, 566
Nociceptors, 565
Non-A, non-B hepatitis
   epidemiology of, 109
   morbidity and mortality of, 109
   posttransfusion, 109
   prevention, 109
   screening blood for, 109
   test for antibody to, 109
Nondepolarizing relaxants, for myasthenic patients, 408
Non-Hodgkin's lymphomas, with AIDS, 101
Nonspecific interstitial pneumonitis, in AIDS, 101
Nonsteroidal anti-inflammatory drugs, as adjuvants to opioid analgesics, 578
Norepinephrine, 229
   action of, in lung, 129
   handling of, in lungs, 115–116, 127
   indications for, 153
   metabolism of, 127, 128f
      in pulmonary endothelium, 119
   structure of, 227f
   uptake, in pulmonary endothelium, 119
Nosocomial infection(s), risk of
   with chronic pulmonary disease, 88–89
   perioperative management, 91
Noxious stimulus, definition of, 564
5'-Nucleotidase, 128
   in pulmonary endothelial cells, 118–119

Nutrients, caloric content of, 682
Nutrition, and respiratory system, 691–701
Nutritional status, and risk of infection, 91
Nutritional support
   catheter-related infections with, 702–703
   enteral versus parenteral, 701–703
   goals of, 690–691
   with hypercatabolism, 690–691
   postoperative, 689–691
      goals of, 690–691
      requirements for, 691
   preoperative, 685–689
      and postoperative course, 687–688
   of thoracic surgical patient, 681–703
   of uncomplicated postoperative patient, 690–691
   during weaning from mechanical ventilation, 701

Oat cell carcinoma, 1–2
Obesity
   effects of, on functional residual capacity, 621
   respiratory mechanics in, during anesthesia, 172
Obstructive lung disease. *See also* Chronic obstructive pulmonary disease
   functional residual capacity in, 168
   lung transplantation for, 556, 559t, 561
   physical signs of, 322
Obstructive ventilatory defects, 7–8
Occlusion pressure, 182
   in chronic obstructive pulmonary disease, 183
Oliguria, after major trauma, 480
One-lung intubation. *See* Endobronchial intubation
One-lung ventilation, 193
   arterial oxygenation in, 204–205, 314, 350
   blood flow distribution, shunt flow, and arterial oxygen tension in
      effects of isoflurane on, 209–210
      factors affecting, 208–209, 209f
   blood flow distribution during, 204–211, 205f, 357
      to dependent, ventilated lung, 211

to nondependent, nonventilated lung, 205–211

carbon dioxide elimination in, 204–205

continuous positive airway pressure (CPAP) in, selective application of, 213f, 214–215

differential lung CPAP (nondependent lung)/PEEP (dependent lung), 213f, 215–217

differential lung management in, 212–216, 356

in esophageal surgery, 396

hypercapnia in, 210–211

hypocapnia in, 210

hypoxemia during, causes of, 211

indications for, 371–372, 372t

inspired oxygen concentration in, 212

intrapulmonary shunting during, 204–206, 205f, 208–209, 209f, 350, 355, 356f

management of, 211–217

monitoring of ventilation during, 314–315

need for, 371

physiology of, 204–217

positive end-expiratory pressure in, selective dependent-lung, 212–214, 213f

pulse oximetry during, 312, 313f

recommended protocol for, 216f, 216–217

respiratory rate in, 212

tidal volume in, 212

transcutaneous carbon dioxide monitoring in, 312, 313f

ventilation-perfusion relationships in, 16, 355–356

Open chest

paradoxical respiration with, 203f, 204

and spontaneous ventilation, physiology of, 203f, 203–204

Opioids, 258

analgesia with, 265

and ataractic drugs, combined effects of, 268, 269f

effects of, on ventilatory control, 357–358

epidural

for postoperative analgesia, 574

respiratory depression with, 575–576

side effects of, 575

and euphoria, 266–267

front-loading, 579, 579t

and hydroxyzine, combined effects of, 270, 270f

minimum effective analgesic concentration, 579

premedication, 258, 261, 265–267

effects on incidence of anesthetic convulsions, 271

PRN depot administration, versus patient-controlled analgesia, 580–581, 580f

respiratory depression with, 265–266, 266f

spinal

complications of, 362

for postoperative analgesia, 573–577

dosage and administration of, 574, 575t

respiratory effects of, 362

respiratory monitoring with, guidelines for, 576, 576t

systemic

dosage and administration of, 579t, 579–580

pharmacology of, 579–580

for postoperative analgesia, 579–580

Opportunistic infection(s), in AIDS, 100–101

Optode arterial oxygen tension, with endobronchial intubation, 312–314, 314f

Oropharyngeal bougie, in esophageal surgery, 396

Orotracheal intubation, in pediatric patient, 553–554

for thoracic surgery, 503

Orthopnea, diagnostic significance of, 338–339

Otolaryngologic surgery, ventilation during, 676

Oximeter, 296

Oxygenation. *See also* Arterial oxygenation; Extracorporeal membrane oxygenation

in acute respiratory failure, 620

during bronchopulmonary lavage, 427

in bronchoscopy, 326–327

during bullectomy, 424

with endobronchial intubation, 312–313, 314f

evaluation of, 15

features in common with ventilation, 649–653

measurement of, 285–287

monitoring of, 156–157

applications in thoracic surgery, 311–314

importance of, 285

postoperative

factors affecting, 630

principles of, 606

preoperative assessment of, 322–324

provision of fresh gas into circuits, 649–650

provision of medication via airways in, 652–653, 653f

provision of water vapor in, 650–652

support of, 649, 653–660

Oxygen capacity, definition of, 294

Oxygen conformity, 154

definition of, 163

Oxygen consumption. *See also* Maximal oxygen consumption

calculation of, 286

definition of, 286

effects of carbohydrates on, 696

effects of malnutrition and refeeding on, 694f

measurement of, 682–683

to predict morbidity and mortality, 12–14

Oxygen debt, 155–156

Oxygen delivery, 145–153. *See also* Oxygen transport

in anemia, 150

calculation of, 286

definition of, 286

in hypovolemia, 150–151

in sickle cell disease, 150

Oxygen delivery index, 286

Oxygen extraction ratio, 286–287

definition of, 163

Oxygen free radicals, in acute respiratory failure, 629

Oxygen-hemoglobin dissociation, 146–148

factors affecting, 148, 148t

Oxygen mask(s), 654t, 654–658

aerosol, 654t, 655, 655f

for closed systems, 654t, 657f, 657–658, 658f

face shield, 654t, 655

hoods, 654t, 656–657

incubators, 654t, 656–657

non-rebreathing mask, 654t, 655

partial rebreathing mask, 654t, 655

simple, 654t, 654–655

tents, 654t, 656–657

tracheostomy collar, 654t, 655

Oxygen mask(s) (*Continued*)
  T tube, 654t, 655–656
Oxygen pulse, 14–15
Oxygen saturation, definition of, 294
Oxygen tension, 145–146, 285. *See also*
    Alveolar oxygen tension
  continuous monitoring of, 287–294
    invasive, 287–290
    noninvasive, 290–294
  measurement of, 287
  relationship of, to saturation of
    hemoglobin, 146–147,
    147f
Oxygen therapy
  for acute respiratory failure,
    632–633
  delivery devices, 608–610, 653–658,
    654t
    for infant/neonate, 656–657
  for hypercyanotic episodes with
    tetralogy of Fallot, 497
  indications for, 146
  post-thoracotomy, delivery systems
    for, 608–610
  precautions with, 606–607
  in premature infant, and retrolental
    fibroplasia, 490–491
  supplemental, 649
    provision of, 653–658
Oxygen toxicity, pulmonary, 130
Oxygen transport. *See also* Oxygen
    delivery
  abbreviations and definitions for,
    162
  calculation of, 154, 285–287
  components of, 143
  with high-frequency ventilation, 675
  in sepsis, 154
  in septic shock, 144
  systemic, 143–157
Oxygen uptake
  calculation of, 154
  measurement of, 154
  in sepsis, 154
  supply dependency of, 154–155
Oxygen utilization. *See also* Oxygen
    uptake
Oxyhemoglobin, 294
  light absorbance spectrum of, 295f
Oxyhemoglobin dissociation curve, 147f
  loading part of, 147, 147f
  P_{50}, 147–148
  right shift, 147
  unloading part of, 147, 147f
Oxyhemoglobin fraction, definition of,
    294

Oxymorphone, effects of, on airway
    resistance, 349
$P_{0.1}$. *See* Occlusion pressure
Pacemaker(s)
  atrioventricular sequential, proper
    placement of, 78, 78f
  cardiac, complications of, 78
  complications of, radiographic evi-
    dence of, 78
  for infant/neonate, implantation
    anesthetic and perioperative con-
      siderations with, 524t
    description of, 524t
  transvenous
    aberrant location of, radiograph-
      ic evaluation of, 76f,
      76–78, 77f
    malplacement of, 78, 80f
    proper placement of, 76
    vessel perforation, 78, 80f
P_ACO_2. *See* Alveolar carbon dioxide ten-
    sion
$PaCO_2$. *See* Arterial carbon dioxide ten-
    sion
Pain. *See also* Postoperative pain; Post-
    thoracotomy pain syn-
    drome
  acute
    definition of, 564
    model of, 566, 566f
    natural history of, 565–566
    principles of management,
      566–567
  approaches to therapy for, 567–568
  definition of, 564
  grading scale for, 567, 567t
  investigation of, 567
  perception, in infant/neonate,
    493–494
  reflex responses to, 565
Pain pathway, 565, 565f
Pain-related behavior, definition of, 565
Pain relief. *See also* Postoperative anal-
    gesia
  with flail chest, 469
  with rib fractures, 465
P_{alv}. *See* Alveolus, pressure in
Pancoast's syndrome, 413
Pancreas, blood flow to, in shock, 151
Pancuronium
  effects of, on airway resistance, 350
  for myasthenic patients, 408
  precautions for, in trauma patient,
    467
P_AO_2. *See* Alveolar oxygen tension

PaO_2/SaO_2, in differentiation of cardiac
    versus pulmonary impair-
    ment, 14t
Paradoxical respiration
  with open chest, 203f, 204
  postoperative, 714
Paraldehyde, 256
Parallel beam CO_2 analyzer, 304–306,
    306f
Paraquat, pulmonary damage induced
    by, 131
Paravertebral block, for postoperative
    analgesia, 569–570
Paravertebral catheter, for analgesia,
    570
Paravertebral injection, needle direc-
    tion for, 569, 570f
Parenteral nutrition, versus enteral
    nutrition, 701–703
Passive exhalation method, for estimat-
    ing resistance, 171f,
    171–172
Patent ductus arteriosus, 487
  clinical manifestations of, 540
  and gestational age, 540
  hemoglobin levels with, 541
  ligation and/or division of
    anesthetic and perioperative con-
      siderations with, 524t,
      539–541
    description of, 524t
  medical therapy for, 540
  pathophysiology with, 529
Patient-controlled analgesia, 580–581,
    596
  dosage and administration of, 581
  for pediatric patient, 507, 564
  safety of, 581
PCO_2. *See* Carbon dioxide tension
Peak expiratory flow rate, 2f, 4, 4f
Peak negative pressure measurement,
    616
Pectus carinatum, in infant/neonate,
    anesthetic and periopera-
    tive considerations with,
    518t
Pectus excavatum
  in infant/neonate, anesthetic and
    perioperative considera-
    tions with, 518t
  radiographic findings with, 26
Pediatric patient. *See also*
    Infant/neonate
  age- and size-related differences in,
    486, 486t
  AIDS in, 103

anesthetic management for
　advances in, 485
　challenges of, 485–486
bronchopulmonary lavage in,
　427–428
capnography in, 310, 311f
endotracheal reintubation, 615
esophagoscopy in, anesthetic and
　perioperative considera-
　tions with, 525
oral versus tracheal intubation for,
　553–554
patient-controlled analgesia for,
　581
postoperative pain in, 563–564
prevention of bacterial endocarditis
　in, during diagnostic and
　therapeutic procedures,
　542–544, 544t
respiratory care for, 552–554
respiratory support for, parameters
　used in determining need
　for, 553
unique characteristics of, 486–
　494
PEEP. *See* Positive end-expiratory pres-
　sure
PEFR. *See* Peak expiratory flow rate
P_{el}. *See* Lung, elastic recoil pressure of
Pendelluft phenomenon, 468
Pentamidine
　indications for, in AIDS, 104
　prophylaxis, for *P. carinii* pneumo-
　　nia, 104
　side effects of, 104
Pentazocine, front-loading, 579t
Pentobarbital
　effects of
　　on airway resistance, 349
　　on incidence of anesthetic con-
　　　vulsions, 271t
　　on lung metabolism, 132
　premedication, for infant/neonate,
　　dosage and administration
　　of, 497t
　sedative effect, 259
　ventilatory response to, 267, 268f
Pentothal. *See* Thiopental
Peptides
　bioactive, in lung, 125t, 125–127
　in lungs, vasoactive and bron-
　　choconstrictive properties,
　　127
Percussion, therapeutic, 596
Perfusion scanning, 11
Peribronchial cuffing, 20

Pericardial cysts, in infant/neonate,
　anesthetic and periopera-
　tive considerations with,
　518t
Pericardial effusion
　in infant/neonate, anesthetic and
　　perioperative considera-
　　tions with, 519t
　radiographic findings with, 59–61,
　　64f
Pericardiocentesis, 473
Pericarditis, in infant/neonate
　acute, anesthetic and perioperative
　　considerations with, 518t
　chronic constrictive, anesthetic and
　　perioperative considera-
　　tions with, 518t
Pericardium, absent, in infant/neonate,
　anesthetic and periopera-
　tive considerations with,
　518t
Peripheral nerve vasculitis, with AIDS,
　102
Peripheral neuropathies, with AIDS,
　102
Peritonitis, acute respiratory failure
　with, 629–630
Perivascular cuffing, 20
Peroxide, in acute respiratory failure,
　629
Persistent fetal circulation, 487–488,
　529–530
Persistent pulmonary hypertension of
　the newborn, 487–488
　leukotrienes in, 122
Phenergan. *See* Promethazine
Phenolsulfonephthalein, intramuscular
　route for, 275
Phenothiazines
　indications for, 578
　and opioids, combined effects of,
　　268, 269f
　premedication with, 267–268
　side effects of, 268
Phenylephrine
　effects on hypoxic pulmonary vaso-
　　constriction, 210
　for heart failure, 562
Phosphodiesterase(s), 226–227
Phosphodiesterase inhibitors, postoper-
　ative administration of,
　613
Phospholipase A_2, 120
Photoluminescence quenching, 287
Phrenic electromyography, 183
Phrenic nerve, 165–166

effect of topical cooling on, 27
　injury, 719
　in mediastinoscopy, 340
Phrenic nerve palsy, in infant/neonate,
　anesthetic and periopera-
　tive considerations with,
　519t
Physiologic dead space, 300–301
Physiologic shunt, 144
Pierre-Robin syndrome, 503–504
P_IO_2. *See* Inspired oxygen tension
Pirbuterol, 227
　dosage and administration of, 228t,
　　231
　duration of action, 228t
　mechanism of action, 228t
　pharmacology of, 231
　relative potency of, 231
　structure of, 227f
P_{isf}. *See* Pulmonary interstitial fluid
　pressure
Plasma, with high anti-HIV antibody
　titers, therapy with, in
　AIDS, 105
Plasma oncotic pressure, decrease in,
　37
Plasmapheresis, for myasthenia gravis,
　404
　preoperative, 411
Platelet-activating factor
　and acute lung injury, 133
　pathophysiologic effects on lung,
　　125
Platelet aggregation, in acute respirato-
　ry failure, 629
Pleural drainage, 611–613
　management of, 612–613
　postoperative, 593
　systems for, 611–612, 611f–612f
　tube placement for, radiographic
　　evaluation of, 70, 70f–71f
　underwater seal system, 611f,
　　611–612
Pleural effusions, 36
　computed tomography scan of, 62f
　diagnosis of, 340
　drainage of, 341
　with esophageal perforation, 393
　with heart failure, 56
　postoperative, 713–714
　with pulmonary embolization, 39,
　　56
　radiographic appearance of, 56–57,
　　59f
Pleural fluids
　loculations, as pseudotumor, 59, 61f

Pleural fluids (*Continued*)
  radiographic appearance of, 55–59
  rapid or significant accumulation of, 55
  subpulmonic, radiographic assessment of, 57, 60f
Pleural infection, postoperative, 713–714
Pleural needle biopsy, complications of, 720–721
Pleural pressure, 3, 3f
  gradient of, 187
    in lateral decubitus position, 198–200, 199f
    in upright position, 196, 196f–197f
  with lung dependency, 196, 196f
  in upright position, 195
Pleural reaction, along tube tracts, 71f, 75
Pleural space, air-fluid level in, 56, 59
  postoperative studies, 61–62, 66f–67f
Plexus myentericus, 394
Pneumatocele, in infant/neonate, anesthetic and perioperative considerations with, 519t
Pneumocystis carinii, 31
Pneumocystis carinii pneumonia
  in AIDS, 95–96, 100
  anesthetic management with, 107
  prophylaxis against, 104
  radiographic patterns of, 31
  treatment of, 104
  ventilation with, 108
Pneumomediastinum, 48–49, 714
  causes of, 49
  with esophageal perforation, 393
  in infant/neonate, anesthetic and perioperative considerations with, 517t
  in newborns, 48
Pneumonectomy. *See also* Pulmonary resection
  dysrhythmias with, 420
  left, cardiac herniation after, 717
  predicted postoperative FEV$_1$ with, 11
  radiographic findings after, 61–63
  right, cardiac herniation after, 717
Pneumonia
  acute respiratory failure with, 630
  in adult respiratory distress syndrome, 39
  bacterial, 630
  bronchopneumonia pattern, 32, 33f
  community-acquired, 31

hospital-acquired, 88–89
  causes of, 31
  radiographic findings with, 32
Klebsiella
  characteristic feature of, 32
  radiographic patterns of, 32f
lobar, 630
  radiographic patterns of, 31, 32f
mycoplasma, radiographic patterns of, 31
P. aeruginosa, 31–32
P. carinii. See Pneumocystis carinii pneumonia
postoperative
  correlation with nutritional status, 685–686
  and preoperative TPN, 688
  prevention of, 710
  risk factors for, 686, 693
radiographic findings with, 27, 31–32, 45
systemic oxygen uptake in, 154–155
viral, 630
  radiographic patterns of, 31
Pneumonitis. *See also* Aspiration pneumonitis
  in AIDS, 101
Pneumopericardium, 48
  in infant/neonate, 48
    anesthetic and perioperative considerations with, 519t
Pneumoperitoneum, 48, 714
  with esophageal perforation, 393
Pneumoretroperitoneum, 48
Pneumothorax, 30f, 48, 85
  after esophageal surgery, 397
  after thoracic trauma, 447
  after thymectomy, 406
  after tracheostomy, 70
  after tube removal, 75
  with associated lobar atelectasis, 51
  with bronchoscopy, 326
  in bullous disease, 423–424
  diagnosis of, 50–51, 469
  with hemothorax, 471
  iatrogenic, 75
  in infant/neonate, anesthetic and perioperative considerations with, 519t
  with intercostal block, 568
  loculated, 51
  management of, 469
  mediastinal shift with, 711
  with mediastinoscopy, 720
  open, 469
    management of, 469

with pleural needle biopsy, 720
postoperative, in infant/neonate, management of, 508–509
radiographic appearance of, 50–52, 51f–52f
recurrent, chemical pleurodesis for, 340
with subclavian puncture, 470
subcutaneous air present after, 49
in unoperated cavity, in infant/neonate, 509
PNI. *See* Prognostic nutritional index
PO$_2$. *See* Oxygen tension
Poiseuille's law, 332–333
Poland's syndrome, in infant/neonate, anesthetic and perioperative considerations with, 520t
Polarogram, 288f
Polyhydramnios, 534
Polyvinylchloride endobronchial tube, 377, 378t, 383
  malpositioning of, 387
Polyvinylchloride endotracheal tube, flammability of, during laser resection, 435
PO$_2$ optode, 287, 289f
  in continuous oxygen tension monitoring, 290, 291f
Position. *See also* Lateral decubitus position; Upright position
  effects of
    on distribution of pulmonary perfusion, 596, 640–641
    on distribution of ventilation, 596, 640
    on functional residual capacity, 621
  requirements, for postural drainage, 597f–599f
Positive end-expiratory pressure. *See also* One-lung ventilation, differential lung CPAP (nondependent lung)/PEEP (dependent lung)
  application of, with lateral decubitus position, 201
  with bronchopleural fistula, 422
  versus continuous positive airway pressure, 635–637
  and hypoxic pulmonary vasoconstriction, 211
  for near-drowning, 630
  newborn infant on, for hyaline

membrane disease, interstitial air with, 48, 49f
in one-lung ventilation, selective dependent-lung, 212–214, 213f, 217
for respiratory distress syndrome, 490
selective, in lateral decubitus position, 202–203
Positive end-expiratory pressure/CPAP
in acute respiratory failure, 636–637
optimal, 636–638
complications of, 638–640
for near-drowning, 631
therapeutic end-point of, 636–638
Positive-pressure ventilation
in acute respiratory failure, 620
in bullous disease, 424
with fiberoptic bronchoscopy, 333
gas exchange in, 634–635, 635f
selective, during acute respiratory failure, 371–372
during thoracotomy, principles of, 203f, 203–204
Postanesthetic apnea, in infant/neonate, 491–492
Postoperative analgesia, 563–585, 595–596, 710
after thymectomy, 411–412
combined local anesthetic-opioid infusions, 577–578
conceptual framework of, 566–568
contribution of premedication to, 261
effectiveness of, comparison of techniques, 575
effects of
on endocrine-metabolic stress response, 583–584
on gastrointestinal function, 584
on hemodynamic stability, 584
on length of hospital stay, 584
on patient outcome, 584–585
on pulmonary complications, 582–583
on pulmonary function, 582–583
epidural block for, 595
local anesthetics for, 595–596
morphine for, 596
with esophageal surgery, 397
historical development of, 564t
for infant/neonate, 505–508
intercostal block for, 568–569, 595
interpleural block for, 570–572
local and regional techniques
central, 572–578

peripheral, 568–572
paravertebral block for, 569–570
patient-controlled analgesia for, 580–581, 596
and pulmonary hygiene, 92
for pulmonary resection, 421
spinal opioids for, 573–577
systemic, 578–582
nonopioid, 578–579
opioids for, 579t, 579–580
transcutaneous electrical nerve stimulation for, 595
transdermal delivery system for, 581–582
Postoperative metabolic responses, 689–690
Postoperative pain
in children, 563–564
with thoracotomy, 715
undertreatment of, 563, 564t
Postoperative respiratory care, 593–617
drug therapy in, 613–615, 614t–615t
Post-thoracotomy pain syndrome, 719
Postural drainage
indications for, 596
position requirements for, 597f–599f
Posture. *See also* Position
and functional residual capacity, 582
Potassium balance
after massive transfusion of stored blood, 479
and dysrhythmias, 88
P_{pl}. *See* Pleural pressure
Precision, definition of, 288
Prednisolone, 241
pharmacology of, 242t
structure of, 241f
Prednisone, 241
bioavailability of, 243
pharmacology of, 242t
structure of, 241f
Premature infant
characteristics of, 489–490
postanesthetic apnea in, 491–492
pulmonary disease in, 490, 491f
retrolental fibroplasia in, 490–491
Premedication, 255–278
administration routes, 275–276
for amnesia, 277t
for analgesia, 277t
antisialagogue activity, 259–260
for anxiety relief, 277t
for bronchoscopy, 333–334
buccal route for, 276

cardiovascular considerations with, 277t
central nervous system effects, 277t
dosage and administration of, 278
drug selection for, 277t
gastrointestinal considerations with, 273–274, 277t
goals of, 258–261
for heart rate regulation, 277t
historical development of, 256–257
for hypertension, 277t
for hypotension, 277t
for infant/neonate, 496–498
intramuscular route for, 275
intravenous route for, 275–276
nasal route for, 276
oral route for, 276
pharmacology of, 261–273
regimen for, synthesis of, 276–279
respiratory considerations with, 277t
and sleep apnea, 266
and surgical aims and expectations, 257–258
for thymectomy, 405
for tracheal reconstruction, 452
transdermal route for, 276
Preoperative assessment, 90
for diagnostic procedures, 321–324
for esophageal surgery, 395
of infant/neonate, 494–496
for mediastinoscopy, 338–339
of patient with AIDS, 107
of pulmonary circulation, 716
for thoracoscopy, 341
for thymectomy, 405
Preoperative preparation, and prevention of postoperative complications, 710
Pressure generator(s), 663, 664f
Pressure-support ventilation, 666–668, 668f
in acute respiratory failure, 643
nebulization with, 653
Prognostic nutritional index, 686–687
Promethazine, 268
anxiolytic effect, 258
premedication, for infant/neonate, dosage and administration of, 497t
Propanidid, effects of, on airway resistance, 349
Propiomazine, 268
Propofol
effects of, on airway resistance, 349–350

Propofol (*Continued*)
  and hypoxic pulmonary vasocon-
    striction, clinical studies
    of, 354
  indications for, 271
Propranolol
  for atrial dysrhythmias, 716
  for hypercyanotic episodes with
    tetralogy of Fallot,
    497–498
  pulmonary uptake of, 132
Prostacyclin
  actions, in pulmonary vasculature
    and airways, 120
  handling of, in lungs, 116
  as modulator of acute lung injury, 133
  release
    from lung, 120
    role of angiotensin II, 125
Prostaglandin(s)
  actions, in pulmonary vasculature
    and airways, 120
  pulmonary synthesis, release, and
    metabolism of, 120–
    122
  receptors, in airway smooth muscle,
    226t, 226–227
Prostaglandin E$_1$
  effects of, on capillary permeability,
    626
  and hypoxic pulmonary vasocon-
    striction, 357
Prostaglandin E$_2$, in acute respiratory
    failure, 629
Prostaglandin F$_{2\alpha}$, and hypoxic pul-
    monary vasoconstriction,
    357
Prostigmin. *See* Neostigmine
Protein
  caloric content of, 682
  metabolism, 683–684
    anabolic phase, 684
    catabolic phase, 683–684
  oxidation, respiratory quotient for,
    682
  respiratory effects of, 697–700
    in malnourished patients, 699,
    699f
Proteolysis, in hypercatabolic patients,
    690
Proxyphylline, 237
Pseudomonas, 39
Pseudomonas aeruginosa, 31–32
  airway colonization, and nutritional
    status, 693
Pseudotumor(s)

of hemorrhage, postoperative, 61,
    65f
  pleural fluid, 59, 61f
Psychological preparation, for thoracic
    surgery, 261
Psychosis, in AIDS, 102
Psychosocial management, with chron-
    ic pulmonary disease, 92
Pulmonary arteriovenous fistula, in
    infant/neonate, anesthetic
    and perioperative consid-
    erations with, 520t
Pulmonary artery(ies), 224
  absolute pressure in, in upright posi-
    tion, 194–196
  compression of, with mediastinal
    mass, 400–401
  injury, in mediastinoscopy, 340
  left, aberrant, 446
  perforation, hemoptysis with, 428
  rupture, hemoptysis with, 428
Pulmonary artery banding
  anesthetic and perioperative consid-
    erations with, 523t
  description of, 523t
Pulmonary artery catheterization
  bleeding after, 716
  catheter placement, 75–76
    radiographic evaluation of,
    72f–73f, 76
  complications with, 76
  for patients at risk for right heart
    failure, 717
  rupture or perforation with, 428
Pulmonary artery diastolic pressure,
    717
Pulmonary artery hypertension
  cardiac failure secondary to, 87
  conditions producing, 87t
  definition of, 87
Pulmonary artery pressure
  elevation in, 86
  postresection, prognostic evaluation
    of, 11
  preoperative assessment of, 716–717
Pulmonary artery sling, 446
  in pediatric patient, anesthetic and
    perioperative considera-
    tions with, 520t, 542
Pulmonary artery wedge pressure, 717
Pulmonary blood flow
  during anesthesia, 350–357
  with right-to-left shunts, monitoring,
    500
Pulmonary capillary wedge pressure,
    623

measurement, during mechanical
    ventilation, 639–640
  during volume infusion, 476
Pulmonary circulation
  bleeding from, 715
  preoperative assessment of, 716
Pulmonary complications, 710–714
  postoperative
    incidence of, 83
    prevention and treatment of,
    594–605
  prediction of, 324
  and preoperative pulmonary prepa-
    ration, 83–84, 84t
  risk factors for, 321
Pulmonary defense mechanisms, effects
    of malnutrition and
    refeeding on, 693
Pulmonary dysfunction
  during and after thoracotomy and
    upper abdominal surgery,
    89
  in AIDS, 101
  with intravenous fat emulsions,
    696–697
  preoperative assessment of, 223
  preoperative treatment of, 223
Pulmonary edema, 27
  after surgery for mediastinal mass,
    399
  and aspiration, 37
  atypical patterns of, 36–37
  cardiac, 34
  with chronic lung disease, 36–37
  developing, radiographic findings
    with, 34–37
  iatrogenic, 91
  mechanisms of, 32–34, 35t
  pathophysiology of, 88
  preoperative therapy, 88
  radiographic findings with, 32–37,
    45
  re-expansion, 52
  during volume infusion, 476
Pulmonary embolism
  acute respiratory failure with, 632
  versus adult respiratory distress syn-
    drome, 38–39
  diagnosis of, 718
  differential diagnosis, 718
  effects of, on lung water, 624, 626
  hemoptysis with, 428
  hypoxia with, 86, 86t
  manifestations of, 718
  metabolic effects during, 133
  mortality with, 718

pathophysiology of, 86
pleural effusion with, 39, 56
prevention of, 718
pulmonary vascular response to, 133
radiographic findings with, 37,
40–45, 46f–47f
treatment of, 718
Pulmonary emphysema. *See*
Emphysema, pulmonary
Pulmonary endothelium
damage, metabolic effects of, 130
metabolic function of, 130
nucleotide metabolism by, 128
role in HPV, 132
Pulmonary fibrosis, 85
after adult respiratory distress syndrome, 39, 40t
after hemorrhage, 40
with bleomycin therapy, 392
Pulmonary function, postoperative,
effects of postoperative
analgesia on, 582–583
Pulmonary function tests
with airway obstruction, 450
in evaluation for thoracotomy, 9–11
indications for, 91, 710
interpretation of, 7–9
methods of, 2–7
preoperative, 324
Pulmonary gas exchange, impairment
of, during anesthesia,
185–188
Pulmonary hemodynamics, effects of
PEEP on, 638–639
Pulmonary hemorrhage, radiographic
findings with, 39–40, 44f
Pulmonary host defense, 88
Pulmonary hygiene, perioperative, 92
Pulmonary hypertension. *See also*
Pulmonary artery hyper-
tension; Pulmonary
venous hypertension
and acute respiratory failure, 634
after lung resection, predicting, 13
with congenital diaphragmatic hernia, 529–530
lung transplantation for, 556, 561
of newborn, extracorporeal membrane oxygenation for, 676
postoperative, 716–717
primary, 86
with pulmonary embolism, 718
reduction of, 92
Pulmonary hypoplasia, with congenital
diaphragmatic hernia, 530,
533

survival with, 533
Pulmonary infarction, 40–44
postoperative, 711–713
radiographic resolution of, 44, 47f
secondary to direct arterial occlusion by catheter, 73f, 76
Pulmonary infection, treatment of, 92
Pulmonary insufficiency
postoperative, 710
preoperative
prevention of postoperative complications of, 594
quantitation of, 593–594
Pulmonary interstitial fluid, transudation, and pulmonary per-
fusion, 195–196
Pulmonary interstitial fluid pressure,
effect of, on extra-alveolar
vessels, 195f, 195–196
Pulmonary mechanics, in fiberoptic
bronchoscopy, 327
Pulmonary occlusion test, predictive
value of, 717
Pulmonary perfusion, distribution of
effects of position on, 596
in lateral decubitus position,
197–203, 199f
in supine position, 641
in upright position, 193–196, 194f,
640–641
Pulmonary preparation
preoperative, effects on surgical
recovery, 83–84
10-step outline for, 84, 91–92
therapeutic regimen, 90t, 91–92
Pulmonary rehabilitation, postoperative, 91–92
Pulmonary resection (lung resection)
anesthetic management of, 419–422
annual numbers of, 419
complications of, 710
dysrhythmias with, 419–420
endotracheal tubes for, 420
indications for, 419
intraoperative considerations and
management, 420–421
monitoring for, 420
pathophysiologic effects of, 89
postoperative analgesia for, 421
potential effects of, perioperative
assessment of, 91
preoperative bronchoscopy with,
325
radiographic findings after, 61–63
Pulmonary sequestration, in
infant/neonate, anesthetic

and perioperative consid-
erations with, 520t
Pulmonary thromboembolism, postoperative, 718
Pulmonary tissue resistance, during
anesthesia, 174
Pulmonary vascular disease(s), 84
lung transplantation for, 556, 559t,
561
pathophysiology of, 86
Pulmonary vascular pressure, effects on
hypoxic pulmonary vaso-
constriction, 210
Pulmonary vascular resistance
during exercise, and postoperative
outcome, 13
postnatal, 487
Pulmonary vasculature
barrier function, 116
cytochrome P-450 system, 131
radiographic evaluation of, 47
Pulmonary venous hypertension, radiographic findings with,
34–35
Pulmonary venous pressure, in upright
position, 194–196
Pulse oximeter, 297
Pulse oximetry, 156, 296–300, 709–710
accuracy of, 299
ambient light interference in, 298
clinical applications of, 299–300
for infant/neonate, during thoracic
operations, 500
limitations of, 300
motion artifacts, 298–299
in neonate, 298
during one-lung ventilation, 312,
313f
physiologic limitations of, 297–298
probe-to-probe variability in, 299
range of cardiac output for, 298
response times of, 299
technical development of, 296–297
technical difficulties in, 298, 300
theory of, 297
Pulsus paradoxus, 473
Pump lung, definition of, 619
Pyridostigmine (Mestinon)
effects of, on airway resistance, 350
for myasthenia gravis, 403, 403t, 406

Quiet lung, 371

Radial artery catheterization
in infant/neonate, for blood pressure
monitoring, 500–501

Radial artery catheterization (*Continued*)
during tracheal reconstruction, 452–453
Radiographic density, 20, 21f
definition of, 19
and tissue interface, 19–20
Radioimmunoprecipitation assay, for HIV, 97
Radiologic evaluation
of esophageal perforation or rupture, 393
principles of, 19–27
of tracheal lesions, 450, 451f–452f
Radionuclide lung scan, with pulmonary embolization, 40, 44, 47f
Radiospirometry, 11
Rales, clinical implications of, 322
Raman spectrometry, for carbon dioxide measurement, 304, 305f
Ranitidine
dosage and administration of, 391
effects of, on airway resistance, 350
gastrointestinal actions of, 274–275
indications for, 391
side effects of, 391
Reactive airway
of chronic obstructive pulmonary disease, 85
management of, 92
Rebreathing, 601–602
Recurrent laryngeal nerve
dysfunction, with tumor extension, 395
injury, 719–720
in mediastinoscopy, 340
REE. *See* Resting energy expenditure
Refeeding
carbohydrate-based, ventilatory and metabolic effects of, 695, 697f
clinical effects of, 687–688
complications of, 689
fat-based, ventilatory and metabolic effects of, 695, 697f
of malnourished patients, 687–689
nutritional requirements for, 688–689
respiratory effects of, 691–695
standard TPN formula for, 689, 689t
Reflection coefficient, 624
Regional analgesia/anesthesia
effect on respiratory mechanics, 172

intravenous, for AIDS patients, 108
for postoperative analgesia, 570
in infant/neonate, 507–508
respiratory effects of, 362
for thoracoscopy, 341–342
Relative flow metering, 650
Relaxation volume, of respiratory system, 168
Renal blood flow, monitoring of, 156
Renal circulation, autoregulation of, 153
Renal failure
in AIDS, 102–103
posttraumatic, diagnosis and management of, 480–481
Renal function
with mechanical ventilation, 640
neonatal, 488
preoperative evaluation of, with AIDS, 107
Reperfusion syndrome, 709
Resectability
diagnosis of, 2
evaluation of, 2
Residual volume, 2, 621f
in acute respiratory failure, 622
during anesthesia, 348f
definition of, 621
determinants of, 166–167
Resistance, 169
in normalcy and disease, in ventilatory support, 668–669
pulmonary, 170, 661, 662f
changes in, during anesthesia, 173–174
Resonant frequency, of respiratory system, 171
Resorcinols
dosage and administration of, 228t
duration of action, 228t
mechanism of action, 228t
metabolism of, 229
structure of, 227f
Respiratory acidosis, postoperative, 616
Respiratory alkalosis, in acute respiratory failure, 620, 634
Respiratory control, effects of anesthesia on, 183–188
Respiratory depression
with epidural opioids, 575–576
with hydroxyzine and opioids, 270, 270f
in infant/neonate, with postoperative analgesia, 507–508
with inhalation anesthesia, 184
late, 574

with opioids, 265–266, 266f, 358, 362
treatment of, 576
with sedatives, 363
Respiratory distress syndrome. *See also* Adult respiratory distress syndrome
infant
CPAP in, 604
extracorporeal membrane oxygenation for, 676
management of, 490, 491f
pathophysiology of, 490, 491f
Respiratory failure. *See also* Acute respiratory failure
after massive transfusion, 478
during and after thoracotomy and upper abdominal surgery, 89
with flail chest, 468
postoperative
correlation with nutritional status, 685–686
risk factors for, 684
risk factors of, 91
with thymectomy, 409–411
Respiratory frequency, effects of malnutrition and refeeding on, 694f
Respiratory inhalant products, 614t–615t
Respiratory insufficiency
acute. *See also* Acute respiratory failure
definition of, 620
chronic
management of, 92
preoperative evaluation, 90–91
Respiratory mechanics, 165–172
Respiratory monitoring, with intraspinal opioids, guidelines for, 576, 576t
Respiratory muscle(s), 165–166
effects of malnutrition on, 691–693
effects of refeeding on, 693
inspiratory resistance loading, 605
inspiratory threshold loading, 605
retraining, 92
strength
and electrolyte imbalance, 700
evaluation of, 166
training, 605
Respiratory paradox, postoperative, 714
Respiratory physiology, during anesthesia, 165–188
Respiratory quotient, 682

definition of, 163
effects of malnutrition and refeeding on, 694f
Respiratory rate
age- and size-related differences in, 486, 486t
during and following thoracotomy and upper abdominal surgery, 89
in one-lung ventilation, 212
Respiratory stimulants, postoperative administration of, 613
Respiratory system
dynamics, 170–172
equilibrium position of, 168
nutrition and, 691–701
pressure-flow relationships in, 175
pressure-volume relationships of, postural alterations of, 168
recoil pressure of, 168
relaxation pressure volume characteristics of, 167, 167f, 168
statics, 169–170
transmural pressures in, 169, 169t
Resting energy expenditure, 681
changes in, in pathologic states, 682f
in chronic obstructive pulmonary disease, 694
effects of carbohydrates on, 696
effects of diet on, 683f
effects of disease on, 683f
effects of malnutrition and refeeding on, 694f
estimation of, 683, 683t
with injury, 689–690
in intensive care patients, 683
in malnourished patients, 688
measured versus predicted, 682–683
with sepsis, 689–690
Resting ventilation, as index of ventilatory controls, 180
Resting volume, of respiratory system, 168
Restrictive pulmonary disease, 84
etiology of, 85
extrinsic, 85
intrinsic, 85
acute, 85
chronic, 85
lung transplantation for, 556, 559t, 561
pathophysiology of, 85
Restrictive ventilatory defects, 7–8
Retinopathy of prematurity, 490–491
Retrolental fibroplasia, in premature infant, 490–491

Retrovirus, 97
Reverse transcriptase, 97
Reverse transcriptase inhibitor, 105
Reynaud's phenomenon, and primary pulmonary hypertension, 86
Rhonchi, clinical implications of, 322
Rib fractures, 464–465
Ribs
bucket-handle motion, 166
pump-handle motion, 166
Rifampin, indications for, in AIDS, 104
Right middle lobe syndrome, in infant/neonate, anesthetic and perioperative considerations with, 520t
Right ventricular dysfunction, in chronic obstructive pulmonary disease, 716
Right ventricular failure, 86
pharmacotherapy for, 561–562
Right ventricular function, in lung transplantation, support for, 561
Right ventricular hypertrophy, with chronic cor pulmonale, 88
Rigid bronchoscopy. *See* Bronchoscopy, rigid
Ro 15-1788, 271
Robertshaw double-lumen endobronchial tube, 377, 378t, 381–383, 382f
Robertshaw double-lumen endotracheal tube, proper placement of, 69, 69f
Robinul. *See* Glycopyrrolate
RQ. *See* Respiratory quotient
Ruby laser, characteristics of, 430t
RV/TLC ratio, to predict postoperative lung function and survival, 10

Safe sex techniques, 99
Salbutamol. *See* Albuterol
Saligenins
dosage and administration of, 228t
duration of action, 228t
mechanism of action, 228t
metabolism of, 229
structure of, 227f
Saline, effects on incidence of anesthetic convulsions, 271t
Salivation, effects of antimuscarinic drugs on, 265t
Salmeterol, 227
dosage and administration of, 232

duration of action, 232
mechanism of action, 232
pharmacology of, 231
relative potency of, 231–232
structure of, 227f
Sanders injector, 329–331, 330f–331f, 433
Sanders Venturi principle, 329–331
SaO$_2$. *See* Fractional hemoglobin saturation
Sarcoidosis, diagnosis of, 720
Scalene muscles, 166
Scalene node biopsy, complications of, 720
Schizophrenia, in AIDS, 102
Scimitar syndrome, in infant/neonate, anesthetic and perioperative considerations with, 520t
Scopolamine
amnestic effect, 259
anticholinergic effect, dose-response for, 264f
antisialagogue effect, 259, 263
bronchodilator effect, 263f
effects of, 265t
pharmacology of, 261–262
premedication
for bronchoscopy, 334
dosage and administration of, 263
duration of action, 263
for infant/neonate, dosage and administration of, 497t
side effects of, 263
Sedation
definition of, 255
premedication for, 259
Sedative(s)
definition of, 256
dose-response after, 260, 260f
effects of, on ventilatory control, 357–363
indications for, 578
respiratory effects of, 362–363
Sepsis
complicating lobectomy, 713
correlation with nutritional status, 685–686
metabolic response to, 689–690
nutritional implications of, 690–691
nutritional support for, 690–691
nitrogen balance in, 691, 692f
oxygen delivery in, 154
oxygen uptake in, 154

Sepsis (*Continued*)
  peripheral oxygen transport in, 154
  and preoperative TPN, 688
Septic shock, oxygen transport in, 144
Series dead space, 301f
Serotonin, metabolism of, 128
Serum oncotic pressure, 624
Severinghaus-Stowe PCO$_2$ electrode, 302–303, 303f
Sevoflurane, 359–361
Sheridan YAG Tracheal Tube, 435
Shock. *See also* Hemorrhagic shock
  anesthetic management with, 466–467
  induction technique with, 466
  resuscitation for, 152
Shock lung, definition of, 619
Shock phase, of metabolic response to injury, 689–690
Shortness of breath, diagnostic significance of, 339
Sickle cell anemia, rheologic properties of blood in, 150
Sickle cell disease
  oxygen delivery in, 150
  transfusion therapy in, 150
Siemans-Elema PEEP valve, 660
Silhouette sign, 20
  in lobar atelectasis, 28
Silhouetting, on radiographs, 19–20, 20f–21f
Sleep apnea, 84
  pathophysiology of, 86
  and premedication, 266
Sleeve resection, one-lung ventilation with, 371
Slow-reacting substance of anaphylaxis, 122
Slow vital capacity, 3
Sluice effect, 194–195
Smoking, and risk of perioperative complications, 321–322
Smoking cessation, 710
  and risk of perioperative complications, 322
  before surgery, 92
Smooth muscle, airway. *See* Airway(s), smooth muscle of
Snoring, and sleep apnea, 266
Sodium, urinary, and lung cancer, 89
Sodium bicarbonate, for metabolic acidosis, with congenital diaphragmatic hernia, 530
Sodium citrate (Bicitra), indications for, 391
Sodium nitroprusside

effect on blood flow and oxygen delivery, 153
  and hypoxic pulmonary vasoconstriction, 357
Spasmogenic lung peptide, actions of, in lung, 127
Spinal analgesia/anesthesia
  effect on respiratory mechanics, 172
  intravenous, for AIDS patients, 108
  for postoperative pain, 572
Spirogram tracing, normal, 621, 621f–622f
Spirometry, 2–5
  with airway obstruction, 450
  interpretation of, 7–8, 8f
  preoperative, predictive value of, 324
Splanchnic blood flow
  monitoring of, 156
  in reflex control of cardiovascular system, 151
Split lung function, evaluation of, 10–11
Squamous cell carcinoma, of trachea, 446t, 446–447
Stab wound(s), 464
  cardiac, 472
Starling equation, 624
Starling forces, 624–625, 625f
  effects of, on water movement, 629
Starling resistor, 194–195
Starvation, adaptive mechanisms in, 685
Steal syndrome, 145
  in hyperdynamic state, 154
Sternal clefts, in infant/neonate, anesthetic and perioperative considerations with, 520t
Sternocleidomastoid muscles, 166
Stern-Volmer equation, 287
Steroid analogs, metabolism of, 242*
Steroid therapy. *See also* Corticosteroids
  effects of, on venous admixture, 607–608, 608f, 610f
  for myasthenia gravis, 404
  preoperative, for thymectomy, 411
Streptococcus pneumoniae, 31
Stress-related mucosal damage, prevention of, 273–274
Stress response
  effects of postoperative analgesia on, 583–584
  of neonates, to surgery, 493–494
Stridor, clinical implications of, 322
Subacute encephalitis, in AIDS, 101

Subacute necrotizing myelopathy, with lung cancer, 89
Subarachnoid anesthesia, respiratory effects of, 361–362
Subclavian vein cannulation
  complications of, 470
  misplaced catheter in, pleural fluid caused by, 55–56, 58f
  and pneumothorax, 470
Subcutaneous air, 48
  causes of, 49
  radiographic appearance of, 49, 50f
Subglottic edema, in children, 522
Subglottic stenosis, 324
  in infant/neonate, anesthetic and perioperative considerations with, 521t
  postintubation, 448
Subpleural air, 48
Substance P, action of
  in airways, 224
  in lung, 127, 129
Substances of abuse, 256
Succinylcholine
  for myasthenic patients, 408
  precautions with, in trauma patient, 467
  respiratory sparing action, 174
Sucking chest wound, 469
Suctioning
  after left upper lobectomy, 711
  of endotracheal tubes and tracheotomies, in pediatric patient, 552
  nasotracheal, 600–601
  in repair of esophageal atresia/tracheoesophageal fistula, 536–537
  tracheobronchial, 600–601
Sufentanil
  and bupivacaine, combined infusions of, for postoperative analgesia, 578
  effects of
    on airway resistance, 350
    on ventilatory control, 358
  epidural, for postoperative analgesia
    dosage and administration of, 575
    duration of action, 575t
  nasal instillation, 276
  for postoperative analgesia, in infant/neonate, 507
    dosage and administration of, 507t
  respiratory effects of, 362

time course of blood levels, and administration route, 276f
Suffering, definition of, 565
Summation, on radiograph, 20, 21f
Superficial temporal artery, catheterization, in infant/neonate, for blood pressure monitoring, 501
Superior laryngeal nerve, blockade, 335, 336f
Superior vena cava syndrome, 338–339
following pacer insertion, 78
with mediastinal mass, 400–401, 401f
Superoxide, in acute respiratory failure, 629
Supply dependency, 144
definition of, 163
pathologic, 154–155
Surfactant
deficiency, 490
inactivation of
in acute respiratory failure, 628, 628f
in near-drowning, 630
production, 117
Surgical lesion
assessment of, 91
pathophysiologic effects of, 89
Surgical procedure
pathophysiologic changes associated with, 89
potential effects of, perioperative assessment of, 91
Surgical risk factors, 83
Sustained inflation, for treatment of atelectasis, 601
Swan-Ganz catheter
malplacement of, 72f
peripherally placed, 73f
tethered in heart, 74f, 76
Swyer-James syndrome, 37
Sympathomimetic bronchodilators, 227–233
structure of, 227f
Sympathomimetics
inhalant products, 614t–615t
nonbronchodilator actions of, 232–233
Synchronized intermittent mandatory ventilation, 666
Syncope, with thoracocentesis, 721

Tachyphylaxis
with beta-adrenergics, 233
to bupivacaine, 573

T cell(s)
failure, in AIDS, 100
T4 (helper), 97
T8 (suppressor), 97
Teeth, aspiration or ingestion of, 68
Temazepam, oral, 276
Temperature
effect on oxyhemoglobin dissociation, 148, 148t
monitoring, in infant/neonate, during thoracic operations, 502
Temporary unilateral pulmonary artery occlusion, 11, 13
TENS. *See* Transcutaneous electrical nerve stimulation
Tensilon test, 402–404
Tension pneumomediastinum, 48
Tension pneumothorax, 39, 49, 51–52
in infant/neonate
anesthetic and perioperative considerations with, 521t
management of, 508–509
loculated, 52
management of, 469–470, 470f
in premature infant, 491f
radiographic evaluation with, 469–470, 470f
radiographic evidence of, 52, 53f
signs of, 469, 469t
Teratoma, mediastinal, computed tomography scan of, 56f
Terbutaline, 227
dosage and administration of, 228t, 230
duration of action, 228t, 230
mechanism of action, 228t
postoperative administration of, 613
relative potency of, 229
side effects of, 230
structure of, 227f
Tetracaine
anesthesia, for flexible fiberoptic bronchoscopy, 334
respiratory effects of, 361
toxic reaction to, 326
Tetralogy of Fallot
induction technique with, 498–499
and premedication, 497–498
radiologic findings with, 496f
Theobromine, structure of, 234f
Theophylline
cardiovascular response to, 233
clearance, factors affecting, 234, 235t
dosage and administration of, 235

mechanism of action, 233
nonbronchodilator actions of, 232t, 232–233, 236
pharmacology of, 233–234
serum level
monitoring, 236
therapeutic, 235–236
side effects of, 234–235
structure of, 234f
Thermal dye method, for measurement of lung water, 625
Thermic effect, definition of, 681
Thermodilution cardiac output catheter, 154
Thermoregulation, for infant/neonate, 493
Thiamylal, effects of, on airway resistance, 349
Thiobarbiturates, precautions with, in patient in shock, 466
Thiopental
effects of
on airway resistance, 349–350
on functional residual capacity, 173
on lung elastic recoil, 348
effects on incidence of anesthetic convulsions, 271t
and hypoxic pulmonary vasoconstriction, clinical studies of, 355
induction, for infant/neonate, 498
premedication, for infant/neonate, dosage and administration of, 497t
respiratory effects of, 364t
Thoracocentesis, complications of, 720–721
Thoracic blood volume, and anesthesia, 173
Thoracic cage deformities, radiographic findings with, 26
Thoracic surgery
history of, 257–258
pathophysiologic changes associated with, 89
pharmacologic preparation of patient for, 255–278
psychological preparation for, 261
respiratory complications associated with, 90
risk of morbidity and mortality, 83
Thoracoscope(s), 340f, 341, 341f
Thoracoscopy
historical development of, 340
indications for, 340–341

Thoracoscopy (*Continued*)
  postoperative care for, 342
  preoperative assessment for, 341
  safety of, 341
  technique for, 341
  therapeutic, 340–341
Thoracostomy tube(s), 611
  indications for
    after pulmonary resection, 421
    in hemothorax, 470
  management of, 612–613
Thoracotomy
  complications of, 710
  for esophageal surgery, 395–396
    complications of, 397
  evaluation for. *See also* Resectability
    pulmonary function tests in, 9–11
  in evaluation of resectability of cancer, 2
  with hemothorax, 471, 471t
  limited, in evaluation of resectability of cancer, 2
  pulmonary function criteria indicating increased risk in, 10t
Thrombin, action of, in lung, 129
Thrombocytopenia, dilutional, after massive transfusion, 478–479, 479t
Thromboxane, lung metabolism of, 122
Thromboxane A$_2$
  actions, in pulmonary vasculature and airways, 120
  in acute respiratory failure, 629
Thymectomy
  anesthetic management for, 405–406
  anesthetic technique for, choice of, 406–409
  complications of, 406
  effects of, 412
  general anesthesia for, 405–406
  induction technique for, 405–406
  management of drug therapy with, 405
  monitoring in, 405
  optimization of patient's physical condition for, 405
  postoperative considerations, 411–412
  postoperative ventilatory requirement with, 409–411
  premedication for, 405
  preoperative assessment for, 405
  surgical approaches for, 404–405
  for treatment of myasthenia gravis, 401, 404–405

Thymus conditions, in infant/neonate, anesthetic and perioperative considerations with, 521t
Tidal volume, 6
  effects of malnutrition and refeeding on, 694f
  in one-lung ventilation, 212
  for support of ventilation, 670
TLC. *See* Total lung capacity
Tolazoline
  mechanism of action, 530
  for pulmonary vasodilation, 530–531
Topical anesthesia, for flexible fiberoptic bronchoscopy, 334–336
Toronto Lung Transplant group, 555
  experience with lung transplantation, 561–562
Total body water, 684
Total lung capacity, 2
  determinants of, 166
  during and following thoracotomy and upper abdominal surgery, 89
Total parenteral nutrition
  gas exchange and breathing patterns during, 698f
  immediate, for uncomplicated postoperative patient, 690–691
  mechanical complications of, 702
  metabolic complications of, 701–702
  monitoring during, 701–702, 702t
  practical considerations with, 701
  preoperative, and postoperative course, 687–688
Toxoplasmosis, in AIDS, 101
Trace elements
  in nutritional protocols, 689
  requirements for, in nutritional protocols, 689, 689t
Trachea. *See also* Transtracheal catheterization
  lesions of
    congenital, 446
    neoplastic
      primary, 446t, 446–447
      secondary, 447
      surgical mortality with, 447
    radiographic findings with, 450, 451f–452f
  trauma to, 447, 471–472. *See also* Tracheal injury
    blunt, 447
    penetrating, 447
Tracheal collapse, after mediastinoscopy, 340

Tracheal compression
  with mediastinal mass, 397–398
  by vascular ring, 542
Tracheal injury
  complications of, 449
  etiologies of, 445–449, 446t
  postintubation, 448f, 448–449
  in tracheostomy, 444, 448f, 448–449
Tracheal reconstruction, 445–460
  airway equipment for, 453
  anastomotic technique, 456, 457f
  anesthetic management for, 450–454
  bronchoscopy in, 453–454
  complications of, postoperative, 459–460
  endotracheal intubation in, 454
  extubation after, 459
  incisions for, 454, 455f
  induction technique for, 453
  for lower trachea, 454, 456–459, 458f
  monitoring during, 452–453
  postoperative care with, 459–460
  premedication for, 452
  preoperative assessment for, 450–452
  for upper trachea, 454–456, 455f, 457f
Tracheal rings, 446
Tracheal rupture, 49
Tracheal stenosis
  after tracheostomy, 69f–70f, 444
  congenital, 446
  at stoma, 449
Tracheal stricture(s)
  in infant/neonate, anesthetic and perioperative considerations with, 521t
  in infection, 448
Tracheobronchial irritation, after bronchoscopy, 720
Tracheobronchial obstruction
  by mediastinal mass, anesthetic management of, 397–400
  postoperative, 710–711
Tracheobronchial rupture
  with endobronchial intubation, 384
  traumatic, 471–472
Tracheobronchial suction, 600–601
Tracheobronchial tree, bleeding into, postoperative, 716
Tracheoesophageal fistula, 324, 449
  after tracheostomy, 444
  associated anomalies, 495
  diagnosis of, 534–535
  incidence of, 534

intubation with, 503
mortality with, 535
pulmonary complications of, 535–536
repair
anesthetic and perioperative considerations with, 534–537
complications of, 537
testing integrity of, 537
Tracheoinnominate artery fistula, 449
Tracheomalacia, 324
with cuff-related injury, 449
in infant/neonate, anesthetic and perioperative considerations with, 521t
Tracheostomy
air leakage with, 70
anesthetic requirements, 441
care and maintenance of, 445
complications of, 441, 443
emergency, 443–444
indications for, 441
with flail chest, 468
monitoring during, 441
for myasthenic patients, 409
operative conditions for, 441
for pediatric patient
anesthetic and perioperative considerations with, 541–542
complications of, 554
indications for, 554
in management of persistent atelectasis, 510
surgical procedure for, 441–443, 442f
tracheal injury in, 448f, 448–449
Tracheostomy tube(s)
cuffs, 444, 444f
design of, 444–445
for pediatric patient, 541
placement of, 442f, 442–443
proper placement of, 70
removal and reinsertion, 445
sizes of, 443, 443t
Tranquilizer premedication, for infant/neonate, dosage and administration of, 497t
Trans-airway pressure, 169
Transcutaneous carbon dioxide monitoring, 303
applications in thoracic surgery, 311–312, 312f–313f
for continuous carbon dioxide monitoring, 308

Transcutaneous electrical nerve stimulation, for postoperative analgesia, 595
Transcutaneous oxygen index, 291, 293t
Transcutaneous oxygen monitoring, 290–293, 292f
effects of site of measurement, 293
potential pitfalls, 292–293
Transcutaneous oxygen tension
with endobronchial intubation, 312–314, 314f
for monitoring oxygenation, 151
Transpulmonary pressure, 169, 594f, 594–595
Transthoracic atrial catheters, in infant/neonate, 502
Transtracheal catheterization, 599–600
complications of, 600
Trauma
acute respiratory failure with, 629
flail chest with, 632
laryngeal, with endobronchial intubation, 384
subcutaneous air present after, 49
thoracic, 463–481
blunt, 463, 464t, 464–465
cardiac injuries resulting from, 475, 475t
penetrating, 463–464, 464t
resuscitation with, 466–467
surgery for, premedication for, 258
tracheal, 447, 471–472
Trauma care
anesthesia requirements for, 465–467
basic requirements for, 465, 465t
induction technique in, 466
maintenance of anesthesia in, 466–467
monitoring in, 466
preanesthetic evaluation and preparation in, 465–466
priorities for, 465
regionalization of, 463–464
Triamcinolone acetonide, 241
aerosolized (topical) therapy, 243
dosage and administration of, 244
pharmacology of, 242t
structure of, 241f
Trimethoprim-sulfamethoxazole, prophylaxis, for *P. carinii* pneumonia, 104
Triple-lumen catheters, for nutritional support, 703
Trypsin, action of, in lung, 129

Tube feeding. *See* Enteral nutrition
Tuberculosis
in AIDS, 100–101
hemoptysis with, 428
surgical, 257
Tubes. *See also specific type of tube*
radiographic monitoring of, 63
d-Tubocurarine
effects of, on airway resistance, 349
for myasthenic patients, 408
precautions for, in trauma patient, 467
Tumor(s)
airway, laser therapy for, 429–437
mediastinal, diagnosis of, 338
Tumor necrosis factor, in acute respiratory failure, 629
Two-lung ventilation, blood flow distribution in, factors affecting, 208
Type II pneumocyte(s), 117
cytochrome P-450 enzymes, 131

Umbilical artery, catheterization, in infant/neonate, 501
Underwater seal, for distending airway pressure therapy, 659
Univent endotracheal tube and blocker, 374, 374f
Universal precautions, 106–107
Upright position
distribution of pulmonary perfusion in, 193–196, 194f, 640–641
distribution of ventilation in, 196, 196f–197f, 596, 640
ventilation-perfusion relationship in, 196–197, 198f
Uric acid, structure of, 234f
Urinary output, 156
monitoring, in infant/neonate, during thoracic operations, 502
Utilization ratio, definition of, 163

ΔV40, 181, 181f
Vagal activity, decreasing, premedication for, 260–261
Vagus nerve, injury, 719
Valium. *See* Diazepam
Variable-flow generator, 663, 663f
Vascular endothelium, of human lung parenchyma, 115–116
Vascular rings
clinical manifestations of, 542
division of

Vascular rings (*Continued*)
    anesthetic and perioperative con-
        siderations with, 522t,
        524t, 542
    description of, 524t
Vasoactive compounds, released from
        lung, 119
Vasoactive intestinal polypeptide
    action of
        in airways, 224
        in lung, 126–127, 129
    as modulator of acute lung injury,
        133
Vasoconstrictors, effects on hypoxic
        pulmonary vasoconstric-
        tion, 210
Vasodilators
    in hemorrhagic shock, 480
    and hypoxic pulmonary vasocon-
        striction, 356–357
Vasopressin, action of, in lung, 129
VC. *See* Vital capacity
V_E60, 181, 181f
Vecuronium
    effects of, on airway resistance, 350
    indications for, in trauma patient,
        467
    for myasthenic patients, 408
$V_E$max/MVV, in differentiation of car-
        diac versus pulmonary
        impairment, 14t
Vena cava filter, indications for, 718
Venereal disease, and HIV transmis-
        sion, 99
Venous admixture, 606
    postoperative
        effects of CPAP on, 608,
            609f–610f
        effects of steroid therapy on,
            607–608, 608f, 610f
        evaluation of, 606, 607f
        reduction of, for treatment of acute
            respiratory failure, 637
Venous carbon dioxide content, 300
Ventilating bronchoscope, 328–329,
        329f–330f
Ventilation. *See also* High-frequency
        ventilation; Mechanical
        ventilation; One-lung ven-
        tilation; Pressure support
        ventilation
    adequacy of, with neuromuscular
        blockade, 174
    and arterial carbon dioxide tension,
        699f–700f
    in bronchoscopy, 326

    methods of, 328–333
    chemical regulation of, 177–183. *See
        also* Hypercapnia;
        Hypoxia; Metabolic acido-
        sis; Metabolic alkalosis
    control of, effects of anesthetics on,
        357–363
    distribution of
        effects of position on, 596
        in lateral decubitus position,
            197–203, 200f
        in supine position, 641
        in upright position, 196,
            196f–197f, 640
    features in common with oxygena-
        tion, 649–653
    during fiberoptic bronchoscopy, 336
        methods of, 332–333
    inadequate, during anesthesia, 709
    intraoperative, in infant/neonate,
        505
    during laser therapy, 433, 436
    monitoring of, 300–311
        importance of, 285
        during one-lung ventilation,
            314–315
    muscles of, 165–166
    neural control system, 177
    with *Pneumocystis* pneumonia, 108
    preoperative assessment of, 322–324
    provision of fresh gas into circuits,
        649–650
    provision of medication via airways
        in, 652–653, 653f
    provision of water vapor in, 650–652
    reciprocal relationship with $PaCO_2$,
        177, 177f
    response to standard stimuli, mea-
        surement of, 179–180
    during rigid bronchoscopy, 433–434
        assessment of, 331–332
    support of, 649, 661–670
        with air leakage, 711
        with flail chest, 468
        postoperative, in infant/neonate,
            506
        routine application of, 670
        weaning of, 670–671
    for surgical repair of congenital
        diaphragmatic hernia, 532
    in surgical treatment of
        esophagorespiratory tract
        fistula, 396–397
Ventilation-perfusion mismatch, 16
    in acute respiratory failure, 620,
        628, 633

    during anesthesia, 350, 351f
    with anesthesia and paralysis, 187f,
        187–188
Ventilation-perfusion relationship
    positional effects on, 187f, 187–188
        in lateral decubitus position,
            198–202, 202f
        in upright position, 196–197,
            198f
    and regional composition of alveolar
        gas, 198f
Ventilatory drive, 616
    effects of malnutrition and refeeding
        on, 693, 694f
    hereditary aspects of, 182
    measurement of, 181–182
Ventilatory timing, measurement of,
        182
Ventricular function, effects of PEEP
        on, 639, 639f
Ventricular septal defect, radiographic
        findings with, 495f
Venturi injector, 329, 332, 436
    Carden modification of, 331, 332f
Venturi mask, 654t, 656
Venturi principle, 329, 331f, 650, 650f,
        656
Verapamil
    for atrial dysrhythmias, 716
    and hypoxic pulmonary vasocon-
        striction, 357
Versed. *See* Midazolam
Vidarabine, indications for, in AIDS,
        104
Vistaril. *See* Hydroxyzine
Vital capacity, 2, 6, 166
    during and following thoracotomy
        and upper abdominal
        surgery, 89
    measurement, 616
Vital Signs Facemask, 657, 657f
Vital Signs PEEP valve, 660
Vitamin K_1, for neonate, 488
Vitamins, requirements for, in nutri-
        tional protocols, 689,
        689t
Vocal cord edema, after bronchoscopy,
        720
Vocal cord paralysis, in infant/neonate,
        anesthetic and perioperae-
        tive considerations with,
        522t
Volatile anesthetics
    effects of, on ventilatory control,
        358–361
    respiratory effects of, 364t

Volume loading, in treatment of right
    heart failure, 717
VO$_2$max/AT, in differentiation of car-
    diac versus pulmonary
    impairment, 14t

Water, radiographic density, 20, 20f–21f
Water density, 19
Waterfall effect, 194–195
Waterston shunt
    anesthetic and perioperative consid-
        erations with, 523t
    description of, 523t
Water vapor content, 651, 652f
Water vapor pressure, 651, 652f
Weight gain, as index of nutritional sta-
    tus, 684
Weight loss
    in AIDS, 101
    with cancer, 685

in chronic obstructive pulmonary
    disease, 694
as index of nutritional status,
    684–686
Weir effect, 194–195
Western blot assays, for HIV, 97
Wet lung syndrome, definition of, 619
Wheezing
    clinical implications of, 322
    diagnostic significance of, 324
White double-lumen endobronchial
    tube, 377, 378t, 380–381,
    381f
Wound dehiscence, 715
    postoperative, correlation with
        nutritional status, 685–686
    risk factors for, 684
Wound fistula, postoperative, correla-
    tion with nutritional sta-
    tus, 685–686

Wound healing, and nutritional sup-
    port, 687–688
Wound hematoma, with medi-
    astinoscopy, 340
Wound infection, postoperative, corre-
    lation with nutritional sta-
    tus, 685–686
Wrap-around procedures, for repair of
    hiatus hernias, 391

Xanthine, structure of, 234f
Xanthine bronchodilators, 233–237
X-ray, 19

ZEEP. *See* Zero end-expiratory pressure
Zero end-expiratory pressure
    in lateral decubitus position,
        202–203
    in nondependent lung, 216
Zidovudine. *See* Azidothymidine